CURRENT OCULAR THERAPY 3

FREDERICK T. FRAUNFELDER, M.D.

Professor and Chairman, Department of Ophthalmology,
Oregon Health Sciences University,
Portland, Oregon

F. HAMPTON ROY, M.D., F.A.C.S.

Clinical Associate Professor, Department of Ophthalmology,
University of Arkansas for Medical Sciences;
Baptist Medical Center, Arkansas Children's Hospital;
Doctors Hospital, St. Vincent Infirmary,
Little Rock, Arkansas

Associate Editor:

S. MARTHA MEYER

Research Associate, Department of Ophthalmology,
Oregon Health Sciences University,
Portland, Oregon

1990

W. B. SAUNDERS COMPANY
Harcourt Brace Jovanovich, Inc.

Philadelphia, London, Toronto, Montreal, Sydney, Tokyo

W.B. SAUNDERS COMPANY
Harcourt Brace Jovanovich, Inc.

The Curtis Center
Independence Square West
Philadelphia, PA 19106

NOTICE

The authors and editors of this book have been careful to ensure that dosage recommendations are precise and in agreement with standards officially accepted at the time of publication.

It does happen, however, that dosage schedules are changed from time to time in the light of accumulating clinical experience and continuing laboratory studies. This is most likely to occur in the case of recently introduced products.

It is essential that you check the manufacturer's warnings and recommendations for dosage, especially if the drug to be administered or prescribed is one that you use only infrequently or have not used for some time.

THE PUBLISHER

Library of Congress Cataloging in Publication Data

Fraunfelder, FT

Current ocular therapy.

1. Therapeutics Ophthalmological. 2. Ocular
    pharmacology.   I. Roy, Frederick Hampton, joint author.
    II. Meyer, S. Martha.   III. Title [DNLM: 1. Eye
    diseases—Complications.   2. Eye diseases—Therapy.
    3. Eye manifestations. WW140 F845c]
RE991.F75   617.7'06   79-66715
ISBN   0-7216-3848-1

Listed here is the latest translated edition of this book together with the language of the translation and the publisher:

Current Ocular Therapy, 2—*Portuguese*—Novos Tempos Livros de Medicina Ltda., Rua
    Santa Clara, 50- SALA 416, CEP 22041
    Copacabana, Rio de Janeiro, Brazil

Acquisition Editor: Richard Zorab

CURRENT OCULAR THERAPY 3   ISBN 0-7216-3848-1

Copyright © 1990, 1985, 1980 by W.B. Saunders Company

All rights reserved. No part of this publication may be reproduced or transmitted in any form or by any means, electronic, or mechanical, including photocopy, recording, or any information storage and retrieval system, without permission in writing from the publisher.

Printed in the United States of America.

Last digit is the print number: 9   8   7   6   5   4   3   2   1

CONTRIBUTORS

RICHARD L. ABBOTT, M.D.
Consultant, Corneal and External Disease Service, Department of Ophthalmology, Pacific Presbyterian Medical Center, San Francisco, California.
Erysipelas

ROBERT ABEL, JR., M.D.
Assistant Professor of Ophthalmology, Jefferson Medical College of Thomas Jefferson University, Philadelphia, Pennsylvania. Director, Department of Ophthalmology, Wilmington Medical Center, Wilmington, Delaware.
Epidemic Keratoconjunctivitis

IRA A. ABRAHAMSON, M.D.
Associate Clinical Professor of Ophthalmology, Assistant Clinical Professor of Family Medicine, University of Cincinnati Medical Center, Cincinnati, Ohio.
Mucocele

WILLIAM A. AGGER, M.D.
Internal Medicine and Infectious Diseases, Gundersen Clinic. Director, Microbiology Laboratory, La Crosse Lutheran Hospital, La Crosse, Wisconsin.
Sporotrichosis

MATHEA R. ALLANSMITH, M.D.
Associate Professor of Ophthalmology, Harvard Medical School Institute Scientist, Eye Research Institute, Boston, Massachusetts.
Allergic Conjunctivitis; Giant Papillary Conjunctivitis; Phlyctenulosis

DUNCAN P. ANDERSON, M.D.C.M., F.R.C.S. (C)
Associate Professor of Ophthalmology, McGill University. Director of Neuro-Ophthalmology Service, Montreal General Hospital, Montreal, Quebec, Canada.
Meningioma

RICHARD L. ANDERSON, M.D., F.A.C.S.
Professor of Ophthalmology, Director of Oculoplastic Surgery Division, University of Utah School of Medicine, Salt Lake City, Utah.
Distichiasis; Hypertrichosis

DAVID J. APPLE, M.D.
Professor and Chairman, Department of Ophthalmology, Vallotton Chair of Biomedical Engineering, Albert Florens Storm Eye Institute and Center for Intraocular Lens Research, Medical University of South Carolina, Charleston, South Carolina.
Histiocytosis X

BUDD APPLETON, M.D.
Clinical Professor of Ophthalmology, University of Minnesota School of Medicine, Minneapolis, Minnesota. On active staff of United Hospital, St. Paul, Minnesota.
Radiation

LEONARD APT, M.D.
Professor of Ophthalmology, Director Emeritus of the Division of Pediatric Ophthalmology, Jules Stein Eye Institute, University of California School of Medicine, Los Angeles, California.
Medulloepithelioma

JAMES V. AQUAVELLA, M.D.
Clinical Professor of Ophthalmology, University of Rochester Medical Center, Rochester, New York.
Scleromalacia Perforans

JUAN J. ARENTSEN, M.D.
Professor of Ophthalmology, Jefferson Medical College of Thomas Jefferson University. Attending Surgeon, Wills Eye Hospital, Philadelphia, Pennsylvania.
Molluscum Contagiosum

FELICIA B. AXELROD, M.D.
Professor of Pediatrics, New York University Medical Center, New York, New York.
Familial Dysautonomia

ANN M. BAJART, M.D.
Clinical Instructor in Ophthalmology, Harvard Medical School, Boston, Massachusetts.
Phlyctenulosis

PETER H. BALLEN, M.D.
Clinical Professor of Ophthalmology, State University of New York Health Science Center, Stony Brook, New York. Visiting Professor, University of Puerto Rico School of Medicine, San Juan, Puerto Rico.
Listeriosis

ANTHONY L. BARBATO, M.D.
Professor of Medicine, Vice President for Health Affairs and Dean, Loyola University Stritch School of Medicine, Maywood, Illinois.
Hypocalcemia

SUSAN BARKAY, M.D.
Head, Department of Ophthalmology, Central Emek Hospital, Afula, Israel.
Leptospirosis

iv / CONTRIBUTORS

SOREN S. BARNER, M.D., M.D.O.S.

Professor of Ophthalmology, Institute for Experimental Research in Surgery, University of Copenhagen. Lecturer in Ophthalmology, Gentofte University Hospital, Copenhagen, Denmark.

Astigmatism

JAMES M. BARNETT, M.D.

Ophthalmologist, Hackley Hospital. Staff, Mercy Hospital, Muskegon, Michigan.

Loaisis

GARY P. BARTH, M.D.

Assistant Clinical Professor, University of California School of Medicine, San Francisco, California.

Aspergillosis

WILLIAM L. BASUK, M.D.

Senior Resident in Ophthalmology, Albert Einstein College of Medicine, Montefiore Medical Center, Bronx, New York.

Benign Intracranial Hypertension and Pseudotumor Cerebri

JULES BAUM, M.D.

Professor of Ophthalmology, Tufts-New England Medical Center, Boston, Massachusetts.

Moraxella

CROWELL BEARD, M.D.

Clinical Professor Emeritus of Ophthalmology, University of California School of Medicine, San Francisco, California. On active staff of University of California Hospitals, San Francisco, California.

Blepharochalasis

ROBERT H. BEDROSSIAN, M.D., M.Sc.

Senior Clinical Instructor in Ophthalmology, Oregon Health Sciences University, Portland, Oregon.

Myopia

A. ROBERT BELLOWS, M.D.

Assistant Clinical Professor of Ophthalmology, Harvard Medical School. Surgeon, Massachusetts Eye and Ear Infirmary, Boston, Massachusetts.

Choroidal Detachment

SUSAN C. BENES, M.D.

Assistant Professor of Ophthalmology, Ohio State University College of Medicine, Columbus, Ohio.

Tolosa-Hunt Syndrome

ELAINE R. BERMAN, Ph.D.

Professor of Experimental Ophthalmology. Head, Eye Biochemistry Unit, Department of Ophthalmology, Hadassah University Hospital, Jerusalem, Israel.

Mucopolysaccharidosis II; Mucopolysaccharidosis III

VITALIANO B. BERNARDINO, JR., M.D.

Professor of Ophthalmology, Jefferson Medical College of Thomas Jefferson University. Attending Surgeon, Wills Eye Hospital, Philadelphia, Pennsylvania.

Melanocytic Lesions of the Eyelids

ROBERT L. BERRY, M.D.

Ophthalmologist, Baptist Medical Center, St. Vincent Infirmary, Doctors Hospital, Little Rock, Arkansas.

Blindness; Scrub Typhus

ALBERT W. BIGLAN, M.D., F.A.C.S.

Adjunct Associate Professor of Ophthalmology, University of Pittsburgh School of Medicine, Eye and Ear Hospital, Children's Hospital, Pittsburgh, Pennsylvania.

Tetanus

ALAN C. BIRD, M.D., F.R.C.S.

Professor of Ophthalmology, Institute of Ophthalmology, London University, and Honorary Consultant Moorfields Eye Hospital, London, England.

Onchoceriasis

PETER BLACK, B.Sc., M.B., F.R.C.S., D.O.

Consultant Ophthalmic Surgeon, Great Yarmouth and Waveney District Hospitals, James Paget Hospital, Gorleston, Great Yarmouth, England.

Cerebral Palsy

RAPHAEL S. BLOCH, M.D., F.A.C.S.

Assistant Clinical Professor of Ophthalmology, Albert Einstein College of Medicine, New York, New York. Chief of Ophthalmology, Northern Westchester Hospital Center, Mount Kisco, New York.

Homocystinuria

MARK S. BLUMENKRANZ, M.D.

Associate Clinical Professor of Ophthalmology, Kresge Eye Institute, Wayne State University, Detroit Michigan and Oakland University, Rochester, Michigan.

Acute Retinal Necrosis

MILTON BONIUK, M.D.

Professor of Ophthalmology, Cullen Eye Institute, Baylor College of Medicine, Houston, Texas.

Cavernous Sinus Thrombosis

VIVIEN BONIUK, M.D.

Associate Professor of Ophthalmology, State University of New York Health Science Center, Stony Brook, New York.

Rubella

S. ARTHUR BORUCHOFF, M.D.

Associate Clinical Professor of Ophthalmology, Harvard Medical School, Boston, Massachusetts.

Posterior Polymorphous Corneal Dystrophy

CONTRIBUTORS / v

WILLIAM M. BOURNE, M.D.
Professor of Ophthalmology, Mayo Medical School, Consultant in Ophthalmology, Mayo Clinic, Rochester, Minnesota.
Fuchs' Corneal Dystrophy

BENJAMIN F. BOYD, M.D., F.A.C.S.
Founder and Director, Clinica Boyd, Panama, Republic of Panama.
Aphakia

LAURENCE S. BRAUDE, M.D., F.A.C.S., F.R.C.S. (C)
Clinical Assistant Professor of Ophthalmology, The University of Illinois College of Medicine at Chicago, Chicago, Illinois.
Diphtheria

GLEN O. BRINDLEY, M.D.
Associate Professor of Ophthalmology, Department of Surgery, Texas A & M University College of Medicine, Temple, Texas.
Lacrimal Gland Tumors

ROBERT J. BROCKHURST, M.D.
Associate Clinical Professor of Ophthalmology, Harvard Medical School, Surgeon, Massachusetts Eye and Ear Infirmary, Boston, Massachusetts.
Nanophthalmos

MARK A. BRONSTEIN, M.D.
Clinical Instructor in Ophthalmology, University of California School of Medicine, Irvine, California.
Macular Hole

H. LOGAN BROOKS, M.D.
Retinal Fellow, Wills Eye Hospital, Jefferson Medical College of Thomas Jefferson University, Philadelphia, Pennsylvania.
Retinal Vein Obstruction

MARION H. BROOKS, M.D.
Professor of Medicine, Chief, Section of Endocrinology and Metabolism, Loyola University Medical Center, Maywood, Illinois.
Hypocalcemia

DONNA DODSON BROWN, M.D.
Assistant Clinical Instructor, Department of Ophthalmology, University of Texas, Southwestern Medical School, Dallas, Texas.
Staphylococcal and Mixed Staphylococcal/Seborrheic Blepharoconjunctivitis

STUART I. BROWN, M.D.
Professor, Department of Ophthalmology, University of California School of Medicine, San Diego, California.
Ocular Rosacea

JOHN D. BULLOCK, M.D., M.S., F.A.C.S.
Professor and Chairman, Department of Ophthalmology, Wright State University School of Medicine, Dayton, Ohio.
Eyelid Coloboma; Nocardia; Werner's Syndrome

RAYMOND BUNCIC, M.D., F.R.C.S. (C)
Associate Professor of Ophthalmology, University of Toronto. Staff Ophthalmologist, Hospital for Sick Children. Staff Ophthalmologist, Toronto General Hospital, Toronto, Ontario, Canada.
Orbital Hypertelorism

RONALD M. BURDE, M.D.
Professor and Chairman, Department of Ophthalmology, Professor of Neurology and Neurosurgery, Albert Einstein College of Medicine, Montefiore Medical Center, Bronx, New York.
Benign Intracranial Hypertension and Pseudotumor Cerebri

ROBERT P. BURNS, M.D.
Roy E. Mason Distinguished Professor and Chairman, Department of Ophthalmology, University of Missouri Health Sciences Center, Columbia, Missouri.
Juvenile Corneal Epithelial Dystrophy; Tyrosinemia II

THOMAS C. BURTON, M.D.
Professor of Ophthalmology, Eye Institute, Medical College of Wisconsin, Milwaukee, Wisconsin.
Rocky Mountain Spotted Fever

J. DOUGLAS CAMERON, M.D.
Chief, Department of Ophthalmology, Hennepin County Medical Center, Minneapolis, Minnesota.
Acrodermatitis Enteropathica

DAVID G. CAMPBELL, M.D.
Professor of Ophthalmology, Dartmouth-Hitchcock Medical Center, Hanover, New Hampshire.
Ghost Cell Glaucoma; Pigmentary Glaucoma

LUISELLA CASU, M.D.
Assistant Professor, Institute of Ophthalmology, University of Sassari. Assistant, Ophthalmology Service, University Hospital, Sassari, Italy.
Drug-Induced Optic Atrophy

VICKY CEVALLOS, M.T. (A.S.C.P.)
Ocular Microbiologist, Procter Foundation, San Francisco, California.
Pneumococcus

JOHN W. CHANDLER, M.D.
Professor and Chairman, Department of Ophthalmology, University of Wisconsin Center for Health Sciences, Madison, Wisconsin.
Diphtheria

vi / CONTRIBUTORS

SURESH R. CHANDRA, M.D.
Professor of Ophthalmology, University of Wisconsin Center for Health Sciences, Madison, Wisconsin.
Diabetes Mellitus

DEVRON H. CHAR, M.D.
Director, Ocular Oncology Unit. Professor of Ophthalmology and Radiation Oncology, and the Francis I. Proctor Foundation for Research in Ophthalmology, University of California School of Medicine, San Francisco, California.
Neuroblastoma; Orbital Metastases

STEVE CHARLES, M.D.
Co-Director, Vitreo-Retinal Research Foundation. Clinical Assistant Professor of Ophthalmology, University of Tennessee Center for the Health Sciences, Memphis, Tennessee.
Proliferative Vitreoretinopathy

RICHARD M. CHAVIS, M.D.
Clinical Assistant Professor of Ophthalmology, Georgetown University Medical Center, Washington, District of Columbia. Consultant, National Naval Hospital, Bethesda, Maryland.
Liposarcoma

MICHAEL CHERINGTON, M.D.
Clinical Professor of Neurology, University of Colorado Health Sciences Center, Denver, Colorado.
Botulism

GEORGE N. CHIN, M.D., F.A.C.S.
Director, Ophthalmology Service, Northwest Hospital, Seattle, Washington.
Typhoid Fever

STEVEN S. T. CHING, M.D.
Assistant Professor of Ophthalmology, University of Rochester School of Medicine and Dentistry, Rochester, New York.
Infectious Mononucleosis

LEONARD CHRISTENSEN, M.D.
Clinical Professor of Ophthalmology, Oregon Health Sciences Center, Portland, Oregon.
Iris Bombé

STEVEN B. COHEN, M.D.
Assistant Professor of Ophthalmology, Director, Sickle Cell Eye Center, University of Illinois College of Medicine, Chicago, Illinois.
Sickle Cell Disease

WILLIAM H. COLES, M.D., M.S.
Professor and Chairman, Department of Ophthalmology, State University of New York Health Science Center, Buffalo, New York.
Cockayne's Syndrome; Indirect Global Ruptures and Sharp Scleral Injuries

DOUGLAS J. COSTER, F.R.C.S.
Professor of Ophthalmology, Flinders Medical Center, Bedford Park, Adelaide, South Australia.
Bacterial Conjunctivitis; Bacterial Corneal Ulcers

J. BROOKS CRAWFORD, M.D.
Clinical Professor of Ophthalmology, University of California School of Medicine, San Francisco, California.
Keratoacanthoma

JOHN S. CRAWFORD, M.D., F.R.C.S. (C)
Professor and Head, Department of Ophthalmology, Staff Surgeon, Department of Ophthalmology, University of Toronto, Toronto, Ontario, Canada.
Brown's Syndrome; Marcus Gunn Syndrome

R. PITTS CRICK, F.R.C.S.
Emeritus Lecturer in Ophthalmology, School of Medicine and Dentistry of King's College and Honorary Consultant Ophthalmic Surgeon, Kings College Hospital, London, England.
Uveoparotid Fever

HAROLD E. CROSS, M.D., Ph.D.
Clinical Professor of Surgery, University of Arizona Health Sciences Center, Tucson, Arizona.
Microspherophakia

LUIZ CARLOS CUCE, M.D.
Associate Professor of Dermatology, São Paulo University School of Medicine, São Paulo, Brazil.
American Mucocutaneous Leishmaniasis

RICHARD D. CUNNINGHAM, M.D., M.S.
Professor and Director, Division of Ophthalmology, Texas A & M University College of Medicine, Temple, Texas.
Lacrimal Gland Tumors

ROGER A. DAILEY, M.D.
Clinical Instructor in Ophthalmology, University of Washington School of Medicine, Oculoplastic Surgeon, Eye Associates, Seattle, Washington.
Dacryocystitis; Entropion; Epicanthus

LOUIS DAILY, M.D., Ph.D. (Ophth.)
Associate Clinical Professor of Ophthalmology, Baylor College of Medicine. Senior Attending (in Ophthalmology), Methodist Hospital, Houston, Texas.
Retinoschisis

ROBERT D'AMICO, M.D.
Chairman of Ophthalmology, St. Vincent's Hospital and Medical Center of New York, New York, New York.
Familial Dysautonomia

CONTRIBUTORS / vii

STUART R. DANKNER, M.D.
Clinical Professor of Ophthalmology, University of Maryland Hospital. Director of Pediatric Ophthalmology, Sinai Hospital, Baltimore, Maryland.
Acquired Nonaccommodative Esotropia

S. DAROUGAR, M.D., D.T.M.&H., M.R.C.Path.
Professor of Virology, Institute of Ophthalmology, University of London, London, England.
Trachoma

FREDERICK H. DAVIDORF, M.D.
Professor of Ophthalmology, Ohio State University College of Medicine, Columbus, Ohio.
Ocular Metastatic Tumors

CHANDLER R. DAWSON, M.D.
Director, Francis I. Proctor Foundation for Research in Ophthalmology. Professor of Ophthalmology, University of California School of Medicine, San Francisco, California.
Inclusion Conjunctivitis; Pharyngoconjunctival Fever

N. W. H. M. DEKKERS, M.D.
Ophthalmologist, St. Elizabeth Hospital, Tilburg, The Netherlands.
Rubeola

ROBERT C. DELLA ROCCA, M.D., F.A.C.S.
Surgeon Director, Ophthalmic Plastic, Reconstructive, and Orbital Service, New York Eye and Ear Infirmary, New York. Associate Clinical Professor of Ophthalmology, Albert Einstein College of Medicine, Montefiore Medical Center, Bronx, New York.
Eyelid Contusions, Lacerations, and Avulsions

ANGELO M. DIGEORGE, M.D.
Professor of Pediatrics, Temple University Health Sciences Center. Chief, Section of Endocrinology and Metabolism, St. Christopher's Hospital for Children, Philadelphia, Pennsylvania.
Waardenburg's Syndrome

GEORGE N. DONNELL, M.D.
Winzer Professor and Chairman of Pediatrics, University of Southern California School of Medicine, Pediatrician-In-Chief, Children's Hospital of Los Angeles, Los Angeles, California.
Galactosemias

JOHN J. DONNELLY, Ph.D.
Research Fellow, Department of Immunology Cancer Research, Merck Sharp & Dohme Research Laboratory, Philadelphia, Pennsylvania.
Ascariasis

T. W. DOUCET, M.D.
Ophthalmologist, Doctor's Hospital, Conroe, Texas. Hermann Hospital, Houston, Texas.
Marcus Gunn Syndrome

DONALD J. DOUGHMAN, M.D.
Professor and Chairman, Department of Ophthalmology, University of Minnesota Health Sciences Center, Minneapolis, Minnesota.
Acrodermatitis Enteropathica

STEPHEN M. DRANCE, M.D.
Professor and Head, Department of Ophthalmology, University of British Columbia, Vancouver General Hospital, Vancouver, British Columbia, Canada.
Low-Tension Glaucoma

MARK S. DRESNER, M.D.
Corneal/External Disease Instructor of Ophthalmology, Bethesda Eye Institute, St. Louis University Medical Center, St. Louis, Missouri.
Corneal and Conjunctival Calcifications; Herpes Simplex; Pellucid Marginal Corneal Degeneration

ROBERT C. DREWS, M.D.
Professor of Clinical Ophthalmology, Washington University Medical Center, St. Louis, Missouri.
Adult Cataracts

ROBERT M. DRYDEN, M.D., F.A.C.S.
Clinical Professor, Department of Ophthalmology, College of Medicine, University of Arizona, Tucson, Arizona.
Periocular Squamous Cell Carcinoma

STEVEN P. DUNN, M.D.
Clinical Associate Professor of Ophthalmology, Michigan State University, Lansing, Michigan.
Amyloidosis

HOWARD EGGERS, M.D.
Associate Professor of Ophthalmology, Columbia University College of Physicians and Surgeons. Attending Surgeon Columbia Presbyterian Medical Center, New York, New York.
Oculomotor (Third Nerve) Paralysis

MATTHEW EHRLICH, M.D.
Ophthalmologist, Los Angeles, California.
Fungal Keratitis

RICHARD ELANDER, M.D.
Associate Clinical Professor of Ophthalmology, Jules Stein Eye Institute, University of California School of Medicine, Los Angeles, California.
Myopia

M. M. EL HENNAWI, M.Ch.
Professor of Ophthalmology, Faculty of Medicine, University of Alexandria, Alexandria, Egypt.
Vernal Keratoconjunctivitis

viii / CONTRIBUTORS

PHILIP P. ELLIS, M.D.

Professor and Chairman, Department of Ophthalmology, University of Colorado Health Sciences Center, Denver, Colorado.

Intraocular Foreign Body—Steel or Iron

ROBERT M. ELLSWORTH, M.D.

Professor of Ophthalmology, Cornell Medical Center. Attending Ophthalmologist, New York Hospital, New York, New York.

Retinoblastoma

ROY J. ELLSWORTH, M.D.

Ophthalmologist, St. Alphonsus Hospital, St. Luke's Hospital. Consultant, Veterans Administration Medical Center, Boise, Idaho.

Rabies

FRANK P. ENGLISH, F.R.A.C.O., F.R.C.S.

Australian Government Consultant Ophthalmologist. Visiting Ophthalmic Surgeon, St. Andrews Hospital, Brisbane, Australia.

Demodicosis

DAVID L. EPSTEIN, M.D.

Associate Professor of Ophthalmology, Harvard Medical School. Surgeon in Ophthalmology, Massachusetts Eye and Ear Infirmary, Boston, Massachusetts.

Lens-Induced Glaucoma

EDWARD EPSTEIN, M.B., B.Ch., D.O.M.S.

Consultant Ophthalmologist, Boksburg Hospital, Johannesburg, South Africa.

Coenurosis

WILLIAM L. EPSTEIN, M.D.

Professor, Department of Dermatology, University of California School of Medicine, San Francisco, California.

Poison Ivy, Oak, and Sumac Dermatitis

JOSEPH ESHAGIAN, M.D.

Ophthalmologist, Hollywood Presbyterian Hospital, Los Angeles, California.

Chronic Progressive External Ophthalmoplegia

ROGER A. EWALD, M.D.

Clinical Assistant Professor of Ophthalmology, University of Illinois College of Medicine, Urbana-Champaign, Illinois.

Solar Retinopathy

FUAH S. FARAH, M.D.

Professor of Medicine, Chief of the Section of Dermatology, State University of New York Health Science Center, Syracuse, New York.

Cutaneous Leishmaniasis

BISHARA FARIS, M.D.

Chief, Department of Ophthalmology, American University of Beirut, Beirut, Lebanon. Now in Boston, Massachusetts.

Scleral Staphyloma and Dehiscences

MARIANNE E. FEITL, M.D.

Instructor, Department of Ophthalmology, Scheie Eye Institute, Presbyterian-University of Pennsylvania Medical Center, Philadelphia, Pennsylvania.

Juvenile Glaucoma

STEVEN S. FEMAN, M.D.

Professor of Ophthalmology, Vanderbilt University Medical Center, Nashville, Tennessee.

Thalassemia

T. J. FFYTCHE, F.R.C.S., D.O.

Consultant Ophthalmologist, St. Thomas's Hospital, Moorfields Eye Hospital, and Hospital for Tropical Diseases, London, England.

Leprosy

JAMES C. FOLK, M.D.

Professor of Ophthalmology, Director, Vitreoretinal Service, University of Iowa Hospitals and Clinics, Iowa City, Iowa.

Central Serous Chorioretinopathy

RICHARD K. FORSTER, M.D.

Medical Director, King Khaled Eye Specialist Hospital, Riyadh, Saudi Arabia

Bacterial Endophthalmitis

C. STEPHEN FOSTER, M.D., F.A.C.S.

Director, Immunology and Uveitis Unit, Massachusetts Eye and Ear Infirmary. Associate Adjunct Clinical Scientist, Eye Research Institute of Retina Foundation. Associate Professor of Ophthalmology, Harvard Medical School, Boston, Massachusetts.

Candidiasis

JULES FRANCOIS, M.D., F.A.C.S., F.R.S.M.

Professor of Ophthalmology, University of Ghent, Ghent, Belgium.

Ligneous Conjunctivitis

F. T. FRAUNFELDER, M.D.

Professor and Chairman, Department of Ophthalmology, Oregon Health Sciences University, Portland, Oregon.

Conjunctival, Corneal or Scleral Cysts; Conjunctival Melanotic Lesions; Conjunctival or Corneal Intraepithelial Neoplasia (CIN) and Squamous Cell Carcinoma; Echinococcosis; Electrical Injury; Ewing's Sarcoma; Hemophilus Influenzae; Hordeolum; Lyme Disease; Lymphoid Tumors; Trichiasis; Xanthelasma

JEFFREY FREEDMAN, M.B., B.Ch., Ph.D., F.R.C.S.E.
Professor of Clinical Ophthalmology, State University of New York Health Science Center, Brooklyn, New York.
Xeroderma Pigmentosa

H. MACKENZIE FREEMAN, M.D.
Associate Clinical Professor of Ophthalmology, Harvard Medical School. Vice-President, Eye Research Institute of Retina Foundation, Boston, Massachusetts.
Peripheral Retinal Breaks and Degeneration; Scleral Staphyloma and Dehiscences

MITCHELL H. FRIEDLAENDER, M.D.
Department of Ophthalmology, Scripps Clinic and Research Foundation, La Jolla, California.
Atopic Dermatitis; Contact Dermatitis; Urticaria and Hereditary Angioedema

ALAN H. FRIEDMAN, M.D.
Clinical Professor of Ophthalmology and Pathology, Mount Sinai School of Medicine, New York, New York.
Vogt-Koyanagi-Harada Syndrome

JOSEPH FRUCHT, M.D.
Corneal Department in Department of Ophthalmology, Hadassah University, Jerusalem, Israel.
Ocular Rosacea

WAYNE E. FUNG, M.D.
Consultant, Vitreoretinal Service, Department of Ophthalmology, Pacific Presbyterian Medical Center, San Francisco, California.
Cystoid Macular Edema

WESLEY KING GALEN, M.D.
Associate Clinical Professor of Dermatology, Tulane Medical Center, New Orleans, Louisiana.
Neurodermatitis

STEVEN GANCHER, M.D.
Assistant Professor of Neurology, Oregon Health Sciences University, Portland, Oregon.
Parkinson's Disease

JAMES P. GANLEY, M.D., Dr. P.H.
Professor and Chairman, Department of Ophthalmology, Louisiana State University Medical Center, Shreveport, Louisiana.
Coccidioidomycosis

HERBERT J. GERSHEN, M.D.
Active Staff, St. Mary's Hospital, San Francisco, California. Mills-Peninsula Hospitals, San Mateo, California.
Chalazion

WILLIAM B. GLEW, M.D.
President, Washington National Eye Center. Chairman, Department of Ophthalmology, Washington Hospital Center, Washington, District of Columbia.
Psoriasis

DANIEL H. GOLD, M.D.
Associate Clinical Professor, Department of Ophthalmology, University of Texas Medical Branch, Galveston, Texas.
Sarcoidosis

MICHAEL H. GOLDBAUM, M.D.
Associate Professor of Surgery and Medicine, Treatment of Retina and Vitreous, Diabetic Retinopathy and Macular Degeneration, University of California School of Medicine, San Diego, California.
Central or Branch Retinal Artery Occlusion

MORTON F. GOLDBERG, M.D.
Professor and Head, Department of Ophthalmology, Eye and Ear Infirmary of the University of Illinois Hospital, Chicago, Illinois.
Sickle Cell Disease

STUART H. GOLDBERG, M.D.
Assistant Professor, Department of Ophthalmology, Penn State University College of Medicine, Hershey, Pennsylvania.
Eyelid Coloboma; Nocardia; Werner's Syndrome

JEROME N. GOLDMAN, M.D.
Clinical Associate Professor of Ophthalmology, Center for Sight, Georgetown University Medical Center, Washington, District of Columbia.
Acquired Syphilis; Congenital Syphilis

GEORGE M. GOMBOS, M.D., F.A.C.S.
Professor of Ophthalmology, State University of New York Health Science Center. Chief, Department of Ophthalmology, Veterans Administration Medical Center, Brooklyn, New York.
Traumatic Cataract

J. GRAVELINE, M.D.
Ophthalmologist, Armed Forces Hospital, Marseille, France.
Schistosomiasis

BAIRD S. GRIMSON, M.D.
Professor of Ophthalmology, University of North Carolina School of Medicine, Chapel Hill, North Carolina.
Cluster Headache; Trigeminal Neuralgia

LEWIS R. GRODEN, M.D.
Associate Professor of Ophthalmology, Vice-Chairman Department of Ophthalmology, Director of External Disease, USF Eye Institute, Tampa, Florida.
Molluscum Contagiosum

x / CONTRIBUTORS

STUART A. GROSSMAN, M.D.

Assistant Professor of Oncology, Medicine, and Neurologic Surgery, Johns Hopkins University School of Medicine, Baltimore, Maryland.

Hodgkin's Disease

ARTHUR S. GROVE, JR., M.D.

Assistant Professor of Ophthalmology, Harvard Medical School. Director of Orbital and Plastic Surgery, Massachusetts Eye and Ear Infirmary, Boston, Massachusetts.

Dermoid

ROBERTO GUERRA, M.D.

Professor and Chairman, Institute of Ophthalmology, University of Modena, Modena, Italy.

Drug-Induced Optic Atrophy

YEZID GUTIERREZ, M.D., Ph.D.

Associate Professor of Pathology, Case Western Reserve University School of Medicine, University Hospitals of Cleveland, Cleveland, Ohio.

Dirofilariasis

FRONCIE A. GUTMAN, M.D.

Chairman, Department of Ophthalmology, Cleveland Clinic Foundation. Associate Clinical Professor of Ophthalmology, Case Western Reserve University School of Medicine, Cleveland, Ohio.

Branch Retinal Vein Occlusion

HESKEL M. HADDAD, M.D.

Clinical Professor of Ophthalmology, New York Medical College, New York, New York.

Hypothyroidism

WILLIAM S. HAGLER, M.D.

Clinical Associate Professor of Ophthalmology, Emory University School of Medicine, Atlanta, Georgia. Clinical Associate Professor of Ophthalmology, Medical College of Georgia, Augusta, Georgia.

Toxocariasis

BARRETT G. HAIK, M.D.

Professor of Ophthalmology, Tulane Medical Center, New Orleans, Louisiana.

Capillary Hemangioma; Cavernous Hemangioma

MICHAEL HALSTED, M.D.

Assistant Instructor, Department of Ophthalmology, University of Texas Southwestern Medical Center, Dallas, Texas.

Seborrheic Blepharitis

KAY-UWE HAMANN, M.D.

Private Lecturer in Neuro-Ophthalmology, Eye Clinic, University Hospital, Hamburg, West Germany.

Acute Idiopathic Polyneuritis

HIRAM H. HARDESTY, M.D.

Associate Clinical Professor of Ophthalmology, Case Western Reserve University School of Medicine, Cleveland, Ohio.

Intermittent Exotropia

R. D. HARLEY, M.D., Ph.D., F.A.C.S.

Professor Emeritus and Former Chairman, Department of Ophthalmology, Temple University Health Sciences Center. Attending Surgeon, St. Christopher's Hospital for Children. Consulting Surgeon, Department of Pediatric Ophthalmology, Wills Eye Hospital, Philadelphia, Pennsylvania.

Congenital Fibrosis of the Extraocular Muscles

WILLIAM H. HAVENER, M.D.

Professor Department of Ophthalmology, Ohio State University College of Medicine. Attending Staff, The Ohio State University Hospitals, Grant Hospital, Columbus, Ohio.

Intraocular Foreign Body—Nonmagnetic Chemically Inert

BARTON F. HAYNES, M.D.

Frederic M. Hanes Professor of Medicine, Professor of Microbiology and Immunology. Chief, Division of Rheumatology and Immunology, Duke University Medical Center, Durham, North Carolina.

Cogan's Syndrome

SOHAN SINGH HAYREH, M.D., Ph.D., D.Sc., F.R.C.S.

Professor of Ophthalmology, University of Iowa Hospitals and Clinics, Iowa City, Iowa.

Ischemic Optic Neuropathy

THOMAS R. HEDGES, JR., M.D.

Professor of Ophthalmology, Presbyterian-University of Pennsylvania Medical Center, Philadelphia, Pennsylvania.

Bell's Palsy; Headache

THOMAS R. HEDGES, III, M.D.

Associate Professor of Ophthalmology and Neurology, Tufts University School of Medicine, Boston, Massachusetts.

Bell's Palsy

J. TIMOTHY HEFFERNAN, M.D.

Clinical Instructor Department of Ophthalmology, University of Washington, Seattle, Washington.

Lid Retraction

EUGENE M. HELVESTON, M.D.

Coleman Professor and Chairman, Department of Ophthalmology, Indiana University School of Medicine, Indianapolis, Indiana.

Abducens (Sixth Nerve) Paralysis; Essential-Infantile Esotropia; Extraocular Muscle Lacerations; Superior Oblique Palsy

CONTRIBUTORS / xi

HUGH L. HENNIS, M.D., Ph.D.

Resident in Ophthalmology, Medical College of South Carolina, Charleston, South Carolina.

Histiocytosis X

ROBERT S. HEPLER, M.D.

Professor of Ophthalmology, Chief, Division of Neuro-Ophthalmology, Jules Stein Eye Institute, University of California School of Medicine, Los Angeles, California.

Multiple Sclerosis

ROGER L. HIATT, M.D.

Professor and Chairman, Department of Ophthalmology, University of Tennessee Center for the Health Sciences, Memphis, Tennessee.

Corneal Abrasions, Contusions, Lacerations, and Perforations

DAVID A. HILES, M.D.

Clinical Professor of Ophthalmology, University of Pittsburgh School of Medicine. Chief of Ophthalmology, Children's Hospital. Director, Fight for Sight, Children's Eye Clinic, Children's Hospital, Pittsburgh, Pennsylvania.

Congenital and Infantile Cataracts

BARTON L. HODES, M.D.

Professor and Head, Department Ophthalmology, University of Arizona Health Sciences Center, Tucson, Arizona.

Phacoanaphylactic Endophthalmitis

HAROLD J. HOFFMAN, M.D., B.Sc. (Med.), F.R.C.S. (C)

Professor of Surgery, Division of Neurosurgery, University of Toronto. Chief of Staff, The Hospital for Sick Children, Toronto, Ontario, Canada.

Craniopharyngioma

JAMES D. HOGAN, M.D.

Department of Dermatology, Gundersen Clinic, La Crosse, Wisconsin.

Pruritus

JOHN B. HOLDS, M.D.

Fellow, Department of Ophthalmology, University of Utah Medical Center, Salt Lake City, Utah

Distichiasis

GARY N. HOLLAND, M.D.

Assistant Professor of Ophthalmology, Medical Director, Uveitis Center, Jules Stein Eye Institute, University of California School of Medicine, Los Angeles, California.

Acquired Immunodeficiency Syndrome (AIDS)

DAVID J. HOPKINS, M.B., F.R.C.S., D.O.

Consultant Ophthalmic Surgeon, Bradford Royal Infirmary, Bradford, West Yorkshire, England.

Hallermann-Streiff-Francois Syndrome

RICHARD B. HORNICK, M.D.

Professor of Clinical Medicine, University of Florida School of Medicine, Gainesville, Florida.

Q Fever

GEORGE M. HOWARD, M.D.

Associate Professor of Clinical Ophthalmology, College of Physicians and Surgeons, Columbia University, New York, New York.

Erythema Multiforme

DAVID S. HULL, M.D.

Professor of Ophthalmology, Department of Ophthalmology, Medical College of Georgia, Augusta, Georgia.

Proteus; Pseudoxanthoma Elasticum

WILLIAM E. HUNT, M.D.

Professor and Director, Division of Neurologic Surgery, Ohio State University College of Medicine, Columbus, Ohio.

Tolosa-Hunt Syndrome

J. J. HURWITZ, M.D., F.R.C.S. (C)

Assistant Professor of Ophthalmology, University of Toronto, Toronto, Ontario, Canada.

Alacrima

B. THOMAS HUTCHINSON, M.D.

Associate Clinical Professor of Ophthalmology, Harvard Medical School, Boston, Massachusetts.

Aphakic and Pseudophakic Pupillary Block

ROBERT A. HYNDIUK, M.D.

Professor of Ophthalmology, Eye Institute, Medical College of Wisconsin, Milwaukee, Wisconsin.

Bacillus Subtilis; Granular Corneal Dystrophy; Lattice Corneal Dystrophy; Ocular Vaccinia

D. ROGER ILLINGWORTH, M.D., Ph.D.

Associate Professor of Medicine, Research Associate Professor of Biochemistry, Oregon Health Sciences University, Portland, Oregon.

Abetalipoproteinemia and Homozygous Familial Hypobetalipoproteinemia

DOUGLAS A. JABS, M.D.

Associate Professor of Ophthalmology, Assistant Professor of Medicine, Johns Hopkins University School of Medicine, Baltimore, Maryland.

Ankylosing Spondylitis; Systemic Sclerosis

JERRY C. JACOBS, M.D.

Professor of Clinical Pediatrics, Columbia University College of Physicians and Surgeons, New York, New York.

Juvenile Rheumatoid Arthritis

xii / CONTRIBUTORS

EDWARD A. JAEGER, M.D.

Professor of Ophthalmology, Jefferson Medical College of Thomas Jefferson University, Attending Surgeon, Wills Eye Hospital, Philadelphia, Pennsylvania.

Down's Syndrome

NORMAN S. JAFFE, M.D.

Clinical Professor of Ophthalmology, Bascom Palmer Eye Institute, University of Miami School of Medicine, Miami, Florida.

Lid Myokymia

LEE M. JAMPOL, M.D.

Professor of Ophthalmology, University of Illinois College of Medicine. Director, Sickle Cell Eye Clinic, Eye and Ear Infirmary of the University of Illinois Hospital, Chicago, Illinois.

Sickle Cell Disease

RICHARD P. JOBE, M.D.

Clinical Professor of Surgery (Plastic), Stanford University School of Medicine, Stanford, California.

Lagophthalmos

THOMAS JOHN, M.D.

Director of Cornea and Contact Lens Service, Assistant Professor Department of Ophthalmology, University of Chicago, Chicago, Illinois.

Ascariasis

IRA SNOW JONES, M.D.

Clinical Professor Emeritus of Ophthalmology, Columbia University College of Physicians and Surgeons, New York, New York.

Lymphangioma; Rhabdomyosarcoma

G. FRANK JUDISCH, M.D.

Professor of Ophthalmology, University of Iowa College of Medicine, Iowa City, Iowa.

Robin Sequence

ROBERT E. KALINA, M.D.

Professor and Chairman, Department of Ophthalmology, University of Washington School of Medicine, Seattle, Washington.

Choroidal Neovascular Membranes; Retinopathy of Prematurity

SATOSHI KASHII, M.D.

Neuro Ophthalmology Fellow, Albert Einstein College of Medicine, Montefiore Medical Center, Bronx, New York.

Benign Intracranial Hypertension and Pseudotumor Cerebri

MICHAEL A. KASS, M.D.

Professor of Ophthalmology, Washington University Medical Center, St. Louis, Missouri.

Corticosteroid-Induced Glaucoma

FUMIO KAYAZAWA, M.D.

Vice-President, Shōzankai Medical Foundation Miyake Eye Clinic Hospital, Osaka, Japan.

Angioid Streaks

JEROME KAZDAN, M.D., F.R.C.S. (C)

Associate Professor of Ophthalmology, University of Toronto, Toronto, Ontario, Canada.

Ligneous Conjunctivitis

B. H. KEAN, M.D.

Clinical Professor Emeritus of Tropical Medicine and Public Health, Cornell University Medical College. Attending Physician, The New York Hospital, New York, New York.

Trichinosis

RONALD V. KEECH, M.D.

Assistant Professor of Ophthalmology, College of Medicine and University of Iowa Hospitals and Clinics, Iowa City, Iowa.

Dissociated Vertical Deviation; Functional Amblyopia

T. E. KELLY, M.D., Ph.D.

Director, Division of Medical Genetics, University of Virginia Medical Center, Charlottesville, Virginia.

Mucopolysaccharidosis I-H; Mucopolysaccharidosis I-H/S

NANCY G. KENNAWAY, D. Phil.

Professor of Medical Genetics, Oregon Health Sciences University, Portland, Oregon.

Gyrate Atrophy of the Choroid and Retina with Hyperornithinemia

JOHN S. KENNERDELL, M.D.

Clinical Professor of Ophthalmology, University of Pittsburgh School of Medicine. Chairman, Department of Ophthalmology, Allegheney General Hospital, Pittsburgh, Pennsylvania.

Orbital Graves' Disease

MARSHALL P. KEYS, M.D.

Clinical Associate Professor, Department of Ophthalmology, Clinical Assistant Professor of Pediatrics, Department of Pediatrics, Georgetown University Medical Center, Washington, District of Columbia.

Dylexia

ROBERT C. KIMBROUGH, III, M.D., F.A.C.P.

Chief, Division of Infectious Diseases, Good Samaritan Hospital and Medical Center. Assistant Professor of Medicine, Oregon Health Sciences University, Portland, Oregon.

Staphylococcus

MARILYN C. KINCAID, M.D.

Assistant Professor Ophthalmology and Pathology, St. Louis University School of Medicine, St. Louis, Missouri.

Pediculosis and Phthiriasis

JAMES L. KINYOUN, M.D.
Associate Professor of Ophthalmology, University of Washington School of Medicine, Seattle, Washington.
Wegener's Granulomatosis

TREVOR H. KIRKHAM, M.D., F.R.C.S.
Professor of Neurology and Neurosurgery, McGill University, Montreal, Quebec, Canada.
Mandibulofacial Dysostosis

YOSHIAKI KITAZAWA, M.D.
Professor and Chairman, Department of Ophthalmology, Gifu University School of Medicine, Gifu, Japan.
Primary Angle-Closure Glaucoma

MICHAEL L. KLEIN, M.D.
Associate Professor of Ophthalmology, Oregon Health Sciences University, Portland, Oregon.
Age-Related Macular Degeneration; Eales' Disease

STEPHEN A. KLOTZ, M.D.
Associate Professor of Medicine and Ophthalmology, Louisiana State University School of Medicine, Shreveport, Louisiana.
Coccidioidomycosis

PHILIP KNAPP, M.D.
Professor Emeritus of Clinical Ophthalmology, Columbia University College of Physicians and Surgeons, New York, New York.
Oculomotor (Third Nerve) Paralysis

DAVID L. KNOX, M.D.
Associate Professor of Ophthalmology, Wilmer Ophthalmological Institute, Johns Hopkins University School of Medicine, Baltimore, Maryland.
Crohn's Disease

FELIX O. KOLB, M.D.
Clinical Professor of Medicine, University of California School of Medicine, San Francisco, California.
Hypoparathyroidism

J. SCOTT KORTVELESY, M.D.
Department of Ophthalmology, Straub Clinic and Hospital, Honolulu, Hawaii.
Oribital Graves' Disease

JAY H. KRACHMER, M.D.
Professor of Ophthalmology, University of Iowa Hospitals and Clinics, Iowa City, Iowa.
Amyloidosis; Infectious Mononucleosis

RICHARD P. KRATZ, M.D.
Clinical Professor of Ophthalmology, University of Southern California. Clinical Professor of Ophthalmology, University of California, Irvine, California.
Stripping or Detachment of Descemet's Membrane

INGRID KREISSIG, M.D.
Professor of Ophthalmology, University of Tübingen and Chairman (Retina) University Eye Clinic, Tubingen, West Germany.
Retinal Detachment

GREGORY B. KROHEL, M.D.
Clinical Professor of Ophthalmology, Albany Medical Center, Albany, New York.
Orbital Cellulitis and Abscess

THEODORE KRUPIN, M.D.
Professor of Ophthalmology, Scheie Eye Institute, Presbyterian-University of Pennsylvania Medical Center, Philadelphia, Pennsylvania.
Juvenile Glaucoma

GEOFFREY M. KWITKO, M.D.
Oculoplastic, Orbital, and Neuro-ophthalmic Fellow, Kresge Eye Institute, Wayne State University School of Medicine, Detroit, Michigan.
Optic Neuritis

F. LAGOUTTE, M.D.
Professor of Ophthalmology, Medical University. Bordeaux, France.
Fuchs' Dellen

PETER R. LAIBSON, M.D.
Director, Cornea Service, Wills Eye Hospital. Professor of Ophthalmology, Jefferson Medical College of Thomas Jefferson University, Philadelphia, Pennsylvania.
Epithelial Basement Membrane Dystrophy and Recurrent Corneal Erosion; Pseudomonas Aeruginosa

LAURENT LAMER, M.D., F.R.C.S. (C)
Associate Professor of Ophthalmology, University of Montreal, Montreal, Quebec, Canada.
Newcastle Disease

ROGER H. S. LANGSTON, M.D., C.M.
Cornea Service, Department of Ophthalmology, Cleveland Clinic Foundation, Cleveland, Ohio.
Infectious Crystalline Keratopathy

A. LARMANDE, M.D.
Professor of Ophthalmology, University of Tours, Tours, France.
Brucellosis

CYRIL P. LEGUM, M.D.
Assistant Professor of Pediatrics and Medical Genetics, Tel Aviv University, Sachler School of Medicine, Tel Aviv, Israel.
Mucopolysaccharidosis IV

MICHAEL A. LEMP, M.D.

Professor and Chairman, Department of Ophthalmology, Clinical Director, Director of the Cornea Service, Center for Sight, Georgetown University Medical Center, Washington, District of Columbia.

Lacrimal Hypersecretion; Lacrimal Hyposecretion; Sjögren's Syndrome

CHARLES R. LEONE, JR., M.D.

Clinical Professor of Ophthalmology, University of Texas Health Science Center, San Antonio, Texas.

Oculoauriculovertebral Dysplasia

SIDNEY LERMAN, M.D.

Professor of Ophthalmology, New York Medical College, Valhalla, New York.

Direct and Photosensitized Ultraviolet Radiation; Gout

ROBERT L. LESSER, M.D.

Associate Clinical Professor, Department of Ophthalmology and Visual Science, Yale University School of Medicine, New Haven, Connecticut.

Creutzfeldt-Jakob Disease

MARK R. LEVINE, M.D.

Associate Clinical Professor of Ophthalmology, Case Western Reserve University School of Medicine. Chief of Ophthalmology, Mount Sinai Medical Center, Cleveland, Ohio.

Orbital Implant Extrusion

NORMAN S. LEVY, M.D., Ph.D., F.A.C.S.

Clinical Assistant Professor, Department of Community Health and Family Medicine, University of Florida-Health Center, College of Medicine, Gainesville, Florida.

Neurilemmoma

RICHARD A. LEWIS, M.D., M.S.

Associate Professor of Ophthalmology, Departments of Medicine, and Pediatrics, Cullen Eye Institute, Institute for Molecular Genetics, Baylor College of Medicine, Houston, Texas.

Neurofibromatosis

THOMAS J. LIESEGANG, M.D.

Associate Professor, Division of Ophthalmology, Mayo Clinic, Jacksonville, Florida.

Azotobacter; Fuchs' Heterochromic Iridocyclitis

HARVEY LINCOFF, M.D.

Professor of Clinical Ophthalmology, New York Hospital, Cornell Medical Center, New York, New York.

Retinal Detachment

RICHARD D. LISMAN, M.D.

Surgeon Director and Clinic Co-Chief Ophthalmic Plastic Surgery, Manhattan Eye, Ear, and Throat Hospital. Professor of Ophthalmology, New York Medical College (Lisman), New York, New York.

Ectropion; External Orbital Fractures; Internal Orbital Fractures

HUNTER L. LITTLE, M.D., F.A.C.S.

Clinical Professor of Surgery (Ophthalmology), Stanford University Medical Center, Stanford, California. Palo Alto Retinal Group, Menlo Park, California.

Subretinal Neovascular Membranes

LOIS A. LLOYD, M.D., F.R.C.S. (C)

Associate Professor in Ophthalmology, University of Toronto. Active Staff in Ophthalmology; The Toronto Hospital; and The Hospital for Sick Children, Toronto, Ontario, Canada.

Orbital Hypertelorism

WILLIAM C. LLOYD III, M.D., F.A.C.S.

Clinical Assistant Professor of Surgery, Uniformed Services University of the Health Sciences, Bethesda, Maryland.

Melanocytic Lesions of the Eyelids

RONALD R. LUBRITZ, M.D.

Clinical Professor of Medicine (Dermatology). Tulane University School of Medicine, New Orleans, Louisiana.

Actinic and Seborrheic Keratosis

MALCOLM N. LUXENBERG, M.D.

Professor and Chairman, Department of Ophthalmology, Medical College of Georgia, Augusta, Georgia.

Crystalline Corneal Dystrophy; Hyperlipoproteinemia; Tularemia

JAMES P. McCULLEY, M.D.

David Bruton Jr. Professor and Chairman, Department of Ophthalmology, University of Texas Health Science Center, Dallas, Texas.

Seborrheic Blepharitis; Staphylococcal and Mixed Staphylococcal/Seborrheic Blepharoconjunctivitis

CLEMENT McCULLOCH, M.D., F.R.C.S. (C)

Emeritus Professor of Ophthalmology, University of Toronto, Toronto, Ontario, Canada.

Macular Corneal Dystrophy

DAVID J. McINTYRE, M.D., F.A.C.S.

Consultant in Ophthalmology, University of Washington School of Medicine, Seattle, Washington.

After-Cataracts

VICTOR A. McKUSICK, M.D.

Chairman, Department of Medicine, Johns Hopkins University School of Medicine, Physician-in-Chief, Johns Hopkins Hospital, Baltimore, Maryland.

Mucopolysaccharidosis I-H

IAN A. MACKIE, M.B., F.R.C.S.

Associate Specialist, External Eye Diseases Clinic, Moorfields Eye Hospital, London, England.

Neuroparalytic Keratitis

SCOTT M. MAC RAE, M.D.
Assistant Professor of Ophthalmology, Director, Oregon Eye Bank, Director, Contact Lens Service, Oregon Health Sciences University, Portland, Oregon
Cat-Scratch Disease

LARRY E. MAGARGAL, M.D.
Co-Director, Retina Vascular Unit, Wills Eye Hospital. Associate Surgeon, Retina Service, Wills Eye Hospital. Clinical Associate Professor of Ophthalmology, Jefferson Medical College of Thomas Jefferson University, Philadelphia, Pennsylvania.
Retinal Vein Obstruction

MUNEERA A. MAHMOOD, M.D.
Clinical Instructor in Ophthalmology, Georgetown University Medical Center, Washington, District of Columbia.
Lacrimal Hypersecretion

SID MANDELBAUM, M.D.
Assistant Professor of Ophthalmology, Bascom Palmer Eye Institute, University of Miami School of Medicine, Miami, Florida.
Bacterial Endophthalmitis

MARK J. MANNIS, M.D., F.A.C.S.
Associate Professor of Ophthalmology, Director, Cornea and External Disease Service, Department of Ophthalmology, University of California, Davis, Sacramento, California.
Keratoconus; Terrien's Marginal Degeneration

GEORGE E. MARAK, JR., M.D.
Clinical Professor of Ophthalmology, Georgetown University Medical Center, Washington, District of Columbia.
Sympathetic Ophthalmia

DANIEL MARCHAC, M.D.
Consultant Plastic Surgeon, Hopital des Enfant-Malades, Paris, France.
Anophthalmos

R. J. MARSH, F.R.C.S.
Consultant Ophthalmic Surgeon, St. Mary's Hospital. Honorary Consultant, Moorfields Eye Hospital, London, England.
Herpes Zoster

BRUCE M. MASSARO, M.D., M.P.H.
Assistant Professor of Ophthalmology Oculoplastic Section, Medical College of Wisconsin, Milwaukee, Wisconsin.
Ocular Vaccinia

KANJIRO MASUDA, M.D.
Chairman and Professor, Department of Ophthalmology, University of Tokyo School of Medicine, Tokyo, Japan.
Behçets Disease

IRENE H. MAUMENEE, M.D.
Professor of Ophthalmology and Medicine, Johns Hopkins University School of Medicine, Baltimore, Maryland
Congenital Hereditary Endothelial Dystrophy; Mucopolysaccharidosis I-S

WALTER MAYER, M.D.
Associate Clinical Professor of Ophthalmology, Medical College of Virginia of Virginia Commonwealth University, Richmond, Virginia.
Corneal Neovascularization

MALCOLM L. MAZOW, M.D.
Clinical Professor of Ophthalmology and Pediatrics, Director of Pediatric Ophthalmology, University of Texas, Houston, Texas.
Convergence Insufficiency Syndrome

SAUL MERIN, M.D.
Professor of Ophthalmology, Hebrew University of Jerusalem. Head, Unit of Ophthalmology, Hadassa University Hospital, Jerusalem, Israel.
Retinitis Pigmentosa

HENRY S. METZ, M.D.
Professor and Chairman, Department of Ophthalmology, University of Rochester School of Medicine and Dentistry, Rochester, New York.
A-Pattern Esotropia; A-Pattern Exotropia; Duane's Retraction Syndrome; V-Pattern Esotropia; V-Pattern Exotropia

ROGER F. MEYER, M.D.
Professor of Ophthalmology, University of Michigan School of Medicine, Ann Arbor, Michigan.
Mumps

RONALD G. MICHELS, M.D.
Professor of Ophthalmology, Wilmer Ophthalmological Institute, Johns Hopkins University School of Medicine, Baltimore, Maryland.
Epithelial Ingrowth; Macular Pucker

BENJAMIN MILDER, M.D.
Professor of Clinical Ophthalmology, Washington University Medical Center, St. Louis, Missouri.
Actinomycosis; Dacryolith; Lacrimal System Contusions and Lacerations

COLETTA M. MILLER, D.D.S.
Zoller Dental Clinic, University of Chicago Hospitals and Clinics, Chicago, Illinois.
Engelmann's Disease

KEVIN N. MILLER, M.D.
Ophthalmologist, Las Vegas, Nevada
Histiocytosis X

NEIL R. MILLER, M.D.
Frank B. Walsh Professor of Neuro-Ophthalmology, Professor of Ophthalmology, Neurology, and Neurosurgery, Johns Hopkins University School of Medicine, Baltimore, Maryland.
Hodgkin's Disease; Myasthenia Gravis; Temporal Arteritis

JOHN A. MILLS, M.D.
Associate Professor of Medicine, Harvard Medical School, Boston, Massachusetts.
Polyarteritis Nodosa

MARY BETH MOORE, M.D.
Assistant Professor of Ophthalmology, Department of Ophthalmology, University of Texas Southwestern Medical School, Dallas, Texas.
Acanthamoebae

JOHN C. MORRISON, M.D.
Assistant Professor of Ophthalmology, Oregon Health Sciences University, Portland, Oregon.
Glaucoma After Ocular Contusion; Malignant Glaucoma

LYNNE H. MORRISON, M.D.
Assistant Professor of Dermatology, Oregon Health Sciences University, Portland, Oregon.
Cicatricial Pemphigoid

PETER H. MORSE, M.D., F.A.C.S.
Professor of Ophthalmology, University of Chicago Hospitals and Clinics, Pritzker School of Medicine, Chicago, Illinois.
Engelmann's Disease

P. K. MUKHERJEE, M.S.
Professor of Ophthalmology, Pt. J.N.M. Medical College, D.K. Hospital, Raipur, (M.P.) India.
Rhinosporidiosis; Thelaziasis

RALPH MULLER, Ph.D.
Director, CAB Commonwealth Institute of Parasitology, St. Albans, Herts, England. Senior Lecturer (honorary) London School of Hygiene and Topical Medicine, London, England.
Dracunculiasis

K. J. MURPHY, F.R.A.C.P.
Emeritus Clinical Tutor, University of Queensland, Emeritus Medical Superintendent and Medical Director, Princess Alexandra Hospital, Wooloongabba, Queensland, Australia.
Hyperparathyroidism

AIDAN MURRAY, F.R.C.S.
Senior Ophthalmic Registrar, Department of Ophthalmology, King's College Hospital, London, England.
Uveoparotid Fever

MICHAEL A. NAIDOFF, M.D.
Associate Professor of Ophthalmology, Jefferson Medical College of Thomas Jefferson University. Associate Surgeon, Wills Eye Hospital, Philadelphia, Pennsylvania.
Melanotic Lesions of the Eyelids

JOHN NASSIF, M.D.
Fellow, Ophthalmic Plastic, Reconstructive, and Orbital Surgery, New York Eye and Ear Infirmary, New York, New York.
Eyelid Contusions, Lacerations, and Avulsions

KAMAL F. NASSIF, M.D.
Associate Clinical Professor of Ophthalmology, Eye Institute, Medical College of Wisconsin, Milwaukee, Wisconsin.
Granular Corneal Dystrophy

HELLMUT F. NEUBAUER, M.D.
Professor Emeritus of Ophthalmology, Department of Ophthalmology, University of Cologne, Cologne, West Germany.
Iris Lacerations, Holes, and Iridodialysis

THOMAS P. NIGRA, M.D.
Clinical Professor and Chairman, Department of Dermatology, Washington Hospital Center, Washington, District of Columbia.
Psoriasis

MOGENS S. NORN, M.D., Ph.D.
Professor of Ophthalmology, University of Copenhagen. Chief Surgeon, Ophthalmology Department, Copenhagen Municipal Hospital in Hvidovre, Copenhagen, Denmark.
Keratoconjunctivitis Sicca

JULIAN J. NUSSBAUM, M.D.
Clinical Associate Professor of Ophthalmology, University of Michigan Medical Center, Ann Arbor, Michigan. Associate Professor of Ophthalmology, Wayne State University of Medicine, Detroit, Michigan.
Peripheral Retinal Breaks and Degeneration

DENIS M. O'DAY, M.D.
Professor of Ophthalmology, Vanderbilt University Medical Center, Nashville, Tennessee.
Bacillus Cereus; Blastomycosis

EAMON P. O'DONOGHUE, M.B., B.Ch., B.A.O., F.R.C.S. (Ed.)
Ophthalmic Surgeon, Moorfields Eye Hospital, London, England.
Relapsing Polychondritis

JAY JUSTIN OLDER, M.D.
Associate Professor of Ophthalmology, Director Oculoplastic Service, University of South Florida Medical Center, Tampa, Florida.
Blepharophimosis

H. BRUCE OSTLER, M.D.
Clinical Professor of Ophthalmology, Francis I. Proctor Foundation for Research in Ophthalmology, University of California School of Medicine, San Francisco, California.
Pneumococcus

EARL A. PALMER, M.D.
Associate Professor of Ophthalmology and Pediatrics, Director of Pediatric Ophthalmology, Oregon Health Sciences University, Portland, Oregon.
Ophthalmia Neonatorum

FRANK PARKER, M.D.
Professor and Chairman, Department of Dermatology, Oregon Health Sciences University, Portland, Oregon.
Vitiligo

MARSHALL M. PARKS, M.D.
Clinical Professor of Ophthalmology, George Washington University Medical Center. Senior Attending, Children's National Medical Center, Washington, District of Columbia.
Lenticonus and Lentiglobus; Monofixation Syndrome

JOHN A. PARRISH, M.D.
Professor and Chairman, Department of Dermatology, Director, Wellman Laboratories of Photomedicine, Harvard Medical School, Boston, Massachusetts.
Photosensitivity and Sunburn

HAROLD C. PATTERSON, M.D.
Clinical Assistant Professor of Ophthalmology (Retired), Yale University School of Medicine, New Haven, Connecticut. Chairman of the Ophthalmology Section (Past), Attending Ophthalmologist (Present), Danbury Hospital, Danbury, Connecticut.
Iris Prolapse

BARRY S. PAUL, M.D.
Clinical Instructor in Dermatology, Harvard Medical School. Clinical Associate in Dermatology, Massachusetts General Hospital, Boston, Massachusetts.
Photosensitivity and Sunburn

ALAN PESTRONK, M.D.
Assistant Professor of Neurology, Johns Hopkins University School of Medicine, Baltimore, Maryland.
Myasthenia Gravis

THOMAS H. PETTIT, M.D.
Professor of Ophthalmology, University of California School of Medicine, Los Angeles, California.
Fungal Keratitis

GISSUR J. PETURSSON, M.D.
Professor of Ophthalmology, University of Arkansas for Medical Sciences, Little Rock, Arkansas.
Filtering Blebs

ROSWELL R. PFISTER, M.D.
Director, Brookwood Eye Research Laboratories. Professor of Ophthalmology, University of Alabama Medical Center, Birmingham, Alabama.
Alkaline Injury

STEVEN M. PODOS, M.D.
Professor and Chairman, Department of Ophthalmology, Mount Sinai School of Medicine, New York, New York.
Ocular Hypertension; Plateau Iris

FRANK M. POLACK, M.D., F.A.C.S.
Consultant in Ophthalmology, University of South Florida, Tampa, Florida. Veterans Administration Medical Center, Lake City, Florida.
Reis-Bucklers' Superficial Corneal Dystrophy

J. POLETTI, M.D.
Chief of Ophthalmology, Hospital of Tarbes, Tarbes, France.
Brucellosis

ZANE F. POLLARD, M.D.
Chief of Ophthalmology, Scottish Rite Hospital for Crippled Children, Atlanta, Georgia.
Toxocariasis

RONALD C. PRUETT, M.D.
Assistant Clinical Professor of Ophthalmology, Harvard Medical School. Surgeon in Ophthalmology, Massachusetts Eye and Ear Infirmary. Boston, Massachusetts.
Persistent Hyperplastic Primary Vitreous

ALLEN M. PUTTERMAN, M.D.
Professor of Clinical Ophthalmology and Chief, Oculoplastic Service, University of Illinois College of Medicine. Professor and Director of Oculoplastic Surgery, Eye and Ear Infirmary of the University of Illinois Hospital, Chicago, Illinois.
Madarosis; Orbital Fat Herniation

P. QUEGUINER, M.D.
Ophthalmologist, Armed Forces Hospital, Marseille, France.
Schistosomiasis

EDWARD L. RAAB, M.D.
Professor of Ophthalmology, Associate Professor of Pediatrics, Director of Pediatric Ophthalmology and Strabismus, Mount Sinai School of Medicine, New York, New York.
Accommodative Esotropia

JOHN M. RAMOCKI, M.D.
Clinical Instructor in Ophthalmology, Kresge Eye Institute, Wayne State University School of Medicine, Detroit, Michigan.
Optic Neuritis

xviii / CONTRIBUTORS

NARSING A. RAO, M.D.

Professor of Ophthalmology and Pathology, University of Southern California School of Medicine, Los Angeles, California.

Sebaceous Gland Carcinoma

LAWRENCE A. RAYMOND, M.D.

Associate Professor of Ophthalmology, Director, Retina and Vitreous Service, University of Cincinnati Medical Center, Cincinnati, Ohio.

Dirofilariasis

JOHN E. READ, M.D.

Assistant Clinical Professor of Ophthalmology, Eye and Ear Infirmary of the University of Illinois Hospitals, University of Illinois College of Medicine, Chicago, Illinois.

Ciliary Body Concussions and Lacerations

AUGUST L. READER, III, M.D., F.A.C.S.

Associate Clinical Professor of Ophthalmology, University of Southern California School of Medicine. Attending Surgeon, Cedars-Sinai Medical Center, Los Angeles, California.

Hysteria, Malingering, and Anxiety States

L. F. RICH, M.S., M.D.

Associate Professor of Ophthalmology, Director, Cornea and External Disease Service, Oregon Health Sciences University. Chief of Ophthalmology, Veterans Administration Medical Center, Portland, Oregon.

Conjunctival Lacerations and Contusions; Pterygium and Pseudopterygium; Relapsing Fever

CLAUDIA U. RICHTER, M.D.

Clinical Assistant in Ophthalmology, Harvard Medical School, Assistant Surgeon in Ophthalmology, Massachusetts Eye and Ear Infirmary, Boston, Massachusetts.

Aphakic and Pseudophakic Pupillary Block

ROBERT RITCH, M.D.

Professor of Clinical Ophthalmology, New York Medical College, Valhalla, New York. Chief, Glaucoma Service, New York Eye and Ear Infirmary, New York, New York.

Ocular Hypertension; Plateau Iris

JOSEPH E. ROBERTSON, JR., M.D.

Assistant Professor of Ophthalmology, Oregon Health Sciences University, Portland, Oregon.

Diffuse Unilateral Subacute Neuroretinitis; Familial Exudative Vitreoretinopathy

JEFFREY B. ROBIN, M.D.

Associate Professor, Eye Center, Department of Ophthalmology, University of Illinois College of Medicine, Chicago, Illinois.

Gonococcal Ocular Disease

JOHN H. ROCKEY, M.D., Ph.D.

Professor of Ophthalmology, Scheie Eye Institute, Presbyterian-University of Pennsylvania Medical Center, Philadelphia, Pennsylvania.

Ascariasis

JAIME ROIZENBLATT, M.D.

Assistant Professor of Ophthalmology, São Paulo University School of Medicine, São Paulo, Brazil.

American Mucocutaneous Leishmaniasis

PAUL E. ROMANO, M.D., M.S.O.

Formerly Professor of Ophthalmology and Pediatrics, University of Florida School of Medicine, Gainesville, Florida.

Juvenile Xanthogranuloma; Traumatic Hyphema

HILARY J. RONNER, M.D.

Assistant Attending Ophthalmologist, Manhattan Eye, Ear, and Throat Hospital. Assistant Adjunct in Ophthalmology, Lenox Hill Hospital, New York, New York.

Lymphangioma; Rhabdomyosarcoma

ARTHUR L. ROSENBAUM, M.D.

Professor of Ophthalmology, Jules Stein Eye Institute, University of California School of Medicine, Los Angeles, California.

Esotropia—High AC/A Ratio

JAMES T. ROSENBAUM, M.D.

Associate Professor of Medicine, Ophthalmology and Cell Biology, Director, The Uveitis Clinic, Oregon Health Sciences University, Portland, Oregon.

Rheumatoid Arthritis; Systemic Lupus Erythematosus; Uveitis

TED ROSENSTOCK, M.D.

Ophthalmologist, Sunnybrook Hospital, Eye Clinic, Toronto, Ontario, Canada.

Alacrima

ROBERT N. ROSS, Ph.D.

Staff Associate at the Eye Research Institute of the Retina Foundation, Boston, Massachusetts.

Allergic Conjunctivitis; Giant Papillary Conjunctivitis

F. HAMPTON ROY, M.D., F.A.C.S.

Clinical Associate Professor of Ophthalmology, University of Arkansas for Medical Sciences, Baptist Medical Center, Arkansas Children's Hospital, Doctors Hospital, St. Vincent Infirmary, Little Rock, Arkansas.

Fibrosarcoma; Mikulicz's Syndrome; Spider Bites; Sturge-Weber Syndrome

MELVIN L. RUBIN, M.D.

Professor and Chairman, Department of Ophthalmology, University of Florida School of Medicine, J. Hillis Miller Health Center, Gainesville, Florida.

Anisometropia

RICHARD S. RUIZ, M.D.
Professor and Chairman, Department of Ophthalmology, University of Texas Health Science Center, Houston, Texas.
Vitreous Wick Syndrome

THOMAS E. RUNYAN, M.D., F.A.C.S.
Associate Professor of Ophthalmology, Texas A & M University College of Medicine. Senior Staff, Scott and White Clinic, Temple, Texas.
Malaria

K. MATTI SAARI, M.D.
Professor of Ophthalmology, University of Turku. Head, Department of Ophthalmology, Turku University Hospital, Turku, Finland.
Reiter's Disease; Yersiniosis

BIJAN SAFAI, M.D., D.S.C.
Attending Physician and Chief, Dermatology Service, Memorial Sloan-Kettering Cancer Center. Professor of Medicine (Dermatology), Cornell Medical Center. Adjunct Member, Rockefeller University School of Medicine, New York, New York.
Kaposi's Sarcoma

S. Y. SALIH, M.D., M.R.C.P., D.C.M.T.
Professor of Medicine, University of Khartoum, Khartoum, Sudan.
Relapsing Fever

JOHN R. SAMPLES, M.D.
Assistant Professor of Ophthalmology, Oregon Health Sciences University, Portland, Oregon.
Bengin Essential Blepharospasm; Glaucoma Associated With Elevated Venous Pressure; Hemifacial Spasm; Rubeosis Iridis; Streptococcus

DAVID J. SCHANZLIN, M.D.
Professor and Chairman, Department of Ophthalmology, Bethesda Eye Institute, St. Louis University Medical Center, St. Louis, Missouri.
Corneal and Conjunctival Calcifications; Herpes Simplex; Pellucid Marginal Corneal Degeneration

ABRAHAM SCHLOSSMAN, M.D., F.A.C.S.
Clinical Associate Professor of Ophthalmology, State University of New York Health Science Center, Brooklyn, New York. Director of Ocular Motility Service, Manhattan Eye, Ear, and Throat Hospital, New York, New York.
Glaucomatocyclitic Crises

LEE K. SCHWARTZ, M.D.
Consultant, Corneal and External Disease Service, Department of Ophthalmology, Pacific Presbyterian Medical Center, San Francisco, California.
Floppy Eyelid Syndrome

WILLIAM E. SCOTT, M.D.
Professor of Ophthalmology, University of Iowa Hospitals and Clinics, Iowa City, Iowa.
Accommodative Spasm

LYN A SEDWICK, M.D.
Neuro Ophthalmologist, Private Practice, Orlando, Florida.
Juvenile Xanthogranuloma

DAVID SEVEL, M.D., Ph.D., F.A.C.S.
Division of Ophthalmology, Scripps Clinic and Research Foundation, La Jolla, California.
Clostridium Perfringens; Leiomyoma

RAYMOND J. SEVER, M.D.
Clinical Assistant Professor of Ophthalmology, University of South Florida Medical Center, Tampa, Florida.
Ichthyosis

ROBERT N. SHAFFER, M.D., F.A.C.S.
Clinical Professor Emeritus of Ophthalmology, University of California School of Medicine, San Francisco, California.
Open-Angle Glaucoma

H. JOHN SHAMMAS, M.D.
Associate Clinical Professor of Ophthalmology, University of Southern California School of Medicine, Los Angeles, California.
Escherichia Coli; Iris Melanoma

CAROL L. SHIELDS, M.D.
Clinical Fellow, Ocular Oncology Service, Wills Eye Hospital, Jefferson Medical College of Thomas Jefferson University, Philadelphia, Pennsylvania.
Glaucoma Associated With Intraocular Tumors; Malignant Melanoma of the Posterior Uvea

JERRY A. SHIELDS, M.D.
Director, Ocular Oncology Service, Wills Eye Hospital. Professor of Ophthalmology, Jefferson Medical College of Thomas Jefferson University, Philadelphia, Pennsylvania.
Glaucoma Associated With Intraocular Tumors; Malignant Melanoma of the Posterior Uvea

M. BRUCE SHIELDS, M.D.
Professor of Ophthalmology, Duke University Medical Center, Durham, North Carolina.
Glaucoma Associated with Anterior Uveitis; Iridocorneal Endothelial Syndrome

WILLIAM T. SHULTS, M.D.
Associate Professor of Ophthalmology, Clinical Associate Professor of Neurology, Oregon Health Sciences University, Portland, Oregon.
Lid Myokymia; Superior Oblique Myokymia

xx / CONTRIBUTORS

JERRY N. SHUSTER, M.D.

Glaucomologist. Private Practice, Orlando, Florida.

Traumatic Hyphema

HARVEY H. SLANSKY, M.D.

Clinical Instructor in Ophthalmology, Harvard Medical School, Boston, Massachusetts.

Acid Burns

WILLIAM S. SLY, M.D.

Alice Doisy Professor of Biochemistry. Chairman, E.A. Doisy Department of Biochemistry and Nuclear Biology, St. Louis University Medical Center, Professor of Pediatrics, Genetics, and Internal Medicine, Washington University Medical Center.

Mucopolysaccharidosis VII

BYRON C. SMITH, M.D.

Professor of Ophthalmology, New York Medical College. Emeritus Chariman, Manhattan Eye, Ear, and Throat Hospital, New York, New York.

Ectropion; External Orbital Fractures; Internal Orbital Fractures

PATRICIA W. SMITH, M.D.

Assistant Professor of Ophthalmology and Pathology, University of Virginia Medical Health Sciences Center, Charlottesville, Virginia.

Epithelial Ingrowth; Intraocular Epithelial Cysts

RONALD E. SMITH, M.D.

Professor of Ophthalmology, University of Southern California School of Medicine, Estelle Doheny Eye Foundation, Los Angeles, California.

Choroidal Ruptures; Irritative Conjunctivitis; Ocular Histoplasmosis; Proprionibacterium Acnes

GILBERT SMOLIN, M.D.

Clinical Professor of Ophthalmology, University of California School of Medicine. Research Ophthalmologist, Francis I. Proctor Foundation for Research in Ophthalmology, San Francisco, California.

Bee Sting of the Cornea

DAVID B. SOLL, M.D., F.A.C.S.

Clinical Professor of Surgery (Ophthalmology), University of Medicine and Dentistry of New Jersey, Robert Wood Johnson Medical School, Camden, New Jersey.

Enophthalmos

ALFRED SOMMER, M.D., M.H.Sc.

Professor of Ophthalmology, Epidemiology, and International Health, Johns Hopkins University School of Medicine, Baltimore, Maryland.

Hypovitaminosis A

HAROLD F. SPALTER, M.D.

Professor of Clinical Ophthalmology, Columbia University College of Physicians and Surgeons, New York, New York.

Juvenile Rheumatoid Arthritis

DAVID J. SPENCE, M.D.

Corneal Specialist, Kaiser Permanente Hospital, Los Angeles, California.

Corneal and Conjunctival Calcifications; Herpes Simplex

DANIEL H. SPITZBERG, M.D.

Clinical Associate Professor of Ophthalmology, Indiana University School of Medicine, Indianapolis, Indiana.

Influenza; Pars Planitis; Toxoplasmosis

THOMAS C. SPOOR, M.D., M.S., F.A.C.S.

Associate Professor of Ophthalmology, Kresge Eye Institute, Wayne State University School of Medicine, Detroit, Michigan.

Optic Neuritis; Tuberculosis

ROBERT L. STAMPER, M.D.

Chairman, Department of Ophthalmology, Pacific Presbyterian Medical Center, San Francisco, California.

Ankyloblepharon; Symblepharon

WALTER J. STARK, M.D.

Professor of Ophthalmology, Wilmer Ophthalmological Institute, Johns Hopkins University School of Medicine, Baltimore, Maryland.

Epithelial Ingrowth; Intraocular Epithelial Cysts

ROGER F. STEINERT, M.D.

Clinical Assistant in Ophthalmology, Harvard Medical School, Boston, Massachusetts.

Posterior Polymorphous Corneal Dystrophy

WALTER H. STERN, M.D.

Professor of Ophthalmology, University of California School of Medicine, San Francisco, California.

Fungal Endophthalmitis

PAUL STERNBERG, JR., M.D.

Assistant Professor of Ophthalmology, Emory University School of Medicine, Atlanta, Georgia.

Dislocation of the Lens

ALAN SUGAR, M.D.

Professor of Ophthalmology, W. K. Kellogg Eye Center, University of Michigan Medical Center, Ann Arbor, Michigan.

Dermatophytosis; Impetigo; Koch-Weeks Bacillus

JOEL SUGAR, M.D.

Professor of Ophthalmology, University of Illinois College of Medicine. Director of Corneal Service, Eye and Ear Infirmary of the University of Illinois Hospital, Chicago, Illinois.

Corneal Edema

CONTRIBUTORS / xxi

JOHN H. SULLIVAN, M.D.

Clinical Professor of Ophthalmology, University of California School of Medicine, San Francisco, California.

Blepharochalasis; Ptosis

KENNETH C. SWAN, M.D.

Professor of Ophthalmology, Oregon Health Sciences University, Portland, Oregon.

Cicatricial Pemphigoid; Fibrous Ingrowth; Iris Cysts; Recurrent Late Hyphema From Focal Wound Vascularization

THOMAS E. TALBOT, M.D.

Clinical Associate Professor of Ophthalmology, Oregon Health Science University, Portland, Oregon.

Low Vision

K. NOLEN TANNER, M.D., Ph.D.

Assistant Clinical Professor of Ophthalmology, Oregon Health Sciences University. Teaching Associate, Devers Memorial Eye Clinic, Good Samaritan Hospital and Medical Center, Portland, Oregon.

Accommodative Insufficiency; Low Vision

AHTI TARKKANEN, M.D.

Professor and Chairman, Department of Ophthalmology, University of Helsinki. Director, Helsinki University Eye Hospital. Vice-Dean, Faculty of Medicine, University of Helsinki, Helsinki, Finland.

Exfoliation Syndrome

WILLIAM TASMAN, M.D.

Professor and Chairman, Department of Ophthalmology, Jefferson Medical College of Thomas Jefferson University. Ophthalmologist-In-Chief, Wills Eye Hospital. Attending Surgeon, Chestnut Hill Hospital. Consultant, Children's Hospital of Philadelphia, Philadelphia, Pennsylvania.

Coats' Disease

BRUCE C. TAYLOR, M.D.

Associate Clinical Professor of Ophthalmology, University of Texas Health Science Center, Dallas, Texas.

Vitreous Hemorrhage

DANIEL M. TAYLOR, M.D., F.A.C.S.

John and Florence M. Solomon Professor of Ophthalmology, Co-Chairman of Ophthalmology, University of Connecticut Health Center, Farmington, Connecticut.

Expulsive Hemorrhage

KLAUS D. TEICHMANN, M.D., F.R.C.S. (C), F.R.A.C.O.

Consultant Ophthalmic Surgeon, Uthoff Eye Hospital, Kiel-Bellevue, West Germany.

Orbital Hemorrhages

RICHARD R. TENZEL, M.D.

Clinical Professor of Ophthalmology, Bascom Palmer Eye Institute, University of Miami School of Medicine, Miami, Florida.

Lid Retraction

PAUL TESSIER, M.D.

Head, Department of Plastic Surgery, Foch Hospital. Honorary Fellow of the American College of Surgeons, Paris, France.

Crouzon's Disease

THOM S. THOMASSEN, M.D.

Director, Anterior Segment Surgery Unit, Ophthalmology Service, Walter Reed Army Medical Center, Washington, District of Columbia. Instructor of Surgery, Division of Ophthalmology, Uniformed Services University of the Health Sciences, Bethesda, Maryland.

Intraocular Foreign Body—Copper

KRISTIAN THOMSEN, M.D.

Associate Professor University Hospital. Assistant Professor, Department of Dermatology, Rigshospitalet, Copenhagen, Denmark.

Mycosis Fungoides

LAWRENCE G. TOMASI, M.D., Ph.D.

Associate Professor of Pediatrics and Neurology, Loma Linda University School of Medicine, Loma Linda, California.

Maple Syrup Urine Disease

ANDREA CIBIS TONGUE, M.D.

Clinical Associate Professor of Ophthalmology, Oregon Health Sciences University, Portland, Oregon.

Basic Exotropia; Oculocerebrorenal Syndrome

HARVEY W. TOPILOW, M.D.

Associate Clinical Professor of Ophthalmology, Albert Einstein College of Medicine, Montefiore Medical Center, Bronx, New York.

Cysticerosis

RAMESH C. TRIPATHI, M.D., Ph.D.

Professor of Ophthalmology and Visual Science, and Professor in The College, University of Chicago Hospitals and Clinics, Pritzker School of Medicine, Chicago, Illinois.

Corneal Mucous Plaques

DAVID T. TSE, M.D., F.A.C.S.

Associate Professor of Ophthalmology, Bascom Palmer Eye Institute, Miami, Florida.

Hypertrichosis

AUDREY W. TUBERVILLE, M.D.

Associate Professor of Ophthalmology, University of Tennessee Center for the Health Sciences, Memphis, Tennessee.

Filamentary Keratitis; Mooren's Ulcer

YUKIO UCHIDA, M.D.

Professor and Chairman, Department of Ophthalmology, Tokyo Women's Medical College, Tokyo, Japan.

Varicella

xxii / CONTRIBUTORS

E. MICHAEL VAN BUSKIRK, M.D.

Professor of Ophthalmology, Oregon Health Sciences University, Portland, Oregon.

Glaucoma Associated With Intraocular Lenses; Postoperative Flat Anterior Chamber

A. J. M. Van Der WERF, M.D.

Professor of Neurosurgery, Academisch Ziekenhuis, University of Amsterdam, Amsterdam, The Netherlands.

Optic Foramen Fractures

HENRY J. L. VAN DYK, M.D.

Deceased.

Orbital Graves' Disease

DAVID W. VASTINE, M.D.

Chief of Ophthalmology, Highland General Hospital. San Francisco, California.

Ankyloblepharon; Symblepharon

J. VÉDY, M.D.

Docteur en Médicine, Professeur, Ophthalmologiste des Hopitaux, Institut de Médecine Tropicale, Marseille, France.

Schistosomiasis

JACLYN VIDGOFF, Ph.D.

Assistant Professor of Medical Genetics, Oregon Health Sciences University, Portland, Oregon.

Mucopolysaccharidosis VI

N. VISWALINGAM, M.D., D.O.

Research Associate, Institute of Ophthalmology, University of London, London, England.

Trachoma

MICHAEL D. WAGONER, M.D.

Assistant Professor of Ophthalmology, Harvard Medical School. Cornea Service, Massachusetts Eye and Ear Infirmary, Boston, Massachusetts.

Phlyctenulosis

THOMAS J. WALSH, M.D.

Professor of Ophthalmology Visual Science and Neurology, Yale University School of Medicine, New Haven, Connecticut.

Papilledema

DAVID S. WALTON, M.D.

Assistant Clinical Professor of Ophthalmology, Harvard Medical School. Associate Surgeon in Ophthalmology, Massachusetts Eye and Ear Infirmary, Boston, Massachusetts.

Aniridia; Infantile Glaucoma; Weill-Marchesani Syndrome

MARTIN WAND, M.D.

Assistant Clinical Professor of Ophthalmology, University of Connecticut Health Center, Farmington, Connecticut. Senior Staff, Department of Ophthalmology, Hartford Hospital, Hartford, Connecticut.

Acinetobacter

ARDEN H. WANDER, M.D.

Associate Professor of Clinical Ophthalmology, University of Cincinnati Medical Center, Cincinnati, Ohio.

Superior Limbic Keratoconjunctivitis; Thermal Burns

PETER G. WATSON, M.A., M.B., B.Chir., F.R.C.S., D.O.

Consultant Ophthalmic Surgeon, Addenbrooke's Hospital, Cambridge, England. Honorary Consultant Ophthalmic Surgeon, Moorfields Eye Hospital, London, England.

Episcleritis; Relapsing Polychondritis; Scleritis

RICHARD J. WEINBERG, M.D.

Clinical Assistant Professor of Ophthalmology, Georgetown University. Active Staff, Georgetown University Hospital, Washington, District of Columbia.

Fusobacterium

THOMAS A. WEINGEIST, M.D., Ph.D.

Professor and Head, Department of Ophthalmology, University of Iowa Hospitals and Clinics, Iowa City, Iowa.

Angiokeratoma Corporis Diffusum Universale

GEORGE W. WEINSTEIN, M.D.

Professor and Jane McDermott Shott Chairman, Department of Ophthalmology, West Virginia University Medical Center, Morgantown, West Virginia.

Hyperopia

JOHN J. WEITER, M.D., Ph.D.

Assistant Clinical Professor of Ophthalmology, Harvard Medical School. Associate Clinical Professor, Tufts University. Senior Scientist, Eye Research Institute of Retina Foundation, Boston, Massachusetts.

Angiomatosis Retinae; Polyarteritis Nodosa

RICHARD G. WELEBER, M.D.

Professor of Ophthalmology and Medical Genetics, Oregon Health Sciences University, Portland, Oregon.

Abetalipoproteinemia and Homozygous Familial Hypobetalipoproteinemia; Gyrate Atrophy of the Choroid and Retina with Hyperornithinemia; Mucopolysaccharidosis VI; Refsum's Disease

FLEMING D. WERTZ, M.D.

Director, Retina Unit, Ophthalmology Service, Walter Reed Army Medical Center, Washington, District of Columbia. Assistant Professor, Department of Surgery Division of Ophthalmology, Uniformed Services University of the Health Sciences, Bethesda, Maryland.

Intraocular Foreign Body—Copper

JOHN P. WHITCHER, M.D.
Associate Clinical Professor Department of Ophthalmology, University of California School of Medicine. Associate Research Ophthalmologist, Francis I. Proctor Foundation for Research in Ophthalmology, San Francisco, California.
Acute Hemorrhagic Conjunctivitis

GEORGE A. WILLIAMS, M.D.
Clinical Associate Professor of Ophthalmology, Kresge Eye Institute, University, Detroit, Michigan.
Bacillus Subtilis

HUGH P. WILLIAMS, F.R.C.S., D.O.
Consultant Ophthalmic Surgeon, North Middlesex Hospital, Edmonton, London, England.
Thygeson's Superficial Punctate Keratopathy

DAVID J. WILSON, M.D.
Assistant Professor of Ophthalmology, Director, Ophthalmic Pathology Laboratory, Oregon Health Sciences University, Portland, Oregon.
Chorioretinal Concussions and Lacerations; Mucormycosis; Ocular Hypotony; Retinal Emboli

FRED M. WILSON II, M.D.
Professor of Ophthalmology, Department of Ophthalmology, Indiana University School of Medicine, Indianapolis, Indiana.
Papilloma

WARREN A. WILSON, M.D.
Deceased.
Galactosemias

DENNIS L. WINGFIELD, M.D.
Ophthalmologist, Rebsamen Memorial Hospital, North Little Rock, Arkansas. Staff, Baptist Medical Center, Doctors Hospital, St. Vincent Infirmary, Little Rock, Arkansas. Staff, Jacksonville Memorial Hospital, Jacksonville, Arkansas.
Hypothermal Injury

RICHARD L. WINSLOW, M.D.
Associate Clinical Professor of Ophthalmology, University of Texas Southwestern Medical Center, Dallas, Texas.
Vitreous Hemorrhage

JONATHAN D. WIRTSCHAFTER, M.D., F.A.C.S.
Professor of Ophthalmology, Neurology, and Neurosurgery, University of Minnesota Medical School. Director, Neuro-ophthalmology-Orbit Service, University of Minnesota Hospital, Minneapolis, Minnesota.
Osteopetrosis

JOHN L. WOBIG, M.D.
Clinical Associate Professor of Ophthalmology, Oregon Health Sciences University. Chief, Oculoplastic Service, Good Samaritan Hospital and Medical Center, Portland, Oregon.
Basal Cell Carcinoma; Congenital Anomalies of the Lacrimal System; Dacryoadenitis; Epiphora

J. REIMER WOLTER, M.D.
Professor of Ophthalmology and Pathology, University of Michigan Medical Center, Ann Arbor, Michigan.
Arteriovenous Fistula

IRA G. WONG, M.D.
Chief, Department of Ophthalmology, Kaiser Foundation Hospital, Redwood City, California. Associate Research Ophthalmologist, Francis I. Proctor Foundation for Research in Ophthalmology, University of California School of Medicine, San Francisco, California.
Bee Sting of the Cornea

RANDALL V. WONG, M.D.
Washington, District of Columbia.
Cystinosis

VERNON G. WONG, M.D.
Professor of Ophthalmology, Georgetown University Medical Center, Washington, District of Columbia.
Cystinosis

THOMAS O. WOOD, M.D.
Professor of Ophthalmology, University of Tennessee. Active Staff, Baptist Memorial Hospital, The Regional Medical Center, Memphis, Tennessee.
Filamentary Keratitis; Mooren's Ulcer

ROBERT D. YEE, M.D.
Professor and Chairman, Department of Ophthalmology, Indiana University School of Medicine, Indianapolis, Indiana.
Nystagmus

BRIAN R. YOUNGE, M.D.
Consultant, Department of Ophthalmology, Mayo Clinic and Mayo Foundation. Associate Professor of Ophthalmology, Mayo Medical School, Rochester, Minnesota.
Carotid Cavernous Fistulas and Cavernous Sinus Arteriovenous Malformations; Optic Gliomas

EDWIN OLMOS ZAPATA, M.D.
Ophthalmologist, San Juan Hospital, Medical Director of the Eye Bank, Medical Director of the Eye Center "Ojitos Olmos", Oruro Bolivia.
Sparganosis

PREFACE

Current Ocular Therapy is intended for the busy practitioner who needs a concise outline of therapy for a particular ocular condition. The consultants were chosen on the basis of experience and recent publications. Each has explained his method of treatment in a concise format with emphasis on recent developments in therapy. In this way, we have made available to the user an authoritative method of management with the most recent clinical advances.

Although we have dealt primarily with specific ocular diseases, discussions of disorders encountered in general medicine are also included. Chapters on generalized infectious diseases, metabolic disorders, dermatologic disorders, and neoplasms are intended to serve as medically oriented introductory discussions of these fields, with emphasis on ocular implications and specific ocular treatment.

In addition to therapy, drug dosages and methods of administration are included in the text. Drug dosages and methods of administration have been checked against officially accepted standards. However, clinical experience, new data, differences in opinion among authorities, and individual clinical situations require that the physician exercise his own judgment in the choice and use of a drug. In particular, the physician is advised to check the product information included in the drug's package insert prior to drug administration, especially if the drug is one with which he is unfamiliar.

Throughout this book we have used nonproprietary or "generic" names. However, these drugs are listed in alphabetical order, followed by many of their proprietary or trade names, in the Drug Roster at the end of this book. If a particular proprietary drug is not manufactured in the United States, the country of origin is given in parentheses after its name. Combination drugs are seldom included.

The preparations available and usual dosages indicate routes of administration for these drugs. The inclusion of a drug in this list does not indicate approval or disapproval of its use in any category, nor does it imply efficacy or safety of action. When various indications have dictated different dosage ranges, a broad range from lowest to highest dosage has been given, regardless of indications.

A few of these drugs have been given special symbols in the book. An asterisk (*) denotes the particular route of administration as unapproved by the F.D.A. A few drugs are included which are investigational or presently not approved by the F.D.A. for any indication; these drugs are represented by a dagger (†). If a drug has not been approved by the F.D.A. for the specific indication, the drug is labeled with a double dagger (‡). Indicated dosages above the manufacturer's recommendation have been noted with a section mark (§). Some of these drugs may subsequently be released as approved new drugs or with new indications for use. For the reader's convenience, efforts have been made to include in the Drug Roster those drugs not sanctioned by the F.D.A. for specific dosage, method of use, or indication. Information concerning preparation or administration of these drugs has been collected from published data or provided by the consultant.

We have had contributions from more than 400 consultants throughout the world. In sincere gratitude for their time and effort, we have acknowledged the contributors in the front of the book. This third edition has added a few new subjects and deleted a few subjects as well. In the main, new authors for past subjects were obtained.

We wish to express appreciation and pay special tribute to our Associate Editor, Mrs. Martha Meyer, who has worked long and hard with devotion and skill to create this book.

F.T. Fraunfelder
F. Hampton Roy

CONTENTS

Part 1 GENERALIZED DISORDERS

SECTION 1 INFECTIOUS DISEASES

BACTERIAL INFECTIONS

ACINETOBACTER 3
(Herellea Vaginicola, Mima Polymorpha)
  Martin Wand, M.D.

ACQUIRED SYPHILIS 4
(Acquired Lues, Lues Venera, Malum Venereum)
  Jerome N. Goldman, M.D.

AZOTOBACTER 6
  Thomas J. Liesengang, M.D.

BACILLUS CEREUS 7
  Denis M. O'Day, M.D.

BACILLUS SUBTILIS 8
  George A. Williams, M.D.
  Robert A. Hyndiuk, M.D.

BOTULISM 10
  Michael Cherington, M.D.

BRUCELLOSIS 11
(Malta Fever, Mediterranean Fever, Melitococcosis, Undulant Fever)
  J. Poletti, M.D.
  A. Larmande, M.D.

CLOSTRIDIUM PERFRINGENS 12
  David Sevel, M.D., Ph.D, F.A.C.S.

CONGENITAL SYPHILIS 13
  Jerome N. Goldman, M.D.

DIPHTHERIA 15
  Laurence S. Braude, M.D., F.A.C.S., F.A.C.S.(C)
  John W. Chandler, M.D.

ERYSIPELAS 17
(St. Anthony's Fire)
  Richard L. Abbott, M.D.

ESCHERICHIA COLI 18
  H. John Shammas, M.D.

FUSOBACTERIUM 19
  Richard J. Weinberg, M.D.

GONOCOCCAL OCULAR DISEASE 20
  Jeffrey B. Robin, M.D.

HEMOPHILUS INFLUENZAE 22
  F. T. Fraunfelder, M.D.

KOCH-WEEKS BACILLUS 24
(Hemophilus Aegyptius)
  Allan Sugar, M.D.

LEPROSY 24
(Hansen's Disease)
  T. J. ffytche, F.R.C.S., D.O.

LEPTOSPIROSIS 26
  Susan Barkay, M.D.

LISTERIOSIS 28
(Listerellosis)
  Peter H. Ballen, M.D.

MORAXELLA 29
  Jules Baum, M.D.

NOCARDIA 30
  John D. Bullock, M.D., M.S., F.A.C.S.
  Stuart H. Goldberg, M.D.

PNEUMOCOCCUS 31
(Streptococcus Pneumoniae)
  H. Bruce Ostler, M.D.
  Vicky Cevallos, M.T. (A.S.C.P.)

PROPIONIBACTERIUM ACNES 33
  Ronald E. Smith, M.D.

PROTEUS 34
  David S. Hull, M.D.

PSEUDOMONAS AERUGINOSA 35
  Peter R. Laibson, M.D.

RELAPSING FEVER 37
(Recurrent Fever)
  S. Y. Salih, M.D., M.R.C.P., D.C.M.T.
  L. F. Rich, M.S., M.D.

STAPHYLOCOCCUS 38
  Robert C. Kimbrough, III, M.D., F.A.C.P.

STREPTOCOCCUS 39
  John R. Samples, M.D.

xxviii / CONTENTS

TETANUS 42
(Lockjaw)
 ALBERT W. BIGLAN, M.D., F.A.C.S.

TUBERCULOSIS 43
 THOMAS C. SPOOR, M.D., M.S., F.A.C.S.

TULAREMIA 45
(Deerfly Tularemia, Pahvant Valley Plague,
Rabbit Fever)
 MALCOLM N. LUXENBERG, M.D.

TYPHOID FEVER 46
 GEORGE N. CHIN, M.D., F.A.C.S.

YERSINIOSIS 48
 K. MATTI SAARI, M.D.

CHLAMYDIAL INFECTIONS

INCLUSION CONJUNCTIVITIS 50
(Paratrachoma, Chlamydia)
 CHANDLER R. DAWSON, M.D.

TRACHOMA 51
 S. DAROUGAR, M.D., D.T.M.&H.,
 M.R.C.Path.
 N. VISWALINGAM, M.D., D.O.

MYCOTIC INFECTIONS

ACTINOMYCOSIS 53
 BENJAMIN MILDER, M.D.

ASPERGILLOSIS 54
 GARY P. BARTH, M.D.

BLASTOMYCOSIS 55
 DENIS M. O'DAY, M.D.

CANDIDIASIS 56
 C. STEPHEN FOSTER, M.D., F.A.C.S.

COCCIDIOIDOMYCOSIS 59
 JAMES P. GANLEY, M.D., Dr. P.H.
 STEPHEN A. KLOTZ, M.D.

DERMATOPHYTOSIS 61
(Epidermophytosis, Epidermomycosis,
Rubrophytia, Tinea, Trichophytosis)
 ALAN SUGAR, M.D.

MUCORMYCOSIS 62
(Phycomycosis)
 DAVID J. WILSON, M.D.

OCULAR HISTOPLASMOSIS 63
(Presumed Ocular Histoplasmosis Syndrome)
 RONALD E. SMITH, M.D.

RHINOSPORIDIOSIS 65
(Oculosporidiosis)
 P. K. MUKHERJEE, M.S.

SPOROTRICHOSIS 66
 WILLIAM A. AGGER, M.D.

RICKETTSIAL INFECTIONS

Q FEVER 68
(Query Fever)
 RICHARD B. HORNICK, M.D.

ROCKY MOUNTAIN SPOTTED FEVER   69
 THOMAS C. BURTON, M.D.

SCRUB TYPHUS 70
(Japanese River Fever, Mite-Borne Typhus,
Rural Typhus, Tropical Typhus, Tsutsugamushi
Disease)
 ROBERT L. BERRY, M.D.

VIRAL INFECTIONS

ACQUIRED IMMUNODEFICIENCY
SYNDROME (AIDS) 72
 GARY N. HOLLAND, M.D.

ACUTE HEMORRHAGIC
CONJUNCTIVITIS 76
(AHC, Epidemic Hemorrhagic
Keratoconjunctivitis)
 JOHN P. WHITCHER, M.D.

CAT-SCRATCH DISEASE 77
 SCOTT M. MACRAE, M.D.

EPIDEMIC
KERATOCONJUNCTIVITIS 78
(EKC)
 ROBERT ABEL, JR., M.D.

HERPES SIMPLEX 79
 MARK S. DRESNER, M.D.
 DAVID J. SPENCE, M.D.
 DAVID J. SCHANZLIN, M.D.

HERPES ZOSTER 82
 R. J. MARSH, F.R.C.S.

INFECTIOUS MONONUCLEOSIS 84
 JAY H. KRACHMER, M.D.
 STEVEN S. T. CHING, M.D.

INFLUENZA 85
 DANIEL H. SPITZBERG, M.D.

LYME DISEASE 86
 F. T. FRAUNFELDER, M.D.

MOLLUSCUM CONTAGIOSUM 87
 LEWIS R. GRODEN, M.D.
 JUAN J. ARENTSEN, M.D.

MUMPS 88
 ROGER F. MEYER, M.D.

NEWCASTLE DISEASE 89
 LAURENT LAMER, M.D., F.R.C.S.(C)

OCULAR VACCINIA.................................. 90
    Bruce M. Massaro, M.D., M.P.H.
    Robert A. Hyndiuk, M.D.

PHARYNGOCONJUNCTIVAL FEVER ... 92
(Acute Follicular Conjunctivitis, Adenovirus
Conjunctivitis, PCF, Syndrome of Beal)
    Chandler R. Dawson, M.D.

RABIES.. 93
(Hydrophobia)
    Roy J. Ellsworth, M.D.

RUBELLA 94
(German Measles)
    Vivien Boniuk, M.D.

RUBEOLA 95
(Measles, Morbilli)
    N. W. H. M. Dekkers, M.D.

VARICELLA 96
(Chickenpox)
    Yukio Uchida, M.D.

SECTION 2 PARASITIC DISEASES

ACANTHAMOEBAE 98
    Mary Beth Moore, M.D.

**AMERICAN MUCOCUTANEOUS
LEISHMANIASIS** 100
    Jaime Roizenblatt, M.D.
    Luiz Carlos Cuce, M.D.

ASCARIASIS 101
    Thomas John, M.D.
    John J. Donnelly, Ph.D.
    John H. Rockey, M.D., Ph.D.

COENUROSIS 103
    Edward Epstein, M.B., B.Ch., D.O.M.S.

CUTANEOUS LEISHMANIASIS 104
(Old World Leishmaniasis, Oriental Sore,
Tropical Sore)
    Fuad S. Farah, M.D.

CYSTICERCOSIS...................................... 105
    Harvey W. Topilow, M.D.

DEMODICOSIS 106
    Frank P. English, F.R.A.C.O., F.R.C.S.

DIROFILARIASIS..................................... 108
    Lawrence A. Raymond, M.D.
    Yezid Gutierrez, M.D., Ph.D.

DRACUNCULIASIS 109
(Dracontiasis, Dracunculosis, Guinea Worm
Infection)
    Ralph Muller, Ph.D.

ECHINOCOCCOSIS 110
(Echinococciasis, Hydatid Cyst, Hydatidosis)
    F. T. Fraunfelder, M.D.

LOIASIS 111
(African *Loa loa* Eye-Worm Disease)
    James M. Barnett, M.D.

MALARIA.. 112
    Thomas E. Runyan, M.D., F.A.C.S.

ONCHOCERCIASIS 114
    Alan C. Bird, M.D., F.R.C.S.

PEDICULOSIS AND PHTHIRIASIS........ 115
    Marilyn C. Kincaid, M.D.

SCHISTOSOMIASIS.................................. 117
(Bilharziasis)
    J. Védy, M.D.
    P. Queguiner, M.D.
    J. Graveline, M.D.

SPARGANOSIS... 118
    Edwin Olmos Zapata, M.D.

THELAZIASIS.. 119
    P. K. Mukherjee, M.S.

TOXOCARIASIS....................................... 120
    Zane F. Pollard, M.D.
    William S. Hagler, M.D.

TOXOPLASMOSIS.................................... 121
(Ocular Toxoplasmosis, Toxoplasmic
Iridocyclitis, Toxoplasmic Retinochoroiditis)
    Daniel H. Spitzberg, M.D.

TRICHINOSIS.. 123
(Trichinellosis)
    B. H. Kean, M.D.

SECTION 3 ENDOCRINE DISORDERS

HYPERPARATHYROIDISM...................... 125
    K. J. Murphy, F.R.A.C.P.

HYPOCALCEMIA..................................... 126
    Marion H. Brooks, M.D.
    Anthony L. Barbato, M.D.

HYPOPARATHYROIDISM 129
    Felix O. Kolb, M.D.

HYPOTHYROIDISM 130
(Cretinism, Hypothyroid Goiter, Juvenile
Hypothyroidism, Myxedema)
    Heskel M. Haddad, M.D.

SECTION 4 NUTRITIONAL DISORDERS

CROHN'S DISEASE.................... 132
(Granulomatous Ileocolitis, Regional Enteritis,
Terminal Ileitis)
  DAVID L. KNOX, M.D.

HYPOVITAMINOSIS A............................ 134
(Xerophthalmia)
  ALFRED SOMMER, M.D., M.H.Sc.

SECTION 5 DISORDERS OF PROTEIN METABOLISM

CYSTINOSIS.............................. 136
  RANDALL V. WONG, M.D.
  VERNON G. WONG, M.D.

HOMOCYSTINURIA.............................. 137
  RAPHAEL S. BLOCH, M.D.

MAPLE SYRUP URINE DISEASE........... 138
(Branched-Chain Ketoaciduria, MSUD)
  LAWRENCE G. TOMASI, M.D., Ph.D

OCULOCEREBRORENAL SYNDROME 141
(Lowe's Syndrome)
  ANDREA CIBIS TONGUE, M.D.

TYROSINEMIA II.................................... 142
(Pseudodendritic Keratitis, Recessive Keratosis
Palmoplantaris, Richner-Hanhart Syndrome,
Tyrosinosis)
  ROBERT P. BURNS, M.D.

SECTION 6 DISORDERS OF CARBOHYDRATE METABOLISM

DIABETES MELLITUS............................ 144
  SURESH R. CHANDRA, M.D.

GALACTOSEMIAS 146
  WARREN A. WILSON, M.D. (Deceased)
  GEORGE N. DONNELL, M.D.

MUCOPOLYSACCHARIDOSIS I-H......... 147
(Dysostosis Multiplex, Hurler Syndrome, MPS
I-H, Pfaundler-Hurler Syndrome)
  T. E. KELLY, M.D., Ph.D.
  VICTOR A. MCKUSICK, M.D.

MUCOPOLYSACCHARIDOSIS I-H/S 148
(Hurler/Scheie Syndrome, MPS I-H/S)
  T. E. KELLY, M.D., Ph.D.

MUCOPOLYSACCHARIDOSIS I-S.......... 149
(MPS I-S, Scheie Syndrome)
  IRENE H. MAUMENEE, M.D.

MUCOPOLYSACCHARIDOSIS II............ 150
(Hunter Syndrome, MPS II)
  ELAINE R. BERMAN, Ph.D.

MUCOPOLYSACCHARIDOSIS III.......... 151
(MPS III, Sanfilippo Syndrome)
  ELAINE R. BERMAN, Ph.D.

MUCOPOLYSACCHARIDOSIS IV.......... 152
(Chondro-Osteodystrophy, Keratosulfaturia,
Morquio-Brailsford Syndrome, Morquio
Syndrome, MPS IV)
  CYRIL P. LEGUM, M.D.

MUCOPOLYSACCHARIDOSIS VI.......... 153
(Maroteaux-Lamy Syndrome)
  RICHARD G. WELEBER, M.D.
  JACLYN VIDGOFF, Ph.D.

MUCOPOLYSACCHARIDOSIS VII......... 154
(B-Glucuronidase Deficiency, MPS VII)
  WILLIAM S. SLY, M.D.

SECTION 7 DISORDERS OF LIPID METABOLISM

**ANGIOKERATOMA CORPORIS DIFFUSUM
UNIVERSALE** 156
(Anderson-Fabry Disease, Fabry's Disease,
Glycolipid Lipidosis)
  THOMAS A. WEINGEIST, M.D., Ph.D.

HYPERLIPOPROTEINEMIA.................... 157
  MALCOLM N. LUXENBERG, M.D.

SECTION 8 OTHER METABOLIC DISORDERS

GOUT 160
(Hyperuricemia)
  SIDNEY LERMAN, M.D.

XERODERMA PIGMENTOSUM.............. 161
  JEFFREY FREEDMAN, M.D., B.Ch., Ph.D.,
  F.R.C.S.E.

SECTION 9 HEMATOLOGIC AND CARDIOVASCULAR DISORDERS

ARTERIOVENOUS FISTULA 164
(Arteriovenous Aneurysm, Arteriovenous
Angioma, Arteriovenous Malformation, Cirsoid
Aneurysm, Racemose Hemangioma, Varicose
Aneurysm)
    J. REIMER WOLTER, M.D.

**CAROTID CAVERNOUS FISTULAS AND
CAVERNOUS SINUS ARTERIOVENOUS
MALFORMATIONS**.................................. 165
    BRIAN R. YOUNGE, M.D.

CAVERNOUS SINUS THROMBOSIS...... 166
    MILTON BONIUK, M.D.

SICKLE CELL DISEASE.......................... 167
    STEVEN B. COHEN, M.D.
    LEE M. JAMPOL, M.D.
    MORTON F. GOLDBERG, M.D.

TEMPORAL ARTERITIS.......................... 169
(Giant Cell Arteritis)
    NEIL R. MILLER, M.D.

THALESSEMIA 171
    STEPHEN S. FEMAN, M.D.

WEGENER'S GRANULOMATOSIS.......... 172
    JAMES L. KINYOUN, M.D.

SECTION 10 DERMATOLOGIC DISORDERS

**ACRODERMATITIS
ENTEROPATHICA**.................................... 174
    J. DOUGLAS CAMERON, M.D.
    DONALD J. DOUGHMAN, M.D.

ATOPIC DERMATITIS............................. 175
(Atopic Eczema, Besnier's Prurigo)
    MITCHELL H. FRIEDLAENDER, M.D.

CONTACT DERMATITIS 176
(Dermatitis Venenata)
    MITCHELL H. FRIEDLAENDER, M.D.

ERYTHEMA MULTIFORME 177
(Erythema Multiforme Exudativum,
Stevens-Johnson Syndrome)
    GEORGE M. HOWARD, M.D.

HYPERTRICHOSIS.................................. 179
(Hirsutism)
    DAVID T. TSE, M.D., F.A.C.S.
    RICHARD L. ANDERSON, M.D., F.A.C.S.

ICHTHYOSIS 181
(Epidermolytic Hyperkeratosis, Ichthyosis
Vulgaris, Lamellar Ichthyosis, X-Linked
Ichthyosis)
    RAYMOND J. SEVER, M.D.

IMPETIGO... 182
    ALAN SUGAR, M.D.

NEURODERMATITIS 183
(Lichen Simplex Chronicus)
    WESLEY KING GALEN, M.D.

OCULAR ROSACEA................................. 184
    JOSEPH FRUCHT, M.D.
    STUART I. BROWN, M.D.

PHOTOSENSITIVITY AND SUNBURN   185
    JOHN A. PARRISH, M.D.
    BARRY S. PAUL, M.D.

**POISON IVY, OAK, OR SUMAC
DERMATITIS**.. 187
(*Rhus* Dermatitis)
    WILLIAM L. EPSTEIN, M.D.

PRURITUS.. 188
    JAMES D. HOGAN, M.D.

PSORIASIS.. 191
    WILLIAM B. GLEW, M.D.
    THOMAS P. NIGRA, M.D.

**URTICARIA AND HEREDITARY
ANGIOEDEMA**... 192
Urticaria, Hives, Nettle Rash, Quincke's
Disease)
    MITCHELL H. FRIEDLAENDER, M.D.

VITILIGO 194
    FRANK PARKER, M.D.

SECTION 11 CONNECTIVE TISSUE DISORDERS

**JUVENILE RHEUMATOID
ARTHRITIS** 197
(JA, JRA, Juvenile Arthritis, Still's Disease)
    JERRY C. JACOBS, M.D.
    HAROLD F. SPALTER, M.D.

POLYARTERITIS NODOSA 198
(Necrotizing Angiitis, PAN, Periarteritis
Nodosa)
    JOHN J. WEITER, M.D., Ph.D.
    JOHN A. MILLS, M.D.

PSEUDOXANTHOMA ELASTICUM....... 200
(Gronblad-Strandberg Syndrome, PXE)
    DAVID S. HULL, M.D.

RELAPSING POLYCHONDRITIS 201
    PETER G. WATSON, M.A., M.B., B.Chir.,
    F.R.C.S., D.O.
    EAMON P. O'DONOGHUE, M.B., B.Ch.,
    B.A.O., F.R.C.S. (Ed.)

RHEUMATOID ARTHRITIS 203
    JAMES T. ROSENBAUM, M.D.

xxxii / CONTENTS

SJÖGREN'S SYNDROME........................ 205
(Gougerot-Sjögren's Syndrome)
MICHAEL A. LEMP, M.D.

SYSTEMIC LUPUS ERYTHEMATOSUS 206
JAMES T. ROSENBAUM, M.D.

SYSTEMIC SCLEROSIS........................... 208
(Scleroderma)
DOUGLAS A. JABS, M.D.

WEILL-MARCHESANI SYNDROME...... 209
DAVID S. WALTON, M.D.

SECTION 12 SKELETAL DISORDERS

CRANIOSTENOSIS

CROUZON'S DISEASE 211
(Craniofacial Dysostosis, Dysostosis
Craniofacialis)
PAUL TESSIER, M.D.

ENGELMANN'S DISEASE 212
(Camurati-Engelmann's Disease, Diaphyseal
Dysplasia, Hereditary Diaphyseal Dysplasia,
Hereditary Multiple Diaphyseal Sclerosis,
Hyperostosis Corticalis Generalisata Familiaris,
Juvenile Paget's Disease, Osteopathia
Hyperostotica Sclerotisans Multiplex Infantilis,
Progressive Hyperostosis)
PETER H. MORSE, M.D., F.A.C.S.
COLETTA M. MILLER, D.D.S.

ORBITAL HYPERTELORISM 213
(Greig's Syndrome)
LOIS A. LLOYD, M.D., F.R.C.S.(C)
RAYMOND BUNCIC, M.D., F.R.C.S.(C)

DWARFISM

COCKAYNE'S SYNDROME 215
WILLIAM H. COLES, M.D., M.S.

DOWN'S SYNDROME 216
(Mongolism, Trisomy 21)
EDWARD A. JAEGER, M.D.

WERNER'S SYNDROME.......................... 218
JOHN D. BULLOCK, M.D., M.S., F.A.C.S.
STUART H. GOLDBERG, M.D.

FRAGILE BONE DISEASE

ANKYLOSING SPONDYLITIS 219
(Marie Strumpell Disease)
DOUGLAS A. JABS, M.D.

OSTEOPETROSIS 220
(Albers-Schönberg Disease, Marble Bone
Disease, Osteosclerosis Congenita Diffusa,
Osteosclerosis Fragilis Generalisata)
JONATHAN D. WIRTSCHAFTER, M.D.

MANDIBULOFACIAL DYSOSTOSIS

**HALLERMANN-STREIFF-FRANCOIS
SYNDROME** 222
(Francois-Hallermann-Streiff Syndrome,
Francois Syndrome, Hallermann-Streiff
Syndrome, Mandibulo-Oculofacial Dyscephaly,
Mandibulo-Oculofacial Dysmorphia)
DAVID J. HOPKINS, M.B., F.R.C.S., D.O.

MANDIBULOFACIAL DYSOSTOSIS...... 223
(Berry Syndrome, Franceschetti Syndrome,
Treacher Collins Syndrome)
TREVOR H. KIRKHAM, M.D., F.R.C.S

**OCULOAURICULOVERTEBRAL
DYSPLASIA** 224
(Goldenhar's Syndrome)
CHARLES R. LEONE, JR., M.D.

ROBIN SEQUENCE................................. 225
(Pierre Robin Syndrome, Robin Anomalad)
G. FRANK JUDISCH, M.D.

WAARDENBURG'S SYNDROME............. 226
(Klein-Waardenburg Syndrome)
ANGELO M. DiGEORGE, M.D.

SECTION 13 PHAKOMATOSES

ANGIOMATOSIS RETINAE 228
(Angiomatosis of the Retina and Central
Nervous System, Retinal and Optic Disc
Capillary Hemangiomas, Retinal Capillary
Hamartoma, Retinal Hemangioblastoma, von
Hippel-Lindau Disease, von Hippel's Disease)
JOHN J. WEITER, M.D.

NEUROFIBROMATOSIS............................ 229
(von Recklinghausen Disease, NF-1)
RICHARD A. LEWIS, M.D., M.S.

STURGE-WEBER SYNDROME................ 231
(Encephalotrigeminal Syndrome)
F. HAMPTON ROY, M.D.

SECTION 14   NEUROLOGIC DISORDERS

ACUTE IDIOPATHIC POLYNEURITIS 233
(Acute Febrile Polyneuritis, Acute Infectious Polyneuritis, Fisher's Syndrome, Guillain-Barré Syndrome, Inflammatory Polyradiculoneuropathy, Landry-Guillain-Barré-Strohl Syndrome, Landry's Paralysis, Postinfectious Polyneuritis)
    Kay-Uwe Hamann, M.D.

BELL'S PALSY 234
(Idiopathic Facial Paralysis)
    Thomas R. Hedges, Jr., M.D.
    Thomas R. Hedges, III, M.D.

BENIGN INTRACRANIAL HYPERTENSION AND PSEUDOTUMOR CEREBRI 236
    Satoshi Kashii, M.D.
    William L. Basuk, M.D.
    Ronald M. Burde, M.D.

BLINDNESS 240
    Robert L. Berry, M.D.

CEREBRAL PALSY 241
(Brain Damage Syndrome, Perinatal Encephalopathy)
    Peter Black, B.Sc., M.B., F.R.C.S., D.O.

CHRONIC PROGRESSIVE EXTERNAL OPHTHALMOPLEGIA 243
(Abiotrophic Ophthalmoplegia, Chronic Progressive External Ophthalmoplegia with Ragged Red Fibers, Chronic Progressive Muscular Dystrophy, Kearns-Sayre-Daroff Syndrome, Kearns-Sayre Syndrome, Kearns-Shy Syndrome, Ocular Myopathy, Oculocraniosomatic Neuromuscular Disease, Oculopharyngeal Muscular Dystrophy Syndrome, Oculoskeletal Myopathy, Ophthalmoplegia Plus, Progressive Dystrophy of the Extraocular Muscles)
    Joseph Eshagian, M.D.

CLUSTER HEADACHE 246
(Benign Type of Raeder's Paratrigeminal Syndrome, Ciliary Neuralgia, Histamine Headache, Horton's Headache, Paroxysmal Nocturnal Cephalalgia, Periodic Migrainous Neuralgia)
    Baird S. Grimson, M.D.

CREUTZFELDT-JAKOB DISEASE 247
    Robert L. Lesser, M.D.

DYSLEXIA 248
    Marshall P. Keys, M.D.

FUNCTIONAL AMBLYOPIA 250
    Ronald V. Keech, M.D.

HEADACHE 251
    Thomas R. Hedges, Jr., M.D.

HYSTERIA, MALINGERING, AND ANXIETY STATES 255
    August L. Reader, III, M.D., F.A.C.S.

LOW VISION 256
    Thomas E. Talbot, M.D.
    K. Nolen Tanner, M.D., Ph.D.

MULTIPLE SCLEROSIS 259
    Robert S. Hepler, M.D.

MYASTHENIA GRAVIS 261
    Neil R. Miller, M.D.
    Alan Pestronk, M.D.

PARKINSON'S DISEASE 263
    Steven Gancher, M.D.

TOLOSA-HUNT SYNDROME 264
(Painful Ophthalmoplegia)
    William E. Hunt, M.D.
    Susan C. Benes, M.D.

TRIGEMINAL NEURALGIA 265
(Tic Douloureux)
    Baird S. Grimson, M.D.

SECTION 15   NEOPLASMS

BENIGN

ACTINIC AND SEBORRHEIC KERATOSIS 267
    Ronald R. Lubritz, M.D.

CAPILLARY HEMANGIOMA 268
(Angioblastic Hemangioma, Benign Hemangio-Endothelioma, Hemangioblastoma, Strawberry Hemangioma)
    Barrett G. Haik, M.D.

CAVERNOUS HEMANGIOMA 270
    Barrett G. Haik, M.D.

CRANIOPHARYNGIOMA 271
    Harold J. Hoffman, M.D., B.Sc.(Med.), F.R.C.S.(C)

DERMOID 273
(Dermoid Choristoma, Dermoid Cyst, Dermolipoma, Lipodermoid)
    Arthus S. Grove, Jr., M.D.

JUVENILE XANTHOGRANULOMA 274
(JXG, Nevoxanthoendothelioma)
    Paul E. Romano, M.D., M.S.O.
    Lyn A. Sedwick, M.D.

KERATOACANTHOMA 275
    J. Brooks Crawford, M.D.

xxxiv / CONTENTS

LEIOMYOMA 277
DAVID SEVEL, M.D., Ph.D., F.A.S.C.

LYMPHANGIOMA 278
IRA SNOW JONES, M.D.
HILARY J. RONNER, M.D.

MEDULLOEPITHELIOMA 279
(Diktyoma)
LEONARD APT, M.D.

MENINGIOMA 280
DUNCAN P. ANDERSON, M.D.C.M.,
F.R.C.S.(C)

MUCOCELE 282
(Pyocele)
IRA A. ABRAHAMSON, M.D.

NEURILEMMOMA 283
(Neurinoma, Schwannoma)
NORMAN S. LEVY, M.D., Ph.D., F.A.C.S.

OPTIC GLIOMAS 284
BRIAN R. YOUNGE, M.D.

PAPILLOMA 286
(Verruca, Wart)
FRED M. WILSON II, M.D.

MALIGNANT

BASAL CELL CARCINOMA 288
JOHN L. WOBIG, M.D.

CONJUNCTIVAL OR CORNEAL
INTRAEPITHELIAL NEOPLASIA (CIN)
AND SQUAMOUS CELL CARCINOMA   289
(Invasive Neoplasm)
F. T. FRAUNFELDER, M.D.

EWING'S SARCOMA 291
F. T. FRAUNFELDER, M.D.

FIBROSARCOMA 292
F. HAMPTON ROY, M.D.

HODGKIN'S DISEASE 293
STUART A. GROSSMAN, M.D.
NEIL R. MILLER, M.D.

KAPOSI'S SARCOMA 294
(Idiopathic Multiple Pigmented Sarcoma)
BIJAN SAFAI, M.D., D.S.C.

LIPOSARCOMA 296
RICHARD M. CHAVIS, M.D.

LYMPHOID TUMORS 297
(Inflammatory Pseudotumor, Malignant
Lymphoma, Neoplastic
Angioendotheliomatosis, Pseudolymphoma,
Pseudotumor, Reactive Lymphoid Hyperplasia)
F. T. FRAUNFELDER, M.D.

MYCOSIS FUNGOIDES 300
(Cutaneous T-Cell Lymphoma, Lymphomatoid
Papulosis, Sézary Syndrome, T-Cell
Lymphoma-Leukemia)
KRISTIAN THOMSEN, M.D.

NEUROBLASTOMA 301
DEVRON H. CHAR, M.D.

OCULAR METASTATIC TUMORS 302
FREDERICK H. DAVIDORF, M.D.

ORBITAL METASTASES 304
DEVRON H. CHAR, M.D.

PERIOCULAR SQUAMOUS CELL
CARCINOMA 305
ROBERT M. DRYDEN, M.D.

RETINOBLASTOMA 306
ROBERT M. ELLSWORTH, M.D.

RHABDOMYOSARCOMA 309
HILARY J. RONNER, M.D.
IRA SNOW JONES, M.D.

SEBACEOUS GLAND CARCINOMA 310
NARSING A. RAO, M.D.

SECTION 16   MECHANICAL AND NONMECHANICAL INJURIES

BURNS

ACID BURNS 312
HARVEY H. SLANSKY, M.D.

ALKALINE INJURY 313
ROSWELL R. PFISTER, M.D.

DIRECT AND PHOTOSENSITIZED
ULTRAVIOLET RADIATION 315
SIDNEY LERMAN, M.D.

ELECTRICAL INJURY 320
F. T. FRAUNFELDER, M.D.

HYPOTHERMAL INJURY 322
(Cryoinjury, Frostbite)
DENNIS L. WINGFIELD, M.D.

RADIATION 323
(Gamma Rays, Infrared Rays, Microwaves,
Radiowaves, X-rays)
BUDD APPLETON, M.D.

THERMAL BURNS 324
ARDEN H. WANDER, M.D.

FOREIGN BODY

INTRAOCULAR FOREIGN
BODY—COPPER 326
(Chalcosis)
FLEMING D. WERTZ, M.D.
THOM S. THOMASSEN, M.D.

INTRAOCULAR FOREIGN
BODY—NONMAGNETIC CHEMICALLY
INERT 329
   William H. Havener, M.D.

INTRAOCULAR FOREIGN BODY—STEEL
OR IRON 330
(Siderosis)
   Philip P. Ellis, M.D.

ORBITAL IMPLANT EXTRUSION.......... 332
   Mark R. Levine, M.D.

FRACTURES

EXTERNAL ORBITAL FRACTURES...... 333
   Byron Smith, M.D.
   Richard D. Lisman, M.D.

INTERNAL ORBITAL FRACTURES....... 335
(Blowout Fractures)
   Byron Smith, M.D.
   Richard D. Lisman, M.D.

OPTIC FORAMEN FRACTURES............. 337
   A. J. M. van der Werf, M.D.

LACERATION, TEAR, OR CONTUSION

CHORIORETINAL CONCUSSIONS AND
LACERATIONS.. 338
   David J. Wilson, M.D.

CILIARY BODY CONCUSSIONS AND
LACERATIONS.. 339
   John E. Read, M.D.

CONJUNCTIVAL LACERATIONS AND
CONTUSIONS.. 342
   L. F. Rich, M.S., M.D.

CORNEAL ABRASIONS, CONTUSIONS,
LACERATIONS, AND PERFORATIONS 343
   Roger L. Hiatt, M.D.

EXTRAOCULAR MUSCLE
LACERATIONS.. 344
   Eugene M. Helveston, M.D.

EYELID CONTUSIONS, LACERATIONS,
AND AVULSIONS 345
   Robert C. Della Rocca, M.D., F.A.C.S.
   John Nassif, M.D.

INDIRECT GLOBAL RUPTURES AND
SHARP SCLERAL INJURIES 348
   William H. Coles, M.D., M.S.

IRIS LACERATIONS, HOLES, AND
IRIDODIALYSIS.. 349
   Hellmut F. Neubauer, M.D.

LACRIMAL SYSTEM CONTUSIONS AND
LACERATIONS.. 351
   Benjamin Milder, M.D.

STRIPPING OR DETACHMENT OF
DESCEMET'S MEMBRANE 352
   Richard P. Kratz, M.D.

TRAUMATIC CATARACT......................... 354
   George M. Gombos, M.D.

VENOM

BEE STING OF THE CORNEA................ 355
   Ira G. Wong, M.D.
   Gilbert Smolin, M.D.

SPIDER BITES 356
   F. Hampton Roy, M.D.

SECTION 17   UNCLASSIFIED DISEASES OR CONDITIONS

AMYLOIDOSIS 358
   Jay H. Krachmer, M.D.
   Steven P. Dunn, M.D.

BEHÇET'S DISEASE................................ 359
(Silk Road Disease)
   Kanjiro Masuda, M.D.

COGAN'S SYNDROME............................ 360
   Barton F. Haynes, M.D.

FAMILIAL DYSAUTONOMIA 362
(Riley Day Syndrome)
   Felicia B. Axelrod, M.D.
   Robert D'Amico, M.D.

HISTIOCYTOSIS X 364
(Eosinophilic Granuloma,

Hand-Schüller-Christian Disease,
Letterer-Siwe Disease)
   David J. Apple, M.D.
   Hugh L. Hennis, M.D., Ph.D.
   Kevin Miller, M.D.

REITER'S DISEASE 367
   K. Matti Saari, M.D.

SARCOIDOSIS 369
   Daniel H. Gold, M.D.

VOGT-KOYANAGI-HARADA
SYNDROME 372
(Harada's Syndrome,
Uveitis-Vitiligo-Alopecia-Poliosis Syndrome,
Vogt-Koyanagi Syndrome)
   Alan H. Friedman, M.D.

Part 2 EYE AND ADNEXA

SECTION 18 ANTERIOR CHAMBER

EPITHELIAL INGROWTH 377
(Epithelial Downgrowth)
 Patricia W. Smith, M.D.
 Walter J. Stark, M.D.
 Ronald G. Michels, M.D.

FIBROUS INGROWTH 378
(Fibroblastic Ingrowth, Fibrocytic Ingrowth, Fibrous Metaplasia, Stromal Ingrowth, Stromal Overgrowth)
 Kenneth C. Swan, M.D.

INTRAOCULAR EPITHELIAL CYSTS ... 379
 Patricia W. Smith, M.D.
 Walter J. Stark, M.D.

POSTOPERATIVE FLAT ANTERIOR CHAMBER 380
 E. Michael Van Buskirk, M.D.

RECURRENT LATE HYPHEMA FROM FOCAL WOUND VASCULARIZATION 383
 Kenneth C. Swan, M.D.

TRAUMATIC HYPHEMA 384
 Paul E. Romano, M.D., M.S.O.
 Jerry N. Shuster, M.D.

SECTION 19 CHOROID

ANGIOID STREAKS 387
 Fumio Kayazawa, M.D.

CHOROIDAL DETACHMENT 388
(Ciliochoroidal Detachment)
 A. Robert Bellows, M.D.

CHOROIDAL NEOVASCULAR MEMBRANES 390
(Disciform Macular Degeneration, Hemorrhagic Disciform Detachment, Subretinal Neovascularization)
 Robert E. Kalina, M.D.

CHOROIDAL RUPTURES 392
 Ronald E. Smith, M.D.

EXPULSIVE HEMORRHAGE 392
(Subchoroidal Expulsive Hemorrhage)
 Daniel M. Taylor, M.D.

MALIGNANT MELANOMA OF THE POSTERIOR UVEA 394
(Choroidal Melanoma, Ciliary Body Melanoma)
 Jerry A. Shields, M.D.
 Carol L. Shields, M.D.

SYMPATHETIC OPHTHALMIA 398
(Sympathetic Uveitis)
 George E. Marak, Jr., M.D.

SECTION 20 CONJUNCTIVA

ALLERGIC CONJUNCTIVITIS 400
(Atopic Conjunctivitis, Hay Fever Conjunctivitis)
 Mathea R. Allansmith, M.D.
 Robert N. Ross, Ph.D.

BACTERIAL CONJUNCTIVITIS 402
(Mucopurulent Conjunctivitis, Purulent Conjunctivitis)
 Douglas J. Coster, F.R.C.S.

CICATRICIAL PEMPHIGOID 403
(Benign Mucous Membrane Pemphigoid, Ocular Cicatricial Pemphigoid)
 Lynne H. Morrison, M.D.
 Kenneth C. Swan, M.D.

CONJUNCTIVAL MELANOTIC LESIONS 406
(Benign Congenital Melanosis, Benign Nevi, Melanoma, PAM, Precancerous and Cancerous Melanosis, Primary Acquired Melanosis)
 F. T. Fraunfelder, M.D.

CORNEAL AND CONJUNCTIVAL CALCIFICATIONS 408
(Band Keratopathy)
 Mark S. Dresner, M.D.
 David J. Spence, M.D.
 David J. Schanzlin, M.D.

FILTERING BLEBS 410
(Leaking and Inadvertent Nonleaking)
 Gissur J. Petursson, M.D.

GIANT PAPILLARY CONJUNCTIVITIS 411
 Mathea R. Allansmith, M.D.
 Robert N. Ross, Ph.D.

IRRITATIVE CONJUNCTIVITIS 413
(Toxic Conjunctivitis)
 Ronald E. Smith, M.D.

LIGNEOUS CONJUNCTIVITIS............... 414
JULES FRANCOIS, M.D., F.A.C.S., F.R.S.M.
JEROME KAZDAN, M.D., F.R.C.S.(C)

OPHTHALMIA NEONATORUM............. 416
(Conjunctivitis of Newborns, Neonatal Ophthalmia)
EARL A. PALMER, M.D.

PTERYGIUM AND PSEUDOPTERYGIUM............................. 418
L. F. RICH, M.S., M.D.

VERNAL KERATOCONJUNCTIVITIS.... 420
M. M. EL HENNAWI, M.CH.

SECTION 21   CORNEA

DEGENERATIVE CHANGES

CORNEAL MUCOUS PLAQUES............. 422
(Keratitis Mucosa)
RAMESH C. TRIPATHI, M.D., Ph.D.

FUCHS' DELLEN..................................... 423
(Facets, Fuchs' Dimples)
F. LAGOUTTE, M.D.

MOOREN'S ULCER.................................. 424
THOMAS O. WOOD, M.D.
AUDREY W. TUBERVILLE, M.D.

PELLUCID MARGINAL CORNEAL DEGENERATION...................................... 425
(Corneal Piriformis)
MARK S. DRESNER, M.D.
DAVID J. SCHANZLIN, M.D.

TERRIEN'S MARGINAL DEGENERATION...................................... 426
(Furrow Dystrophy, Marginal Ectasia, Peripheral Furrow Keratitis)
MARK J. MANNIS, M.D.

DYSTROPHIES AFFECTING PRIMARILY THE CORNEAL EPITHELIUM

EPITHELIAL BASEMENT MEMBRANE DYSTROPHY... 427
(Cogan's Microcystic Corneal Dystrophy, Map, Dot, Fingerprint Dystrophy)

AND RECURRENT EROSION
(Recurrent Epithelial Erosion)
PETER R. LAIBSON, M.D.

JUVENILE CORNEAL EPITHELIAL DYSTROPHY... 428
(Meesman's Corneal Dystrophy)
ROBERT P. BURNS, M.D.

REIS-BÜCKLERS' SUPERFICIAL CORNEAL DYSTROPHY... 429
Bücklers' Annular Corneal Dystrophy)
FRANK M. POLACK, M.D., F.A.S.C.

DYSTROPHIES AFECTING PRIMARILY THE CORNEAL STROMA

CRYSTALLINE CORNEAL DYSTROPHY... 430
(Schnyder's Crystalline Corneal Dystrophy)
MALCOLM N. LUXENBERG, M.D.

GRANULAR CORNEAL DYSTROPHY.... 431
(Bücklers' Type I; Groenouw's Type I)
KAMAL F. NASSIF, M.D.
ROBERT A. HYNDIUK, M.D.

LATTICE CORNEAL DYSTROPHY........ 432
(Lattice Dystrophy Type I, Lattice Dystrophy Type II, LCD-I, LCD-II, Meretoja's Syndrome)
ROBERT A. HYNDIUK, M.D.

MACULAR CORNEAL DYSTROPHY...... 433
(Fehr's Macular Dystrophy, Groenouw's Type II)
CLEMENT MCCULLOCH, M.D., F.R.C.S.(C)

DYSTROPHIES AFFECTING PRIMARILY THE CORNEAL ENDOTHELIUM

CONGENITAL HEREDITARY ENDOTHELIAL DYSTROPHY................ 435
(Ched)
IRENE H. MAUMENEE, M.D.

FUCHS' CORNEAL DYSTROPHY........... 435
(Combined Dystrophy of Fuchs, Endothelial Dystrophy of the Cornea, Epithelial Dystrophy of Fuchs, Fuchs' Epithelial-Endothelial Dystrophy)
WILLIAM M. BOURNE, M.D.

POSTERIOR POLYMORPHOUS CORNEAL DYSTROPHY... 437
(Hereditary Deep Dystrophy, Hereditary Mesodermal Dystrophy, Keratitis Bullosa Interna, Koeppe's Posterior Polymorphous Degeneration, Schlichting's Dystrophy)
S. ARTHUR BORUCHOFF, M.D.
ROGER F. STEINERT, M.D.

ECTATIC CONDITIONS

KERATOCONUS....................................... 438
MARK J. MANNIS, M.D.

OTHER CORNEAL DISEASES

BACTERIAL CORNEAL ULCERS........... 439
(Bacterial Keratitis)
DOUGLAS J. COSTER, F.R.C.S.

xxxviii / CONTENTS

CONJUNCTIVAL, CORNEAL, OR SCLERAL
CYSTS.. 440
(Acquired Epithelial Inclusion Cysts,
Epithelial Cysts)
    F. T. FRAUNFELDER, M.D.

CORNEAL EDEMA.................................... 442
(Bullous Keratopathy, Epithelial Edema,
Stromal Edema)
    JOEL SUGAR, M.D.

CORNEAL NEOVASCULARIZATION 443
    WALTER MAYER, M.D.

FILAMENTARY KERATITIS.................... 444
    THOMAS O. WOOD, M.D.
    AUDREY W. TUBERVILLE, M.D.

FUNGAL KERATITIS................................ 445
(Fungal Corneal Ulcer, Keratomycosis)
    THOMAS H. PETTIT, M.D.
    MATTHEW EHRLICH, M.D.

INFECTIOUS CRYSTALLINE
KERATOPATHY.. 448
    ROGER H. S. LANGSTON, M.D., C.M.

KERATOCONJUNCTIVITIS SICCA........ 449
(Dry Eye Syndrome, KCS, Keratitis Sicca,
Sjogren's Syndrome)
    MOGENS S. NORN, M.D., Ph.D

NEUROPARALYTIC KERATITIS 452
(Neurotrophic Keratitis, Trigeminal
Neuropathic Keratopathy)
    IAN A. MACKIE, M.B., F.R.C.S.

PHLYCTENULOSIS.................................... 454
(Phlyctenular Keratoconjunctivitis)
    MICHAEL D. WAGONER, M.D.
    ANN M. BAJART, M.D.
    MATHEA R. ALLANSMITH, M.D.

SUPERIOR LIMBIC
KERATOCONJUNCTIVITIS 457
(SLK, Theodore's Superior Limbic
Keratoconjunctivitis)
    ARDEN H. WANDER, M.D.

THYGESON'S SUPERFICIAL PUNCTATE
KERATOPATHY.. 458
    HUGH P. WILLIAMS, F.R.C.S., D.O.

SECTION 22 EXTRAOCULAR MUSCLES

ABDUCENS (SIXTH NERVE)
PARALYSIS 460
    EUGENE M. HELVESTON, M.D.

ACCOMMODATIVE ESOTROPIA........... 461
    EDWARD L. RAAB, M.D.

ACCOMMODATIVE INSUFFICIENCY   464
(Accommodative Effort Syndrome,
Ill-Sustained Accommodation)
    K. NOLEN TANNER, M.D., Ph.D.

ACQUIRED NONACCOMMODATIVE
ESOTROPIA 465
    STUART R. DANKNER, M.D.

A-PATTERN ESOTROPIA......................... 466
    HENRY S. METZ, M.D.

A-PATTERN EXOTROPIA 467
    HENRY S. METZ, M.D.

BASIC EXOTROPIA 468
    ANDREA CIBIS TONGUE, M.D.

BROWN'S SYNDROME 469
(formerly also called Brown's Superior Oblique
Tendon Sheath Syndrome)
    JOHN S. CRAWFORD, M.D., F.A.C.S.(C)

CONGENITAL FIBROSIS OF THE
EXTRAOCULAR MUSCLES 470
(Congenital Enophthalmos with Ocular Muscle
Fibrosis and Ptosis, Congenital Fibrosis of the
Inferior Rectus with Ptosis, General Fibrosis
Syndrome, Strabismus Fixus, Vertical
Retraction Syndrome)
    R. D. HARLEY, M.D., Ph.D., F.A.C.S.

CONVERGENCE INSUFFICIENCY
SYNDROME 471
(Asthenovergence of Stutterheim)
    MALCOLM L. MAZOW, M.D.

DISSOCIATED VERTICAL
DEVIATION 472
(Alternating Sursumduction, Dissociated
Vertical Divergence, Double-Dissociated
Hypertropia, Occlusion Hypertropia)
    RONALD V. KEECH, M.D.

DUANE'S RETRACTION SYNDROME .. 474
    HENRY S. METZ, M.D.

ESOTROPIA–HIGH AC/A RATIO.......... 475
    ARTHUR L. ROSENBAUM, M.D.

ESSENTIAL-INFANTILE ESOTROPIA   476
    EUGENE M. HELVESTON, M.D.

INTERMITTENT EXOTROPIA 478
    HIRAM H. HARDESTY, M.D.

MONOFIXATION SYNDROME 481
(Microstrabismus, Microtropia, Monofixational
Orthophoria, Monofixational Phoria)
    MARSHALL M. PARKS, M.D.

NYSTAGMUS.. 482
(Acquired Fixation Nystagmus, Congenital
Nystagmus, Dissociated Nystagmus, Downbeat
Nystagmus, Gaze-Evoked Nystagmus, Periodic
Alternating Nystagmus, Rebound Nystagmus,
Saccadic Oscillations, Vestibular Nystagmus)
    ROBERT D. YEE, M.D.

OCULOMOTOR (THIRD NERVE)
PARALYSIS 486
    Howard Eggers, M.D.
    Philip Knapp, M.D.

SUPERIOR OBLIQUE MYOKYMIA 488
    William T. Shults, M.D.

SUPERIOR OBLIQUE PALSY 488
    Eugene M. Helveston, M.D.

V-PATTERN ESOTROPIA 490
    Henry S. Metz, M.D.

V-PATTERN EXOTROPIA 491
    Henry S. Metz, M.D.

SECTION 23 EYELIDS

ANKYLOBELPHARON 493
    David W. Vastine, M.D.
    Robert L. Stamper, M.D.

BENIGN ESSENTIAL
BLEPHAROSPASM 494
    John R. Samples, M.D.

BLEPHAROCHALASIS 495
    Crowell Beard, M.D.
    John H. Sullivan, M.D.

BLEPHAROPHIMOSIS 496
    Jay Justin Older, M.D.

CHALAZION 497
    Herbert J. Gershen, M.D.

DISTICHIASIS 498
(Districhiasis)
    Richard L. Anderson, M.D., F.A.C.S.
    John B. Holds, M.D.

ECTROPION 500
    Byron Smith, M.D.
    Richard D. Lisman, M.D.

ENTROPION 502
    Roger A. Dailey, M.D.

EPICANTHUS 505
    Roger A. Dailey, M.D.

EYELID COLOBOMA 507
    John D. Bullock, M.D., M.S., F.A.C.S.
    Stuart H. Goldberg, M.D.

FLOPPY EYELID SYNDROME 507
    Lee K. Schwartz, M.D.

HEMIFACIAL SPASM 509
    John R. Samples, M.D.

HORDEOLUM 510
(Stye)
    F. T. Fraunfelder, M.D.

LAGOPHTHALMOS 511
    Richard P. Jobe, M.D.

LID MYOKYMIA 513
    Norman S. Jaffe, M.D.
    William T. Shults, M.D.

LID RETRACTION 514
    J. Timothy Heffernan, M.D.
    Richard R. Tenzel, M.D.

MADAROSIS 515
(Loss of Eyelashes)
    Allen M. Putterman, M.D.

MARCUS GUNN SYNDROME 516
(Jaw-Winking Syndrome)
    John S. Crawford, M.D., F.R.C.S.(C)
    T. W. Doucet, M.D.

MELANOTIC LESIONS OF THE
EYELIDS 517
(Melanoma, Nevi, Oculodermal Melanocytosis)
    Vitalino B. Bernardino, Jr., M.D.
    William C. Lloyd III, M.D.
    Michael A. Naidoff, M.D.

ORBITAL FAT HERNIATION 520
(Adipose Palpebral Bags, Baggy Eyelids)
    Allen M. Putterman, M.D.

PTOSIS 520
(Blepharoptosis)
    John H. Sullivan, M.D.

SEBORRHEIC BLEPHARITIS 522
    Michael Halstead, M.D.
    James P. McCulley, M.D.

STAPHYLOCOCCAL AND MIXED
STAPHYLOCOCCAL/SEBORRHEIC
BLEPHAROCONJUNCTIVITIS 525
    Donna Dodson Brown, M.D.
    James P. McCulley, M.D.

SYMBLEPHARON 527
    Robert L. Stamper, M.D.
    David W. Vastine, M.D.

TRICHIASIS 529
    F. T. Fraunfelder, M.D.

XANTHELASMA 530
(Xanthelasma Palpebrarum, Xanthoma
Palpebrarum)
    F. T. Fraunfelder, M.D.

SECTION 24 GLOBE

ANOPHTHALMOS 532
DANIEL MARCHAC, M.D.

BACTERIAL ENDOPHTHALMITIS 533
SID MANDELBAUM, M.D.
RICHARD K. FORSTER, M.D.

FUNGAL ENDOPHTHALMITIS 535
WALTER H. STERN, M.D.

NANOPHTHALMOS 537
ROBERT J. BROCKHURST, M.D.

SECTION 25 INTRAOCULAR PRESSURE

**APHAKIC AND PSEUDOPHAKIC
PUPILLARY BLOCK** 539
CLAUDIA U. RICHTER, M.D.
B. THOMAS HUTCHINSON, M.D.

**CORTICOSTEROID-INDUCED
GLAUCOMA** 542
MICHAEL A. KASS, M.D.

EXFOLIATION SYNDROME 543
(Capsular Glaucoma, Pseudoexfoliation of the
Lens Capsule)
AHTI TARKKANEN, M.D.

GHOST CELL GLAUCOMA 545
DAVID G. CAMPBELL, M.D.

**GLAUCOMA AFTER OCULAR
CONTUSION** 547
(Angle Recession)
JOHN C. MORRISON, M.D.

**GLAUCOMA ASSOCIATED WITH
ANTERIOR UVEITIS** 548
M. BRUCE SHIELDS, M.D.

**GLAUCOMA ASSOCIATED WITH
ELEVATED VENOUS PRESSURE** 550
JOHN R. SAMPLES, M.D.

**GLAUCOMA ASSOCIATED WITH
INTRAOCULAR LENSES** 551
E. MICHAEL VAN BUSKIRK, M.D.

**GLAUCOMA ASSOCIATED WITH
INTRAOCULAR TUMORS** 554
CAROL L. SHIELDS, M.D.
JERRY A. SHIELDS, M.D.

GLAUCOMATOCYCLITIC CRISIS 558
(Posner-Schlossman Syndrome)
ABRAHAM SCHLOSSMAN, M.D.

INFANTILE GLAUCOMA 559
(Primary Congenital Open-Angle Glaucoma)
DAVID S. WALTON, M.D.

JUVENILE GLAUCOMA 559
MARIANNE E. FEITL, M.D.
THEODORE KRUPIN, M.D.

LENS-INDUCED GLAUCOMA 562
(Phacolytic Glaucoma)
DAVID L. EPSTEIN, M.D.

LOW-TENSION GLAUCOMA 564
STEPHEN M. DRANCE, M.D.

MALIGNANT GLAUCOMA 565
(Ciliary Block, Iridovitreal Block, Posterior
Aqueous Diversion, Vitreolenticular Ciliary
Block)
JOHN C. MORRISON, M.D.

OCULAR HYPERTENSION 567
STEVEN M. PODOS, M.D.
ROBERT RITCH, M.D.

OCULAR HYPOTONY 569
DAVID J. WILSON, M.D.

OPEN-ANGLE GLAUCOMA 570
ROBERT N. SHAFFER, M.D., F.A.C.S.

**PHACOANAPHYLACTIC
ENDOPHTHALMITIS** 573
(Endophthalmitis Phacoanaphylactica,
Phacoanaphylactic Uveitis, Phacoantigenic
Uveitis)
BARTON L. HODES, M.D.

PIGMENTARY GLAUCOMA 574
(Pigment Dispersion Syndrome)
DAVID G. CAMPBELL, M.D.

PLATEAU IRIS 575
ROBERT RITCH, M.D.
STEVEN M. PODOS, M.D.

**PRIMARY ANGLE-CLOSURE
GLAUCOMA** 577
(Primary Closed-Angle Glaucoma, Primary
Narrow-Angle Glaucoma)
YOSHIAKI KITAZAWA, M.D.

CONTENTS / xli

SECTION 26 IRIS AND CILIARY BODY

ACCOMMODATIVE SPASM 580
WILLIAM E. SCOTT, M.D.

ANIRIDIA 580
DAVID S. WALTON, M.D.

**FUCHS' HETEROCHROMIC
IRIDOCYCLITIS** 582
THOMAS J. LIESEGANG, M.D.

**IRIDOCORNEAL ENDOTHELIAL
SYNDROME** 584
(Chandler's Syndrome, Cogan-Reese
Syndrome, ICE Syndrome, Progressive
"Essential" Iris Atrophy)
M. BRUCE SHIELDS, M.D.

IRIS BOMBÉ 586
LEONARD CHRISTENSEN, M.D.

IRIS CYSTS 587
(Epithelial Cysts, Epithelial Implantation
Cysts, Spontaneous Congenital Iris Cysts)
KENNETH C. SWAN, M.D.

IRIS MELANOMA 588
H. JOHN SHAMMAS, M.D.

IRIS PROLAPSE 589
HAROLD C. PATTERSON, M.D.

PARS PLANITIS 590
(Angiohyalitis, Chronic Cyclitis, Cyclitis,
Peripheral Uveitis, Peripheral Uveoretinitis,
Vitreitis)
DANIEL H. SPITZBERG, M.D.

RUBEOSIS IRIDIS 592
(Neovascular Glaucoma)
JOHN R. SAMPLES, M.D.

UVEITIS 594
JAMES T. ROSENBAUM, M.D.

SECTION 27 LACRIMAL SYSTEM

LACRIMAL GLAND

DACRYOADENITIS 597
JOHN L. WOBIG, M.D.

LACRIMAL GLAND TUMORS 598
(Benign Epithelial Tumors, Inflammatory or
Lymphoid Tumors, Malignant Epithelial
Tumors)
RICHARD D. CUNNINGHAM, M.D., M.S.
GLEN O. BRINDLEY, M.D.

MIKULICZ'S SYNDROME 600
(Dacryosialoadenopathy, Mikulicz-Radecki
Syndrome, Mikulicz-Sjogren Syndrome)
F. HAMPTON ROY, M.D.

UVEOPAROTID FEVER 601
(Heerfordt's Syndrome, Uveoparotitis)
R. PITTS CRICK, F.R.C.S.
AIDAN MURRAY, F.R.C.S.

OUTFLOW SYSTEM

ALACRIMA 603
TED ROSENSTOCK, M.D.
J. J. HURWITZ, M.D., F.R.C.S.(C)

**CONGENITAL ANOMALIES OF THE
LACRIMAL SYSTEM** 604
(Anlage Duct, Closed Nasolacrimal Duct)
JOHN L. WOBIG, M.D.

DACRYOCYSTITIS 605
ROGER A. DAILEY, M.D.

DACRYOLITH 608
BENJAMIN MILDER, M.D.

EPIPHORA 609
JOHN L. WOBIG, M.D.

LACRIMAL HYPERSECRETION 610
MICHAEL A. LEMP, M.D.
MUNEERA A. MAHMOOD, M.D.

LACRIMAL HYPOSECRETION 611
MICHAEL A. LEMP, M.D.

SECTION 28 LENS

ADULT CATARACTS 613
ROBERT C. DREWS, M.D.

AFTER-CATARACTS 614
DAVID J. MCINTYRE, M.D., F.A.C.S.

**CONGENITAL AND INFANTILE
CATARACTS** 616
DAVID A. HILES, M.D.

DISLOCATION OF THE LENS 618
(Ectopia Lentis, Luxation of the Lens,
Subluxation of the Lens)
PAUL STERNBERG, JR., M.D.

LENTICONUS AND LENTIGLOBUS 620
MARSHALL M. PARKS, M.D.

MICROSPHEROPHAKIA 621
HAROLD E. CROSS, M.D., Ph.D.

xlii / CONTENTS

SECTION 29 MACULA

AGE-RELATED MACULAR DEGENERATION 623
MICHAEL L. KLEIN, M.D.

CYSTOID MACULAR EDEMA 624
(CME, Cystoid Maculopathy, Irvine-Gass Syndrome)
WAYNE E. FUNG, M.D.

MACULAR HOLE 627
MARK A. BRONSTEIN, M.D.

MACULAR PUCKER 628
(Cellophane Maculopathy, Preretinal Macular Fibrosis, Surface-Wrinkling Retinopathy)
RONALD G. MICHELS, M.D.

SOLAR RETINOPATHY 630
(Eclipse Burn, Foveomacular Retinitis, Photoretinitis, Solar Burn, Solar Retinitis, Sun Blindness)
ROGER A. EWALD, M.D.

SECTION 30 OPTIC NERVE

DRUG-INDUCED OPTIC ATROPHY 632
ROBERTO GUERRA, M.D.
LUISELLA CASU, M.D.

ISCHEMIC OPTIC NEUROPATHY 633
SOHAN SINGH HAYREH, M.D., Ph.D., D.Sc., F.R.C.S.

OPTIC NEURITIS 635
(Papillitis, Retrobulbar Neuritis)
THOMAS C. SPOOR, M.D., M.S., F.A.C.S.
GEOFFREY M. KWITKO, M.D.
JOHN M. RAMOCKI, M.D.

PAPILLEDEMA 637
(Choked Disc)
THOMAS J. WALSH, M.D.

SECTION 31 ORBIT

ENOPHTHALMOS 640
DAVID B. SOLL, M.D.

ORBITAL CELLULITIS AND ABSCESS 641
GREGORY B. KROHEL, M.D.

ORBITAL GRAVES' DISEASE 643
(Autoimmune Endocrine Exophthalmos, Dysthyroid Exophthalmos, Ophthalmopathy of Graves' Disease)

J. SCOTT KORTVELESY, M.D.
JOHN S. KENNERDELL, M.D.
HENRY J. L. VAN DYK, M.D., (Deceased)

ORBITAL HEMORRHAGES 646
KLAUS D. TEICHMANN, M.D., F.R.C.S.(C), F.R.A.C.O.

SECTION 32 REFRACTIVE DISORDERS

ANISOMETROPIA 648
(Asymmetropia)
MELVIN L. RUBIN, M.D.

APHAKIA 649
BENJAMIN F. BOYD, M.D.

ASTIGMATISM 651
SOREN S. BARNER, M.D., M.D.O.S.

HYPEROPIA 652
(Far-Sightedness, Hypermetropia)
GEORGE W. WEINSTEIN, M.D.

MYOPIA 653
ROBERT H. BEDROSSIAN, M.D., M.Sc.
RICHARD ELANDER, M.D.

SECTION 33 RETINA

ABETALIPOPROTEINEMIA 657
(Bassen-Kornzweig Syndrome)

AND HOMOZYGOUS FAMILIAL HYPOBETALIPOPROTEINEMIA
RICHARD G. WELEBER, M.D.
D. ROGER ILLINGWORTH, M.D., Ph.D.

ACUTE RETINAL NECROSIS 659
MARK S. BLUMENKRANZ, M.D.

BRANCH RETINAL VEIN OCCLUSION 661
FRONCIE A. GUTMAN, M.D.

CENTRAL OR BRANCH RETINAL ARTERY OCCLUSION 663
(BRAO, CRAO)
MICHAEL H. GOLDBAUM, M.D.

CENTRAL SEROUS CHORIORETINOPATHY 665
(Central Serous Retinopathy)
JAMES C. FOLK, M.D.

COATS' DISEASE 667
(Massive Exudative Retinitis, Retinal Telangiectasia)
WILLIAM TASMAN, M.D.

DIFFUSE UNILATERAL SUBACUTE NEURORETINITIS 668
(DUSN)
JOSEPH E. ROBERTSON, JR., M.D.

EALES' DISEASE 669
(Angiopathia Retinae Juvenilis, Inflammatory Disease of the Retinal Veins, Primary Perivasculitis of the Retina, Primary Retinal Hemorrhage in Young Men, Retinal Periphlebitis, Vasculitis Retinae, Vitreous Hemorrhage of Unknown Etiology)
MICHAEL L. KLEIN, M.D.

GYRATE ATROPHY OF THE CHOROID AND RETINA WITH HYPERORNITHINEMIA 670
(Ornithine-δ-amino Transaminase Deficiency)
RICHARD G. WELEBER, M.D.
NANCY G. KENNAWAY, D.Phil

PERIPHERAL RETINAL BREAKS AND DEGENERATION 671
JULIAN J. NUSSBAUM, M.D.
H. MACKENZIE FREEMAN, M.D.

REFSUM'S DISEASE 674
(Heredopathia Atactica Polyneuritiformis, Phytanic Acid Oxidase Deficiency)
RICHARD G. WELEBER, M.D.

RETINAL DETACHMENT 675
HARVEY LINCOFF, M.D.
INGRID KREISSIG, M.D.

RETINAL EMBOLI 678
DAVID J. WILSON, M.D.

RETINAL VEIN OBSTRUCTION 679
LARRY E. MAGARGAL, M.D.
H. LOGAN BROOKS, M.D.

RETINITIS PIGMENTOSA 682
SAUL MERIN, M.D.

RETINOPATHY OF PREMATURITY 683
(Retrolental Fibroplasia, RLF, ROP)
ROBERT E. KALINA, M.D.

RETINOSCHISIS 685
LOUIS DAILY, M.D., Ph.D., (Ophth)

SUBRETINAL NEOVASCULAR MEMBRANES 687
HUNTER L. LITTLE, M.D., F.A.C.S.

SECTION 34 SCLERA

EPISCLERITIS 689
PETER G. WATSON, M.A., M.B., B.Chir., F.R.C.S., D.O.

SCLERAL STAPHYLOMA AND DEHISCENCES 690
BISHARA FARIS, M.D.
H. MACKENZIE FREEMAN, M.D.

SCLERITIS 691
PETER G. WATSON, M.A., M.B., B.Chir., F.R.C.S., D.O.

SCLEROMALACIA PERFORANS 692
JAMES V. AQUAVELLA, M.D.

SECTION 35 VITREOUS

FAMILIAL EXUDATIVE VITREORETINOPATHY 694
(Autosomal Dominant Exudative Vitreoretinopathy, Criswick-Schepens Syndrome, FEVR)
JOSEPH E. ROBERTSON, JR., M.D.

PERSISTENT HYPERPLASTIC PRIMARY VITREOUS 695
(PHPV)
RONALD C. PRUETT, M.D.

PROLIFERATIVE VITREORETINOPATHY 696
(Massive Preretinal Proliferation, Massive Preretinal Gliosis, Massive Preretinal Organization, Massive Vitreous Retraction, Vitreoretinal Membrane Shrinkage)
STEVE CHARLES, M.D.

VITREOUS HEMORRHAGE 698
RICHARD L. WINSLOW, M.D.
BRUCE C. TAYLOR, M.D.

VITREOUS WICK SYNDROME 700
RICHARD S. RUIZ, M.D.

DRUG ROSTER 702

INDEX 773

Part 1

GENERALIZED DISORDERS

SECTION 1

INFECTIOUS DISEASES

Bacterial Infections

ACINETOBACTER
(Herellea vaginicola, Mima polymorpha)

Martin Wand, M.D.
Hartford, Connecticut

The taxonomy of *Acinetobacter calcoaceticus* is still changing at such a rapid pace that following the evolving nomenclature of this gram-negative bacteria is akin to watching a visiting sports team without a scorecard. As originally conceived in 1904, the genus *Acinetobacter* included both oxidase-positive (*Moraxella*) and oxidase-negative strains. Subsequently, only the oxidase-negative strains were included in the genus *Acinetobacter*, which is in the family Neisseriaceae. With newer methods of identification, including cell-envelope protein gel electrophoresis, phase typing, and bacteriocin typing, at least 11 distinct species, with numerous as yet unnamed species, have been isolated. The two clinically most important species are probably still better known by their older names, *Mima polymorpha* and *Herellea vaginicola*, rather than their correct taxonomic names, *A. calcoaceticus var. lwoffi* and *A. calcoaceticus var. anitratus*, respectively. In fact, the newest name for the latter is *Acinetobacter baumanii*. Undoubtedly, this is not the last chapter of this unfolding taxonomic story. Suffice it to say that *Acinetobacter* is an aerobic, oxidase, and gram-negative coccobacillus. Because it is an ubiquitous opportunistic organism that cannot be distinguished on gram stain from other gram-negative coccobacillus (hence the original name *Mima*), its clinical importance is clear.

Recent studies have shown that *Acinetobacter* strains can be found in 100 per cent of soil and fresh water samples and that it is part of the normal flora of fresh meats. It has been found to be part of the normal bacterial flora of almost every part of the human body, especially the skin, and has also been isolated from many inanimate objects in the hospital setting. Although generally a rather avirulent organism, it has of late been causing an increasing number of nosocomial infections, with special predeliction for the old and young and for patients with chronic debilitating diseases. The true incidence of *Acinetobacter* infections, including ocular involvement, is still unknown and probably greatly underestimated because it has been difficult to recognize it or attach any significance to this organism in a mixed culture. Because ocular involvement can range from mild keratoconjunctivitis to corneal perforation and because detailed culture identification is necessary, the most important and almost only diagnostic aid for the ophthalmologist is a high index of suspicion.

Acinetobacter species have shown multiple antibiotic resistance. This resistance can be acquired through the presence of transposable elements or plasmids from either other *Acinetobacter* species of the family Enterobactericeae. As new antibiotics have been introduced and been more widely used, multiple resistance to these antibiotics has appeared. At the present time, *Acinetobacter* species are generally resistant to penicillin, ampicillin, and most cephalosporins. *A. baumanii* is generally resistant to chloramphenicol, whereas *A. calcoaceticus var. lwoffi* is generally sensitive to this antibiotic; this trait is often used to differentiate the two species. Tetracycline, especially minocycline and ticarcillin, and several aminoglycosides, particularly tobramycin and amikicin, are still generally effective antibiotics. More recently, imipenem, a thienamycin broad-spectrum antibiotic; ceftazidime, a semisynthetic broad-spectrum beta-lactam; and cefotaxime, a semisynthetic broad-spectrum cephalosporin, have been found to be effective against this bacteria. However, recently a transferable gene for amikicin resistance has been detected, which emphasizes the importance of doing antibiotic sensitivity studies when treating an *Acinetobacter* infection.

THERAPY

Systemic. Systemic infections require systemic therapy. Intravenous tobramycin and/or ceftazidime are indicated pending results of culture and sensitivity studies.

Ocular. The topical ophthalmic antibiotic of choice is 0.3% tobramycin solution or ointment, administered every 1 to 6 hours depending on the severity of the ocular involvement. Tetracycline ophthalmic ointment, administered at least every 6 hours, is the second choice. Unfortunately, the newer effective antibiotics have not been formulated for topical use yet. Other usual treatment modalities include warm compresses and mydriatic/cycloplegics where appropriate.

4 / ACINETOBACTER

The above recommendations are only for diagnosed cases of *Acinetobacter* infections. Because these organisms are great mimickers of gramnegative rods, especially *Neisseria gonococcus*, a severe ocular infection must be treated with broad-spectrum antibiotics until the diagnosis is bacteriologically confirmed and the antibiotic sensitivity known.

Ocular or Periocular Manifestations

Conjunctiva: Follicular conjunctivitis; keratoconjunctivitis resembling keratitis sicca; ophthalmia neonatorum; purulent conjunctivitis.

Cornea: Marginal ulcers; perforations; superficial punctate staining.

Eyelids: Blepharitis; edema.

Other: Iris prolapse.

PRECAUTIONS

There is no clinical or microscopic way to differentiate a hyperacute *Acinetobacter* eye infection from one caused by *Neisseria gonococcus*. On smear, both organisms appear as gram-negative intra- and extracellular diplococci. Since gonococcal conjunctivitis is a systemic disease requiring systemic and topical therapy with penicillin and since *Acinetobacter* is resistant to penicillin, it is critical to keep *Acinetobacter* in mind in the differential diagnosis of a hyperacute ocular infection. A bacterial culture and sensitivity must be performed in every case of hyperacute conjunctivitis, and treatment should be initiated with broad-spectrum antibiotics until the cause of the infection is known. Because transferable resistance factors to antibiotics have been shown in *Acinetobacter*, antibiotic sensitivity must be determined before starting single specific therapy.

COMMENTS

Previous literature on ocular involvement by *Acinetobacter* has been scanty and unreliable because of the taxonomic confusion. No thorough clinical study employing acceptable diagnostic criteria has yet been performed. Until such a study is performed, one must assume that this ubiquitous opportunistic bacteria can manifest itself in protean ocular infections.

References

Bergogne-Berezin E, Joly-Guillou ML, Vieu JF: Epidemiology of nosocomial infections due to *Acinetobacter calcoaceticus*. J Hosp Infection *10*:105–113, 1987.

Bouvet PJM, Grimont PAD: Taxonomy of the genus Acinetobacter with the recognition of *Acinetobacter baumanni* sp. nov., *Acinetobacter haemolyticus* sp. nov., *Acinetobacter johnsonii* sp. nov., and *Acinetobacter junii* sp. nov., and emended descriptions of *Acinetobacter calcoaceticus* and *Acinetobacter lwoffi*. Int J Syst Bacteriol 36:228–240, 1986.

Burns RP, Florey MJ: Conjunctivitis caused by *Mimeae*. Am J Ophthalmol 56:386–391, 1963.

Maudgal PC, Missotten L: Acinetobacter keratoconjunctivitis clinically resembling keratitis sicca. *Bull Soc Belge Ophtalmol* 182:25–32, 1978.

Wand M, Olive GM, Jr, Mangiaracine AB: Corneal perforation and iris prolapse due to *Mima polymorpha*. Arch Ophthalmol 93:239–241, 1975.

ACQUIRED SYPHILIS
(Acquired Lues, Lues Venera, Malum Venereum)

JEROME N. GOLDMAN, M.D.
Washington, District of Columbia

Acquired syphilis is an infectious disease that is usually transmitted sexually by the fastidious spirochete, *Treponema pallidum*, which produces a typical localized lesion, a chancre, in the region of contact about 3 weeks following inoculation. The chancre remains for several weeks and disappears without treatment. It is frequently intravaginal and therefore unrecognized in women. Associated regional lymphadenopathy is typical. Transmission probably takes place during this period of *primary syphilis*.

Secondary syphilis has its onset within weeks to months after infection. During this stage, the organism is disseminated hematogenously with potential distribution even by way of the smallest blood vessels to every known portion of the human anatomy. Generalized eruptions of the skin and mucous membranes, fever, and diffuse lymphadenopathy characterize this stage. Such episodes may be recurrent.

Latent syphilis follows the secondary stage. By definition, it is devoid of clinical manifestations; there is no anatomic or cerebrospinal evidence of syphilis. A positive serologic test for syphilis is the only indication of the disease.

Late (tertiary) syphilis may be asymptomatic or may have symptoms relative to any part of the body invaded by *T. pallidum* during dissemination. Clinical manifestations of late syphilis occur 20 or more years after the original infection. For the purposes of this review, comments are confined to consideration of ocular syphilis and neurosyphilis as they affect the visual system.

THERAPY

Systemic. *T. pallidum* remains exquisitely sensitive to penicillin in vitro after years of clinical use, and no failures of penicillin therapy in clinical or experimental syphilis have been attributed to intrinsic resistance of the organism to penicillin. Penicillin acts upon the cell walls of *T. pallidum* during growth and division. After a treponemicidal level of penicillin makes contact with the organism in vitro, increasing the concentration is not more effective. Longer periods of exposure in the spirochete to these levels do have greater efficacy, however.

The preferred penicillin regimen for primary, secondary, or latent syphilis of less than one year's duration is 2.4 million units of benzathine penicillin G, administered by intramuscular injection at a single visit. For patients who are allergic to penicillin, 500 mg of oral tetracycline four times a day may be given for 15 days. Because of interference with absorption by food, oral tetracycline should be given 1 hour before and 2 hours after meals. After confirmation of penicillin allergy in patients who cannot tolerate tetracycline, two options are described. If there is assurance of compliance and serologic follow-up, 500 mg of oral erythromycin, four times daily for 15 days is recommended. If there is no such assurance, the patient should be managed in consultation with an expert.

For 1) latent syphilis of indeterminate or more than one year's duration, 2) late benign syphilis without the complication of neurosyphilis, and 3) cardiovascular syphilis, the most efficacious therapy regimen is not as well established as for early syphilis. Often, more prolonged treatment is given for syphilis of longer duration. Benzathine penicillin G is the preferred penicillin regimen. A weekly intramuscular injection of 2.4 million units should be administered for 3 consecutive weeks. A daily dosage of 2 gm of oral tetracycline divided into four doses may be administered for 30 days to those patients allergic to penicillin. Tetracycline should be given 1 hour before or 2 hours after meals. Erythromycin, 500 mg orally four times daily for 30 days, or management in consultation with an expert as described in the treatment of early syphilis is advised.

Treatment of neurosyphilis requires a more rigorous treatment schedule. Crystalline penicillin G is the preferred penicillin treatment. A daily dosage of 12 to 24 million units daily is required; 2 to 4 million units should be administered intravenously every four hours for 10 days, followed by 2.4 million units of intramuscular benzathine penicillin G at weekly intervals for 3 weeks. Another potentially successful regimen is the daily regimen of 2.4 million units of aqueous procaine penicillin G intramuscularly plus 500 mg of probenecid orally four times daily for 10 successive days, followed by 2.4 million units of intramuscular benzathine penicillin G at weekly intervals for 3 weeks.

No treatment for ocular syphilis is currently endorsed by the Centers for Disease Control, but the treatment schedule for neurosyphilis is usually followed. In clinical practice, intravenous infusion of as much as 24 to 36 million units daily has been reported as curative in recently described cases. The combined use of probenecid‡ and ampicillin‡ results in high serum levels of antibiotic activity, which in turn produce higher achievable aqueous humor levels. In addition, it is believed that probenecid also blocks the reabsorption of penicillin from the aqueous humor and maintains higher intra-ocular levels of that antibiotic. Therefore, a regimen of 1.5 gm of ampicillin and 0.5 gm of probenecid given orally every 6 hours is recommended for a 30-day period. Because of interference with absorption by food, oral ampicillin should be given 1 hour before or 2 hours after meals. Because of the known dissemination of *Treponema* in the secondary stage, the failure of the aqueous humor and the cerebrospinal fluid to achieve or maintain treponemicidal levels with conventional penicillin administration, and the natural course of the disease in which ocular and central nervous system manifestations appear many years later, it is also reasonable to administer this ampicillin-probenecid combination in the secondary and any subsequent stages of syphilis. Many patients thought to be allergic to intramuscular or intravenous penicillin will tolerate oral ampicillin with probenecid. If this proves not to be the case, desensitization to penicillin should be considered.

Ocular. Topical cycloplegics and steroids may be necessary for anterior segment inflammations. One or two applications of prednisolone or dexamethasone eyedrops or ointment should be administered as for most anterior segment inflammations. Atropine, homatropine, or cyclopentolate may be instilled two to four times daily during acute attacks of iritis. Glaucoma medications that do not stimulate inflammation, such as an epinephrine derivative or a beta blocker, may be used when indicated for elevated intraocular pressure.

In acute, subacute, or chronic ocular inflammation for which local and systemic treatment does not appear to be effective, subconjunctival injections of dexamethasone* should be given for 3 to 5 days. Following topical anesthesia with 0.5 per cent proparacaine, 0.5 to 1.0 ml of 0.1 per cent dexamethasone and 0.25 ml of 1 per cent lidocaine in the same syringe are injected subconjunctivally.

Ocular or Periocular Manifestations

(P) indicates manifestations of primary syphilis; (S) indicates those of secondary syphilis; and (T) indicates signs of tertiary, late, or neurosyphilis.

Conjunctiva: Chancre (P); conjunctivitis (S).
Cornea: Interstitial keratitis (usually monocular) (S).
Extraocular Muscles: Gumma (T); palsy (T); ptosis (T).
Eyelids: Chancre (P); exanthem (S).
Iris: Gumma (T); iritis (S); posterior uveitis (S).
Lacrimal System: Dacryoadenitis (S); dacryocystitis (S).
Optic Nerve: Atrophy (T); gumma (T); optic neuritis (S); papilledema (S); optic perineuritis (S).
Pupil: Abnormalities (T).
Retina: Arteritis (S); gumma (T); pigmentary degeneration (T); retinitis (S); choroiditis (S); macular scars (S, T).
Sclera: Episcleritis (S); gumma (T); scleritis (S).
Vitreous: Vitreitis (S).
Other: Visual field defects (T).

6 / ACQUIRED SYPHILIS

PRECAUTIONS

When confronted with the history of penicillin allergy, documentation and/or clinical testing should be pursued before choosing alternative antibiotics. Oral ampicillin has fewer serious side effects than systemic administration of any penicillin, even in patients with penicillin allergy. Common side effects experienced with combination use of oral ampicillin and probenecid have been pruritic exanthems and loose stools. Antipruritics or antihistamines, such as diphenhydramine, have been effective in treating the rash without interruption of therapy; the rash usually disappears in 3 to 5 days. The loose stools are never disabling and are tolerated well by the patients. Patients should be encouraged to eat yogurt or to drink acidophilus milk. The occasional vaginitis associated with long-time antibiotic therapy is treated symptomatically.

No less than the recommended doses of antibiotics should be used because inadequate treatment may leave surviving pathogenic treponemal organisms, and this is more likely to result in late ocular or neurosyphilis. Several recent clinical reports demonstrate the failure of intramuscular benzathine penicillin G and tetracycline, followed by apparently successful treatment of ocular or neurosyphilis with the use of very high doses of intravenous aqueous penicillin G for 10 or more days with or without probenecid. A nontreponemal serologic test for syphilis, as well as a FTA-ABS test, should be obtained prior to treatment and 4 to 6 weeks after the termination of treatment. Reinfection should always be considered. Patients with syphilis of indeterminate or of more than one year's duration should have cerebrospinal fluid examination for cells, protein, and VDRL-CSF reaction. Patients with asymptomatic neurosyphilis should be treated and followed as are patients with symptomatic neurosyphilis.

COMMENTS

Despite the well-documented successful treatment of infectious syphilis, the prevention and treatment of ocular and central nervous system syphilis are still in dispute. Fifty to 70 per cent of untreated syphilis patients go through life without inconvenience, despite lack of treatment. Although untreated syphilitics have an excess number of deaths compared to the general population, 90 per cent of deaths are from causes other than syphilis.

These statistics should not undervalue the morbidity resulting from lack of treatment, because prior to the introduction of the heavy metals and, subsequently, penicillin, the scourge of syphilis affected every part of the human body and mimicked nearly every other disease. The manifestations of late syphilis resulting in paresis and blindness particularly were common and feared by all.

References

Arruga J, et al: Neuroretinitis in acquired syphilis. Ophthalmology 92:262–270, 1985.

Brooks AM, et al: Interstitial keratitis in untreated latent (late) syphilis. Aust NZ J Ophthalmol 14:127–132, 1986.
de Souza EC, et al: Unusual central chorioretinitis as the first manifestation of early secondary syphilis. Am J Ophthalmol 105:271–276, 1988.
Dunlop EM: Survival of treponemes after treatment: Comments, clinical conclusions, and recommendations. Genitourin Med 61:293–301, 1985.
Folk JC, et al: Syphilitic neuroretinitis. Am J Ophthalmol 95:480–486, 1983.
Mendelsohn AD, Jampol LM: Syphilitic retinitis. A cause of necrotizing retinitis. Retina 4:221–224, 1984.
Poitevin M, et al: Syphilis in 1986. J Clin Neuro-Ophthalmol 7:11–19, 1987.
Sacks JG, et al: Progressive visual loss in syphilitic optic atrophy. 3:5–8, 1983.
Spoor TC, et al: Ocular syphilis. J Clin Neuro-Ophthalmol. 3:197–202, 1983.
1985 STD Treatment Guidelines. MMWR 34(Suppl 4):75S–108S, 1985.
Veldman E: Neuroretinitis in secondary syphilis. Doc Ophthalmol: 23–29, 1986.
Wilhelmus KR, Yokoyama CM: Syphilitic episcleritis and scleritis. Am J Ophthalmol 104:595–597, 1987.

AZOTOBACTER

THOMAS J. LIESEGANG, M.D.
Jacksonville, Florida

Azotobacter is a large gram-negative aerobic rod belonging to the family Azotobacteraceae. It is ubiquitous in aerobic soil and water throughout the world in both temperate and tropical zones. The organism has many distinctive features, including large size, pleomorphism, gram stain variability, a distinctive cyst stage, and occasionally extensive production of a slime layer. It can appear as rods, cocci, or yeast-like cells within nature or under certain culture conditions. Even a single pure clone of *Azotobacter* may show varying morphologic characteristics. When grown in a nitrogen-free medium, the organism appears gram negative, but becomes more pleomorphic as the culture ages. The organism does not form spores, but has a characteristic thick-walled spherical, dormant cyst under certain circumstances. The cysts are resistant to ultraviolet radiation and drying and, under suitable conditions, can germinate into the vegetative cells from which they arose. Vegetative cells are mobile by means of flagella, but on induction of encystment, these cells lose motility and become spherical.

The genus comprises four species differentiated by their predominant shape, motility, ratio of amino acids, presence of fluorescent pigment, and various biochemical tests. All four species (*A. beijerinckii, A. chroococcum, A. paspali, A. vinelandii*) grow readily on routine culture media at 35° C. On blood agar, colonies are small, waxy, and slightly opaque. As the culture ages, colonies turn yellow or light tan. On carbohydrate media, extensive capsule or slide layers are produced.

Azotobacter is unique in its high respiratory rate and ability to fix atmospheric nitrogen and synthesize plant hormones. It plays an important role in the terrestrial ecosystem because of its ability to fix substantial amounts of nitrogen, especially in established grasslands and forests. It has been applied as a "bacterial fertilizer" for plants. In the laboratory *Azobacter* grows best over a free nitrogen media.

A series of ten cases of *Azotobacter* keratitis was reported from Houston over an 8-year period. During the same period, this ocular microbiology laboratory reported the recovery of *Azotobacter* from the conjunctiva on three other occasions, although they were not isolated from the area of pathologic infection. There were no distinctive biomicroscopic signs characteristic of *Azotobacter* keratitis; some of the cases were characterized by a considerable corneal suppuration and subsequent scarring after resolution of the infection. Some patients had predisposing factors and some had foreign body injury, but others had no recognized predisposing factor. All four species have been isolated in association with keratitis. Plentiful large pleomorphic gram-negative rods were detected in the corneal smears, with some smears demonstrating gram-positive rods or the distinctive cysts as well. Two of the ten cases had a mixed bacterial infection. The organism grew on blood and chocolate agar, as well as thyoglycolate and brain heart infusion broth, within a few days of innoculation. Standard disc-diffusion tests have demonstrated uniform sensitivity to gentamicin, neomycin, chloramphenicol, erythromycin, bacitracin, cephalothin, and ampicillin. The clinical response in these cases suggests that gentamicin or another aminoglycoside should be effective against the various species. An animal model and extensive antimicrobial testing have not been done.

On the basis of the similarity of the organisms, some cases of *Azotobacter* have probably been incorrectly identified as *Moraxella*. The large pleomorphic size, the gram-negative forms, and the presence of cysts usually distinguish the *Azotobacter* on corneal smears. The colonial features, motility, biochemical tests, and inducement of the characteristic cyst stage confirm the presence of *Azotobacter*.

THERAPY

Ocular. The organisms appear to be sensitive to most antimicrobial therapy, although this has not been extensively tested. The microbial keratitis has been treated with topical and subconjunctival* gentamicin with subsequent resolution of the infection, although corneal scarring has limited the vision of most patients.

Ocular or Periocular Manifestations

Cornea: Suppurative corneal infection with subsequent scarring.

PRECAUTIONS

Azobacter is probably misdiagnosed as *Moraxella* keratitis frequently. Careful review of the gram stain should enable differentiation.

COMMENTS

Azotobacter has never been reported as a pathogenic organism in any other organ system in man. There are distinctive morphologic features of *Azotobacter keratitis*, but it has probably not been recognized in microbiology laboratories. The organisms are usually plentiful on the gram stain and search of the smear should confirm the variable morphologic appearance, and perhaps the cyst. The organism grows readily on all media. The definitive characterization of the organism requires growth in a nitrogen-free media or the demonstration of the dormant cyst stage. The organism has been sensitive to all antibiotics.

References

Jensen HL: The Azotobacteriaciae. Bact Rev. *18*:195–214, 1954.
Kennedy C, Toukdarian A: Genetics of *Azotobacter*: Application to nitrogen fixation and related aspects of metabolism. Ann Rev Microbiol *41*:227–258, 1987.
Liesegang TJ, Jones DB, Robinson NM: *Azotobacter* keratitis. Arch Ophthalmol 99:1587–1590, 1981.
Norris JR, Chapman HM: Classification of *Azotobacter*. In Gibbs GM, Shapton DA (eds): Identification Methods For Microbiologists. New York, Academic Press, 1968, pp 19–27.

BACILLUS CEREUS
DENIS M. O'DAY, M.D.
Nashville, Tennessee.

Bacillus cereus is an aerobic gram-positive bacillus that is now recognized as a highly virulent pathogen. The organism enters the eye either as a result of penetrating trauma with a contaminated metallic foreign body or as a metastatic infection that occurs most frequently in drug addiction. In one study, *B. cereus* was noted to be the most common contaminant of injection paraphernalia.

Infection with *B. cereus* leads to the development of a fulminating panophthalmitis, accompanied by fever and leukocytosis. The course is extremely rapid. Characteristically, a ring abscess of the cornea develops as the eye becomes progressively proptosed. In most reported cases, the eye is blind within 72 hours of the onset of infection. These disastrous effects on ocular tissue appear to be related to a specific exotoxin elaborated by the organism, and the virulence of a particular strain may be related to the amount of toxin produced.

8 / BACILLUS CEREUS

THERAPY

Systemic. Unlike most gram-positive bacilli, *B. cereus* is resistant to the natural and semisynthetic penicillins, as well as the cephalosporins. However, because there may be difficulty initially with the specific identification of *B. cereus* as opposed to other gram-positive bacilli, penicillin or cephalosporin should be administered concurrently with clindamycin and gentamicin, to which *B. cereus* is susceptible. Daily intravenous administration of 40 mg/kg of clindamycin and 4 mg/kg of gentamicin is given in divided doses. Initially, 250,000 units/kg of aqueous penicillin G is also administered daily intravenously. Antibiotic therapy should be continued systemically for at least 7 days.

Ocular. In view of the grave nature of the infection, periocular, intravitreal, and topical ophthalmic antibiotics are recommended in addition to intravenous therapy. Clindamycin may be particularly useful because of the therapeutic levels achievable in the eye after systemic and periocular administration. Separate subconjunctival injections of 34 mg of clindamycin* and 40 mg of gentamicin* are recommended daily. This periocular antibiotic therapy should be continued for several weeks. In addition, fortified gentamicin§ (13 mg/ml) and clindamycin* (50 mg/ml) eyedrops should be given every 30 minutes. Recently, the combination of 1 mg of vancomycin* with 100 µg of gentamicin* has been suggested for intravitreal use.

Topical and periocular corticosteroids should be administered concurrently with the antibiotics in an attempt to control the host inflammatory response. Subconjunctival injection of 4 mg of dexamethasone* daily is recommended. Topical ocular 1 per cent prednisolone acetate§ may be used hourly. Corticosteroid and topical antibiotic therapy may be needed for several months.

Surgical. In light of the fulminating course of this disease, an extensive vitrectomy should be performed as soon as infection is suspected. At this time, intravitreal injection of 450 µg of clindamycin* and 250 µg of gentamicin* should be used. Serious consideration should be given to further intravitreal antibiotic therapy in the next 48 hours.

Ocular or Periocular Manifestations

Anterior Chamber: Hypopyon.
Choroid or Retina: Extensive necrosis.
Cornea: Ring abscess.
Globe: Panophthalmitis, progressing to phthisis.
Orbit: Cellulitis with proptosis.
Vitreous: Abscess.

PRECAUTIONS

There is a small but definite risk of pseudomembranous colitis caused by an overgrowth of *Clostridium difficile* in the small bowel that is associated with the systemic administration of clindamycin. However, local administration of clindamycin in the doses recommended has not been known to give rise to this adverse side effect.

Systemic gentamicin is potentially nephrotoxic and should be administered with caution in patients with renal impairment. The actual dose should be calculated on the basis of lean body weight, aiming for a peak level of 6 to 8 µg/ml and a trough of 2 µg/ml. Gentamicin blood levels should be checked 24 hours after the initial dose. Once these levels are stabilized, gentamicin levels can be monitored every 4 to 5 days. Serum creatinine levels can be used to check renal function every 2 to 3 days.

The concurrent administration of corticosteroid and antibiotics carries with it the risk of enhancing microbial proliferation. However, this risk appears justified in the face of the speed and destructive nature of this infection.

COMMENTS

The best hope of salvaging eyes infected with *B. cereus* appears to lie with early diagnosis and prompt treatment. Thus, penetrating trauma with a metallic foreign body occurring in a dirty environment or an apparent metastatic infection in a suspected drug addict should always suggest the possibility of an infection by this organism. In such circumstances, an immediate diagnostic and therapeutic vitrectomy is indicated, with antibiotic therapy being initiated before surgery if an undue delay is anticipated. Although the prognosis is extremely poor, several eyes have now been saved with useful vision by following the above approach.

References

Affeldt JC, et al: Microbial endophthalmitis resulting from ocular trauma. Ophthalmology 94:407–413, 1987.

Mandelbaum S, Forster RK: Postoperative endophthalmitis. Int Ophthalmol Clin 27:95–106, 1987.

O'Day DM, et al: The problem of Bacillus species infection with special emphasis on the virulence of *Bacillus cereus*. Ophthalmology 88:833–838, 1981.

Shamsuddin D, et al: *Bacillus cereus* panophthalmitis: Source of the organism. Rev Infect Dis 4:97–103, 1982.

Tuazon CU, et al: Serious infections with *Bacillus* sp. JAMA 241:1137–1140, 1979.

BACILLUS SUBTILIS
GEORGE A. WILLIAMS, M.D.,
and ROBERT A. HYNDIUK, M.D.
Milwaukee, Wisconsin

The aerobic, spore-bearing, gram-positive rods comprising the genus *Bacillus* most commonly are found in association with soil and vegetation. Although *Bacillus anthracis* is of great historical importance, it very rarely involves the eye. However, other species of *Bacillus* may infect the eye. Because of the difficulty in differentiating among the various *Bacillus* species, some laboratories have labeled them all *B. subtilis*. Recently, several *Bacillus* species have been identified as virulent ocular pathogens, including *B. cereus*. Because of imprecise speciation it is likely that many cases of ocular infection reported to be due to *B. subtilis* were actually the result of other *Bacillus* species.

Ocular infection by *B. subtilis* or other *Bacillus* species manifests most typically as posttraumatic endophthalmitis or occasionally after surgery. Approximately 20 to 40 per cent of posttraumatic endophthalmitis cases are caused by the *Bacillus* species. There have also been reports of purulent and pseudomembranous conjunctivitis and corneal ulcers (classically a ring ulcer after penetrating trauma), as well as dacryocystitis and orbital abscesses, caused by the *Bacillus* species. Normal conjunctival flora occasionally includes *Bacillus* species in persons who are farmers or laboratory workers.

THERAPY

Ocular. *B. subtilis* and the other *Bacillus* species are usually sensitive to gentamicin, tobramycin, and clindamycin. A synergistic effect using both gentamicin and clindamycin has been noted. This combination has been demonstrated to be effective in treating ocular *Bacillus* sp. infections. More recently, vancomycin has been recommended as an effective antimicrobial.

ENDOPHTHALMITIS. In cases of proven *Bacillus* species endophthalmitis, prompt aggressive therapy should be instituted with intravitreal, topical, and subconjunctival antibiotics. Intravitreal gentamicin* (100 µg) is used in combination with either clindamycin* (0.45 to 1.0 mg) or vancomycin* (1 mg). In addition, topical clindamycin§ (50 mg/ml) or vancomycin§ (50 mg/ml), in conjunction with topical gentamicin§ (20 mg/ml), is administered every 30 to 60 minutes along with subconjunctival clindamycin* (34 mg), gentamicin* (20 mg), or vancomycin* (25 mg). Although the efficacy of systemic antibiotics in the treatment of *Bacillus* endophthalmitis remains to be established, if systemic antibiotics are to be used intravenous clindamycin (600 to 900 mg every 6 to 8 hours) is a reasonable choice because of its documented ocular penetration.

CORNEAL ULCERS. *Bacillus* corneal ulcers are treated with topical clindamycin§ (50 mg/ml) or vancomycin§ (50 mg/ml), in conjunction with topical gentamicin§ (20 mg/ml), administered initially every 30 minutes and then adjusted according to clinical response. Initial serial "loading" doses of fortified topical antibiotic are given every 2 minutes times five to achieve tissue level peaks more quickly, and serial topical loading doses are given at times of possible tissue level troughs during the course of therapy. In patients with deep corneal abscess, impending perforation or sclerolimbal involvement, adjunctive subconjunctival injections of clindamycin*, gentamicin*, or vancomycin* may also be given.

Surgical. Vitrectomy should be considered in all eyes with endophthalmitis and significant media opacification. In eyes with *Bacillus* endophthalmitis, vitrectomy provides the theoretical advantage of diluting or washing out the potent tissue-destructive toxins that all *Bacillus* species, but particularly *B. subtilis* and *B. cereus*, produce.

Ocular or Periocular Manifestations

Conjunctiva: Purulent or pseudomembranous conjunctivitis.
Cornea: Ring abscess; ulcer.
Globe: Endophthalmitis; panophthalmitis.
Lacrimal System: Dacryocystitis.
Orbit: Abscess

PRECAUTIONS

If systemic antibiotic therapy is administered, potential toxicities must be considered. For example, systemic clindamycin may cause pseudomembranous colitis and systemic aminoglycosides may result in nephrotoxicity even when administered at appropriate dosages.

Bacillus species other than *B. anthracis* have in the past been considered nonpathogenic laboratory contaminants. The ophthalmologist therefore must be certain that positive cultures are not ignored by laboratory personnel.

COMMENTS

Despite the recommended antibiotic regimens the treatment of established *Bacillus* endophthalmitis rarely preserves useful vision. The virulent nature and dismal natural course of ocular *Bacillus* infections require both a high degree of clinical suspicion and aggressive therapy if vision or even the eye is to be salvaged. For this reason, aggressive prophylaxis, including intravitreal antibiotics, should be considered in high-risk situations for *Bacillus* infections, such as eyes with intraocular foreign bodies or soil-contaminated wounds.

References

Affeldt JC, Flynn HW Jr, Forster RK, et al: Microbial endophthalmitis resulting from ocular trauma. Ophthalmology 94:407–413, 1987.
Brinton GS, Hyndiuk RA, Abrams G, et al: Post-traumatic endophthalmitis. Arch Ophthalmol 102:547–550, 1984.
O'Day DM, Smith RS, Gregg CR: The problem of *Bacillus* species infection with special emphasis on the virulence of *Bacillus cereus*. Ophthalmology 88:833–838, 1981.
Parke DW II, Brinton GS: Endophthalmitis. *In* Tabbara K, Hyndiuk R (eds): Infections of the Eye: Diag-

---

This work was supported in part by an unrestricted grant from Research to Prevent Blindness and by Ophthalmic Research Center Grant EY01931.

nosis and Management. Boston, Little, Brown and Co, 1986, pp 563–585.

Schemmer GB, Driebe WT: Posttraumatic *Bacillus cereus* endophthalmitis. Arch Ophthalmol 105:342–344, 1987.

Williams GA, Hyndiuk RA: Prevention and management of posttraumatic endophthalmitis. *In* Miller D, Stegmann R (eds): Treatment of Anterior Segment Ocular Trauma. Montreal, Medicopea, 1986, pp 175–186.

BOTULISM

MICHAEL CHERINGTON, M.D.

Denver, Colorado

Botulism is a paralyzing disease caused by the most toxic substance known to humans. The toxin is produced by the bacterium *Clostridium botulinum*. Eight immunologically distinct toxins have been identified. Human cases are almost always due to type A, B, or E. When contaminated seafood is found to be responsible, the toxin present is often type E.

Botulism toxin is heat labile and thus is often destroyed by the cooking process. By contrast, the spores of *C. botulinum* are heat resistant. When spores are present in food, actively multiplying bacilli produce the toxin at room temperature under anaerobic conditions at a pH of 6 or above. The toxin causes paralysis of skeletal muscles by interfering with release of acetylcholine.

The clinical symptoms of botulism usually occur within 12 to 36 hours after ingestion of contaminated food. The signs and symptoms begin in the cranial nerve territory (blurred vision, dysarthria, dysphagia) and then descend. This distinguishes botulism from the Guillain-Barré syndrome, which is characterized by ascending paralysis.

In botulism, respiratory paralysis can follow quickly and is often fatal unless treated. Alertness, mentation, and the sensory system remain normal. The pupils are usually normal, particularly early in the disease. Patients with severe botulism almost always have marked extraocular muscle weakness, including ptosis. Weakness of the face, tongue, pharynx, neck, and sometimes the limbs (to a lesser degree) occurs. Weakness progresses until it reaches a plateau at about 4 to 5 days. Although the weakness is bilateral, it is often asymmetric. Severe respiratory paralysis can occur within the first day. Symptoms of parasympathetic dysfunction may include gastrointestinal ileus and dryness of the mouth and eyes. Deep tendon reflexes are reduced in proportion to the degree of muscular weakness. Recovery, if it occurs, is prolonged but nearly total. Laboratory confirmation usually requires the detection of toxin in the contaminated food or in the patient's serum or stool.

THERAPY

Systemic. The role of guanidine[‡] in the treatment of botulism remains that of an adjunct to therapy and not that of a cure. It has helped some but not all patients. The initial oral daily dose is 15 mg/kg administered in divided doses.

Supportive. The major treatment of botulism is good medical care. This consists of providing artificial ventilation for the patients with respiratory paralysis. Tracheotomy and positive pressure support are usually required. Mechanical assistance to respiration may be needed for as long as weeks or months. Early administration of antitoxin may be of value in cases of type E botulism. The literature and experience suggest that antitoxin is less effective in types A and B botulism. Corticosteroid treatment has not been beneficial.

Ocular or Periocular Manifestations

Extraocular Muscles: External ophthalmoplegia.
Eyelids: Ptosis.
Pupil: Variable response.

PRECAUTIONS

Increasing the dose of guanidine may result in considerable epigastric distress and nausea. This is a problem because guanidine has not been approved for parenteral administration and must be given orally. Another problem in treatment with guanidine is failure of its absorption because of the ileus. Serious side effects of guanidine include bone marrow suppression and renal toxicity.

Recently, another drug, 4-aminopyridine[†], has been reported to be effective in reversing the neuromuscular block of botulism. Unfortunately, the drug has little or no benefit in reversing the paralysis of respiratory muscles. In this, it is similar to the action of guanidine. Both guanidine and 4-aminopyridine have serious side effects that may be encountered, particularly with prolonged usage. The clinicians must weigh risk-benefit ratios. Both of these drugs should be considered experimental at this time.

COMMENTS

In some clinical situations the diagnosis cannot be confirmed by serologic means because of delay in diagnosis. In these situations particularly, electrophysiologic studies can often provide additional diagnostic information. The most often-noted electrophysiologic abnormality is a reduced amplitude of muscle action potentials.

The treatment of botulism remains good medical and nursing intensive care. Both guanidine and 4-aminopyridine have serious side effects that must be weighed by the clinician. The most serious side effects seen with guanidine have occurred when its use has been prolonged, usually in illnesses such as myasthenia syndrome.

A relatively new and increasingly frequently recognized form of botulism is infant botulism. A form of botulism that has been reported only rarely and usually in adults, in contrast, is wound botulism.

A very recent development in the history of this disease has been the use of the neurotoxin as a therapeutic tool. Botulinum toxin A was first reported in 1981 as a treatment for strabismus and has since been used in the treatment of hemifacial spasm, blepharospasm, and cervical dystonia.

References

Cherington M: Botulism. Ten-year experience. Arch Neurol 30:432–437, 1974.
Jenzer G, et al: Autonomic dysfunction in botulism B: A clinical report. Neurology 25:150–153, 1975.
Konig H, Gassman HB, Jenzer G: Ocular involvement in benign botulism B. Am J Ophthalmol 80:430–432, 1975.
Pickett J, et al: Syndrome of botulism in infancy: Clinical and electrophysiologic study. N Engl J Med 295:770–772, 1976.
Scott AB: Botulinum toxin injection into extraocular muscles as an alternative to strabismus surgery. Ophthalmology 87:1044–1049, 1980.
Terranova W, Palumbo JN, Breman JG: Ocular findings in botulism type B. JAMA 241:475–477, 1979.

BRUCELLOSIS
(Malta Fever, Mediterranean Fever, Melitococcosis, Undulant Fever)

J. POLETTI, M.D.,
Tarbes, France

and A. LARMANDE, M.D.
Tours, France

Brucellosis is an infectious disease common to animals and humans. The responsible bacteria are nonmotile, gram-negative aerobic coccobacilli. For humans, the common sources of infection are ingestion of milk products and occupational contact with infected animals.

Brucellosis is very polymorphous. The acute septicemic phase does not result in many ocular symptoms. During the subacute form of focal brucellosis, osteo-articular, hepatosplenic, glandular, cardiac, respiratory, nephric, and neuromeningeal localizations may occur. Most of the ocular manifestations noticed at this time are related to neuromeningeal involvement. However, during the chronic phase, uveitis and other allergic ocular manifestations are seen more frequently, often isolated from any general context of malaise, pain, neurovegetative disorders, or localized foci. The iridocyclitis is frequently of rapid onset, evanescent, and recurrent. After some relapses, a granulomatous uveitis may develop. Posterior uveitis is often masked by a vitreous opacity; multiple nodular exudates with weak inflammatory or hemorrhagic reactions may also result. At this stage of infection, the Wright's sero-agglutination reaction is often negative, and the skin reaction to Brucella antigen is usually positive but contraindicated due to a syndromal reaction risk.

THERAPY

Systemic. In the acute phase, rest and antibiotic therapy for 45 to 60 days are recommended.

In the subacute and chronic phases, antibiotic therapy may be useful to erase quiet foci and persistent bacteria. The usual daily adult dose is 0.2 gm of doxycycline and 0.9 gm of rifampicine, administered for 3 to 6 months. A short course of oral corticosteroid therapy may be necessary prior to this treatment. Following remission of chronic brucellosis, specific desensitizing antigen[†] therapy may be administered by intradermal or subcutaneous route. Very small initial doses of the inactivated vaccines should be used, and a slow progression in administration should be made to avoid syndromal reactions.

Ocular. During the uveitis phase, topical ophthalmic atropine and corticosteroids minimize the damage to the eye during an attack and lessen the duration of the ocular disease. Local corticosteroids are also helpful during desensitization to prevent syndromal ocular reaction.

Ocular or Periocular Manifestations

Conjunctiva: Conjunctivitis.
Cornea: Annular keratitis with rounded subepithelial infiltrates; other keratitis; ulcer.
Extraocular Muscles: Paralysis.
Eyelids: Blepharitis.
Lacrimal System: Dacryoadenitis.
Optic Nerve: Papilledema; retrobulbar or optic neuritis.
Retina: Edema; hemorrhages; venous disorders; retinal detachment.
Sclera: Episcleritis; scleritis.
Uvea: Anterior; intermediate, posterior, pan uveitis.
Other: Cataract; decreased intraocular pressure (early); secondary glaucoma (late).

PRECAUTIONS

The thrust of treatment must be essentially preventive. Hygiene systemic animal vaccination and human vaccination* (after sensitizing test) of professionally or geographically exposed individuals are effective control measures.

The treatment of chronic brucellosis and of its ocular allergic manifestations is difficult. It is based upon a specific antigen therapy not approved in many countries. It requires a special

---

* "Vaccin inactivé brucellique PI" and "Test brucellique PS" Mérieux Institute (France, Portugal, Brazil).

control and is not usually given to elderly patients or to others with visceral weaknesses. Its efficiency must be checked with repeated dosages, until a normalization of Witmer's relation is achieved.

COMMENTS

The ocular brucellosis diagnosis must be authenticated by the calculation of Witmer's relation between ocular and serous specific antibodies. If this dosage is not available, a presumptive diagnosis will be given by significant values of serologic tests (buffered antigen, indirect immunofluorescence, passive hemagglutination, specific agglutination test; detection of circulating immune complexes) and by the cell immunity test (lymphocyte transformation, inhibition of leukocyte migration), showing a retarded hypersensitivity.

References

Comité mixte FAO-OMS d'experts de la brucellose, 6ème rapport—WHO, Technical report number 740–1986.

Poletti J, Poletti A, Larmande A: Diagnostic and therapeutic problems in brucellosis uveitis. Med Trop 41:523–525, 1981.

Renoux GM, Larmande A, Poletti JA: Le diagnostic biologique de la brucellose oculaire. Arch Ophthalmol 37:767–769, 1977.

Renoux M, et al: Hémagglutination passive, transformation lymphoblastique et migration des leucocytes appliquées au diagnostic des brucelloses. Dev Biol Stand 31:145–156, 1976.

Rolando IM, Carbone AO: Circulating immune complexes in the pathogenesis of human brucellar uveitis. Chibret Intern J Ophthalmol 3:30–38, 1985.

CLOSTRIDIUM PERFRINGENS

DAVID SEVEL, M.D., Ph.D., F.A.C.S.

La Jolla, California

Clostridium perfringens is a gram-positive, rod-shaped, anaerobic bacillus. It is the most important cause of gas gangrene infection, which occurs predominantly in traumatized, ischemic skeletal muscle but has also been described in the abdominal wall and uterus.

C. perfringens endophthalmitis is rare and occurs as an opportunistic infection. It is associated with a perforating injury, frequently with an intraocular foreign body. *C. perfringens* septicemia may also cause metastatic endophthalmitis. The infection characteristically develops within 24 hours of a penetrating injury. Severe ocular pain, marked edema of the lids, chemosis, and early elevation of the intraocular pressure are the hallmarks of this infection. Bloody or coffee-colored discharge is noted, and hypopyon and air bubbles are characteristically present in the anterior chamber. Intraocular necrosis rapidly ensues, and the patient becomes febrile as systemic toxicity develops. *C. perfringens* orbital cellulitis may occur as an extension of the eye infection or either primarily in the orbit and is then associated with a retained intraorbital foreign body.

THERAPY

Systemic. The successful treatment of *C. perfringens* is dependent on early diagnosis. A major prerequisite is the correct collection and transportation of the ocular exudate or orbital specimen to the laboratory. The fluid specimen is kept in the syringe and either inoculated without delay into thioglycolate broth or placed in an anaerobic jar (Gaspak). By far, the most satisfactory method of inoculation is in a prereduced anaerobic bottle. The latter provides a flat agar surface for evaluation of the number and morphologic characteristics of the colonies.

The gram stain determines the initial choice of antibiotic. If large, uniform gram-positive rods are noted, 1 to 3 million units of sodium penicillin G are administered intravenously every 3 to 4 hours. These massive doses of penicillin serve the purpose of prolonging the period during which surgical intervention can be successful. Although systemic antibiotics cannot control the relentless destruction of the eye associated with *C. perfringens* endophthalmitis, they can prevent orbital extension of the condition. If the patient is sensitive to penicillin, 1 gm of cefazolin every 4 hours should be given intravenously. The latter antibiotic is effective against penicillinase-producing staphylococci, but can cause renal complications.

If gram-positive and gram-negative organisms are observed on gram stain, a combination of 3 million units of sodium penicillin G every 4 hours and 1 gm of chloramphenicol every 6 hours is administered intravenously.

It takes 24 hours or longer to culture the anaerobes. In the interim period, 1 gm of intravenous chloramphenicol is given every 6 to 8 hours so as to cover other anaerobes that may be present.

Once the infection is controlled either by vitrectomy, evisceration, or orbital surgery, 500 mg of ampicillin are given orally every 6 hours. In addition, chloramphenicol is administered orally in a dosage of 500 mg every 8 hours for 1 week and reduced to 250 mg every 6 hours for a further week.

The indications for gas-gangrene antitoxin are shock and hemolytic anemia. The dosage is 50,000 units intravenously every 6 hours for 1 to 2 days. Gas-gangrene antitoxin is of little use in the prophylaxis of gas gangrene and is of questionable value in treatment.

Hyperbaric oxygen treatment does not appear to be efficacious for *C. perfringens* ophthalmitis, but may be of use if there is orbital involvement. Before hyperbaric oxygen is administered, myringotomy tubes are inserted into the eardrums, and the patient is given two 2-hour treatments in a hyperbaric oxygen chamber filled and ventilated with 100 per cent oxygen at a pressure of 3 atmospheres (approximately 30 pounds per square inch).

Ocular. Antibiotic therapy is of prophylactic value and is usually combined with a surgical procedure. Subconjunctival injections of 0.5 to 1.0 million units of sodium penicillin G* or 100 mg of cephaloridine* and 20 mg of gentamicin* are given to cover a mixed infection.

Surgical. A prerequisite for the treatment of *C. perfringens* infection is excision of the necrotic, highly toxic tissue. In the early stages (within 24 hours) of *C. perfringens* endophthalmitis, vitrectomy and instillation of intravitreal antibiotics are indicated. For mixed infection, the dosage of intravitreal infusion fluid is 10 µg of cephaloridine* and 8 µg of gentamicin.*

It appears that, once *C. perfringens* endophthalmitis is established, treatment will not salvage vision because of the severe toxicity generated by the organism. If the infection is confined to the eye, evisceration is indicated. However, if there is obvious evidence of extension of the reaction beyond the confines of the eye into the orbital tissue, enucleation combined with a partial exenteration of the necrotic and macroscopically involved orbital tissue is indicated. Any intraocular or intraorbital foreign bodies should be removed. These steps are essential to prevent the systemic syndrome of gas gangrene, which is a life-threatening condition.

Ocular or Periocular Manifestations

Anterior Chamber: Gas bubbles; hypopyon.
Cornea: Penetrating wound.
Globe: Endophthalmitis; proptosis.
Other: Acute rise of intraocular pressure; chemosis; coffee-colored discharge; eyelid edema; severe ocular pain.

PRECAUTIONS

Once *C. perfringens* endophthalmitis gains a foothold, the destructive process appears to be irreversible. Rapid necrosis of the intraocular tissue ensues, and neither antibiotics nor gas gangrene antitoxin is of any use. Although hyperbaric oxygen may be of avail if there is orbital involvement, it is unlikely to be efficacious for the intraocular infection.

COMMENTS

Vitrectomy with intravitreal injection of antibiotics could theoretically be of value in gas-gangrene endophthalmitis, as involved toxic and infected tissue are excised.

References

Bristow JH, Kassar B, Sevel D: Gas gangrene panophthalmitis treated with hyperbaric oxygen. Br J Ophthalmol 55:139–142, 1971.
Davis CE, et al: Simple method for culturing anaerobes. Appl Microbiol 25:216–221, 1973.
Frantz JF, et al: Acute endogenous panophthalmitis caused by *Clostridium perfringens*. Am J Ophthalmol 78:295–303, 1974.
Levitt JM, Stam J: *Clostridium perfringens* panophthalmitis. Arch Ophthalmol 84:227–228, 1970.
Obertynski H, Dyson C: *Clostridium perfringens* panophthalmitis. Can J Ophthalmol 9:258–259, 1974.
Sevel D, et al: Gas in the orbit associated with orbital cellulitis and paranasal sinusitis. Br J Ophthalmol 57:133–137, 1973.

CONGENITAL SYPHILIS
JEROME N. GOLDMAN, M.D.
Washington, District of Columbia

Congenital syphilis occurs when *Treponema pallidum* passes across the placenta from a mother whose infection is in the primary, secondary, or early latent stage. The condition may become clinically apparent in utero, at birth, shortly after birth, or between late childhood and middle adolescence (7 to 17 years of age).

Typically, the ophthalmologist is consulted in late childhood because of binocular interstitial keratitis that is invariably associated with anterior uveitis. Before penicillin was available, the ocular inflammation lasted for months. Superficial and deep corneal neovascularization may develop but ultimately resolves, leaving the characteristic sheath of translucent scar tissue immediately anterior to Descemet's membrane. A network of relatively clear, branching, linear canals may weave through the opalescent scar as a hallmark of the inflammatory process. After adolescence, the scarred, irregularly thinned corneas with interstitial keratitis typically remain quiescent.

The anterior chamber activity usually damages the chamber angle sufficiently so that secondary glaucoma frequently appears many years later in a quiet eye. The onset of inner ear inflammation, resulting in bilateral deafness, may occur at this time, although it more typically presents later in adolescence or even 3 decades later.

Also appearing in these late periods are chorioretinitis, retinal periphlebitis, or posterior uveitis, which is sometimes associated with anterior uveitis. The residua seen in the inner eye are the "pepper-and-salt" fundus or the typical "bone corpuscular" pigmented and atrophic areas in the midperiphery with ring scotomata mimicking retinitis pigmentosa. Optic atrophy is also seen in congenital syphilis.

Only very early congenital syphilis (intrauterine through 10 weeks postpartum) is infectious. The cases of interstitial keratitis in children and adults that are usually seen by the ophthalmologist are not considered to be infectious.

THERAPY

Systemic. Penicillin is the drug of choice because it is considered effective and incurs no risk

14 / CONGENITAL SYPHILIS

to the fetus. However, detection of many cases of congenital syphilis is difficult because the infant may be asymptomatic and serologically nonreactive to nontreponemal tests. Unless the mother's serology is monitored throughout gestation, syphilis contracted by the mother during pregnancy may remain undetected and therefore untreated. Discovery of the condition in the mother and appropriate treatment of the infected mother are the best preventive measures.

Both symptomatic and asymptomatic infants with congenital syphilis are treated as having neurosyphilis, regardless of cerebrospinal fluid (CSF) serology. A daily dosage of 50,000 units/kg of aqueous potassium penicillin G may be administered intramuscularly or intravenously in two divided doses for at least 10 days. Alternatively, 50,000 units/kg of aqueous procaine penicillin G may be administered daily in intramuscular injections for at least 10 days. However, even with such a rigorous regimen, congenital ocular or neurosyphilis may not be successfully treated. There are no published reports of the use of ampicillin-probenecid combinations in children born with clinically apparent congenital syphilis.

For patients who demonstrate a definite penicillin allergy, 30 to 50 mg/kg of erythromycin or 30 to 40 mg/kg of tetracycline daily may be used in four divided oral doses for 15 days. Tetracycline should not be used in children under 8 years of age. However, successful treatment of congenital syphilis with antibiotics other than aqueous potassium penicillin G or aqueous procaine penicillin G has not been verified.

Children with acute interstitial keratitis secondary to congenital syphilis may require systemic medication in addition to local treatment. Although use of 1.5 gm of oral ampicillin in combination with 500 mg of oral probenecid‡ every 6 hours for 30 days is suggested for adults and older children, the efficacy of such concurrent or antecedent treatment has not been documented. Because of interference with absorption by food, oral ampicillin should be given 1 hour before or 2 hours after meals.

Ocular. Topical ophthalmic corticosteroids and cycloplegics may also be useful in relieving the symptomatology of the acute inflammatory interstitial keratitis. Subconjunctival steroids* are occasionally administered when there has been no dramatic clinical response within a week.

Surgical. Keratoplasty may be required if the interstitial keratitis results in a severe corneal opacity in adult life. Experimentally, it has been shown that spiral organisms that take on fluorescent antibody markers in the aqueous humor are frequently found in such cases. Practically speaking, a history of syphilis and/or a positive FTA-ABA (fluorescent treponemal antibody-absorption) test is an indication for treatment. When patients with a quiescent, old interstitial keratitis undergo penetrating keratoplasty, there frequently occurs a more inflammatory, postoperative intracameral reaction, which requires more frequent and higher doses of topical, subconjunctival, and systemic steroids.

PRECAUTIONS

The loss of the fetus as the result of "placental shock," which may be part of the Jarish-Herxheimer reaction in the mother, is often mentioned but poorly documented in regard to the treatment of the pregnant woman with syphilis. Its possible occurrence does not warrant withholding or modifying treatment. Nor is the modification of treatment of the mother warranted for fear that the fetus will be adversely affected by large doses of penicillin. There is no evidence that this can occur.

The question of whether the mother of a congenitally luetic child should be *retreated* in a subsequent pregnancy has been hotly debated in the past. A reasonable approach is to retreat only if reinfection or previous inadequate treatment is suspected.

Because the tetracyclines affect dental pigmentation in children less than 8 years old, they should be withheld in this age group.

COMMENTS

The best treatment for congenital syphilis is its prevention through the adequate treatment of syphilis during pregnancy. Pregnancies should be followed with serologic testing, since syphilis may be subclinical and nonetheless still affect the fetus. Where there is serologic conversion of the mother, treatment of the pregnant mother is indicated if adequate treatment of the child is not assured. Children of such mothers should be treated if symptomatic or serologically positive and closely followed if serologically negative.

The treatment of the ocular manifestations of congenital syphilis in older children and adults should be guided by the knowledge that the usual regimen for treating syphilis may not be adequate. There is no evidence that the progression of disease is affected when optic atrophy, pupillary abnormalities, or constriction of visual fields are recognized and treated with any single antibiotic or combination of medications or any other treatment.

References

Budell JW: Treatment of congenital syphilis. J Am Vener Dis Assoc 3:168–171, 1976.

Collart P, et al: Significance of spiral organisms found, after treatment, in late human and experimental syphilis. Br J Vener Dis 40:81–89, 1964.

Duke-Elder S (ed): System of Ophthalmology. St. Louis, CV Mosby, 1965, Vol. VIII, pp. 815–832.

Goldman JN: Clinical experience with ampicillin and probenecid in the management of treponeme-associated uveitis. Trans Am Acad Ophthalmol Otolaryngol 74:509–514, 1970.

Goldman JN, Girard KF: Intraocular treponemes in treated congenital syphilis. Arch Ophthalmol 78:47–50, 1967.

Goldman JN, Klein JO: Penetration of ampicillin and penicillin G into the aqueous humor. Ann Ophthalmol 2:35–42, 1970.
Smith JL, Israel CW: Spirochetes in the aqueous humor is seronegative ocular syphilis. Persistence after penicillin therapy. Arch Ophthalmol 77:474–477, 1967.
Smith JL, Israel CW: The presence of spirochetes in late seronegative syphilis. JAMA *199*:126–130, 1967.
Thompson SE III: Treatment of syphilis in pregnancy. J Am Vener Dis Assoc 3:159–167, 1976.

DIPHTHERIA

LAURENCE S. BRAUDE, M.D., F.A.C.S., F.A.C.S.(C)
Chicago, Illinois
and JOHN W. CHANDLER, M.D.
Madison, Wisconsin

Diphtheria is an acute infectious disease caused by *Corynebacterium diphtheriae*, a gram-positive, club-shaped organism. Only those strains that are latently infected by a bacterial virus, diphtheria phage B, produce exotoxin and are capable of producing diphtheria. The toxin is responsible for the most common systemic complications of diphtheria affecting the heart and nervous system. Cranial nerve involvement can include the third, fourth, and sixth nerves. *C. diphtheriae* is essentially a surface saprophyte, most commonly affecting the nasopharyngeal area. Cutaneous diphtheria seems to be more frequently associated with external ocular involvement. External ocular disease includes tender, red, swollen eyelids; membranous or pseudomembranous conjunctivitis; and corneal ulcers and perforation.

THERAPY

Systemic. In addition to topical therapy, 10,000 to 100,000 units of diphtheria antitoxin are also given systemically after appropriate testing for sensitivity has been done. This total dose should be given at one time, rather than in split doses over a long period. For doses less than 20,000 units, the intramuscular route is convenient. When this method is used, only one-half of the dose should be given intramuscularly and the remainder intravenously. Alternatively, the entire amount of antitoxin may be given intravenously in 100 or 200 ml of isotonic saline over 30 minutes.

Antibiotics are believed to have little effect on the clinical course of diphtheria involving the respiratory tract, but they may be of benefit in terminating the toxin production. Antibiotic therapy is of value because this infection is typically mixed with other bacteria, including staphylococci and pneumococci, and many other organisms. In the very severe cases, streptococci are often present, and there is evidence that tissue damage is due to the mixed infection, rather than to the diphtheria bacillus toxin alone. Additional benefits of antibiotics are hastening clearance of the carrier state and prevention of spread of the organism to others.

Penicillin is the drug of choice. Intramuscular administration of 600,000 units of procaine penicillin G twice daily for 7 to 16 days is usually adequate. Oral penicillin V may be substituted after the third day in patients with uncomplicated infections. Intravenous penicillin G in a daily dose of 4 to 6 million units divided into four doses may be used with intravenous solutions. In patients allergic to penicillin, intravenous erythromycin may be used in a daily dose of 25 to 50 mg/kg for 10 to 14 days. It should be noted that erythromycin resistance has been seen in some recent outbreaks. In addition, *C. diphtheriae* is frequently resistant to cephalexin, colistin, lincomycin, and oxacillin. The organism is usually sensitive to ampicillin, clindamycin, tetracycline, and rifampin. Regardless of the antibiotic, therapy should be continued for at least 7 days.

Steroids have been used to prevent or ameliorate myocarditis, but Harnisch feels corticosteroids or corticotrophins are not of value in the treatment of diphtheria or any of its complications.

Ocular. If there is clinical suspicion that the disease is due to *C. diphtheriae*, therapy should be instituted immediately and not withheld until laboratory confirmation is obtained, because the severity of the disease is dependent upon the amount of exotoxin absorbed prior to initiation of specific therapy. Treatment of external ocular diphtheria has two goals: neutralization of toxin and eradication of live organisms.

Since the diphtheria toxins irreversibly bind to tissue, antitoxin is effective only against circulatory toxins: once the clinical manifestations of the toxins appear, they cannot be reversed by antitoxin administration. Antitoxin treatment thus blocks only circulating toxins and toxins still to be formed. There are several regimens for the topical and systemic administration of antitoxin, and the amount given is often based on an empiric decision. In general, the more severe the disease or the more extensive the membrane formation, the greater is the amount of antitoxin required.

After giving a test dose to rule out anaphylactic reactions, 10,000 to 100,000 units of diphtheria antitoxin* are topically applied to the involved eye every 4 to 6 hours for 24 to 48 hours. Diphtheria antitoxin* may also be considered for subconjunctival injection as an alternative to topical application.

Commercially available immune and hyperimmune globulin preparations have low diphtheria antitoxin titers and are not useful. However, there is an investigational preparation that may be useful in special circumstances. It consists of a high-titer gamma globulin preparation[‡] made from the blood of persons with high titers of antitoxin. It was intended for use in prophylaxis, but should be considered for treatment of markedly allergic individuals. It may be given solely to persons who are allergic to horse serum. It is obtainable from the Communicable Disease Division, State Department of Public Health, Lansing, Michigan. The dose for treatment has not been established. This preparation should never be given intravenously.

Antibiotics are not effective against the toxin, but are indicated for the eradication of the bacilli and superinfections. Repeated instillations of 1000 units/gm of sodium penicillin G or 0.5 per cent erythromycin ointment are administered in addition to systemic antibiotics.

If the disease involves the eyelid skin, cutaneous diphtheria responds well to local application of compresses soaked in penicillin solution (250 to 500 units/ml) and intramuscular injection of 20,000 units of diphtheria antitoxin. A canthotomy should not be done to facilitate opening the lids; since the raw wound invariably becomes infected, the canthotomy actually increases the area of toxin absorption.

The diphtheria membrane usually sloughs away spontaneously during convalescence. Membranes should not be peeled off, as this leaves a raw, bleeding surface and hastens absorption of toxin. With this caveat, a glass rod or cotton-tipped applicator may be used intermittently to break early symblepharon formation in the fornices.

Supportive. Patients with diphtheria should be isolated and hospitalized. Bedrest is important for 3 weeks because of the frequency of myocardial involvement. Aspirin and codeine may be indicated for relief of pain.

Ocular or Periocular Manifestations

Conjunctiva: Catarrhal, membranous, pseudomembranous, or purulent conjunctivitis; hyperemia; petechiae, symblepharon; xerophthalmia.
Cornea: Keratitis; perforation; ulcer.
Extraocular Muscles: Accommodative spasm or paralysis; convergence paralysis; divergence paralysis; paralysis of third, fourth, or sixth nerve.
Eyelids: Blepharitis; cellulitis; cicatrization; edema; entropion; meibomianitis; necrosis; ptosis; trichiasis.
Lacrimal System: Dacryoadenitis; dacryocystitis.
Other: Cataract; central retinal artery occlusion; optic neuritis; preauricular lymphadenopathy.

Precautions

Before antitoxin administration, tests for hypersensitivity to horse serum are mandatory. If the patient is allergic to horse serum, antitoxin may be administered following desensitization, or if available, human diphtheria immune globulin may be substituted. Rarely, a patient may exhibit such marked hypersensitivity that antiserum cannot be administered without the risk of death. The heart rate of all patients should be carefully monitored during administration of diphtheria antitoxin because anaphylaxis may occur. In addition, all diphtheria patients should receive careful cardiac monitoring for developing myocarditis. Drugs with depressant effects on the heart must be used with extreme caution in diphtheria patients.

Patients with diphtheria should be quarantined until two successive cultures of the eye, skin, or other infected areas, taken at 24-hours intervals, are negative. If antibiotics have been given, cultural studies should not be initiated until at least 24 hours after cessation of therapy.

Comments

Approximately 200 cases of nonocular diphtheria are reported annually in the United States. The newborn is usually protected by transplacental globulin from the mother, although a few nonocular severe infections in newborns have been reported. Healthy carriers of the organisms, who are themselves not susceptible, are a source of infection to others, but this means of spreading diphtheria has become less important in populations with widespread immunization. However, recent outbreaks of diphtheria in the United States have involved groups of individuals without adequate immunization histories. The disease may be seen in fully immunized persons, in whom it is usually mild and rarely fatal. Death is most frequent in the very young and elderly. As a rule, the longer the delay in the administration of antitoxin, the greater the incidence of complications and death.

References

Chandler JW, Milam DF: Diphtheria corneal ulcers. Arch Ophthalmol 96:53–56, 1978.
Duke-Elder S (ed): System of Ophthalmology. St. Louis, CV Mosby, 1976, Vol. XV, p 46.
Eller JJ: Diphtheria. *In* Conn HF (ed): Current Therapy. Philadelphia, WB Saunders, 1982, pp 15–19.
Harnisch JP: Diphtheria. *In* Isselbacher KJ, et al (eds): Harrison's Principles of Internal Medicine, 9th ed. New York, McGraw-Hill, 1980, pp 671–675.
Rogell G: Infectious and inflammatory diseases. *In* Duane TD (ed): Clinical Ophthalmology. Hagerstown, MD, Harper & Row, 1982, Vol. V, pp 33:9–10.
Shaw EB: Diphtheria. *In* Conn HF, Conn RB Jr (eds): Current Diagnosis 6. Philadelphia, WB Saunders, 1980, pp 167–170.
Top FH, Wehrle PF: Diphtheria. *In* Wehrle PF, Top FH Sr (eds): Communicable and Infectious Diseases, 9th ed. St. Louis, CV Mosby, 1981, pp 197–210.

ERYSIPELAS
(St. Anthony's Fire)

RICHARD L. ABBOTT, M.D.
San Francisco, California

Erysipelas is an acute, localized inflammation of the skin and subcutaneous tissue, characterized by redness, edema, and induration. The pathogenic organisms are usually group A beta-hemolytic streptococci, although an occasional group C strain has been identified. The site of infection is usually the face or extremities. The primary facial infection is often a nasopharyngitis from which the organism is transferred to the skin through an abrasion or a minute wound.

Erysipelas may begin with an abrupt onset of fever and rigor. A definite zone of redness soon appears, with edema, tenderness, and a well-defined, advancing border. In the more severe cases, vesicles may form on the surface. Typically, the infection involves the lymphatic spaces and is spread through these channels to neighboring areas. Constitutional symptoms include high temperature, headache, vomiting, and localized pain. Without treatment, the disease is usually self-limited and runs its course in 4 days to several weeks. As the facial lesions spread, ocular involvement consisting of marked edema and erythema of the lids often occurs. The edema is frequently extensive enough to prevent opening of the eyes. The disease may also progress to gangrene of the eyelids. Although less common, inflammation spreads from the lids to the conjunctiva, producing chemosis and external ophthalmoplegia. Other complications include dacryoadenitis, orbital thrombophlebitis, cellulitis, abscess, and cavernous sinus thrombosis. A late result in chronic infections may be a solid edema or elephantiasis of the eyelids.

THERAPY

Systemic. Penicillin G is the drug of choice in treating erysipelas. Treatment should be instituted promptly and continued for 10 to 14 days to prevent the possibility of systemic spread. Intravenous penicillin G should be given in a minimum divided daily dosage of 6 million units. Once there is evidence of clinical improvement, the route of administration can be changed to oral medication. Potassium penicillin V should be given daily in four divided doses of 250 mg for the duration of the 10- to 14-day therapy period.

In patients sensitive to penicillin, erythromycin may be substituted. Erythromycin may be given orally in an initial dosage of 500 mg four times daily for several days and then reduced to 250 mg four times daily for 10 days. In severely ill patients, 500 mg of the drug should be given intravenously twice a day for the first 2 or 3 days before oral therapy is begun.

Ocular. In severe cases resulting in tissue destruction and lid necrosis, meticulous cleaning and débridement of the wounds on a daily basis should be the mainstay of local therapy. The wounds are surgically débrided and cleansed with a 1 : 1 solution of hydrogen peroxide and sterile saline and repacked daily with iodoform gauze. The use of warm saline compresses and topical broad-spectrum antibiotic ointments helps accelerate the healing process and may prevent secondary bacterial contamination. The application of topical erythromycin ointment within the cul-de-sac helps prevent the occurrence of a secondary bacterial conjunctivitis.

If there is a significant degree of lid contracture in the healing process, exposure keratitis may develop. This condition is best treated initially with tear substitutes and lubricating ointments. Surgical repair of a cicatricial ectropion or other lid deformities may be required. It is prudent, however, to wait a minimum of 3 to 6 months before considering surgical intervention to allow the healing process to stabilize and reduce the likelihood of an under- or over-correction.

Supportive. Attention should be given to the patient's physical, nutritional, emotional, and diversional activity needs. Hospitalization is usually indicated, with the patient on bedrest. The patient should be isolated until fever subsides, and strict hygienic measures should be employed by all hospital personnel who have contact with an infected patient. Alcohol and tepid sponge baths may be used to reduce high temperature. Aspirin with codeine may be needed for pain. Diet should be light with a high fluid intake. Vital signs should be monitored regularly.

Ocular or Periocular Manifestations

Conjunctiva: Chemosis; exudative or membranous conjunctivitis.

Cornea: Superficial punctate keratitis secondary to bacterial toxins or exposure with lid ectropion (late); ulcerative keratitis.

Eyelids: Abscess; blepharitis; ectropion; elephantiasis; erythema; gangrene; madarosis; marked edema; necrosis; trichiasis.

Iris: Iridocyclitis.

Lacrimal System: Dacryoadenitis; dacryocystitis.

Orbit: Abscess; cellulitis; thrombophlebitis.

Vitreous or Retina: Chorioretinitis; metastatic vitreous abscess.

PRECAUTIONS

Because erysipelas usually begins abruptly and may progress rapidly, appropriate antimicrobial therapy must be instituted as soon as possible. The diagnosis may be made on the basis of the clinical presentation of the illness and intravenous penicillin G or its substitute started immediately. Regardless of which drug is used, it is

18 / ERYSIPELAS

essential that treatment in full doses be given over a period of at least 10 days because relapses are relatively common.

Cultures and sensitivities should be obtained for confirmation of the diagnosis only if there is exudate readily available for these studies. Needle aspiration from the lids or orbit is contraindicated in patients with erysipelas because of the possibility of spread of the infection and injury to other structures.

The differential diagnosis must include ophthalmic herpes zoster, allergic contact dermatitis, myositis of collagen diseases, trichinosis, and angioneurotic edema.

COMMENTS

The erysipelas exanthem most frequently appears in the region of the eye, with the sites of predilection being the eyelid and the inner canthus. The pathophysiology of lid necrosis seems to be related to the release of proteolytic enzymes by the streptococcal organisms, which dissolve connective tissue bridges and allow rapid spread of the bacteria. Because the skin of the lid is so thin, large amounts of fluid can accumulate, thereby raising the tissue pressure and shutting off capillary circulation. Thus, the combination of diffuse bacterial spread and diminished blood supply leads to destruction and necrosis of the lid tissue.

For treatment to be effective, one must make an early diagnosis and institute maximum parenteral antibiotic therapy combined with local débridement and topical antibiotic application. It is recommended that this therapy be continued for a minimum of 10 to 14 days until all evidence of the infection has resolved. Long-term therapy consists of lid plastic surgery after all healing processes have stabilized.

References

Abbott RL, Shekter WB: Necrotizing erysipelas of the eyelids. Ann Ophthalmol 11:381–384, 1979.
Bellows J: Ocular complications of erysipelas. Arch Ophthalmol 11:678–683, 1934.
Bellows JG: Acute bacterial infections. In Sorsby A (ed): Modern Ophthalmology, 2nd ed. Philadelphia, JB Lippincott, 1972, Vol 2, pp 90–91.
Scott PM, Bloome MA: Lid necrosis secondary to streptococcal periorbital cellulitis. Ann Ophthalmol 13:461–465, 1981.
Stewart WD, Danto JL, Maddin S: Dermatology: Diagnosis and Treatment of Cutaneous Disorders, 3rd ed. St. Louis, CV Mosby, 1974, p 218.

ESCHERICHIA COLI
H. JOHN SHAMMAS, M.D.
Los Angeles, California

Escherichia coli is a gram-negative rod found as a normal commensal in the gastrointestinal tract from which it may spread to infect contiguous structures when normal anatomic barriers are interrupted. This bacillus can also be found in association with other pathogenic organisms in perforated or inflamed conditions. The urinary tract is the usual portal of entry; however, once infection has occurred in a primary focus, further spread to distant organs may occur by means of the bloodstream. Septicemia is the most serious complication of *E. coli* infections. It occurs frequently in debilitated elderly patients with diabetes mellitus, in patients with urinary tract infection or biliary or intraperitoneal sepsis, and following abortions or pelvic surgery. Enterotoxigenic *E. coli* may cause a gastroenteritis, most commonly in children under 2 years of age.

Ocular involvement is rare and may result in a mucopurulent conjunctivitis. Metastatic endophthalmitis may occur from *E. coli* septicemia, and the usual portal of entry is the central retinal artery. The course of the endophthalmitis is acute; necrosis of the intraocular tissues and loss of vision can occur in less than 24 hours.

THERAPY

Systemic. Choice of an appropriate antimicrobial in *E. coli* infections depends upon the site and type of infection, as well as its severity. A number of antibiotics are effective against the bacillus, but no particular drug is uniformly active against all strains of *E. coli*, so sensitivity testing should guide the choice of antibiotics.

For less severe *E. coli* infections, the initial treatment of choice may be 2 to 4 gm of ampicillin a day administered intramuscularly or intravenously. For more severe infections, the dose could be 6 to 12 gm daily.

Kanamycin is generally indicated for the initial treatment of serious *E. coli* infections. Severe urinary tract infections that seem to be resistant to other antimicrobials have responded to daily doses of 15 mg/kg of kanamycin intramuscularly in divided doses every 6 to 8 hours.

Alternative treatment may be with 3 to 5 mg/kg of parenteral gentamicin, administered in divided doses every 8 hours. In severe infections that appear to be resistant to kanamycin and gentamicin, amikacin is indicated. Amikacin is given in daily doses of 15 mg/kg in two or three equally divided doses.

Neomycin appears to be most effective against *E. coli* gastroenteritis. An oral daily dosage of 25 mg/kg is usually indicated for 1 or 2 days.

Ocular. In *E. coli* conjunctivitis, 0.5 per cent chloramphenicol, 0.3 per cent gentamicin, or 0.3 per cent tobramycin solutions are applied topically every 4 hours until the infection appears to be resolved.

Early systemic and local antibiotic therapy is essential for E. coli endophthalmitis. Blanket local antibiotic therapy should consist of 20 mg of subconjunctival gentamicin,* 0.3 per cent gentamicin or tobramycin, and 0.5 percent chloramphenicol solutions every 2 hours. In very severe cases, intravitreal injection of 100 to 300 µg of gentamicin* can be used.

Steroids administered in combination with antibiotics may reduce the massive inflammatory response of the eye, which is often as destructive as the infection. Two mg of dexamethasone* may be injected subconjunctivally and repeated when necessary.

Secondary involvement of the uveal tract may necessitate use of a cycloplegic/mydriatic. One per cent cyclopentolate drops may be applied topically twice daily to aid in the relief of uveitis.

Supportive. Hospitalization is necessary for more severe forms of E. coli infection. Infants with E. coli gastroenteritis should be isolated and monitored carefully; fluid and electrolyte levels must be maintained, since dehydration can occur rapidly in these patients.

Surgical. Subcutaneous infections are not uncommon in debilitated patients. Drainage of pus and removal of foreign bodies may be necessary.

Ocular or Periocular Manifestations

Anterior Chamber: Cells and flare; gas bubbles; hyphema; hypopyon.
Conjunctiva: Chemosis; hyperemia, pseudomembranous or purulent conjunctivitis.
Cornea: Edema; keratitis; ulcers.
Globe: Panophthalmitis; purulent endophthalmitis.
Other: Increased intraocular pressure; ocular pain; uveitis; visual loss.

PRECAUTIONS

It is advisable to check the serum levels of the aminoglycosides to ensure therapeutic levels and avoid toxicity, since the therapeutic to toxic ratio is very narrow. Monitoring of renal and eighth nerve functions is recommended during therapy with these drugs, particularly for patients with reduced renal function. Concurrent and/or sequential systemic use of potentially neurotoxic or nephrotoxic drugs should be avoided. Cephalosporins, tetracyclines, chloramphenicol, and polymyxin B are still widely used in the treatment of E. coli infections; however, more effective drugs are available.

Isolation and antimicrobial therapy of contacts are essential to abort epidemic infantile diarrhea. Many E. coli infections are hospital acquired, so strict hygienic measures are essential.

COMMENTS

E. coli is rarely found in the normal flora of the conjunctiva. It is most commonly seen as a source of infection in ophthalmia neonatorum. E. coli endophthalmitis is a rare complication of E. coli septicemia. It has a poor prognosis, and early diagnosis and treatment are essential if useful vision is to be retained.

References

Aronson SB, Elliott JH: Ocular Inflammation. St. Louis, CV Mosby, 1972, pp 103–105, 112–114, 228–230.
Asbell P, Stenson S: Ulcerative keratitis, survey of 30 years laboratory experience. Arch Ophthalmol 100:77–83, 1982.
Baum JL: Initial therapy of suspected microbial corneal ulcers. I. Broad antibiotic therapy based on prevalence of organisms. Surv Ophthalmol 24:97–116, 1979.
Jones DB: Initial therapy of suspected microbial corneal ulcers. II. Specific antibiotic therapy based on corneal smears. Surv Ophthalmol 24:97–116, 1979.
Jones DB: Decision making in the management of microbial keratitis. Ophthalmology 88: 814–820, 1981.
Krachmer JH, Purcell JJ Jr: Bacterial corneal ulcers in cosmetic soft contact lens wearers. Arch Ophthalmol 96:57–61, 1978.
Lissner GS, Romano PE: Pneumatosis oculi and spontaneous hyphema in association with pneumatosis intestinalis. Am J Ophthalmol 88:708–713, 1979.
Shammas HF: Endogenous E. coli endophthalmitis. Surv Ophthalmol 21:429–435, 1977.
Turck M, Schaberg D: Infections due to enterobacteriaceae. In Isselbacher KJ, et al. (eds): Harrison's Principles of Internal Medicine, 9th ed. New York, McGraw-Hill, 1980, pp 629–634.

FUSOBACTERIUM
RICHARD J. WEINBERG, M.D.
Washington, District of Columbia

Fusobacterium is a gram-negative, non-spore forming, anaerobic bacillus that is a normal inhabitant of the mouth and respiratory, intestinal, and urogenital tracts. Infection is usually secondary to an underlying disease, surgical procedure, or therapy that impairs the normal defense of the host. *Fusobacterium* infection of the skin may also occur following animal or human bites. It is often found in association with spirochetes. The clinical manifestations of *Fusobacterium* infections include tissue necrosis, abscess formation, and septic thrombophlebitis, as well as foul odor and gas in tissue or discharges. *Fusobacterium* infections may cause abscess formation in the brain, lung, liver, or intra-abdominal area; empyema; and necrotizing pneumonia. Ocular manifestations in the more acute cases may include a purulent conjunctivitis, but ulcerative and even gangrenous manifestations may also occur. Acute or chronic infection in the lacrimal system may be present as dacryocystitis or suppurative canaliculitis. Rarely, cellulitis, tenonitis, or metastatic panophthalmitis may also occur in *Fusobacterium* infections. Corneal ulceration is possibly associated with, but is usually secondary to combined infections.

THERAPY

Systemic. Antimicrobial therapy may be indicated in *Fusobacterium* infections involving

20 / FUSOBACTERIUM

vital organs or when systemic manifestations are present. Chloramphenicol and clindamycin are the antibiotics of choice; however, chloramphenicol is preferred for patients with infections of the central nervous system because clindamycin does not effectively penetrate the blood-brain barrier. Both antibiotics can be administered orally, but parenteral therapy is advisable for patients with severe infection. Chloramphenicol should be administered parenterally or orally in a daily dose of 50 mg/kg divided into four equal portions, and parenteral clindamycin should be administered in a daily dose of 0.6 to 2.7 gm divided into two to four equal doses. The oral adult dosage for clindamycin is 150 to 450 mg every 6 hours.

Penicillin is also active against most anaerobes other than *Bacteroides fragilis* and occasional strains of *Fusobacterium varium*. The dosage of penicillin G should be at least 6 to 8 million units daily in seriously ill patients or in infections with relatively resistant strains. Ampicillin and cephaloridine are usually comparable to penicillin G, but several other penicillins and cephalosporins are less active. Fusobacteria are generally resistant to the aminoglycosides.

Ocular. Topical antibiotic therapy may be necessary in ocular *Fusobacterium* infections. Topical penicillin G ointment in a concentration of 1000 units/gm may be used every 3 hours. One per cent chlortetracycline ointment or 10 or 15 per cent sulfacetamide drops may also be used several times daily for conjunctivitis or canaliculitis. In canaliculitis, however, a definitive cure may not be effected until all concretions that may be present are removed either by surgery or mechanical expression.

Supportive. In *Fusobacterium* infections, anticoagulant therapy and venous ligation should be considered in patients with thrombophlebitis and multiple septic pulmonary infarctions. If shock or disseminated intravascular coagulation occurs, general supportive measures are important aspects of therapy.

Surgical. Drainage of abscess cavities or local suppurative lesions is of prime importance in the management of patients with *Fusobacterium* infections. The perforation should be closed promptly and devitalized tissues and foreign bodies removed as soon as possible. This is often all that is required for cure in many patients.

Ocular or Periocular Manifestations

Conjunctiva: Chemosis; follicular or purulent conjunctivitis; gangrene.

Lacrimal System: Canaliculitis; dacryocystitis.

Orbit: Abscess; cellulitis; fistula.

Other: Corneal ulcer(?); extraocular muscle tenonitis; eyelid edema; panophthalmitis.

PRECAUTIONS

Since most strains of *Fusobacterium* are highly sensitive to penicillin, chloramphenicol,

tetracycline, and clindamycin, susceptibility tests generally serve as a good guide to drug therapy. However, chloramphenicol or clindamycin therapy should be administered with care, since both drugs may cause serious adverse drug-related effects. Chloramphenicol may cause nausea and vomiting, and serious, even fatal blood dyscrasias may occur. Likewise, clindamycin can cause severe colitis, which may end fatally. Precautions to minimize the possibility of aspiration will also be helpful in preventing anaerobic pulmonary infection.

COMMENTS

Therapy with antimicrobial agents in *Fusobacterium* infections must be intensive and prolonged. These infections have a considerable tendency to relapse. If the diagnosis is suspected early and appropriate therapy instituted promptly, the prognosis for recovery is good. The prognosis will vary with the site and extent of lesion; a high mortality may occur in patients with brain abscess, necrotizing pneumonia, liver abscess, endocarditis, or sepsis. Gram-stained specimens may be confused with *Actinomyces* because of similar morphology and variable gram-staining characteristics.

References

Bowers BT, Simmons JR: Surgical management of diverticulum of the canaliculus. Arch Ophthalmol 83:61–62, 1970.

Burns RP, et al: Unilateral conjunctivitis and canaliculitis due to Fusospirochetal infection. Arch Ophthalmol 59:235–242, 1958.

Finegold SM: Disease due to non-spore-forming anaerobic bacteria. *In* Wyngaarden JB, Smith LH Jr (eds): Textbook of Medicine, 16th ed. Philadelphia, WB Saunders, 1982, pp 1503–1507.

Lin RG, Arcala AE: Fusobacterium septicemia with otitis media and mastoiditis. Postgrad Med 57:159–160, 1975.

Ormerod D, et al: Anaerobic bacterial endophthalmitis in the rabbit. Invest Ophthalmol 27:115–117, 1986.

Weinberg RJ, et al: Fusobacterium in presumed *Actinomyces* canaliculitis. Am J Ophthalmol 84:371–374, 1977.

GONOCOCCAL OCULAR DISEASE

JEFFREY B. ROBIN, M.D.

Chicago, Illinois

Gonorrhea is one of the oldest described infectious diseases affecting humans. Caused by the gram-negative diplococcus, *Neisseria gonorrhoeae*, gonorrhea is a major cause of morbidity throughout the world and is presently the most common reportable disease in the United States (over 800,000 reported cases in 1985). The incidence of gonorrhea, once thought to be on the decline, has been steadily rising since 1984. Epidemiologic risk factors for gonorrhea include age, sex, sexual preference, race, socioeconomic status, marital status, and accessibility to health care. The spread of gonorrhea is difficult to control because the main vector for the disease is the asymptomatic carrier.

Gonorrhea primarily affects two patient populations: young, sexually active adults and neonates born to infected mothers. In fact, *N. gonorrhoeae* was, until recently, the major cause of ophthalmia neonatorum. Unlike the adult population, the incidence of gonococcal infections in newborns has been markedly decreasing; this is believed to be the result of more widespread antenatal screening and the use of prophylactic antibiotics.

The gonococcal organism, first identified by Neisser in 1879, primarily attacks mucosal epithelium. Gonorrhea is relatively easy to diagnose, given the characteristic appearance of gram-negative diplococci, many of which can be found inside epithelial and leukocytic cells. The introduction of specific culture medium for *Neisseriae*, developed in 1964 by Thayer and Martin, has further facilitated laboratory diagnosis. Differentiation from *N. meningitidis* is accomplished on the basis of sugar fermentation reactions.

Gonorrhea is a potentially multisystem disease, affecting not only the genitourinary tract but also the joints, skin, pharynx, meninges, heart, liver, and eye. Extragenitourinary involvement may occur via hematogenous spread or direct inoculation. Ocular involvement in adults is usually the result of direct hand-eye inoculation; cases have also occurred from laboratory contamination and from the use of urine as a folk-remedy eye wash. Additionally, rare cases of gonococcal conjunctivitis have been associated with direct hematogenous spread from the genitourinary tract. Gonococcal ophthalmia neonatorum is nearly always caused by direct inoculation of the neonate's eyes during passage through an infected birth canal. Ocular involvement in both adults and neonates is characterized by an acute, copiously purulent conjunctivitis. Involvement may start unilaterally, but may eventually involve both eyes. The *N. gonorrheae* organism is one of the few bacteria that is capable of penetrating the intact corneal epithelium. Therefore, corneal ulcerations, abscesses, and perforations commonly occur in untreated gonococcal ocular infections.

The history of gonorrhea therapy has been marked by landmark discoveries and by the ongoing development of antibacterial resistance. Credé, in 1881, introduced silver nitrate for the prophylaxis of gonococcal ophthalmia neonatorum, thereby rapidly reducing the incidence of this neonatal infection. Sulfonamides, introduced in 1939, were the first agents identified to treat established gonococcal infections successfully. Resistance rapidly developed to sulfonamides, however, and penicillin became the drug of choice. Recently, beta-lactamase-producing gonococci, resistant to both penicillin and ampicillin, have become worldwide in distribution. These penicillinase-producing strains of *N. gonorrheae* (PPNG) have become predominant in several areas of the world, including several cities in the United States. Additionally, some strains of *N. gonorrheae* have chromosomally mediated resistance to penicillin and tetracycline; these chromosomally resistant *N. gonorrheae* (CMRNG) strains can be quite difficult to treat. The continued development of antimicrobial resistance by this organism has forced an ongoing evaluation of treatment regimens.

THERAPY

Systemic. The mainstay of systemic therapy for gonorrhea has been the use of parenteral antibiotics, most commonly penicillin. However, because of the continuing development of antimicrobial resistance, the treatment of gonorrhea has recently been re-evaluated. In 1985, for the treatment of gonococcal ophthalmia in adults, the Centers for Disease Control (CDC) recommended 10 million units of aqueous penicillin G daily administered intravenously for 5 days. All penicillin regimens were accompanied by oral probenecid (1.0 gm), an agent that reduces penicillin secretion by renal tubules and thus increases plasma concentration of the antibiotic. Since 1985, this regimen has been shown in multiple studies to be effective for the treatment of penicillin-sensitive gonococcal keratoconjunctivitis. For those cases involving documented PPNG strains, the CDC recommended the use of "third-generation" cephalosporins, such as 500 mg of intravenous cefotaxime four times daily for 5 days or 1.0 gm of ceftriaxone intramuscularly or intravenously for 5 days.

For gonococcal ophthalmia neonatorum, the CDC in 1985 recommended 100,000 units/kg of intravenous aqueous penicillin G daily in four divided doses for 7 days. For PPNG infections, intravenous administration of cefotaxime or gentamicin is used in appropriate neonatal doses. As with adults, effective treatment of gonococcal ophthalmia in neonates has been recently achieved with single-dose ceftriaxone therapy.

Recently, gonococcal conjunctivitis without keratitis has been successfully treated with a single-dose regimen of intramuscular antibiotics on an outpatient basis. Of course, an assessment of the patient's capability for follow-up and compliance is an essential component in making the decision for outpatient therapy. Many studies have effectively used single-dose ceftriaxone for the treatment of adult gonococcal ophthalmia involving both PPNG and non-PPNG strains.

Based on the above recommendations and recent trends, the following systemic treatment regimen is recommended. For uncomplicated gonococcal conjunctivitis, a single dose of 1.0 gm of intramuscular ceftriaxone together with a 7-day oral course of tetracycline (250 mg four times daily) or doxycycline (100 mg twice daily) is an effective combination to treat both gonococcal and chlamydial infections. Alternative therapy for those patients with documented penicillin allergy should involve spectinomycin 2.0 gm in one intramuscular dose. In more severe cases, particularly with corneal involvement, the patient should be hospitalized and treated with 1.0 gm of ceftriaxone intravenously two times daily for 3 to 5 days; penicillin-allergic patients should receive 2.0 gm of spectinomycin intramuscularly twice daily over a 3 to 5 day course. For neonatal infections, a single intramuscular dose of 125 mg of ceftriaxone is used. If ceftriaxone is contraindicated, gentamicin should be used intravenously in appropriate pediatric doses.

Ocular. Topical antimicrobial agents appear to be ineffective in completely treating gonococcal ophthalmia. They can be used, however, as adjuncts to systemic antibiotics. Topical gentamicin, erythromycin, or bacitracin can be used four times daily. The final choice should be based upon antibiotic sensitivities.

An essential aspect of topical therapy is copious irrigation of the purulent exudate. The gonococcal exudate may contain toxins of live bacteria. It is produced at such a rate that irrigation with 50 ml of sterile saline may be required as often as every hour. Frequent, copious irrigation is especially important for the treatment of gonococcal ophthalmia neonatorum.

Ocular or Periocular Manifestations

Anterior Chamber: Cellular reaction; hypopyon; endophthalmitis.
Conjunctiva: Chemosis; acute purulent exudate; hemorrhages.
Cornea: Punctate epithelial keratitis; marginal, sterile stromal infiltrates; epithelial defects; infectious stromal infiltrates; stromal ulcerations; descemetocele; perforation; opacification.
Eyelids: Erythema; edema.

PRECAUTIONS

The changing face of microbial sensitivity and resistance has forced continual re-evaluation of therapy for gonococcal ophthalmia. Because of the increasing frequency of PPNG infections and also because gonococcal ocular infections can rapidly progress and threaten vision, it is now justifiable to begin appropriate therapy while awaiting the results of antimicrobial sensitivities. It is recommended therefore to avoid agents to which *N. gonorrheae* has demonstrated documented resistance, such as penicillin, erythromycin, ampicillin, and tetracycline) and instead to use a third-generation cephalosporin as the first-line systemic antibiotic. These agents, such as ceftriaxone, have a broad spectrum of sensitivity, are effective against *N. gonorrheae*, do not appear to be affected by beta-lactamase, and appear to be relatively safe. When administered intravenously, ceftriaxone rapidly achieves high blood levels; this therapeutic route appears to be ideal for gonococcal ophthalmia with corneal involvement. Because of the excellent results produced by therapy with third-generation cephalosporins, penicillin allergy should be appropriately documented before using potentially less effective agents, such as spectinomycin.

COMMENTS

Appropriate systemic therapy is the mainstay of treatment for gonococcal ocular infections. In all cases, patients must be evaluated on a daily basis. Complete follow-up examinations, with negative cultures, are essential to confirm treatment efficacy. If follow-up is questionable or if there is corneal involvement, patients should be hospitalized. Additionally, treatment regimens should be supplemented with appropriate patient counseling and education, as well as contact tracing.

Gonococcal ophthalmia is frequently accompanied by other venereally transmitted diseases. All patients therefore should have serologic tests for syphilis. Additionally, because laboratory confirmation of chlamydial infections is difficult, it is reasonable to include anti-chlamydial treatment in the therapeutic regimen, especially in heterosexuals. In most cases, a 7- to 14-day course of oral tetracycline or doxycycline is effective; in tetracycline-allergic patients, neonates, or lactating women, oral erythromycin stearate is an appropriate alternative.

References

Centers for Disease Control: 1985 STD treatment guidelines MMWR 34:81S–90S, 1985.
Centers for Disease Control: Table 1 Summary—Cases specified notable diseases, United States. MMWR 35:810, 1987.
Haase DA, et al: Single-dose therapy of gonococcal ophthalmia neonatorum with ceftriaxone. N Engl J Med 315:1382–1385, 1986.
Judson FN: Treatment of uncomplicated gonorrhea with ceftriaxone: A review. Sex Transm Dis 13:199–202, 1986.
Pareek SS: Conjunctivitis caused by beta-lactamase-producing *Neisseria gonorrhoeae*. Sex Transm Dis 12:159–160, 1985.
Ullman S, Roussel RJ, Forster RK: Gonococcal keratoconjunctivitis. Surv Ophthalmol 32:199–208, 1987.
Wan WL, et al: The clinical characteristics and course of adult gonococcal conjunctivitis. Am J Ophthalmol 102:575–583, 1986.
Zajdowicz TR, et al: Laboratory-acquired gonococcal conjunctivitis: Successful treatment with single-dose ceftriaxone. Sex Transm Dis 11:28–29, 1983.

HEMOPHILUS INFLUENZAE

F.T. FRAUNFELDER, M.D.
Portland, Oregon

Hemophilus influenzae is one of the most important and serious bacterial infections in children; in the United States, it is the leading cause of childhood bacterial meningitis. The most common site of infection for most diseases is the upper respiratory tract. Otitis media, sinusitis, epiglottitus, bronchitis, and pneumonia may occur by contiguous spread from that focus. Type b is the most common strain associated with most *Hemophilus* infections, except in ocular infections when type d is usually identified.

The *Hemophilus* species usually associated with conjunctivitis is the Koch-Weeks bacillus, *H. aegyptius*, which often causes a primary conjunctivitis without other foci of *Hemophilus* infections. Although primary ocular infections with *H. influenzae* have been reported, the eye is usually involved secondarily to systemic bacterial infection with this species. *Hemophilus* types a, b, and d have been cultured from conjunctival inflammations; however, this organism can be cultured from eyes without clinical evidence of a conjunctivitis. Typically, however, the conjunctivitis is worse in the fornices and palpebral areas. In most instances, it is a self-limiting disease, usually lasting a week. It can, however, cause a periorbital cellulitis and even endophthalmitis.

THERAPY

Systemic. Systemic therapy will be dictated by a physician other than an ophthalmologist because it is only an indication for secondary ocular infection, such as cellulitis and corneal or intraocular inflammation. Usual initial therapy consists of ampicillin in a daily dose of 400 mg/kg and 100 mg/kg of chloramphenicol given intravenously. If the strain does not have beta-lactamase present or is inhibited by ampicillin at 2.5 μg/ml with use of a large inoculum, chloramphenicol can be discontinued. Therapy may need to be continued for 2 weeks.

Ocular. Topical ocular antibiotic therapy varies with the severity of the ocular and/or systemic disease. For routine conjunctivitis, application of topical ophthalmic sulfonamides is recommended four times daily. Chloramphenicol eyedrops are probably the treatment of choice only in severe infections, as is true for treatment in other parts of the body. If high doses of systemic chloramphenicol have already been given in treatment of systemic infection, topical ocular chloramphenicol may also be indicated, since hemopoietic exposure will have already occurred.

The conjunctival sac may be irrigated with a saline solution or a boric acid eyewash a few times daily to remove conjunctival secretions. Cold compresses applied for 15 minutes three times daily may provide some comfort. The eyelids should otherwise be kept open, and the eyelashes should be coated with an antibiotic ointment at night to prevent the eyelids from sticking together.

Ocular or Periocular Manifestations

Anterior Chamber: Exudates.
Conjunctiva: Chemosis; follicles; hyperemia; mucopurulent conjunctivitis.
Cornea: Infiltration; opacity; pannus.
Other: Cellulitis; dacryoadenitis; extraocular muscle tenonitis; exudative anterior uveitis; eyelid edema; vitreous opacity.

PRECAUTIONS

Topical ocular chloramphenicol is not without risk and should not be used unless specifically indicated. Because of the well-known hemopoietic effects of chloramphenicol, conjunctivitis without other complications rarely requires the use of this drug, unless chloramphenicol has already been given systemically. Ampicillin, like penicillin, can cause allergic reactions, including anaphylaxis; gastrointestinal effects and eosinophilia are also common adverse effects.

COMMENTS

Other antibiotics, such as newer penicillins, nafcillin, cephalosporins, and rifampin, are also advocated for topical ocular and systemic use. Many of these antibiotics are satisfactory, depending on the severity and site of infection. In vitro sensitivities are indicated and even mandatory for most infections. A significant increase in antibiotic resistance has been noted in *Hemophilus influenzae* infections, especially with ampicillin and chloramphenicol.

Prophylaxis is debatable, since antibiotics alone are not always successful. In the future, a combination of chemoprophylaxis and immunoprophylaxis will be forthcoming. Vaccines are effective in patients above 15 years of age, but ineffective below this age group. Administration of 20 mg/kg of rifampin once daily for 4 days (maximum dose, 600 mg) has been claimed to eradicate carriers in 90 per cent or more of contacts.

References

Fraunfelder FT, Bagby GC Jr, Kelly DJ: Fatal aplastic anemia following topical administration of ophthalmic chloramphenicol. Am J Ophthalmol 93:356–360, 1982.
Gigliotti F, et al: Efficacy of topical antibiotic therapy in acute conjunctivitis in children. J Pediatr 104:623–626, 1984.
Granoff DM, Daum RS: Spread of *Haemophilus influenzae* tybe b: Recent epidemiologic and therapeutic considerations. J Pediatr 97:854–860, 1980.
Millard DD: *Haemophilus influenzae* type b: A rare case of congenital conjunctivitis. Pediatr Inf Dis J 7:363–364, 1988.
Newton NL Jr, Reynolds JD, Woody RC: Cortical blindness following *Hemophilus influenzae* meningitis. Ann Ophthalmol 17:193–194, 1985.
Walterspiel JN, et al: Ampicillin and chloramphenicol resistance in systemic *Hemophilus influenzae* disease. JAMA 251:884–885, 1984.

KOCH-WEEKS BACILLUS
(Hemophilus Aegyptius)

ALAN SUGAR, M.D.

Ann Arbor, Michigan

Koch-Weeks bacillus, *Hemophilus aegyptius*, is a small gram-negative coccobacillus or slender rod. It was initially recovered as a secondary invader in trachoma and as a cause of epidemic "pink eye." It is closely related to *H. influenzae* and may not be a distinct species, but it rarely causes systemic illness. It is cultured on blood or chocolate agar, and growth is enhanced around *Staphylococcus* colonies and in a high carbon dioxide atmosphere.

The typical illness is an acute conjunctivitis with a brief incubation period, often less than 24 hours, in children or young adults. The onset is usually in the warmer months; it is most common in the tropical and subtropical climates of the Middle East and North Africa, where it may be spread by ocular secretions and flies. Severe conjunctival injection, frequently with chemosis and bulbar conjunctival hemorrhage, occurs with increasing mucoid or mucopurulent discharge for the first 3 days. Lid edema may be present for about 5 days. Preauricular node swelling and tenderness occur. Without treatment, the conjunctivitis usually clears in 10 to 14 days, but it may relapse or become a chronic papillary conjunctivitis. In infants, the course may be mild and chronic or acute and severe with pseudomembranes. The cornea may be involved with inferior limbal ulcers beginning on the second or third day; central ulcers with possible perforation may rarely develop. Phlyctenular keratoconjunctivitis with potential corneal scarring may follow healing. It has been postulated that Koch-Weeks infections are often superimposed on trachoma and increase scarring. Although systemic illness is unusual, a fulminant and often fatal bacteremia with purpuric skin lesions, following resolution of the conjunctivitis, has recently been recognized and is known as Brazilian purpuric fever.

THERAPY

Systemic. Intravenous antibiotic therapy is indicated for orbital cellulitis and Brazilian purpuric fever.

Ocular. *H. aegyptius* conjunctivitis responds rapidly to treatment with most ophthalmic antibiotics, including sulfacetamide, chloramphenicol, polymyxin B, gentamicin, tobramycin, and tetracycline. The administration of hourly drops during the day with ointment used at bedtime leads to resolution in 3 days.

Ocular or Periocular Manifestations

Conjunctiva: Acute or chronic conjunctivitis; chemosis; injection; mucoid, mucopurulent, or purulent discharge; pseudomembrane; subconjunctival hemorrhage; phlyctenules.

Cornea: Infiltrates; marginal ulcer; phlyctenule; scarring; perforation.
Eyelids: Edema; cellulitis.
Other: Orbital or periorbital cellulitis; tearing; photophobia; iritis.

PRECAUTIONS

Adequate therapy is necessary to prevent recurrence or development of chronic conjunctivitis. Repeated reinfection is common in endemic regions. Antibiotic resistance may develop. Culture and sensitivity testing should be performed in severe or prolonged cases.

COMMENTS

The relationship between *H. aegyptius* infection and trachoma infection is unclear, but the two may coexist. Systemic illness—Brazilian purpuric fever—while rare, is cause for future concern.

References

Brazilian Purpuric Fever Study Group: *Haemophilus aegyptius* bacteremia in Brazilian purpuric fever. Lancet 2:761–763, 1987.
Dawson CR: Epidemic Koch-Weeks conjunctivitis and trachoma in the Coachilla Valley of California. Am J Ophthalmol 49:801–808, 1960.
Fedukowicz HB, Stetson S: External Infections of the Eye, 3rd ed. New York, Appleton-Century-Crofts, 1985, pp. 66–69.
Taylor HR, Kolarczyk RA, Johnson SL, Schachter J, Prendergast RA: Effect of bacterial secondary infection in an animal model of trachoma. Infect Immun 44:614–616, 1984.

LEPROSY
(Hansen's Disease)

T. J. FFYTCHE, F.R.C.S., D.O.

London, England

Leprosy is a disease caused by the acid-fast bacillus *Mycobacterium leprae;* although it is communicable, its method of spread is still unknown. The skin, peripheral nerves, mucous membranes, testes, and eyes are primarily affected because the organisms have an affinity for neural tissue in those parts of the body where the temperature is relatively low. In addition to the visual impairment, disfigurement, and loss of mobility caused by the effects of the disease on the limbs, patients with leprosy in many countries still carry a social stigma that has persisted through ignorance for centuries.

The clinical picture of the disease depends on the immunity of the host, which is highest in the tuberculoid form and lowest in the lepromatous form. Ocular involvement may occur indirectly in all types of the disease through the combined effects of paralysis of the facial and trigeminal nerve, with consequent corneal hypesthesia and exposure keratopathy. Direct invasion of the anterior part of the globe, which is susceptible because of its relatively low temperature, occurs in lepromatous leprosy, with insidious symptoms and a chronic course. An acute and often severe iridocyclitis may occur as part of an exaggerated immune response in lepromatous leprosy that is known as erythema nodosum leprosum (ENL); ENL may develop spontaneously or as a result of changes in therapy, an intercurrent infection, or stress.

THERAPY

Systemic. The development of resistant organisms to the standard antileprosy drugs has led to a reappraisal of the therapeutic approach to the disease and the introduction of multidrug therapy (MDT) in many centers. In tuberculoid leprosy, the regime recommended by the WHO consists of 100 mg of dapsone daily and 600 mg of rifampin[‡] once a month, with treatment continued for at least 6 months. In lepromatous cases, the WHO recommends 100 mg of dapsone and 50 mg of clofazimine daily, with once-monthly doses of 600 mg of rifampin[‡] and 300 mg of clofazimine. Doses are reduced proportionally for children. Treatment in these multibacillary cases should be continued for at least 2 years and preferably until negative skin smears are obtained. All monthly medication should be given under medical supervision.

Acute reactions in leprosy require energetic therapy in order to avoid permanent neural and ocular damage. Treatment includes the use of analgesics and systemic corticosteroid preparations. In addition, control of the reaction can be facilitated by the use of clofazimine, chloroquine,[‡] and thalidomide[†] (if available).

More traditional therapies, such as chaulmoogra oil and herbal remedies, are still used in many parts of the world. Attempts to improve cell-mediated immunity by means of a vaccine derived from the armadillo are undergoing clinical trials, and prophylactic BCG vaccination has been found to give some protection in areas where the disease is endemic.

Ocular. The acute iridocyclitis that occurs in ENL responds to conventional anti-inflammatory treatment with local mydriatic and steroid drops. During the attack, 1 per cent atropine two to three times daily together with dexamethasone every 2 hours should be used; the dosage can be reduced as the inflammation subsides. In severe cases, subconjunctival injections of steroids* and mydriatics may be necessary. If secondary glaucoma develops, oral hypotensive agents, such as 250 mg of acetazolamide four times daily, should be added to this regime.

In lepromatous leprosy, a chronic iridocyclitis resulting in iris atrophy and pronounced miosis may occur and cause significant visual loss. This condition does not respond to local mydriatic or steroid therapy in the late stages. Attempts should be made to dilate the pupils with daily instillations of 5 per cent phenylephrine or 1 per cent atropine before atrophy becomes too advanced.

Exposure keratopathy resulting from facial nerve involvement combined with corneal hypesthesia may lead to corneal ulceration and secondary infection. It should be treated by measures to protect the cornea with lubricating eye drops and broad-spectrum antibiotic drops and ointment.

Surgical. Lid surgery is designed to prevent corneal damage from exposure caused by facial nerve paralysis; procedures range from simple lateral tarsorrhaphy to more elaborate operations, such as temporalis transfer. Malpositions of the lids also require surgical correction to avoid secondary corneal disease, and an infected lacrimal sac should be removed. The leprous eye tolerates intraocular surgery reasonably well, provided that there is no active inflammation, and such procedures as optical iridectomy, cataract extraction, and keratoplasty may be performed where indicated.

Ocular or Periocular Manifestations

Cornea: Band-shaped degeneration; corneal ulcer; exposure keratopathy; hypesthesia; interstitial keratitis; leproma; pannus; superficial stromal keratitis; thickened corneal nerves.

Episclera and Sclera: Episcleritis; scleritis; staphyloma.

Eyebrows: Madarosis; nodules; thickening of the skin.

Eyelids: Blepharochalasis; distichiasis; ectropion; entropion; lagophthalmos; madarosis; nodules; trichiasis.

Iris: Iridocyclitis, acute or chronic; atrophy; iris pearls; nodular leproma; synechiae.

Lacrimal System: Dacryocystitis, acute or chronic; epiphora; nasolacrimal duct occlusion.

Pupil: Anisocoria; corectopia; diminished or absent response to light; miosis; occlusio pupillae; polycoria; seclusio pupillae.

Other: Cataract; decreased intraocular pressure; paralysis of seventh nerve; phthisis bulbi; secondary glaucoma.

PRECAUTIONS

Patients on dapsone should be watched closely for signs of toxicity, which may include anorexia, nausea and vomiting, neuropathy, anemia, and agranulocytosis. Clofazimine may produce diarrhea and causes a disturbing red-black discoloration of the skin and urine. Rifampin may give rise to gastrointestinal and respiratory symptoms, acute renal failure, thrombocytopenic purpura, hepatic reactions, and skin rashes. The use of topical steroids should be monitored carefully to avoid steroid-induced glaucoma and possible secondary cataract.

26 / LEPROSY

COMMENTS

Visual impairment in leprosy is caused mainly by the effects on the cornea of facial and trigeminal nerve paralysis, by cataract, and by the chronic iridocyclitis that occurs in the lepromatous form of the disease. The complications of acute iridocyclitis in ENL reactions also account for a considerable proportion of cases of blindness if the condition is not treated adequately at its onset. Patients are often unaware of ocular involvement, and education in seeking early advice and drug compliance is fundamentally important. The aim of therapy should be the prevention of ocular changes by attention to eye protection and hygiene and to the early diagnosis of intraocular disease. Once the eye is affected, continuous supervision should be the goal. When late complications develop, attempts should be made to preserve useful vision by medical and surgical means, since blindness is especially tragic in these already disabled and disadvantaged individuals.

References

Brand M: The care of the eye. The Star, Carville, LA, 1980.
Brand M, ffytche TJ: Eye complications of leprosy. *In* Hastings R (ed): Leprosy. Churchill Livingstone 1985.
ffytche TJ: The eye in leprosy. Lepr Rev 52:111–122, 1981.
ffytche TJ: Ocular leprosy. Trop Doct 15:118–127, 1985.
Tharangaraj RH, Yawalkar SJ: Leprosy. Basel, Ciba-Geigy, 1986.

LEPTOSPIROSIS

SUSAN BARKAY, M.D.
Afula, Israel

Leptospirosis is an acute systemic disease with endemic or epidemic occurrence. It is caused by the smallest pathogenic spirochete, the *Leptospira interrogans,* which comprises some 170 serovars (serotypes). These serovars have been differentiated on the basis of distinct agglutinogenic properties, but they are indistinguishable by morphologic, cultural, or physiologic properties. These 170 serovars fall into about 20 serogroups on the basis of common, overlapping antigenic components.

Leptospira organisms are harbored by animal hosts among the lower mammalians: rats, mice, racoons, but also domestic animals, cattle, swine, and dogs. These infected animals seldom show an overt illness, although in some countries they come to the attention of veterinarians frequently. Most carrier animals have asymptomatic infection of the renal tubules with long-lasting leptospiruria, which serves as the source of the disease in humans. In warm seasons the leptospire can survive for weeks in moist soil or alkaline water. Most cases of infection occur during the summer and autumn months.

Humans can acquire the disease through contact with urine or tissues of the infected animals via abraded skin or mucous membranes. Direct transmission from person to person is possible, but rare.

Leptospires penetrate tissues mechanically. After peritoneal inoculation in animal experiments, there is a rapid invasion of the leptospires into the bloodstream. After 24 hours, they are present in virtually all organs and can be recovered from the blood, CSF, the brain, and also from the anterior chamber of the eyes. Similar observations were made in several cases of human disease. The tissue damage caused by *Leptospira* is probably of toxic nature, and the degree of virulence seems to depend on toxin production.

Leptospirosis is a biphasic illness. After an incubation period of 3 to 26 days, leptospires invade the bloodstream and CSF, causing an acute, febrile illness, occasionally in a very severe form, with high temperatures, chills, muscular pains, pulmonary manifestations, gastrointestinal disturbance, and a skin rash, either petechial or purpuric. In this stage, jaundice is not a usual finding. A characteristic sign is an almost asymptomatic conjunctival effusion.

During this "leptospiremic" phase, *Leptospira* organisms can be cultured with semisolid (Fletcher's or Stuart's) mediums from blood or CSF. After the tenth day they disappear from the blood and CSF, and they are excreted with the urine (sometimes until the eleventh month). The leptospiremic phase ceases.

An almost asymptomatic interval of some days follows, after which the immune phase sets in. The immune phase is highly variable, with some patients being almost asymptomatic and others becoming severely ill. About 50 per cent of the patients have a high fever state with meningismus; 25 per cent within the 50 per cent have meningitis with elevated protein values and pleocytosis in the CSF. Encephalitis; Guillain-Barré syndrome; affections of the optic, abducens, facial, and auditory nerve; radiculitis; peripheral nerve lesions; and myocarditis are other complications. The second phase may last from a few days to as long as several weeks.

In some cases, in Weil's syndrome the course is extremely serious. Jaundice appears after the first days with hepatic enlargement, and fever is high and persistent. Pyuria, hematuria, and peak elevations of blood urea nitrogen occur as signs of acute tubular necrosis. There is a diffuse vasculitis with general hemorrhagic manifestations, such as epistaxis, hemoptysis, gastrointestinal bleedings, and subarachnoidal hemorrhage.

The clinical signs of the immune phase are manifested in parallel with the appearance of *Leptospira* antibodies in the blood at the end of the first week. The antibody level peaks in the third or fourth week. During this period of the disease serologic tests should be done. They are theoretically complicated owing to the large number of antigenically distinct leptospiral serotypes, but very often it is sufficient to test only for the organism known to be present in the endemic area.

The microscopic agglutination-lysis test using living *Leptospira* organisms has the highest sensitivity. The simple agglutination test using killed leptospires is a good diagnostic aid, but less accurate because nonspecific reactions occur. Complement-fixing antibodies are present from 10 days until three months in the serum, the complement-fixation test is also an excellent diagnostic aid.

Blood for serologic tests should be examined during the acute illness and also during the convalescence period. A fourfold titer rise is considered diagnostic. If only one specimen is available, a titer of 1 : 1600 gives strong presumptive evidence of infection by *Leptospira* organisms.

Incidence of ocular findings has been reported in 3 to 92 percent of cases of leptospirosis. This wide range probably is due to varying degrees of enthusiasm and knowledge of the clinical observers.

In the first days of the disease a conjunctival injection involving the anterior part of the globe and the conjunctiva of the lower lid may be seen. There is a characteristic clinical picture during this phase of the illness. The conjunctiva is pink in color, except in jaundiced patients, whose conjunctiva is yellow. The engorged conjunctival and episcleral vessels anastamose with dilated pericorneal vessels, thus giving the impression of a reticulum. Usually there are no subjective complaints, lacrimation, or discharge. However, the discharge, if present, contains leptospires and may be the source of further infection. This picture tends to disappear during convalescence.

In the immune phase, as part of the central nervous system involvement, palpebral herpes and optic neuritis may develop with or without iridocyclitis. The complication is usually self-limited and of short duration.

Most important are, however, the late uveitis cases. These occur long after the general features of the disease have subsided in an apparently healthy person. Indeed, cases 5 years after the initial infection have been reported. There is usually an acute, moderate, bilateral irido-cyclitis with hyperemia of the iris. Yet, severe exudative inflammation with mutton-fat precipitates, dense posterior synechiae between the iris and lens, and even hypopyon and secondary glaucoma are quite common findings. Choroiditis, retinal hemorrhages and exudates, and peculiar vitreous membranes running from the optic disc toward the anterior segment have also been described, with a course of absorption lasting for years. Blindness as a final outcome has been reported.

The pathogenesis of the uveitis as a late complication is not clear. *Leptospira* organisms have been isolated from the anterior chamber, but antibodies have also been found in other similar uveitis cases. It has been suggested that the leptospires can survive for a long time in the eye, as they do in the pelvis of the kidney, despite high levels of antibodies in the general circulation. It is possible that those organisms that survive can excite an inflammation in the form of late uveitis only after systemic immunity has faded.

THERAPY

Systemic. There is no specific treatment for leptospirosis, but there is general agreement that treatment with high doses of antimicrobials reduces complications. They must be administered in the first 2 to 4 days of the illness during the phase of leptospiremia. It is not considered worthwhile to initiate antimicrobial treatment after the fifth day of the disease.

Penicillin G, 2.4 million units intravenously a day, or tetracycline, 0.5 gm orally every 6 hours, is recommended for a period of 7 days. Within a few hours of the initial dose of penicillin, a Jarisch-Herxheimer type of reaction may occur, indicating that the drug possesses some in vivo antileptospiral activity. Doxycycline, 0.1 gm orally, twice a day for 7 days, may favorably affect the course of leptospirosis.

Careful management of fluid and electrolyte balance is required in cases of renal failure. In severe cases of tubular necrosis, hemodialysis or peritoneal dialysis is indicated.

Ocular. In cases of iridocyclitis, 1 per cent atropine should be administered three times daily, and 0.5 per cent ophthalmic prednisolone drops should be given three to six times daily. If this treatment fails, subconjunctival betamethasone* injections, 1.0 to 1.5 mg, may be given. In severe cases, 40 to 80 mg of oral prednisone daily is indicated.

Ocular or Periocular Manifestations

Anterior Chamber: Cells, flare, hypopyon.
Conjunctiva: Conjunctivitis, hemorrhages.
Cornea: Keratic precipitates.
Extraocular Muscles: Muscular palsies.
Eyelids: Herpes.
Iris: Posterior synechiae.
Lens: Cataract.
Optic Nerve: Neuritis.
Pupil: Seclusion.
Retina: Hemorrhages, exudates.
Vitreous: Peculiar vitreous strands.
Other: Secondary glaucoma, visual loss.

PRECAUTIONS

From the etiologic point of view, diagnosis of leptospirosis uveitis is not simple. In endemic areas and in cases of short interval between the general disease and uveitis, it is not difficult to find the connection. However, in many cases of severe uveitis, the forerunner is an uncomplicated febrile disease of short duration that occurred months or sometimes years before. In those cases diagnosis is difficult and often presumptive. It must rest on the history of systemic

28 / LEPTOSPIROSIS

illness with characteristic anamnestic data and clinical signs of leptospirosis that occurred before, sometimes long previously, on exclusion of other causes, and on positive serologic tests.

The prognosis of the disease in its anicteric form is mostly good. Recovery is complete except for the rare cases with residual renal tubular dysfunction. Still, there is a case fatality rate of 3 to 6 per cent. In jaundiced patients with Weil syndrome, mortality ranges from 25 to 40 per cent in untreated cases.

Most uveitis cases respond well to treatment, and even in the severe forms there is mostly a complete recovery. However, some cases have a long-lasting course, resulting in cataract formation or secondary glaucoma and thus severe visual impairment.

COMMENTS

Leptospirosis was once regarded primarily as an occupational disease of farmers, dairy workers, veterinarians, rice and sugar cane field workers, and the like. However, it is also a growing recreational hazard to hunters, fishermen, and swimmers in infected areas. In the past decade, infection from contact with dogs has occurred more frequently, particularly among children.

Leptospirosis is a preventable disease that can be avoided with adequate prophylactic methods. Until safe polyvalent vaccines are developed, hygienic precautions should be taken in cooperation with veterinary services and public health authorities.

References

Barkay S, Garzozi H: Leptospirosis and uveitis. Ann Ophthalmol 16:164–168, 1984.
Braude AI: Medical Microbiology and Infectious Diseases. Philadelphia, WB Saunders, 1980, pp 437–441, 1143–1146, 1839–1847.
Duke-Elder S (ed): System of Ophthalmology. London, Henry Kimpton, 1965, Vol VIII, pp 201–203; 1966, Vol IX, pp 322–325.
Infectious diseases VII. Leptospirosis, Scientific American, pp 1–3, 1988.
Jawetz E, Melnick JL, Adelberg EA: Review of Medical Microbiology, 14th ed. Los Altos, CA, Lange, pp 259–260.
Sanford JP: In Braunwald, et al (eds): Harrison's Principles of Internal Medicine, 11th ed. New York, McGraw-Hill, 1987, pp 652–655.
Walsh, Hoyt: Clinical Neuro-Ophthalmology, 3rd ed. Baltimore, Williams & Wilkins, 1969, Vol II, pp 1548–1551.

LISTERIOSIS
(Listerellosis)

PETER H. BALLEN, M.D.

Stony Brook, New York

Listeria monocytogenes is a small, gram-positive, non-spore-forming, non-acid-fast, diphtheroid-like rod with a peculiar tumbling motility at room temperature. It resembles *Corynebacterium* and is found in soil, plants, and vegetation of all sorts. Abortion in pregnant women and neonatal death are common in listeriosis septicemia.

This organism is known to cause ocular involvement in general or meningitic listeriosis infections, as a conjunctivitis that may be purulent or nonpurulent. The purulent form is more commonly seen in newborn infants with listeric septicemia whose eyes have been exposed to contaminated amniotic fluid. The nonpurulent form is associated with listeriosis meningitis or encephalitis.

L. monocytogenes keratitis in the form of a central ulcer has been reported in two cases. Heavy fibrinous reactions were noted in the anterior chamber leading, in one case, to pupillary block glaucoma. Treatment of the glaucoma with laser iridotomy was unsuccessful. The ulcer responded in both cases to cephalosporins and gentamicin in the form of subconjunctival injection* and fortified drops[§]. No paracentesis was performed in these cases, and the diagnosis was made from a surface smear and culture.

Endophthalmitis caused by *L. monocytogenes* is unusual. Three cases were reported in the English literature from 1967 to 1980 and one case in Czechoslovakia. Although the organism appears commonly in immunosuppressed individuals, endophthalmitis in an otherwise healthy individual has been reported. The patient with *L. monocytogenes* endophthalmitis may report a sudden onset of discomfort in an otherwise normal eye. Severe uveitis is present, usually accompanied by elevated intraocular pressure. Biomicroscopic examination of the eye reveals large pigmented precipitates over the posterior surface of the cornea. An extensive fibrinous hypopyon may be tan to brown to black in color. This is a striking clinical feature of *Listeria* endophthalmitis. In addition, severe fibrinous changes in the aqueous may result.

THERAPY

Systemic. A marked synergistic effect against *L. monocytogenes* exists between ampicillin and gentamicin. Intravenous administration of 2 gm of ampicillin every 4 to 6 hours and 100 mg of gentamicin every 8 hours may be given for 5 days.

After discharge from the hospital, the patient may be maintained on oral ampicillin and tetracycline and topical ophthalmic gentamicin. Oral tetracyclines should be used only for adults.

Ocular. Anterior chamber tap should be done as soon as hypopyon is noted. Although this may result in a paracentesis being performed in aseptic endophthalmitis, early diagnosis and treatment are of paramount importance. Intravitreal injection of 200 to 400 µg of gentamicin* should be administered at the time of parecentesis.

Combination systemic and ocular therapy is recommended in the treatment of endophthalmitis. Subtenon injection of 100 mg of ampicillin* may be administered for 7 days. Following the initial intraocular treatment, no further intraocular therapy is required.

Gentamicin drops should be used every hour for the first 3 days. For the remainder of the hospitalization, gentamicin solution may be reduced to every 2 hours while the patient is awake, and gentamicin ointment can be applied at night. Atropine may be instilled for cycloplegia.

PRECAUTIONS

The use of steroids after diagnosis of *L. monocytogenes* is questionable. Small doses of steroids have been shown experimentally to reduce considerably the minimal lethal dose of *Listeria* in rats.

It is not yet clear what specific disturbance in the immune mechanism accounts for the relative ease with which *Listeria* can affect the immunosuppressed individual. In immune-compromised patients, endogenous endophthalmitis caused by organisms with a very rare prevalence must be suspected. Uveitis in such patients must be considered a possible endogenous endophthalmitis. *L. monocytogenes* must be considered, especially if there is a tan to brown hypopyon that acquires a browner color as the infection proceeds. The extreme fibrinous reaction is deposited on the lens and may remain for a long period in the anterior chamber, reducing the visual acuity despite normal function of the retina. The cellular response of *Listeria* is polymorphonuclear in the anterior chamber. It is important that the laboratory not mistake *L. monocytogenes* for a nonpathogenic diphtheroid in the paracentesis specimen.

COMMENTS

Early institution of antibiotic therapy for general *Listeria* infections is extremely important, since a delay of appropriate therapy may result in death. Vision after endophthalmitis secondary to virulent organisms is very poor; unless the organism's effect can be reduced to a minimum early in the course of the disease, the vision will likely be lost. In order to obtain a reasonable expectation of retention of the eye or possibly useful vision, early diagnosis must be made with the institution of proper antibiotic therapy.

References

Abbott RL, Forster RK, Rebell G: *Listeria monocytogenes* endophthalmitis with a black hypopyon. Am J Ophthalmol 86:715–719, 1978.
Azimi PH, Koranyi K, Lindsey KD: *Listeria monocytogenes*. Synergistic effects of ampicillin and gentamicin. Am J Clin Pathol 72:974–977, 1979.
Bagnarello AG, et al: *Listeria monocytogenes* endophthalmitis. Arch Ophthalmol 95:1004–1005, 1977.
Ballen PH, Loffredo FR, Painter B: *Listeria* endophthalmitis. Arch. Ophthalmol 97:101–102, 1979.
Forster RK, et al: Further observations on the diagnosis, etiology, and treatment of endophthalmitis. Trans Am Ophthalmol Soc 73:221–230, 1975.
Goodner EK, Okumoto M: Intraocular listeriosis. Am J Ophthalmol 64:682–686, 1967.
Gray ML, Killinger AH: *Listeria monocytogenes* and listeric infections. Bacteriol Rev 30:309–382, 1966.
Holland S, Alfonso E, Gelender H, Heidemann D, Mendelsohn A, Ullman S, Miller D: Corneal ulcer due to *Listeria monocytogenes*. Cornea 6:144–146, 1987.
Moellering RC, Jr, et al: Antibiotic synergism against *Listeria monocytogenes*. Antimicrob Agents Chemother 1:30–34, 1972.
Murray EGD, Webb RA, Swann MBR: A disease of rabbits characterized by a large mononuclear leucocytosis, caused by a hitherto undescribed bacillus *Bacterium monocytogenes*. J Pathol Bacteriol 29:407–439, 1926.
Zimianski MC, Dawson CR, Togni B: Epithelial cell phagocytosis of *Listeria monocytogenes* in the conjunctiva. Ophthalmol 13:623–626, 1974.

MORAXELLA
JULES BAUM, M.D.
Boston, Massachusetts

Formerly called the diplobacillus of Morax-Axenfeld, *Moraxella lacunata* induces either an angular blepharoconjunctivitis or an infectious corneal ulcer. It is a gram-negative aerobic rod-shaped or coccoid diplobacillus. Organisms formerly called *M. liquefaciens* are indistinguishable from *M. lacunata* and have been incorporated into the latter species.

At the turn of the century, many investigators found the *Moraxella* diplobacillus to be the most commonly diagnosed cause of conjunctivitis. More recently, the reported incidence of *Moraxella* conjunctivitis and blepharoconjunctivitis has decreased dramatically and has ranged from 0.1 to 1.0 per cent of all forms of conjunctivitis in the Western world. *Moraxella* characteristically induces a chronic angular (outer angle) blepharoconjunctivitis with follicles and a typical erythematous eczematoid appearance of the skin at the lateral canthus. *Moraxella* ocular infection is rarely seen in young children. Without treatment, the disease may persist for months or even years. This is also true of staphylococcal blepharoconjunctivitis, now the most frequent cause of angular blepharoconjunctivitis. Rarely, *Moraxella* produces an acute severe conjunctivitis.

M. lacunata may also induce a severe corneal ulcer that is usually associated with a hypopyron. The ulcer may be superficial or deep, central or peripheral. Similar ulcers produced by *M. nonliquefaciens* cannot be distinguished clinically from ulcers induced by *M. lacunata* (or *M. lacunata* subsp *liquefaciens*).

THERAPY

Ocular. *Moraxella* is sensitive to most antibiotics, including penicillin, and treatment of the blepharoconjunctivitis is relatively simple. Proteases produced by the organism cause the maceration of the skin at the canthus, and 0.25 to 0.5 per cent zinc sulfate eyedrops or ointment counteracts the effect of the proteases. After cultures have been obtained, both topical antibiotic and zinc sulfate therapy should be given three to four times daily until the disease process has resolved. The choice of antibiotic may be modified on the basis of in vitro susceptibility results. Treatment of a *Moraxella* corneal ulcer should conform to the initial treatment of any suspected corneal ulcer (see Bacterial corneal ulcers).

Ocular or Periocular Manifestations

Conjunctiva: Chronic catarrhal angular conjunctivitis; follicles; mucopurulent discharge.

Cornea: Central or peripheral ulcer with or without hypopyon.

Eyelids: Chronic blepharitis; eczema and maceration; lateral canthal skin erythema.

Other: Iridocyclitis secondary to corneal ulcer.

PRECAUTIONS

Since *Moraxella* ocular disease usually occurs in a poor and alcoholic population, compliance is often a problem; every effort should be made to impress on the patient the importance of compliance.

COMMENTS

Moraxella ocular infections tend to occur most frequently, but not exclusively, in a derelict, malnourished, alcoholic population. Nasal and conjunctival cultures for *Moraxella* were positive in 12.9 per cent and 0.3 per cent, respectively, of normal subjects in a recent series, whereas similar cultures taken from a derelict alcoholic population yielded positive cultures in 35 per cent and 5.5 per cent, respectively. Although *Moraxella* is part of the normal flora of the respiratory tract, its incidence may be higher in a derelict population. It is curious that, whereas *M. liquefaciens* is the species most often part of the normal nasal flora, the more frequent ocular pathogen is *M. lacunata*.

References

Baum J, Fedukowicz HB, Jordan A: A survey of *Moraxella* corneal ulcers in a derelict population. Am J Ophthalmol 90:476–480, 1980.

Baum JL, Jones DB: Initial therapy of suspected microbial corneal ulcers. Surv Ophthalmol 24:97–116, 1979.

Chandler RL, Bird RG, Smith MD, Anger HS, Turfrey BA: Scanning electron microscope studies on preparations of bovine cornea exposed to *Moraxella bovis*. J Comp Pathol 93:1–8, 1983.

Fedukowicz HB: External Infections of the Eye: Bacterial, Viral and Mycotic, 2nd ed. New York, Appleton-Century-Crofts, 1978.

Jackman SH, Rosenbusch RF: In vitro adherence of *Moraxella bovis* to intact corneal epithelium. Curr Eye Res 3:1107–1112, 1984.

Lennette EH, et al (eds): Manual of Clinical Microbiology, 3rd ed. Washington, DC, American Society for Microbiology, 1980.

Ringvold A, Vik E, Bevanger LS: *Moraxella lacunata* isolated from epidemic conjunctivitis among teen-aged females. Acta Ophthalmol (Copehn) 63:427–431, 1985.

van Bijsterveld OP: Acute conjunctivitis and *Moraxella*. Am J Ophthalmol 63:1702–1705, 1968.

van Bijsterveld OP: The incidence of *Moraxella* on mucous membranes and the skin. Am J Ophthalmol 74:72–76, 1972.

van Bijsterveld OP: Host-parasite relationship and taxonomic position of *Moraxella* and morphologically related organisms. Am J Ophthalmol 77:545–554, 1973.

NOCARDIA

JOHN D. BULLOCK, M.D., M.S., F.A.C.S., *and* STUART H. GOLDBERG, M.D.

Dayton, Ohio

Nocardiosis is typically caused by *Nocardia asteroides,* which is named for the star-like appearance of the colonies on agar plate. Once thought to be a fungus, it is now classified in the bacterial family Nocardiaceae, which includes aerobic *Actinomycetes* having a complex cell wall. The organism reproduces by fragmentation of its hyphae into bacillary and coccoid elements. It is distinguished by a propensity for filamentous growth with true branching. A natural soil saprophyte, it is often found in decaying organic matter. The organisms are gram positive and often show an intermittent or beaded staining pattern with gram stain. Gomori methenamine-silver stain also demonstrates the organisms well. In culture, they tend to grow slowly, but will grow within a wide temperature range on virtually any bacterial, fungal, or mycobacterial medium that lacks antibiotics.

Systemic nocardiosis is a chronic, progressive, localized, or disseminated infection that usually invades the body via the respiratory tract. When the lung is involved, the clinical picture can resemble bronchitis or pneumonia similar to that seen with tuberculosis or other bacterial or fungal infections. Nocardial organisms can also cause mycetoma (maduromycosis or Madura foot), a chronic, deep subcutaneous tissue and bone infection usually of the lower extremity. Between 20 to 50 per cent of cases of nocardiosis are in otherwise healthy patients, but it is much more common in debilitated, immunosuppressed patients. The patient presents with cough and low-grade fever. Malaise, weight loss, and night sweats may occur. The radiologic appearance is that of a rapidly developing lobar or segmental infiltrate. Central nervous system dissemination occurs in 25 to 40 per cent of cases. Other sites of dissemination include the skin and subcutaneous tissues, kidney, liver, and lymph nodes. Ocular involvement has been reported in 3 per cent of cases of systemic nocardiosis. Diagnosis can be made by blood culture, sputum culture, or direct aspiration of material.

Ophthalmic *N. asteroides* infection occurs either exogenously or endogenously. Exogenous ocular disease arises as a superficial infection, usually following trauma, with or without intraocular extension. In endogenous ocular nocardiosis, the organisms reach the eye hematogenously in an immunologically normal, immunosuppressed, or immunocompromised patient. Endogenous ocular nocardiosis occurs at a mean age of 46 years with a male-to-female ratio of 4 : 1 and is bilateral in 30 percent of patients.

THERAPY

Systemic. Most strains of *N. asteroides* are sensitive to sulfonamides. The treatment of choice is 6 to 10 gm of sulfadiazine[§] or sulfisoxazole[§] administered daily. Treatment must be prolonged. Immunologically intact patients require a minimum of 6 weeks of therapy, whereas immunosuppressed patients are treated for a year.

Ocular. Nocardial keratitis may be treated with hourly 15 to 30 per cent sulfacetamide eyedrops with or without hourly topical ampicillin[*] (40 to 100 mg/ml), or topical trimethoprim (16 mg/ml)/sulfamethoxazole[*] (80 mg/ml) given every half-hour initially. Oral administration of trimethoprim/sulfamethoxazole[‡] in a dosage of 320 mg of trimethoprim and 1.6 gm of sulfamethoxazole should be given twice a day. The use of steroids[‡] in the treatment of nocardial keratitis is controversial. Treatment of nocardial endophthalmitis with a variety of systemic and topical antibiotics is frequently unsuccessful. Many reported cases have been eviscerated or enucleated. One reported case of exogenous endophthalmitis in an immunocompetent patient was successfully treated with vitrectomy, penetrating keratoplasty, and intraocular,[*] topical, and systemic antibiotics.

Ocular or Periocular Manifestations

Anterior Chamber: Hypopyon.
Cornea: Keratoconjunctivitis; ulcerative keratitis.
Globe: Endophthalmitis.
Iris: Anterior uveitis.
Lacrimal System: Dacryocystitis.
Orbit: Chronic cellulitis.
Sclera: Scleritis.
Vitreous or Retina: Chorioretinitis.

Precautions

Immunosuppressive medications should be reduced in patients with nocardiosis. In primary isolation from clinical material, the colonies of *N. asteroides* can take as long as 2 to 4 weeks to appear. Because of this long time interval, a high index of suspicion is necessary to make the diagnosis microbiologically. Culture plates tend to be overgrown by contaminants and may be discarded before *Nocardia* colonies grow.

Comments

Healthy individuals have only a 15 per cent mortality from nocardiosis. Nonimmunosuppressed patients with an underlying disease have a mortality of approximately 20 per cent from nocardiosis, whereas patients who are taking immunosuppressive medications and have nocardiosis have a mortality of 80–100 per cent. The probability of surviving nocardiosis is increased by rapid diagnosis, discontinuation or marked reduction of immunosuppressive medication, and prolonged, aggressive, and accurate antimicrobial therapy.

N. asteroides is a facultative, intracellular parasite that can persist and grow within macrophages. The basis of nocardial pathogenicity is its cell wall, which is composed of complex lipids, peptides, and polysaccharides.

Common histopathologic features of nocardial endophthalmitis include a suppurative and necrotizing inflammatory response in the choroid and retina, along with subretinal abscesses.

References

Bullock JD: Endogenous ocular nocardiosis: A clinical and experimental study. Trans Am Ophthalmol Soc 81:451–531, 1983.
Chen CJ: *Nocardia asteroides* endophthalmitis. Ophthalmic Surg 14:502–505, 1983.
Climenhaga DB, Tokarewicz AC, Willis NR: Nocardia keratitis. Can J Ophthalmol 19:284–286, 1984.
Donnenfeld ED, Cohen EJ, Barza M, Baum J: Treatment of *Nocardia* keratitis with topical trimethoprim-sulfamethoxazole. Am J Ophthalmol 99:601–602, 1985.
Ferry AP, Font RL, Weinberg RS, Boniuk M, Schaffer CL: Nocardial endophthalmitis: Report of two cases studied histopathologically. Br J Ophthalmol 72:55–61, 1988.
Srinivason M, Sharma S: *Nocardia asteroides* as a cause of corneal ulcer. Arch Ophthalmol 105:464, 1987.

PNEUMOCOCCUS
(Streptococcus Pneumoniae)

H. BRUCE OSTLER, M.D.,
and VICKY CEVALLOS, M.T. (A.S.C.P.)
San Francisco, California

Commonly known as pneumococcus, *Streptococcus pneumoniae* is a gram-positive lancet-shaped coccus characteristically appearing as diplococcus occasionally singly or in short chains. The normal habitat of the pneumococcus is the upper respiratory tract of humans. They are also present in the eyes of a small percentage of healthy individuals.

The pneumococcus is the primary etiologic

agent in all types of pneumonias in the United States and the most frequent cause of otitis media in children. Pneumococcus has also been implicated in meningitis and septicemia. Infections with pneumococcus occur through droplets released from infected patients.

Pneumonia is often preceded by an upper respiratory infection. The infection is usually sudden, with a shaking chill, sharp pain in the involved hemithorax, cough with early sputum production, fever, and headache. Gastrointestinal symptoms are often present.

Ocular disease occurs from direct invasion by the organism. In newborns, the pneumococcus may cause ophthalmia neonatorum. In the adult, the organism is a common cause of dacryocystitis *S. pneumoniae* is a true corneal pathogen. It also frequently causes an acute catarrhal conjunctivitis.

THERAPY

Systemic. It is inadvisable to rely on oral therapy for acutely ill patients. Patients with mild infection, who are otherwise healthy, however, can be safely treated with an initial intramuscular injection of 300,000 to 600,000 units of procaine penicillin G, followed by 250 mg of oral penicillin V every 6 hours for 10 days. Aqueous potassium penicillin G (40,000 to 50,000 units/kg divided into four equal portions every 6 hours) may be administered intravenously to patients with overwhelming disease and potential cardiovascular collapse. Alternate drugs that may be used for the patient allergic to penicillin include 250 mg of erythromycin every 6 hours or 500 mg of vancomycin every 12 hours. Cephalosporins, such as 1 gm of cefazolin every 8 hours, are effective; however, clinical cross-sensitivity reactions to penicillin occur in about 8 to 15 per cent of patients.

Ocular. Topical ophthalmic antibiotics normally suffice for the treatment of a conjunctivitis caused by pneumococcus. Fortified bacitracin§ eyedrops (10,000 units/ml) may be given every hour during the first day and then four times daily for 1 week. Topical ophthalmic 0.5 per cent erythromycin ointment may be substituted for the bacitracin.

For suppurative keratitis (central corneal ulcers) caused by *S. pneumoniae*, topical fortified aqueous sodium penicillin G* (100,000 units/ml) may be given every 30 minutes during the day and every hour during the night. Bacitracin§ (10,000 units/ml) or cefazolin* (50 mg/ml) topically may be substituted for the penicillin. Subconjunctival cefazolin* (50 to 100 mg) or penicillin* (0.5 to 1.0 million units) should also be given every 12 to 24 hours for the first few days. If perforation appears imminent, systemic antibiotics as outlined below for endophthalmitis should be started.

For treatment of endophthalmitis caused by pneumococcus, intravitreal cefazolin* (2.25 mg) should be administered immediately following aspiration of vitreous or vitrectomy. A daily dosage of 20 to 40 million units of aqueous penicillin G divided into four equal portions should be administered intravenously. In patients with a history of hypersensitivity to penicillin, cefazolin (15 mg/kg/day divided into three equal doses) intravenously, erythromycin (15 to 20 mg/kg/day divided into four equal doses) intravenously, or lincomycin (600 mg three times daily) may be substituted for the penicillin. Subconjunctival injections, as outlined above for treatment of corneal ulcers, should also be given.

Cycloplegics are indicated in order to prevent posterior synechiae and reduce pain in patients with suppurative keratitis or endophthalmitis. One or two drops of 1 per cent atropine or 1 per cent cyclopentolate may be instilled one to three times daily.

Orbital cellulitis caused by pneumococcal infection should be treated with aqueous penicillin G intravenously as outlined above. An otolaryngologist should evaluate and treat the paranasal sinuses, if indicated.

Acute dacryocystitis caused by pneumococcus requires adequate and prompt drainage of the lacrimal sac. When the dacryocystitis is no longer acute, the patency of the nasolacrimal system should be re-established. If periodacryocystitis has occurred, either 250 mg of oral penicillin V every 6 hours or 600,000 units of intramuscular aqueous procaine penicillin G daily may be used. In addition, drainage of the nasolacrimal sac should be re-established. In instances of hypersensitivity to penicillin, 250 to 500 mg of oral erythromycin four times daily may be substituted.

Secondary glaucoma, which can occur in central corneal ulcers or endophthalmitis, may require the use of a systemic carbonic anhydrase inhibitor or a topical beta blocker. The usual oral adult dosage is 250 mg of acetazolamide four times daily.

Supportive. A new pneumococcal capsular polysaccharide vaccine is recommended for the prevention of pneumococcal infection in high-risk patients. Such high-risk patients include the elderly, patients with an underlying disease that adversely affects pulmonary function, and immunosuppressed patients. The vaccine is not indicated for more widespread use at this time, but may be indicated in the future if penicillin-resistant pneumococci become more common.

Ocular or Periocular Manifestations

Anterior Chamber: Hypopyon.
Conjunctiva: Acute catarrhal conjunctivitis; chemosis; hyperemia; membranous, pseudomembranous, purulent, or ulcerative conjunctivitis; petechial subconjunctival hemorrhages (superiorly).

Cornea: Anterior staphyloma; epithelial keratitis; leukoma; perforation; serpiginous ulcer.
Globe: Endophthalmitis; panophthalmitis.
Other: Dacryocystitis; exudative anterior uveitis; orbital cellulitis; palpebral edema; preauricular lymphadenopathy; secondary glaucoma.

Precautions

Systemic therapy for ocular pneumococcal infection, except for endophthalmitis and orbital cellulitis, offers little or no advantage over topical and subconjunctival therapy. In addition to a risk of toxicity, systemic therapy yields comparatively low levels of the appropriate drug in the affected ocular tissues. Although pneumococci are generally regarded as being highly susceptible to most antibiotics and sulfonamides, resistance to penicillin, tetracycline, and erythromycin has nevertheless occurred. Moreover, the organism is usually resistant to neomycin, gentamicin, and polymyxin B. Thus, Neosporin, the principal constituents of which are neomycin and polymyxin B, is a poor choice in the treatment of pneumococcal infections. Strict guidelines for the use of corticosteroids in the treatment of pneumococcal infections are not currently available, and one is cautioned in the use of this drug.

References

Applebaum PC: World-wide development of antibiotic resistance in Pneumococci. Eur J Clin Microbiol 6:367–373, 1987.
Conte JE, Barriere SL: Manual of Antibiotics and Infectious Diseases, 5th ed. Philadelphia, Lea and Febiger, 1984, pp 25–26.
Hoeprich PD: Bacterial pneumonias. In Hoeprich PD (ed): Infectious Diseases, 3rd ed. Hagerstown, MD, Harper and Row, 1983, pp 347–360.
Jones DB: Early diagnosis and therapy of bacterial corneal ulcers. Int Ophthalmol Clin 13:1–29, 1973.
Lauer BA, Reller LB: Serotypes and penicillin susceptibility of pneumococci isolated from blood. J Clin Microbiol 11:242–244, 1980.
Lentnek A, LeFrock JL, Molavi A: *Streptococcus pneumoniae.* In Levison, ME (ed): The Pneumonias: Clinical Approaches to Infectious Diseases of the Lower Respiratory Tract. Littleton, MA, John Wright, 1984, pp 261–271.
Mandell GL, Sande MA: Antimicrobial agents: Penicillins and cephalosporins. In Gilman AG, Goodman LS, Gilman A (eds): The Pharmacological Basis of Therapeutics, 7th ed. New York, Macmillan, 1985, pp 1115–1145.
Okumoto M, Smolin G: Pneumococcal infections of the eye. Am J Ophthalmol 77:346–352, 1974.
Robins-Brown RM, et al: Resistance mechanisms of multiply resistant pneumococci: Antibiotic degradation studies. Antimicrob Agents Chemother 15:470–474, 1979.
Sande MA, Mandell GL: Antimicrobial agents: Tetracyclines, chloramphenicol, erythromycin, and miscellaneous antibacterial agents. In Gilman AG, Goodman LS, Gilman A (eds): The Pharmacological Basis of Therapeutics, 7th ed. New York, Macmillan, 1985, pp 1170–1198.

PROPIONIBACTERIUM ACNES
RONALD E. SMITH, M.D.
Los Angeles, California

Propionibacterium acnes is a fastidious gram-positive non-spore-forming, pleomorphic, anaerobic bacteria that has been associated with a wide variety of ocular infections. Infectious corneal ulcers, conjunctivitis, dacryocystitis, and frank bacterial endophthalmitis have been reported. More recently, a new syndrome possibly related to *P. acnes* has emerged. This postcataract extraction syndrome includes chronic recurrent postoperative uveitis with large keratic precipitates. Infiltrates occur in the capsular bag with recurrent hypopyon. There may be gradual progression to more typical signs of infectious endophthalmitis. It is possible that *P. acnes*, in addition to producing disease as a replication infectious agent, may act as an immunopotentiater in the presence of residual lens material and an intraocular lens in such cases.

THERAPY

Systemic. Cases of corneal ulceration and frank infectious endophthalmitis due to *P. acnes* require appropriate intensive antibiotic therapy as in any such case. Culturing the organism may be difficult, and culture techniques that take into consideration the anaerobic culture requirements of the organism are necessary. Penicillin derivatives are usually effective.

Ocular. Therapy of the postcataract extraction/intraocular lens (IOL) "*P. acnes* syndrome" is less well established. There is usually a favorable response to high-dose topical steroids in early phases with resolution of keratic precipitates and hypopyon and return of good vision. However, this form of postoperative inflammation often returns or remains chronic and may gradually progress to more frank endophthalmitis in the vitreous cavity. At this stage, vitreous aspiration and culture with antimicrobial therapy by systemic, intravitreal,* and subconjunctival* routes are probably indicated.

Surgical. If frank infectious endophthalmitis is present due to *P. acnes*, intravitreal* antibiotics and possible vitrectomy are indicated. The usual criteria for vitrectomy in microbial endophthalmitis may be employed. The role of capsulectomy and removal of residual lens material and the removal of the intraocular lens itself are controversial at this time. In some instances, recurrence of inflammation is a clinical problem because residual lens material in the presence of the intraocular lens may encourage further inflammation related to immunopotentiation by the *P. acnes* organism itself.

34 / PROPIONIBACTERIUM ACNES

Ocular or Periocular Manifestations

Cornea: Corneal edema with large keratic precipitates.

Anterior Chamber: Recurrent hypopyon; precipitates in the capsular bag and on the intraocular lens.

Vitreous Cavity (advanced cases): Cells in the vitreous; other evidence of bacterial endophthalmitis.

PRECAUTIONS

It is very difficult to culture *P. acnes*. Consultation with a microbiology laboratory may be necessary to ensure proper identification of this organism.

The diagnosis and therapy of the newly described "*P. acnes* syndrome" remain controversial. It is not clear what role the removal of the intraocular lens or the posterior capsule may play in the management of this entity. The rationale for removal of the capsule relates to the possible role of residual lens material that remains after extracapsular cataract extraction.

COMMENTS

In the treatment of the postcataract extraction/IOL "*P. acnes* syndrome," some authorities have recommended immediate removal of the posterior capsule and residual lens material and the intraocular lens. Others favor a staged approach consisting of posterior vitrectomy and partial capsulectomy. The importance of intravitreal antibiotics that are effective against the organism is generally accepted, along with a vitrectomy if the infectious inflammatory condition has progressed. Topical and systemic corticosteroids are also helpful to reduce the phacoantigenic component of this ocular inflammatory condition.

References

Beatty RF, Robin JB, Trousdale MD, Smith RE: Anaerobic endophthalmitis caused by *Propionibacterium acnes.* Am J Ophthalmol *101*:114–116, 1986.

Jones DB, Robinson NM: Anaerobic ocular infections. Trans Am Acad Ophthalmol Otolaryngol 83:309–331, 1977.

Meisler DM, Palestine AG, Vastine DW, Demartini DR, Murphy BF, Reinhart WJ, Zakov N, McMahon JT, Cliffel TP: Chronic *Propionibacterium* endophthalmitis after extracapsular cataract extraction and intraocular lens implantation. Am J Ophthalmol *102*:733–739, 1986.

Meisler DM, Zakov ZN, Bruner WE, Hall GS, McMahon JT, Zachary AA, Barna BP. Endophthalmitis associated with sequestered intraocular *Propionibacterium acnes.* Am J Ophthalmol *104*:428–429, 1987.

Smith RE: Inflammation after cataract surgery. Am J Ophthalmol *102*:788–790, 1986.

PROTEUS
DAVID S. HULL, M.D.
Augusta, Georgia

Proteus organisms are gram-negative bacilli found as free-living saprophytes in water, soil, and dead or decaying organic substances. They are enterobacteria and a component of the normal flora of the mammalian intestine; they may cause an opportunistic infection in a weakened host. The pathogenic species in humans include *P. mirabilis, P. vulgaris,* and *P. penneri;* of these, *P. mirabilis* is implicated most frequently in human infections. A former *Proteus* species, *P. morganii* has been reclassified as *Morganella morganii.* A third genus is called *Providencia* and includes the former *Proteus rettgeri,* which is now classified as *Providencia rettgeri.*

Parts of the body that may be affected by *Proteus* infection include the skin, ears, mastoid sinuses, eyes, peritoneal cavity, bone, urinary tract, meninges, lungs, and bloodstream. The majority of *Proteus* infections are hospital acquired, and patients with long-term indwelling urinary tract catheters are particularly at risk. Cutaneous infections occur most often in surgical wounds, particularly after antimicrobial therapy. *Proteus* species have been recovered from 2.6 per cent of normal eyes, with *P. mirabilis* being the most common. Ocular infection by *Proteus* organisms is uncommon, but when it occurs it is usually severe and carries a relatively poor prognosis. Most *Proteus* infections of the eye occur following trauma to the eye; however, *Proteus* bacteremia may result in secondary ocular involvement. Postoperative *Proteus* infection can be particularly troublesome, since the *Proteus* bacilli replace the more susceptible flora eradicated by postoperative antibiotics. Ocular infections in which *Proteus* organisms have been implicated include · keratitis, corneal ulcers, necrotic inflammation of the eyelid, and panophthalmitis. As in other types of bacterial endophthalmitis, panophthalmitis often results in loss of the eye.

THERAPY

Systemic. For *Proteus* infections, ampicillin, gentamicin, and tobramycin are frequently effective. However, because of the emergence of multiple drug-resistant strains of *Proteus*, a complete microbiologic evaluation with drug testing is necessary to rationally formulate effective chemotherapy. *Proteus* organisms are becoming increasingly resistant to gentamicin; however, tobramycin and, especially, amikacin are useful alternatives. Amikacin, cefoxitin, piperacillin, or third-generation cephalosporins may be of value in the treatment of multiple drug-resistant organisms. *P. mirabilis* is almost always susceptible to ampicillin and cephalosporins, whereas *P. vulgaris* is frequently resistant to ampicillin and cephalosporins. *P. penneri* is typically resistant to chloramphenicol.

Ocular. For severe *Proteus* infections of the external eye, suggested treatment includes subconjunctival injections of 20 mg of gentamicin* or 20 mg of tobramycin* daily. In addition, topical fortified 14 mg/ml gentamicin§ ophthalmic drops or fortified 14 mg/ml tobramycin§ ophthalmic drops may also be applied two or three times hourly.

Ocular or Periocular Manifestations

Conjunctiva: Conjunctivitis; edema; exudates.
Cornea: Abscess; descemetocele; edema, exudates; folds in Descemet's membrane; keratitis; perforation; ulcer.
Eyelids: Edema; infiltration; gangrene; necrosis.
Globe: Endophthalmitis; panophthalmitis.
Other: Anterior uveitis; dacryocystitis; hypopyon; paralysis of seventh nerve.

PRECAUTIONS

Proteus organisms, as with other enteric species, may carry resistant factors, and antibiotic susceptibility tests should be done on clinical isolates. *Proteus* corneal ulceration may rapidly lead to perforation and require surgical intervention.

Renal function of all patients must be monitored carefully during administration of aminoglycoside antibiotics. If renal failure should occur, dosage must be adjusted downward to prevent nephrotoxicity. Aminoglycosides have been implicated in severe vestibular and auditory dysfunction, particularly in patients with impaired kidney function. Patients should be carefully observed for signs of damage to the eighth nerve.

Because of the similarity of structure of penicillins and cephalosporins, patients may manifest cross-reactive allergic reactions.

COMMENTS

Proteus organisms have a tendency to produce infection in locations previously infected by other bacilli. These organisms are frequently cultured from superficial wounds, draining ears, and sputum. *Proteus* infection, especially *P. vulgaris,* may occur as a sequela to previous antibiotic treatment.

References

Glasser DB, Hyndiuk RA: Antibacterial agents. *In* Tabbara KF, Hyndiuk RA (eds): Infections of the Eye. Boston, Little, Brown, 1986, pp 211–238.
Hickman FW et al: Identification of *Proteus penneri* sp. nov., Formerly known as *Proteus vulgaris* indole negative or as *Proteus vulgaris* Biogroup 1. J Clin Microbiol 15:1097–1102, 1982.
Okumoto M, et al: *Proteus* species isolated from human eyes. Am J Ophthalmol 81:495–501, 1976.
Parunovic A: *Proteus mirabilis* causing necrotic inflammation of the eyelid. Am J Ophthalmol 76:543–544, 1973.
Smolin G: *Proteus* endophthalmitis. Arch Ophthalmol 91:419–420, 1974.
Yoshikawa TT, et al: Outbreak of multiply drug-resistant *Proteus mirabilis* originating in surgical intensive care unit: In vitro susceptibility pattern. Antimicrob Agents Chemother 13:177–179, 1978.

PSEUDOMONAS AERUGINOSA
PETER R. LAIBSON, M.D.
Philadelphia, Pennsylvania

Pseudomonas aeruginosa, an opportunistic, gram-negative, motile rod, is the bacterial organism that can cause the most serious infection of the cornea. *Pseudomonas* infections of the cornea cause severe damage because of their ability to produce stromal necrosis rapidly, with resultant corneal thinning and perforation. *Pseudomonas* corneal ulcers can cause corneal perforation in only 24 hours, whereas infections due to staphylococci, streptococci, and *Hemophilus* take days to weeks to cause similar corneal thinning and possible perforation. In the past 8 years the incidence of corneal ulcers caused by *Pseudomonas* has significantly increased compared to previous years. This increase is directly linked to the use of daily-wear soft contact lenses and, over the past 5 years, particularly to extended-wear soft contact lenses. *Staphylococcus* is probably still the most common bacteria to infect the cornea, although the most severe infections are undoubtedly caused by *P. aeruginosa.* The *Pseudomonas* infection characteristically starts in a small central or paracentral area and spreads rapidly. When *Pseudomonas* infection occurs near the limbus and in the sclera, the prognosis for ocular recovery is very poor.

Pseudomonas is the most common bacterial organism isolated from infections related to soft and hard contact lens use. Approximately 50 per cent of the corneal ulcers occurring with daily-wear and extended-wear soft contact lens use are caused by *Pseudomonas* infection. These ulcerations are usually the result of the patient's failure to follow the manufacturer's advice concerning sterilization and change of solutions. In addition to obtaining positive cultures from the corneal ulcer itself, the organisms can often be recovered from the contact lens solutions, the contact lens containers, and the soft contact lens itself.

THERAPY

Systemic. Usually, systemic therapy is not necessary for bacterial corneal ulcers. However, with extensive involvement of the cornea, particularly when *P. aeruginosa* involves the limbus and sclera, systemic medication is indicated. In

36 / PSEUDOMONAS AERUGINOSA

this case, daily injections of 4 mg/kg of either tobramycin or gentamicin should be used. For more resistant, severe infections with poor response, tobramycin and piperacillin or tobramycin and ticarcillin may be used. When the sclera is involved, the use of topical and systemic antibiotics, as well as cryotherapy, has been advocated by some ophthalmologists.

Ocular. A corneal ulcer caused by *P. aeruginosa* must be diagnosed and treated as soon as possible because of the rapid destruction of stromal collagen by enzymes produced with this infection. In the past, subconjunctival injections* of fortified aminoglycosides were commonly used, but today, the frequent application of fortified topical medication§ is preferred. These fortified medications are now readily available from most pharmacies that dispense ophthalmic drugs, particularly at eye centers, because most pharmacists know how to change regular-strength aminoglycoside to fortified concentrations. The drug of choice for known *Pseudomonas* infection is fortified tobramycin,§ rather than gentamicin.§ In studies performed on *Pseudomonas* corneal ulcers at Wills Eye Hospital almost 30 per cent of the *Pseudomonas* isolates were intermediately affected by gentamicin, whereas they were strongly inhibited by tobramycin. In our experience at Wills Eye Hospital, all *Pseudomonas* isolates were sensitive to tobramycin.

Since fortified medications are readily available, use of topical drops every 15 minutes for the first several hours and then every 30 minutes for the next 24 hours is indicated, rather than subconjunctival medications.

Corneal ulcerations with or without hypopyon should be scraped first before instituting antibiotics. These scrapings should be looked at with gram stain for bacterial organisms and with giemsa stain for cell type. After the scrapings and cultures are performed, topical antibiotics are applied. The antibiotic of choice is fortified tobramycin§ (15 mg/ml) every 15 minutes if the ulcer is severe or every 30 minutes for the first day or two. This medication should be given around the clock. If it is unclear whether this is a gram-positive or gram-negative organism, the use of fortified cefazolin* (100 mg/ml) is also recommended either every 30 minutes, 1 hour, or 2 hours around the clock between applications of the fortified tobramycin. In addition to the antibiotics, atropine should be applied for cycloplegia and antiglaucoma medications instituted if the pressure is elevated. Under no circumstances should steroids be used in the early stages of any *Pseudomonas* infection. Once the ulcer shows signs of response, the topical drops can be tapered slowly.

If one is sure that *P. aeruginosa* alone is responsible for the corneal ulcer, then tobramycin is usually sufficient for appropriate therapy. Topical antibiotics may be tapered according to the response of the bacterial ulcer, but should be continued for at least 1 to 2 months after the epithelial ulceration has healed. Once the epithelial ulceration has healed, the judicious use of topical steroids may be employed to limit the stromal inflammation and eventual scarring. Although steroids have been used following epithelial healing, tobramycin drops should also be used as a prophylactic medication to prevent recurrence of *Pseudomonas* infection. Recurrent *Pseudomonas* infection is common if the antibiotic is tapered too quickly while steroids are being used even in very low doses.

The use of a collagenase inhibitor is still controversial, and very few ophthalmologists use these medications today in conjunction with stromal melting caused by *Pseudomonas* infections. In the past, 10 or 20 percent solutions of acetylcysteine* have been employed four or five times a day.

Surgical. When endophthalmitis occurs secondary to cataract extraction, filtering blebs, or corneal or retinal surgery and this infection is caused by *P. aeruginosa*, the visual outcome is very poor. Immediate vitrectomy is indicated along with intravitreal injection* of antibiotics and corticosteroids, depending upon the severity of the infection. Early vitrectomy with intravitreal antibiotics is essential if there is any hope of salvaging vision in these severe postoperative infections caused by *Pseudomonas*.

PRECAUTIONS

Although one must carefully monitor the systemic levels of tobramycin or gentamicin when systemic therapy is being used, treatment with topical fortified drops to the cornea does not require close monitoring. For this reason, most bacterial corneal ulcers alone are treated with topical medication, which is highly effective in reaching the site of bacterial growth rapidly. The use of frequent topical drops every 15 or 30 minutes is far more effective in treating a corneal ulcer caused by *Pseudomonas* than is systemic medication. If systemic medication is needed for endophthalmitis or scleral involvement, one must obtain peak and trough antibiotic levels 30 minutes before and 30 minutes after antibiotic infusion. If the systemic levels are satisfactory every other day, serum creatinine levels should be obtained because systemic aminoglycosides, such as tobramycin and gentamicin, can cause kidney failure. The patient on long-term systemic antibiotics should also be followed by an internist.

The use of corticosteroids in bacterial corneal ulcers or endophthalmitis is very controversial. Once the *Pseudomonas* corneal ulcer seems to be brought under control with appropriate local therapy, steroids may be used judiciously. The rule is that steroids are to be used very cautiously in any patient with corneal ulcer caused by *Pseudomonas* because of the problem of recurrent infections, as mentioned previously. Corticosteroids should be used in the lowest effective dosage and accompanied by antibiotics.

COMMENTS

Serious infections caused by *Pseudomonas* have become a problem because of their increasing frequency, particularly in soft daily-wear and extended-wear contact lens users. The chief characteristics of this organism are its antibiotic resistance and rapid and deep spread with resulting corneal thinning and perforation. Corneal perforation has been seen within 24 hours of the onset of a *Pseudomonas* corneal ulcer. All suspicious corneal ulcers should be treated with fortified preparations of either tobramycin or gentamicin until the culture definitely shows the absence of a gram-negative organism.

The prognosis is very grave for scleral involvement and *P. aeruginosa* endophthalmitis.

References

Clemmons CS, et al: Pseudomonas ulcers following patching of corneal abrasions associated with contact lens wear. CLAO J 13:3, 1987.
Donnenfeld ER, et al: Changing trends in contact lens associated corneal ulcers: An overview of 116 cases. CLAO J 12:145–149, 1986.
Hassman G, Sugar J: Pseudomonas corneal ulcer with extended wear soft lens for myopia. Arch Ophthalmol 101:1549–1560, 1983.
Stern GA, et al: Adherence to *Pseudomonas aeruginosa* to the mouse cornea. Epithelial stromal adherence. Arch Ophthalmol 100:1956–1958, 1982.

RELAPSING FEVER
(Recurrent Fever)

S.Y. SALIH, M.D., M.R.C.P., D.C.M.T.,
Khartoum, Sudan

and L.F. RICH, M.S., M.D.
Portland, Oregon

Relapsing fever is an acute infectious disease caused by spirochetes of the genus *Borrelia* that are transmitted in humans by lice (causing an endemic form of the disease) and by ticks (causing an epidemic form of the disease). The clinical course of infection transmitted by either vector tends to be similar. It is characterized by toxemia and recurring febrile paroxysms separated by afebrile periods. Relapses duplicating the original attack recur at intervals of 1 to 2 weeks and become progressively less severe. Recovery usually occurs after two to ten relapses. Ocular involvement in relapsing fever is not uncommon, particularly in the tick-borne form of the disease. The ocular symptoms usually occur during periods of relapse, rather than in the initial febrile attack. Common ocular manifestations may include extraocular muscle paralysis, uveitis, conjunctivitis, a transient interstitial keratitis, palpebral edema, and visual impairment. Retrobulbar neuritis and optic atrophy may be produced if there has been meningeal involvement.

THERAPY

Systemic. The medication of choice is tetracycline, given orally in an adult dosage of 0.5 gm every 6 hours for 7 days and followed by 1 gm daily for another 5 days. This treatment usually clears all infection and prevents the occurrence of relapses. Alternative treatment may be with aqueous procaine penicillin G, which is given in a dosage of 600,000 units daily by intramuscular injection for 10 days.

Recent information suggests that combination therapy with both tetracycline and aqueous procaine penicillin G may be even more effective than use of either drug singly. Such combination treatment avoids the severe reaction that invariably follows tetracycline treatment and clears any residual brain infection. In this therapy, 400,000 units of aqueous procaine penicillin G are given by intramuscular injection on the first day. This treatment is followed the next 7 days by 500 mg of oral tetracycline, given every 6 hours.

Ocular. For uveitis, 2 per cent homatropine or 0.25 per cent scopolamine eyedrops may be applied twice daily to keep the pupil dilated and produce cycloplegia. Topical corticosteroid eyedrops may be used during waking hours to reduce inflammation, and an ointment containing 0.05 per cent dexamethasone may be applied at night before retiring.

Supportive. The patient with relapsing fever is extremely ill; therefore, careful nursing is essential. Bedrest is indicated for all patients with this infection. Liberal fluids and proper nutrition are necessary. Since relapses may lead to the false assumption that the infection has run its course, the patient should not be allowed to undertake strenuous work until complete recovery is certain.

Ocular or Periocular Manifestations

Anterior Chamber: Hypopyon.
Conjunctiva: Conjunctivitis; discharge; hemorrhages.
Cornea: Band-shaped keratopathy; dendritic keratitis; interstitial keratitis.
Optic Nerve: Atrophy (secondary to meningeal involvement); retrobulbar neuritis (secondary or meningeal involvement).
Retina: Exudates; hemorrhages; venous engorgement.
Vitreous: Exudates; opacity.
Other: Decreased visual acuity; icterus; ocular pain; paralysis of sixth or seventh cranial nerve; photophobia; ptosis, uveitis; visual loss.

Precautions

A Jarisch-Herxheimer reaction occurs quite commonly after administration of high doses of tetracycline or penicillin. Recent evidence indicates that the Jarisch-Herxheimer reaction with tetracycline may be greatly diminished if penicillin is given prior to administration of the tetracycline. Therefore, combination therapy may produce better results than use of either drug by itself. Complete bedrest for at least 48 hours after treatment with tetracycline or penicillin is recommended.

COMMENTS

Louse-borne relapsing fever has been reported from all continents, occurring most frequently in overcrowded areas where unhygienic conditions prevail. This disease is still a serious problem in the Near East, the Mediterranean Basin, and tropical America.

The prognosis is serious in both forms of the disease if no treatment is given. Tick-borne relapsing fever is an especially grave disease, since neurologic and ophthalmologic involvement often occurs in this type of relapsing fever. Death has occurred from hyperpyrexia with convulsions, myocardial failure, or hepatic coma; however, treatment of relapsing fever has greatly reduced mortality from the disease.

References

Bryceson ADM, et al: Louse-borne relapsing fever. A clinical and laboratory study of 62 cases in Ethiopia and a reconsideration of the literature. Q J Med 39:129–170, 1970.
Burgdorfer W: The relapsing fevers. In Hunter GW III, Swartzwelder JC, Clyde DF: Tropical Medicine, 5th ed. Philadelphia, WB Saunders, 1976, pp 137–146.
Duke-Elder S (ed.): System of Ophthalmology. St. Louis, CV Mosby, 1976, Vol XV, p 138.
Ginsberg SP: Corneal problems in systemic disease. In Duane T (ed): Clinical Ophthalmology. Hagerstown, MD, Harper & Row, 1982, Vol V, pp 43:1–23.
Magnarelli LA: Serologic diagnosis of Lyme disease. Ann NY Acad Sci 539:154–161, 1988.
Rogell G: Infectious and inflammatory diseases. In Duane TD (ed): Clinical Ophthalmology. Hagerstown, MD, Harper & Row, 1982, Vol V, pp 33:14–15.
Salih SY, Mustafa D: Louse-borne relapsing fever. II. Combined penicillin and tetracycline therapy in 160 Sudanese patients. Trans R Soc Trop Med Hyg 71:49–51, 1977.
Southern PM Jr, Sanford JP: Relapsing fever. A clinical and microbiological review. Medicine 48:129–149, 1969.
Warrell DA, et al: Pathophysiology and immunology of the Jarisch-Herxheimer-like reaction in louse-borne relapsing fever: comparison of tetracycline and slow-release penicillin. J Infect Dis 147:898–909, 1983.

STAPHYLOCOCCUS

ROBERT C. KIMBROUGH, III, M.D., F.A.C.P.

Portland, Oregon

Staphylococci are gram-positive, aerobic (facultatively anaerobic), nonmotile bacteria that tend to grow in clusters. Most of the staphylococci isolated from skin infections are *Staphylococcus aureus*. These organisms produce coagulase and a golden pigment and elaborate a number of exotoxins. The cell walls of these coagulase-positive cocci contain protein A and teichoic acid antigens. Rarely does *S. epidermidis*, which is coagulase-negative and generally nonhemolytic, cause skin infections. The staphylococci may produce serious infections of any organ and may cause bacteremia. These ubiquitous organisms frequently colonize the nose, the umbilicus in neonates, and less often the perineum or the gut. Chronic skin colonization and infection may begin early in childhood and continue throughout life.

The hallmark of staphylococcal infection is abscess formation and local disease. Chronic localized infections are caused by the organism's ability to live in partially anaerobic environments, to protect itself from host defense mechanisms by microabscess formation, and to survive inside of phagocytes. Multiple host factors predispose to more serious staphylococcal disease: breakdown in skin defense, as with intravenous catheters; pulmonary injury, as with influenza and numerous leukocyte-related and humoral defects; antibiotic and steroid therapy; implantation of foreign bodies; and a host of underlying debilitating diseases, ranging from diabetes mellitus to hypogammaglobulinemia. Disseminated staphylococcal diseases may be due to direct invasion, as with bacteremias, or be secondary to toxin production, as in the scalded skin syndrome and staphylococcal gastroenteritis.

Staphylococci may infect any portion of the eye or orbital structures. Marginal blepharitis, conjunctivitis, and corneal problems are common disorders. Orbital cellulitis and endophthalmitis are the more serious ophthalmic infections.

THERAPY

Systemic. Specific antimicrobial therapy is chosen based on the site and severity of the infection and the particular antimicrobial sensitivities of the organism involved. Fewer than 20 per cent of staphylococci are still sensitive to penicillin. Indeed, resistance to the semisynthetic penicillinase-resistant penicillins has occurred with increasing frequency in the past decade. Because of numerous clinical failures, these resistant staphylococci must be treated with vancomycin.

Methicillin and nafcillin are equally efficacious parenteral penicillinase-resistant penicillins. Both should be given in daily dosages of 150 to 175 mg/kg. Methicillin has the disadvantage of possibly causing interstitial nephritis, whereas nafcillin may produce neutropenia. Oxacillin may be used in the same dose. None of these drugs should be administered at less than every 6 hours and preferably at every 4-hour intervals.

Cephalosporins are acceptable alternatives to semisynthetic penicillinase-resistant penicillin in patients who have had prior reactions to penicillin. The newer cephalosporins, "second- and third-generation" cephalosporins, are much less effective against staphylococci than are the "first-generation" drugs. For serious infections, the choice should be limited to cephalothin, cephapirin, cephradine, or cefazolin. Intravenous doses of cephalothin or cephapirin should be 150 to 175 mg/kg per day for serious infections. Cefazolin has the advantage of being given intramuscularly or intravenously in a maximum dose of 1 gm every 6 hours. Oral preparations of the semisynthetic penicillinase-resistant penicillins and cephalosporins are available for less serious infections. The usual oral dosage schedule is 250 to 500 mg every 6 hours.

No staphylococci have yet been found resistant to vancomycin. This drug is available only or parenteral administration in intravenous dosages of 500 mg every 6 hours given over a 1-hour period. High levels of vancomycin, greater than 30 μg/ml, should be avoided because of ototoxicity.

Erythromycin, clindamycin, and tetracycline are oral and parenteral alternatives to the above antibiotics. Tetracycline may not be used in pregnant women or growing children. Clindamycin usage may be complicated by pseudomembranous colitis. Rifampin kills the staphylococci intracellularly; however, emergence of resistance is rapid, and this drug should not be used as a single antistaphylococcal agent. In combination with either parenteral or local therapy, rifampin may be useful in oral dosages of 300 to 600 mg every 12 hours. Rifampin may be particularly useful in combination regimes for the elimination of the staphylococcal carrier state.

Ocular. Staphylococcal infections of the lid may be treated with applications of various antibiotic ointments, including sulfacetamide, aminoglycosides (gentamicin or tobramycin), erythromycin, or bacitracin. The severity of the illness will dictate the frequency of application. Conjunctivitis or keratitis will respond to the same drugs delivered by eyedrops.

Corneal complications that may not be primarily infectious may be treated with numerous anti-inflammatory steroid preparations. In addition to steroid preparations, anterior uveitis may be improved by the application of 1 per cent atropine solution. Intraocular infections should be treated with both systemic, subconjunctival,* and intraocular* antimicrobial agents.

Supportive. Localized abscesses that do not spontaneously drain with moist heat require incision and drainage. Occluded secretions of the Meibomian gland may be gently expressed by squeezing the lid between two cotton-tipped applicators, after scaling has been removed with a mild shampoo of the lids. If lid seborrhea is an associated problem, it should be treated with a mild antiseborrheic product.

The anterior nares, the nasolabial fold, and the hands and fingernails all harbor staphylococci. In vigorous attempts to overcome the carrier state, antibiotic ointment must be applied to these areas. Bacitracin is recommended; however, aminoglycoside ointments are also effective.

Ocular of Periocular Manifestations

Anterior Chamber: Cells and flare; hypopyon.
Conjunctiva: Chemosis, hyperemia; phlyctenules; purulent conjunctivitis.
Cornea: Keratitis; marginal ulcerative abscess; perforation, phlyctenules.
Eyelids: Abscess; cellulitis; ectropion; edema; entropion; granuloma; hordeolum; madarosis; meibomianitis; ptosis; seborrheic blepharitis.
Globe: Endophthalmitis; panophthalmitis.
Iris: Nongranulomatous anterior uveitis; posterior synechiae.
Orbit: Cellulitis; osteomyelitis; periosteitis.
Other: Dacryocystitis; increased intraocular pressure; ocular pain; photophobia.

PRECAUTIONS

Emergence of methicillin-resistant *S. aureus* and penicillin- and methicillin-resistant *S. epidermidis* is a concern in nosocomial infections. For this reason, vigorous attempts should be made to isolate the organisms and perform sensitivities to a wide range of antimicrobials. Sensitivity patterns may differ from hospital to hospital, particularly from the teaching hospital setting to the community hospital.

COMMENTS

The most likely gram-positive cocci to produce central corneal ulcers are *S. aureus*. In the past, *S. aureus* was implicated as the single most responsible organism for causing endophthalmitis. Although *S. epidermidis* is not usually considered a pathogen, it has also been responsible for endophthalmitis.

References

Bryan CS, et al: Topical antibiotic ointments for staphylococcal nasal carriers: Survey of current practices and comparison of bacitracin and vancomycin ointments. Infection Control 1:153–156, 1980.
Kaplan MH, Tenebaum MJ: Staphylococcus aureus: Cellular biology and clinical application. Am J Med 72:248–258, 1982.
Musher DM, McKenzie SO: Infections due to *Staphylococcus aureus*. Medicine 56:383–409, 1977.
Smith IM: *Staphylococcus aureus. In* Mandell GL, Douglas RG Jr, Bennet JE: Principles and Practice of Infectious Diseases. New York, John Wiley & Sons, 1979, pp 1530–1552.
Waldvogel FA: *Staphylococcus aureus. In* Mandell GL, Douglas RG Jr, Bennet JE: Principles and Practice of Infectious Diseases, 2nd ed. New York, John Wiley & Sons, 1985, pp 1097–1117.
Zinner SH, Lagast H, Klastersky J: Antistaphylococcal activity of rifampin with other antibiotics. J Infect Dis 144:365–371, 1981.

STREPTOCOCCUS
JOHN R. SAMPLES, M.D.
Portland, Oregon

Streptococci and aerococci are gram-positive, catylase-negative cocci that may appear singly, in pairs, in short chains, or in long chains. These organisms are facultative anaerobes, although some strains can grow poorly under aerobic conditions. *Streptococcus* is a ubiquitous organism and is part of the normal flora of the mouth, pharynx, and the intestinal tract of humans.

Streptococci may be classified according to a serologic system based upon antigenic carbohydrate extracted from the cell wall. Based on both the chemical composition and immunologic reactivity of this carbohydrate, streptococci can be divided into 18 groups (A through H and K through T). The organisms within each of these groups are similar.

Some streptococci are not grouped on the basis of carbohydrate antigenicity, including the anaerobes, but according to their ability to produce hemolysis. Alpha-hemolysis is denoted by a greenish color of the sheep red blood cells that surround the colony, which indicates the incomplete or partial lysis of red blood cells. Beta-hemolysis is denoted by a clear zone surrounding the colony, which indicates the complete lysis of blood cells. Gamma-hemolysis indicates that there is no lysis of erythrocytes surrounding the colony. Two compounds, termed hemolysins, cause beta-hemolysis. One is streptolysin-O, which is antigenic and oxygen-sensitive. The other is streptolysin-S, which is nonantigenic and resistant to oxygen. If only aerobic incubation is used when streptococci are identified, oxygen will neutralize the activity of streptolysin-O and cause beta-hemolytic colonies to be overlooked.

The alpha-hemolytic *Streptococcus* that is the most common and important human pathogen is *Streptococcus pneumonia.* Although there is only one species of this organism, frequently termed pneumococcus, there are 83 distinct serotypes. On gram stain, this organism appears as oval or spherical gram-positive diplococci with distal ends that are pointed or lancet shaped. This organism is responsible for conjunctivitis, endophthalmitis, and dacryocystitis and is becoming increasingly resistant to penicillin. As a result, when the organism is isolated, antimicrobial susceptibility testing may be helpful. Alpha-hemolytic streptococci are found as part of the normal flora of the mouth and pharynx. Nonetheless, they may be pathologic agents as in acute or subacute bacterial endocarditis.

Beta-hemolytic streptococci are probably the most common streptococcus to cause human disease. *S. pyrogenese*, a group A organism, has been isolated from the eyelids in conjunctivitis, in periorbital cellulitis, in endophthalmitis, and keratitis. Its normal habitat is the nasopharynx, skin, and rectum. These organisms are harmful in three ways: through direct invasion, through the elaboration of erythogenic toxin that is an exotoxin responsible for scarlet fever, and by provoking immunoresponses resulting in delayed postinfectious syndromes, such as acute rheumatic fever and acute glomerulonephritis. *S. agalactiae* (Group B) has been isolated in neonatal conjunctivitis, endophthalmitis accompanying meningitis, and adult endophthalmitis. *S.* *equisimilis* (Group C) has been identified as a cause of endophthalmitis and conjunctivitis.

Aerococci are alpha-hemolytic gram-positive cocci that have been identified in subacute bacterial endocarditis and urinary tract infections. They are not known to be pathogens in the eye.

THERAPY

Systemic. Traditionally, penicillin has been regarded as the drug of choice for streptococcal infections. However, with the emergence of penicillin resistance, therapy needs to be tailored to the antibiotic sensitivity of the infecting organism. Generally, the alpha-streptococci, including pneumococcus, are resistant to aminoglycosides and polymyxin B, but are susceptible to cephalosporins, erythromycin, clindamycin, bacitracin, vancomycin, and chloramphenicol. The beta-streptococci, excluding enterococci, are susceptible to penicillin, cephalosporins, erythromycin, bacitracin, vancomycin, clindamycin, and chloramphenicol. Enterococci usually respond to a combined therapy that includes both penicillin or vancomycin, as well as an aminoglycoside.

Penicillin is the drug of choice for pneumococcal pneumonia. Unless complications are present, the presently advocated high-dose regimes provide little advantage over the standard daily dose of 1.2 to 2.4 million units. The many alternative drugs available for the treatment of pneumococcal infections include erythromycin, clindamycin, cephaloridine, and other cephalosporins. Although cephalosporins have excellent bactericidal activity against pneumococci, they must be used with caution in a penicillin-allergic patient. It should be kept in mind that first- and second-generation cephalosporins are ineffective in the treatment of meningitis. Clindamycin is also ineffective against meningitis, but chloramphenicol is an acceptable alternative for pneumococcal meningitis. A mutation pneumococcal gene that includes penicillin-binding proteins groups I and II decreases the affinity of these proteins for penicillin and leads to the increase in penicillin resistance. A type 57 pneumococcus has been identified in Durbin, South Africa, which is completely resistant to penicillin, ampicillin, cephaloridine, erythromycin, chloramphenicol, and clindamycin. The strain has remained sensitive to vancomycin, rifampin, and bacitracin. This organism has produced at least 15 cases of pneumonia and meningitis. A multiple resistant Type 6-B pneumococcus was identified in Colorado in 1980. This organism was resistant to penicillin G, chloramphenicol, and tetracycline and was isolated from the cerebrospinal fluid of an infant who had meningitis. The organism was sensitive to rifampin, ampicillin, and chloramphenicol. Penicillin-resistant pneumococci have also been isolated in cases from Brooklyn, New York.

Pneumococcal vaccines are excellent, safe immunogens that produce long-lasting antibody titers. However, children younger than 2 years of age respond poorly to the vaccine. There have been few side effects reported, except for mild erythema and pain at the injection site. The efficacy of the vaccine remains controversial largely because of an ongoing failure to demonstrate its effectiveness. For this reason, it has not been well accepted for clinical use, with less than 25 percent of vaccine candidates being immunized. The vaccine is generally recommended in healthy adults older than 65 years and in adults with chronic respiratory disease, immunosuppression, cirrhosis, alcoholism, renal failure, Hodgkin's disease, myeloma, and those who are asplenic or have a splenic dysfunction.

Group A streptococci continue to be uniformly sensitive to penicillin, which remains the drug of choice. The dosage and duration vary enormously, ranging from 10 days of low-dose therapy for pharyngitis to prolonged high-dose intravenous therapy for osteomyelitis. Cephalosporins are effective substitutes in penicillin-allergic patients, but they must be used with caution because of the risk of an allergic cross-reactivity. As mentioned above, other alternatives include erythromycin, vancomycin, and clindamycin. Group B streptococci are sensitive to clinically achievable levels of penicillin, but the minimum inhibitory concentrations are somewhat higher than those for group A streptococci. Other streptococci, including anaerobes, are almost uniformly penicillin sensitive.

Ocular. Patients with conjunctivitis or eyelid involvement by *Streptococcus* should be treated systemically, as well as locally. Topical treatment may consist of the use of bacitracin or erythromycin ointment. Hot compresses and the removal of any impetiginous crust may be helpful.

Streptococcal conjunctivitis can usually be successfully treated with erythromycin or bacitracin alone.

When a streptococcal ulcer is evident, both topical and systemic therapy are indicated. Topical ophthalmic antibiotics, including erythromycin, bacitracin, or cefazolin,* should be given every hour while awake and every 2 hours at night. Subconjunctival injection of sodium penicillin G,* 0.5 to 1.0 million units, or 50 to 100 mg of methicillin* should be considered. Since this type of injection is painful, analgesia is advocated.

Streptococcal endophthalmitis requires prompt initiation of vigorous treatment with systemic, local, intraocular, and subconjunctival injections of antibiotics and steroids. At the time of vitrectomy or vitreous tap for culture, intracameral instillation of 250 μg of cephaloridine* or 1 mg of methicillin* with 0.1 mg of subconjunctival dexamethasone* is initiated. This is supplemented with topical application of 250 to 1,000 units/ml of bacitracin[§] or 100,000 units/ml of sodium penicillin G.[§] Orbital cellulitis secondary to *Streptococcus* should be treated with systemic antibiotics.

Supportive. Treatment of symptoms is important in patients with streptococcal sore throat. Analgesia for relief of headache, adequate hydration, and treatment of other symptoms are all necessary.

Ocular and Periocular Manifestations

Eyelids: Blepharitis; dermatitis; impetigo; madarosis; scarletina rash.
Conjunctiva: Chemosis; mucopurulent or purulent conjunctivitis; hyperemia.
Cornea: Hyperesthesia infiltration; ring ulcer; central ulcer.
Globe: Endophthalmitis; proptosis; lacrimal system dacroadenitis; dacrocystitis.
Optic Nerve: Optic neuritis.
Orbit: Abscess; cellulitis; thrombophlebitis.

Precautions

Penicillin must always be used with caution in patients who have a history of allergy or asthma. Cephalosporins must be used with the understanding that they may be cross-reactive with penicillin.

Comments

Streptococci are common bacterial pathogens in humans that produce infections in many tissues of the body. Because transmission may occur, vigorous hygiene is well advised in caring for these patients.

References

Abbott RL, Shekter WB: Necrotizing erysipelas of the eyelids. Ann Ophthalmol 11:381–384, 1979.
Brinser JH: Ocular bacteriology. In Tabbara KF, Hyndiuk RA (eds): Infections of the Eye. Boston, Little, Brown and Co, 1986.
Jacobs MR, Kornahof HJ, Robbins-Browne et al: Emergence of multiply resistant pneumococci. N Engl J Med 299:735, 1978.
Leveille AS, McMullan FD, Cavanaugh HD: Endophthalmitis following penetrating keratoplasty. Ophthalmology 83:38–39, 1977.
Liesegang TJ, Samples JR, Waller RR: Suppurative interstitial ring keratitis due to streptococcus. Ann Ophthalmol 16:392–396, 1984.
Multiply resistant pneumococcus—Colorado. MMWR 30:197, 1981.
Okumoto M, Smolin G: Pneumoccocal infections of the eye. Am J Ophthalmol 77:345–352, 1974.
Scott PM, Bloome MA: Lid necrosis secondary to streptococcal periorbital cellulitis. Ann Ophthalmol 13:461–465, 1981.
Wannamaker LW, Ferrieri P: Streptococcal infections—updated. DM; Disease–A–Month. Oct: 1–40, 1975.

TETANUS
(Lockjaw)

ALBERT W. BIGLAN, M.D., F.A.C.S.
Pittsburgh, Pennsylvania

Tetanus is an acute neuromuscular disease that results from the exotoxin produced by the anaerobic spore-forming bacteria, *Clostridium tetani*. Symptoms may be local or systemic and are characterized by uncontrolled spasms of voluntary muscles following the production, transport, and fixation of the exotoxin tetanospasmin on the cell membranes of the striated muscle and the central nervous system. The symptoms of dysphagia, trismus, facial palsy, muscle stiffness, autonomic dysfunction sweating, urine retention, and irritability may occur shortly following a soil-contaminated penetrating wound. The incubation period may be 3 to 21 days. Complete recovery can be expected if the patient survives the acute episode.

Cephalic tetanus is a rare form of tetanus occurring in 1.1 per cent of the patients with generalized tetanus. Cephalic tetanus produces a paradoxic development of a cranial nerve palsy with uncontrolled spasms. Unlike generalized tetanus, cephalic tetanus may leave a residual weakness of the affected nerve.

THERAPY

Systemic.
TETANUS PROPHYLAXIS. Most children complete an active immunization against tetanus by receiving one dose of diphtheria and tetanus toxoids and pertussis vaccine (DTP) on four occasions starting at 6 weeks of age. The first three doses are given at 4- to 8-week intervals. The fourth or reinforcing dose is given 1 year after the third dose.

In persons 7 years of age and older, a series of three doses of tetanus and diphtheria toxoids adsorbed (TD) is given intramuscularly. The second dose should be given intramuscularly 4 to 8 weeks after the first and the third dose 6 months to a year after the second. TD is the preferred agent in this age group, because side effects from the higher dose of diphtheria toxoid in DTP are more common in older children and adults and because pertussis in these age groups is infrequent.

TETANUS PROPHYLAXIS IN ROUTINE WOUND MANAGEMENT. The need for active immunization with or without passive immunization depends on the condition of the wound. Complete primary immunization with tetanus toxoid (DTP or DT) provides long-lasting protection for 10 years or more. If a fresh wound is tetanus prone (deep or severe puncture), a booster is appropriate if the patient has not received tetanus toxoid within the preceding 5 years.

Patients who have not completed a full immunization series may require tetanus toxoid and passive immunization with 250 units of intramuscular human tetanus immune globulin (TIG). When TIG is used with tetanus toxoid (DTP or TD), separate syringes and injection sites should be used.

TREATMENT OF PATIENTS WITH CLINICAL TETANUS. Treatment of tetanus consists of meticulous surgical débridement of the wound, antibiotics to eliminate the causative organism, antitoxin to bind the circulating clostridial toxin, and supportive measures. Antitoxin, available as human tetanus immune globulin (TIG), is given intramuscularly in doses of 3000 to 6000 units. Recommended antibiotic administration includes 1 million units of aqueous penicillin G intravenously every 6 hours or 1.2 million units of aqueous procaine penicillin G intramuscularly every 6 hours for 10 days. Two grams of tetracycline daily are sufficient for patients who have an allergy to penicillin.

In mild cases of generalized tetanus or cases with dysphagia or respiratory difficulties, supportive care consists of management with titrated doses of 5 to 10 mg of diazepam every three to four hours. Moderate cases, those with pronounced spasticity, dysphagia, and respiratory problems, require tracheostomy in addition to sedation. Severe cases with gross spasticity and major spasms require paralysis with curare agents and artificial ventilation. Very severe cases with sympathetic overactivity require very heavy sedation, general anesthesia, and adrenergic blockade.

Simultaneous with management of the acute episode, active immunization should be started using 0.5 ml of tetanus toxoid intramuscularly with subsequent doses to complete the active immunization series.

Ocular. Tetracycline ointment should be applied to the eye every 2 to 6 hours. Cycloplegia with atropine may be used to manage uveitis following trauma. In patients receiving prolonged respirator therapy, care for the globe with frequent lubrication is essential. Temporary tarsorrhaphy may be necessary in patients with accompanying seventh cranial nerve palsy.

Surgical. Careful débridement and removal of all foreign material, both intraocular and periocular, in any tetanus-prone wound should be accomplished. Primary closure of the wound or wounds is recommended.

Ocular or Periocular Manifestations

Conjunctiva: Chemosis; hyperemia; necrosis.
Cornea: Exposure keratitis and ulcer (secondary to seventh cranial nerve palsy or prolonged respirator care).
Extraocular Muscles: Nystagmus; palsy of the sixth, third, and fourth cranial nerves (in decreasing frequency); spasm.
Eyelids: Blepharospasm; ptosis (may be asso-

ciated with a third nerve palsy); tonic spasm (pseudoptosis).

Orbit: Abscess; panophthalmitis; trauma changes.

Precautions

The extent of injury does not seem to have any relationship to susceptibility to tetanus. A trivial wound or an insect bite can produce tetanus, although most cases arise from severe globe or orbital trauma. Time from the injury to the onset of symptoms may be as long as 2 weeks. Patients without prior immunization should be observed closely during this period. Local reactions to DTP are common and do not indicate sensitization; however, severe and fatal adverse reactions can occur.

Immunosuppressive therapy may suppress the immune response, and routine vaccinations should be deferred if possible during such therapy. In addition, a severe febrile illness is reason to defer routine vaccinations.

Comments

Tetanus is a preventable disease; its incidence has declined to approximately 90 cases annually in the United States, and two thirds of the cases are 50 years of age or older. Tetanus cases occur almost exclusively in unimmunized or inadequately immunized patients. Mortality is high, ranging from 15 to 46 per cent, and the coexistence of cephalic tetanus does not adversely affect the mortality. Spores of *C. tetani* are ubiquitous, and there is no natural immunity to tetanus toxin. Therefore, all patients with penetrating injuries should be given appropriate prophylaxis. If a severe case of clinical tetanus develops intensive medical care is required, and referral to a tertiary care center should be considered.

References

Biglan AW, Ellis FD, Wade TA: Supranuclear oculomotor palsy and exotropia after tetanus. Am J Ophthalmol 86:666–668, 1978.
Bleck TP: Pharmacology of tetanus. Clin Neuropharmacol 9:103–120, 1986.
Edmondson RS, Flowers MW: Intensive care in tetanus: Management, complications, and mortality in 100 cases. Br Med J 1:1401–1404, 1979.
Immunization Practices Advisory Committee: Diphtheria, tetanus, and pertussis. Guidelines for vaccine prophylaxis and other preventive measures. Ann Intern Med 95:723–728, 1981.
Recommendation of The Immunization Practices Advisory Committee: Diphtheria, Tetanus and Pertussis Guidelines for Vaccine Prophylaxis and Other Preventive Measures. MMWR 34:405–426, 1985.
Rothstein RJ, Baker FJ II: Tetanus. Prevention and treatment. JAMA 240:675–676, 1978.
Wetzel JO: Tetanus following eye injury. Report of case: Review of literature. Am J Ophthalmol 25:933–944, 1942.

TUBERCULOSIS
THOMAS C. SPOOR, M.D., M.S., F.A.C.S.
Detroit, Michigan

Tuberculosis is a communicable disease caused by the acid-fast bacillus, *Mycobacterium tuberculosis*. It occurs primarily as a pulmonary infection; however, the bacillus may be widely disseminated hematogenously. Tuberculosis infection of the eye is rare and may occur as either a primary or secondary infection. Primary ocular infection is often a conjunctivitis, probably introduced into the eye by contaminated hands, fomites, or exposure to dust or sputum particles containing tubercle bacilli. In secondary infection (hematogenously spread), tubercles may be present in or on any part of the eye. Tuberculous allergic manifestations (phlyctenular keratitis and conjunctivitis) are more common than ocular infection. Ocular symptoms may also result from infection of adjacent structures (sinuses and orbit) or from intracranial involvement of the optic pathways.

In the United States, tuberculosis affects 28,000 persons annually (13/100,000), causing 2800 deaths. The incidence may increase due to recrudescence of disease in the elderly population, growth of immigration from endemic areas (Southeast Asia, Mexico), and the increased number of cases of acquired immunodeficiency syndrome (AIDS). Indeed, in 1986, a 1.7 per cent increase in the number of cases occurred after years of steady decline.

THERAPY

Systemic. Curative short-course therapy is available for tuberculosis using fully bactericidal drugs. The major barrier to effective therapy is premature cessation of treatment, which results in inadequate treatment and emergence of resistant organisms.

The specific drug regimen is usually chosen by the infectious disease consultant. One successful regimen consists of 300 mg of isoniazid and 600 mg of rifampin daily for 1 month, followed by 900 mg of isoniazid and 600 mg of rifampin given twice weekly for 8 additional months, or the daily regimen may be continued for 9 months. Ethambutol in a dosage of 15 to 25 mg/kg may be substituted for rifampin in resistant cases. However, a recent report describes several cases of irreversible, bilateral optic neuritis with resultant optic atrophy and permanent visual loss irrespective of ethambutol dosage. Thus, from an ophthalmologist's standpoint, ethambutol is a drug of last resort. Therefore, if primary drug resistance is suspected, 30 mg/kg of pyrazinamide per day may be added to the isoniazid/rifampin regimen. Resistance to pyrazinamide is rare. Addition of a third or fourth drug, such as 1 gm of intramuscular streptomycin daily for 2 months or 1 gm of pyrazinamide twice daily, is necessary in previously treated cases or

44 / TUBERCULOSIS

in cases thought to be acquired in countries where isoniazid resistance is common, such as in Southeast Asia, Mexico, and the Philippines. Such treatment may be continued for 6 to 8 weeks or until drug sensitivities are known. Addition of a third and fourth drug is of no advantage in cases sensitive to isoniazid and rifampin. Patients with AIDs and tuberculosis are treated initially with standard doses of a three-drug regimen.

Ocular. Systemic treatment is necessary for metastatic ocular tuberculosis and may also be necessary for primary ocular tuberculosis. Topical ophthalmic corticosteroids and cycloplegics may be necessary to control inflammation and prevent scarring due to keratitis and iritis. Secondary infection should be treated vigorously with topical antibiotics as sensitivities warrant. Localized lid lesions may be excised surgically.

Supportive. Rest, good diet, and improved general hygiene may be used as supportive measures to increase the patient's resistance.

Ocular or Periocular Manifestations

Choroid: Disseminated choroiditis; isolated tubercles.

Conjunctiva: Follicular, hypertrophic granulomatous, papillary, or purulent conjunctivitis; hyperemia; miliary ulcer; phlyctenules; polypoid "fibroma"; subconjunctival nodules (tuberculomas).

Cornea: Interstitial or sclerosing keratitis; mutton-fat keratic precipitates; pannus; phlyctenules; ulcer.

Eyelids: Blepharitis, cellulitis, edema; hyperemia; lupus tuberculosis; meibomianitis.

Iris: Granulomatous anterior uveitis; nodules.

Lacrimal System: Chronic dacryoadenitis; dacryocystitis; tuberculous pericystitis.

Motility: Internuclear ophthalmoplegia, gaze palsies.

Optic Nerve: Atrophy; optic neuritis (associated with tuberculous meningitis); optochiasmic arachnoiditis.

Orbit: Chronic cellulitis; fistula formation; periosteitis; primary abscess (extension from lacrimal gland or sinuses).

Retina: Exudative retinitis; periphlebitis.

Sclera: Perforation; scleritis; ulcer.

Other: Hypopyon; preauricular, submaxillary, or cervical lymphadenopathy; tuberculous panophthalmitis; vitreous hemorrhages.

PRECAUTIONS

Treatment with a single drug usually results in early emergence of resistant organisms. Combination drug therapy helps avoid this problem and should be supervised by physicians trained in this area. If drug toxicities occur, they may be controlled by altering the drug dosage or varying the antitubercular agents. Isoniazid is known to deplete pyridoxine and may induce a peripheral or optic neuropathy. This side effect may be ob-

viated by adding 50 mg of pyridoxine daily to the therapeutic regimen. Ethambutol may induce a dose-related optic neuritis, which has recently been shown to be *irreversible* upon discontinuation of the drug. Disadvantages of streptomycin use include intramuscular administration and eighth nerve dysfunction, which is a troublesome complication, especially in patients over 50 years of age who may be unable to compensate for loss of vestibular function. Pyrazinamide use has a very significant incidence of hepatotoxicity. Likewise, hepatic toxicity may occur secondary to isoniazid, but is reversible in its early stage. Long-term treatment with corticosteroids or immunosuppressants lowers host resistance and may cause reactivation of quiescent lesions.

COMMENTS

Phlyctenular keratoconjunctivitis is the most common form of external ocular tuberculosis. Conjunctival lesions are more commonly found on the palpebral than the bulbar conjunctiva and may be diagnosed by biopsy with appropriate stains and cultures. Orbital and sinus involvement are also reported infrequently.

The diagnosis of tuberculosis by the ophthalmologist is often indirect and is based upon the clinical picture, a positive purified protein derivative, and response to therapy. The ophthalmologist must consider tuberculosis as a possible etiology for any chronic anterior uveitis or disseminated choroiditis. One must also be aware that ophthalmic complications can occur secondary to treatment of systemic tuberculosis.

References

Cangemi FE, Friedman AH, Josephberg R: Tubercloma of the choroid. Ophthalmology 87:252–258, 1980.

De Vita EG, Maio M, Sadun A: Optic neuropathy in ethambutol-treated renal tuberculosis. J Clin Neuro-Ophthalmol 7:77–83, 1987.

DeVoe AG, Locatcher-Khorazo D: The external manifestations of ocular tuberculosis. Trans Am Ophthalmol Soc 62:203–212, 1964.

Fedukowicz HB: External infections of the Eye: Bacterial, Viral, and Mycotic, 2nd ed. New York, Appleton-Century-Crofts, 1978, pp. 136–141.

Goodwin RA Jr: Pulmonary tuberculosis. *In* Wyngaarden JB, Smith LH Jr (eds): Textbook of Medicine, 16th ed. Philadelphia, WB Saunders, 1982, pp 1542–1548.

Inocencio FP, Ballecer R: Tuberculosis granuloma in the midbrain causing wall-eyed bilateral intranuclear ophthalmoplegia. J Clin Neuro-Ophthalmol 5:31–35, 1985.

Locatcher-Khorazo D, Seegal BC: Microbiology of the Eye. St. Louis, CV Mosby, 1972, pp 119–130.

Prichard JG, Raleigh J: Tuberculosis and other mycobacterial diseases *In* Conn's Current Therapy. Philadelphia, WB Saunders, 1986, pp 167–174.

Schlaegel TF Jr, O'Connor GR: Tuberculosis and syphilis. Arch Ophthalmol 99:2206–2207, 1981.

Smith JL: Should ethambutol be barred? Editorial. J Clin Neuro-Ophthalmol 7:84–86, 1987.

Spoor TC, Harding SA: Orbital tuberculosis. Am J Ophthalmol 91:644–647, 1981.

Stead WW, Dutt AK: What's new in tuberculosis? Am J Med 71:1–4, 1981.

TULAREMIA
(Deerfly Tularemia, Pahvant Valley Plague, Rabbit Fever)

MALCOLM N. LUXENBERG, M.D.
Augusta, Georgia

Tularemia is an acute infectious disease caused by *Francisella tularensis*, a gram-negative coccobacillus. The disease occurs throughout the United States, but is most common in the Southeast. The organism has been recovered from many wild mammals, some domestic animals (such as the cat), and many insects. The most important reservoir hosts in the United States are rabbits and ticks. The route of entry is through the skin or mucous membranes, with human infection most frequently occurring after contact with tissues or body fluids of an infected animal or from the bite of an infected insect. Less frequently, infection can be acquired by inhalation of infectious aerosols, by ingestion of contaminated water, or by eating inadequately cooked meat from an affected animal. Infection can occur throughout the year and at any age, but is seen most frequently in adult males who are outdoorsmen or hunters.

The incubation period is approximately 3 to 5 days, after which a nodular ulcerated lesion develops at the site of entry. Most patients then have a rapid onset of fever, chills, malaise, and headache, followed by one of several clinical syndromes of which the ulceroglandular form is most common and the oculoglandular type least common. The portal of entry in the latter type is usually via the conjunctiva. The oculoglandular form is most frequently unilateral and is characterized by purulent conjunctivitis, nodular-ulcerative lesions of the conjunctiva, chemosis and periorbital edema, pain, and lymphadenopathy. Less commonly seen are corneal infiltrates, ulceration, scarring, and vascularization. Dacryocystitis occasionally occurs. In rare instances, there may be perforation of the cornea and endophthalmitis with loss of the eye. Laboratory diagnosis is difficult as gram stains of exudate are usually negative, the organism does not grow on routine media, and biopsies of lesions with standard stains rarely reveal the organism. Most cases are diagnosed by serologic testing with a fourfold rise in the tularemia agglutination titer considered to be diagnostic. Unfortunately, the agglutination titers are usually negative for the first 2 weeks after the initial infection and do not reach their maximum for 2 to 3 months.

THERAPY

Systemic. Streptomycin, which is bactericidal for the organism, is the drug of choice for the treatment of tularemia, and a rapid response to treatment, often within 48 hours, is seen in most cases. A daily dose of 15 to 20 mg/kg is given intramuscularly in divided doses for up to 14 days. In selected cases, gentamicin, which is also bactericidal, may be used in a daily dose of 5 mg/kg as a therapeutic alternative to streptomycin. Relapses are uncommon. Tetracycline may be used but is bacteriostatic for *F. tularensis*, and relapses occur more frequently with this drug, especially if it is used for less than 14 days. A loading dose of 30 mg/kg of tetracycline is given orally, followed by 30 mg/kg in divided doses for 14 days. There has been limited clinical experience with tobramycin.[‡]

Ocular. Topical gentamicin or tetracycline eyedrops should be used along with the systemic therapy. Administration every 2 to 3 hours for 1 to 2 days may be decreased to four times a day for 7 to 10 days if the infection is responding adequately. Cycloplegic drops should be used as needed. Cool compresses may provide symptomatic relief, especially in the acute phases.

Supportive. Medical consultation, preferably from a specialist in infectious diseases, should be obtained to help with the overall management, including selection and dosage of antibiotics, as this is a serious systemic illness.

Ocular or Periocular Manifestations

Conjunctiva: Chemosis; marked hyperemia; nodular ulcerative granuloma; purulent conjunctivitis.
Cornea: Infiltrates; opacity; perforation; ulcer; vascularization.
Eyelids: Edema; nodular ulcerative lesions.
Globe: Endophthalmitis.
Lacrimal System: Dacryocystitis.
Other: Ocular pain; periorbital edema; preauricular or cervical lymphadenopathy.

PRECAUTIONS

The dosage of streptomycin and gentamicin must be carefully adjusted depending on the patient's renal function and age. The patient should be properly monitored for possible development of toxicity from medications, such as streptomycin, which can damage the labyrinthine system.

COMMENTS

The diagnosis of tularemia infection of the eye can be difficult as the condition is uncommon and routine laboratory tests are usually negative, especially in the earlier stages. Therefore, a high index of suspicion is important, and a careful history for exposure to known vectors must be obtained. Once the diagnosis is made or strongly suspected, treatment should be started as quickly as possible, preferably with streptomycin, as the response to treatment is better and relapses less frequent if therapy is initiated within the first 2 weeks of illness.

References

Bloom ME, Shearer WT, Barton LL: Oculoglandular tularemia in an inner city child. Pediatrics 51:564–566, 1973.

Boyce JM: Francisella tularensis (Tularemia). *In* Mandell GL, Douglas RG Jr, Bennett JE: Principles and Practice of Infectious Diseases. New York, John Wiley & Sons, 1979, pp 1784–1788.

Evans ME, et al: Tularemia and the tomcat. JAMA *246*:1343, 1981.

Evans ME, et al: Tularemia: A 30-year experience with 88 cases. Medicine *64*:251–269, 1985.

Francis E: Oculoglandular tularemia. Arch Ophthalmol *28*:711–741, 1942.

Guerrant RL, et al: Tickborne oculoglandular tularemia. Arch Intern Med *136*:811–813, 1976.

Hanna C, Lyford JH: Tularemia infection of the eye. Ann Ophthalmol *3*:1321–1325, 1971.

Mason WL, et al: Treatment of tularemia, including pulmonary tularemia, with gentamicin. Am Rev Respir Dis *121*:39–45, 1980.

TYPHOID FEVER

GEORGE N. CHIN, M.D., F.A.C.S.
Seattle, Washington

Typhoid fever is an acute febrile illness caused by the ingestion of and the intestinal invasion by *Salmonella typhi*, a gram-negative bacillus found only in humans. Prevalent in those regions of the world lacking sanitary water and sewage systems, its transmission can occur through ingestion of contaminated food or water, contact with an acute case of typhoid fever, or contact with a chronic asymptomatic carrier. Transmission through direct fecal-oral contact is more common among children.

Typhoid fever is characterized by sustained fever, headache, chills, sore throat, coughing, nausea, vomiting, diarrhea, constipation, abdominal pain, anorexia, muscle pain, weakness, dizziness, and, occasionally, seizures. The onset is usually gradual, and the illness achieves maximum severity during the second or third week, with marked weakness, abdominal discomfort and distention, "rose spots" rash, cervical adenopathy, hepatomegaly, splenomegaly, rales, and occasional neurologic manifestations, such as mental dullness. Recovery, characterized by declining fever, begins by the end of the third or fourth week. The most prominent major complications are intestinal hemorrhage and perforation, which can occur during the third week, often heralded by a sudden drop in temperature and increased pulse.

Ocular manifestations of typhoid fever are rare and may include lid abscesses, corneal ulcers, uveitis, vitreous hemorrhage, retinal hemorrhage and detachment, panophthalmitis, optic neuritis, extraocular muscle palsies, orbital thrombosis, and orbital abscesses. Ocular complications of this nature are probably a result of direct invasion by the organism into the ocular tissues, but some such as vitreous hemorrhage following typhoid vaccination, may be hypersensitivity phenomena.

THERAPY

Systemic. Diagnosis of typhoid fever is made through isolation of *Salmonella* organisms from cultures of blood, urine, stool, bone marrow aspirates, or skin biopsies of "rose spots." Once the illness is confirmed, prompt antimicrobial therapy should begin. Chloramphenicol is the preferred antibiotic, given orally or intravenously in daily dosages of 50 mg/kg divided into four doses for at least 14 days. A general sense of improvement and well-being can be expected within 48 hours. The febrile episode may continue for 5 to 7 days and should not be interpreted as treatment failure.

Numerous reports over the last 15 years have documented the presence of chloramphenicol-resistant strains of typhoid fever. When these are present, ampicillin should be administered orally or intravenously in dosages of 100 mg/kg per day in four divided doses for at least 14 days. Most of the *S. typhi* chloramphenicol-resistant strains have been found in Mexico, India, and southeast Asia.

When isolates are shown to be resistant to both chloramphenicol and ampicillin, a trimethoprim-sulfamethoxazole[‡] combination has proven to be a reasonably effective alternative. This combination of 320 to 640 mg of trimethoprim with 1.6 to 3.2 gm of sulfamethoxazole may be given orally or intravenously in two divided doses for 2 weeks. Slow intravenous infusion of 160 mg of trimethoprim and 800 mg of sulfamethoxazole diluted in 250 ml of 5 per cent dextrose in water may be administered every 12 hours. Rapid infusion or bolus injection should be avoided.

Severely toxemic patients may benefit from a short course of systemic corticosteroids, such as 60 mg of intravenous prednisolone. Corticosteroid therapy should be rapidly tapered and discontinued after the third day.

Treatment of chronic carriers of *S. typhi* consists of oral ampicillin in daily doses of 3 to 6 gm for 4 to 6 weeks. Chloramphenicol has no influence on the chronic typhoid fever carrier state. Radiographic examination of the biliary tract is essential during the initial assessment, since the gallbladder is the nidus of the chronic carrier state in the majority of such patients. If gallbladder disease is not evident, prolonged administration of ampicillin may end the carrier state. All chronic carriers should be discouraged from handling food and must be carefully instructed in the importance of hand washing. The appropriate public health officials should be notified.

Ocular. In addition to systemic antibiotics, ocular infection with salmonellosis should be treated with frequent topical chloramphenicol and/or periocular injection of ampicillin* when indicated. Lid abscesses should be drained and specimens carefully handled for culture. Topical application of a chloramphenicol ointment may be applied to the wound. All purulent conjunctival discharges should be irrigated with saline. Conjunctivitis and corneal ulcers should be treated with an hourly application of 0.5 per cent chloramphenicol ophthalmic solution, with appropriate smears and cultures taken to rule out secondary invaders. If corneal perforation occurs, the general method of treatment includes pressure bandage, tissue adhesives, or blowout patch.

Uveitis can be treated with 1 per cent atropine ophthalmic solution three times a day to keep the pupil dilated and prevent synechiae. Prednisolone, 1 percent ophthalmic suspension, should also be instilled hourly to control the inflammation and should be tapered according to its response.

Orbital infection and vitreous, retinal, optic nerve, and intraocular muscle involvement are much more difficult to treat. Since their pathogenesis is unknown, no effective treatment has been found. Exudative nonrhegmatogenous retinal detachment has been shown to respond to oral administration of 40 to 60 mg of prednisone for 3 days, which controls the exudative fluid. When endophthalmitis or panophthalmitis is present, the prognosis for visual recovery is poor. To relieve ocular pain, hot packs or compresses 10 to 15 minutes three times a day may be effective.

Supportive. Supportive care with particular attention given to nutritional requirements, adequate hydration, and correction of electrolyte disorders is of utmost importance during the initial phase of managing typhoid fever patients. All patients should be hospitalized under enteric isolation precaution in order to prevent spreading the disease to other patients and hospital personnel. Vital signs and white blood cell count must be carefully monitored. Bedrest during the initial phase is essential; ambulation should be gradual. Tepid sponge baths or cooling blankets can reduce the temperature of individuals with severe hyperpyrexia. Codeine rather than aspirin should be used in treating headache, since salicylates can produce wide swings in temperature with very uncomfortable chills and sweats, in addition to their effects on blood platelets and irritating action on the bowels. Hypothermia and hypotension occur in some patients after administration of salicylates. A high caloric liquid diet should be provided to those capable of oral intake. Those who cannot eat should be given intravenous infusion supplemented with vitamins.

Transfusion is indicated if significant intestinal hemorrhaging occurs. Typing and cross-matching should be done at the time of initial diagnosis of typhoid fever. If perforation is suspected, emphasis should be placed on efforts to combat shock and decompression of the bowels. Additional antimicrobials may be added to control peritonitis. Small perforations may localize and can be managed without surgical intervention. Typhoid patients are considered poor surgical risks.

Ocular or Periocular Manifestations

Conjunctiva: Chemosis; conjunctivitis; subconjunctival hemorrhages.
Cornea: Ulcer.

Extraocular Muscles: Conjugate gaze paralysis; paralysis; tenonitis.
Eyelids: Abscess; hemorrhages.
Globe: Endophthalmitis; panophthalmitis.
Iris: Iritis; uveitis.
Optic Nerve: Disc edema; optic neuritis.
Orbit: Abscess; cellulitis; orbital vein thrombosis.
Retina: Central retinal artery emboli; edema; exudative detachment; hemorrhages; venous engorgement.
Vitreous: Hemorrhages.
Other: Central scotoma; choroiditis; dacryoadenitis; hypopyon; ocular pain; paralysis of accommodation; visual loss.

PRECAUTIONS

Because salicylates can produce severe hypothermia and vascular collapse, they should be avoided in patients with typhoid fever. Laxatives and enemas should be avoided despite constipation, since they may precipitate intestinal hemorrhage and ulcer perforation.

All patients receiving chloramphenicol should be monitored for bone marrow toxicity, and a complete blood count should be obtained. Chloramphenicol-induced granulocytopenia may occur and is reversible with discontinuation of the antibiotic. Aplastic anemia is rare, but may follow the use of chloramphenicol.

Renal function should be monitored in patients receiving trimethoprim and sulfamethoxazole, and a creatinine clearance should be done. The most frequent clinical side effects seen with these drugs are rash, nausea, and vomiting; megaloblastic anemia may also occur. In any event, the drugs should be reduced or discontinued if these adverse reactions occur. Patients receiving trimethoprim, sulfamethoxazole, or ampicillin should be monitored for hypersensitivity reactions.

Although immunization with typhoid vaccine provides significant immunity against typhoid infection, protection is not complete and can be readily overcome by a large dose of organisms. Nevertheless, immunization is recommended for those individuals living or traveling in areas where the disease is endemic and for persons working with the organism in the laboratory. Family members of a chronic carrier should also be vaccinated. Immunization of a person living within the United States is not necessary. Because of the extremely low prevalence of the disease and of carriers in the United States, mass vaccination against typhoid, even in such disasters as floods, is rarely needed. Adults should receive 0.5 ml of vaccine on two separate occasions 1 to 2 weeks apart. The vaccine causes a transient titer elevation of agglutinins against typhoid O antigens for several months and a persistent elevated titer for H antigens. The yearly booster is required to maintain immunity.

Local health authorities should be made aware of all typhoid fever patients so that appropriate field investigation can begin to determine the source of infection. Precautions should be ob-

48 / TYPHOID FEVER

served to prevent the spread of infection from persons with active cases or from carriers. Stool specimens should be cultured during convalescence at weekly intervals. Three consecutive negative stool cultures usually indicate that a carrier state does not exist. On the other hand, a positive culture 4 months after treatment indicates a carrier state may have developed. Chronic or convalescing carriers should not be allowed to prepare food until clear documentation shows that at least three or more stool cultures are negative for typhoid bacilli. Carriers should be cautioned regarding routine sanitary techniques.

COMMENTS

As many as 20 per cent of all patients with typhoid fever who are successfully treated with chloramphenicol may relapse. In most cases, relapse appears as a brief febrile illness 2 to 4 weeks after the completion of antimicrobial therapy. Relapses usually do not require treatment due to the self-limiting nature of the illness, but retreatment with antibiotics for 1 week may be necessary if symptoms persist longer than 36 to 48 hours. Therapy is identical to that of the initial episode.

The mortality rate of typhoid fever prior to the introduction of chloramphenicol was about 12 per cent. Mortality presently stands at 2 to 3 per cent in patients treated with proper antibiotic therapy and 10 per cent in untreated patients. Causes of death include toxemia, inanition, pneumonia, and intestinal perforation and hemorrhage. Death is primarily observed in infants, the aged, or individuals with malnutrition or other underlying diseases.

References

Bajpai PC, Dikshit SK: Bilateral optic neuritis and encephalitis complicating typhoid fever. J Indian Med Assoc 30:54–57, 1958.
Calhoun FP: Ocular complications due to typhoid inoculations. Arch Ophthalmol 48:553–558, 1919.
Dhir SP, et al: *Salmonella* lid abscess. Indian J Ophthalmol 24:27–28, 1977.
Doughman DJ: Treatment of corneal thinning and perforation. JCE Ophthalmol, January, 1978, pp 15–23.
Foote SC, Hook EW: *Salmonella* species (including typhoid fever). *In* Mandell GL, Douglas RG Jr, Bennett JE: Principles and Practice of Infectious Diseases. New York, John Wiley & Sons, 1979, pp 1730–1750.
Herzog C: Chemotherapy of typhoid fever: A review of literature. Infection 4:166–173, 1976.
Hook EW, Guerrant RL: *Salmonella* infections. *In* Isselbacher KJ, et al (eds): Harrison's Principles of Internal Medicine, 9th ed. New York, McGraw-Hill, 1980, pp 641–648.
Lewis PJ, Jones BL: Vitreous haemorrhage after typhoid cholera inoculation. Med J Aust 2:914, 1974.
Mathur JS, et al: Post typhoid retinal detachment. J All-India Ophthalmol Soc 18:135–137, 1970.
Prélat: Un cas d'iridocyclite bilatérale au cours de la vaccination antityphoidique (T.A.B.). Arch Ophthalmol 35:742–746, 1916–1917.
Warren JW, Hornick RB: Immunization against typhoid fever. Annu Rev Med 30:457–472, 1979.

YERSINIOSIS
K. MATTI SAARI, M.D.
Turku, Finland

Yersiniosis is a disease caused by infection with the gram-negative bacilli *Yersinia enterocolitica* or *Y. pseudotuberculosis*. Plague bacterium has been reclassified as *Y. pestis*. A wide range of clinical manifestations have been attributed to these bacilli, and they vary according to the age and condition of the patient. In the infant, gastroenteritis with high fever is common. Older children often experience acute abdominal symptoms, which may include acute terminal ileitis or mesenteric adenitis. Adults may present with enteritis, including diarrhea, nonspecific abdominal pain, nausea, vomiting, and fever. Nonpurulent reactive arthritis, often with myalgia, is more common in young and middle-aged adults, and erythema nodosum is more usual in women in late middle age. Less common symptoms include carditis, septicemia, glomerulonephritis, hepatitis, and hemolytic anemia.

Pyogenic ocular involvement (microbial invasion of the eye) is very rare in patients with yersiniosis; however, Parinaud's oculoglandular syndrome with ensuing corneal perforation and panophthalmitis leading to visual loss has been reported. Reactive ocular inflammation (the causative agent cannot be isolated from the eye), including acute anterior uveitis, conjunctivitis, and Reiter's syndrome, are occasionally associated with *Yersinia* infection in patients with HLA-B27 antigen.

THERAPY

Systemic. Most *Y. enterocolitica* strains are resistant in vitro to ampicillin, amoxicillin, carbenicillin, and penicillin, and are sensitive to gentamicin, kanamycin, tobramycin, tetracycline, chloramphenicol, and to the combination of sulfamethoxazole and trimethoprim. However, success with these drugs is not uniform. Drug therapy must be started promptly when the diagnosis of yersiniosis is suspected. Usually, 250 to 500 mg of tetracycline are given orally every 6 hours for 10 days. If chloramphenicol is given, the dosage should be 250 to 500 mg orally every 4 to 6 hours or 500 mg every 6 hours by intravenous injection. Alternatively, 160 mg of trimethoprim and 800 mg of sulfamethoxazole may be given orally two to three times daily. Gentamicin is given by intramuscular injection in an initial dosage of 0.8 mg/kg, followed by 0.4 mg/kg every 6 hours. Therapy should be continued for at least 24 to 48 hours after symptoms and fever have subsided.

Ocular. With conjunctival *infections*, fortified gentamicin§ (14 mg/ml) eyedrops should be given hourly for 8 days, and then one drop should be given every 6 hours until the infection appears to be resolved. With corneal involvement, subtenon injection of 20 to 40 mg of gentamicin* daily for 4 to 5 days, followed by two more injections on alternate days, may be indicated. If corneal perforation occurs, a corneal patch graft may be indicated to seal the perforation.

Topical 1 per cent atropine solution may be used for uveitis, and one drop may be given every 6 hours. If the patient is sensitive to atropine, 0.25 per cent scopolamine may be substituted.

Reactive conjunctivitis associated with *Yersinia* infection usually resolves in 1 week without treatment. Reactive iritis should be treated with topically administered corticosteroids (0.1 per cent dexamethasone or 0.5 to 1 per cent prednisolone) every hour daily, corticosteroid ointment for the night, and 0.25 per cent scopolamine three times a day. In cases with fulminant onset of intraocular inflammation, systemic corticosteroids, beginning with 40 to 60 mg of oral prednisolone daily and followed by reduction of the dosage, may be used. Associated *Yersinia* infection should be treated with 250 mg of tetracycline orally every 6 hours for 10 days.

Surgical. The management of *Y. enterocolitica* endophthalmitis and panophthalmitis is extremely difficult, and most eyes are lost at this stage of the disease. Emergency pars plana vitrectomy may be indicated to remove the infectious organisms, to confirm their antibiotic sensitivity by vitreous culture, and to enable intravitreal injection of 0.1 mg of gentamicin.* The postoperative therapeutic regimen should include systemic antibiotics, daily subtenon injections of 20 to 40 mg of gentamicin* or 20 to 40 mg of tobramycin,* and topical instillation of fortified gentamicin§ (14 mg/ml) or tobramycin§ (11 mg/ml) eyedrops every 30 minutes for the first few days and then tapered.

Supportive. Supportive care may consist of intravenous fluid, pressor drugs, and oxygen, when required.

Ocular or Periocular Manifestations

(P) indicates pyogenic manifestations; (R) indicates reactive manifestations.

Anterior Chamber: Cells and flare (P,R); fibrinous exudates (R).
Conjunctiva: Chemosis (R); edema (P); follicles (R); granulomatous conjunctivitis (Parinaud's) (P); hyperemia (P,R); mucopurulent conjunctivitis (P,R); necrosis (P); ulcer (P).
Cornea: Clouding (P); perforation (P); ulcer (P).
Globe: Endophthalmitis (P); panophthalmitis (P).
Iris: Acute anterior uveitis (P,R); posterior synechiae (P,R); vasodilation of iris vessels (R).
Retina: Disc edema (R); hemorrhages (P); macular edema (R); vascular constriction (P).
Vitreous: Cells (R).
Other: Cataract (P); hypopyon (P); ocular pain (P,R); photophobia (P,R); visual loss (P).

Precautions

Since yersiniosis may present with such a wide spectrum of symptoms, diagnosis may easily be missed. This infection should always be considered in patients with fever of unknown origin. This fact is underlined by the possibility of fatal complications from the disease, especially in malnourished patients and those who develop sepsis. When a diagnosis of yersiniosis is suspected, stool and conjunctival discharges should be cultured. Serologic diagnosis is available at reference laboratories. An elevated erythrocyte sedimentation rate is characteristic for yersiniosis in patients of all ages.

Adverse effects caused by tetracyclines include nausea, enterocolitis, superinfections, and photosensitivity. Patients taking tetracyclines should not sunbathe. Products containing aluminum, magnesium, or calcium ions (antacids, milk, and milk products) decrease the absorption and should not be taken during the hour before or 2 hours after an oral dose of tetracycline. Tetracyclines should be avoided during pregnancy and in children below 8 years because of irreversible deposition of the substance in growing teeth and bones.

Gentamicin should be used with caution in patients who have renal impairment. Both nephrotoxicity and neurotoxicity with involvement of the eighth cranial nerve have been reported with the use of gentamicin.

Chloramphenicol may have severe side effects, although these are rather uncommon. Adverse effects reported with this drug include skin rashes, fever, gastrointestinal disturbance, bone marrow depression, and the gray-baby syndrome.

Comments

The mode of transmission of *Yersinia* bacilli is not fully understood. The bacilli have been isolated from a wide number of wild and domestic animals, and transmission to humans by contact with infected animals may occur in some instances. However, the primary mode of transmission appears to be fecally contaminated food and water. It also seems likely that the disease may be spread by contact with infected persons.

Although serious complications may occur in debilitated and older patients, the prognosis in *Yersinia* infections is generally good, especially if diagnosis can be made and treatment started relatively early. In children, *Y. enterocolitica* diarrhea is often self-limiting, and the role of antibiotic therapy is unclear. Subacute localizing forms of infection sometimes appear in patients with *Y. pseudotuberculosis* infection, particularly those with concurrent underlying disease.

References

Bottone EJ (ed): Yersinia enterocolitica. Boca Raton, FL, CRC Press, 1981.
Butler T: Plague and other yersinia infections. New York, Plenum Medical Book Co., 1983.
Chin GN, Noble RC: Ocular involvement in *Yersinia enterocolitica* infection presenting as Parinaud's oculoglandular syndrome. Am J Ophthalmol 83:19–23, 1977.

Mäki M et al: Yersiniosis in children. Arch Dis Child 55:861–865, 1980.

Mattila L et al: Acute anterior uveitis after yersinia infection. Br J Ophthalmol 66:209–212, 1982.

Saari, KM, et al: Acute anterior uveitis and conjunctivitis following yersinia infection in children. Int Ophthalmol 9:237–241, 1986.

Saari KM: The eye and reactive arthritis. *In* Toivanen A and Toivanen P (eds): Reactive arthritis. Boca Raton, FL, CRC Press, Inc, 1988, pp 113–124.

Saari KM, et al: Ocular inflammation associated with *Yersinia* infection. Am J Ophthalmol 89:84–95, 1980.

Chlamydial Infections

INCLUSION CONJUNCTIVITIS
(Paratrachoma, Chlamydia)

CHANDLER R. DAWSON, M.D.

San Francisco, California

The chlamydiae are obligate intracellular organisms derived from bacteria and comprise only two species: *Chlamydia trachomatis* and *C. psittaci*. *C. trachomatis* is almost exclusively a human pathogen and includes the agents of classic trachoma (always associated with serotypes A, B, Ba, and C) and of inclusion conjunctivitis or paratrachoma (serotypes D, E, F, G, H, I, J, and K). These organisms infect the epithelium of mucoid surfaces and were once identified as the TRIC (trachoma-inclusion conjunctivitis) agents. The *C. trachomatis* agents also include the agents of lymphogranuloma venereum (serotypes L1, L2, and L3) that infect deeper tissues but not epithelial surfaces and are more pathogenic in animal systems.

As with lymphogranuloma venereum, serotypes D through K are sexually transmitted, and the secondary eye involvement in adults occurs in about 1 in 300 genital cases. Exposure of the infant in the birth canal causes ocular infection in 35 to 50 per cent of exposed newborns, resulting in chlamydial ophthalmia neonatorum. Infection of the eyes of adults occurs from sexual partners or from autoinoculation of infective genital discharges into the eye. Genitally transmitted chlamydial infections are the major cause of nongonococcal urethritis in males and of cervicitis and salpingitis in females, and they cause a number of other diseases as well.

Infants exposed to chlamydial infection from the mother's cervix during birth develop ophthalmia neonatorum at 5 to 12 days of age. Of infants exposed during delivery, 10 to 20 per cent also develop chlamydial respiratory disease with pneumonia as late as 6 months postpartum; the infection involves the gastrointestinal tract as well. Neonatal ophthalmia presents as tearing with moderate discharge and swelling of the lids. The eyes are usually red and inflamed, and there is infiltration and swelling of the conjunctiva. If untreated, chlamydial conjunctivitis in newborns may resolve spontaneously in 5 to 9 months, but has been known to persist for years with development of chronic follicular conjunctivitis, corneal neovascularization (vascular pannus), and conjunctival scarring. Infants with chlamydial respiratory disease may present from 2 to 6 months of age with rhinitis, cough, and a pertussis-like inspiratory whoop and frequently have eosinophilia.

In adults, ocular chlamydial infection produces chronic follicular conjunctivitis with keratitis. Because this adult disease is difficult to distinguish from the clinical findings in early trachoma, the term "paratrachoma" is used to describe the whole spectrum of eye disease with genitally transmitted chlamydial infection. Ocular chlamydial disease occurs most frequently in adults between the ages of 18 and 30 years. The eye disease usually has an acute onset in one eye, with watering and mucoid discharge, sticking of lids in the morning, foreign body sensation, hyperemia of the conjunctiva, and sometimes swelling of the lids. Examination reveals a swollen preauricular node, follicular conjunctivitis with easily visible conjunctival lymphoid follicles, and a diffuse inflammatory response with fine tarsal papillae and diffuse infiltration. Superficial keratitis includes fine and larger macropunctate epithelial erosions, subepithelial infiltrates similar to those of epidemic keratoconjunctivitis, limbal infiltration, and superficial neovascularization.

Laboratory procedures to identify chlamydial infections include the following: Giemsa staining of smears, isolation in cell culture, direct fluorescent monoclonal antibodies (DFA) staining of smears, enzyme labeled immunoassay (ELISA) test, DNA probes (under development in 1989), and serum antibody levels measured by complement-fixation (CF) or microimmunofluorescent (MIF) tests. Microscopic examination of Giemsa-stained conjunctival smears is very effective in detecting neonatal chlamydial infections because the inclusions are so numerous, but it is less sensitive in adult inclusion conjunctivitis. The DFA and ELISA tests are now widely available and are highly sensitive for identifying chlamydial infection in the conjunctiva of both adults and neonates. Cell culture techniques are less available, but are highly sensitive. The presence of serum IgM antibody against chlamydia in newborns suggests a systemic infection, particularly pneumonia.

THERAPY

Systemic. Because infection is not limited to the eye in either neonatal infants or adults, it is necessary to use systemic antimicrobial treatment. Moreover, the sexual consorts of adults or parents of infants must also receive a full course of therapy. For infants, effective therapy is provided by oral erythromycin, 40 mg/kg daily in four divided dosages for a minimum of 2 weeks. Adults with chlamydial eye infections should receive tetracycline or erythromycin. Daily administration of 1 to 2 gm of tetracycline should be given in four divided doses for 2 or preferably 3 weeks; doxycycline, 100 mg twice daily, is also effective; erythromycin is effective at doses of 1 to 1.5 gm given daily in four divided doses for 2 to 3 weeks. The use of erythromycin estolate or ethylsuccinate is known to carry a high risk of toxic hepatitis, and erythromycin is also generally less well tolerated than oral tetracyclines. As a distant third choice, sulfonamides may be used in the full doses necessary to maintain adequate blood levels (5 to 10 mg per cent). The sulfonamides must be given for at least 3 weeks in full doses, but they carry a high risk of systemic sensitivity.

Ocular. Local antimicrobial treatment with tetracycline or erythromycin ointment to the eye is not necessary for patients on full oral therapeutic doses of antibiotic. It has been shown that the topical treatment alone is extremely slow and only partially effective in treating adult or neonatal inclusion conjunctivitis, and relapses are frequent. Topical sulfonamide alone is even less effective than topical tetracyclines or erythromycin. Moreover, because the infection is systemic, local therapy alone should be discouraged. For the occasional adult patient who develops an anterior iritis with inclusion conjunctivitis, the use of topical corticosteroids carries no more risk than to any other patient, as long as the patient is under systemic treatment with antimicrobials or has received a full course of systemic treatment. When used without systemic antichlamydials, topical corticosteroids are definitely contraindicated for the treatment of the conjunctivitis or keratitis, even when combined with topical antimicrobial therapy, such as sulfonamide, because they simply prolong the disease.

Topical rifampin* ointment has been used in the treatment of ocular chlamydial infections but, as with all topical antimicrobials, is of limited use. Moreover, rifampin and its derivatives are available only for investigational use in the eye in the United States.

Ocular or Periocular Manifestations

Conjunctiva: Cicatrization (rare); follicular conjunctivitis, hyperemia; marked papillary infiltration.
Cornea: Anterior stromal opacities; diffuse, fine punctate, or macropunctate keratitis; marginal infiltration; pannus ulcer (rare); vascularization.
Eyelids: Edema.
Other: Anterior uveitis; irritation.

PRECAUTIONS

Anterior uveitis that is nongranulomatous and self-limited may develop in patients with HLA B27 positive lymphocytes, apparently as a response to chlamydial infection. The uveitis does not respond to antimicrobial treatment for the conjunctival disease, but can be readily suppressed with adequate doses of topical corticosteroids. Recurrent episodes of uveitis occur with this syndrome, but they are unrelated to chlamydial infection.

Conjunctival scar formation may occur in patients who receive prolonged courses of topical corticosteroids without appropriate antimicrobial therapy.

COMMENTS

The recommended prophylaxis for neonates to prevent both gonococcal neonatal ophthalmia and chlamydial ophthalmia is a single application of tetracycline or erythromycin ointment within 1 hour after delivery. Credé prophylaxis with 1 per cent silver nitrate does not prevent chlamydial eye infection of the newborn.

References

Beem MO, Saxon EM: Respiratory-tract colonization and a distinctive pneumonia syndrome in infants infected with *Chlamydia trachomatis.* N Engl J Med 296:306–310, 1977.

Dawson CR, et al: Inclusion conjunctivitis and Reiter's syndrome in a married couple. *Chlamydia* infections in a series of both diseases. Arch Ophthalmol 83:300–306, 1970.

Grossman M, et al: Prospective studies in chlamydia in newborns. *In* Mardh P, et al (eds): Chlamydial Infections. Amsterdam, Elsevier Biomedical, pp 213–216, 1982.

Mordhorst CH, Dawson C: Sequelae of neonatal inclusion conjunctivitis and associated disease in parents. Am J Ophthalmol 71:861–867, 1971.

Schachter J, Dawson CR: Human Chlamydial Infections. Littleton, MA, Publishing Sciences Group, 1978.

Schachter J, et al: Nonculture methods for diagnosing chlamydial infection in patients with trachoma: A clue to the pathogenesis of the disease? J Infect Dis 158:1347–1352, 1988.

Sexually transmitted diseases. Treatment guidelines 1985. MMWR 34(4S):75S–108S, 1985.

TRACHOMA

S. DAROUGAR, M.D., D.T.M.&H.,
M.R.C. Path.,
and N. VISWALINGAM, M.D., D.O.
London, England

Trachoma, a chronic keratoconjunctivitis, is most common in rural communities of the Middle East, Africa, Asia, and South and Central America. It is estimated that 500 million people have trachoma, and approximately 5 million are blind because of its complications. Trachoma is caused by *Chlamydia trachomatis* serotypes A, B, and C. Common clinical features of the disease are papillae, follicles, and scars in the palpebral conjunctiva and pannus, keratitis, and opacities in the cornea. The majority of patients are asymptomatic, but some present with ptosis, mild tearing, and discharge, redness, and swelling of lids in one or both eyes. Trachoma is occasionally accompanied by rhinitis, otitis media, upper respiratory tract infection, and preauricular lymphadenopathy.

Trachoma presents in various clinical forms. In infants, it may present as a moderate to severe papillary conjunctivitis, with some follicles in the lower lid and upper fornix but no pannus. In young children, the disease presents in its classical form, with follicles and papillae in the upper tarsal conjunctiva and active pannus. In older children and young adults, papillae and follicles may be present together with scars.

The potentially blinding complications of trachoma are severe conjunctival scarring, leading to trichiasis, entropion, and corneal scarring. These complications generally occur in older patients, although they are occasionally found in younger patients, particularly in mothers who have young children with severe trachoma.

Trachoma can be divided epidemiologically into blinding and nonblinding disease. Blinding trachoma is associated with a high prevalence of severe disease and blinding trachomatous complications. Nonblinding trachoma is also endemic and common, but it is a mild disease that does not usually produce blinding complications.

Blinding trachoma is associated with overcrowding, poor sanitation, and poor standards of living and medical care. Under these conditions, infants may become infected 1 to 2 months after birth. At 3 to 5 years of age, most of these children have moderate to severe disease, shedding large numbers of infectious particles in their eye secretions. In these communities, the duration of active trachoma is protracted because of the continuing transmission of infectious agent from one patient to another. This repeated reinfection and the burden of associated bacterial conjunctivitis can lead to a high prevalence of severe scarring, trichiasis, entropion, and corneal scarring. The distinction between blinding and nonblinding trachoma is important in determining priority areas for prevention of blindness.

THERAPY

Systemic. Trachoma is effectively treated with oral antibiotics. A 3-week course of 15 mg/kg of tetracyclines or erythromycin, 1.5 mg/kg of doxycycline, or 30 mg/kg of sulfamethoxazole daily is recommended for systemic infections.

Ocular. *C. trachomatis* is highly sensitive to tetracyclines, erythromycin and related macrolides, rifampin, and, to a lesser degree, sulfonamides. Topical therapy with tetracyclines (chlortetracycline, oxytetracycline,* or tetracycline), rifampin, or erythromycin eye ointment or 10 per cent sulfacetamide solution is effective. The ophthalmic ointment may be applied three times daily for 6 weeks, and the ophthalmic solution may be applied three times daily for 8 weeks.

Surgical. Trichiasis and entropion are the major blinding complications of trachoma. An essential part of the preventive blindness program is to make corrective lid operations available to those living in rural communities.

PRECAUTIONS

Topical tetracycline or rifampin eye ointment may cause irritation and allergic responses. Concurrent topical application of corticosteroids is not recommended because it masks signs and symptoms, and rebound of the disease may occur when they are discontinued. Corticosteroids may also reactivate herpes virus infections.

Oral tetracyclines should not be given to children under 8 years old and pregnant women.

COMMENTS

In rural communities with a high prevalence of blinding trachoma, continuous topical or systemic treatment of all individuals is not feasible. The World Health Organization recommends an intermittent topical treatment with tetracycline eye ointment twice daily for 5 consecutive days each month for 6 months. This method of therapy is designed to reduce the severity of the disease and the shedding of infectious agents, hence interrupting the transmission of trachoma. However, in recent studies on prevention and control of trachoma, the failure rate of the intermittent topical therapy of mass population was found to be very high. This may have been due to the inability or apathy of parents in using the eye ointment properly and regularly in their own eyes and in the eyes of their children, lack of supervision in most villages, spoilage of ointment due to excessive heat and melting of the base, and exchange of ointment with other families. For moderate to severe trachoma, the results of pilot projects using an oral dosage of 5 mg/kg of doxycycline or 35 mg/kg of sulfalene† once monthly for 6 to 8 months or once weekly for 3 weeks were as effective as the intermittent therapy using tetracycline eye ointment. These drugs were administered by health workers who treated considerable numbers of patients daily. Although the initial cost of the drug was rather high, the reduction of follow-up surveys and the very low failure rate make this regimen cost effective. In these studies, there were no serious side effects, but minor side effects, such as nausea, vomiting, and skin rashes, were observed in about 5 per cent of patients.

References

Al-Rifai KM: Trachoma through history. Int Ophthalmol 12:9–14, 1988.

Darougar S, et al: Family-based suppressive intermittent therapy of hyperendemic trachoma with topical oxytetracycline or oral doxycycline. Br J Ophthalmol 64:291–295, 1980.

Darougar S, et al: Topical therapy of hyperendemic trachoma using rifampicin, oxytetracycline, or spiramycin eye ointments. Br J Ophthalmol 64:37–42, 1980.

Darougar S, et al: A double-blind comparison of topical therapy of chlamydial ocular infection (TRIC infection) with rifampicin or chlortetracycline. Br J Ophthalmol 65:549–552, 1981.

Dawson CR, Jones BR, Tarizzo ML: Guide to Trachoma Control. Geneva, World Health Organization, 1981.

Jones BR: The prevention of blindness from trachoma. Trans Ophthalmol Soc UK 95:16–33, 1975.

Olson CM: In herpes or chlamydial infections, immune response may be key factor in lost vision [news]. JAMA 261:819–820, 1989.

Schachter J, Moncada J, Dawson CR, Sheppard J, Courtright P, Said ME, Zaki S, Hafez SF, Lorincz A: Nonculture methods for diagnosing chlamydial infection in patients with trachoma: a clue to the pathogenesis of the disease? J Infect Dis 158:1347–1352, 1988.

Tabbara KF, Cooper H: Minocycline levels in tears of patients with active trachoma. Arch Ophthalmol 107:93–95, 1989.

Treharne JD: The microbial epidemiology of trachoma. Int Ophthalmol 12:25–29, 1988.

Mycotic Infections

ACTINOMYCOSIS
BENJAMIN MILDER, M.D.
St. Louis, Missouri

Actinomycosis is a noncontagious infection caused by a group of organisms, the *Actinomyces*. The disease is generally described as a mycotic infection, although this anaerobic organism is not a true fungus. The species most often identified in ocular disease is the *Actinomyces israelii*.

Actinomycosis is usually acquired by chewing on or otherwise making contact with contaminated straw or hay. Thus, it is a disease of rural settings and is transmitted to the orbit and ocular structures by way of the mouth or nasal passages.

The principal sites of actinomycosis are cutaneous, cervicofacial, thoracic, and abdominal. In the facial area, involvement of the buccal cavity, teeth, and mandible is most common. Involvement of the lacrimal system is usually unaccompanied by other concurrent clinical manifestations of actinomycosis.

THERAPY

Systemic. Significant improvement in actinomycosis patients may be expected when either penicillin or tetracycline antibiotics are administered in high doses over long periods of time. The tetracyclines are the drugs of choice for oral administration, administered in dosages of 500 mg every 6 hours. A suitable alternative is penicillin G, which may be administered topically,* subconjunctivally,* or systemically. In severe infections, adequate therapeutic levels require intramuscular or intravenous administration. Daily recommended dosages are 25,000 to 50,000 units/kg in divided doses every 4 hours. Treatment should be continued for several weeks after clinical cure.

Ocular. For corneal ulcers, therapeutic concentrations can be obtained rapidly by the subconjunctival route. The recommended dosage is 0.5 to 1 million units of penicillin G.*

Natamycin has been used for topical treatment of blepharitis, conjunctivitis, and keratitis of mycotic origin, particularly if the fungus has not been identified. However, if *Actinomyces* is known to be the causative agent, the drug of choice is sodium penicillin G, used as eye drops* in a concentration of 500,000 units/ml.

Surgical. Aspiration or surgical drainage is a valuable adjunct to the chemotherapy of actinomycotic lesions of the lids and orbit. Since the larger orbital lesions tend to be "honeycombed," care must be taken to ensure that the incision is adequate and pockets of abscess are opened.

In *Actinomyces* canaliculitis, small concretions can be expressed through the punctum by massaging the canaliculus. However, since this form of canaliculitis tends to be resistant to therapy, the definitive cure may require slitting the canaliculus to remove the concretions and the infected mucosal lining. It is essential that the slitting be limited to the horizontal limb of the canaliculus as far as the ampulla and that this be performed on the conjunctival aspect of the lid, not on the lid margin. The punctum should never be included in such an incision. The canaliculus, thus opened, is curetted to remove infected mucosa. It is not necessary to close the canaliculotomy wound with sutures. Surgical excision of firm nodules in the subconjunctival tissues may also be indicated.

Ocular or Periocular Manifestations

Anterior Chamber: Hypopyon.
Conjunctiva: Angular, catarrhal, or pseudomembranous conjunctivitis; mucopurulent discharge; ulcer; yellow nodules.

Eyelids: Abscess; fibrosis; yellow nodules.

Iris: Anterior uveitis secondary to keratitis and corneal ulceration.

Lacrimal System: Canaliculitis with fullness in the region of the canaliculus, pouting of the punctum and creamy pus exuding from the punctum, often with "sulfur granules"; dacryocystitis (rare).

Orbit: Abscess; infiltration; proptosis.

PRECAUTIONS

Older methods, such as irradiation and sulfonamides, have not been shown to be effective in the treatment of actinomycosis. Amphotericin B also is of no value. When the canaliculus has been opened and curetted, one "old-fashioned" remedy that may still be of value is the application of tincture of iodine to destroy the remaining canalicular mucosa.

COMMENTS

Actinomycosis is disappearing because of the wide use of modern therapeutic agents. Such drugs as the penicillins and tetracyclines are now used prophylactically after dental extraction and in other conditions that might evolve into actinomycosis. However, the disease still exists, especially in the rural Midwest.

Actinomycosis tends to run an extremely chronic course, but spontaneous resolution has been reported even after many months. Favorable prognosis in the cervicofacial forms is directly related to early diagnosis and specific therapy based on microscopic confirmation of the organism.

References

Bennett JE: Actinomycosis. *In* Isselbacher KJ, et al (eds): Harrison's Principles of Internal Medicine, 9th ed. New York, McGraw-Hill, 1980, pp 734–735.

Blanksma LJ, Slijper J: Actinomycotic dacryocystitis. Ophthalmologica 176:145–149, 1978.

Bohigian GM: Handbook of External Diseases of the Eye. Fort Worth, Alcon, 1980, p 163.

Korting GW: The Skin and Eye: A Dermatologic Correlation of Diseases of the Periorbital Region. Philadelphia, WB Saunders, 1973, pp 52–54.

Leigh RJ, Good EF, Rudy RP: Ophthalmoplegia due to actinomycosis. J Clin Neuro Ophthalmol 6:157–159, 1986.

Seal DV, et al: Lacrimal canaliculitis due to *Arachnia* (*Actinomyces*) *propionica*. Br J Ophthalmol 65:10–13, 1981.

ASPERGILLOSIS

GARY P. BARTH, M.D.

Santa Rosa, California

Aspergillosis is a systemic infection caused by the ubiquitous saprophytic, *Aspergillus* fungi. In most cases, the respiratory system serves as the portal of entry.

The disease is prevalent in the southern United States, India, and Africa. Its frequency is highest among grain farmers and feeders or breeders of poultry or pigeons. Ocular and orbital involvement is rare and may be associated with complications of infected sinuses, trauma, surgery, intravenous drug abuse, or immunosuppression. Occasionally, it has no known cause. Infection reaches the orbit by direct extension and is characterized by chronic nonnecrotizing, granulomatous inflammation and fibrosis. Orbital aspergillosis is characterized by slowly progressive unilateral proptosis, ocular pain, and decreased vision. Keratomycosis due to *Aspergillus* accounts for nearly 50 per cent of all reported cases of oculomycosis.

THERAPY

Systemic. Amphotericin B is the most reliable drug for the treatment of aspergillosis. However, because of its toxicity, an intravenous test dose of 1.0 mg dissolved in 50 to 150 ml of 5 per cent dextrose in water should be given. The dose can then be progressively increased in 5- to 10-mg increments to a daily maximum of 0.5 to 0.6 mg/kg. Fulminant infections can be treated with daily doses as high as 0.8 to 1.0 mg/kg during the first 2 weeks.

Rifampin‡ has shown activity against *Aspergillus* when used in combination with the detergent effects of amphotericin B. The antimetabolite flucytosine also acts synergistically with amphotericin B. An oral dose of 37.5 mg/kg of flucytosine‡ every 6 hours may be used in combination with 0.3 mg/kg of intravenous amphotericin B daily.

Synthetic imidazoles have been found to be variably effective against many *Aspergillus* infections. A single daily dose of 0.4 to 1.0 gm of ketoconazole‡ may be administered orally. Miconazole‡ may be given intravenously in doses of 10 to 15 mg/kg every 8 hours.

Systemic steroids may be necessary in visual loss and proptosis caused by allergic *Aspergillus* sinusitis.

Ocular. Five per cent natamycin ophthalmic suspension is available for the treatment of *Aspergillus* corneal infection. Natamycin is similar to amphotericin B in its activity against *Aspergillus*, but is more stable in suspension and much less irritating to the conjunctiva. Amphotericin B* in a 0.1 to 0.3 per cent suspension can be used until natamycin can be obtained. In severe cases, either drug can be used hourly for the first 48 hours.

In cases refractory to natamycin therapy, 1 or 2 per cent miconazole* can be substituted. Four per cent thiabendazole* or 1 per cent clotrimazole* has also been reported to be effective against *Aspergillus* infections.

Subconjunctival injection of 1 mg of amphotericin B* and intravitreal doses of 5 µg of amphotericin B* have been used in *Aspergillus* endophthalmitis, but the risk of retinal toxicity has not been established.

Surgical. Orbital involvement with *Aspergillus* is a life-threatening problem. Prompt medical therapy should be combined with surgical drainage. In a corneal ulcer caused by *Aspergillus*, débridement of the fungal growth that raises up above the corneal epithelium may allow better penetration of antifungal drops. A penetrating keratoplasty may be required in cases that are refractory to medical therapy. With intraocular extension of *Aspergillus* keratomycosis, an iridotomy or a lensectomy and vitrectomy may be needed to prevent pupillary-block glaucoma.

Ocular or Periocular Manifestations

Cornea: Abscess; keratitis; keratoconjunctivitis.
Globe: Endophthalmitis; proptosis.
Lacrimal System: Canaliculitis; dacryocystitis.
Other: Cataracts; cranial nerve palsy; hypopyon; ocular pain; secondary glaucoma.

PRECAUTIONS

Proper diagnostic procedures are essential for establishing the diagnosis of *Aspergillus* infection. In suspected *Aspergillus* keratitis, at least six to eight scrappings with a Kimura spatula from the bed of the infection are needed. Intravitreal and anterior chamber aspirates should be concentrated by the use of a filter or by centrifugation. Orbital biopsy material should be plated soon after collection, since *Aspergillus* is a ubiquitous organism and false-positive results could occur if the specimen were to remain unnecessarily exposed. If the organism can be cultured, either Sabouraud's media (Emmon's modification) or blood agar will usually be positive within 48 hours. Gram, giemsa, and Grocett's methanemine-silver stains are better than potassium hydroxide for detecting the branching septated hyphae. Specific antifungal treatment should be withheld until a diagnosis of a fungal infection can be established. Once antifungal therapy has been initiated, negative scrapings do not indicate elimination of the infection.

Medical therapy of aspergillosis is made more difficult by the poor ocular penetration of most drugs, the toxicity associated with their use, the length of time that therapy must be continued, and the lack of published studies documenting their effectiveness. The poor ocular penetration and toxicity preclude systemic use of drugs in *Aspergillus* keratitis. Side effects may include a dose-related febrile reaction, anorexia, nausea, decreased weight, hypokalemia, thrombophlebitis, bone marrow depression, and nephrotoxicity. Natamycin in drop form is well tolerated, but may produce necrosis and granulomas following subconjunctival injection. Flucytosine can cause rash, gastrointestinal intolerance, hepatic dysfunction, and leukopenia. Ketoconazole has been known to cause nausea, rash, pruritus, and severe hepatitis. Patients treated with ketoconazole should have their liver enzymes and liver function tests monitored regularly. Miconazole can cause pruritus, phlebitis, thrombocytosis, hyperlipidemia, and hyponatremia. Since cardiorespiratory arrest has been associated with the first intravenous dose of miconazole, the initial dose is best administered by the physician.

COMMENTS

Therapy of *Aspergillus* infections is often complicated by a delay in diagnosis, the previous use of corticosteroids, and the long-term use of the antifungal medications. In vitro sensitivity tests are not completely reliable and should serve only as a guide to the clinical response. When a penetrating keratoplasty is performed, the subsequent use of corticosteroids should be delayed as long as possible to prevent reactivation of the fungus.

References

Boldrey EE: Bilateral endogenous *Aspergillus* endophthalmitis. Retina *1*:171–174, 1981.
Dunlop IS, Billson FA: Visual failure in allergic *Aspergillus* sinusitis: Case report. Br J Ophthalmol 72:127–130, 1988.
Foster CS: Miconazole therapy for keratomycosis. Am J Ophthalmol *91*:622–629, 1981.
Jones DB: Chemotherapy of fungal infections. In Srinivasan D: Ocular Therapeutics. New York, Masson, 1980, pp 35–50.
Roney P, et al: Endogenous *Aspergillus* endophthalmitis. Rev Infect Dis 8:955–958, 1986.
Searl SS, et al: *Aspergillus* keratitis with intraocular invasion. Ophthalmology 88:1244–1250, 1981.
Sihota R, et al: *Aspergillus* endophthalmitis. Br J Ophthalmol 71:611–613, 1987.

BLASTOMYCOSIS
DENIS M. O'DAY, M.D.
Nashville, Tennessee

Blastomycosis, a chronic fungal disease caused by *Blastomyces dermatitidis*, produces granulomatous lesions that may involve any part of the body, with a predilection for the skin, lung, and bones. Ocular involvement can occur by direct extension from lesions involving the face and eyelids or by hematogenous dissemination from a primary pulmonlesion. The lids appear to be the ocular structure that is most commonly involved in blastomycosis. Intraocular involvement is rare.

THERAPY

Systemic. Three antifungal agents have been recommended for the treatment of blastomycosis: amphotericin B, hydroxystilbamidine, and

56 / BLASTOMYCOSIS

miconazole. Before intravenous administration of amphotericin B, an initial test injection should be given over a period of 2 to 4 hours in a dosage of 1 mg in 250 ml of 5 per cent dextrose in water. This dose is then gradually increased in 2- to 5-mg increments every 24 hours until a daily dose of 30 to 40 mg is reached. This dosage is then administered until a total dose of 2 gm is achieved.

Because hydroxystilbamidine is probably less toxic than amphotericin B, it has been proposed as an alternative to amphotericin B therapy. Therapy is begun with 25 to 50 mg given intravenously as a test dose. The usual daily dose is 225 mg, given by slow intravenous drip during a 2- to 4-hour period. Total dosage should be determined by the extent of the disease and the rapidity of the response. In most cases, however, a maximum of 8 gm is recommended.

Miconazole has shown promise in the treatment of a variety of deep mycoses in humans, including some ocular infections. This drug is administered intravenously in a daily dose of 30 mg/kg.

Ocular. Of these three antifungal drugs used systemically, only miconazole is tolerated by subconjunctival injection. A daily dose of 5 mg of undiluted intravenous preparation of miconazole* may be injected subconjunctivally. Topical ophthalmic administration of 1 per cent miconazole,* prepared from the undiluted intravenous form of the drug, can be given hourly.

Surgical. Surgical drainage of lid or orbital abscesses may be indicated, with antifungal therapy given before and after surgery.

Ocular or Periocular Manifestations

Anterior Chamber: Hypopyon.
Choroid: Focal choroiditis.
Cornea: Descemetocele; perforation; stromal keratitis; ulcer.
Eyelids: Abscess leading to cicatrization; entropion; papules; pustules.
Iris: Anterior uveitis; nodules.
Orbit: Abscess; cellulitis.

PRECAUTIONS

Intravenous usage of amphotericin B may result in two types of reactions: idiosyncratic and dose related. Idiosyncratic reactions occur rarely, but can be lethal and include grand mal seizures, vertigo, flushing and anaphylaxis, thrombocytopenia, acute liver failure, generalized pain, ventricular fibrillation, and cardiac arrest. Dose-related side effects, which are more common, include anemia, hypokalemia, fever, and chills. Less commonly, leukopenia, thrombocytopenia, renal failure, thrombophlebitis, nausea and vomiting, anorexia, and headaches may occur. Direct topical ocular application of amphotericin B is toxic to the cornea, and periocular injection is poorly tolerated.

The toxic effects of hydroxystilbamidine are less severe and less common than amphotericin B; they consist mainly of occasional elevations of hepatic transaminase levels, nausea, vomiting, chills and fever and, rarely, a hypotensive or idiosyncratic reaction.

The adverse reactions to miconazole include chills, fever, nausea, anorexia, anemia, altered sensorium, and transient increase in serum lipids; there are also reports of immediate severe cardiopulmonary reactions.

COMMENTS

Ocular infection with blastomycosis is so rare that the most appropriate therapy remains an unsettled question. In those instances where corneal involvement occurs, consideration should be given to the topical administration of miconazole in combination with systemic therapy. Experience with infection in other tissue indicates that treatment should be for a prolonged period. There is some evidence of an impaired cell-mediated immunity facilitating infection with *B. dermatitidis.* This has been observed especially in children. In such circumstances, attention to appropriate parenteral alimentation is an important prerequisite for a return to normal immunologic function.

References

Barr CC, Gamel JW: Blastomycosis of the eyelid. Arch Ophthalmol *104*:96–97, 1986.
Chesney JC, et al: Pulmonary blastomycosis in children. Amphotericin B therapy and a review. Am J Dis Child *133*:1134–1139, 1979.
Fitzsimons RB, Ferguson AC: Cellular immunity and nutrition in refractory disseminated blastomycosis. Can Med Assoc J *119*:343–346, 1978.
Lewis H, et al: Latent disseminated blastomycosis with choroidal involvement. Arch Ophthalmol *106*:527–530, 1988.
Margo CE, Bombardier T: The diagnostic value of fungal autofluorescence. Surv Ophthalmol *29*:374–376, 1985.
Rodrigues MM, Laibson P, Kaplan W: Exogenous mycotic keratitis caused by *Blastomyces dermatitidis.* Am J Ophthalmol *75*:782–789, 1973.
Rose HD, Varkey B: Miconazole treatment of relapsed pulmonary blastomycosis. Am Rev Respir Dis *118*:403–408, 1978.
Vida L, Moel SA: Systemic North American blastomycosis with orbital involvement. Am J Ophthalmol *77*:240–242, 1974.

CANDIDIASIS

C. STEPHEN FOSTER, M.D., F.A.C.S.
Boston, Massachusetts

Candidiasis, an infection caused by the yeast fungus family of *Candida,* may occur as a result of local or generalized infection by any member of this family; *Candida albicans* is by far the most common species identified in cases of human candidiasis. When the infection is local in such sites as the vagina, mouth, or skin, the clinical problem is not usually life threatening and frequently responds rapidly to local, appropriate antifungal therapy. However, local candidiasis in vital structures and in the eye or systemic infections caused by *Candida* are frequently considerably more devastating.

Generalized candidiasis is uncommon but may occur in two settings: 1) systemic dissemination in drug addicts, in the debilitated patient, or in the immunosuppressed patient; and 2) chronic mucocutaneous candidiasis (CMCC), a distinct clinical entity involving immune and/or immunoregulatory dysfunctions. Four subgroups of chronic mucocutaneous candidiasis have been described: 1) early CMCC, 2) late-onset CMCC, 3) familial CMCC, and 4) juvenile familial polyendocrinopathy with candidiasis. Early CMCC is the most severe form; in addition to the persistent *Candida* colonization of the skin, hair, nails, and mucous membranes, *Candida* granulomata form and produce substantial disfiguring of the patient. Approximately half of the patients with early CMCC also have some form of endocrinopathy, such as hypoparathyroidism, diabetes mellitus, Addison's disease, or hypothyroidism. Late-onset CMCC is the mildest form of chronic mucocutaneous candidiasis, with clinical involvement usually only of the oral cavity and occasionally the nails. As the name implies, this form of the disease typically is seen in elderly individuals. Familial CMCC is transmitted as an autosomal recessive trait and is usually not associated with endocrinopathy. The disease is mild to moderate in severity. Juvenile familial polyendocrinopathy with candidiasis is characterized by mild to moderate candidiasis and endocrinopathy, usually in the form of hypoparathyroidism or Addison's disease. Other disorders not infrequently seen in patients with CMCC are pernicious anemia, iron-deficiency anemia, chronic active hepatitis, ovarian dysfunction, and keratoconjunctivitis.

The immunologic defects most commonly found in patients with CMCC include anergy to *Candida* antigen, impaired in vitro lymphocyte responsiveness to stimulation with *Candida* antigens (impaired blastogenic transformation and impaired lymphokine production), and occasional elaboration of serum factors (usually antibodies) that inhibit lymphocyte responsiveness to *Candida* antigens in vitro, even from normal donors.

Ocular involvement with *Candida* infestation may occur as a result of local inoculation or from endogenous colonization. Any part of the eye may be affected. Local inoculation most typically results in *Candida* keratitis, although *Candida* conjunctivitis, blepharitis, canaliculitis, or dacryocystitis may occur. Endogenous spread usually results in retinitis, uveitis, and/or endophthalmitis.

THERAPY

Systemic. Ketoconazole is the current therapy of choice for chronic mucocutaneous candidiasis, is probably also a useful component in the therapeutic management of patients with disseminated systemic candidiasis, and is a useful adjunct in the treatment of patients with keratomycosis. Oral administration of 200 to 400 mg of ketoconazole daily results in relatively high levels of penetration into the cornea and aqueous humor.

Flucytosine likewise penetrates the ocular structures relatively well after oral administration. The usual oral daily dose of flucytosine is 150 mg/kg in divided doses. Most *Candida* isolates are usually quite sensitive to flucytosine, but resistance can develop relatively rapidly, particularly if the administered dose is suboptimal.

Miconazole and amphotericin B are additional agents that may be used systemically in candidiasis therapy. Miconazole is usually administered intravenously every 8 hours, with a total daily dosage of 0.6 to 1.8 gm being the usually effective dose range for candidiasis. Amphotericin B may be given by slow intravenous infusion under specific guidelines, primarily for patients with progressive and potentially fatal infections.

Ocular. A 5 per cent suspension of natamycin may be administered every 1 to 2 hours for the treatment of a *Candida* corneal ulcer. However, two major problems confront the ophthalmologist who must rely on natamycin. Many *Candida* isolates are not highly sensitive to this drug, and none of the polyene antibiotics, including natamycin, penetrates the ocular structures well. Although these drugs may be effective in curing very superficial ocular surface infections with *Candida*, deeper corneal ulcers frequently do not respond adequately to this therapy.

Two other classes of antifungal agents are considerably more effective in treating infections caused by *Candida:* the imidazoles and flucytosine.

The imidazole agents are usually highly effective against ophthalmic *Candida* infections. Clotrimazole has been successfully used to treat patients with *Candida* corneal ulcers, without evidence of significant ocular toxicity; clotrimazole* cream may be applied eight to twelve times a day for 6 weeks. Miconazole penetrates well into the cornea and anterior chamber after topical or subconjunctival administration. Undiluted 1 per cent intravenous miconazole* solution may be topically applied every hour for the treatment of *Candida* keratitis. In addition, subconjunctival injection of 10 mg of miconazole* every 48 hours may also be used for deep *Candida* keratitis. Although intense conjunctival inflammation has been reported after subconjunctival injection of this drug, significant evidence of toxicity was not present.

None of the antifungal agents penetrates into the vitreous cavity well after systemic administration, and the intravenous administration of amphotericin B can be associated with substantial undesirable side effects. Intravitreal administration of antifungal agents is controversial, but limited data suggest that up to 5 μg of amphotericin B* or 40 μg of miconazole* administered intravitreally may be a reasonable therapeutic choice for management of *Candida* endophthalmitis with vitreal involvement.

The preferred regimen for the management of *Candida* corneal ulcers and external ocular infections caused by *Candida* includes 1 per cent flucytosine* administered every hour on the hour, alternating with 1 per cent miconazole* every hour on the half hour.

Management of intraocular *Candida* infections may include 150 mg/kg of oral flucytosine and intravenous therapy of 1.8 gm of miconazole combined with surgical therapy and intraocular antifungal administration.

Surgical. The surgical management of ocular *Candida* infections may range from a procedure as mild as periodic expression of the Meibomian glands for *Candida* meibomianitis, periodic curettage of the canaliculus for *Candida* canaliculitis, and daily scraping débridement of *Candida* corneal ulcer, to therapeutic penetrating keratoplasty or therapeutic vitrectomy. Each of these surgical modalities is important in the adequate care of patients with *Candida* infections of the eye. Curettage of an infected canaliculus, irrigation of an infected lacrimal sac, and frequent expression of infected Meibomian glands are essential to the successful eradication of *Candida* infections in these regions. Daily débridement of a *Candida* corneal ulcer not only removes necrotic and infected material but also enhances the penetration of topically applied antifungal agents.

The decision about the need for and technique of therapeutic penetrating keratoplasty in a case of advanced or progressing *Candida* keratitis is as complex as the decisions surrounding the appropriate use of corticosteroids in such infections. Most ophthalmologists probably delay too long in the face of a worsening case of *Candida* corneal ulcer before proceeding with therapeutic penetrating keratoplasty. The decision to proceed with this therapeutic modality should be made before progression of the process into the anterior chamber and before the process extends to the corneal periphery, where total excision of the affected area would be extremely difficult. Intraocular extension or the development of "malignant fungal glaucoma" or both are absolute indications for surgical intervention.

The safety and efficacy of therapeutic vitrectomy for infectious endophthalmitis have not been proven, but there are some obvious theoretical attractions to this therapeutic modality. Some surgeons feel that it is important to remove as much of the "abscess" of infected material in the vitreous cavity as possible and to instill antifungal agents locally into the vitreous cavity when *Candida* endophthalmitis with vitreous involvement is present.

Ocular or Periocular Manifestations

Anterior Chamber: Cells and flare; hypopyon.

Conjunctiva: Cicatrization; follicular, pseudomembranous, or purulent conjunctivitis; necrotic ulcer; phlyctenulosis.

Cornea: Dendritic, epithelial, or superficial punctate keratitis; opacity; stromal infiltrate, with or without feathery edges and "satellite" lesions; stromal vascularization.

Eyelids: Blepharitis; cheesy material expressible from Meibomian glands; eczema; edema; granuloma; hyperemia; pustules.

Globe: Atrophy; endophthalmitis; panophthalmitis.

Lacrimal System: Calcareous cast; dacryocystitis; epiphora; occlusion of lacrimal canaliculi.

Optic Nerve: Granulation; Hyperemia; infiltration; papillitis; perivasculitis.

Retina: Atrophy; embolism; exudative detachment; perivasculitis; Roth's spot; vascular engorgement.

Vitreous: Abscess; cellular reaction; condensation; fluffy, white exudates.

Other: Decreased visual acuity; hemorrhages; retrobulbar abscess.

PRECAUTIONS

Although fungi rank behind bacteria and viruses in overall incidence as causes of ocular infections, they often produce greater structural and functional damage to the eye. This is partly due to the fact that fungal infections often develop slower and the diagnosis may be delayed. Also, their propensity to mimic other infections or neoplastic diseases is often a problem to the ophthalmologist, and effective treatment may be missed or delayed thereby. Deficiencies of current ocular antifungal agents also limit the opportunity for specific treatment of these microorganisms. Amphotericin B is not a good ocular antifungal agent. As with other polyene antibiotics, it is highly irritating and does not reach the anterior chamber in effective levels following parenteral, subconjunctival, or topical administration. There is no evidence to indicate that nystatin is more effective than amphotericin B against *Candida*. Natamycin penetrates the eye so poorly that it is useful only for superficial infections, and it is not the most effective antifungal agents against *Candida*.

It is usually unwise to initiate broad-spectrum antifungal therapy for a suspected fungal ulcer or suspected fungal endophthalmitis. The best defense against eventual confusion in the face of a deteriorating clinical picture in a patient with infectious keratitis or endophthalmitis is an adequate initial diagnostic effort that guarantees the successful isolation of the causative organism, so that ultimate identification and selection of specific therapy are possible. Therefore, for a corneal ulcer, adequate corneal scrapings for smears and for cultures on multiple media are essential. In suspected endophthalmitis, aqueous or vitreous samples are similarly essential; in any case of aphakic endophthalmitis or vitreal involvement in endophthalmitis, a vitreous tap should be considered mandatory.

COMMENTS

The use of systemic and/or topical corticosteroids in the management of patients with infectious keratitis or endophthalmitis, including those cases caused by *Candida*, is controversial. It is clear that corticosteroids can inhibit the host response to the infecting organism and can thereby promote undesirable progression of the infectious process. It also seems clear, however, that excessive inflammatory host responses can be highly destructive and can produce undesirable permanent structural alterations in the eye. Some clinicians believe that it is possible and desirable to modify such excessive host responses with corticosteroids while simultaneously not overdepressing the host immune response, so that adequate eradication of the organism occurs without excessive inflammatory-response-induced tissue destruction. In an animal model, it would appear that dosages of topical corticosteroids considerably less than those commercially available might be required to achieve such a balance. Decisions regarding the appropriate use of corticosteroids in these settings are complex and extremely tricky. At the very least, it should be strongly emphasized that steroid therapy has no place in the management of an ocular infection, unless the causative organism has been isolated and definitively identified and specific therapy to which the organism is sensitive has been instituted.

References

Foster CS: Miconazole therapy for keratomycosis. Am J Ophthalmol 91:622–629, 1981.
Foster CS, et al: Ocular toxicity of topical antifungal agents. Arch Ophthalmol 99:1081–1084, 1981.
Heinemann MH, Bloom AF, Horowitz J: Candida albicans endophthalmitis in a patient with AIDS. Case report. Arch Ophthalmol 105:1172–1173, 1987.
Insler MS, Urso LF: Candida albicans endophthalmitis after penetrating keratoplasty. Am J Ophthalmol 104:57–60, 1987.
Malecaze F, Bessieres MH, Bec P, Fleutiaux S, Mathis A, Seguela JP: Immunological analysis of the aqueous humour in candida endophthalmitis. I: Experimental study. Br J Ophthalmol 72:309–312, 1988.
Mathis A, Malecaze F, Bessieres MH, Arne JL, Seguela JP, Bec P: Immunological analysis of the aqueous humour in candida endophthalmitis. II: Clinical study. Br J Ophthalmol 72:313–316, 1988.
Parrish CM, O'Day DM, Hoyle TC: Spontaneous fungal corneal ulcer as an ocular manifestation of AIDS. Am J Ophthalmol 104:302–303, 1987.
Tolentino F et al: Retinal and lens toxicity studies of intravitreal miconazole. Invest Ophthalmol Vis Sci (Suppl) 19:114, 1980.

COCCIDIOIDOMYCOSIS
JAMES P. GANLEY, M.D., Dr. P.H.,
and STEPHEN A. KLOTZ, M.D.
Shreveport, Louisiana

Coccidioidomycosis is an infectious disease caused by *Coccidioides immitis*, a dimorphic fungus whose free-living or saprobic state is restricted to the semi-arid Lower Sonoran Life Zone. Hence, in the United States, it is endemic to southeast California, southern Arizona and New Mexico, and southwestern Texas. Elsewhere in the Western hemisphere, *C. immitis* can be found in Mexico, Central America, and parts of South America. Primary infection occurs following the inhalation of air-borne arthroconidia and is usually asymptomatic. White women are particularly prone to develop a characteristic syndrome known as valley fever or desert rheumatism. Conjunctivitis or episcleritis, along with erythema nodosum or erythema multiforme and arthritis, is prominent in this syndrome; a positive skin test reaction and tube precipitin antibodies in the serum characteristically develop simultaneously. Uncommonly, primary infection is not contained by the host, and progressive cavitary pulmonary disease (typically in men with pre-existing lung disease) or extrapulmonary dissemination of the fungus may occur (in pregnant women, in persons with diabetes mellitus, or in men of dark-skinned races). Patients with impaired cell-mediated immunity caused either by such drugs as corticosteroids or concurrent infection with the human immunodeficiency virus are at particular risk for relapsing infection and/or extrapulmonary dissemination.

Chorioretinal lesions occur in up to 9 per cent of individuals with documented disease; the majority of these lesions are asymptomatic and resolve spontaneously without therapy. No relationship has been associated between the presence of these asymptomatic lesions and the severity of systemic disease. Most documented cases of symptomatic intraocular involvement cause significant visual loss and ocular morbidity; these cases tend to be associated with progressive systemic coccidioidomycosis. The major symptomatic intraocular manifestations are chronic granulomatous iridocyclitis, choroiditis, and retinitis; endophthalmitis has also been described. Posterior ocular involvement is usually focal, but may be diffuse; overlying vitreous reaction varies from only mild involvement to marked turbidity.

Granulomatous lesions of eyebrow, lids, and palpebral conjunctiva have been reported. Anterior segment manifestations, including phlyctenular conjunctivitis, episcleritis, and scleritis, usually occur with primary pulmonary infection and are often associated with erythema nodosum. These manifestations are considered to be hypersensitivity responses to the coccidioidal antigen and usually subside along with the primary infection without treatment. Rarer ocular manifestations of *C. immitis* infection include

60 / COCCIDIOIDOMYCOSIS

orbital and optic nerve granulomas and extraocular nerve palsies secondary to intracerebral infection.

THERAPY

Systemic. Amphotericin B remains the drug of choice in the initial treatment of life-threatening disease. Intravenous therapy is indicated in disseminated diseases, including progressive periocular and intraocular involvement. Lid granulomata are often associated with other granulomata of the skin and often resolve with amphotericin B therapy. The penetration of amphotericin B into the cerebral spinal fluid occurs at levels below the minimal inhibitory concentration of the drug, but unlike cryptococcal meningitis, which responds to intravenous therapy alone, coccidioidal meningitis requires intrathecal,* intracisternal,* or intraventricular* therapy as well.

Amphotericin B binds to ergosterol contained within fungal plasma membranes and in so doing induces membrane defects. It possesses considerable immunoadjuvant effects, as well as antifungal properties. Amphotericin B is administered intravenously in dextrose and water; it will precipitate in saline. Premedication with aspirin and diphenhydramine (or meperidine, if reactions are severe) reduces or eliminates uncomfortable reactions that commonly occur during administration. It is customary to administer a 1 mg test dose in 100 to 200 ml of 5 per cent dextrose in water over 1 to 2 hours; this should be followed with therapeutic doses (up to 0.6 mg/kg) administered over 4 to 6 hours. If nausea, headache, or fever is particularly troublesome, extending the time of infusion to 8 hours is often helpful. Following stabilization of the patient's condition, a double dose may then be given on alternate days, thus allowing outpatient treatment. A total dose of 2 to 2.5 gm, or frequently more is required. Total doses of 9 gm or more, lifelong intrathecal injections, or permanent oral imidazole therapy may be required in patients in whom remission is slow, those with meningitis, or those with AIDS. The duration of therapy depends on the patient's extent of disease, response to therapy, and reduction in the complement-fixation antibody titers, not by the total amount of amphotericin B administered.

The efficacy and safety of a new formulation of amphotericin B administered intravenously in liposomes have been demonstrated with other fungi. Liposomes are cleared by the reticuloendothelial system, thus sparing amphotericin B-induced toxicity to such target organs as the kidney. This is a particularly attractive strategy in treating such diseases as histoplasmosis in which the reticuloendothelial system is characteristically parasitized by the fungus. However, the short shelf-life of the liposome preparation limits its current usefulness, and its efficacy in coccidioidomycosis is unknown.

Azoles are an alternative therapy to amphotericin B. Their mode of action is by inhibition of the cytochrome P-450 enzyme system, resulting in a reduction of ergosterol in fungal cell membranes. Ketoconazole in daily doses of 400 mg orally has been successful in the treatment of disseminated disease without meningitis. Using extremely stringent criteria, cure was established in 30 to 40 per cent of patients treated with ketoconazole. It has been used concurrently with amphotericin B for the treatment of coccidioidomycosis in AIDS patients. It is useful in limited pulmonary disease caused by *C. immitis*, as well as in the treatment of such deep-seated infections as arthritis or osteomyelitis.

Itraconazole[†], a newer imidazole, shows promise of activity comparable to amphotericin B. In initial trials of 400 mg daily, about 50 per cent of patients became culture-negative or improved their clinical status. Fluconazole[†] at low doses (50 mg) was ineffective in the treatment of coccidioidomycosis, although higher doses will be tried in future trials. Neither of these third-generation imidazoles is currently available. Miconazole, an approved first-generation imidazole, remains an alternative intravenous drug to amphotericin B for disseminated coccidioidomycosis. It has been used successfully for the treatment of central nervous system disease as well.

Ocular. Amphotericin B has poor intraocular (aqueous humor and vitreous) penetration when administered intravenously, unless large doses are used, which increases the risk of renal toxicity. Subconjunctival injection of amphotericin B* is sometimes used for severe fungal endophthalmitis in a dosage of 0.75 to 5.0 mg in 1.0 ml aqueous suspension, but its efficacy in coccidioidal endophthalmitis is unknown. However, subconjunctival injections likewise result in poor penetration into the vitreous of experimentally inflamed eyes. In severe anterior uveitis, intracameral injection* has been used with intravenous therapy without benefit and experimentally produces a severe vitritis with scarring.

Ocular or Periocular Manifestations

Anterior Chamber: Cells; flare; hypopyon.

Choroid: Atrophic scars; diffuse chorioretinitis; focal choroiditis; granulomas.

Conjunctiva: Conjunctivitis (bulbar); granulomas (palpebral); phlyctenules (bulbar); ulcer (palpebral).

Cornea: Mutton-fat keratic precipitates; necrotic inflammatory foci; perforation; superficial infiltrate.

Extraocular Muscles: Abducens paralysis; diplopia.

Eyelids: Edema; granuloma.

Globe: Endophthalmitis.

Iris or Ciliary Body: Granulomatous iridocyclitis; peripheral anterior synechia; posterior synechia.

Optic Nerve: Atrophy; juxtapapillary granuloma; neuritis; optic nerve granuloma; papilledema.

Orbit: Granuloma.

Retina: Edema; exudates; focal retinitis; hemorrhages; perivascular sheathing.
Sclera and Episclera: Episcleritis; scleritis.
Vitreous: Exudates; vitritis.

Precautions

Immunosuppressive therapy, especially corticosteroids, is a primary factor in increasing the risk of dissemination and should be reduced or discontinued where possible. An initial improvement of ocular lesions may be seen with topical and systemic corticosteroids, but an exacerbation of ocular inflammation usually follows their continued use and results in progressive destruction of the eye.

Treatment with amphotericin B results in significant but predictable toxicity that can be managed with modest dose reduction if necessary. Nephrotoxicity causes a reduction in the glomerular filtration rate and therefore an elevation of blood urea nitrogen. To avoid uremic symptoms, reduction in dose and interval is recommended in patients with a serum creatinine greater than 3.0 mg/dl. Both reversible and permanent nephrotoxicity occur, but the latter is rarely clinically apparent. Hypokalemia develops as a consequence of renal tubular acidosis and can be treated with oral potassium supplements. A reversible normocytic, normochromic anemia is an expected complication, but usually does not require transfusion. Amphotericin B should be infused slowly. Rapid administration (in less than 60 minutes) is associated with potentially lethal hyperkalemia that is presumably caused by cell death associated with binding of amphotericin B to cholesterol in host plasma membranes.

Ketaconazole requires an acid pH in the stomach for absorption. Therefore, patients with achlorhydria or who are receiving antacids or histamine H_2 blockers are not suitable candidates for treatment with this drug. It interferes with steroidogenesis in humans as well. Testicular and adrenal dysfunction occur, manifesting clinically as gynecomastia and oligospermia; minor elevations in liver function tests also occur. Idiosyncratic hepatic failure is a rare but fatal reaction.

Miconazole, because of its Cremaphor carrier, induces intense pruritus in one half of patients, as well as occasional anaphylactoid reactions. Because of these and other adverse reactions and the fact that it is available only as an intravenous drug, miconazole has fallen into disfavor.

Comments

Measurement of serum tube precipitin and complement-fixation antibody titers, radiographs, and geographic exposure are important in diagnosing coccidioidomycosis. Coccidioidin and spherulin skin testing are valuable epidemiologic tools; the former is important in judging response to therapy. Therapy is best supervised by clinicians experienced in the vagaries of this disease. A full and complete ophthalmic examination is indicated in anyone with ocular symptoms or signs. Confirmation of the diagnosis should be sought by culture or, if possible, by tissue diagnosis. Anterior chamber or vitreous paracentesis may be indicated in some cases.

The detection of acute peripheral chorioretinal lesions associated with coccidioidomycosis does not necessarily imply the presence of active disseminated disease requiring treatment. Frequently, these lesions are self-limiting, leaving asymptomatic, atrophic chorioretinal scars. They should be followed periodically, and the decision regarding treatment should depend on ocular disease progression, as well as the overall coccidioidal disease status.

References

Blumenkranz MS, Stevens DA: Endogenous coccidioidal endophthalmitis. Ophthalmology 87:974–984, 1980.

Blumenkranz MS, Stevens DA: Therapy of endogenous fungal endophthalmitis. Miconzaole or amphotericin B for coccidioidal and candidal infection. Arch Ophthalmol 98:1216–1220, 1980.

Danetta A, et al: Coccidioidomycosis in the acquired immunodeficiency syndrome. Ann Intern Med 106:372–379, 1987.

Drutz DJ: Amphotericin B in the treatment of coccidioidomycosis. Drugs 26:337–346, 1983.

Drutz DJ, Catanzaro A: Coccidioidomycosis. Am Rev Resp Dis 117:559–585, 727–771, 1978.

Galgiani JN, et al: Ketoconazole therapy of progressive coccidioidomycosis. Comparison of 400- and 800-mg doses and observations at higher doses. Am J Med 85:603–610, 1988.

Glasgow BJ, et al: Miliary retinitis in coccidioidomycosis. Am J Ophthalmol 104:24–27, 1987.

Graybill JR: Azole antifungal drugs in treatment of coccidioidomycosis. Sem Resp Infect 1:53–60, 1986.

Graybill JR, Craven PC: Antifungal agents used in systemic mycoses. Activity and therapeutic use. Drugs 25:41–62, 1983.

Rodenbiker HT, Ganley JP: Ocular coccidioidomycosis. Surv Ophthalmol 24:263–290, 1980.

Rodenbiker HT, et al: Prevalence of chorioretinal scars associated with coccidioidomycosis. Arch Ophthalmol 99:71–75, 1981.

Ross JB, et al: Ketoconazole for treatment of chronic pulmonary coccidioidomycosis. Ann Intern Med 96:440–443, 1982.

Stevens DA: *Coccidioides immitis. In* Mandel GL, Douglas RG Jr, Bennett JE (eds): Principles and Practice of Infectious Diseases. New York, John Wiley and Sons, 1985, pp 1485–1493.

DERMATOPHYTOSIS
(Epidermophytosis, Epidermomycosis, Rubrophytia, Tinea, Trichophytosis)

ALAN SUGAR, M.D.

Ann Arbor, Michigan

Dermatophytosis refers to superficial infection of the skin by the ringworm fungi; *Trichophyton, Epidermophyton,* and *Microsporum* are among the common species causing cutaneous infection. Clinically, dermatophytoses are classified by the involved skin area, such as tinea capitis (ringworm of the scalp), tinea corporis (of body skin), and tinea pedis (athlete's foot). Ocular or periocular involvement usually is rare and a result of facial infection. This group of fungi affects only keratinized tissue and is therefore usually limited to superficial infection. Lesions begin as red papules that become red, circular, scaly patches. As the lesions enlarge centrifugally, the center may clear, leaving a typical ringworm pattern. There is usually very little underlying inflammation. Marginal blepharitis, lid ulcers, and loss of lashes or brow hair may occur secondary to facial or scalp involvement. Allergy to fungi—dermatophytid reactions—can occur causing noninfected vesicular lesions on the hands and rarely allergic conjunctivitis. The diagnosis can be confirmed by examination of skin scrapings under the microscope after adding a drop of 10 per cent potassium hydroxide. Cultures on Sabouraud's medium, kept at room temperature, grow in 2 to 3 weeks.

THERAPY

Systemic. Extensive involvement or lesions unresponsive to topical treatment may be treated with oral griseofulvin. A dosage of 125 to 250 mg for children or 500 mg for adults of the microsize crystalline form is given in a single dose after a meal. The ultramicrosize crystalline form requires half of the above dosage. Because the drug is incorporated into keratin slowly and is fungistatic, at least 4 to 6 weeks of treatment are required. For severe infections or in patients allergic to griseofulvin, daily administration of ketoconazole in a dosage of 50 to 200 mg for children or 200 to 400 mg for adults may be used.

Topical. Antifungal creams can be successful in treating milder lesions of the face, scalp, and lids. The available agents include 1 per cent clotrimazole, 2 per cent miconazole, 1 per cent tolnaftate, and 1 per cent haloprogin. The medication should be applied twice daily after the involved skin is gently cleansed, and treatment should be continued for 1 week after the lesion clears. Care should be taken in the application of these antifungal agents because they are irritating if applied to the eye. Involved lashes should be epilated.

Ocular or Periocular Manifestations

Conjunctiva: Infectious or allergic conjunctivitis.
Cornea: Fungal ulcer (very rare).
Eyebrows: Folliculitis; madarosis; scaly rash.
Eyelids: Blepharitis; dermatitis; edema; madarosis; ulcer.

PRECAUTIONS

As in other fungal infections, corticosteroids may mask the nature of the dermatophytosis, may increase its severity, and may prolong its course. Premature discontinuation of topical or systemic antifungals may be followed by relapse of infection.

COMMENTS

Ocular and periocular involvement with dermatophytosis is rare and usually is an extension from involved scalp or facial skin. Tinea capitis, scalp ringworm, occurs most frequently in children in hot humid weather. Other forms occur in adult men. As in other fungal infections, such systemic diseases as malignancy or diabetes and systemic steroids may be predisposing factors.

References

Duke-Elder S: System of Ophthalmology. St. Louis, CV Mosby, 1974, Vol XIII, pp 175–179.
Fedukowicz HB, Stetson S: External Infections of the Eye: Bacterial, Viral, and Mycotic, 3rd ed. East Norwalk, Appleton-Century-Crofts, 1985, pp 194–196.
Francois J, Rysselaere M: Oculomycoses. Springfield, IL, Charles Thomas, 1972, pp 229–245.
Korting GW: The Skin and Eye. A Dermatologic Correlation of Diseases of the Periorbital Region. Philadelphia, WB Saunders, 1973, pp 50–54.
Ostler HB, Okumoto M, Halde C: Dermatophytosis affecting the periorbital region. Am J Ophthalmol 72:934–938, 1971.

MUCORMYCOSIS
(Phycomycosis)
DAVID J. WILSON, M.D.
Portland, Oregon

Mucormycosis is an acute, severe infection caused by fungi of the order Mucorales and the class Phycomycetes. Some authors prefer the term *phycomycosis* to describe this disease because fungi of orders other than Mucorales are pathogenic to humans. Several terms have been used in the ophthalmic literature to describe this entity, including rhino-orbitocerebral, rhinocerebral, craniofacial, spheno-orbital, and orbital mucormycosis or phycomycosis.

Mucormycosis represents an opportunistic infection in which a ubiquitous organism (normally found in soil, air, and as a common bread mold) becomes a pathogen in humans under a variety of metabolic situations. Diabetes, particularly when ketoacidosis is present, is by far the most common predisposing condition; it is present in 40 to 80 per cent of patients. Other predisposing conditions include chronic renal failure, leukemia, lymphoma, metabolic acidosis, and cirrhosis. Mucormycosis with no underlying disease has been reported, but these cases are quite rare.

The classic presentation of mucormycosis is a diabetic patient who initially complains of rhinitis, sinusitis, and facial pain with rapid progression to signs and symptoms of orbital cellulitis and orbital apex syndrome. With cerebral involvement, severe headache, altered mental status, and signs of cavernous sinus or internal carotid artery thrombosis become manifest. The diagnosis of mucormycosis requires the demonstration of the characteristic broad, nonseptate, branching hyphae in tissue, as well as culture of the fungi. These fungi have a marked predilection for invading arteries, which characteristically produces thrombosis with extensive coagulative necrosis and gangrene.

THERAPY

Early diagnosis is critical and has been credited with the tremendous improvement in mortality seen in this disease since 1979. A combination of surgical débridement of necrotic tissue, systemic and local antifungal (amphotericin B) administration, and correction of the underlying metabolic defect is essential for successful management of this disease.

Systemic. Amphotericin B is the antifungal agent of choice. Because of the numerous systemic side effects of this medication, it should be administered under the direction of a physician familiar with its use. After administration of a test dose, a regimen of 0.3 mg/kg dissolved in 500 ml of 5 per cent dextrose in water has been recommended for intravenous administration over a 1- to 3-hour period each day. This should be advanced to a daily dose of 0.5 to 0.6 mg/kg. Amphotericin B is continued as indicated by the patient's clinical course, and total doses of over 4 gm are often required.

Ocular. Histologic evaluation of débrided tissue may give some indication of adequacy of therapy. Local irrigation and packing of the orbit with gauze containing 1 mg/ml of amphotericin B have been advocated as measures to limit the amount of disfiguring débridement that must be done.

Surgical. Complete débridement of all necrotic tissue must be performed. Since mucormycosis begins as an infection of the sinuses and may spread to the orbit and brain, débridement may require the combined efforts of an ophthalmologist, otolaryngologist, and neurosurgeon.

Supportive. Standard medical techniques are employed to correct the basic metabolic defect. It is usually advisable to admit the patient to a medical service where the metabolic defect can be managed and the patient can be monitored for toxicity from amphotericin B.

Ocular or Periocular Manifestations

Conjunctiva: Chemosis; hyperemia; suppuration.
Cornea: Clouding; ulcer; anesthesia.
Eyelids: Ptosis; edema; discoloration; necrosis.
Globe: Proptosis.
Pupil: Dilation; absent reaction to light.
Other: Decreased visual acuity; orbital and facial pain; diplopia; paralysis of extraocular muscles; nasal or palatal eschar or ulcer; headache; altered mental status; orbital apex syndrome; cavernous sinus thrombosis; internal carotid artery occlusion.

PRECAUTIONS

Mucormycosis is a life-threatening disease, and early diagnosis is essential in its successful management. Mucormycosis can be mistaken for bacterial orbital cellulitis or sinusitis with cavernous sinus thrombosis. Awareness of the epidemiology is helpful in alerting the clinician to the possibility of mucormycosis. Corticosteroids do not have a role in the management of mucormycosis and may exacerbate the condition. Amphotericin B is an extremely toxic drug and should be administered under the guidance of a physician skilled in its use.

COMMENTS

Three principles should guide the treatment of patients with mucormycosis: correction of predisposing metabolic abnormalities, surgical débridement of nonviable tissues, and use of systemic amphotericin B.

References

Castelli JB, Pallin JL: Lethal rhinocerebral phycomycosis in a healthy adult: A case report and review of the literature. Ophthalmology 86:696–703, 1978.
Kohn R, Hepler R: Management of limited rhino-orbital mucormycosis without exenteration. Ophthalmology 92:1440–1444, 1985.
Lie K-J, et al: Phycomycosis of the central nervous system associated with diabetes mellitus in Indonesia. Am J Clin Pathol 32:62–70, 1959.
Parfrey NA: Improved diagnosis and prognosis of mucormycosis: A clinicopathologic study of 33 cases. Medicine 65:113–123, 1986.
Schwartz JN, Donnelly EH, Klintworth GK: Ocular and orbital phycomycosis. Surv Ophthalmol 22:3–28, 1977.

OCULAR HISTOPLASMOSIS
(Presumed Ocular Histoplasmosis Syndrome)
RONALD E. SMITH, M.D.
Los Angeles, California

Ocular histoplasmosis or the presumed ocular histoplasmosis syndrome consists of macular dis-

64 / OCULAR HISTOPLASMOSIS

ciform lesions (hemorrhagic or nonhemorrhagic), atrophic peripheral chorioretinal scars, and peripapillary scars; the vitreous is clear and there is no anterior segment reaction. This disorder is felt to be associated with a previous benign infection with the fungus, *Histoplasma capsulatum*, which is endemic to the Ohio and middle Mississippi River valleys of the United States. The organism itself does not appear to be actively replicating in the ocular lesions, although the patients do have evidence of prior exposure to and infection with the organism. The organism initially causes a mild pulmonary infection with the typically vague and mild systemic symptoms of an upper respiratory tract infection; asymptomatic multifocal active choroiditis probably also occurs at this early stage. The acute ocular lesions, along with those elsewhere in the body, resolve spontaneously, leaving small chorioretinal scars at the posterior pole and around the nerve head or in the periphery. As long as 10 to 20 years after the initial fungemia and spontaneous healing, active disciform lesions, consisting of hemorrhage and edema, occur around the old scars. Thus, "reactivation" of old histoplasmosis chorioretinal scars accounts for this macula-threatening ocular lesion.

THERAPY

Ocular. Because the exact pathogenesis of the late macular lesion of ocular histoplasmosis is unknown, therapy has been empiric and remains controversial. In any event, fluorescein angiography is most important in the evaluation of such patients to determine the presence of subretinal neovascularization, which may occur in areas adjacent to inactive small scars, usually in the macula.

In general, if early active lesions have not hemorrhaged and there is no clear-cut evidence of subretinal neovascularization, high-dose systemic corticosteroid therapy with short-acting agents, such as prednisone, prednisolone, or methylprednisolone, is suggested in doses of 80 to 100 mg every morning. Patients should be followed carefully with repeat fluorescein angiography several days after initiation of therapy to determine if subretinal neovascularization has occurred or progressed.

If neovascularization has occurred or progressed under such conditions or if the patient has developed hemorrhage in association with the active lesion, photocoagulation should be performed. Argon laser photocoagulation is currently the best treatment to destroy a neovascular net that is outside the capillary-free zone of the macula. Photocoagulation should be moderate to heavy, with the goal being complete destruction of the neovascularization, incomplete or partial photocoagulation can result in rapid progression of the subretinal net. Krypton laser therapy may allow photocoagulation even closer to the fovea.

Evaluation of the "second eye" is most important in patients with active lesions in the macula of one eye. A complete ocular examination, including fluorescein angiography, is most important to determine if small scars are present, as such foci are a potential source of later activity. In fact, it is estimated that 20 to 30 per cent of such small scars may become active over a period of several years.

Ocular or Periocular Manifestations

Choroid or Retina: Atrophic scars at the posterior pole, periphery, and around the nerve head; choroiditis; subretinal neovascularization.

Macula: Edema; hemorrhages.

Precautions

Since the organism is no longer actively replicating, treatment with amphotericin B or other antifungal agents is not indicated in the management of presumed ocular histoplasmosis. Similarly, histoplasmin desensitization has not been found to be effective and is not recommended.

Patients on corticosteroid therapy should be followed closely to rule out systemic or ocular side effects of medication.

Prophylactic photocoagulation of inactive scars in the macula or peripapillary region is not recommended and, in fact, may cause reactivation of an inactive process.

Comments

The pathophysiology and precise etiology of reactivation of previously inactive small atrophic choroidal scars in presumed ocular histoplasmosis are unknown, although nonspecific events, such as emotional or physical stress, may be implicated. At the present time, there is no known therapy that will decrease the incidence or preclude the recurrence of ocular histoplasmosis.

References

Lewis ML, Van Newkirk MR, Gass JDM: Follow-up study of presumed ocular histoplasmosis syndrome. Ophthalmology 87:390–399, 1980.

Schlaegel TF Jr: Histoplasmic choroiditis. Ann Ophthalmol 6:237–252, 1974.

Schlaegel TF Jr: Ocular Histoplasmosis. New York, Grune & Stratton, 1977.

Smith RE: Ocular histoplasmosis. *In* Ryan SJ Jr, Smith RE (eds): Selected Topics on the Eye in Systemic Disease. New York, Grune & Stratton, 1974, pp 135–165.

Watzke RC, Claussen RW: The long-term course of multifocal choroiditis (presumed ocular histoplasmosis). Am J Ophthalmol 91:750–760, 1981.

RHINOSPORIDIOSIS
(Oculosporidiosis)

P.K. MUKHERJEE, M.S.
Raipur, India

Rhinosporidiosis is a chronic infective granuloma most commonly affecting nasal mucosa. Because the nose is frequently involved and the first reported case was a chronic granuloma of nostril, the name rhinosporidiosis was given to this condition. It may also involve the nasopharynx, lacrimal sac, conjunctiva, and the postnasal space by direct continuity. It may be seen in the larynx, palate trachea, bronchus, and maxillary sinus as well. Rhinosporidiosis can infect other parts of the body far from the nose, such as the urethra, vulva, vagina, and rectum. Lesions of skin and bone have also been reported. It seems that only few organs, such as the brain and heart, are immune to the disease. The disease occurs naturally both in humans and animals independently or may spread from one to the other.

The organism, once believed to be a sporozoan, is now considered to be a fungus belonging to class Phycomycetes. The organism starts its life cycle as a parasite measuring 8 μ, but grows by nuclear division until it reaches a size about 200 to 300 μ and contains 40,000 nuclei that form 16,000 spores. The spores appear round or oval and measure 2–10 μ in size. After implantation in mucosa or a mucocutaneous area, the infective spores enter deeper and lead a parasitic life. They increase in size by asexual multiplication and, in course, develop into a sporangium.

The sporangium measures about 300 to 500 μ in diameter and has a double-walled envelope; the outer one is chitinous and the inner one consists of cellulose. The mature sporangium may contain as many as 16,000 spores. It bursts at a weak spot in its wall, and spores are discharged into the tissue to begin the cycle again.

The disease has a wide distribution, mostly in the tropics. Cases reported from nontropical countries are sporadic and have a history of migration from the tropics. It is seen more commonly in tropical countries in part because of their moderate to heavy annual rainfall, which results in a humid climate. The countries most affected are India, Ceylon, Indonesia, and the Phillipines. The greatest number of cases are found in India and Ceylon. In India, the distribution is not uniform; it is seen mostly in the South Central and Southern states. Surprisingly, no case has been reported from Australia or New Zealand.

The mode of infection is not well understood. Males are more frequently affected, with 75 per cent of cases seen in males under 20 years of age. Almost all infected patients have a habit of bathing in common village pools along with cattle. The cattle in the endemic area show frequent involvement. Yet, the fungus has neither been cultured under artificial conditions nor have experiment lesions been produced in animals. The possible mode of infection could be water-borne or air-borne. One hypothesis is that the spore reaches the person's mucous membrane while bathing in an infected pond and becomes lodged in natural recesses in the mucosal fold (conjunctival fornices) or pathologic strictures (nasolacrimal duct stenosis) where it proliferates to produce a typical lesion. Wide systemic dissemination may be blood-borne or by continuity of the mucous membrane (from the nasal mucosa down to the trachea, bronchus, and lungs or spread from the oropharynx to gastrointestinal tract). Genitourinary tract involvement is most probably retrograde from the external genitals to the bladder or pelvic organs.

The typical lesion is a pedunculated fleshy mass ranging from few millimeters to few inches in size; occasionally, it is sessile. The mass is red in color due to the abundance of vascularity, and the surface is rough and shows fine capillaries on it. On the surface are multiple brown or white dots representing old and immature sporangia, respectively. The tissue is friable, and slightest trauma causes bleeding, resulting in epistaxis, hemoptysis, hematuria, or bleeding from conjunctiva.

The diagnosis in endemic areas is not difficult, but in nonendemic areas it may be confused with chronic granuloma-like tuberculosis, syphilis, burst chalazia, or a new growth, that is hemangioma, papilloma, or malignancy. However, the reverse is also true, as the above-mentioned conditions are often confused with rhinosporidiosis in endemic areas.

The diagnosis is best confirmed by histopathology of the excised tissue. Under high power of the microscope, sporangia in wet preparation of small tissue removed from the growth have been demonstrated in most of the ocular cases.

The ocular lesion has two modes of presentation, one being spread from the nose and the other being involvement of the ocular structure without nasal or systemic involvement. The latter type of lesion is designated as primary rhinosporidiosis of eye or oculosporidiosis, which accounts for 10 per cent of all cases.

Patients with conjunctival involvement seek medical help earlier than those with an affected lacrimal sac, because the fleshy red growth attracts attention earlier. A conjunctival growth overhanging the cornea may cause foreign body sensation and lacrimation. The conjunctival growth is a solitary chronic granuloma that can be sessile or pedunculated. Growth arising from fornices are more likely to develop long pedicles than those arising from tarsal conjunctiva or the limbus. The pedunculated growth is a flat, leaf-like, red mass with crenated edges. The surface is rough and has multiple white dots that represent sporangia, it bleeds on manipulation.

The sclera is very rarely involved, although a scleral staphyloma may result. Generally, a conjunctival growth overlies the staphyloma.

The lacrimal sac is most commonly affected in the form of chronic dacryocystitis. The sac presents a typical appearance. The skin over the swelling has an orange peel appearance; the

66 / RHINOSPORIDIOSIS

swelling is soft, nontender, and compressible. There is no regurgitation, and complete block of the nasolacrimal duct is rare. Erosion of the surrounding bone is common. The sac may be secondarily infected, presenting as cellulitis. Bilateral involvement is rare.

THERAPY

Ocular. Ocular involvement does not require any specific drug therapy. No known drug is effective against rhinosporidiosis. However, associated conjunctivitis may be treated with appropriate broad-spectrum antibiotics.

Surgical. The most satisfactory results are obtained by complete surgical removal of the growth. Surgery can be undertaken under topical anesthesia, but children may require general anesthesia. The conjunctival growth is grasped with blunt and flat forceps without trauma to the growth and is pulled away from the conjunctiva. The pedicle is cut by sharp scissors, and the cut distal stump retracts immediately. Because of profuse hemorrhage, it may be necessary to tie the stump or use thermal cautery. In most cases, using a firm-pressure bandage is sufficient. For small conjunctival growths, cryoapplication is sufficient to convert the whole mass into an ice ball, resulting in shrinkage of the growth.

In scleral staphyloma, best results are obtained by applying cryo all around the staphyloma. The overlying conjunctiva is dissected clear from the staphyloma, and the scleral bulges is indented with silicone or a silastic sponge of a suitable size. The buckle must overlap the staphyloma by about 1 mm on each side. A posteriorly placed scleral staphyloma is clearly visible with an indirect ophthalmoscope. The conjunctiva is replaced over the buckle. The eye may be made soft by use of intravenous mannitol during manipulation. Diathermy is contraindicated as this may perforate the staphyloma and cause intractable bleeding.

Management of chronic dacryocystitis due to rhinosporidiosis is less satisfactory than that of conjunctival growth. Unless meticulous care is taken to remove the growth in one sitting, recurrence is frequent, especially if nasal growth is not taken care of simultaneously. The procedure consists of dissection of the friable growth, mostly by blunt dissection from the surrounding structure without rupture. If the mass is ruptured, there is profuse hemorrhage that obscures the field and promotes recurrence, which is more difficult to manage.

Ocular or Periocular Manifestation

Conjunctiva: Sessile or pedunculated granuloma bleeding from the growth.
Lacrimal System: Chronic dacryocystitis.
Sclera: Scleral staphyloma.
Other: Lacrimation due to growth rubbing over the cornea.

PRECAUTIONS

Precaution should be taken not to rupture the sac while removing it. Doing so leads to intractable bleeding.

COMMENTS

Involvement of ocular adnexa is very common. In endemic areas, rhinosporidiosis may be confused with other chronic granuloma or malignancy.

References

Acharya PV, Gupta RL, Darbari BS: Cutaneous rhinosporidiosis. Indian Dermatol Vener 39:22–23, 1973.
Darbari BS, Gupta RL, Shukla IM, Arora MM: Rhinosporidiosis in Raipur. A clinicopathological study of 348 cases. Indian J Pathol Bact 15:105–107, 1972.
Gupta RL, Darbari BS, Dwevedi MP, Billore OP, Arora MM: An epidemiological study of rhinosporidiosis in and around Raipur. Indian J Med Res 64:1293–1299, 1976.
Krishnan MM, Kawatra VK, Rao VA, Ratnakar C: Diverticulum of the lacrimal sac associated with rhinosporidiosis. Br J Ophthalmol 70:867–868, 1986.
Mukherjee PK, Shukla IM, Despande M, Pravenna K: Rhinosporidiosis of the lacrimal sac. Indian J Ophthalmol 30:513–514, 1982.
Naik RS, Siddiqui RA, Naik V: Urethronasal rhinosporidiosis. J Indian Med Assoc 72:238–239, 1979.
Savino DF, Margo CE: Conjunctival Rhinosporidiosis. Light and electron microscopic study. Ophthalmology 90:1482–1489, 1983.
Shukla IM, Darbari BS, Arora MM, Gupta RL, Arora NP: Ocular rhinosporidiosis. Proc All-India Ophthalmol 21:133–137, 1970.

SPOROTRICHOSIS

WILLIAM A. AGGER, M.D.
La Crosse, Wisconsin

Sporotrichosis is a chronic fungal infection caused by *Sporothrix schenckii*. Infection usually occurs when the spores are traumatically inoculated into the skin, often on the extremities and occasionally about the eyes. The most common form of the disease is the localized subcutaneous variety. This lesion usually occurs on exposed skin and is characterized by nodules or pustules that may develop into small ulcers. If the condition is not treated, similar nodules may develop along the lymphatics draining the area. The disease often becomes chronic, resulting in enlargement of the regional lymph nodes.

Rarely, a systemic form of the disease may develop. This most commonly occurs in compromised hosts, such as alcoholics, or patients with human immunodeficiency virus infection, and probably develops after inhalation of spores. Following an initial pulmonary lesion, hematogenous spread can occur but is extremely rare. In this form of the disease, the pathogen may metastasize widely, causing granulomas in the joints, genitourinary system, skin, or eyes.

Ocular involvement in sporotrichosis is uncommon. It usually occurs as a result of a primary infection, often on the eyelids, and rarely as a result of a disseminated infection. When the eyelid is the site of a primary or rarely secondary lesion, one or more nodules appear subcutaneously, producing a purulent and ulcerative blepharitis. Secondary to the palpebral infection, preauricular adenopathy, dacryocystitis, and orbital abscesses may develop. Other rare instances of primary ocular sporotrichosis include sporotrichotic keratitis, conjunctivitis, and scleritis. Intraocular sporotrichosis may occur following perforation of a corneal ulcer, trauma to the eye, or metastasis. The usual intraocular form of the disease is a granulomatous tumor on the iris.

THERAPY

Systemic. The drug of choice in cutaneous sporotrichosis is potassium iodide. Ten drops of a saturated solution of potassium iodide are given orally three times daily in progressively increasing doses as tolerated, to a total daily dose of 120 drops. This regimen should be continued for one month after the skin lesions have cleared.

In disseminated sporotrichosis, an initial intravenous dose of 0.25 mg/kg of amphotericin B is indicated. Daily dosage may then be increased to 0.4 mg/kg and continued to a total dose of between 1.5 and 2.5 gm. Only if unusual circumstances occur, such as renal insufficiency, should the dose be reduced.

Flucytosine‡ is not effective in sporotrichosis. Ketoconazole‡ has produced inconsistent results, and itraconazole† therapy has been successful in nonocular disease in small numbers of patients but has not yet been released for general use.

Ocular. Primary ocular treatment usually consists of systemic potassium iodide, in addition to ophthalmic administration of natamycin or amphotericin B. For patients with sporotrichotic corneal ulcers, systemic treatment should be supplemented with topical 5.0 per cent natamycin or 0.25 to 0.50 per cent amphotericin B ophthalmic solution, administered hourly during the day and every other hour at nighttime. Adjunctive therapy includes subconjunctival injection of amphotericin B* and cycloplegics.

In sporotrichotic endophthalmitis, subconjunctival injection of 2 to 5 mg of amphotericin B* may be added to the systemic treatment. Anterior chamber irrigation of 10 to 25 μg of amphotericin B* in a volume of 0.1 to 0.2 ml may follow paracentesis. In a fulminant primary intravitreal infection, vitrectomy is probably the treatment of choice. Intravitreal injection of 5 to 10 μg of amphotericin B* has been recommended by some authorities.

Depending on the severity of the disease, natamycin or amphotericin B eyedrops may be sufficient to treat sporotrichotic conjunctivitis. In patients with sporotrichosis of the lacrimal canaliculi or sac, local irrigation and topical administration of amphotericin B may be effective.

Ocular or Periocular Manifestations

Conjunctiva: Granulomatous or purulent conjunctivitis; ulcerative oculoglandular conjunctivitis.

Cornea: Keratitis; perforation; ulcer.

Eyelids: Purulent or ulcerative blepharitis; subcutaneous abscess.

Globe: Endophthalmitis; panophthalmitis.

Iris: Atrophy; granuloma.

Lacrimal System: Dacryocanaliculitis; dacryocystitis; fistula.

Orbit: Abscess; erosion of bony walls; fistula; osteitis; periosteitis.

Sclera: Abscess; scleritis.

Other: Preauricular lymphadenopathy; visual loss.

PRECAUTIONS

Saline solution should not be used to dilute amphotericin B because it may cause amphotericin B to precipitate. Surgery is usually contraindicated in patients with sporotrichosis, except for simple aspiration of secondary nodules, which is often done for diagnosis.

The patient receiving potassium iodide treatment should be observed for evidence of iodism; if it appears, dosage should be reduced or discontinued. Reactions may include acneiform rashes, coryza, bronchitis, stomatitis, gastritis, parotid swelling, conjunctivitis, and eyelid edema. Iodide sensitivity may lessen or disappear, despite continued therapy.

Because of the well-known toxicity of amphotericin B, dosage with this drug must be individualized. Fever, nausea, nephrotoxic reactions, and electrolyte disturbances are common side effects of this drug. Topical ophthalmic concentrations greater than 5 per cent are irritating and can cause corneal erosions, and subconjunctival injections greater than 300 mg have been reported to cause tissue necrosis. The ophthalmologist should note that intraocular penetration of topical and subconjunctival amphotericin B is poor.

COMMENTS

If endophthalmitis or anterior uveitis fails to respond to steroid therapy, the ophthalmologist should consider paracentesis of the anterior chamber or vitreous aspiration to confirm fungal infection. Appropriate microscopy and cultures for bacteria, mycobacteria, and fungi should be done. If left untreated, sporotrichosis will develop into a chronic condition. Once intraocular sporotrichosis has developed, the prognosis for useful vision is very grave, even with treatment. Although iodide treatment is successful in the subcutaneous forms of sporotrichosis, it is unfortunately not effective in the treatment of deep tissue disease. In these cases, amphotericin B is required.

68 / SPOROTRICHOSIS

References

Agger WA, Caplan RH, Maki DG: Ocular sporotrichosis mimicking mucormycosis in a diabetic. Ann Ophthalmol 10:767–771, 1978.

Allen HF: Amphotericin B and exogenous mycotic endophthalmitis after cataract extraction. Arch Ophthalmol 88:640–644, 1972.

Axelrod AJ, Peymon GA, Apple DJ: Toxicity of intravitreal injection of amphotericin B. Am J Ophthalmol 76:578–583, 1973.

Clarkson JG, Green WR: Endogenous fungal endophthalmitis. In Duane TD (ed): Clinical Ophthalmology. Hagerstown, Md, Harper & Row, 1982, Vol III, pp 11:23–27.

Francois J, Rysselaere M: Oculomycoses. Springfield, IL, Charles C Thomas, 1972, pp 370–386.

Kurosawa A, et al: Sporothrix schenckii endophthalmitis in a patient with human immunodeficiency virus infection. Arch Ophthalmol 88:376–380, 1988.

Roberts SOB, Mackenzie DWR: Mycology. In Rook A, Wilkinson DS, Ebling FJG (eds): Textbook of Dermatology, 3rd ed. St. Louis, CV Mosby, 1979, pp 859–860.

Stern GA, Fetkenhour CL, O'Grady RB: Intravitreal amphotericin B treatment of Candida endophthalmitis. Arch Ophthalmol 95:89–93, 1977.

Rickettsial Infections

Q FEVER
(Query Fever)

RICHARD B. HORNICK, M.D.
Orlando, Florida

Q fever is the name attached to the infections produced by *Coxiella burnetii*. The name comes from the frustration that Derrick encountered when he was unable to isolate a bacterial pathogen from workers in an abattoir who were part of an outbreak of a febrile illness. Thus, he called this Q (for query) fever. Even though the organism continues to be classified as a rickettsia, its intracellular growth characteristics are different from those of the other rickettsia. It is a highly infectious agent; probably infection with only one organism may cause disease in humans. Diagnosis is confirmed by serologic tests because attempts at isolation of the organism are dangerous due to its high infectivity. Reported infections are rare, about 15 to 20 per year. Infections are usually asymptomatic. Serologic surveys indicate as high as 40 per cent of a population exposed to cattle, sheep, and goats may have demonstrable circulating antibodies. Persons who are ill have a mild, self-limiting, febrile illness that is characterized by fever, severe intractable headache, and myalgia. About half of such patients can be shown to have pneumonitis. Ten per cent may develop hepatitis; however, as many as 85 per cent of patients may have abnormal liver function tests. Rarely, chronic infection of the heart valves occurs. Rash is not a manifestation of this infection.

Ocular involvement in Q fever is unusual, and ocular manifestations as the only evidence of the disease are very rare. Lesions involving the eye are probably a consequence of the vasculitis that is the hallmark of rickettsial infections. The organisms multiply in the endothelial cells of small blood vessels. Most patients have a severe headache with associated photophobia, and the pain is frequently retro-orbital in location. The pathogenesis of this pain is probably related to the vasculitis. Conjunctivae are injected, but no exudate occurs. Uveitis occurs very rarely; however, thorough evaluation of *C. burnetii* as a cause of uveitis has not been carried out. Lesions in the retina are also unusual, but evidence of the vasculitis may occur as hemorrhages, edema, and engorgement of veins. As a consequence of immune reactions, episcleritis can conceivably occur.

THERAPY

Systemic. No antibiotic has demonstrated equal in vivo therapeutic effectiveness to tetracycline and chloramphenicol, which remain the drugs of choice for treatment of rickettsial infections. Either tetracycline or chloramphenicol in a dosage of 0.5 gm every 6 hours can produce good therapeutic responses. Antibiotic therapy should be continued for 7 to 10 days for the patient with pneumonitis. Duration of antibiotic therapy for such ocular manifestations as uveitis seen secondary to Q fever is unknown. Steroid therapy for symptoms related to Q fever has not been evaluated; however, in other rickettsial infections, steroids have been used with some success for patients in shock.

Ocular. In those rare patients who develop episcleritis, topical corticosteroid drops can be used to reduce the erythema. These patients must also receive concurrent systemic antibiotic therapy. The steroids will interfere with the host's attempts to contain the *C. burnetii* and thus the need for the antibiotic.

PRECAUTIONS

Adverse effects of antibiotic and steroid treatment need to be kept in mind. Gastrointestinal disturbances, such as nausea, vomiting, and diarrhea, can be associated with tetracycline therapy. The occurrence of diarrhea requires that the drug be stopped immediately and the patient evaluated for the possibility of antibiotic colitis. Chloramphenicol is less likely to cause these same problems, but antibiotic colitis has been reported in patients receiving chloramphenicol.

The risk of blood marrow depression following chloramphenicol administration is about 1 in 20,000 to 40,000. Steroid therapy may interfere with immune mechanisms necessary to suppress the infectious processes.

COMMENTS

Q fever is acquired primarily by inhalation of infected aerosols. Large domestic animals are the usual sources of contamination. To date, these animals have not been demonstrated to be compromised by *C. burnetii* infection, although huge numbers of organisms are shed with the placentas of these animals and the area around some slaughterhouses can be shown to be contaminated with these rickettsiae. *C. burnetii* bacteria are very resistant to environmental decremental forces and will persist for years on surfaces where they have been deposited. After drying, they can be readily transmitted by windborne dust. Ingestion of milk from infected cows may be a source of inapparent infection, as well as overt disease. Infected ticks may be responsible for transmitting the disease among animals, but this mode of transmission has not been proven in humans. Person-to-person spread of the disease is unlikely, but pathologists have acquired such while performing autopsies on infected patients.

References

Clark WH, et al: Q fever in California. Arch Intern Med 88:155–167, 1951.
D'Angelo LJ, Baker EF, Schlosser W: Q fever in the United States, 1948–1977. J Infect Dis *139*:613–615, 1979.
Derrick EH: "Q" fever, A new fever entity: Clinical features, diagnosis and laboratory investigation. Med J Aust 2:281–299, 1937.
Doller G, Doller PC, Gerth H-J: Early diagnosis of Q fever: Detection of immunoglobulin M by radioimmunoassay and enzyme immunoassay. Eur J Clin Microbiol 3:550–553, 1984.
Duke-Elder S (ed): System of Ophthalmology. St. Louis, CV Mosby, 1976, Vol XV, p 135.
Dupont HL, et al: Q fever hepatitis. Ann Intern Med 74:198–206, 1971.

ROCKY MOUNTAIN SPOTTED FEVER

THOMAS C. BURTON, M.D.
Milwaukee, Wisconsin

Rocky Mountain spotted fever is an acute, infectious disease caused by the bacteria *Rickettsia rickettsii* and transmitted through the skin by the bite, excretions, or crushed tissues of infected ticks. Approximately 1000 cases and 40 fatalities are reported annually in the United States, with the majority occurring in the West, South Central, and South Atlantic regions. The organism invades the endothelial and smooth muscle cells of the microvasculature, producing a systemic vasculitis associated with increased capillary permeability. Mural thrombi occur over damaged endothelial cells, resulting in occlusions of the capillary bed, small arteries, and venules.

Following a prodromal period of mild fever, irritability, malaise, and decreased appetite, a macular, then petechial, rash appears on the distal extremities, including the palms and soles, and spreads toward the trunk. Systemic symptoms rapidly progress with the onset of high fever, severe headache, myalgias, abdominal pain, nausea, vomiting, lethargy, confusion, and even seizures or coma. Signs of dehydration often occur. Increased vascular permeability results in loss of serum proteins, decreased blood volume, hypotension, and peripheral circulatory failure. There is an interstitial pneumonitis with increased alveolar capillary permeability.

Ophthalmic manifestations are similar to those observed in scrub typhus, reflecting the systemic vasculitis, increased permeability, and small vessel occlusive process. Catarrhal conjunctivitis, occasionally with petechiae, is the most common ocular involvement. Nongranulomatous uveitis has been reported. The most common fundus changes are increased vascular engorgement and tortuosity, retinal edema, cotton-wool spots, retinal hemorrhages, and optic disc edema. Periorbital edema occurs in the most severely affected cases. Ocular histopathology from a case clinically consistent with Rocky Mountain spotted fever included retinal and choroidal vasculitis, arteriolar occlusions, and focal infiltrates of chronic inflammatory cells.

THERAPY

Systemic. The specific antibiotics are tetracycline or chloramphenicol administered orally in four divided doses at a rate of 50 mg/kg/day, up to 2 gm/day in children and 4 gm/day in adults. Seriously ill patients require a parenteral route of administration. These antibiotics are rickettsiastatic, and final elimination of the organism is achieved by host immune systems. Therapy should be continued for 2 to 3 days after the fever disappears.

Ocular. When systemic antibiotic therapy is instituted, ocular signs and symptoms rapidly resolve. Moderately severe iritis probably should be treated with topical cycloplegics, such as 1 per cent atropine or 0.2 per cent scopolamine solution, once or twice daily. Theoretically, anterior uveitis should be ameliorated by topical application of corticosteroids, although no specific information is available. Similarly, no data are available regarding enhanced resolution of conjunctivitis by topical antibiotics.

Supportive. Supportive therapy is indicated for fever and convulsions. Intravenous fluids may be required to overcome dehydration, to expand the intravascular volume, and to support blood pressure. Pulmonary edema and impaired alveolar gas exchange are managed by digitalization, fluid restriction, diuretics, and oxygen inhalation.

Ocular or Periocular Manifestations

Conjunctiva: Catarrhal conjunctivitis; petechiae.
Cornea: Keratic precipitates.
Iris: Anterior nongranulomatous iritis.
Optic Nerve: Disc edema.
Orbit: Edema.
Retina: Vasculitis; arteriolar occlusions; cotton-wool spots; edema; hemorrhages; vascular engorgement and tortuosity.
Other: Enlarged blind spots.

PRECAUTIONS

Secondary bronchopneumonia is a common complication, resulting in further accumulation of pulmonary fluid and greater impairment of gas exchange. Fluids, whether colloidal or crystalloid, must be administered with caution, as these patients are susceptible to vascular overload and acute pulmonary edema. Thus, orbital edema is an important sign of increased extravascular volume.

Intravascular coagulation accompanies the disease process. Thrombocytopenia should not be regarded arbitrarily as an indication of drug toxicity.

A significant fatality rate of 4 per cent persists, usually attributable to delay in diagnosis and institution of specific antibiotic therapy. Among the commonly employed laboratory tests, the Weil-Felix reaction exhibits too many false-positive and false-negative results, whereas the more specific complement-fixation test does not become positive until the second or third week of illness. Other specific tests, including latex agglutination, rickettsial microagglutination, and microimmunofluorescence of biopsied skin lesions, are not widely available. Therefore, antirickettsial therapy should be administered on the basis of a presumptive diagnosis.

COMMENTS

Ophthalmologists uncommonly participate in the management of patients with Rocky Mountain spotted fever because mild ocular symptoms are masked by the more serious systemic expressions. The ocular changes usually resolve within 3 weeks of initial appropriate antibiotic therapy. Undoubtedly, intraocular manifestations, as determined by slitlamp examination and careful fundus evaluation through a dilated pupil, are underestimated. Papilledema has been described several times; however, optic disc edema (secondary to vasculitis of the anterior portion of the optic nerve) seems to be a preferable description because increased intracranial pressure is not a feature of the disease.

References

Duffey RJ, Hammer E: The ocular manifestations of Rocky Mountain spotted fever. Ann Ophthalmol 19:301–306, 1987.

Grossman M, Jawetz E: Infectious diseases: Viral and rickettsial. *In* Krupp MA, Chatton MJ (eds): Current Medical Diagnosis and Treatment. Los Altos, Lange, 1982, pp 826–828.

Haynes RE, Sanders DY, Cramblett HG: Rocky Mountain spotted fever in children. J Pediatr 76:685–693, 1970.

Helmick CG, Winkler WG: Epidemiology of Rocky Mountain spotted fever, 1975–1979. *In* Burgdorfer W, Anacker RL (eds): Rickettsiae and Rickettsial Diseases. New York, Academic Press, 1981, pp 547–557.

Kaplowitz LG, Fischer JJ, Sparling PF: Rocky Mountain spotted fever: A clinical dilemma. *In* Remington JS, Swartz MN: Current Clinical Topics in Infectious Diseases 2. New York, McGraw-Hill, 1981, pp 89–108.

Presley GD: Fundus changes in Rocky Mountain spotted fever. Am J Ophthalmol 67:263–267, 1969.

Raab EL, Leopold IH, Hodes HL: Retinopathy in Rocky Mountain spotted fever. Am J Ophthalmol 68:42–46, 1969.

Riley HD Jr: Rickettsial diseases and Rocky Mountain spotted fever. Part I. Curr Probl Pediatr 11:1–46, 1981.

Smith TW, Burton TC: The retinal manifestations of Rocky Mountain spotted fever. Am J Ophthalmol 84:259–262, 1977.

Sulewski ME, Green WR: Ocular histopathologic features of a presumed case of Rocky Mountain spotted fever. Retina 6:125–130, 1986.

Walker DH, Mattern WD: Rickettsial vasculitis. Am Heart J 100:896–906, 1980.

SCRUB TYPHUS
(**Japanese River Fever, Mite-Borne Typhus, Rural Typhus, Tropical Typhus, Tsutsugamushi Disease**)

ROBERT L. BERRY, M.D

Little Rock, Arkansas

Scrub typhus is an acute febrile illness caused by *Rickettsia tsutsugamushi* or *R. orientalis.* This organism is endemic to a large area of the Far East bounded by Japan, Pakistan, and Australia. It is transmitted to humans by the larva (chiggers) of several mite (*Leptotrombidium*) species. The name derives from the "scrub" or wasteland favored by the rodent hosts carrying the mites. Tsutsugamushi, the Japanese name, was used much earlier than scrub typhus, but the latter name was widely used by the soldiers of World War II in whom many thousands of cases developed.

The classic presentation, seen in 60 per cent or more of cases, is an initial papule progressing to an ulcer or eschar at the site of the chigger bite. Invariably, there is moderate to high-grade continuous fever, very often accompanied by frontal headache and significant regional lymphadenopathy. Chest pain, blurred vision, conjunctivitis, and maculopapular rash are common. The spectrum of the disease is wide, however, and often the characteristic signs are not present. Mild disease is difficult to diagnose, and the disease is much more common than originally thought. A definite clinical diagnosis of scrub typhus is often difficult to achieve, and specific laboratory confirmation (by immunofluorescent technique) is expensive and rarely available early enough to influence patient management. Some studies of tropical workers show it to be the most common cause of febrile illness requiring hospitalization.

The acute phase of the untreated disease lasts 2 to 3 weeks, followed by a prolonged convalescence. Serious or fatal respiratory, neurologic, cardiovascular, or hematologic complications may develop during the second week of untreated illness. Prompt diagnosis and the use of appropriate antibiotics rapidly alter the clinical course of the disease.

Ocular findings in scrub typhus are particularly striking and may be of diagnostic aid in the early stages of the disease. Although the marked flush, conjunctival hyperemia, conjunctivitis, and periorbital edema are seen with other infectious diseases, a distinguishing feature of scrub typhus is the marked retinal vein engorgement. This retinopathy usually occurs in the second or third week of the disease and persists for many weeks and well into the period of convalescence.

THERAPY

Systemic. Broad-spectrum antibiotics are effective in the treatment of this disease and should be initiated early in the illness. Tetracycline is probably the drug of choice because it eliminates symptoms of scrub typhus more rapidly than chloramphenicol, and relapses are uncommon unless an incomplete course of therapy is administered. A daily adult dosage of 2 gm of tetracycline should be administered in four equal doses. The recommended daily dosage of tetracycline for children is calculated on the basis of 25 to 50 mg/kg.

A single oral dose of a long-acting tetracycline, such as 200 mg of doxycycline, may be as effective as a 7-day course of tetracycline in the treatment of scrub typhus. Doxycycline should not be given on an empty stomach.

Chloramphenicol may also be effective for the treatment of scrub typhus. The daily chloramphenicol dosage should be calculated on the basis of 39 mg/kg.

Antibiotics should be continued for at least 7 to 10 days. Doing so allows time for the patient's immunologic defense to develop appropriate antibodies and to prevent relapses.

Ocular. Cycloplegics are used to put the ciliary body at rest and control the anterior uveitis and photophobia. One drop of 1 per cent atropine, 5 per cent homatropine, or 0.25 per cent scopolamine may be used in the involved eye two to four times daily. Local corticosteroid eyedrops are also effective for control of inflammation. One drop of 0.1 per cent dexamethasone, 0.12 per cent prednisolone acetate, or 1 per cent prednisolone phosphate may be used two to four times daily.

Supportive. Adjunctive therapy includes bedrest, fluid and electrolyte replacement, and adequate protein intake. The patient should be hospitalized and observed for potential complications secondary to inadequate or delayed therapy, such as circulatory collapse, renal failure, anemia, or hypoproteinemia. These patients should also be carefully observed for disseminated intravascular coagulation.

Ocular or Periocular Manifestations

Conjunctiva: Hemorrhages; hyperemia.
Cornea: Keratic precipitates; ulcers.
Eyelids: Cicatrization; ecchymosis; edema; madarosis.
Iris: Anterior uveitis; synechiae.
Retina: Edema; exudates, hemorrhages, venous engorgement.
Vitreous: Haze.
Other: Decreased visual acuity; enlarged blind spot; fixation nystagmus; irritation; lacrimation; paracentral scotoma; photophobia.

PRECAUTIONS

In addition to its greater potential for bone marrow toxicity, chloramphenicol is somewhat slower than tetracycline in reducing the fever and other clinical manifestations of scrub typhus. Therefore, chloramphenicol should be restricted to only those patients in whom there is a contraindication to tetracycline administration.

All tetracyclines have relatively low toxicity at usual dosage levels. However, tetracycline use in children under 8 years of age is contraindicated because of possible temporary depression of bone growth and permanent changes in teeth. Gastrointestinal disturbances occur in about 10 per cent of patients receiving 2 gm or more of tetracycline daily. Gastric irritation and vomiting following single-dose administration of doxycycline may necessitate that some doses be repeated. Strict adherence to the instructions that the drug should be taken after a meal usually eliminates gastric irritation and vomiting. Intolerance to doxycycline may be more marked than to tetracycline.

COMMENTS

Single-dose therapy for scrub typhus would shorten the time that patients spend in the hospital and might allow treatment to be given on an outpatient basis because consumption of the antibiotic could be assured.

References

Brown GW: Recent studies in scrub typhus: A review. J Roy Soc Med 71:507–510, 1978.
Brown GW, et al: Scrub typhus: A common cause of

illness in indigenous populations. Trans Roy Soc Trop Med Hyg 70:444–448, 1977.
Brown GW et al: Single-dose doxycycline therapy for scrub typhus, Trans Roy Soc Trop Med Hyg 72:412–416, 1978.
Chamberlain WP Jr: Ocular findings in scrub typhus. Arch Ophthalmol 48:313–321, 1952.
Kitagawa M: A rare case of acute neuroretinitis due to tsutsugamushi disease. Jpn J Clin Ophthalmol 33:1047–1052, 1979.
Paul SR, Karanth S, Dickson D: Scrub typhus along the Thai-Kampuchean border; new treatment regimen, Trop Doc 17:104–107, 1987.
Pogge RC: Tsutsugamushi fever in Arizona, Ariz Med 31:832–833, 1974.
Ramanathan M, Abidin M, Balachand V: The diagnosis of scrub typhus: An evaluation. Med J Malaysia 42:61–64, 1987.
Scheie HG: Ocular changes associated with scrub typhus: Study of 451 patients. Arch Ophthalmol 40:245–267, 1948.
Sheehy TW, Hazlett D, Turk RE: Scrub typhus. A comparison of chloramphenicol and tetracycline in its treatment. Arch Intern Med 132:77–80, 1973.
Twartz JC, et al: Doxycycline prophylaxis for human scrub typhus. J Infect Dis 146:811–818, 1982.

Viral Infections

ACQUIRED IMMUNODEFICIENCY SYNDROME (AIDS)

GARY N. HOLLAND, M.D.
Los Angeles, California

AIDS is the most severe condition in a spectrum of clinical disorders caused by the recently discovered retrovirus human immunodeficiency virus, type 1 (HIV-1). HIV-1 can infect a variety of cells, but its most serious effects are caused by infection of CD4+ ("helper") T-lymphocytes. The resulting immunologic abnormalities make patients susceptible to life-threatening opportunistic infections and lead to the development of unusual neoplasms through unknown mechanisms. HIV-2 is a related retrovirus that causes AIDS among African patients.

The term *AIDS* was created by the Centers for Disease Control for epidemiologic purposes to describe the most serious cases of HIV infection; individuals are given a diagnosis of AIDS if they have one or more specific "indicator diseases" that result from HIV infection, including serious opportunistic infections such as *Pneumocystis carinii* pneumonia, unusual neoplasms such as Kaposi sarcoma, and HIV encephalopathy. The spectrum of HIV-associated conditions also includes the acute, transient mononucleosis-like syndrome that can follow initial infection; a syndrome of persistent generalized lymphadenopathy, chronic fever, weight loss, and diarrhea (commonly referred to as AIDS-related complex [ARC]); and asymptomatic infections. It is not known how many HIV—infected individuals will eventually develop AIDS.

Infection with HIV occurs through sexual intercourse, receipt of contaminated blood products, or congenital transmission from an infected mother to her unborn child. Groups at high risk for HIV infection include homosexual and bisexual males, intravenous drug abusers, and heterosexual partners of HIV-infected individuals. Routine testing of blood donors for HIV antibodies has reduced the risk of infection for hemophiliacs and recipients of whole blood transfusions.

Ocular disorders are among the common manifestations of AIDS. The majority of patients develop one or more ophthalmic disorders during the course of their illness. Most disorders fall into four categories: lesions related to microvascular disease (cotton-wool spots, retinal hemorrhages, conjunctival microvasculopathy); opportunistic ocular infections; neoplasms of the ocular surface, adnexa, and orbit; and neuro-ophthalmic abnormalities related to intracranial infections and neoplasms. Cytomegalovirus (CMV) retinopathy is the most common sight-threatening lesion associated with AIDS.

THERAPY

Systemic. Zidovudine is the only drug currently approved for use in the treatment of HIV infection. A prospective, randomized, placebo-controlled study showed that zidovudine increased patient survival and decreased the incidence of secondary opportunistic infections. The currently recommended dosage is 200 mg orally every 4 hours.

There have been several anecdotal reports that zidovudine will alter the course of CMV retinopathy or halt its progression, presumably through its immunopotentiating effect because it has no in vitro activity against CMV. It is doubtful that zidovudine therapy alone will be effective treatment for CMV retinopathy in the vast majority of patients, however. The role of zidovudine as an adjunct to specific anti-CMV therapy remains to be determined.

It has been hypothesized that HIV infection of ocular tissues can cause uveitis in the absence of secondary opportunistic infections. Zidovudine therapy has been reported anecdotally to cause resolution of anterior chamber and vitreous inflammatory reactions. Zidovudine should never be used as initial therapy, however, until a thorough examination and laboratory investigation rule out a secondary infectious cause.

Despite the use of zidovudine, AIDS therapy

is primarily directed toward treatment of secondary opportunistic infections and neoplasms. Patients are best treated by a team of physicians that may include infectious disease specialists, immunologists, oncologists, neurologists, radiation oncologists, pediatricians, and ophthalmologists. The evaluation and systemic treatment of ocular infections should be conducted with the assistance of infectious disease specialists, since autopsy studies indicate that intraocular infections always are associated with widely disseminated disease.

The treatment of CMV retinopathy has been a particularly difficult problem. The use of currently available antiviral agents (vidarabine‡, acyclovir‡) and immunomodulating drugs (interleukin-2†, interferon-alfa‡, and interferon gamma‡) has had no effect on CMV retinopathy in AIDS patients. In non-AIDS patients, the only truly effective treatment for CMV retinopathy is to restore immunocompetence by discontinuing or reducing the dosage of immunosuppressive drugs. There is as yet no way to restore immunocompetence to AIDS patients, however.

Recently, it has been shown that an investigational antiviral drug, ganciclovir,† can halt or slow the progression of CMV retinopathy in immunocompromised patients. It does not eradicate virus from the eye; virus can be recovered from the retina after treatment, and reactivation of the retinopathy occurs after cessation of drug therapy. Therefore, patients must receive chronic low-dose therapy to prevent disease recurrence. Even with continued treatment, eventual reactivation or slow spread of infection is common.

Based on clinical experience with ganciclovir, a dosing regimen has been established empirically that consists of an "induction" phase (5 mg/kg intravenously twice daily for 14 days) followed by a "maintenance" phase (5 mg/kg intravenously in one infusion daily). The drug is available only in an intravenous preparation. A permanent indwelling catheter is usually placed in patients receiving maintenance therapy.

The use of ganciclovir is limited by its bone marrow toxicity; as many as 38 per cent of AIDS patients receiving the drug will become neutropenic. Patients who cannot tolerate systemic administration of the drug due to neutropenia may benefit from intravitreal* administration of drug (see "Ocular" section).

Foscarnet (trisodium phosphonoformate hexahydrate)† is another antiviral drug with activity against CMV that is being investigated for the treatment of CMV retinopathy. Its efficacy appears to be similar to that of ganciclovir, and it also must be given as maintenance therapy to prevent reactivation of infection. Its major toxicity is renal. The best dosing regimen has not yet been established.

There is no consensus on the indications for initiation of antiviral therapy for CMV retinopathy. Successful treatment will preserve vision, but cannot restore vision already lost because of retinal necrosis. The author therefore recommends that ganciclovir or foscarnet therapy begin immediately in patients with vision-threatening lesions in one or both eyes—those adjacent to or inside the major temporal vascular arcades and those adjacent to the optic nerve head. Because of the toxic effects of drug therapy and an incomplete understanding of the natural history of CMV retinopathy, it currently is appropriate to delay treatment of more anterior lesions until progression is documented. In cases of unilateral disease where treatment is not indicated because extensive infection has already caused blindness, prophylactic treatment to protect the opposite eye is not given. Such patients are observed closely and informed of the symptoms of infection, which include floaters, visual field changes, and blurring.

Retinal destruction in CMV retinopathy is due to productive viral infection of retinal cells. It is not a secondary effect of inflammation. Steroids therefore should play no role in the treatment of CMV retinopathy.

Toxoplasmic retinochoroiditis responds to treatment with antiparasitic drugs, but the best therapy has not been established. The author and his colleagues recommend the use of pyrimethamine‡ in combination with one of the following antibiotics: sulfadiazine‡, clindamycin‡, tetracycline‡ (if other drugs cannot be tolerated), or spiramycin.† With treatment, lesions will involute and scar, and inflammation will resolve. Reactivation of lesions is common unless at least one drug is continued on a chronic basis. The majority of retinal destruction in immunocompromised patients with toxoplasmosis results from the proliferation of parasites, rather than from inflammation. Steroid therapy is probably of little value in these patients.

All patients suspected of having ocular syphilis should be referred for evaluation of the cerebrospinal fluid to rule out neurosyphilis. Drug regimens appropriate for the treatment of neurosyphilis should be used in all patients with ocular disease: at least 10 days of aqueous crystalline penicillin G (2 to 4 million units intravenously every 4 hours) or aqueous procaine penicillin G (2.4 million units intramuscularly each day) with probenecid (500 mg orally 4 times daily). The efficacy of penicillin therapy may be altered in HIV-infected patients; it is believed that the rate of treatment failures is increased. Patients should be observed closely after treatment for evidence of disease recurrence.

Systemic corticosteroids should be used with caution in patients with HIV infection. Although commonly used in the treatment of zoster ophthalmicus, ocular toxoplasmosis, and other uveitic disorders in immunocompetent individuals, their use in patients with AIDS may result in additional, unacceptable immunosuppression. Furthermore, they probably contribute little to the management of most sight-threatening lesions. As stated above, retinal necrosis in CMV retinopathy and ocular toxoplasmosis results primarily from cellular destruction by the proliferating pathogens, rather than from the associated inflammatory response.

Chemotherapy is the first line of defense

against multifocal Kaposi sarcoma and should be administered under the direction of an oncologist. Drugs used successfully to induce regression of tumors (including ophthalmic lesions) are doxorubicin, bleomycin, and vinblastine. Local therapy to ophthalmic lesions (see "irradiation" section) is necessary only if systemic therapy is unsuccessful or cannot be tolerated or if the patient has isolated ophthalmic lesions.

Ocular. Intravitreal injections of ganciclovir* have been used in patients with CMV retinopathy who are neutropenic and therefore cannot receive intravenous ganciclovir. A dose of 200 μg in 0.1 ml is delivered via the pars plana to the midvitreous. Injections are given twice weekly until the disease is brought under control; maintenance of quiescent lesions with one injection per week then can be considered. Experience with this treatment is limited, and issues regarding drug toxicity after repeated injections have not been resolved. Intravitreal ganciclovir therapy should be reserved only for those patients with progressive, sight-threatening infections who cannot tolerate systemic administration of the drug.

Laser therapy of CMV retinopathy has been attempted, but does not appear to be capable of preventing the spread of CMV retinopathy.

Surgical. Repair of retinal detachments in patients with CMV retinopathy is the most commonly performed ophthalmic surgical procedure in patients with AIDS. Detachments occur in as many as 25 per cent of patients. Because of extensive hole formation in areas of necrotic retina, vitrectomy and use of silicone oil or long-acting gases may be necessary to tamponade the reattached retina. Recurrent detachments are common.

As in immunocompetent hosts, vitrectomy may be necessary for treatment of those rare cases of fungal endophthalmitis that occur in patients with AIDS.

Large molluscum contagiosum lesions of the eyelids that result in a follicular conjunctivitis may require complete surgical excision. Curettage is far less effective for treatment of lesions in AIDS patients than in immunocompetent hosts.

Surgical excision of Kaposi sarcoma lesions of the conjunctiva or eyelids is rarely necessary because of their good response to systemic chemotherapy or irradiation. If surgery is necessary for diagnostic examination or to debulk large tumors, they can be excised easily without excessive bleeding despite their vascular nature. Even total excision of isolated tumors is not curative because of the multifocal nature of this neoplasm.

Topical. Herpes simplex virus epithelial keratitis associated with AIDS tends to be more severe and to recur more frequently than in immunocompetent patients. Lesions appear to respond to topical antiviral therapy (1 per cent trifluridine administered every 2 hours, up to nine times daily), but resolution of lesions, even with treatment, may take 3 weeks or longer. Lesions should be treated until the dendriform or geographic lesions have completely resolved. Continued use of topical antiviral medication to prevent recurrences is not indicated.

Persistent dendriform keratitis resembling herpes simplex virus keratitis but caused by a productive herpes zoster virus infection has been reported in a patient without severe zoster lesions of the skin. This infection appears to respond to treatment with topical ophthalmic acyclovir* ointment but not to topical trifluridine.

Vigorous topical antibiotic therapy for secondary bacterial infections of the cornea, based on culture results and sensitivity testing, may be curative in selected cases despite the severe immunosuppression of AIDS.

Topical steroid therapy for the mild iridocyclitis that accompanies necrotizing viral infections of the retina is not necessary.

Irradiation. Local irradiation may be effective palliative treatment for Kaposi sarcoma lesions that involve the conjunctiva and/or eyelids in lieu of systemic chemotherapy. Appropriate indications for treatment of conjunctival tumors include the presence of large bulky lesions that are cosmetically disturbing, interfere with eyelid function (rare), or produce discomfort because of mass effect (the tumors themselves are not painful). Appropriate indications for treatment of eyelid tumors are entropion formation and trichiasis resulting from large indurated tumors, ulceration of tumor-involved eyelid margins, and enlarging tumors that may eventually result in these complications.

Administration of 2000 to 3000 centigrays (cGy) in 200- to 300-cGy fractions over a 3-week period by means of a 6-MeV linear accelerator (while shielding the eye) or a 100-kvp superficial radiation unit has been reported to cause total or near-total resolution of lesions with minimal side effects for 4 months or longer. Recurrences after 6 months are common.

Radiation therapy to decrease tumor mass also may be a useful adjunct to chemotherapy of Burkitt's lymphoma involving the orbit.

Ocular or Periocular Manifestations

Anterior Segment: Iridocyclitis (syphilitic, secondary to retinal infections, idiopathic).

Choroid: Infections (pathogens that affect primarily the choroid but may have retinal involvement include *Mycobacterium avium* complex, *Mycobacterium tuberculosis, Cryptococcus neoformans, Candida albicans, Histoplasma capsulatum, Pneumocystis carinii*); choroidal effusion of unknown cause with forward displacement of ciliary body and angle-closure glaucoma.

Conjunctiva: Microvascular changes (dilated capillaries, isolated vascular fragments, vessel segments of irregular caliber, microaneurysms, sludging of blood flow); conjunctivitis (*Chlamydia trachomatis*, serotype L2 [lymphogranuloma venereum], molluscum contagiosum, idiopathic).

Cornea: Dendriform keratitis (herpes simplex virus, herpes zoster virus); spontaneous fungal ulcers (*Candida species*); secondary bacterial ulcers.

Eyelids and Periocular Skin: Molluscum contagiosum; zoster ophthalmicus; Kaposi sarcoma.

Optic Nerve: Ischemic optic neuropathy; infection (CMV); papilledema (frequently associated with cryptococcal meningitis); optic atrophy.

Orbit: Neoplasms (Kaposi sarcoma, Burkitt's lymphoma); pseudotumor.

Retina: Lesions attributable to retinal microvasculopathy (cotton-wool spots, retinal hemorrhages, microaneurysms, ischemic maculopathy); infections (pathogens that affect primarily the retina include CMV, *Toxoplasma gondii*, herpes simplex virus, herpes zoster virus, *Treponema pallidum*); isolated retinal vasculitis of unknown cause.

Other: Neuro-ophthalmic signs of intracranial disease (cranial nerve palsies, visual field defects, pupillary abnormalities); vitritis of unknown cause.

Precautions

Physicians administering treatment must be aware of the risks associated with some antimicrobial therapies. Allergic reactions to sulfonamides occur commonly in patients with AIDS. Patients given sulfadiazine for treatment of toxoplasmosis should be observed closely for the development of rashes. Neutropenia occurs in as many as 38 per cent of patients who receive ganciclovir. Absolute neutrophil counts usually rise with cessation of treatment, but irreversible neutropenia and death have been associated rarely with ganciclovir use. Ganciclovir-resistant strains of CMV have been isolated from patients receiving long-term treatment. Foscarnet may cause reversible azotemia, anemia, and abnormalities in calcium metabolism.

Care should be taken to minimize factors predisposing to opportunistic infections. Maintenance of nonspecific natural defenses, such as normal eyelid function and an intact corneal epithelium, are the most important means of decreasing serious infections of the ocular surface. Careful attention should be directed to the lid margins, looking for development or progression of Kaposi sarcoma lesions, which can cause entropion formation and trichiasis. Patients whose corneas have been compromised by previous disease should be observed carefully; neurotrophic keratitis following herpetic infections, for example, may be more susceptible to secondary bacterial ulcers. HIV-infected patients who develop contact-lens-associated infections may be less able to combat these infections than their immunocompetent counterparts.

Iatrogenic factors can increase the risk of certain infections. Intraocular fungal infections are rare unless patients develop candidemia, which can occur from contaminated indwelling catheters.

Health care workers' patient care activities put them at very low risk for HIV infection, although infection has occurred following needlestick accidents or prolonged exposure of open skin lesions to contaminated blood. The risk of such infection appears to be less than 1 per cent. Nevertheless, all physicians, including ophthalmologists, should take great care to avoid such exposures. Care should be taken when handling sharp instruments during ocular surgery. Needles should be placed in puncture-resistant containers immediately after use; resheathing of needles before disposal is not necessary and may result in needlestick injuries.

HIV has been identified in tears and ocular fluids, but there is no evidence that virus transmission has ever occurred by exposure to tears or contaminated instruments. However, our understanding of HIV transmission remains incomplete, and, therefore, precautions are warranted to prevent virus transmission during ophthalmic examinations and procedures. Precautions should be employed with all patients because HIV infection may not be apparent.

Gowns, masks, and eye goggles are recommended if there is a possibility of contact with splashed blood or infected body fluids during examinations, invasive procedures, or laboratory studies. They are not necessary for routine ophthalmic examinations. Gloves may be worn if excessive lacrimation is expected or if the examiner has open lesions on the hands. Gloves should be worn when touching mucous membranes, open skin lesions, or body fluids. Although gloves will not prevent needlestick injuries, their use during fluorescein and retrobulbar anesthesia injections will prevent exposure to blood from the injection site or dripping from the needle. Coughing patients may be asked to wear masks to prevent the air-borne spread of secondary pathogens.

Disposable items contaminated by blood or body fluids should be placed in water-tight containers. Reusable instruments should be sterilized by standard techniques. Other contaminated devices, including tonometer tips, should be wiped clean after direct contact with the ocular surface and then soaked in one of the following solutions for 10 minutes or longer: a *fresh* solution of 3 per cent hydrogen peroxide, 0.525 per cent sodium hypochlorite (1:10 dilution of household bleach), 70 per cent ethyl alcohol, or 70 per cent isopropyl alcohol. Instruments then should be thoroughly rinsed with water and dried before reuse. Surfaces contaminated with blood or body fluids may be cleaned with a 2 per cent phenolic solution.

Contact lenses from trial fitting sets should be disinfected after every patient use by either of the following methods: commercially available hydrogen peroxide contact lens disinfecting solution or heat disinfection (78 to 80° C, 172 to 176° F) for at least 10 minutes. Some contact lenses will not tolerate heat disinfection. Specific recommendations for a given lens can be obtained from its manufacturer. Various commercially available chemical sterilizing solutions for contact lenses have not been fully eval-

76 / ACQUIRED IMMUNODEFICIENCY SYNDROME (AIDS)

uated for their ability to inactivate HIV in clinical situations.

HIV also has been identified in corneal tissue. Currently, all cornea donors are screened for the presence of HIV antibodies, and tissue is not accepted from individuals known to be members of high-risk groups, regardless of their antibody status. There is no evidence, however, that HIV transmission by penetrating keratoplasty occurs, despite the fact that tissue has been used from donors discovered in retrospect to be HIV infected.

COMMENTS

Accurate diagnosis of HIV-related ophthalmic disorders may have important implications for the overall care of patients. Disseminated infections, for example, may be apparent first in the eye. Early referral to specialists in other fields will allow more successful treatment of nonocular disorders.

AIDS is a uniformly fatal disease. Treatment of its secondary ophthalmic disorders is generally palliative because neoplasms are rarely cured and infections are rarely eliminated after they develop. Instead, therapy is aimed at controlling existing disease. Prolonged therapy may be required to prevent recurrences, but chronic prophylactic treatment to prevent infection is not recommended. Such treatment might be selective for antibiotic-resistant organisms or fungi.

The goal of therapy is to improve or maintain quality of life for patients before they die. Clinicians must weigh the morbidity of various medications or operations against their potential benefits before beginning treatment. Factors to consider include visual potential, life expectancy for a given patient, and need for other medications that may interfere with treatment. Some patients may decide against certain treatments, such as prolonged intravenous therapy for extensive unilateral retinal infections, because of the associated cost and inconvenience.

The understanding of AIDS and its treatment is evolving rapidly. The findings and recommendations contained herein are based on experience with the syndrome through early 1989. Additional ocular disorders will undoubtedly be identified, and knowledge about disease pathophysiology will improve as the epidemic spreads. Existing therapies will be refined, and new drugs will become available. To provide appropriate care for patients, practicing ophthalmologists will need to remain abreast of these developments.

References

Cantrill HL, et al: Treatment of cytomegalovirus retinitis with intravitreal ganciclovir. Ophthalmology 96:367–374, 1989.

Centers for Disease Control: Recommendations for preventing possible transmission of human T-lymphotropic virus type III/lymphadenopathy-associated virus from tears. MMWR 34:533–534, 1985.

Collaborative DHPG Treatment Study Group: Treatment of serious cytomegalovirus infections with 9-(1,3-dihydroxy-2propoxymethyl)guanine in patients with AIDS and other immunodeficiencies. N Engl J Med 314:801–805, 1986.

Freeman WR, et al: Prevalence, pathophysiology, and treatment of rhegmatogenous retinal detachment in treated cytomegalovirus retinitis. Am J Ophthalmol 103:527–536, 1987.

Fischl MA, et al: The effect of azidothymidine (AZT) in the treatment of patients with AIDS and AIDS-related complex. A double-blind, placebo controlled trial. N Engl J Med 317:185–91, 1987.

Holland GN, et al: Treatment of cytomegalovirus retinopathy with ganciclovir. Ophthalmology 94:815–823, 1987.

Holland GN, et al: Ocular toxoplasmosis in patients with the acquired immunodeficiency syndrome. Am J Ophthalmol 106:653–667, 1988.

Palestine AG, et al: Ophthalmic involvement in acquired immune deficiency syndrome. Ophthalmology 91:1092–1099, 1984.

Pepose JS, et al: Acquired immunodeficiency syndrome: Pathogenic mechanisms of ocular disease. Ophthalmology 92:472–484, 1985.

Schuman JS, Orellana J, Friedman AH, Teich SA: Acquired immunodeficiency syndrome (AIDS). Surv Ophthalmol 31:384–410, 1987.

Shuler JD, et al: Kaposi sarcoma of the conjunctiva and eyelids associated with the acquired immunodeficiency syndrome. (submitted)

Walmsley SL, et al: Treatment of cytomegalovirus retinitis with trisodium phosphonoformate hexahydrate (Foscarnet). J Infect Dis 157:569–572, 1988.

ACUTE HEMORRHAGIC CONJUNCTIVITIS
(AHC, Epidemic Hemorrhagic Keratoconjunctivitis)

JOHN P. WHITCHER, M.D.
San Francisco, California

Acute hemorrhagic conjunctivitis, a new disease entity first reported in 1969 in Ghana, has since become pandemic, with the first epidemic in the United States occurring September, 1981, in Key West, Florida. The etiologic agent, which has been isolated from patients worldwide including one patient in Florida, has been designated as enterovirus type 70, a new member of the enterovirus group.

After a short incubation period of 24 to 48 hours, patients experience an explosive onset of irritation, foreign body sensation, and periorbital pain. In several hours, a full-blown conjunctivitis develops with lid edema, chemosis, seromucous discharge, and complaints of photophobia and tearing. Both eyes are usually involved, and preauricular lymphoadenopathy with variable tenderness is present. Subconjunctival hemorrhages are invariably present, beginning as small petechiae on the bulbar conjunctiva and quickly spreading to cover both the bulbar and palpebral conjunctiva. Moderate follicular hypertrophy is present, as well as a fine, diffuse, epithelial keratitis. In the majority of patients, the acute conjunctivitis subsides spontaneously in 3 or 4 days, with residual conjunctival hemorrhages and corneal epithelial staining remaining as long as 7 to 14 days. Systemic symptoms are rare, although several cases of lumbosacral radiculomyelitis have been reported late in the course of the disease.

THERAPY

Ocular. Topical broad-spectrum antibiotics, such as 10 per cent sulfacetamide eyedrops, may be used to prevent secondary bacterial infection. One drop instilled into both eyes four times daily is sufficient.

Topical corticosteroids are not usually indicated. The rapid course of the infection leads to quick resolution without complications in most cases.

Supportive. Because acute hemorrhagic conjunctivitis is extremely contagious, strict hygiene should be observed. Family members are especially at high risk of infection.

Ocular or Periocular Manifestations

Conjunctiva: Chemosis; follicular conjunctivitis; petechial bulbar hemorrhages (which rapidly coalesce on the palpebral conjunctiva also); seromucous discharge.

Cornea: Fine, diffuse, epithelial keratitis present centrally or superiorly.

Other: Lacrimation; lid edema; periorbital pain; photophobia; preauricular lymphadenopathy with variable tenderness.

PRECAUTIONS

As in the case of epidemic keratoconjunctivitis, transmission of acute hemorrhagic conjunctivitis appears to be mainly by eye-to-hand-to-eye contact. Contaminated instruments or medications may also be implicated, and great care should be taken by the physician examining patients with the disease not to unwittingly transmit it to other individuals. Careful hand washing and cleansing of instruments are essential.

It is likely that acute hemorrhagic conjunctivitis is now endemic in many populations where there were previous epidemics. The presence of continuing sporadic infections has been demonstrated by significant titers of virus neutralizing antibody to enterovirus type 70 in many young children in Ghana, even though a major epidemic has not occurred there in over 15 years.

COMMENTS

Even though acute hemorrhagic conjunctivitis is an extremely symptomatic and highly visible ocular disease occurring in epidemic proportions, complications are fortunately rare. Prolonged visual disability does not occur as in some cases of epidemic keratoconjunctivitis, and patients recover with remarkably few sequelae.

Because of the relatively benign course of the disease, overtreatment with topical antibiotics and corticosteroids should be avoided.

References

Acute hemorrhagic conjunctivitis caused by coxsackievirus A24-Caribbean. MMWR 36:245–251, 1987.
Acute hemorrhagic conjunctivitis—Key West, Florida. MMWR 30:463–464, 1981.
Asbell PA, de la Pena W, Harms D, et al: Acute hemorrhagic conjunctivitis in central America: First enterovirus epidemic in the western hemisphere. Ann Ophthalmol 17:205–209, 1985.
Chatterjee S, Quarcoopome CO, Apenteng A: Unusual type of epidemic conjunctivitis in Ghana. Br J Ophthalmol 54:628–630, 1970.
Isolation of enterovirus 70 from a patient with acute hemorrhagic conjunctivitis—Key West, Florida. MMWR 30:497, 1981.
Kuritsky JN, Weaver JH, Bernard KW, et al: An outbreak of acute hemorrhagic conjunctivitis in central Minnesota. Am J Ophthalmol 96:449–452, 1983.
Minami K, et al: Seroepidemiologic studies of acute hemorrhagic conjunctivitis virus (enterovirus type 70) in West Africa. I. Studies with human sera from Ghana collected eight years after the first outbreak. Am J Epidemiol 114:267–273, 1981.
Sklar VE, Patriarca PA, Onorato IM, et al: Clinical findings and results of treatment in an outbreak of acute hemorrhagic conjunctivitis in Southern Florida. Am J Ophthalmol 95:45–54, 1983.
Whitcher JP, et al: Acute hemorrhagic conjunctivitis in Tunisia. Report of viral isolations. Arch Ophthalmol 94:51–55, 1976.
Wulff H, Anderson LJ, Pallansch MA, et al: Diagnosis of enterovirus 70 infection by demonstration of IgM antibodies J Med Virol 21:321–327, 1987.

CAT-SCRATCH DISEASE
SCOTT M. MACRAE, M.D.
Portland, Oregon

Cat-scratch disease is a self-limited disease most often seen in children and characterized by localized lymphadenopathy. The disease is usually preceded by a history of a cat scratch, bite, or lick. Less commonly, the disease may result from exposure to another animal, such as a rabbit or monkey. Typically, from 1 to 4 weeks after exposure, a red papule or rash or both occur at the inoculation site with subsequent occurrence of lymphadenopathy. Low-grade fever, malaise, and lymph node discomfort may be present. Although complications are rare, thrombocytopenic purpura, encephalitis, and osteolytic lesions have been documented. A skin test in which cat-scratch (Hanger-Rose) antigen is injected intradermally into the volar surface of the forearm confirms the diagnosis, although false-negative results may occur early in the course of the disease. Other causes of regional lymphadenopathy, such as tularemia, sporotrichosis, tuberculosis, syphilis, and coccidioidomycosis, should be considered. Parinaud's oculoglandular syndrome occurs in 5 per cent of all cases. This syndrome is characterized by unilateral palpebral conjunctival involvement with granulomatous nodules surrounded by follicles, chemosis, and injection, as well as preauricular lymph node enlargement. The conjunctival nodules may occasionally ulcerate. Recently, a gram-negative intracellular rod similar to leptothrix has been noted in conjunctiva, skin and lymph nodes using a Warthin-Starry silver impregnation stain.

THERAPY

Supportive. The treatment of cat-scratch disease is palliative. If discomfort or fever occurs, analgesics, warm compresses, and antipyretics are warranted. A conjunctival biopsy of the granuloma may shorten the course of the disease and provides a specimen to rule out the infectious agents noted earlier. Excisional biopsy of the lymph node usually is not indicated, since it may lead to a persistent draining sinus. Lymph node needle aspiration may be necessary if there is marked suppuration and painful adenopathy. Systemic and topical antibiotics and steroids do not seem to affect the course of the disease and are of dubious value.

Ocular or Periocular Manifestations

Conjunctiva: Acute and chronic conjunctivitis; granuloma or nodules; serous (nonpurulent) discharge.
Other: Tender or nontender preauricular or cervical lymphadenopathy.

Precautions

Familial outbreaks of cat-scratch disease have been reported but are unusual. The cats appear to be infectious only for several weeks. Transmission of the disease between humans has never been documented.

Comments

Cat-scratch disease is a diagnosis of exclusion in which other more debilitating diseases should be ruled out. The diagnosis is based on a history of exposure to cats, the identification of the inoculum site, lymphadenopathy, and a positive cat-scratch skin test. Patients usually experience only mild discomfort, and the lymphadenopathy usually resolves in 30 to 90 days without sequelae.

References

Carithers HA: Oculoglandular disease of Parinaud. A manifestation of cat-scratch disease. Am J Dis Child *132*:1195–1200, 1978.
Carithers HA, Carithers CM, Edwards RO Jr: Cat-scratch disease: Its natural history. JAMA *207*:312–316, 1969.
Chin GN, Hyndiuk RA: Parinaud oculoglandular conjunctivitis. *In* Duane TD (ed): Clinical Ophthalmol-

ogy. Hagerstown, MD, Harper & Row, 1982, Vol IV, pp 4:1–8.
Marcy SM, Kibrick S: Cat-scratch disease. *In* Top FH Sr, and Wehrle PF (eds): Communicable and Infectious Diseases, 8th ed. St. Louis, CV Mosby, 1976, pp 154–160.
Margileth AM: Cat scratch disease. *In* Wyngaarden JB, Smith LH Jr (eds): Textbook of Medicine, 16th ed. Philadelphia, WB Saunders, 1982, pp 1695–1697.
Wear DJ, et al: Cat scratch disease: A bacterial infection. Science *221*:1403–1405, 1983.
Wear DJ, et al: Cat scratch disease bacilli in the conjunctiva of patients with Paranaud's oculoglandular syndrome. Ophthalmology *92*:1282–1287, 1985.

EPIDEMIC KERATOCONJUNCTIVITIS
(EKC)

ROBERT ABEL, JR., M.D.
Wilmington, Delaware

Epidemic keratoconjunctivitis (EKC) is a highly communicable, acute, external ocular inflammatory disease. The most frequent cause of "pink eye" is adenovirus types 8 and 19, although other serotypes can be responsible. The disease is characterized by acute onset of a unilateral, then bilateral papillary or follicular conjunctival reaction, with focal corneal epithelial lesions and regional lymphadenopathy. A frequent symptom is the lids being stuck together in the morning; marked lid inflammation and serous discharge may also be present. Approximately 2 weeks after the onset, the conjunctivitis subsides and discrete subepithelial opacities slowly appear, presumably at the site of previous epithelial lesions. When these opacities are located centrally, vision may be impaired. If uveitis develops, these opacities may be associated with photophobia and rarely pain. These typical opacities spontaneously regress over a period of months; however, they may rarely persist for as long as several years.

Giemsa staining of conjunctival scrapings demonstrates degenerated epithelial cells with many lymphocytes and few polymorphonuclear cells (PMNS). Cell cultures are frequently positive in the acute phase, whereas a fourfold antibody rise may provide retrospective confirmation. More laboratories are making direct and indirect immunofluorescent techniques and the new immunoperoxidase staining available.

Adenovirus can cause EKC (serotypes 2–4, 7–11, 14, 16, 19 and 29), pharyngoconjunctival fever, hemorrhagic conjunctivitis, chronic papillary conjunctivitis, and recurrent keratitis.

THERAPY

Systemic. Analgesics may be employed for patient comfort, although this is generally not emphasized. In a double-blind trial in England, oral amantadine has been found to be an effective prophylactic agent. Topical 1 per cent silver nitrate has been useful in a number of cases.

Ocular. Artificial tears applied four times daily or even hourly provide symptomatic relief and dilute the desquamative debris. Topical decongestants may decrease conjunctival congestion, but often do not provide as much relief of discomfort as do cold packs applied to the eyes. Topical corticosteroids and cycloplegics are useful in anterior uveitis. Corticosteroids are generally reserved for patients with significant iritis or with corneal opacities in the visual axis. If corticosteroids are used, they should be tapered very gradually.

It has been indicated that convalescent serum[†] eyedrops can provide some relief if they are administered early in the course of the disease. Likewise, one report states that interferon-alfa[‡] appears to reduce the spread of infection in a community epidemic.

Supportive. Since spread occurs readily by hand-to-eye transmission, patients must be instructed to avoid touching their eyes and then touching others. Frequent washing of the hands and use of separate linen are very important to quarantine the infection.

Ocular or Periocular Manifestations

Conjunctiva: Diffuse papillary or follicular, conjunctivitis; hyperemia; marked chemosis; pseudomembrane or true membrane formation; subconjunctival hemorrhages.

Cornea: Discrete subepithelial central opacity (late); punctate epithelial keratitis; scattered epithelial erosions.

Eyelids: Blepharospasm; edema; serous discharge with slight crusting.

Other: Anterior uveitis (rare); epiphora; periocular, submaxillary, or cervical lymphadenopathy; photophobia.

PRECAUTIONS

Although treatment of adenovirus infection has been long awaited, there is still no effective therapy available for this worldwide epidemic disease. Antiviral agents and topical interferon have not been proven to be clinically effective. Topical and systemic antibiotics have been used to eliminate bacterial or chlamydial etiology. Topical corticosteroids are rarely employed, except for iritis, because of the delayed resolution of the corneal opacities; early administration of these agents does not prevent the development of the subepithelial opacity.

Numerous hospital and community outbreaks have been documented in the literature. Spread occurs both by direct hand-to-eye transmission and by contact with tonometers and other eye instruments. It is vital that physicians, patients, and personnel in medical facilities wash their hands frequently to avoid transmission of this potentially epidemic disease. Patients should likewise be instructed in good hygienic techniques.

COMMENTS

Epidemic keratoconjunctivitis and other serotypes of adenovirus are usually limited to ocular disease in adults. With children, there is a greater chance of systemic findings associated with the conjunctivitis. Rarely, epidemic keratoconjunctivitis may be seen in conjunction with a bacterial infection (such as Koch-Weeks bacillus), in which case copious exudate and dissemination of the virus can occur more readily.

References

Abel R Jr: Adenovirus keratoconjunctivitis and new approaches to prophylaxis. Ann Ophthalmol 9:13, 1977.

Dawson C, Darrell R: Infections due to adenovirus type 8 in the United States. I. An outbreak of epidemic keratoconjunctivitis originating in a physician's office. N Engl J Med 268:1031–1034, 1963.

Dawson CR, et al: Adenovirus type 8 keratoconjunctivitis in the United States. III. Epidemiologic, clinical, and microbiologic features. Am J Ophthalmol 69:473–480, 1970.

Dawson CR, Hanna L, Togni B: Adenovirus type 8 infections in the United States. IV. Observations on the pathogenesis of lesions in severe eye disease. Arch Ophthalmol 87:258–268, 1972.

Sprague JB, et al: Epidemic keratoconjunctivitis. A severe industrial outbreak due to adenovirus type 8. N Engl J Med 289:1341–1346, 1973.

Vastine DW: Viral diseases: adenovirus and miscellaneous viral infections. In Smolin G, Thoft RA (eds): Viral Diseases in the Cornea, 2nd ed. Boston, Little, Brown and Co, p. 216, 1987.

Vastine DW, Wilner BI, Anicetti VR: Detection of adenovirus, herpes simplex virus, and chlamydia by an immunoperoxidase staining technique. Presented to the Annual Meeting of ARVO, Sarasota, FL, May 1981.

HERPES SIMPLEX
MARK S. DRESNER, M.D.,
DAVID J. SPENCE, M.D.,
and DAVID J. SCHANZLIN, M.D.
St. Louis, Missouri

Herpes simplex virus, a large complex DNA virus, commonly infects the skin and mucous membranes in the regions of the mouth, genitalia, and eye. The disease usually is minor, and the primary attack is subclinical; however, a wide range of clinical manifestations can result from infection with this agent. Characteristically, herpetic disease is recurrent.

Primary herpes infection of the eye is characterized by vesicles on the skin of the lids, follicular conjunctivitis, and sometimes punctate keratitis. Following primary infection, recurrent disease is usually in the form of dendritic ulceration of the cornea; however, ulceration can occa-

80 / HERPES SIMPLEX

sionally assume an amoebic or geographic form. This more severe form of ulcerative herpetic keratitis frequently occurs in patients using topical corticosteroid preparations. Between 10 and 20 per cent of patients with herpetic ulceration of the cornea subsequently develop underlying stromal inflammation, which may be disciform or irregular in configuration and is usually associated with uveitis. Indolent (metaherpetic) ulceration occurs when healing of the epithelium is compromised by the underlying stromal inflammation.

THERAPY

Ocular. Therapy for *primary herpes infection* of the eye is directed at removal of virus from the cornea and adjacent skin. Cultures of the cornea may be made for virus, but should also be made for bacteria if secondary infection is suspected. To inhibit virus replication and prevent corneal infection, topical idoxuridine, vidarabine, or trifluridine may be used; ointments should be instilled five times a day and eyedrops instilled every hour while the patient is awake. A cycloplegic may also be prescribed to relieve photophobia and ciliary spasm, and frequent follow-up is advised. No topical antiviral medication is effective in the treatment of herpes simplex skin lesions.

Recurrent herpetic epithelial keratitis is best treated initially by débridement combined with trifluridine or trifluridine alone. Débridement, which when used alone is considered suboptimal therapy, is performed after instillation of topical anesthetic (4 per cent cocaine or 0.5 per cent proparacaine) into the conjunctival sac; cocaine has the advantage of loosening the corneal epithelium. The loose epithelium at the edge of the dendritic figure is wiped away with a sterile cotton-tipped applicator or with the edge of a knife blade or platinum spatula. Following débridement, a cycloplegic drug is instilled into the conjunctival sac, and a semipressure patch is applied. The patient is asked to return in 48 hours. If the epithelial defect has an irregular appearance on re-examination or has the branching appearance of a dendritic or geographic ulcer at any point, débridement and patching are repeated or antiviral drug therapy is started.

Triflurothymide, a pyrimidine analog, is the drug of choice for topical ophthalmic antiviral therapy. Although similar in structure to idoxuridine, it is twice as potent, and because of its biphasic solubility, it is tenfold more soluble and can achieve therapeutic intraocular concentrations. It is considered more efficacious than idoxuridine in the treatment of dendritic and geographic ulcers and superior to vidarabine for geographic ulcers. Trifluridine is the least vulnerable of the three antiviral agents to resistant viral strains. There is no cross-allergenicity between trifluridine, idoxuridine, and vidarabine.

One per cent trifluridine is administered nine times daily for 14 days (or one drop each waking hour); 1 per cent idoxuridine can be administered every waking hour and every 2 hours at night. Three per cent vidarabine ointment, a purine analog, is prescribed five times daily.

The most recent topical ophthalmic drug to undergo clinical scrutiny in the treatment of herpes simplex is acyclovir.* It is a prodrug; thymidine kinase, specified by the herpes virus, activates acyclovir by phosphorylation. Host cells have a different phosphorylating enzyme that only minimally activates acyclovir. This gives the drug a 3000 times greater effect against herpes simplex virus than against the host. Its toxicity is equal to trifluridine and less than vidarabine or idoxuridine. Acyclovir and trifluridine heal approximately the same percentage of ulcers, but acyclovir heals dendritic ulcers more rapidly. It is not yet available in the United States for topical ophthalmic use.

The ability to augment or modify the host's immunologic milieu has led some investigators to study the role of interferon-alfa[‡] and thymic factor[†] as an adjunct to standard antiviral therapy. The efficacies of these modalities have not been fully established.

Stromal herpetic keratitis usually occurs in patients who have had previous attacks of epithelial herpes. In the presence of an epithelial defect, no corticosteroids should be used; rather, the patient should be treated with antiviral therapy and a short-acting cycloplegic agent to keep the pupil moving. If no epithelial defect is present and topical corticosteroid therapy is felt to be indicated, therapy should begin with the minimal prescriptive dosage; the dose is then gradually increased until the desired effect is obtained. The least amount of corticosteroid necessary to achieve the desired effect should be used and therapy tapered as soon as clinically feasible. As with all corticosteroid therapy, the patient should be followed closely. Antiviral medication should be continued as long as corticosteroids are utilized. Elevation of intraocular pressure may be treated with timolol and systemic acetazolamide if necessary.

Disciform herpetic disease presents as a pattern of local stromal corneal edema with underlying folds in Descemet's membrane and keratic precipitates. It is almost always accompanied by a moderate to severe anterior chamber reaction. The treatment of disciform keratitis is generally similar to that of stromal herpes. If the lesion is paracentral and does not cause significant visual impairment, the patient can be managed with cycloplegic agents and the lesion will resolve with time; if there is a significant decrease in visual acuity, topical corticosteroids can be used in combination with an antiviral cover and cycloplegic agent. Glaucoma should be treated with timolol and systemic acetazolamide as necessary.

Indolent stromal ulceration is managed with antiviral and corticosteroid therapy along with a soft contact lens to prevent corneal drying. When there is melting of the cornea, care must be taken not to stop corticosteroid therapy abruptly, as this may lead to rebound inflammation and increase the melting process resulting in perforation.

Supportive. Epithelial disease usually runs a short course of several days, and an initial dose of a short-acting cycloplegic, such as 5 per cent homatropine, is usually sufficient. With stromal keratitis and uveitis, the long-acting effect of atropine is preferred.

Bacterial infection complicating herpetic keratitis is sufficiently uncommon to make the routine administration of antibiotics unnecessary. However, any rapid change in the nature of the corneal lesion should arouse suspicion of a bacterial infection, and one should instigate appropriate investigations and treatment.

Surgical. Keratoplasty should be considered when descemetocele formation and perforation are imminent. If the cornea perforates, the best management is keratoplasty, performed as expediently as possible. Sealing of a perforated descemetocele with a tissue adhesive and fitting with a soft contact lens often lead to reformation of the anterior chamber in preparation for definitive corneal transplantation.

Keratoplasty for corneal scarring secondary to stromal herpes simplex virus should be done with caution. Most corneal transplant surgeons wish to have the patient remain without recurrent disease for 6 to 12 months before considering the procedure.

Ocular or Periocular Manifestations

Conjunctiva: Follicular conjunctivitis; hyperemia.
Cornea: Dendritic, geographic, or metaherpetic ulcer; disciform keratitis; hypesthesia; irregular (nondisciform) keratitis; lipid keratopathy; stromal scarring; vascularization.
Iris: Anterior uveitis; atrophy.
Other: Cataract; hypopyon; increased intraocular pressure; occlusion of nasolacrimal canaliculi; preauricular lymphadenopathy; scleritis; vesicular blepharitis.

PRECAUTIONS

The major problems related to therapy include the difficulty in achieving both a precise débridement that does not damage Bowman's layer and the fine balance between the beneficial anti-inflammatory action of these drugs on the balance of virus and host and the toxicity of the antiviral compounds.

Some forms of débridement are particularly injurious. The use of sharp instruments, cryotherapy, or strong chemicals, such as phenol or iodine, should be avoided as unnecessarily damaging. Adequate débridement can usually be achieved by brushing the epithelial lesions with a cotton-tipped applicator, a technique that is not only convenient but effective in that epithelial healing is rapid (usually within 24 hours) with resultant early disappearance of pain and discomfort. Any tendency for recurrent lesions to form in the early period following healing can be overcome by using a topical antiviral for 7 to 10 days after débridement.

Topical corticosteroids are very effective in suppressing the inflammatory response of herpetic keratitis. However, their inappropriate use may result in severe epithelial disease or stromal necrosis, increased tendency to recurrence, elevation of the intraocular pressure, and lens changes. Patients requiring topical corticosteroids for suppression of the inflammatory response usually require the drug for a period of months, and withdrawal is often complicated by recurrence of inflammation. The immunosuppressive complications of steroid administration can largely be avoided by the concurrent administration of topical antiviral therapy. Patient cooperation is a prerequisite for safe administration of corticosteroids in herpetic keratitis.

All antiviral medications currently in clinical use are toxic, with signs of toxicity being similar for all such drugs. Punctate epithelial keratopathy, limbal follicles, a follicular conjunctival response, ptosis, punctal stenosis, and contact dermatitis can occur at any time after 10 to 14 days of therapy. In mild cases of antiviral toxicity, epithelial changes may be the only manifestation. Idoxuridine is the most toxic antiviral agent in clinical use, whereas vidarabine and trifluridine appear to be less toxic.

COMMENTS

The major difficulties in treating herpetic keratitis are related to the tendency for recurrence and the management of stromal diseases. Several mechanisms seem responsible for the recurrences. In latent form, herpes simplex virus can be present in the cells of the cornea and in the central connections of the trigeminal nerve, particularly in the trigeminal ganglion. However, disturbance of the nerve results in activation of the virus and passage of particles centrifugally along the nerve, with shedding from the nerve endings. Lesions tend to occur when the balance between latency and host defenses is disturbed, such as during febrile illnesses, during menses, or on exposure to sunlight.

The toxic potential of antiviral agents should always be considered in cases showing poor healing, as these agents are inhibitors of cell division. Although continuous ocular drug delivery systems are currently under investigation, the limitations of such systems in the prevention of recurrences are related to the unacceptable toxicity from chronic use of currently available medications.

References

Coster DJ, Jones BR, Falcon MG: Role of debridement in the treatment of herpetic keratitis. Trans Ophthalmol Soc UK 97:314–317, 1977.
Falcon MG: Rational acyclovir therapy in herpetic eye disease. Br J Ophthalmol 71:102–106, 1987.
Falcon MG, et al: Management of herpetic eye disease. Trans Ophthalmol Soc UK 97:345–349, 1977.
Herbort CP, Buechi ER, Matter M: Blunt spatula de-

bridement and trifluorothymidine in epithelial herpetic keratitis. Curr Eye Res 6:225–228, 1987.
McGill J, Fraunfelder FT, Jones BR: Current and proposed management of ocular herpes simplex. Surv Ophthalmol 20:358–365, 1976.
Parlato CJ, et al: Role of debridement and trifluridine (trifluorothymidine) in herpes simplex dendritic keratitis. Arch Ophthalmol 103:673–675, 1985.
Pavan-Langston D: Diagnosis and management of herpes simplex ocular infection. Int Ophthalmol Clin 15:19–35, 1975.
Pivetti-Pezzi P, et al: Thymic factor therapy for herpetic keratitis. Ann Ophthalmol 17:327–331, 1985.
Sundmacher R, et al: The potency of interferon-alpha 2 and interferon-gamma in a combination therapy of dendritic keratitis. Curr Eye Res 6:273–276, 1987.
Williams HP, Falcon MG, Jones BR: Corticosteroids in the management of herpetic eye disease. Trans Ophthalmol Soc UK 97:341–344, 1977.

HERPES ZOSTER

R.J. MARSH, F.R.C.S.
London, England

Herpes zoster is an acute vesicular eruption caused by varicella-zoster virus, which is morphologically identical to the virus that causes chickenpox. It may be activated by a local lesion involving the posterior root ganglia, by systemic disease (particularly Hodgkin's disease), recently by early HIV infection, or by immunosuppressive therapy. The disease may occur at any age, but it is more common after 50 years of age. Ophthalmic herpes zoster is a variable disease, ranging from trivial to devastating. Inadequate management may lead to disastrous eyelid scarring, neuralgia, loss of the eye, and even suicide. In about 50 per cent of ophthalmic zoster cases, ocular complications occur. They fall primarily into those associated with inflammatory changes, those resulting from nerve damage, and those secondary to tissue scarring.

THERAPY

Systemic. Acyclovir has been used extensively over the last 3 years. There is good evidence that intravenous administration is effective in preventing severe dissemination of disease in immunosuppressed patients. The role of oral acyclovir in otherwise healthy patients is uncertain. It was first claimed that a dose of 400 mg daily for 5 days reduced the incidence and severity of ocular complications. Now, it is suggested that if the dose is doubled to 800 mg[§] daily for 7 days and administered within 2 days of the rash, better results are achieved. However, there seems to be no effect on postherpetic neuralgia, although there is brief early analgesia.

Although some authorities believe that use of routine systemic steroids results in fewer zoster complications, the increased risk of systemic spread of the disease should be considered. Systemic corticosteroids are indicated only in progressive proptosis with total ophthalmoplegia hemorrhagic bullae of the skin, and at the onset of optic neuritis or contralateral hemiplegia. These conditions are most probably due to occlusive vasculitis that threatens sight and are therefore a logical indication for this means of therapy. An initial oral daily dosage of 60 mg of prednisone may be given, which may be rapidly reduced to a maintenance dose. Oral administration of 50 to 100 mg of flurbiprofen* three times daily is useful in cases of severe scleritis, episcleritis, and sclerokeratitis that have not fully responded to the strongest doses of topical ophthalmic steroids.

Pain is notoriously difficult to treat and is generally the most severe within the first 2 weeks. During this acute phase, patients should be given sufficient drugs to suppress their pain. Mild analgesics, such as acetaminophen or propoxyphene, should be tried initially before stronger analgesics, such as pentazocine or meperidine, are used. The anti-inflammatory content of these drugs is also useful. In addition, the pain and paresthesia of postherpetic neuralgia generally tend to be worse at night and are aggravated by heat and wind. Extra analgesia may be needed at these times. Sublingual buprenophrine* may be particularly useful in cases of refractory intermittent neuralgia.

Depression frequently occurs during the acute phase of herpes zoster and may also be an important component of postherpetic neuralgia. It is important to treat this depression, and amitriptyline is particularly useful.

Ocular. The mainstay of therapy for ocular complications of herpes zoster is steroids. During the acute stage when lid vesicles are discharging and forming crusts or a mucopurulent conjunctivitis is present, antibiotic-steroid solutions may be applied to the eye and continued for at least 3 weeks after the onset of the rash. Tetracycline ointment should be applied twice daily to chronically scarred or inflamed lid margins, since they become a focus for staphylococcal secondary infection if left untreated.

Steroids should be used for all moderate or severe inflammatory lesions and are essential for those linked with vasculitis. At the first evidence of severe episcleritis, scleritis, sclerokeratitis, or iritis, 0.1 per cent dexamethasone suspension should be instilled every 4 hours and ointment applied at night. Prompt treatment at the start of vasculitis reduces the ischemic and fibrotic scarring that usually develops. Once control is achieved, the potency and frequency of administration can be reduced. The iritis of herpes zoster frequently causes elevation of intraocular pressure; this is true even with low-grade anterior uveitis. Fortunately, steroid therapy alone usually controls this pressure elevation within a few days. Although this complication generally occurs at the onset of the disease, it may appear as a late relapsing phenomenon years after the acute attack.

The inflammatory keratitis, of herpes zoster responds well to steroid therapy and does not require such high doses as the above. In fact, very mild keratitis often resolves without any treatment over 2 to 3 months. The dose of topical steroids should be titrated against the degree of disease activity in the eye. This is a slow cautious process and may extend over a period of years. As well as reducing the frequency of administration of the drug, serial logarithmic dilutions or a change to another weaker steroid (from dexamethasone to betamethasone or prednisolone) may be made. Many of the more intelligent patients can titrate their own dose, which may be reduced to as little as 0.03 per cent prednisolone once a day to maintain control.

Fairly common ocular complications in herpes zoster are loss of corneal sensitivity and damage to the mechanisms that produce a stable precorneal tear film. A combination of artificial tears and mucolytics will help stabilize the tear film and improve the health of the corneal epithelium. Bandage lenses are best avoided in all cases of keratitis where there is loss of corneal sensation because of the risk of hypopyon ulcer formation. Acute melting neuroparalytic ulcers have been successfully treated by botulism antitoxin-induced ptosis.

Topical ophthalmic antiviral treatment, including acyclovir,* seems to have no significant value in ocular zoster, and in fact, idoxuridine seems to have an adverse effect on an already compromised corneal epithelium.

Surgical. A lateral half-tarsorrhaphy should be carried out immediately in all cases of neurotrophic ulceration and may be necessary in cases of chronic exposure and neuroparalytic keratitis. It can be difficult to persuade patients to accept this treatment, but it provides rapid healing and security and dramatically reduces outpatient visits. Emergency grafting may have to be done in cases of neurotrophic ulceration with perforation. The prognosis is not as good in these situations as considerable difficulty may be encountered in establishing a stable corneal epithelium over the graft.

Corrective lid surgery may need to be considered for lid margin deformities, such as ectropion and trichiasis. It is urgently required when there is full-thickness loss of the lid margin.

Neglected disciform keratitis or sclerokeratitis frequently gives rise to dense scarring and lipid deposits in the central cornea. These patients tend to do well with perforating corneal grafts, provided that the cornea is not too vascularized.

Topical. Routinely, in the crusting phase, an antibiotic-steroid ointment, such as neomycin and hydrocortisone, is applied to the eyelids and skin two or three times daily. Topical antiviral agents in the form of idoxuridine dissolved in dimethyl sulfoxide have been used for treating the acute skin lesions of ophthalmic zoster. Although the rash tends to heal faster with this treatment, there is some doubt of its effectiveness in preventing postherpetic neuralgia.

Supportive. Patients with acute ophthalmic herpes zoster are often very ill, aged, and infirm. It is very difficult for them to take their treatment, feed themselves, and rest at home, and the kindest course is to admit them for one week to the hospital. The patient should be in partial isolation until the vesicles have dried (usually within 5 days). It is preferable that personnel in contact with the patient at this stage have had chickenpox, since they possibly could acquire varicella from the patient. The converse, however, is not true. Patients should be reassured that the duration of the rash is short and that the neuralgia is usually short-lived.

Ocular or Periocular Manifestations

Conjunctiva: Fatty granuloma; nonspecific conjunctivitis.
Cornea: Dendrites; disciform, neuroparalytic, neurotropic, punctate, or stromal nummularis keratitis; lipoid deposits; mucous plaques; recurrent ulcer; stromal cicatrization; stromal loss; vascularization.
Eyelids: Cicatricial entropion; neuralgia; paralysis; trichiasis; zoster rash.
Iris: Anterior uveitis; atrophy; distortion.
Sclera: Atrophy; episcleritis; scleritis.
Other: Cataract; optic neuritis; paralysis of third, fourth, or sixth nerve; proptosis; secondary glaucoma.

Precautions

The important essentials of steroid management are careful follow-up and examination to detect toxic side effects. A significant number of patients on topical steroids develop glaucoma and cataract following long-term use. Secondary infection may occur when using steroids in patients with neurotrophic keratitis. It may be difficult differentiating steroid glaucoma from hypertensive iritis, particularly in mucous plaque keratitis; a helpful measure is to increase the dose of steroid and review in 2 days. When the steroid is confirmed as the culprit, fluoromethalone drops should be substituted. The dose of steroids should be reduced as soon as possible to avoid lens opacities, although in some cases it is impossible to know whether to attribute the cataracts to the chronic iritis. Regular slitlamp examination and applanation are therefore essential.

It should be emphasized that the acute edema that occurs shortly after the onset of the rash is not due to bacterial cellulitis and will settle without antibiotics within a few days.

Comments

One of the most important aspects of the ocular complications in herpes zoster is their tendency to recur, even years after the rash. It should be remembered that some relapses may occur when the original attack of herpes zoster has either been forgotten or was so mild as to pass unnoticed. The stimulus for the relapse is often unknown, although the precipitate withdrawal of topical steroids is a potent cause. Therefore, follow-up must be long and thorough in those with

84 / HERPES ZOSTER

ocular involvement, and topical steroids must be slowly and cautiously withdrawn (over years, if necessary). Adequate analgesia must be administered. Those patients referred to an ophthalmologist from their family physicians have a much lower incidence of dermatologic nonmetastatic tumors than those referred from a hospital internist.

References

Adams GGW, Kirkness CM, Lee JP: Botulinum toxin A induced protective ptosis. Eye 1:603–608, 1987.

Cobo LM, et al: Oral acyclovir in the therapy of acute herpes zoster ophthalmas: An interim report. Ophthalmology 92:1574–1583, 1985.

Dawber R: Idoxuridine in herpes zoster: Further evaluation of intermittent topical therapy Br Med J 2:526–527, 1974.

Jeul-Jenson BE, MacCallum FO: Herpes Simplex, Varicella and Zoster. Philadelphia, JB Lippincott, 1972, pp 163–171.

Marsh RJ: Current management of ophthalmic herpes zoster. Trans Ophthalmol Soc UK 96:334–337, 1976.

Marsh RJ: Herpes zoster keratitis. Trans Ophthalmol Soc UK 93:181–192, 1973.

Marsh RJ: Idoxuridine (IDU) in dimethyl sulfoxide (DMSO) in the treatment of ophthalmic zoster. Ophthalmic Digest 39:17–19, 1977.

Marsh RJ, Fraunfelder FT, McGill JI: Herpetic corneal epithelial disease. Arch Ophthalmol 94:1899–1902, 1976.

McKendrick HW, et al: Oral acyclovir in acute herpes zoster. Br Med J 293:1529–1532, 1986.

Peterslund NA, et al: Acyclovir in herpes zoster. Lancet 2:827–830, 1981.

Stevens DA, Merigan TC: Interferon, antibody, and other host factors in herpes zoster. J Clin Invest 51:1170–1178, 1972.

INFECTIOUS MONONUCLEOSIS

JAY H. KRACHMER, M.D.,
Iowa City, Iowa

and STEVEN S.T. CHING, M.D.
Rochester, New York

Infectious mononucleosis is a clinical syndrome of adolescents and young adults, which is characterized by malaise, fever, sore throat, and generalized lymphadenopathy. Other systemic involvement may include splenomegaly (50 per cent), hepatomegaly (20 per cent), headache, vomiting, jaundice, palatal petechiae, and skin rash. Complications can be seen in any organ system. The etiologic agent of infectious mononucleosis has been shown to be the Epstein-Barr Virus (EBV). The primary infection with the virus may present clinically with less than the full syndrome; in children, the infection may be indistinguishable from other upper respiratory infections.

The ocular system may be involved directly by the virus or indirectly via the central nervous system. The most common ocular involvement is a follicular conjunctivitis.

Laboratory findings indicative of EBV infection are atypical lymphocytosis and heterophile antibodies to ox or sheep erythrocytes. Because of the possibility of false-negative heterophile antibodies (5 to 10 per cent), specific serologic testing for EBV infection can be performed. Early infection generates early antigen (EA) antibodies and gamma M antibodies to viral capsid antigens (VCA). After several months, anti-EA and gamma M anti-VCA become negative. Evidence of past infection is indicated by the presence of antibodies to Epstein-Barr nuclear antigens (EBNA) and gamma G antibodies to VCA. These latter antibodies may be present for life.

THERAPY

Systemic. The disease is self-limited, and usually only supportive therapy is necessary. Rest during the acute illness and gradual resumption of normal activity are recommended. Acetaminophen or aspirin may be used to decrease fever and sore throat. Systemic corticosteroids have been used to shrink obstructing tonsils.

Ocular. The conjunctivitis may be treated with cool compresses. Topical steroids have been used to treat the stromal keratitis and iritis. One case of epithelial dendritic keratitis appeared to respond to topical ophthalmic acyclovir.* Systemic corticosteroids have been used in cases of extensive neurologic involvement; their efficacy is uncertain. Theoretically, systemic acyclovir may be useful in severe involvement.

Ocular or Periocular Manifestations

Conjunctiva: Follicular, granulomatous, or membranous conjunctivitis; subconjunctival hemorrhages; hyperemia.

Cornea: Punctate epithelial keratitis; dendritic keratitis; stromal keratitis as nummular opacities, subepithelial infiltrates, or ring-shaped opacities.

Lacrimal System: Dacryoadenitis; dacryocystitis.

Neuro-Ophthalmologic: Accommodation paresis; convergence deficiency; hemianopsia; nystagmus; ophthalmoplegia; optic neuritis; papilledema.

Sclera: Episcleritis; scleritis.

Uvea: Iritis; vitritis; multifocal choroiditis with retinal pigment epithelial disturbance; punctate outer retinitis.

PRECAUTIONS

In childhood and adolescence, the disease may present symptoms similar to other upper respiratory illnesses. Aspirin should not be used in this age group because of the association of aspirin, influenza, and Reye's syndrome. The efficacy of corticosteroids and acyclovir in this disease is unproven.

Comment

Almost 100 per cent of individuals over 30 years of age demonstrate evidence of past EBV infection, but few have had the clinical syndrome of infectious mononucleosis. With the availability of specific EBV antibody testing, the practitioner should keep this infection in mind when searching for etiologies of puzzling ocular disease.

References

Aaberg TM, O'Brien WJ: Expanding ophthalmologic recognition of Epstein-Barr virus infections, Am J Ophthalmol 104:420, 1987.
Darrel RW (ed): Viral Diseases of the Eye, Philadelphia, Lea and Febiger, 1985, pp 112–117.
Matoba AY, Jones DB: Corneal subepithelial infiltrates associated with systemic Epstein-Barr viral infection. Ophthalmology 94:1669, 1987.
Raymond LA, et al: Punctate outer retinitis in acute Epstein-Barr virus infection. Am J Ophthalmol 104:424, 1987.
Tiedeman JS: Epstein-Barr viral antibodies in multifocal choroiditis and panuveitis, Am J Ophthalmol 103:659, 1987.
Wong KW, et al: Ocular involvement associated with chronic Epstein-Barr virus disease. Arch Ophthalmol 105:788, 1987.
Wyngaarden JB, Smith LH Jr: Cecil Textbook of Medicine, 18th ed. Philadelphia, WB Saunders, 1988, pp 1786–1788.

INFLUENZA

DANIEL H. SPITZBERG, M.D.
Indianapolis, Indiana

Influenza is an acute respiratory infection of specific viral etiology. There are three distinct antigenic types of influenza virus, designated A, B, and C. Although type C usually produces only a minor illness, antigenic types A and B can cause major epidemics. This disease often occurs sporadically or in localized outbreaks, particularly in schools or military camps and usually in the fall or winter season. The characteristics of influenza include sudden onset of headache, fever, malaise, muscular aching, substernal soreness, nasal stuffiness, and nausea. In this condition, the temperature rises abruptly and usually subsides over 2 to 3 days. Coryza, nonproductive cough, sore throat, mild pharyngeal infection, flushed face, and conjunctival redness are common symptoms. Influenza may cause necrosis of the respiratory epithelium, which predisposes the body to secondary bacterial infections. Influenza early in pregnancy has been said to result in multiple congenital deformities in the fetus, including the occurrence of anencephaly and congenital cataract. Ocular complications may include acute catarrhal conjunctivitis, superficial punctate or interstitial keratitis, palpebral edema, and secondary bacterial infections. A usually bilateral, self-limited nongranulomatous anterior uveitis may occur during convalescence. This can become chronic with exacerbation and remission.

THERAPY

Systemic. Prophylactically, amantadine protects 50 to 70 per cent of recipients exposed to influenza A viruses and is indicated for patients over 1 year of age during influenza A outbreaks, especially individuals for whom influenza would entail a grave risk (such as the elderly). It may be most effective in individuals who already have antibodies against influenza A virus strains; therefore, previous vaccination does not interfere with and may augment its effect. Amantadine also may have therapeutic value if given promptly after the first symptoms of infection appear. Administration of 100 mg of amantadine twice daily should be continued for at least 10 days.

Ocular. In cases of mild uveitis, 5 per cent homatropine solution should be applied topically four times daily to decrease pain. Influenzal uveitis can become chronic, with exacerbations and remissions. Patients with this type of uveitis respond well to topical ocular corticosteroid therapy for short periods of time. Topical ophthalmic 0.12 per cent prednisolone can be added two or three times a day to the regimen for a week to control low-grade uveitis.

Catarrhal marginal ulcers are an immunologic response and should be treated with 0.12 per cent prednisolone solution four times daily.

Supportive. Bedrest and gradual return to full activity are advisable to reduce complications. Codeine in an adult oral dosage of 15 to 60 mg may be used to depress the cough reflex and is more effective than salicylates for the treatment of headache and myalgia. Salicylates often increase discomfort by causing sweats and chills. Antibiotics should be reserved for treatment of bacterial complications.

Ocular or Periocular Manifestations

Conjunctiva: Catarrhal conjunctivitis; hyperemia; subconjunctival hemorrhages.
Cornea: Dendritic ulcer due to herpes simplex; erosion; interstitial or superficial punctate keratitis; marginal ulcer.
Extraocular Muscles: Myalgia; paralysis of third or fourth nerve; tenonitis.

86 / INFLUENZA

Lacrimal System: Dacryoadenitis; dacryocystitis.

Orbit: Cellulitis; panophthalmitis.

Retina: Angiospasm; edema; exudates; hemorrhages; stellate retinopathy; venous thrombosis.

Other: Accommodative spasm; cataract (congenital); episcleritis; mydriasis; myopia; optic neuritis (associated with encephalitis); uveitis.

PRECAUTIONS

If the fever persists for more than 4 days, if cough becomes productive, or if the white count rises about 12,000/cubic millimeter, secondary bacterial infection should be ruled out or verified and treated.

Routine yearly immunization with polyvalent influenza virus vaccine for high-risk groups is strongly recommended. Persons of all ages who suffer from chronic rheumatic heart diseases, other cardiovascular diseases, chronic bronchopulmonary diseases, diabetes mellitus, or Addison's disease should be considered for prophylactic treatment. Pregnant women and persons 65 years or older should also be considered, regardless of their previous state of health.

COMMENTS

The duration of uncomplicated influenza is 1 to 7 days, and complete recovery is the rule. However, pre-existing respiratory disease and secondary bacterial pneumonia can lead to a fatal outcome. Most fatalities are due to bacterial pneumonia. Pneumococcal pneumonia is most common, but staphylococcal pneumonia is most serious.

In general, serious ophthalmic complications are rare; however, secondary bacterial infections must be watched closely. The cornea is usually the site of most serious ocular complications. This area, along with the anterior chamber, is where the main follow-up examinations should be centered.

References

Grossman M, Jawetz E: Infectious diseases: Viral and rickettsial. *In* Krupp MA, Chatton MJ (eds): Current Medical Diagnosis and Treatment. Los Altos, Lange, 1982, pp 821–822.

Knight V: Influenza. *In* Isselbacher KJ et al (eds): Harrison's Principles of Internal Medicine, 9th ed. New York, McGraw-Hill, 1980, pp 785–789.

Rabon RJ, Louis GJ, Zegarra H, Gutman FA: Acute bilateral posterior angiopathy with influenza A viral infection. Am J Ophthalmol 103:289–293, 1987.

Schlaegel TF Jr: Uveitis associated with viral infections. *In* Duane TD (ed): Clinical Ophthalmology. Hagerstown, MD, Harper & Row, 1982, Vol IV, pp 46:1–13.

LYME DISEASE
F. T. FRAUNFELDER, M.D.
Portland, Oregon

Lyme disease is an immune-mediated multisystem disorder caused by the spirochete *Borrelia burgdorferi* transmitted by the Ixodidae ticks. In the United States, three foci of Lyme disease follow the distribution of *Ixodes dammini* in the Northeast and upper Midwest and *Ixodes pacificus* in the West. Lyme disease is the most common tick-transmitted illness and disseminates rapidly, creating joint, neurologic, and cardiac abnormalities. The clinical hallmark is a distinctive expanding skin lesion erythema chronicum migrans, which follows the bite of Ixodidae ticks. Clinical as well as spirochete similarities have been established between Lyme disease in Europe and the United States.

Three clinical stages of Lyme disease have been described, which can occur singly or overlap. Stage 1 includes the characteristic skin lesion and flu-like symptoms. During this period of dissemination, some patients develop conjunctivitis and dermatologic findings not associated with previous tick bite. In the first 3 to 6 weeks, IgM anti-*B. burgdorferi* antibody may develop, followed by a delayed IgM response to a specific *B. burgdorferi* several months to a year after infection.

Stage 2 Lyme disease involves cardiac and neurologic disease. Approximately 8 per cent of patients have cardiac involvement, and approximately 15 per cent of patients develop significant neurologic abnormalities after several weeks to months of the disease. IgG anti-*B. burgdorferi* antibody usually appears in stage 2. A common triad of symptoms is meningitis, radiculoneuropathy, and cranial neuropathy.

The late manifestations of Lyme disease, stage 3, are characterized by arthritis and chronic neurologic syndromes. Within a few weeks to 2 years after infection, approximately 60 per cent of patients develop arthritis. Involvement of large joints may persist chronically, with erosion of cartilage and bone in some of those afflicted with arthritis. Late neurologic symptoms, including neuropsychiatric disease, fatigue syndromes, focal central nervous system disease, and progressive deterioration of persistent spirochetal infection of the central nervous system, may also occur.

Considerable variation may thus occur in the clinical expression of Lyme disease and possibly even in the ophthalmic expression. The most common ocular complication of Lyme disease is conjunctivitis, which may occur during stage 1. Other ocular manifestations of stage 1 and early stage 2 include decreased vision, diffuse choroiditis, exudative retinal detachments, iridocyclitis, retinal vasculitis, and disc edema. Keratitis and diplopia may develop with stage 3 disease.

THERAPY

Systemic. All stages of Lyme disease have been found to respond to antibiotic treatment. In adults and children over 8 years, 250 mg of oral tetracycline[‡] four times daily or 100 mg of doxycycline[‡] two times daily are recommended for 10 to 21 days, depending on the rapidity of response. Penicillin V[‡] or amoxicillin[‡] is also effective for children less than 8 years old and pregnant or lactating females. Penicillin V may be administered in doses of 250 to 500 mg four times daily (pediatric dose, 50 mg/kg daily in four divided doses), and amoxicillin may be given in doses of 250 mg three times daily (pediatric dose, 20 mg/kg daily in three divided doses). For patients allergic to tetracyclines or penicillins, 250 mg of erythromycin[‡] four times daily (pediatric dose, 30 mg/kg daily) can be substituted, but appears to be less effective.

Patients with mild neurologic manifestations, such as Bell's palsy, respond to the tetracycline or doxycycline regimen, but therapy must be prolonged up to 30 days. Severe neurologic or cardiac disease requires 10 to 20 million units of intravenous penicillin G[‡] daily for 10 to 14 days. In nonresponsive patients, 2 gm of ceftriaxone[‡] daily may be substituted; however, variable success in stage 3 neurologic disease has been attained with ceftriaxone.

For Lyme disease arthritis, intravenous penicillin G administered for 2 to 3 weeks has been effective, although the response may be delayed for weeks to months. Recalcitrant arthritis has resolved after retreatment with the same or an alternative antibiotic regimen.

Ocular. For uveitis, 2 per cent homatropine or 0.25 per cent scopolamine may be administered twice daily to keep the pupil dilated.

Ocular or Periocular Manifestations

Choroid: Diffuse choroiditis.
Conjunctiva: Conjunctivitis.
Cornea: Keratitis (involving epithelial basement membrane, superficial and deep stroma).
Extraocular Muscles: Bell's palsy; paresis of third or sixth nerve.
Iris: Iridocyclitis.
Optic Nerve: Papilledema; pseudotumor cerebri.
Retina: Detachment; vasculitis.
Other: Decreased vision; diplopia.

PRECAUTIONS

A Jarisch-Herxheimer reaction occurs frequently after administration of high doses of tetracyclines or penicillins. Tetracyclines should not be administered to pregnant or lactating women or to children under 8 years old.

COMMENTS

Recent surveillance studies have demonstrated that Lyme disease is spreading among individuals in endemic areas, as well as to other geographic areas. Ocular manifestations of Lyme disease may occur in any stage, and ophthalmologists should be alert to unusual forms of conjunctivitis, keratitis, uveitis, retinal vasculitis, or papilledema, especially in those who have been within endemic areas. Early treatment with an oral tetracycline can shorten the duration of symptoms and prevent later disease in most patients.

References

Aaberg TM: The expanding ophthalmologic spectrum of Lyme disease. Am J Ophthalmol 107:77–80, 1989.
Baum J, et al: Bilateral keratitis as a manifestation of Lyme disease. Am J Ophthalmol 105:75–77, 1988.
Bertuch AW, Rocco E, Schwartz EG: Lyme disease: Ocular manifestations. Ann Ophthalmol 20:376–378, 1988.
Bialasiewicz AA, et al: Bilateral diffuse choroiditis and exudative retinal detachments with evidence of Lyme disease. Am J Ophthalmol 105:419, 1988.
Falco RC, Fish D: Prevalence of *Ixodes dammini* near the homes of Lyme disease patients in Westchester County, New York. Am J Epidemiol 127:826, 1988.
Jacobson DM, Frens DB: Pseudotumor cerebri syndrome associated with Lyme disease. Am J Ophthalmol 107:81, 1989.
Raucher HS, et al: Pseudotumor cerebri and Lyme disease, a new association. J Pediatr 107:931, 1985.
Steere AC, Malawista SE: Cases of Lyme disease in the United States. Locations correlated with distribution of *Ixodes dammini.* Ann Intern Med 91:730, 1979.
Steere AC, et al: The clinical spectrum and treatment of Lyme disease. Yale J Biol Med 57:453, 1984.
Steere AC, et al: Unilateral blindness caused by infection with Lyme disease spirochete, *Borrelia burgdorferi.* Ann Intern Med 90:382–384, 1985.
Treatment of Lyme disease. Med Lett Drugs Ther 30:65, 1988.
Wu G, et al: Optic disc edema and Lyme disease. Ann Ophthalmol 18:252–255, 1986.

MOLLUSCUM CONTAGIOSUM

LEWIS R. GRODEN, M.D.,
Tampa, Florida
and JUAN J. ARENTSEN, M.D.
Philadelphia, Pennsylvania

Molluscum contagiosum is a self-limited, mildly contagious skin disease caused by a poxvirus. Typical lesions are small dome-shaped, umbilicated, shiny skin-colored papules. The lesions are usually not inflamed and are most often asymptomatic. Lesions on the eyelid or lid margin can be inconspicuous and hidden by the lashes; less commonly, lesions are found on the conjunctiva and rarely on the cornea. The corneal findings usually involve the superior third of the eye and can progress to a trachoma-like

88 / MOLLUSCUM CONTAGIOSUM

picture. The follicular conjunctivitis and keratitis associated with molluscum contagiosum are toxic reactions to the virus, not infectious processes.

THERAPY

Surgical. Molluscum contagiosum is best managed by simple excision of the lesion. This can be done under local infiltration anesthesia, using scissors or a scalpel blade. Eradication of the lesion can also be achieved using electrocautery.

Incision and curettage effectively remove the viruses that pack the core of the molluscum contagiosum lesion. Curettage can be done with either a curette, needle, or comedo extractor.

Cryosurgery is also effective treatment. Light freezing followed by curettage decreases the risks of cryosurgery and effectively removes the lesion.

The application of chemical caustics, such as liquefied phenol, silver nitrate, or trichloroacetic acid, may also effect a cure.

Ocular or Periocular Manifestations

Conjunctiva: Molluscum contagiosum lesions; scarring; subacute or chronic follicular conjunctivitis.
Cornea: Fine epithelial keratitis; keratinization; molluscum contagiosum lesions; pannus; pseudodendrite; subepithelial infiltration; ulcer.
Lacrimal System: Epiphora; punctal occlusion.
Other: Foreign body sensation; photophobia; visual loss.

PRECAUTIONS

Although cryosurgery is effective in the treatment of molluscum contagiosum, it must be used with caution as it can lead to depigmentation of dark skin. Both cryosurgery and chemical caustics can also cause excess scarring. Although such drugs as cantharidin are valuable for skin lesions, they should not be used around the eyes, as scleral erosion can occur.

At one time, systemic sulfonamides were suggested as adjunctive therapy to surgery. However, such use is no longer recommended.

COMMENTS

The ocular findings clear rapidly after eradication of the molluscum contagiosum lesion. If the lesions are untreated, however, the ocular disease can lead to a trachoma-like picture and visual loss. The ocular and periocular lesions of molluscum contagiosum are often associated with lesions elsewhere, particularly in the genital areas. Venereal contact is a common means of transmission, and contaminated cosmetics can also spread the virus. Although usually a self-limiting disease, molluscum contagiosum can be progressive in an immunosuppressed individual.

References

Cobbold RJC, MacDonald A: Molluscum contagiosum as a sexually transmitted disease. Practitioner *204*:416–419, 1970.
Duke-Elder S (ed): System of Ophthalmology. St. Louis, CV Mosby, 1965, Vol VIII, pp 376–379.
Grayson M: Diseases of the Cornea. St. Louis, CV Mosby, 1979, pp 116–118.
Kohn SR: Molluscum contagiosum in patients with acquired immunodeficiency syndrome [letter]. Arch Ophthalmol *105*:458, 1987.
Rodrigues MR, et al: Methods for rapid detection of human ocular viral infections. Ophthalmology *86*:452–464, 1979.

MUMPS
ROGER F. MEYER, M.D.
Ann Arbor, Michigan

Mumps is an acute contagious disease caused by the mumps virus, which is transmitted by droplet on direct contact. The ports of entry are the nose, mouth, and possibly conjunctiva. The incubation period averages 18 days. One attack usually produces lifelong immunity. A generalized viremia carries the virus to the susceptible tissues. The parotid and other salivary glands are usually affected, but their involvement is only one aspect of a widely disseminated disease. The testicles and ovaries may also be affected. The major systemic complications are those that affect the central nervous system, including mumps meningitis, encephalitis, myelitis, polyradiculitis, and cranial neuritis. They may be present individually or in combination. Deafness can occur after mumps and may be profound. The ocular manifestations of mumps, in approximate order of frequency, include dacryoadenitis, conjunctivitis, scleritis, keratitis, uveitis, optic neuritis, retinitis, and ocular muscle palsies. Mumps in the mother during the early months of pregnancy may result in congenital abnormalities.

THERAPY

Ocular. There is no specific treatment for mumps infection. Warm moist compresses are generally sufficient to improve patient comfort and reduce ocular swelling.

If iritis is present, atropine may be used to put the ciliary body at rest. In normal adults, one or two topical ocular instillations of 1 per cent atropine produce cycloplegia, which begins within 25 minutes and persists for 3 to 5 days.

The course of scleritis, keratitis, and uveitis may be shortened by the use of topical corticosteroids. One or two drops of 1 per cent prednisolone two to four times daily may control the inflammation.

Supportive. The mumps virus has been shown to be present in the saliva as long as 7 days before and 9 days after the appearance of parotid swelling; until the parotid swelling subsides, the patient should be isolated. Bedrest is recommended during the febrile period. Analgesics, such as 300 to 600 mg of aspirin every 6 to 8 hours, may be used for relief of headache and fever. If additional sedation is necessary, codeine in a dosage of 15 to 60 mg every 3 to 4 hours should prove adequate.

Ocular or Periocular Manifestations

Conjunctiva: Chemosis; follicular or papillary conjunctivitis; hyperemia; subconjunctival hemorrhages.

Cornea: Interstitial keratitis with stromal infiltration and edema; opacity (congenital); punctate epithelial keratitis; ulcer.

Extraocular Muscles: Paralysis; tenonitis.

Eyelids: Edema; hyperemia.

Globe: Exophthalmos; microphthalmos (congenital).

Lacrimal System: Dacryoadenitis; epiphora.

Optic Nerve: Atrophy; disc hyperemia; optic neuritis; papillitis.

Sclera: Episcleritis; scleritis.

Other: Anterior uveitis; central retinal vein occlusion; cortical blindness; posterior subcapsular lens opacity (congenital); posterior uveitis (congenital); transient glaucoma; vitreous hemorrhages.

PRECAUTIONS

Since there is no specific treatment for mumps infection, therapy should be directed toward relief of symptoms and prevention of complications. Because of the potential hazards of corticosteroid therapy, its use in mild cases is not recommended. Antimicrobial drugs are of no value, except when secondary bacterial infections are present.

COMMENTS

A live, attenuated mumps virus vaccine was licensed in the United States in 1968. It has been found to be safe and highly effective. Adverse reactions are rare, except for the occasional case of parotitis. It has been used increasingly as a combined vaccine with measles and rubella vaccines (measles, mumps, and rubella virus vaccine live). It is recommended for routine immunization of children over 1 year of age. When used in an outbreak of mumps, the vaccine will not adversely affect an exposed person during the incubation period, and it will provide immunity against infection during subsequent exposures.

References

Hayden GF, et al: Current status of mumps and mumps vaccine in the United States. Pediatrics 62:965–969, 1978.
Krishna N, Lyda W: Acute suppurative dacryoadenitis as a sequel to mumps. Arch Ophthalmol 59:350–351, 1958.
Love A, Malm G, Rydbeck R, Norrby E, Kristensson K: Developmental disturbances in the hamster retina caused by a mutant of mumps virus. Dev Neurosci 7:65–72, 1985.
Meyer RF, Sullivan JH, Oh JO: Mumps conjunctivitis. Am J Ophthalmol 78:1022–1024, 1974.
Polland W, Thorburn W: Transient glaucoma as a manifestation of mumps. A case report. Acta Ophthalmol 54:779–782, 1976.
Riffenburgh RS: Ocular manifestations of mumps. Arch Ophthalmol 66:739–743, 1961.
Strong LE, Henderson JW, Gangitano JL: Bilateral retrobulbar neuritis secondary to mumps. Am J Ophthalmol 78:331–332, 1974.
Swan JW, Penn RF: Scleritis following mumps. Report of a case. Am J Ophthalmol 53:366–368, 1962.

NEWCASTLE DISEASE
LAURENT LAMER, M.D., F.R.C.S.(C)
Montreal, Quebec

Newcastle disease, caused by a paramyxovirus, is primarily a serious epizootic pneumoencephalitic infection of fowls. In humans, the disease is usually transmitted by contact with infected poultry. It produces an acute follicular conjunctivitis with slight serous discharge and enlarged preauricular lymph nodes. Characteristic ocular symptoms include burning, foreign body sensation, pain, redness, tearing, and photophobia. The infection usually has an abrupt onset; the bulbar conjunctivae become injected and chemotic, follicles appear on the tarsus of the caruncle, and the lid may become edematous. The conjunctivitis is usually unilateral. Corneal involvement is rare; however, a fine epithelial keratitis or round subepithelial opacities may develop. In patients who experience systemic involvement, there may be fatigue, a slight elevation of temperature, headaches, and mild arthralgia.

THERAPY

Ocular. There is no specific treatment for Newcastle disease. Therapy should be directed toward preventing complications, reducing secondary bacterial infection, and relieving symptoms. The use of topical ocular broad-spectrum antibiotics, such as a mixture of neomycin, polymyxin B, and bacitracin, may be of some value, although this has not been definitively demonstrated. The application of hot compresses gives some systemic relief.

90 / NEWCASTLE DISEASE

Systemic. Bedrest may be indicated in more severe cases. The patient should be instructed to avoid eyestrain or any activity that might increase the severity of the ocular affections.

Ocular or Periocular Manifestations

Conjunctiva: Chemosis; exudates; follicular conjunctivitis; hemorrhages; hyperemia; mucopurulent discharge.
Cornea: Fine keratic precipitates; round central subepithelial opacity.
Eyelids: Edema; follicles.
Other: Decreased accommodation; decreased visual acuity; irritation; lacrimation; ocular pain; photophobia; preauricular lymphadenopathy.

PRECAUTIONS

Newcastle disease is a benign, self-limited disease that normally runs its course in 7 to 10 days. In rare instances, some blurring of vision or difficulty of accommodation may persist for a short period of time.

COMMENTS

Newcastle disease occurs as a disease of poultry throughout the world. Human infection usually occurs through conjunctival contact, primarily in poultry workers and laboratory personnel. Although human-to-human transmission of the disease has not been documented, it appears likely that this may occur.

There is some concern that the Newcastle disease virus may develop into a more serious human pathogen. The virus, a parainfluenza type, has demonstrated its genetic plasticity by assuming four pathologic forms.

References

Charan S, Mahajan VM, Rai A, Balaya S: Ocular pathogenesis of Newcastle disease virus in rabbits and monkeys. J Comp Pathol 94:159–163, 1984.
Duke-Elder S (ed): System of Ophthalmology. St. Louis, CV Mosby, 1965, Vol VIII, pp 369–372; 1976, Vol XV, p 110.
Hanson RP: Paramyxovirus infections. *In* Hubbert WT, McCulloch WF, Schnurrenberger PR (eds): Diseases Transmitted from Animals to Man, 16th ed. Springfield, IL, Charles C Thomas, 1975, pp 851–858.
Lamer L: Sur un cas de conjonctivite de la maladie de Newcastle. Can J Ophthalmol 4:390–393, 1969.
Schemera B, Toro H, Herbst W, et al: Conjunctivitis and disorders of general health status in humans caused by infection with Newcastle disease virus. DTW 94:383–384, 1987.
Zehetbauer G, Kunz C, Thaler A: Cases of pseudo fowl plague (Newcastle disease) in man in lower Austria. Wien Klin Wochenschr 83:878–880, 1971.

OCULAR VACCINIA
BRUCE M. MASSARO, M.D., M.P.H., *and* ROBERT A. HYNDIUK, M.D.
Milwaukee, Wisconsin

Vaccinia is an infection caused by the DNA-containing laboratory virus used for smallpox prophylaxis. Vaccination with this live virus can result in infection of ocular tissues as a result of hand or fomite transfer from a primary vaccination site (76 per cent) or from the site of another individual (20 per cent). An incubation period of 7 to 10 days precedes development of a severe, typically unilateral blepharoconjunctivitis. Nonimmune patients are generally more severely affected than previously vaccinated patients. The overall incidence of accidental vaccinial infection is 18.8 per million vaccinations.

The eyelid skin is most commonly affected. Single or multiple lesions, initially papulovesicular, become pustular or ulcerated or both. Severe lid edema and erythema, regional lymphadenopathy, and an acute febrile illness with myalgias occur. Scarring is more severe in nonimmune patients and those with eczema. Vaccinial conjunctivitis may occur with or without blepharitis and is often purulent with possible membrane formation or frank ulceration. Orbital cellulitis may develop. Vaccinial infections of the lids and conjunctiva generally last about 10 days and resolve without sequelae.

Corneal infection usually occurs in association with eyelid or conjunctival infection or both. It may range in intensity from a mild superficial punctate keratitis to a disciform necrotizing stromal keratitis with possible corneal perforations. Nonimmune patients with ocular vaccinia develop significant keratitis in 20 to 50 per cent of cases, whereas only 10 per cent of those previously vaccinated suffer this complication. Stromal keratitis may occur as late as 2 to 3 months after the original infection and is felt to be immune in origin, unlike corneal epithelial disease, which presents acutely and reflects replicating virus. Giemsa-stained scrapings of infected tissues display diagnostic eosinophilic intracytoplasmic inclusion bodies (Guarnieri's bodies).

THERAPY

Systemic. Vaccinia immune globulin (VIG) is gamma globulin fractionated from serum in patients vaccinated a few months before blood donation. VIG is effective in modifying the complications of systemic and ocular vaccinia and is especially helpful in cases with orbital cellulitis. It is available from the American Red Cross Regional Blood Centers and the Centers for Disease Control. VIG is given intramuscularly in a

---

Supported in part by an unrestricted grant from Research to Prevent Blindness, Inc. and supported in part by Ophthalmic Research Core Grant EY-01931.

dosage of 0.6 ml/kg. No more than 5 ml should be injected at one site, and no more than 20 ml should be given at one time. The dose may be repeated in 48 hours if no improvement occurs.

Ocular. For vaccinial infection of the lids or conjunctiva without corneal involvement, investigational use of topical antiviral medications may help prevent the development of keratitis. A combination of 3 per cent vidarabine‡ ophthalmic ointment five times daily and 1 per cent trifluridine‡ solution every 2 hours during waking hours is probably more effective than idoxuridine. Idoxuridine‡ can be administered as 0.5 per cent ophthalmic solution every hour during the day and every 2 hours at night.

If corneal involvement has occurred, investigational use of vidarabine, trifluridine, or idoxuridine in the dosages outlined above will probably be effective in the resolution of the epithelial stage of the keratitis (due to multiplying virus). Both vidarabine and trifluridine have been shown to be significantly more effective than idoxuridine for the treatment of vaccinial keratitis. The antivirals should be continued topically for one week after there is an absence of macropunctate epithelial fluorescein staining. Whether acyclovir* or other newer antiviral agents are effective in treating ocular vaccinia is not known. Topically applied interferon-alfa* has been shown to be effective in treating the punctate epithelial and ulcerative keratitis of ocular vaccinia.

Good hygiene should be maintained, with warm, moist compresses applied to the eye as needed. Topical antibiotics should be given twice daily to prevent bacterial superinfection. Topical corticosteroids may be used for significant active stromal keratitis, if the epithelium has healed and topical antiviral coverage is maintained. Cycloplegics should be used as needed for iritis.

Surgical. In cases of progressive necrotizing keratitis, lamellar or penetrating keratoplasty may be indicated.

Ocular or Periocular Manifestations

Conjunctiva: Chemosis; hyperemia; nonfollicular, catarrhal, or purulent conjunctivitis; ulceration of palpebral or bulbar conjunctiva.

Cornea: Epithelial ulceration; fine or coarse punctate epithelial keratitis; interstitial, disciform, or necrotizing stromal keratitis; stromal scarring; vascularization.

Eyelids: Edema; erythema; pustules; ulcers; vesicles.

Other: Anterior uveitis, choroiditis; extraocular muscle palsies secondary to postvaccinial encephalitis; optic neuritis; orbital cellulitis; preauricular lymphadenopathy.

PRECAUTIONS

Although useful in the presence of vaccinial blepharitis or orbital cellulitis, VIG should not be used if keratitis is present. Experimental results show that the use of VIG in the presence of established keratitis may actually result in prolonged, more extensive stromal inflammation and subsequent stromal scarring. Topical corticosteroids may aggravate the acute stage of the disease. However, once the corneal epithelium has healed and significant stromal inflammation or anterior uveitis is present, topical corticosteroids may be used cautiously, along with topical antiviral coverage. Systemic steroids should be avoided.

COMMENTS

Ocular vaccinia is now rarely seen because routine childhood smallpox vaccination ended in the early 1970s. The World Health Organization declared the world free of smallpox in May 1980, and vaccination of civilians is indicated only for laboratory workers directly involved with smallpox-related viruses. Vaccination is no longer recommended for international travel. However, all active military personnel are vaccinated for strategic defensive reasons. As more men and women born after 1970 enter military service, the percentage of those undergoing primary vaccination continues to increase with an attendant increased risk for systemic dissemination. Patients at risk include those with atopic or other forms of dermatitis, those undergoing immunosuppressive therapy, and those with a systemic disease that compromises the immune status, such as acquired immunodeficiency syndrome (AIDS).

References

deLuise VP: Viral conjunctivitis. In Tabbara KF, Hyndiuk RA (eds): Infections of the Eye: Diagnosis and Management. Boston, Little, Brown and Co, 1986, pp 437–460.

Duke-Elder S (ed): System of Ophthalmology. St. Louis, CV Mosby, 1965, Vol VIII, pp 360–367.

Fulginiti VA, et al: Therapy of experimental vaccinial keratitis. Effect of idoxuridine and VIG. Arch Ophthalmol 74:539–544, 1965.

Hyndiuk RA, et al: Treatment of vaccinial keratitis with vidarabine. Arch Ophthalmol 94:1363–1364, 1976.

Hyndiuk RA, et al: Treatment of vaccinial keratitis with trifluorothymidine. Arch Ophthalmol 94:1785–1786, 1976.

O'Brien WJ: Antiviral agents. In Tabbara KF, Hyndiuk RA (eds): Infections of the Eye: Diagnosis and Management. Boston, Little, Brown and Co, 1986, pp 257–274.

Pavan-Langston D: Ocular antiviral therapy. Int Ophthalmol Clin 20:149–161, 1980.

Redfield RR, et al: Disseminated vaccinia in a military recruit with human immunodeficiency virus (HIV) disease. N Engl J Med 316:673–676, 1987.

Ruben FL, Land JM: Ocular vaccinia: An epidemiologic analysis of 348 cases. Arch Ophthalmol 84:45–48, 1970.

PHARYNGOCONJUNCTIVAL FEVER
(Acute Follicular Conjunctivitis, Adenovirus Conjunctivitis, PCF, Syndrome of Beal)

CHANDLER R. DAWSON, M.D.

San Francisco, California

Pharyngoconjunctival fever (PCF) and acute follicular conjunctivitis are the most common manifestations of ocular adenovirus (Ad) infection. Adenovirus follicular conjunctivitis can occur without other signs or as PCF in association with pharyngitis and fever. In either form, the conjunctivitis usually has an acute onset. It is often unilateral at first, with involvement of the second eye within a week, and is frequently accompanied by preauricular lymphadenopathy on the side of the affected eye. The virus probably is transmitted by finger-to-eye spread or by respiratory droplets directly onto the conjunctival surface. After an incubation period of 5 to 12 days, the disease starts with hyperemia, watery discharge, and follicle formation. In PCF, the conjunctivitis is accompanied by pharyngitis and fever and occasionally by gastrointestinal symptoms. Systemic signs occur in about one third of patients with Ad type 4 conjunctivitis and are even less common with Ad type 3. The conjunctivitis subsides gradually in 7 to 15 days, during which time the virus can regularly be found in the conjunctiva and upper respiratory tract. Ad type 3 persists even longer in the conjunctiva, although the conjunctivitis is milder. Epidemics of PCF usually occur in the summer and in association with poorly chlorinated swimming pools.

THERAPY

Ocular. Topical ophthalmic antivirals[‡] and interferon-alpha[†] have not been generally useful for treating adenovirus conjunctivitis. Astringent drops may diminish hyperemia and relieve symptoms. Topical antibiotics may be used to prevent secondary bacterial infections. If the keratitis is particularly severe, mydriatic drops (cyclopentolate, homatropine) may be used to alleviate discomfort. Topical corticosteroids[‡] have not been shown to be effective and carry a certain risk because some cases of follicular conjunctivitis are caused by herpes simplex virus, which is made worse by steroids.

Supportive. Management is primarily supportive. Patients should be reassured that the condition is self-limited (less than 15 days) and rarely results in serious complications. Patients and their families need to be told how to prevent spread of adenovirus on towels, pillows, and hands. Other general supportive measures include antipyretics to control fever.

Ocular or Periocular Manifestations

Conjunctiva: Acute follicular conjunctivitis; chemosis; hyperemia; punctate hemorrhages; serofibrinous exudates.

Cornea: Marginal infiltration; superficial punctate keratitis.

Eyelids: Blepharospasm; edema; pseudoptosis.

Other: Lacrimation; periorbital pain; photophobia; preauricular and submandibular lymphadenopathy.

PRECAUTIONS

There are several reports of *chronic adenovirus ocular infections*. Boniuk et al. isolated Ad type 2 from the eye of a patient with chronic keratitis. Darougar and associates reported a case of recurrent papillary conjunctivitis that persisted for 16 months and from which Ad type 19 was isolated 12 months after onset. Pettit and coworkers described three cases of chronic keratoconjunctivitis associated with Ad types 3, 4, and 5. In two of these three patients, there was active epithelial keratitis; the third patient had purulent conjunctivitis and subepithelial opacities. All three patients received topical corticosteroids early in the course of their diseases. Our group at the Proctor Foundation isolated Ad type 5 from a patient with long-standing superficial punctate keratitis of Thygeson and folliculosis.

Although the role of adenovirus infection was not clear in these patients with long-standing disease, the adenoviruses could well cause chronic disease of the external eye. In addition, unusual forms of adenovirus infection have been reported in patients with immunosuppression.

COMMENTS

There are 42 currently known serotypes of adenovirus that are subdivided into six subgenera (A, B, C, D, E, and F) based upon DNA restriction enzyme analysis genome typing. The causes of PCF and adenovirus conjunctivitis include Ad types 3 and 7, which belong to subgenus B and Ad 4, the only type in subgenus E. All of the types associated with epidemic keratoconjunctivitis are in subgenus D, which has 19 serotypes, including Ad types 8, 19, and 37. Worldwide, Ad types 1, 2, 3, 5, and 7 are isolated most frequently, and types 4, 6, and 8 are found much less frequently.

After the initial infection, the viruses may persist as a latent infection in the lymphoid tissues of the nasopharynx and gastrointestinal tract. Children ar usually infected with the endemic types before the age of 2 years. Types 3 and 7 are associated with "swimming pool conjunctivitis," as well as lower respiratory disease in children younger than 6 years of age. Types 4, 7, and 21 are the major cause of epidemics of acute respiratory disease in military recruits and cause sporadic pneumonia in children. Types 40 and 41 are associated with diarrheal disease in hospitalized pediatric patients. Adenoviruses, as can other latent viruses, can present as active infections in immunosuppressed patients.

References

Aoki K, et al: Clinical and aetiological study of adenoviral conjunctivitis with special reference to adenovirus types 4 and 19 infections. Br J Ophthalmol 66:776–3780, 1982.

Boniuk M, Phillips CA, Friedman JB: Clinic adenovirus type 2 keratitis in man. N Engl J Med 273:924–925, 1965.

Darougar S, et al: Epidemic keratoconjunctivitis and chronic papillary conjunctivitis in London due to adenovirus type 19. Br J Ophthalmol 61:76–85, 1977.

Dawson CR: Follicular conjunctivitis. In Wilson LA (ed): External Diseases of the Eye. Hagerstown, MD, Harper & Row, 1979, pp 57–75.

Ishii K, et al: Comparative studies on aetiology and epidemiology of viral conjunctivitis in three countries of East Asia—Japan, Taiwan and South Korea. Int J Epidemiol 16:98–103, 1987.

Pettit TH, Holland GM: Chronic keratoconjunctivitis associated with ocular adenovirus infection. Am J Ophthalmol 88:748–751, 1979.

Tullo AB: Adenovirus infections. In Easty DL (ed): Virus Disease of the Eye. Philadelphia, WB Saunders, 1985, pp 257–270.

RABIES
(Hydrophobia)

ROY J. ELLSWORTH, M.D.
Boise, Idaho

Rabies is an acute viral zoonosis of the central nervous system. The virus is almost always transmitted by the bite of a rabid animal, which introduces infected saliva through the skin. The disease has rarely been reported by nonbite contamination of saliva through a cut on the skin or inhalation of the virus. Transmission of rabies from human to human has only recently been reported. In 1979, Houff et al. reported human-to-human transmission of rabies virus by corneal transplant. Since that time, three other cases of human-to-human transmission have been reported following corneal transplant of a rabies-infected donor to neurologically normal recipients. There was no history of an animal bite in any of the donor patients, which obscured the diagnosis.

The incubation period is asymptomatic and usually lasts between 20 and 52 days. The initial symptoms are nonspecific, consisting of headache, fever, malaise, and anorexia. These symptoms may occur a few days before the appearance of the neurologic symptoms. The acute neurologic symptoms include paresthesia and pain around the site of the original wound. The patient then develops dysphagia and pharyngeal spasms, followed by sensitivity to light and sound. Weakness of the extremities usually occurs, which in some cases progresses to complete paralysis. Many patients exhibit increased salivation and hydrophobia. During the acute neurologic phase, the patient may develop progressive symptoms that last between 2 and 10 days; the patient may die of cardiac arrest during this time. The cortical phase of the infection manifested by convulsions, delerium, and coma may follow. With modern intensive care, life may be prolonged or even saved. Myocarditis with hypotension and arrhythmias with cardiopulmonary arrest are frequent causes of death. The principal ocular signs of rabies are ocular pain, photophobia, excessive lacrimation, and conjunctival hyperemia, followed in the neurologic phase by oculomotor palsies.

THERAPY

Systemic. Modern intensive care with special cardiovascular and airway support is essential.

Ocular. Ocular therapy for rabies is essentially symptomatic.

Supportive. Treatment for any person bitten by a possible rabid animal depends on the status of the animal. If the animal is domestic and healthy, it should be captured and observed for 10 days; if no symptoms of rabies are present, vaccination can be withheld. If the animal is wild, it should be killed and sent to the Public Health Laboratory for rabies examination.

Vigorous local wound care should be encouraged, including immediate cleansing of the area with soap and water and consideration of tetanus prophylaxis. If immunization is determined to be necessary, a new effective vaccine is now available through the state health departments. A human diploid cell strain rabies vaccine plus human rabies immune globulin (RIG) have been proven to be a safe and effective prophylaxis against rabies. The recommended dose of the rabies vaccine is 1-ml injections on days 0, 3, 7, 14, and 28, with 20 IU/kg of RIG administered on day 0.

Ocular or Periocular Manifestations

Conjunctiva: Hyperemia.
Extraocular Muscles: Paralysis of the third, fourth, or seventh nerve.
Eyelids: Retraction.
Retina: Edema; hemorrhages.
Other: Lacrimation; ocular pain; photophobia.

Precautions

Since the development of human diploid cell strain rabies vaccine, rabies prophylaxis is more rapid and effective with fewer side effects. The rabies duck embryo vaccine is not as effective and causes numerous allergic reactions.

Comments

Rabies prophylaxis should be started as soon as possible in a person known or suspected to have been exposed to the infection. Human-to-human transmission by corneal transplant has

94 / RABIES

now been documented in four cases from three donors who gave no history of animal bites. Rabies symptoms are nonspecific and can mimic other diseases, such as Guillain-Barré encephalitis. These cases along with previously reported transmission of the Creutzfeldt-Jakob virus by corneal transplantation make it important to exclude those corneal donors who die of postinfectious polyneuritis or unexplained encephalopathy.

The diagnosis of rabies can be made from corneal smears or skin biopsies from the back of the neck, which are checked for the presence of rabies antigen by direct fluorescence and assays for rabies antibodies. Postmortem diagnosis is made by demonstrating Negri bodies and isolating the virus or confirming rabies antigen by immunofluorescence techniques.

References

Duffy P, et al: Possible person-to-person transmission of Creutzfeldt-Jacob disease. N Engl J Med 290:692–693, 1974.
Gode GR, Bhide NK: Two rabies deaths after corneal grafts from one donor [letter]. Lancet 2(8614):791, 1988.
Haltia M, Tarkkanen A, Kivelia T: Rabies: ocular pathology. Br J Ophthalmol 73:61–67, 1989.
Houff SA, et al: Human-to-human transmission of rabies virus by corneal transplant. N Engl J Med 300:603–604, 1979.
Human-to-human transmission of rabies by a corneal transplant—Idaho, MMWR 28:109–111, 1979.
Human-to-human transmission of rabies via a corneal transplant—France. MMWR 29:25–26, 1980.
Human-to-human transmission of rabies via corneal transplant—Thailand. MMWR 30:473–475, 1981.
Plotkin SA, Koprowski H: Phobia of hydrophobia justified. N Engl J Med 300:620–622, 1979.
Plotkin SA, Wiktor T: Rabies vaccination. Annu Rev Med 29:583–591, 1978.
Warrel DA: The clinical picture of rabies in man. Trans Roy Soc Trop Med Hyg 70:188–195, 1976.

RUBELLA
(German Measles)
VIVIEN BONIUK, M.D.
Stony Brook, New York

Rubella has been known as a clinical entity for almost 200 years. It is viral in origin, caused by a member of the toga-virus group with one antigenic type. In 1941, Gregg made the astute clinical observation that a peculiar type of congenital cataract was associated with the occurrence of a rubella epidemic 9 to 10 months earlier. This led to the description of the congenital rubella syndrome, which is a well-defined and well-described group of ocular, cardiac, and other organ system abnormalities resulting from exposure to the rubella virus during embryonic life. The rubella epidemic of 1964 to 1965 afforded an opportunity for multidisciplinary study of the effects of the rubella virus and led to development of a vaccine.

Since rubella infrequently causes significant ocular and systemic complications in the postnatal period, attention here is directed only to the congenital rubella syndrome. Although several cases of acute rubella retinal pigment epithelitis have been reported in adults, they have not led to serious sequelae. The effects in utero are explainable by the observation that chronic infection by the rubella virus causes cells to have a prolonged doubling time and shortened survival; therefore, organ systems infected with virus during their active growing period will be underdeveloped and abnormal.

Depending on the stage of gestation during which rubella is acquired, there is a wide spectrum of systemic features ranging from stillbirths to the most minimally detectable damage to the retinal pigment epithelium and the pigmented epithelium in the organ of Corti. Other systemic abnormalities are prematurity by weight and mental and physical developmental retardation that persists into childhood. Also included are thrombocytopenic purpura, pancytopenia, large skull with bulging anterior fontanel, encephalitis, various neurologic anomalies, hepatosplenomegaly, radiologically observable bone changes, pancreatic insufficiency, esophageal atresia, and cleft palate. Various types of cardiac anomalies may be present and are frequently associated with ocular defects.

The most common ocular findings in congenital rubella syndrome are retinopathy; a peculiar central, often eccentric, dense nuclear cataract; and microphthalmos. Less frequent findings are iris hypoplasia with pigment epithelial defect, nystagmus and strabismus, congenital glaucoma, and corneal haze due to transient keratitis (which may leave a permanent scar). The pigmentary changes of the retina may show progression in early childhood, and there have been reported cases of subretinal neovascularization and disciform macular detachment as late complications.

THERAPY

Surgical. As soon as the child's condition permits, the congenital rubella cataract should be treated in a one-stage procedure that removes as much lens material as possible. Postoperative treatment with mydriatics should be intensive and continued for at least 3 months; parents should be cautioned about the importance of punctal occlusion following eyedrop administration. Early optical correction of aphakia is essential.

The glaucoma secondary to the congenital rubella syndrome behaves as a phenotypic congenital glaucoma. Other ocular abnormalities, such as strabismus, are treated in a manner consistent with basic therapeutic principles.

PRECAUTIONS

A multidisciplinary approach to treatment of these children is essential because of the presence of multiple anomalies associated with physical and mental developmental delay. It is essential that they be followed in centers familiar with coordination of therapy in order to maximize development.

COMMENTS

The incidence of rubella in pregnancy is directly related to the pool of susceptible women in that age group and their exposure to those recently infected with rubella virus. Recent epidemiologic data indicate that most cases reported now occur in young adults (those over 15 years of age), which include women of childbearing age who are at a high risk; prior prevalence predominated in the under 14 years of age group. Therefore, the incidence of reported congenital rubella syndrome has not decreased substantially in recent years.

In the United States, laws require vaccination against rubella for school entry, and this should ultimately reduce the adult pool; however, particularly susceptible at this time are those individuals in health care facilities providing care for women of childbearing age. Special attention should be paid to the immunization status of those individuals as a condition for employment. The risk of severe congenital malformation after rubella vaccination is low, even should it be given to a pregnant woman; however, to avoid this risk, women known to be pregnant should not be vaccinated and conception should be avoided for 3 months after vaccination.

References

Boniuk V: Rubella. Int Ophthalmol Clin 15:229–241, 1975.
Collis WJ, Cohen DN: Rubella retinopathy: A progressive disorder. Arch Ophthalmol 84:33, 1970.
Deutman AF, Grizzand WS: Rubella retinopathy and subretinal neovascularization. Am J Ophthalmol 85:22, 1978.
Gerstle C, Zinn KM: Rubella-associated retinitis in an adult: Report of a case. Mt Sinai J Med NY 43:303–308, 1976.
Greaves WL, et al: Prevention of rubella transmission in medical facilities. JAMA 248:861–864, 1982.
Hayashi M, Yoshimura N, Kondo T: Acute rubella retinal pigment epitheliitis in an adult. Am J Ophthalmol 93:285–288, 1982.
Orenstein WA, Greaves WL: Congenital rubella syndrome: A continuing problem. JAMA 247:1174–1175, 1982.
Preblud SR, et al: Fetal risk associated with rubella vaccine. JAMA 246:1413–1418, 1981.

RUBEOLA
(Measles, Morbilli)

N.W.H.M. DEKKERS, M.D.
Tilburg, The Netherlands

Rubeola is an acute, extremely communicable febrile disease, which primarily used to affect young school-aged children. The rapidly increasing rate of immunization has caused a shift toward the older age groups, whereas in developing countries, mainly the very young (6 months to 2 years) are affected. Rubeola is caused by a **paramyxovirus** and is characterized by a catarrhal inflammation of the respiratory tract and subepithelial conjunctivitis in the prodromal phase of the disease, followed by a maculopapular rash. The viral epithelial keratoconjunctivitis, late in the prodromal phase and in the exanthematous stage starts in the exposed parts of the conjunctiva and progresses toward the central cornea. Separate lesions can coalesce into large corneal erosions. Corneal ulcers and perforations, which are rare complications in well-nourished patients, can result from bacterial or viral (herpetic) superinfections and are usually associated with protein energy malnutrition. Infection with the virus in utero has been associated with cataracts, dacryostenosis, pigmentary retinopathy, and cardiopathy.

THERAPY

Systemic. Mild antipyretics and analgesics, such as aspirin, may be indicated for relief of fever, myalgias, and headache. Systemic antibiotics are not indicated, except in cases of secondary bacterial infections.

Ocular. The conjunctivitis and keratitis are usually of a mild and self-limiting nature. Eye care can be restricted to normal cleansing of the eyelids to remove crusts and secretions caused by conjunctivitis. In debilitated children, the application of eye ointment three or four times daily prevents the development of exposure keratitis and the progression of the keratitis into large corneal erosions.

Supportive. Low illumination reduces photophobia.

Ocular or Periocular Manifestations

Rare, apart from conjunctival and corneal signs.

Anterior Chamber: Hypopyon (associated with corneal ulcers and perforations).
Choroid: Posterior uveitis.
Conjunctiva: Kopliks' spots; subepithelial conjunctivitis, sometimes with follicles and hemorrhages (prodromal stage).
Cornea: Viral epithelial keratoconjunctivitis (exanthematous stage) as a common sign; rarely erosion, ulcer, adherent leukoma.
Eyelids: Blepharospasm; cellulitis; edema.
Iris: Prolapse; synechiae.
Lacrimal System: Dacryoadenitis; dacryocystitis; dacryostenosis (congenital).
Optic Nerve: Atrophy; retrobulbar or optic neuritis (associated with visual hallucinations, homonymous hemianopsia, and sixth nerve palsy).
Retina: Edema; pigmentary retinopathy

96 / RUBEOLA

(congenital); vascular constriction (may simulate central retinal artery occlusion).

Other: Accommodative spasm; hemianopsia; mydriasis; orbital cellulitis; paralysis of sixth nerve; secondary glaucoma, strabismus.

PRECAUTIONS

Routine immunization with live, attenuated measles vaccine has considerably changed the epidemiology of measles. This makes the clinical diagnosis a more difficult one than it used to be. In severe immunosuppression as in protein energy malnutrition, the characteristic rash is lacking and the measles infection is clinically not diagnosed.

COMMENTS

In the United States and Europe, measles is a relatively mild disease. On the contrary, measles is associated with high mortality and considerable morbidity in developing countries.

The incidence of blindness after measles can be as high as 1 per cent. This corneal blindness is caused by a combination of factors: measles, malnutrition, vitamin A deficiency, traditional treatment, and secondary bacterial or viral infection.

References

Dekkers NWHM: The cornea in measles. Doc Ophthalmol 52:1–120, 1981.
Dekkers NWHM: The cornea in measles. *In* Darrell RW (ed): Viral Infections of the Eye. Philadelphia, Lea & Febiger, pp 239–250, 1985.
Frederique G, Howard RO, Boniuk V: Corneal ulcers in rubeola. Am J Ophthalmol 68:996–1003, 1969.
Morley DC, Martin WJ, Allen I: Measles in East and Central Africa. E Afr Med J *44*:497–508, 1967.
Sanford-Smith JH, Whittle HC: Corneal ulceration following measles in Nigerian children. Br J Ophthalmol 63:720–724, 1979.

VARICELLA
(Chickenpox)

YUKIO UCHIDA, M.D.

Tokyo, Japan

Varicella is a mild, highly contagious exanthem of childhood characterized by fever and vesicular eruptions in successive crops on the skin and mucous membranes. It is transmitted by droplet infection and caused by the varicella zoster virus, a member of the herpesvirus group. Although the majority of children and nonimmune adults recover promptly without sequela, rare but severe complications, such as pneumonia and encephalitis, have been known to occur. Ophthalmic involvement consists primarily of unilateral, small, papular, phlyctenular eruptions along the lid margin, on the semilunar fold of the conjunctiva, and, most commonly, at the limbus.

THERAPY

Systemic. Systemic antibiotics may be administered when secondary infections occur. Zoster immunoglobulins can be used to prevent the development of the disease in children who are immunologically compromised and have been exposed to varicella. Zoster immunoglobulins work favorably when given within three days after the exposure.

Ocular. There is no specific therapy for varicella. Cool compresses may be used to relieve the pruritus. For photophobia and discomfort caused by keratitis and uveitis, mydriatic-cycloplegics may be used. One drop of 1.0 per cent atropine solution may be instilled into the conjunctival sac once to twice daily. Vesicles or ulcers of the outer eye may become secondarily infected. Therefore, topical antibiotics, such as erythromycin, gentamicin, or tobramycin, should be used prophylactically to prevent infection. Antibiotic ointment may be applied on the skin three times daily, and solution instilled into the conjunctival sac four to six times daily. Antiviral agents, such as vidarabine,‡ trifluridine,‡ or acyclovir,* have not proved of value clinically against stromal keratitis and uveitis; however, they appear to have some therapeutic effect on epithelial lesions. Vidarabine or acyclovir ointment may be administered into the conjunctival sac five times daily, and trifluridine ophthalmic solution may be instilled five to nine times daily.

The use of topical corticosteroids should be avoided, except for severe nonulcerative stromal keratitis with uveitis. In this situation, a minimal amount of corticosteroid (one drop of 0.1 per cent dexamethasone three times daily at most) should be used in combination with topical antibiotics, antivirals, and cycloplegics. The patients should be seen at least twice a week, and the medication must be tapered gradually as a response is attained.

Supportive. Patients should rest in bed while they are febrile and remain at home until cutaneous eruptions become crusted. An antipyretic may be administered while patients are febrile, but the use of salicylates, such as aspirin, should be avoided in children. Because the secondary infection of the cutaneous lesion with *Staphylococcus* or *Streptococcus* is common, the patient's skin should be kept clean. The fingernails of the patient should be trimmed to prevent secondary skin infections caused by scratching. Antipruritic and drying preparation, such as calamine lotion, may be applied to the cutaneous lesions.

Ocular or Periocular Manifestations

Conjunctiva: Hyperemia; phlyctenular lesion at limbus; ulcer; vesicles.
Cornea: Descemetocele; opacity; pseudodendritic epithelial lesion; punctate epithelial

keratitis; stromal discifom or interstitial keratitis; ulcer; vesicles.

Eyelids: Cicatrization of lid margin; distortion of cilia; ulcer; vesicles.

Optic Nerve: Optic neuritis; papilledema.

Retina: Diffuse retinitis; exudative retinitis; hemorrhagic retinopathy; periphlebitis.

Other: Anterior uveitis; cataract; external ophthalmoplegia; internal ophthalmoplegia; phthisis bulbi.

PRECAUTIONS

Treatment of varicella is essentially symptomatic. Systemic corticosteroids are contraindicated, because these drugs are known to cause dissemination of the disease. Once stromal keratitis has been treated with topical corticosteroids, it is difficult to withdraw these drugs without recurrence of the disease, even if the medication is tapered. Therefore, this therapy should be restricted to severe cases.

COMMENTS

The ocular vesicles or ulcers of varicella resolve spontaneously with minimal scarring. Uni-lateral serous iridocyclitis occasionally occurs as a separate entity, but it is self-limited. Rare intra-ocular involvement, such as retinitis or optic neuritis, may cause transient loss of vision; however, recovery of vision is the usual outcome. Stromal keratitis of the disciform type may occur at different periods after the onset, from weeks to several months. When it is treated with topical corticosteroids, pseudodendritic lesions that harbor the virus occasionally appear in the corneal epithelium. This is thought to be a reactivation phenomenon caused by corticosteroids. These lesions, however, do not appear to develop into large ulcers.

References

Duke-Elder S (ed): System of Ophthalmology. St. Louis. CV Mosby, Vol VIII, 1965, pp 337–339.

McGill J, Chapman C: A comparison of topical acyclovir with steroids in the treatment of herpes zoster keratouveitis. Br J Ophthalmol 67:746–750, 1983.

Pavan-Langston D: Varicella-zoster ophthalmicus. Int Ophthalmol Clin 15:171–185, 1975.

Uchida Y, Kaneko M, Hayashi K: Varicella dendritic keratitis. Am J Ophthalmol 89:259–262, 1980.

SECTION 2

PARASITIC DISEASES

ACANTHAMOEBAE

MARY BETH MOORE, M.D.
Dallas, Texas

Two genera of small free-living amoebae can cause infections in humans. Amoebae of the *Naegleria* species are flagellated and gain access to the central nervous system by penetration of the nasal mucosa and direct invasion of the cribiform plate following a swim in contaminated water. The acute, necrotizing encephalitis that follows is rapidly fatal and may last 5 to 7 days. In contrast, amoebae of the *Acanthamoeba* species are nonflagellated and relatively less aggressive. They cause a slowly progressive, usually fatal granulomatous encephalitis that may last weeks or months. The route of infection is thought to be hematogenous.

Corneal infections are also caused by direct contact either with a foreign body contaminated with *Acanthamoeba* or with a contaminated soft or hard contact lens. Contact lenses become contaminated when rinsed or stored in homemade saline solution, distilled water, tap water, or well water. Contamination may also occur when a patient wears contact lenses while swimming in contaminated water or immersing in a contaminated hot tub. Commercially prepared preserved and nonpreserved saline solution can become contaminated once opened, and currently available disinfection methods may not eradicate the organism. Repeated inoculation onto the cornea via a contaminated contact lens results in a chronic, smoldering, painful keratitis.

Species responsible for corneal infections include *A. castellanii, A. polyphaga, A. culbertsoni, A. hatchetti,* and *A. rhysodes.* The organism exists in two forms: the motile, replicating trophozoite and the sessile, dormant cyst. It inhabits soil and water, and the cysts can become air-borne. The trophozoite feeds on bacteria and releases enzymes that may facilitate tissue invasion.

The number of reported cases of *Acanthamoeba* keratitis has increased significantly over the past 5 years. Initially, patients underwent multiple failed grafts or enucleation because of delayed diagnosis, and in some cases, the diagnosis was not made until tissue specimens were examined retrospectively. However, recently, early recognition and appropriate treatment have resulted in medical and surgical eradication of the infection and preservation of good vision. The most common misdiagnosis is *Herpes simplex* keratitis because of the similar ocular pain, pseudodendrites, nonsuppurative keratitis, and initial positive response to topical steroids. The clinical course of *Acanthamoeba* keratitis is characterized by infection in young, healthy individuals, intense ocular pain, waxing and waning keratitis, pseudodendrites, recurrent epithelial defects, anterior stromal ring infiltrate, radial neuritis, and disciform keratitis. Diffuse anterior and posterior scleritis, scleral nodules, and uveitis have also been reported to be caused by *Acanthamoeba.* Organisms have been recovered from an anterior chamber paracentesis and have been seen on the iris surface histopathologically, thus raising the possibility of intraocular invasion. Fundus involvement is rare and thought to be due to hematogenous spread.

THERAPY

Systemic. A single, daily dose of 200 to 600 mg of ketoconazole[‡] may be used for severe infections; however, it is not known if therapeutic levels of this drug are achieved in the cornea. Sulindac, 200 mg or less, four times a day, may be used to relieve ocular pain. Oral narcotics may be required to alleviate severe ocular pain, which may last several weeks or months. However, long-term use of narcotics should be avoided.

Ocular. Medical therapy is evolving as more drugs are tested, found to be effective in vitro, and applied to the clinical situation. Currently, the accepted approach is topical ophthalmic treatment with one or more of the following: 0.1 per cent propamidine,[†] 0.15 per cent dibromopropamidine,[†] 0.1 per cent pentamidine,[‡] 1 per cent miconazole[‡] and 1 per cent clotrimazole, in combination with neomycin/polymyxin B/gramicidin[‡] or paromomycin[‡] solution. Both propamidine and pentamidine are members of the aromatic amines, which have well-documented antiparasitic properties. The antifungal imidazoles and antibacterial aminoglycosides inhibit growth of amoebae in vitro.

Initial treatment is intensive. A typical regimen includes propamidine and neomycin/polymyxin B/gramicidin solutions; each drop is given every hour or more frequently and then tapered over 1 month to four times a day. This maintenance therapy is continued for 1 year in an attempt to eradicate cysts that might persist in the cornea. Reactivations during maintenance therapy are treated as vigorously as initial infections. Because these drops are toxic, some patients develop medicamentosal conjunctivitis.

98

This condition is reversible once the dose is reduced. Therefore, therapy with these drops should not be reduced because of toxicity.

The use of topical steroids[‡] is controversial. Cellular host defense mechanisms against amoebae consist of macrophages and neutrophils. Steroids inhibit that arm of defense and, as with fungal and mycobacterial infections for which drugs alone may be only partially effective, may potentiate or prolong the infection. Unfortunately, patients are usually started on steroids before the correct diagnosis is made, and they then become dependent on them for control of pain and inflammation. It is important to try to wean them off steroids as quickly as possible. A topical mydriatic-cycloplegic may be used to dilate the pupil and prevent ciliary spasm.

Surgical. The timing and role of penetrating keratoplasty are also controversial. Some clinicians advocate medical treatment for 1 year to eradicate the organism before surgery, thus avoiding grafting into an infected host bed. There are several reports of successful medical cures that resulted not only in saving the eye but also in preserving good vision. Others advocate early surgery to remove all organisms before they spread to the periphery. However, the extent of the infection is not always apparent on slitlamp examination, and recurrences in the graft can lead to repeated graft failures, uncontrolled glaucoma, cataract, wound melt and dehiscence, and phthisis.

Other. One method used to prevent recurrences after penetrating keratoplasty is to freeze the recipient bed at the time of surgery. Cryotherapy may kill trophozoites, but it does not eradicate cysts, which survive freezing temperatures and can potentially excyst to reinfect the graft. Cryotherapy may also cause increased intraocular inflammation and retrocorneal fibrous membrane formation, resulting in graft failure. Conjunctival flaps were tried in the first reported cases. However, they failed because of progression of the infection under the flap, which resulted in necrosis and melting of the flap. For therapy of extreme ocular pain that is unresponsive to the treatment described earlier, an absolute alcohol, retrobulbar block (0.3 to 0.6 ml of absolute alcohol, or 1 to 2 ml of 50 percent alcohol, mixed with 1 to 2 ml of .75 percent marcaine) may be given. This block is painful; therefore, intravenous sedation before its administration is recommended.

Ocular or Periocular Manifestations

Anterior Chamber: Cells and flare; fibrin strands; hypopyon.
Conjunctiva: Chemosis; ciliary flush; hyperemia.
Cornea: Pseudodendrite; persistent or recurrent epithelial defects; punctate anterior stromal infiltrates; diffuse patchy anterior stromal infiltrates; full or partial anterior stromal ring infiltrate; disciform keratitis; radial neuritis; double-ring infiltrate; stromal cysts; stromal necrosis; descemetocele; perforation.
Eyelids: Reactive ptosis; hyperemia; edema.
Iris: Nongranulomatous anterior uveitis; posterior synechiae.
Sclera: Nodular scleritis; diffuse anterior and posterior scleritis.
Other: Decreased visual acuity; *severe* ocular pain (out of proportion to the clinical findings); photophobia; epiphora; secondary glaucoma; vitreitis; retinal perivasculitis; papillitis; chorioretinitis.

Precautions

Topical ophthalmic miconazole is acidic and poorly tolerated by patients. Clotrimazole is currently used for infections that do not respond to propamidine, dibromopropamidine, or neomycin/polymyxin B/gramicidin combination.

Liver functions must be monitored in patients administered ketoconazole or sulindac, and neither drug should be used in pregnant women or women of childbearing age.

Comments

The diagnosis of infection by *Acanthamoebae* is difficult. It requires a high index of suspicion, persistence, and an experienced observer and laboratory personnel. In a patient wearing contact lenses, a painful keratitis and a culture that is negative and unresponsive to antibacterial and antiviral therapy should alert the practitioner to the possibility of an amoebic infection. Using calcofluor white and immunofluorescent antibody staining of corneal scrapings and tissue biopsy specimens, and cultures on nonnutrient agar plates precoated with *E. coli* can improve the chances of a positive diagnosis. Positive cultures of contact lenses, contact lens paraphernalia, and saline solutions may lend support for the diagnosis of amoebic keratitis when appropriate laboratory tests are repeatedly negative. Because this can be a devastating infection that is unresponsive to current medical and surgical therapy, prevention is extremely important. Practitioners who fit contact lenses must ensure that patients do not use nonsterile fluids to rinse, store, or disinfect their lenses.

References

Acanthamoeba keratitis associated with contact lenses—United States. MMWR 35:405, 1986.

Auran JD, Starr MB, Jakobiec FA: *Acanthamoeba* keratitis. A review of the literature. Cornea 6:2, 1987.

Moore MB, McCulley JP: *Acanthamoeba* keratitis associated with contact lenses: Six cases of successful medical treatment. Invest Ophthalmol Vis Sci 28:371(Suppl), 1987.

Moore MB, McCulley JP: Letter to the editor. Am J Ophthalmol *104*:310, 1987.

Moore MB, et al: *Acanthamoeba* keratitis associated with soft contact lenses. Am J Ophthalmol *100*:396, 1985.

Moore MB, et al: *Acanthamoeba* keratitis: A growing problem in soft and hard contact lens wearers. Ophthalmology *94*:1654, 1987.

Wright P, Warhurst D, Jones BR: *Acanthamoeba* keratitis successfully treated medically. Br J Ophthalmol 69:778, 1985.

AMERICAN MUCOCUTANEOUS LEISHMANIASIS

JAIME ROIZENBLATT, M.D.,
and LUIZ CARLOS CUCE, M.D.
Saõ Paulo, Brazil

American mucocutaneous leishmaniasis is a zoonosis that occurs endemically in certain areas in Latin America; it is caused by the flagellate protozoa, *Leishmania braziliensis*. The American form of leishmaniasis resembles the oriental cutaneous type in that it is characterized by specific ulcerating granulomas of the skin; however, American leishmaniasis is distinguished from *L. tropica* by the presence of mucocutaneous lesions. Like all types of leishmaniasis, American mucocutaneous leishmaniasis is transmitted to humans by the bite of the infected female *Phlebotomus* sandfly. The initial lesion normally occurs in exposed parts of the body, and those who work in forests are most frequently affected. Reservoirs other than human include wild rodents, such as rats, mice, agoutis, and pacas that are common in the neotropics. The human being is only an accidental member in the biologic cycle of this zoonosis. The incubation period varies from 2 to 8 weeks, after which an erythematous papule develops at the site of inoculation and gradually increases in size by peripheral extension. The papule may vesiculate, ulcerate, or take on a mulberry appearance. Regional adenopathy may be noted in the initial stages.

Generally, the lesions are secondarily infected. The disease may follow an apparently benign and self-limiting course; the ulcer usually heals within a year, leaving a typical scar at the site of the lesion. After a long period of time, mucocutaneous lesions may develop in the nasal mucosa; the nasal cartilage usually is invaded and destroyed, resulting in a deformity known as "tapir's nose." The involvement of the nasal fossae, pharynx, soft palate, floor of the mouth, and tonsils, as well as the upper respiratory tract and larynx, may cause difficulty in breathing, feeding, and deglutition. In its preference for cartilages, the ear may also be invaded and destroyed. The mucocutaneous involvement occurs as a result of direct spread of the original lesion or hematogenous and even lymphatic dissemination. In addition to the previously discussed forms, a disseminated anergic form may occur in which there is widespread involvement of the skin by nodular infiltrative lesions.

Ocular findings associated with American mucocutaneous leishmaniasis involve the eyelids and conjunctiva. Eyelid edema, scarring or even destruction of the tarsus, and nodular granulomas of the tarsal or bulbar conjunctiva may develop. Ulceration of the conjunctiva and cornea as well as interstitial keratitis have also been described. The eye may be involved by contiguous spread to the eyelid and conjunctiva, by hematogenous spread, or by inoculation of the conjunctiva by the patient's own fingers.

THERAPY

Systemic. Only sporadic forms of American mucocutaneous leishmaniasis are self-limiting. If the initial lesion does not heal or there are signs of systemic spread, particularly of mucocutaneous involvement, systemic treatment should be instituted immediately.

The drug of choice is antimony meglumine.[†] It is the most often used antimonate at present due to its low toxicity and good therapeutic results. The daily dose of antimony meglumine is 50 to 100 mg/kg for adults and 4 to 6 mg/kg for children. The drug should be administered intramuscularly or intravenously by slow infusion for 10 to 20 days. This course can be repeated two or more times after 15- to 20-day intervals.

Equally efficient is stibogluconate sodium, given intramuscularly or intravenously in daily doses of 600 mg for 6 to 10 days. In the United State, antimony meglumine and stibogluconate sodium are available from the Centers for Disease Control in Atlanta.

In resistant cases and particularly when there is mucocutaneous involvement, the drug of choice is amphotericin B. Slow infusion of 0.5 mg/kg diluted in 500 ml of a 5 per cent dextrose in water solution may be administered over a 6- to 8-hour period every 1 to 2 days; this may slowly be increased to 1.0 mg/kg. Fresh solutions should be prepared for each injection. The drug should be protected from light during administration. For cutaneous forms, a total dose of 1.5 to 2.0 gm is given; this may be increased up to 3 gm until the patient is clinically cured.

Cycloguanil pamoate[†] has not shown more significant results than the previously discussed drugs. Therefore, its use is not indicated.

Ocular. Topical ocular antibiotics are indicated to prevent secondary bacterial infection of conjunctival or corneal defects. Cool compresses may give symptomatic relief. Sunglasses will aid in the relief of photophobia.

Supportive. Secondary infection in mucocutaneous leishmaniasis should be controlled by use of appropriate antimicrobial drugs. Cauterization of the verrucose lesions and plastic surgery for facial disfigurement may sometimes be necessary. Surgery should only be considered after a long interval has passed after the patient is clinically cured; otherwise, it may have disastrous effects.

Ocular or Periocular Manifestations

Conjunctiva: Papulonecrotic and ulcerative lesions; phlyctenules.
Cornea: Abscess; diffuse keratitis; granulom-

atous and ulcerative lesions; interstitial keratitis.

Eyelids: Cicatrization and destruction of the tarsus; "hard" edema; nodular or ulcerating granuloma.

PRECAUTIONS

American mucocutaneous leishmaniasis is a form of human leishmaniasis that is sometimes very resistant to therapy and has a high relapse rate. The duration of the disease and the patient's immune status are in part responsible for these different responses to medication. Treatment should be continued until an apparent cure is obtained, and the patient should be observed for an extended period. If the drug of choice appears to be ineffective, it is advisable to try a second course of therapy with this same drug before using alternative drugs. Complement-fixing antibody should not be detectable 6 to 12 months after the apparent clinical cure. In chronic leishmaniasis, it is very uncommon to find the parasite. However, the diagnosis can be confirmed with the Montenegro skin test, which is positive in more than 90 per cent of patients with this disease.

Adverse effects with use of antimony meglumine and stibogluconate sodium are not uncommon. These drugs have significant toxicity, and their use should be carefully monitored. The most frequent adverse effects include chills, fever, coughing, vomiting, muscle and joint stiffness, arthralgia, bradycardia, and anaphylactoid reactions. The intravenous administration of amphotericin B usually produces chills, fever, vomiting, headache, and hypersensitivity reactions. Phlebitis is also often a problem with intravenous administration of amphotericin B, and 1000 to 2500 units of heparin in the intravenous solution may be needed to prevent this complication. Intravenous infusion by means of a pediatric scalp vein needle minimizes the risk of thrombophlebitis. Tolerance may be enhanced by temporary lowering of the dose or administration of aspirin, diphenhydramine, phenothiazines, and corticosteroids. Therapeutically active amounts of amphotericin B commonly impair kidney and liver function and produce anemia (impaired iron utilization by bone marrow). Electrolyte disturbances (hypokalemia, distal tubular acidosis), shock, and a variety of neurologic symptoms also may occur.

COMMENTS

American leishmaniasis occurs most frequently in rural areas among forest workers. The disease occurs more often in men than in women, probably because of the greater number of men in these occupations. Prophylactic measures include eradication of the *Phlebotomus* with insecticide, use of repellents and nets, and continuous surveillance in endemic areas.

The patient may also be an incidental source of infection, and prompt treatment will render him or her noninfective to sandflies. A vaccine is not commercially available at this time.

The prognosis in mucocutaneous leishmaniasis is much more serious than in cutaneous leishmaniasis because of the destructiveness of the mucocutaneous lesions and the resistance sometimes found to therapy. The prognosis is good if treatment is begun early, preferably before mucocutaneous lesions develop.

References

Bryceson ADM: Leishmaniasis. *In* Wyngaarden JB, Smith LH Jr (eds): Textbook of Medicine. 16th ed. Philadelphia, WB Saunders, 1982, p 1731.

Drugs for parasitic infections. Med Lett Drugs Therap 24:5–12, 1982.

Duke-Elder S (ed): System of Ophthalmology. St. Louis, CV Mosby, 1976, Vol XV, pp 85–86.

Goldsmith RS: Infectious diseases: Protozoal. *In* Krupp MA, Chatton MJ (eds): Current Medical Diagnosis and Treatment. Los Altos, Lange, 1982, pp 878–880.

Harman RRM: Parasitic worms and protozoa. *In* Rook A, Wilkinson DS, Ebling FJG (eds): Textbook of Dermatology, 2nd ed. Oxford, Blackwell, 1972, pp 839–841.

Marsden PD, Zamith VA: Leishmaniose tegumentar americana. *In* Veronesi R (ed): Doencas Infecciosas e Parasitarias, 7th ed. Rio de Janeiro, Guanabara Koogan, 1982, pp 739–752.

Roizenblatt J: Interstitial keratitis caused by American (mucocutaneous) leishmaniasis. Am J Ophthalmol 87:175–179, 1979.

Rollo IM: Miscellaneous drugs used in the treatment of protozoal infections. *In* Gilman AG, Goodman LS, Gilman A (eds): The Pharmacological Basis of Therapeutics, 6th ed. New York, Macmillan, 1980, pp 1070–1079.

Wilcocks C, Manson-Bahr PEC (eds): Manson's Tropical Diseases, 17th ed. Baltimore, Williams & Wilkins, 1972, pp 140–147.

Woodruff AW: Leishmaniases. *In* Woodruff AW (ed): Medicine in the Tropics. Edinburgh, Churchill Livingstone, 1974, pp 103–109.

ASCARIASIS

THOMAS JOHN, M.D.,
JOHN J. DONNELLY, Ph.D.,
and JOHN H. ROCKEY, M.D., Ph.D.
Philadelphia, Pennsylvania

Ascariasis results from the ingestion of infective eggs of the roundworm, *Ascaris lumbricoides* (or rarely, *A. suum*). Larvae hatch from the ova in the small intestines, penetrate the intestinal wall, and are carried via the portal venous system and lymphatics through the liver to the lungs. There they penetrate into and migrate up the respiratory passages and are swallowed; the adult worms mature in the small intestines. In severe infections, larvae may pass through the lungs into the general circulation and may reach such structures as the eye and periocular tissues. Ascariasis may be asymptomatic, or pulmonary disease (Loeffler's eosinophilic pneumonitis, asthma), abdominal disease (small intestine, biliary duct or pancreatic duct obstruction, intussusception, volvulus, appendicitis, diverticulitis, perforation, hepatic abscess), or type I hypersensitivity reactions (urticaria, acute conjunctivitis, acute laryngeal obstruction, wheal-and-flare dermal reactions) to ascarid antigens mediated by high titer IgE antibody may develop. Intraocular or periocular (within nasolacrimal system) localization of an ascarid larva is rare, being an accident of aberrant larval migration.

THERAPY

Systemic. The drug of choice is mebendazole, which blocks glucose uptake by the parasite. It has a wide antiparasitic spectrum and gives a cure rate of 95 to 100 per cent for *Ascaris, Necator,* and *Enterobius;* hence, it is useful in mixed infections. Mebendazole is administered orally in a dosage of 100 mg twice daily for 3 consecutive days. Pyrantel is an alternative drug of choice for treating ascariasis. A single oral dose of 11 mg/kg (maximum 1 gm) is given for adults and children. Pyrantel paralyzes the worms, which then are expelled intact, and a laxative is usually not required. Piperazine is also very effective and less expensive but more toxic than the previous two agents. It blocks neuromuscular junctions and produces paralysis of the ascarid, leading to expulsion of the worm. For adults, a single daily oral dose of 3.5 gm given on 2 consecutive days is recommended; for children, 75 mg/kg (daily maximum, 3.5 gm) may be administered in the same fashion. Oral thiabendazole in a dose of 25 mg/kg (daily maximum, 3 gm) taken twice daily after meals is also effective in the treatment of ascariasis. Likewise, levamisole,[†] which appears to act by inhibiting succinate dehydrogenase in the muscles of the worm, results in paralysis and expulsion of the worm.

Ocular. Most of the ocular allergic manifestations of ascariasis may be resolved with systemic antiparasitic therapy. Anterior uveitis may be treated with topical corticosteroids and mydriatic/cycloplegics. Depending on the severity of the uveitis, the frequency of steroid drops may range from hourly application to once every other day. Subconjunctival injections[*] of corticosteroids may be used if necessary. The strongest and longest-acting cycloplegic is atropine. It may be used topically one to four times daily, depending on the degree of inflammation. For milder uveitis, 0.5 per cent scopolamine or 2 to 5 per cent homatropine may be used. Systemic corticosteroids are indicated when other forms of corticosteroids have failed or posterior inflammatory reaction of chorioretinitis is present. Photocoagulation has been used to kill intraocular parasites, but may cause an increased allergic reaction because of the release of parasite antigens.

Supportive. Hospitalization is usually limited to patients with severe infections and complications. Such patients may require correction of fluid and electrolytes, transfusions, and high caloric intake. Saline enemas may be useful to remove worms that may be present in the large bowel. Intestinal obstruction, if present, is initially treated conservatively with nasogastric suction and intravenous fluids. After vomiting is controlled, piperazine may be given through the nasogastric tube in a dosage of 65 mg/kg (maximum, 1.0 gm) every 12 to 24 hours for six doses. If there is no improvement, it may be possible to manipulate the bolus of worms into the large bowel during laparotomy. Only if this procedure is unsuccessful should enterotomy and removal of the worms be attempted.

Ocular or Periocular Manifestations

Conjunctiva: Conjunctivitis; subconjunctival parasite; xerosis.
Eyelids: Edema; urticaria.
Iris: Uveitis.
Lacrimal System: Egress of larva via lacrimal punctum.
Lens: Subluxation.
Optic Nerve: Papilledema.
Orbit: Pseudotumor.
Retina: Edema; hemorrhagic macular chorioretinitis; periphlebitis.
Vitreous: Recurrent hemorrhages.
Other: Scotoma; secondary glaucoma; visual loss.

PRECAUTIONS

In multiple intestinal helminthic infections, ascariasis should be treated first in order to prevent migration of ascarids. Before elective surgery, patients should be dewormed because worms can penetrate the intestinal wall, especially in the region of surgical anastomosis.

Pyrantel should be used with caution in patients with pre-existing liver dysfunction. Its safe usage in pregnancy and in children under 2 years of age has not been established. Likewise, mebendazole is contraindicated during pregnancy and has not been investigated extensively in children below the age of 2. Piperazine is contraindicated in renal or hepatic insufficiency and in epileptic patients. Its accumulation in the presence of renal insufficiency may produce neurotoxic signs.

During examination of the feces, fertilized ova are easy to recognize, whereas unfertilized ova assume bizarre shapes and may be mistaken for debris. Rarely, infections may be due only to male worms.

COMMENTS

Ascariasis, a worldwide helminthic infection, is the most common helminthiasis that affects humans. One quarter of the world's population is infected with *A. lubricoides*. Although cosmopolitan, ascariasis is most common in the tropics where sanitation is poor and is endemic in the rural southwestern United States. Susceptibility to infection and serious complications are greatest in childhood. Ascariasis is usually accompanied by minor symptoms, although severe complications can develop. Elevated blood eosinophil levels usually are present only during the tissue migratory phase. Eggs appear in the feces 60 to 75 days after the ingestion of infective eggs. Examination of feces may help establish the diagnosis. Visceral larva migrans due to the related ascarid *Toxocara canis* may be differentiated by the ELISA (enzyme-linked immunosorbent assay) immunoassay. Other ascarids, such as *Baylisascaris procyonis*, also may cause ocular larva migrans. In the United States, the worm load is usually modest. Cure rate is high with adequate therapy. The case fatality rate of intestinal obstruction in the United States is 3 per cent. Treatment of ascariasis may be nutritionally advantageous for children with heavy worm burdens and marginal protein availability.

References

Beck JW, Davies JE: Medical Parasitology, 3rd ed. St. Louis, CV Mosby, 1981, pp 136–140.
Blumenthal DS: Ascariasis. *In* Wyngaarden JB, Smith LH Jr (eds): Textbook of Medicine, 16th ed. Philadelphia, WB Saunders, 1982, pp 1768–1769.
Cook GC: The clinical significance of gastrointestinal helminths: A review. Trans Roy Soc Trop Med Hyg 80:675–685, 1986.
Duke-Elder S (ed): System of Ophthalmology. St. Louis, CV Mosby, 1976, Vol XV, pp 15–16.
Gass JDM, Braunstein RA: Further observations concerning the diffuse unilateral subacute neuroretinitis syndrome. Arch Ophthalmol 101:1689, 1983.
Glickman LT, Schantz PM: Epidemiology and pathogenesis of zoonotic toxocariasis. Epidemiol Rev 3:230–250, 1981.
Most H: Treatment of common parasitic infections of man encountered in the United States. (First of two parts). N Engl J Med 287:495–498, 1972.
Schlaegel TF Jr, Knox DL: Uveitis and parasitoses. *In* Duane TD (ed): Clinical Ophthalmology. Hagerstown, MD, Harper and Row, 1982, Vol IV, pp 52:1–16.
Sharma S: Advances in the treatment and control of tissue-dwelling helminth parasites. Prog Drug Res 30:473–547, 1986.
Turner JA: Drug therapy of gastrointestinal parasitic infections. The ACG Committee of FDA-related matters. Am J Gastroenterol 81:1125–1137, 1986.

COENUROSIS

EDWARD EPSTEIN, M.B., B.Ch., D.O.M.S.
Johannesburg, South Africa

Coenurosis is a rare human infestation of the cystic larval stage of the dog tapeworm *Multiceps*. Three species of *Multiceps* have been associated with human coenurosis: *M. multiceps*, *M. serialis*, and *M. glomeratus*. Humans rarely harbor coenuri, although they occur quite commonly in a variety of wild and domestic animals. When *Coenurus* infestation does develop in humans, it usually occurs in the muscle, subcutaneous tissue, eye, or nervous system. In tropical areas, the brain is usually involved, and the infestation may be fatal. The clinical manifestations of coenurosis are ataxia, headache, loss of weight, somnolence, visual disturbance, and stiffness of the neck and shoulders. *Multiceps coenurus* may involve almost any area of the eye. Subconjunctival infestation may occur in young children, whereas involvement of the globe is more common in older people. Late in the course of the disease, reaction with fibrosis and blindness is the general rule.

THERAPY

Ocular. Cycloplegics, such as 1 per cent atropine solution, should be applied three times daily to decrease ocular pain and manage uveitis.

Surgical. The treatment of choice for systemic and intraocular coenurus cysts is surgical excision of the cyst. This is relatively simple and curative if the cyst is subconjunctival. Systemic and intraocular cysts are more difficult to treat because significant damage may occur from attempted removal. However, because the outcome is almost always devastating if the cyst is left in place, an attempt at removal should be made. Oral corticosteroid therapy, such as 5 to 20 mg of prednisolone a day, should be used to control postoperative inflammation. Enucleation may be necessary in cases of end stage ocular disease.

Ocular or Periocular Manifestations

Anterior Chamber: Cells and flare; hypopyon.
Choroid and Retina: Detachment; edema; granuloma.
Conjunctiva: Coenurus cysts; conjunctivitis.
Cornea: Infiltration; keratic precipitates.
Globe: Pain; proptosis.
Iris: Anterior uveitis; coenurus cysts; posterior synechiae.
Other: Increased intraocular pressure; miosis; visual loss; vitreal haze.

Precautions

Clinical judgment dictates the degree of surgical intervention. If surgery is too late to salvage an eye, then observation or enucleation is indicated.

Comments

Intraocular helminthic infestations occur rarely. When the parasite has ruptured into the vitreous, the diagnosis is fairly simple. However, when the cyst is subretinal, and especially when it is within the uvea, the diagnosis becomes more difficult. Parasitic cysts usually produce signs of iritis, inflammation, and localized swelling. Subconjunctival infestation is seen in young children. Involvement of the globe occurs in older people secondary to spread from the bloodstream.

References

Boase AJ: Coenurus cyst of the eye. Br J Ophthalmol 40:183–185, 1956.
Epstein E, Proctor NSF, Heinz HJ: Intra-ocular coenurus infestation. S Afr Med J 33:602–604, 1959.
Johnstone HG, Jones OW, Jr.: Cerebral coenurosis in an infant. Am J Trop Med 30:431–441, 1950.
Skerritt GC, Stallbaumer MF: Diagnosis and treatment of coenuriasis (gid) in sheep. Vet Rec 115:399–403, 1984.
Williams PH, Templeton AC: Infection of the eye by tapeworm Coenurus. Br J Ophthalmol 55:766–769, 1971.

CUTANEOUS LEISHMANIASIS
(Old World Leishmaniasis, Oriental Sore, Tropical Sore)

FUAD S. FARAH, M.D.
Syracuse, New York

The causative agent of cutaneous leishmaniasis is *Leishmania tropica*, a parasite that causes a specific granuloma of the skin. Cutaneous leishmaniasis does not involve the other tissues of the body, and healing is associated with permanent immunity in the majority of patients. The disease is common in the Middle East and the Mediterranean basin and may occur as epidemics in certain areas. The clinical picture seen in any one patient depends upon the parasite and the immunologic status of the patient. Innate inherited factors may also have a determinant effect as seen in animal studies, but this effect has not yet been demonstrated in human infections.

The clinical manifestations of cutaneous leishmaniasis can generally be divided into localized or disseminated involvement. Acute cutaneous leishmaniasis appears on an exposed area at sites accessible to sandfly bites. The initial lesion is a small papule resembling an insect bite that persists, enlarges, becomes firm and adherent, and is asymptomatic except for mild pruritus. With time, central ulceration develops and is followed by healing with a characteristic scar within 1 year of onset. Although numerous cutaneous lesions resulting from multiple sandfly inoculations may be seen, cutaneous leishmaniasis is usually localized to a single lesion. Chronic cutaneous leishmaniasis is rare and is usually seen in elderly patients. The face is most commonly affected. Although ulceration does not occur, the lesions are persistent and do not heal. *Leishmania* recidiva follows the same course as acute cutaneous leishmaniasis and is indistinguishable from it early in its course. However, after the lesions have healed, usually within a year, there is reactivation of the parasite

and new lesions appear months or years later at the original scar. Disseminated cutaneous leishmaniasis is characterized by the development of multiple lesions rich in organisms. Eyelid manifestations are the most common ocular involvement, but these occur in only approximately 2 to 5 per cent of patients.

THERAPY

Systemic. Cutaneous leishmanial lesions respond to pentavalent antimonials and antimalarials. Stibogluconate sodium and antimony meglumine† are antimonials that are effective in patients with multiple lesions. Antimony meglumine† is administered intramuscularly in daily doses of 60 to 100 mg/kg for 10 to 12 days. These injections may be repeated after an interval of 1 to 2 weeks until the lesion is cured (30 to 40 days). For acute cutaneous leishmaniasis, cycloguanil pamoate administered as a single intramuscular injection of 5 to 6 mg/kg is preferred. Intralesional injection of chloroquine* has also benefited selected patients. In chronic cutaneous leishmaniasis, cryotherapy should be combined with antimonials. Although cryotherapy is destructive, liquid nitrogen or carbon dioxide is very effective in treating localized lesions and results in cosmetically accepted scars.

Amphotericin B may be used, although its effect has been limited to cutaneous leishmaniasis caused by *L. braziliensis*. A slow intravenous drip of 50 mg of amphotericin B in 500 ml may be given over 3 to 4 hours, up to a total of 1.8 gm.

Imidazoles, such as ketoconazole,‡ have been experimentally tried in *L. tropica*-infected macrophage systems with successful elimination of 80 to 95 per cent of the parasites.

Since bacterial infection is a complicating factor in many patients, topical and systemic antibiotics may be necessary.

Surgical. Surgical excision of lesions is not recommended for routine use, but could be used for early, small, single lesions.

PRECAUTIONS

The therapeutic regimens in use for cutaneous leishmaniasis are not ideal. The antimonials are toxic chemicals, and their effects are cumulative. Toxic effects may include headaches, fainting, muscle and joint pains, reversible electrocardiographic changes, and anaphylactic reactions. Antimonials should be avoided in patients with myocarditis, hepatitis, and nephritis. Injection of cycloguanil pamoate is painful, but otherwise this drug is not toxic. If amphotericin B is administered, kidney function should be closely monitored.

COMMENTS

Unfortunately, there is no proven effective treatment for cutaneous leishmaniasis; all treatment should be considered experimental. Uncomplicated acute cutaneous leishmaniasis may best be managed by utilizing the treatment with the least side effects. However, aggressive treatment may be desired in particularly refractory patients or when cosmetic considerations would seem to indicate therapy. Secondary bacterial infection should always be treated if present.

References

Berman JD: Activity of imidazoles against *Leishmania tropica* in human macrophage cultures. Am J Trop Med Hyg *30*:566–569, 1981.
Chu FC, Rodrigues MM, Cogan DG, Neva FA: Leishmaniasis affecting the eyelids. Arch Ophthalmol *101*:84–91, 1983.
Duke-Elder S (ed): System of Ophthalmology. St. Louis, CV Mosby, 1976, Vol XV, pp 85–86.
Farah FS: Protozoan and helminth infections. *In* Fitzpatrick TB, et al (eds): Dermatology in General Medicine. Textbook and Atlas, 2nd ed. New York, McGraw-Hill, 1979, pp 1638–1656.
Farah FS: Leishmaniasis. *In* Demis DJ et al: Clinical Dermatology. Hagerstown, MD, Harper & Row, 1980, pp 1–21.
Francois J, et al: Ocular manifestations of leishmaniasis. Ann Oculist *206*:295–305, 1973
Guerra R, Tosi P, Molinelli G: Leishmaniasis of the lid in Tuscany. Ophthalmologica *168*:193–196, 1974.

CYSTICERCOSIS

HARVEY W. TOPILOW, M.D.
New York, New York

Humans may serve as either the definitive host of the adult pork tapeworm (Cestoda), *Taenia solium*, or the intermediate host, harboring the larval form, *Cysticercus cellulosae*. Taenia solium is endemic in India, South America, Africa, and Asia.

Gravid proglottid segments of the adult worm release eggs in the stool, which are then ingested by the usual intermediate host, the hog. In the hog's intestine, the cestode embryo is released from the egg, penetrates into vascular channels, and is carried to all parts of the body, predominantly to striated muscle. Once the embryo lodges in a small vessel, it transforms into the encysted cysticercus or larval stage. Humans become infected by eating undercooked pork containing viable cysticerci, which mature in the human intestine to the adult worm.

Humans may also ingest the ova either via reverse peristalsis if the adult worm inhabits the intestine or, more commonly, by eating food or water contaminated with cestode ova, thus becoming an intermediate host. Just as in the hog model, the embryo released from the ingested ova penetrates the bowel wall vasculature to embolize throughout the human host, encyst, and develop as cysticerci or "bladder worms". This systemic infestation with the larval organism constitutes cysticercosis.

Cysticerci are commonly found in the brain, muscle, skin, and the eye. They may cause muscular pain and fever and may mimic meningoencephalitis or brain tumor.

Ocular involvement occurs in half of affected patients. Bilateral ocular involvement and multifocal uniocular involvement are extremely rare. The most common intraocular locations for cysticerci are the subretinal space or the vitreous. There are numerous reports of cysticerci invading the anterior chamber, subconjunctival space, orbit, and the eyelids. Optic atrophy due to prolonged papilledema from central nervous system cysticercosis has also been reported.

The embryo reaches the choroid via the posterior ciliary arteries, causing alteration of the overlying pigment epithelium as the cyst develops. Formation of a large cyst in the subretinal space often produces an exudative retinal detachment. Perforation of the retina by the cysticercus results in a free-floating intravitreous cyst. If the inflammatory response in the retinal pigment epithelium is adequate, the small retinal tear created by the entrance of the cyst into the vitreous is sealed, and an atrophic chorioretinal scar results. If the retinal break is larger and remains open, a rhegmatogenous retinal detachment can then occur.

THERAPY

Surgical. The most effective recognized means for preserving function in an eye with subretinal or intravitreous cysticerci is surgical removal of the larva. Severe inflammation caused by toxic products from the dead larva destroys the eye in 80 per cent of cases in which the cyst is not removed. Therefore, every attempt should be made to remove a subretinal or intravitreous cysticercus.

Intravitreous cysticercosis is best treated by removing the parasite using a vitrectomy instrument via the pars plana. This technique provides excellent visualization of the larva by using a precorneal contact lens, operating microscope, and endoillumination. It makes lens extraction, which is required in open-sky vitrectomy, unnecessary. The cyst is soft and pliable and is readily sucked into the cutting port. The specific instrumentation used is not critical as any of the currently available vitrectomy units are adequate. In some designs the suction-cutter and endoillumination and irrigation capabilities are on the same probe, thereby requiring only a single sclerotomy. Others require three separate sclerotomies to accommodate separate probes for suction-cutting, endoillumination, and an infusion cannula. The only advantage of the latter design relates to the fact that the cysticercus is often "photophobic," scurrying away from such sources of bright light as the endoillumination probe. If the endoilluminator and suction-cutter are contained on the same probe, it is often necessary to chase the parasite through the vitreous as it flees from the endoilluminator light. If the light and suction-cutter are separate, it may be

106 / CYSTICERCOSIS

easier to guide the parasite toward the suction-cutter for removal.

A subtotal vitrectomy is performed to remove any toxic products released from the cyst, and a periocular corticosteroid injection is given at the conclusion of surgery. Postoperatively, the mild vitreous inflammation often seen is usually well controlled by topical corticosteroids and mydriatics.

Subretinal cysticercosis is best managed by first carefully localizing the parasite with indirect ophthalmoscopy and scleral depression. A transilluminating diathermy probe is useful in localization. The exact position of the parasite is outlined on the sclera with a marking pen. A lamellar scleral dissection is performed over the cyst, and the scleral bed is treated with diathermy to produce a firm retinal-retinal pigment epithelial adhesion once the retinal is reattached. A radial sclerotomy is performed over the center of the cyst. The exposed choroid is treated with diathermy using confluent applications of low intensity and long duration to coagulate small blood vessels and minimize bleeding.

Transillumination of the sclerotomy site is used to identify patent choroidal vessels that require additional diathermy. It is also used to verify that the cysticercus has not moved. The knuckle of exposed choroid is incised, and the cyst is extruded from the eye by maintaining gentle pressure on the globe. A solid silicone implant is placed within the scleral bed beneath scleral flaps with an encircling band to create a permanent buckling effect and to close any retinal breaks created by the parasite or surgical manipulation.

In certain cases, a posteriorly located subretinal cyst containing a dead parasite may be collapsed and fibrosed to such a degree that it cannot be removed. In such cases, vitreous traction on the retina overlying the cyst can be successfully relieved by a localized buckling procedure. Systemic, periocular*, and topical corticosteroids may be required to control the intraocular inflammation resulting from the dead retained parasite.

Ocular or Periocular Manifestations

Optic Nerve: Atrophy; papilledema.
Retina: Break; chorioretinal scar; exudative or rhegmatogenous retinal detachment.
Other: Cysticerci present almost anywhere in or around the eye; ocular pain; uveitis.

PRECAUTIONS

The gravity of cysticercosis is reflected by the 40 per cent mortality of patients with central nervous system involvement and the fact that in certain underdeveloped nations 2 to 4 per cent of all autopsies reveal cysticercosis as the cause of death. Therefore, once the infection is diagnosed, it is of utmost importance to begin an exhaustive search for the organisms in the central nervous system. In addition, careful fecal examination of the patient and the family members should be undertaken to determine whether the patient harbors the adult cestode or has been infected by a family member.

COMMENTS

Intraocular cysticercosis usually results in blindness unless the parasite is surgically removed from the eye. While the cysticercus is alive, it induces a mild to moderate inflammatory response. A violent inflammatory reaction ensues when the parasite dies, often resulting in destruction of the globe.

References

Bartholomew RS: Subretinal cysticercosis. Am J Ophthalmol 79:670–673, 1975.
Hutton WL, Vaiser A, Snyder WB: pars plana vitrectomy for removal of intravitreous cysticercus. Am J Ophthalmol 81:571–573, 1976.
Kapoor S, Kapoor MS: Ocular cysticercosis. J Pediatr Ophthalmol Strabismus 15:170–172, 1978.
Messner KH, Kammerer WS: Intraocular cysticercosis. Arch Ophthalmol 97:1103–1105, 1979.
Perry HD, Font RL: Cysticercosis of the eyelid. Arch Ophthalmol 96:1255–1257, 1978.
Santos R, et al: Management of subretinal and vitreous cysticercosis: Role of photocoagulation and surgery. Ophthalmology 86:1501–1504, 1979.
Shea M, et al: Intraocular *Taenia crassiceps* (Cestoda). Trans. Am Acad Ophthalmol Otolaryngol 77:778–783, 1973.
Topilow HW, et al: Bilateral multifocal intraocular cysticercosis. Ophthalmology 88:1166–1172, 1981.
Wood TR, Binder PS: Intravitreal and intracameral cysticercosis. Ann Ophthalmol 11:1033–1036, 1979.
Zinn KM, Guillory SL, Friedman AH: Removal of intravitreous cysticerci from the surface of the optic nervehead. A pars plana approach. Arch Ophthalmol 98:714–716, 1980.

DEMODICOSIS

FRANK P. ENGLISH, F.R.A.C.O., F.R.C.S.
Brisbane, Australia

Demodectic infestation of *Homo sapiens* is characterized by the presence of two congeric species on the same host: *Demodex folliculorum*, which is found in the hair and eyelash follicles, and *D. brevis*, which infests the meibomian and sebaceous glands. These metazoans are virtually ubiquitous in the adult population and are predominantly located in the facial area, involving the eyelids, eyebrows, forehead, and nasal region. All phases of their development can be seen, including the immature and mature stages.

D. folliculorum lies in the hair follicle with its head downward and feet facing the epithelial surface. Its sharp chelicerae puncture epithelial cells, allowing evacuation of the cytoplasm by the parasite. Later, its trifid claws shred these damaged cells; this contributes to the bulk of characteristic cuffing seen in this condition.

D. brevis consumes glandular cells in its particular locus. In heavy infestation, it may affect the lipid layer of the tear film coacervate.

Patients complain of itching and burning of the eyelids, with crusting and loss of lashes. This pruritus is episodic and may parallel the activity of the mite in oviposition. Normally, the parasite's existence is torpid; however, in oviposition there is a bout of frenetic activity lasting several hours. This mite may cause a granuloma of the eyelid that is characterized by pain and swelling of tissue.

Many crumpled dead parasites are observed often unwittingly by the ophthalmologist in the daily office routine. They are located in cellular debris on the lid margin and sometimes straddling the cilia. In effect, the observer is scanning a graveyard of mites. These parasites can be observed when the lid is scrubbed with a moist cotton-wool applicator that is soaked in a droplet of saline on a slide and examined with light microscopy.

Demodectic mites undergo two moulting periods in development, and the cast exoskeletons of immature specimens are also seen with the high magnification. The observer is rewarded with an exquisite view of the exoskeleton of the acarid and is able to identify with clarity the body contours and even ruptures in the integument at the time of ecdysis.

THERAPY

Ocular. Assessment of the degree of infestation is mandatory. With high magnification, experienced observers can often identify mites lying in the mouths of follicles. Generally, however, diagnosis is established by examination of epilated lashes with light microscopy.

In heavy infestation, mite nests occur. These conglomerates resemble cuffing, but contain many eggs and parasites in all stages of development. It is important to recognize and remove these colonies that act as a reservoir of infestation.

Although it has been traditional to treat the eyelid margin with an ether scrub, only partial evacuation from follicles occurs and the application needs to be repeated. Ether cleanses the eyelid, but has little effect on this acarid. A suitable substitute for ether is saline. After a drop of anesthetic has been applied to the eye, a saturated cotton-wool applicator is used to cleanse the eyelashes and dislodge nests. This maneuver is less dangerous than ether therapy. Following this procedure, a course of sulfacetamide or neomycin/polymyxin B/bacitracin ophthalmic ointment is applied at nighttime for a few weeks. This reduces concomitant bacterial infection and slows down the migration of parasites. The life cycle is believed to be longer than previously estimated, and it may be necessary to prolong therapy in recalcitrant cases. Patients are prone to recurrence, as it is impossible to eradicate the mite completely. Cryotherapy on isolated mites offers promise, but the real answer will be found in the development of an affective acaricide. Recently an effective agent against the house dust mite has been developed in Australia by Allersearch. The formula contains an alcohol based benzyltannate complex. I have found this substance also destroys Demodectic mites and clinical trial studies are warranted. Tarsal massage is valuable in reducing the population of *D. brevis*, especially when there has been a history of recurrent meibomianitis.

Ocular or Periocular Manifestations

Conjunctiva: Erythema.
Eyebrows or Eyelids: Blepharitis; cuffing; follicular distension and hyperplasia; hyperemia; hyperkeratinization; madarosis; meibomian gland destruction; mite colonies; granuloma; exoskeleton of dead parasites; acarid exuviae; eyelid tumor.
Other: Pruritus.

PRECAUTIONS

Extreme care is necessary in ether application to the lid margin to avoid spillage onto the cornea. The amount of ether necessary to kill an isolated mite is staggering, and realistically, there cannot be a clinical parallel.

In the general management of demodicosis, it is important not to induce the state of symbiophobia. This condition is an entity that is causing increasing concern among dermatologists. It can manifest itself in such bizarre behavior as sleeping with the lights on to avoid nocturnal migration or bathing regularly in a bath filled with gasoline!

COMMENTS

Demodicosis is associated with specific pathology of the eyelids. There is also a potential bacterial vector role. This allows passage of bacteria from the depths of the follicle to the integumentary surface. *D. brevis* may penetrate the dermis with resultant inflammation, producing a granuloma.

A recent study of the feeding habits of these mites raises the suspicion of a viral vector role. This could be particularly significant, especially for the smaller acarid.

References

Ayres S Jr, Ayres S III: Demodectic eruptions (demodicidosis) in the human. Arch Dermatol 83:816–827, 1961.
Coston TO: *Demodex folliculorum* blepharitis. Trans Am Ophthalmol Soc 65:361–392, 1967.
Duke-Elder S (ed): System of Ophthalmology. St. Louis, CV Mosby, 1974, Vol XIII, p 228.
English FP, Nutting WB: Demodicosis of ophthalmic concern. Am J Ophthalmol 91:362–372, 1981.
English FP, Nutting WB: Feeding characteristics in

demodectic mites of the eyelid. Aust J Ophthalmol 9:311–313, 1981.

English FP, Nutting WB: Eyelid mite nests. Aust J Ophthalmol 10:187–189, 1982.

English FP, Cohn D, Groeneveld ER: Demodectic mites and chalazion. Am J Ophthalmol 100:482–483, 1985.

Norn MS: Demodex folliculorum. Incidence, regional distribution, pathogenicity. Dan Med Bull 18:14–17, 1971.

DIROFILARIASIS

LAWRENCE A. RAYMOND, M.D.,
Cincinnati, Ohio

and YEZID GUTIERREZ, M.D., Ph.D.
Cleveland, Ohio

Dirofilariasis is a zoonotic infection caused by several species of Dirofilaria, nematodes that naturally parasitize animals. Their life cycles are complicated. The adults produce microfilariae that circulate in blood. The microfilariae are ingested by mosquitoes wherein they progress to an infective stage. Infective larvae gain access to the new host through the skin, and development starts. There are at least three Dirofilaria species known to occur in the human eye or periocular tissues, but many other filaroids of humans and animals can be found in these locations. Most Dirofilaria infections are in the subcutaneous tissues, usually presenting as painless nodules. When the parasite dies, there is an inflammatory reaction with marked polymorphonuclear cell infiltrate, mostly eosinophils. At this stage, the nodule becomes painful, and the patient may consult the physician.

The incidence of Dirofilaria infections in humans is low; a disproportionate number of cases affecting the eye or periorbital tissues are reported, but the location in the eye or near the eye may cause patients to consult a physician more often. When the parasite is in the conjunctiva or anterior chamber, the patient may see it and seek consultation. If it is in the vitreous or retina, the patient may note a moving shadow. In either case, Dirofilaria and other filarial parasites should be considered in the differential diagnosis. When the parasite is in a nodule, the diagnosis is made by the pathologist examining the specimen removed from the patient.

Species of Dirofilaria found in ocular and periocular tissues are D. repens, D. tenuis, and D. immitis. D. repens, occurring naturally in the subcutaneous tissues of dogs, foxes, and cats in Europe, Africa, the USSR, and Asia, has been referred to as D. conjunctivae when present in humans. D. tenuis, a parasite of the subcutaneous tissues of the raccoon in the southeastern United States, also was referred to as D. conjunctivae until 1965 when its true nature was demonstrated. Both D. repens and D. tenuis are responsible for infections in the conjunctiva, the eyelid,

and rarely the lacrimal canal. These parasitic infections usually present as a nodule, or rarely, the nematode is detected before it encapsulates. D. immitis, a cosmopolitan parasite of the right ventricle and pulmonary arteries of dogs, has an early developmental phase in the subcutaneous tissues. Most infections with D. immitis in humans occur in the lungs where they produce small infarct-like lesions, but the parasite has been recovered from the anterior chamber of the eye on at least two occasions in Australia and from the posterior chamber once in Malaysia. In the United States, a parasite that was morphologically indistinguishable from D. immitis and D. lutrae has been recovered from the orbit at least twice.

In endemic areas of human filarial infections other than from Dirofilaria, such as Brugia malayi and Wuchereria bancrofti, the parasites have been found often in the eye. In the United States, a Dipetalonema arbuta-like worm in pleural and peritoneal cavities of the porcupine has been removed from the anterior chamber of a human eye.

THERAPY

Surgical. If the nematode is migrating in the retina area outside of the macular area, photocoagulation may be used. The purposes of photocoagulation are to prevent damage of the retinal pigment epithelium by Dirofilaria and to avoid migration of the parasite into the optic nerve, macula, or vitreous with resultant uveitis.

Surgical excision of the inflammatory nodule containing the parasite in the eyelid, periorbital region, or subconjunctival area is the treatment of choice. Surgical removal of the living intraocular Dirofilaria from the anterior chamber or vitreous preserves eyesight and decreases the associated uveitis.

Ocular or Periocular Manifestations

Anterior Chamber: Cells and flare; free nematode present.

Conjunctiva: Chemosis; hyperemia; nodules; nonencapsulated parasite beneath bulbar conjunctiva.

Extraocular Muscles: Tenonitis.

Eyelids or Eyebrows: Nodules.

Orbit: Inflammatory pseudotumor; pain; proptosis.

Retina: Macular degeneration; migrating nematode; unilateral pseudoretinitis pigmentosa.

Sclera: Nodules.

Vitreous: Free nematode present.

Other: Diplopia; irritation; itching; lacrimation; lowered amplitudes on electroretinogram; uveitis; visual loss.

PRECAUTIONS

Because the patient is infected with only a single nematode, systemic treatment with diethylcarbamazine is usually not indicated. If diethylcarbamazine is administered to these patients with intraocular location of a living parasite, allergic responses may occur after the death of the nematode. These reactions may include urticaria, fever, gastrointestinal disturbance, and lymphadenitis. Corticosteroids need to be given with caution in patients with secondary bacterial infection.

COMMENTS

Dirofilaria can incite inflammatory reactions in ocular tissues. When the parasite is located within the conjunctiva, eyelid, anterior chamber, or vitreous and can be removed, symptomatic inflammation is relieved. Also, retrieval of the parasite allows for identification of the species. When a filarial worm is migrating in the retina away from the macula, photocoagulation is the treatment of choice.

References

Beaver PC: Intraocular filariasis: A brief review. Am J Trop Med Hyg. *40:*40–45, 1989.
Font RL, Neafie RC, Perry HD: Subcutaneous dirofilariasis of the eyelid and ocular adnexa. Report of six cases. Arch Ophthalmol 98:1079–1082, 1980.
Guterbock WM, Vestre WA, Tood KS Jr: Ocular dirofilariasis in the dog. Mod Vet Pract 62:45–47, 1981.
Moorhouse DE: *Dirofilaria immitis:* A cause of human intra-ocular infection. Infection 6:192–193, 1978.
Orsoni JG, Coggiola G, Minazzi P: Filaria conjunctivae. Ophthalmologica *190:*243–246, 1985.
Raymond LA, et al: Living retinal nematode (filariallike) destroyed with photocoagulation. Ophthalmology 85:944–949, 1978.
Skrjabin KL: Invasions a filariides chez l'homme en l'URSS. Med Parasitol Parasite Dis 9:119–127, 1940.
Thomas D, et al: The *Dirofilaria* parasite in the orbit. Am J Ophthalmol 82:931–933, 1976.
Vodovozov AM, Jarulin GR, Djakonowa SW: *Dirofilaria* im Glaskörper des Menschen. Ophthalmologica *166:*88–93, 1973.

DRACUNCULIASIS
(Dracontiasis, Dracunculosis, Guinea Worm Infection)
RALPH MULLER, Ph.D.
St. Albans, England

Dracunculiasis is an infection of connective and subcutaneous tissues by the nematode, *Dracunculus medinensis.* Clinical effects are produced primarily by the gravid female when she discharges her larvae near the skin surface, usually on the extremities. There are symptoms of local itching, urticaria, and burning pain at the site of a small blister. As the blister bursts, the anterior end of the nematode gradually appears through the ulcerated skin. Secondary infection is common, and invasion of the deeper tissues is a rare complication. These complications may include tetanus, septicemia, arthritis, paraplegia, constrictive pericarditis, or urogenital involvement. Ocular manifestations in dracunculiasis are uncommon, but can include allergic reactions, such as intense eyelid edema and conjunctival hyperemia. The parasite may also be found in the tissues of the eyelid or subconjunctiva, or very rarely, it may localize behind the globe.

THERAPY

Systemic. Several drugs have recently been found to be effective in facilitating expulsion or removal of worms, rapid resolution of symptoms, and healing of ulcers. These drugs include niridazole, thiabendazole, and metronidazole. Niridazole is given orally in a dosage of 25 mg/kg daily for 7 days, and the dosage is normally divided. Thiabendazole should be given orally in a dosage of 25 mg/kg twice daily for 2 days. Metronidazole may be used as an alternative drug and is administered orally in a dosage of 250 mg three times daily for 10 days. Although it is unlikely that any of these drugs will have direct antiparasitic activity, they do reduce tissue reaction.

Supportive. Bedrest is indicated, with the affected part being elevated. Strict hygienic measures should be observed; the ulcer should be kept clean, and secondary infection should be controlled with antibiotics. Guinea worms that have emerged through an ulcer may be wound gradually around a small stick and thus removed over a period of about 1 month. Sterile dressings and acriflavine cream should be applied daily during this procedure in order to prevent secondary infection.

Surgical. Surgical extraction of the worm is recommended only when the worm can be palpated subcutaneously, but has not yet emerged through the skin. Worms should be carefully removed intact; otherwise, severe cellulitis may result.

Abscesses caused by worms bursting in the tissues or secondary infection may be incised and aspirated, if necessary. True guinea worm abscesses caused by the gravid female's expulsion of larvae may require incision, evacuation, and primary closure of the abscess under antibiotic cover. Guinea worm cysts or calcified worms may be extracted by surgery, if necessary.

Ocular or Periocular Manifestations

Conjunctiva: Abscess; conjunctivitis; erythema; hyperemia; nematode present.
Eyelids: Abscess; edema; erythema; nematode present; nodules; urticaria.
Globe: Nematode present; proptosis.
Orbit: Nematode present.

PRECAUTIONS

Niridazole should be taken after meals to minimize gastric irritation. Metronidazole may cause abdominal discomfort and breathlessness. Some

110 / DRACUNCULIASIS

patients object to the bitter taste of the drug, so care should be taken to see that patients actually take it. Simultaneous administration of an antihistamine often blocks uncomfortable side effects.

Surgical extraction of the guinea worm may be very difficult, since the worm may lie very tortuously. Great care should be taken to see that the entire worm is removed intact because sepsis almost always results if the worm is broken and may lead to cellulitis, abscess formation, or septicemia.

COMMENTS

Dracunculiasis is primarily a disease of poverty, particularly in remote rural communities without sanitary supplies. The disease occurs most commonly in India, Pakistan, and Africa. Infection occurs through the ingestion of water containing infected *Cyclops*, the intermediate host of the parasite.

Dracunculiasis is not usually a serious disease, provided that complications do not ensue. However, because infection often occurs during the planting season, it can be economically important to poor rural communities. An international effort to control and finally eradicate this disease is being mounted.

References

Duke-Elder S (ed): System of Ophthalmology. St. Louis, CV Mosby, 1976, Vol XV, p 47.
Hopkins DR: Dracunculiasis eradication: A mid-decade status report. Am J Trop Med Hyg 37:115–118, 1987.
Kale OO: Clinical evaluation of drugs for dracontiasis. Trop Doct 7:15–16, 1977.
Muller R: Guinea worm disease: Epidemiology, control and treatment. Bull WHO 57:683–689, 1979.
Muller R: Pathology of experimental *Dracunculus* infection and its relevance to chemotherapy. *In* Soulsby EJL (ed): Pathophysiology of Parasitic Infections. New York, Academic Press, 1977, pp 133–148.
Solanes MP: Tropical diseases. *In* Dunlap EA (ed): Gordon's Medical Management of Ocular Disease, 2nd ed. Hagerstown, MD, Harper & Row, 1976, pp 290–304.

ECHINOCOCCOSIS
(Echinococciasis, Hydatid Cyst Hydatidosis)

F.T. FRAUNFELDER, M.D.
Portland, Oregon

Echinococcosis is a tissue infection of humans caused by the larval stage of *Echinococcus granulosus, E. vogeli, E. orligarthrus,* or *E. multilocularis.* The natural habitat of *E. granulosus* is most commonly the intestine of a dog. The human is an intermediate host who is infected by ingestion of food containing the eggs of the organism. The ovum hatches in the intestinal tract, and the embryo penetrates the intestinal wall to enter the portal circulation. The life cycle of *E. multilocularis* is similar, except that small rodents serve as the natural intermediate hosts, and the hydatid cyst is always of the alveolar type.

The liver is the most common site for this disorder. In 5 to 10 per cent of cases, the organisms become entrapped in the pulmonary circulation, forming lung cysts. Rarely, the larvae escape the previous two barriers and enter the circulation of the left side of the heart to be distributed to the other body systems—the brain and kidney being the most common.

Although subretinal, vitreous, and anterior chamber hydatid cysts have been reported, the orbit is the primary ophthalmologic location. One to 2 per cent of the cases of human echinococcosis have an orbital location. Inside the orbital, hydatid cysts tend to be located superiorly, and some may erode the orbital roof and become intracranial. Hydatid cysts of the orbit tend to occur most often in persons under 30 years of age. Although there is evidence that infected individuals may not manifest systemic symptoms for long periods of time, this is not usually the case in orbital hydatidosis, where even small cysts can cause serious complications. The ocular history is relatively short, from 1 to 12 months, and is characterized by unilateral, progressive, nonpulsating, firm exophthalmos. Chemosis, lid edema, and orbital cellulitis may develop as a consequence of rupture or secondary infection. Other findings may include mechanical restriction of ocular motion (which may reach total ophthalmoplegia), visual impairment, papilledema or papillitis, retinal striae, and exposure keratitis due to extensive proptosis.

THERAPY

Systemic. There is no established medical therapy. Experimentally, prolonged administration of mebendazole[‡] has been shown to be larvicidal, but this treatment cannot be recommended until more information becomes available. Mebendazole has been given in daily oral doses of 200 mg for the first 3 or 4 days. If no idiosyncratic reactions are encountered, the daily dosage may be increased to 3 or 4 gm for a period of at least 30 days. BCG vaccine[‡] administration has been shown effective in suppressing the growth and metastasis of experimental *E. multilocularis* infections, raising the possibility that effective immunotherapeutic modalities may be available in the future.

Surgical. The major treatment of this lesion is surgical excision of the cyst. The cyst is surgically exposed through a transconjunctival or transpalpebral approach for the anterior cysts, a lateral orbitotomy for the lateral ones, or a Dandy superior orbitotomy after frontal craniectomy for the most frequently encountered cases involving a superior or medial position. Except for the small cysts that can be removed entirely, the usual technique is to puncture the cyst and aspirate the hydatid fluid. Subsequently, the fluid of the cyst is replaced with either 1 per cent formaldehyde in saline or 70 per cent alcohol and left in place for 5 minutes prior to surgical excision of the membrane.

Ocular or Periocular Manifestations

Conjunctiva: Chemosis; conjunctivitis; granuloma; hydatid cysts.
Cornea: Abscess; keratitis.
Eyelids: Edema; granuloma; hydatid cysts; ptosis; widening or asymmetry of palpebral fissure.
Globe: Exophthalmos; pain; phthisis bulbi; proptosis.
Lacrimal System: Hydatid cysts in the lacrimal gland.
Optic Nerve: Atrophy; optic neuritis; papilledema.
Orbit: Abscess; hydatid cysts; erosion of bony walls.
Retina: Hydatid cysts; detachment; hemorrhages.
Vitreous: Hydatid cysts; opacity.
Other: Cataract; disturbances of conjugate movement; hypopyon; ocular pain; secondary glaucoma; visual loss.

PRECAUTIONS

Surgical removal of the cysts must be done with great care so that multiple scolices (hydatid sand) are not scattered into adjacent tissue. Sterilization of the cyst with formaldehyde or alcohol may prevent additional seeding in the event of accidental rupture of the cyst. Accidental rupture of the cyst may produce a severe inflammatory reaction that is responsive to systemic corticosteroid treatment.

COMMENTS

Environmental control measures have been shown to reduce the incidence of echinococcosis. Contact with infected dogs, particularly fecal contamination of hands and food, should be avoided. Infected carcasses should be burned or buried in order to prevent access by animals to material containing scolices. Dogs should also be treated if found to be infected with this organism.

References

Agarwal MB, et al: Splenic and orbital hydatid cysts and treatment with mebendazole. (A case report). J Postgrad Med 28:115–117, 1982.
Apple DJ, et al: Orbital hydatid cyst. J Pediatr Ophthalmol Strabismus 17:380–383, 1980.
Awan KJ: Orbital echinococcosis. Pakistan J Ophthalmol 3:3–4, 1987.
Crompton JL, et al: Hydatid cyst: An unusual cause of diplopia. Aust NZ J Ophthalmol 13:195–203, 1985.
Morales AG, et al: Hydatid cysts of the orbit: A review of 35 cases. Ophthalmology 95:1027–1032, 1988.
Shah A, et al: Hydatid cyst of the orbit (A case report). J Postgrad Med 34:43–44A, 1988.
Sheikh SA, Akram M, Javaid I: Hydatid disease of the orbit in Pakistan. Pakistan J Ophthalmol 3:5–8, 1987.
Williams DF et al: Intraocular *Echinococcus multilocularis.* Arch Ophthalmol 105:1106–1109, 1987.

LOIASIS
(African *Loa loa* Eye-Worm Disease)
JAMES M. BARNETT, M.D.
Muskegon, Michigan

Loiasis is a chronic parasitic infection caused by the filariae *Loa loa*. The larva stage of the *L. loa* worm is transferred to humans by bites of the female deer fly of the genus *Chrysops*. The larva eggs hatch into the human subcutaneous or lymph tissues and develop into microfilariae. These microfilariae migrate into the bloodstream via the lymphatics. The microfilariae can be picked up in the bite of another deer fly, and thus, the circle is complete. Infection may be asymptomatic; however, the most common clinical manifestations are "calabar swellings." These transient swellings are areas of localized subcutaneous edema. They may occur anywhere, but are especially common around medium-sized joints and areas exposed to trauma, such as legs, hands, and orbits. The onset of the lesion is often heralded by local pain and itching. An edematous, nonerythematous swelling 10 to 20 cm in diameter then develops, lasts for several days, and slowly subsides. These swellings recur irregularly either at the same site or in various locations.

The adult worm occasionally migrates under the skin, producing a prickly, crawling sensation. Periocular skin and subconjunctiva are common sites. When the worm passes under the conjunctiva, it may be directly visualized. Often, males will follow a female on her subcutaneous or subconjunctival path. The worms produce an edematous conjunctivitis that may last for several days.

THERAPY

Systemic. Diethylcarbamazine is the drug of choice and is effective against the parasite in all stages of development. The oral dosage in adults and children is 2 mg/kg three times a day after meals for 14 to 21 days. The dosage may be increased to 6 mg/kg if the above dosage fails to eliminate the parasite.

Surgical. Surgical extraction of the worm is advised when it appears superficially in the periocular skin or conjunctiva. Worms typically move directly under the bulbar conjunctiva where they can be seen. A drop of 0.59 per cent proparacaine hydrochloride is used to anesthetize the conjunctiva. The worm is grasped through the conjunctiva with a forcep and held firmly while a suture is placed through the conjunctiva and around the worm and tied in place. Finally, the conjunctiva is buttonholed, and the worm is extracted. Female adult worms measure about 60 mm, whereas males are 30 mm in length.

Ocular or Periocular Manifestations

Conjunctiva: Conjunctivitis; parasites present.
Eyelids: Edema.
Other: Lacrimation.

PRECAUTIONS

Adverse reactions can occur with the administration of diethylcarbamizine in loiasis. These reactions may include headache, dizziness, nausea, and fever. Destruction of the microfilariae may cause serious allergic reactions manifested by severe pedal edema, intense itching, dermatitis, fever, colic, and lymphadenitis. Rarely, an allergic encephalitis reaction has occurred in patients treated with this drug for loiasis. The concomitant administration of antihistamines or corticosteroids is advisable to minimize allergic reactions. If reactions are severe, the dosage of diethylcarbamazine should be reduced or treatment interrupted.

COMMENTS

Loiasis is endemic in western and central Africa. Most cases diagnosed in the United States are in people who have resided in these endemic areas. The infections can last in certain individuals for as long as 30 years. It is necessary that ophthalmologists be aware of loiasis, particularly in this age of global travel. It has been shown that loiasis can be prevented with the use of 5 mg/kg of diethylcarbamazine for 3 days each month while exposure lasts.

The American deer fly, *C. atlanticus* (which is endemic in the Mississippi Gulf Coast), has been shown experimentally to maintain the *Loa loa* parasite in an infective state. Large numbers of infective larvae were commonly recovered from experimentally infected flies. Therefore, *C. atlanticus* could theoretically transmit *Loa loa* from human to human within the United States.

The prognosis of loiasis is good with treatment. Without treatment, loiasis is annoying and uncomfortable but rarely life endangering. Penetration of the worms into the eye is rare, and generally there are no serious sequelae to the subconjunctival parasite.

References

AMA Drug Evaluations, 4th ed. New York, John Wiley & Sons, 1980, pp 1416–1417.

Barnett JM, Wolter JR: *Loa Loa:* The African eye worm observed in Michigan. J Pediatr Ophthalmol 8:23–25, 1971.
Duke-Elder S (ed): System of Ophthalmology. St. Louis, CV Mosby, 1965, Vol VIII, pp 402–405.
Farrer WE, Wittner M, Tanowitz HB: African eye worm (*Loa loa*) in a tourist. Ann Ophthalmol 13:1177–1179, 1981.
Gibbs RD: Loiasis: Reports of three cases and literature review. J Natl Med Assoc 71:853–854, 1979.
Jaccard A, Lortholary O, Visser H: Diethylcarbamazine and human loiasis (letter). N Engl J Med 5:320, 1989.
Kazacos KR, Smith LE Jr: Loiasis (*Loa loa*) in an African student in Indiana. Am J Trop Med Hyg 28:213–215, 1979.
Nutman TB, Miller KO, Mulligan M, Reinhardt GN, Currie BJ, Steel C, Ottese, EA: Diethylcarbamazine prophylaxis for human loiasis. Results of a double-blind study. N Engl J Med 319:752–756, 1988.
Olness K, Franciosi RA, Johnson MM, Freedman DO: Loiasis in an expatriate American child: Diagnostic and treatment difficulties. Pediatrics 80:943–946, 1987.
Rollo IM: Drugs used in the chemotherapy of helminthiasis. In Gilman AG, Goodman LS, Gilman A (eds): The Pharmacological Basis of Therapeutics, 6th ed. New York, Macmillan, 1980, pp 1015–1016.
Sacks HN, Williams DN, Eifrig DE: Loiasis. Report of a case and review of the literature. Arch Intern Med 136:914–915, 1976.

MALARIA
THOMAS E. RUNYAN, M.D., F.A.C.S.
Temple, Texas

Malaria is an acute, sometimes severe, and often chronic protozoan infection. It remains the major infectious disease in the world. Four types of malarial parasites, each having a different biologic pattern, may affect humans: *Plasmodium vitax, P falciparum, P. malariae,* and *P. ovale.*

Malaria often begins with nonspecific malaise, which is followed shortly by a characteristic shaking chill and rapidly rising temperature that are usually accompanied by headache and nausea; the initial episode ends with profuse sweating. After a fever-free interval, the cycle of chills, fever, and sweating is repeated either daily (*P. falciparum*, 36 to 48 hours), every other day (*P. vivax* and *P. ovale*, 48 hours), or every third day (*P. malariae,* 72 hours). Duration of an untreated primary attack varies from a week to a month or longer. Relapses are common in all forms, except *P. falciparum* malaria, and may occur at irregular intervals for several years. *P. falciparum* malaria is also known as pernicious, subtertian, malignant, and estivoautumnal malaria and is the most severe form. Malarial infection occurs in humans (primary host) through the bite of an infected *Anopheles* mosquito (secondary host), transfusion of blood from an infected donor, or use of a common syringe by drug addicts. *P. falciparum* malaria cannot be transmitted by the latter two modes. Chemotherapeutic agents and insecticides have made autochthonous malaria rare in the United States and in many other parts of the world, but visitors from malarious areas may introduce the infection. Returning armed forces personnel have caused small sporadic epidemics.

THERAPY

Systemic. Malaria is treated by chemotherapeutic agents given systemically to suppress the disease, to manage an acute attack, or as curative therapy. Patients with malaria develop a gradual immunity that considerably modifies the clinical course, this immunity has a degree of strain specificity. Attempts to induce immunity by vaccines have failed. Suppressive therapy consists of 500 mg (300-mg base) of oral chloroquine administered once or twice weekly. This therapy protects travelers to malarious areas by suppressing the erythrocytic infection and, thus, the clinical manifestations of malaria. It is started 1 week prior to arrival in an endemic area and should be continued for 4 to 6 weeks after leaving the area, since its continued use results in parasitic eradication of sensitive strains of *P. falciparum*. In *P. vivax*, *P. ovale*, and *P. malariae*, 26.3 mg (15-mg base) of primaquine must be given daily for 14 days in conjunction with or following the discontinuance of chloroquine.

An acute attack of any type of malaria, except drug-resistant *P. falciparum* malaria, can be treated by chloroquine. The dose is 1 gm (600-mg base) of oral chloroquine, followed by 500 mg (300-mg base) in 6 hours and then 500 mg (300-mg base) daily for 2 days. The total dose is 2.5 gm (1.5-gm base). Comatose or vomiting patients may be given 250 to 375 mg (200 to 300-mg base) of intramuscular chloroquine every 6 hours. Oral therapy with chloroquine should be resumed as soon as possible.

Chloroquine-resistant strains of *P. falciparum* should be treated with a combination of quinine, pyrimethamine, and a sulfonamide given concurrently. Oral administration of 650 mg of quinine three times daily is continued for 10 days. If oral therapy is precluded, 600 mg of quinine may be diluted in 300 ml of normal saline and given intravenously over 1 hour. The dose may be repeated every 8 hours, but oral therapy should be restarted as soon as feasible. In cases with renal failure, the dose is limited to 600 mg once a day. Pyrimethamine is given orally in a dosage of 25 mg twice daily for 3 days. Sulfadiazine is administered orally in a dosage of 500 mg twice daily for 5 days.

Curative therapy for *P. falciparum* differs from that of the other three types of malaria. *P. falciparum* parasites do not have a persistent hepatic phase as do *P. vivax*, *P. ovale*, and *P. malariae*, and thus the disease is cured once the attack is adequately treated. In the latter three forms of malaria, the exoerythrocytic and erythrocytic parasites must be eradicated to prevent relapse. In over 80 percent of primary infections, administering 26.3 mg (15-mg base) of oral primaquine daily for 14 days accomplishes this by destruction of forms that persist in the liver. It may be given at the same time as chloroquine or later. A second course of primaquine may be given if relapse occurs. Gametocytes usually appear 2 or 3 days after onset of the erythrocytic phase and may persist for long periods, particularly in *P. falciparum* malaria. They do not produce symptoms, but indicate pre-existing infection and serve as a source of infection for the *Anopheles* mosquito. *P. vivax* and *P. malariae* gametocyte development can be prevented by suppression with chloroquine or by adequate and prompt treatment of the acute attack. *P. falciparum* gametocytes, once developed, are resistant to suppressive drugs, but are susceptible to 26.3 mg (15-mg base) of primaquine daily for 3 days or a single 45-mg base dose will sterilize the gametocyte.

Ocular. The most frequent ocular complication associated with malaria is herpes simplex keratitis, and appropriate topical management should be instituted. Iritis may also accompany an attack of malaria and is treated in a routine manner. Other ophthalmic abnormalities that occur with malaria generally resolve as the disease process subsides, with the exception of ischemic optic nerve lesions and large macular hemorrhages that may result in permanent sequelae.

Ocular or Periocular Manifestations

Choroid or Retina: Hemorrhages with or without edema (small peripheral, large central); vaso-occlusion.
Conjunctiva: Enlarged horizontally oriented conjunctival vessels in the intrapalpebral zones; icterus; pallor; petechiae; subconjunctival hemorrhages.
Cornea: Herpes simplex keratitis; herpes zoster keratitis; interstitial keratitis; nonherpetic keratitis; stromal opacification.
Extraocular Muscles: Paresis of third, fourth, or sixth nerve (transient).
Eyelids: Blepharitis; edema; herpes zoster involvement; neuralgia and hyperalgesia of various ocular sensory nerves (particularly the supraorbital and infraorbital nerves); ptosis.
Iris: Iridocyclitis; iritis.
Lens: Cataracts (rare).
Optic Nerve: Atrophy; hyperemia; papillary hemorrhages; papilledema; retrobulbar or optic neuritis.
Pupil: Anisocoria; reflex disturbances.
Vitreous: Hemorrhages; opacity.

Precautions

Chloroquine is the drug of choice in all types of malaria, except drug-resistant *P. falciparum* malaria. Side effects secondary to chloroquine may include corneal deposits and retinopathy. Infants and children are particularly susceptible to parenteral chloroquine overdosage, and severe reactions and deaths have been reported.

In chloroquine-resistant cases, quinine, pyrimethamine, and a sulfonamide are given concurrently. Quinine may cause tinnitus and occasionally drug fever or allergic purpura. Quinine also constricts the arterioles and thus may cause ischemic damage to the retinal and/or optic nerve. Blackwater fever, a rare complication characterized by intravascular hemolysis and hemoglobinuria, probably occurs exclusively in patients with chronic *P. falciparum* malaria, especially those treated with quinine. Pyrimethamine is a folate antagonist and may cause or accentuate an already present anemia. Primaquine may cause intravascular hemolysis in patients with G6PD deficiency, but this condition is infrequent and generally benign if the recommended therapeutic doses are given. Abdominal cramps and methemoglobinuria may also occur with primaquine.

COMMENTS

From an epidemiologic standpoint, malaria can be controlled with few exceptions by present chemotherapeutic agents and hygienic measures. The major proportion of ocular complications associated with malaria can be attributed to small vessel or capillary obstruction that produces ischemic sequelae in the central nervous system, orbit, or the eye itself. This is particularly true of *P. falciparum* malaria, which has a significant mortality rate if untreated.

Herpes simplex keratitis is probably the most common of all ocular complications seen in conjunction with malaria, but it is an associated disease process and not directly related to the pathophysiology of the malarial parasites. Other ocular problems, such as involvement of the optic nerve, anterior uvea, retina, and choroid, generally resolve with the subsidence of the malarial episode.

References

Bell RW: Ophthalmologic findings in malaria. Ann Ophthalmol 7:1439–1442, 1975.

Grant WM: Ocular complications of malaria. Arch Ophthalmol 35:48–54, 1946.

Looareesuwan S, Warrell DA, White NJ, Chanthavanich P, Warrell MJ, Chantaratherakitti S, Changswek S, Chongmankongcheep L, Kanchanaranya C: Retinal hemorrhage, a common sign of prognostic significance in cerebral malaria. Am J Trop Med Hyg 32:911–915, 1983.

Plorde JJ: Malaria. *In* Isselbacher KJ, et al (eds): Harrison's Principles of Internal Medicine, 9th ed. New York, McGraw-Hill, 1980, pp 867–873.

Poncet F: De la chorio-retinite palustre. Ann Oculist 79:201–218, 1878.

Ross JVM: Ocular complications associated with malaria. Eye Ear Nose Throat Monthly 32:707–711, 1953.

Runyan TE, Ostberg RC: An unusual macular lesion associated with malaria. Ann Ophthalmol 9:1521–1525, 1977.

ONCHOCERCIASIS
ALAN C. BIRD, M.D., F.R.C.S.
London, England

Onchocerciasis results from infection with the nematode, *Onchocerca volvulus*. The human is the definitive host. The transmission of *O. volvulus* requires the intervention of a vector, the blood-sucking black fly of the genus *Simulium*. The fly becomes infected by the intake of microfilariae from humans, and infection occurs by insertion of immature adult worms. Adult worms can be found in fibrous nodules that are characteristically subcutaneous and are most easily identified over bony prominences, such as the rib cage, pelvis, and head. The offspring of the adults—microfilariae—are mobile and migrate in subcutaneous tissue, but can also be found in the blood. In the eye, they can be seen in the cornea, aqueous humor, and vitreous. There are some reports of microfilariae within the neuroretina, and they have also been located by histopathology in the optic nerve. In patients infected within the first year of life, viable microfilariae cause little or no tissue reaction; however, dead microfilariae produce considerable focal inflammation with subsequent tissue destruction. In these patients, microfilariae can be found in large numbers in the skin and eye. In patients infected in later life, the live microfilariae appear to evoke an inflammatory response, and the identifiable population of microfilariae is low.

Dead microfilariae evoke localized corneal stromal disease around the dead worm that resolves spontaneously. A continued high population of microfilariae causes progressive sclerosis of the corneal stroma, which usually begins in the lower part of the cornea and spreads upward. Anterior uveitis is accompanied by downward movement of the pupil. In the fundus, the chorioretinal scarring characteristically is seen temporal to the fovea; it progresses to a ring of change in the peripheral macula. In advanced disease, there is confluent atrophy of the entire macular region. Optic nerve disease is manifest as swelling of the optic nerve that, within months, causes arcuate scotomata. As the disease develops, there occurs the total loss of peripheral field so that the patient may remain with a small central field but normal acuity.

Apart from ocular disease, the major impact of onchocerciasis is on the skin. Chronic generalized dermatitis gives rise to itching and hyperpigmentation. It is also believed that progressive fibrosis may give rise to elephantiasis. There is little good information concerning involvement of other systems. The microfilariae appear to have widespread distribution in the body, although their effects on various internal organs are unknown.

There appears to be significant variation in the expression of the disease in different parts of the world, which may be related to differences in *Onchocerca*, host response, or biting habits of the vector.

Diagnosis can be made on the basis of known history of contact with the disorder and identification of microfilariae in various tissues. These may be identified in the eye or in skin snips. A small dose of diethylcarbamazine causes microfilariae death and a consequent inflammatory response that is manifest as fever, eosinophilia, and skin rash; this is known as the Mazotti test.

THERAPY

Systemic. Two drugs have been used in the past for the treatment of onchocerciasis. Diethylcarbamazine is very effective in causing microfilarial death, but has little effect on the adult worm. Massive microfilarial death generates secondary inflammation, resulting in visual loss, and considerable dermatitis, lymphadenopathy, and arthralgia. Attempts have been made to modify the inflammatory response with systemic corticosteroids, although doing so appears to reduce the microfilaricidal effect of the drug. The severe consequences of diethylcarbamazine treatment have caused this form of treatment to be abandoned. Likewise, suramin causes death of adult worms and is also microfilaricidal. However, this form of treatment is associated with severe systemic disease and, in particular, may induce renal failure.

Over the last 3 years, a new microfilaricidal drug, ivermectin,[†] has been introduced. It appears to be effective in causing reduction of microfilariae within the body over a period of 3 months. It is believed that this drug kills microfilariae, although their disappearance is much slower than with diethylcarbamazine and little inflammatory response is seen. There is also some evidence that ivermectin affects the germinal epithelium of the adult worm, as manifested by large numbers of dysmorphic microfilariae around the adult worms. Phase 3 studies have failed to show any major complications of this form of treatment, although its widespread use must await the completion of phase 4 studies. The form of treatment seems to be eminently practical, since a single oral dose of 12 mg appears to cause disappearance of microfilariae for up to a year. Although this treatment does not eradicate onchocerciasis from the individual, there are high hopes that annual dosing within a population may control the disorder.

Ocular. Local anti-inflammatory agents are effective in controlling ocular inflammation.

Surgical. Excision of subcutaneous nodules containing adult worms has been practiced for some time. It is evident that the load of microfilariae in the eye bears some relationship to the number of subcutaneous nodules in the head. Removal of these subcutaneous nodules reduces the microfilarial load. Although this reduction has some effect, it does not eradicate the infection, and the use of this treatment in a large population is relatively impractical.

Supportive. Vector control has been used in widespread areas of Africa by the World Health Organization. This has proved to be effective, although it requires repeated spraying of the area and is expensive. It is unlikely that vector control represents a practical long-term solution to the problem.

PRECAUTIONS

In the eye, punctate inflammatory disease at the level of the pigmented epithelium may result secondary to diethylcarbamazine treatment. A more important complication is the onset or aggravation of optic neuritis. There are reports of patients suffering visual loss as a result of treatment.

References

Anderson J, Fugslang H: Further studies on the treatment of ocular onchocerciasis with diethylcarbamazine and suramin. Br J Ophthalmol 62:450–457, 1978.

Anderson J, Fugslang H, Marshall TF deC: Effects of suramin on ocular onchocerciasis. Trop Med Parasitol 27:279–296, 1976.

Bird AC, Anderson J, Fugslang H: Morphology of posterior segment lesions of the eye in patients with onchocerciasis. Br J Ophthalmol 60:2–20, 1976.

Dadzie KY, et al: Ocular findings in a double-blind study of ivermectin versus diethylcarbamazine versus placebo in the treatment of onchocerciasis. Br J Ophthalmol 71:78–85, 1987.

Greene BM, et al: Comparison of ivermectin and diethylcarbamazine in the treatment of onchocerciasis. N Engl J Med 313:133–138, 1985.

Newland HS, et al: Effect of single-dose ivermectin therapy on human *Onchocerca volvulus* infection with onchocercal ocular involvement. Br J Ophthalmol 72:561–569, 1988.

Taylor HR, et al: Treatment of onchocerciasis. The ocular effects of ivermectin and diethylcarbamazine. Arch Ophthalmol 104:863–870, 1986.

PEDICULOSIS AND PHTHIRIASIS

MARILYN C. KINCAID, M.D.

St. Louis, Missouri

Pediculosis refers to infestation by *Pediculus humanus* var. *corporis* and *Pediculosis humanus* var. *capitis* body and head lice, respectively. These lice are similar to each other in appearance and interbreed freely. Infestation by *Phthirus pubis*, the pubic louse, is called phthiriasis and is by far the most common type of louse infestation of the ocular region. Both types of lice lay eggs on the hair shafts; the eggs or nits are firmly adherent, resisting both mechanical and chemical removal.

Pediculus organisms are 2 to 4 mm long and have long slender legs that allow them to move about freely to feed. These lice are typically

116 / PEDICULOSIS AND PHTHIRIASIS

passed from person to person by close contact either with another infested person or with contaminated clothing or bedding. Infestation of the cilia is very rare and occurs only when there is massive infestation of the adjacent scalp hair.

Phthirus pubis is also called the crab louse because of its shape. At 2 mm, it is smaller than *Pediculus* and has a broad, shield-like body. This louse is much less mobile than *Pediculus*. Its legs are thicker with claw-like feet, and it prefers sites where the distance between adjacent hairs is similar to its grasping span, particularly the public hair, but also axillary, chest, and beard hair, as well as the eyelashes. *Phthirus* also causes 1 per cent of all lice infestations of scalp hair.

Both types of lice are associated with conditions of crowding or poor personal hygiene, but may occur in all socioeconomic groups.

THERAPY

Topical. In cooperative adults and older children, when the infestation is mild, physical removal of the involved eyelashes under direct visualization may be sufficient. Cryotherapy has been found effective in killing both adult lice and nits and is likewise feasible in older children and adults.

Topical white petrolatum smothers the adult lice and should be applied twice daily for 10 days in order to eradicate the emerging nits. Some authors have found this treatment to be only partially effective, however.

Lindane (gamma benzene hexachloride) 1 per cent shampoo is an effective pediculocide available by prescription. It is used as a single application to the head and body and can be repeated after 7 days if necessary, since it is less effective against the nits. Central nervous system toxicity has been reported from absorption through the skin, particularly in infants. This preparation is also irritating to the eye, and its use on the lashes is not recommended. However, some authors have used it successfully after applying an antibiotic ointment to the eye to act as a mechanical barrier.

A recently available agent, 1 per cent permethrin creme rinse, has been shown to be effective against both *Pediculus* and *Phthirus*. It is not specifically recommended for use around the eye, but is apparently nonirritating to the eye, according to the manufacturer.

A-200 Pyrinate (Norcliff Thayer) is a solution of pyrethrins, piperonyl butoxide, kerosene, and other ingredients available without a prescription. These agents are effective, but are toxic to the corneal epithelium, causing erosions with secondary ulceration and necrosis. The toxic agent may, in fact, be one of the "inert" ingredients.

Recently, 20 per cent fluorescein[‡] was observed to be effective in killing *Phthirus*, but to date there has been no large therapeutic trial of this apparently nontoxic agent. No information is available regarding whether it kills the nits.

One per cent yellow mercuric oxide[‡] and 3 per cent ammoniated mercury[‡] ophthalmic ointments have been recommended as effective when used twice daily for a week.

Cholinesterase inhibitors, including physostigmine ointment,[‡] kill the adult lice but not the nits. These agents cause cholinergic side effects—both local, such as ciliary spasm, and systemic, such as trembling and ataxia. An aqueous solution of the organophosphate insecticide malathion[†] has been described in the British literature as nontoxic and effective against both adult lice and nits, but it is not yet available in the United States.

Supportive. In adult patients, phthiriasis is usually acquired from sexual contacts, so the patient may also have other sexually transmitted diseases. Reinfestation may occur if sex partners are not examined and treated. Phthiriasis is less common in children than in adults, and although it may be contracted from an adult caregiver, the possibility of sexual abuse must be considered when a child has phthiriasis. In all cases, family members should be examined and treated, if necessary. The patient may also have other sites of infestation, so the entire body should be examined. Clothing, bedding, hair brushes, and combs should be sterilized by heating to 50° C, achieved by using the highest available washer and dryer temperature settings. Any cosmetics used around the eyes should be discarded.

Re-examination 7 to 10 days after treatment is important in order to detect inadequate treatment, newly emerging adult lice, or reinfestation.

Ocular or Periocular Manifestations

Conjunctiva: Follicular conjunctivitis (may cause more symptoms than the actual lid infestation, so a high index of suspicion is required for prompt diagnosis).

Cornea: Marginal keratitis (rare).

Eyelids: Infestation (manifest by direct visualization of lice and nits, reddish-brown louse feces, and maculae ceruleae, the blue spots on the skin indicative of louse bites); pruritus; blepharitis; secondary infection with preauricular lymphadenopathy.

PRECAUTIONS

Because most of the pediculocides are much less effective against nits than against adult lice, re-examination at 7 to 10 days is necessary, with retreatment as indicated.

Several of the agents noted above are irritating or toxic to the eye, and should be used cautiously. Agents requiring a prescription should be nonrefillable. Pruritus that persists after the lice are eradicated may indicate hypersensitivity to the pediculocide.

COMMENTS

Pediculosis of the ocular region is extremely rare and is generally an extension of heavy scalp infestation. Phthiriasis is more common and in many circumstances can be considered a venereal disease. Adequate treatment and follow-up are necessary to prevent ongoing or recurrent infestation.

References

Awan KJ: Cryotherapy in phthiriasis palpebrarum. Am J Ophthalmol 83:906–907, 1977.
Burns DA: The treatment of *Pthirus* [sic] *pubis* infestation of the eyelashes. Br J Dermatol 117:741–743, 1987.
Couch JM, et al: Diagnosing and treating *Phthirus pubis* palpebrarum. Surv Ophthalmol 26:219–225, 1982.
Kalter DC, et al: Treatment of pediculosis pubis: Clinical comparison of efficacy and tolerance of 1% lindane shampoo vs. 1% permethrin creme rinse. Arch Dermatol 123:1315–1319, 1987.
Kirschner MH: *Phthirus pubis* infestation of the eyelashes. JAMA 248:428, 1982.
Mathew M, D'Souza P, Mehta DK: A new treatment of Pthiriasis [sic] palpebrarum. Ann Ophthalmol 14:439–441, 1982.
Pe'er J, BenEzra D: Corneal damage following the use of the pediculocide A-200 Pyrinate. Arch Ophthalmol 106:16–17, 1988.

SCHISTOSOMIASIS
(Bilharziasis)

J. VÉDY, M.D.,
P. QUEGUINER, M.D.,
and J. GRAVELINE, M.D.
Marseille, France

Schistosomiasis is a very common epidemic disease; the World Health Organization estimates that about 300 million people are infested. This disease is caused by four species of trematodes that invade the human abdominal venous system and cause urinary or intestinal disorders. *Schistosoma haematobium* is mainly found in Africa and the Middle East and is responsible for urinary schistosomiasis, whereas *S. mansoni* (common in Africa and South America), *S. japonicum* (prevalent in the Far East), and *S. intercalatum* (found only in equatorial Africa) are responsible for intestinal schistosomiasis.

The life cycle of these parasites requires both an aquatic environment and a human vector. The female parasite lays eggs in the perivascular or perintestinal veins of a human and then the eggs move through either intestinal or bladder walls creating urinary or intestinal manifestations 1 to 8 months after infestation. The eggs are disseminated throughout the environment with excreta and develop into aquatic larvae: myracidia. When a myracidium succeeds in penetrating into a snail, it becomes an infesting larva, called cercaria. Emitted in water, a cercaria is able to infest humans by penetrating through their skin. After a maturation phase in the liver, a cercaria develops into an adult worm that finally migrates in the abdominal veins. This disease is contracted following water immersion, and the initial phase lasts a few weeks with characteristic features of fever, arthralgia, cephalgia, "swimmer's itch," bronchitis, and pulmonary disorders.

The seriousness of this disease is complicated by eggs encysting in viscera or migrating in the bloodstream. Consequences of such include superinfection, liver fibrous degenerations, splenic fibrous degeneration with portal hypertension (*S. mansoni* and mainly *S. japonicum*), renal insufficiency (*S. haematobium*), and genital lesions (*S. haematobium*). Canceration is still under review.

Ocular manifestations are mainly caused by *S. haematobium* and rarely by *S. japonicum*. Although allergic ocular manifestations occurring at the same time as infestation are most common, aberrant *Schistosoma* eggs or adults may also develop ocular features. Aberrant eggs are infrequent, but may cause hyperplasia of the lacrimal glands or inflammatory nodules in the conjunctiva or lids. Aberrant adults may result in parasites located in the orbital veins or in the eyeball. During infestation, "cercarian" conjunctivitis and palpebral or orbital edema may develop. Uveitis, chorioretinitis, retinal venous thrombosis, chorioretinal artery occlusion, and optic neuritis have been reported during egg laying.

THERAPY

Systemic. Niridazole is effective mainly on *S. haematobium* trematodes, requires a treatment of 7 days and is often poorly tolerated. Therefore, it has been replaced by more active drugs without toxicity that can be administered in a single dose.

Oxamniquine[†] is effective on *S. mansoni* trematodes only and is administered in a single dose of 15 mg/kg.

Oltipraz[†] is effective on *S. mansoni* in a dose of 15 mg/kg and on *S. haematobium* and *S. intercalatum* using 30 mg/kg in a single dose.

Praziquantel[†] is also very effective, and its spectrum covers the four types of human schistosomiasis. It is administered in a single dose of 40 mg/kg for *S. mansoni*, *S. haematobium*, and *S. intercalatum* and in a dosage of 60 mg/kg in three doses for *S. japonicum*.

Systemic corticosteroids may be needed to treat orbital edema, allergic chorioretinitis, optic neuritis, or ophthalmoplegia. Anticoagulative and antiagglutinative therapy combined with open dissection may be required for retinal phlebitis.

Ocular. Ocular therapy of schistosomiasis is secondary to systemic treatment. Conjunctival or eyelid nodules may need to be excised if they are a nuisance. "Cercarian" conjunctivitis and other allergic reactions may need to be treated with topical coricosteroids. Parasites lodging in the globe or the orbital veins may be removed surgically. Arterial occlusions require mydriatics

TOXOCARIASIS

ZANE F. POLLARD, M.D.,
and WILLIAM S. HAGLER, M.D.
Atlanta, Georgia

Toxocariasis is an infection caused mainly by the dog roundworm, *Toxocara canis*, and rarely by the cat roundworm, *T. cati*. It is acquired by ingesting the ova of *T. canis* or *T. cati*. The larvae hatch in the intestine and penetrate the mucosa to spread throughout the body. When the liver and lung are involved, the term "visceral larva migrans" is used. The organism can also involve the brain, heart, eye, or orbit. When the eye is involved, the disorder is known as ocular toxocariasis. In the past, the diagnosis has been made by demonstrating the presence of larvae in a liver biopsy or in studying enucleated eyes for the presence of larvae or an eosinophilic abscess. The clinical diagnosis for either ocular toxocariasis or visceral larva migrans is confirmed by the ELISA (enzyme-linked immunosorbent assay) test, which is both highly sensitive and specific because the antigen used is the *Toxocara*-embryonated egg. However, occasionally in ocular toxocariasis, the serum titers are normal but aqueous titers are highly elevated. The diagnostic titer for ocular toxocariasis is felt to be 1 : 8 whereas that for visceral larva migrans is 1 : 32. One should not be reluctant to make the diagnosis of ocular *Toxocara* because of a low titer. Eighty-five per cent of cases show a decrease in titers over a period of 6 months to 6 years from the time of the initial examination, ten per cent will show an increase, and 5 per cent show stable titers. It should be remembered that a patient with low titers may be presenting late and may actually have had higher titers in the past. Visceral larva migrans usually presents around the age of 2 years; the average age for ocular toxocariasis is 7.5 years. Elevated white blood count and eosinophilia (as high as 30 per cent) are usually seen with visceral larva migrans but only occasionally with ocular toxocariasis. Likewise, hepatomegaly and splenomegaly are usually seen with visceral larva migrans and only rare with ocular toxocariasis. Ocular lesions are rarely seen in cases of visceral larva migrans, and visceral larva migrans is rarely present in cases of ocular toxocariasis.

The prognosis of ocular toxocariasis is quite poor, and 80 per cent of untreated eyes will become legally blind (20/200 or less). The largest number of cases of ocular toxocariasis have been reported in the United States, followed by Great Britain and Australia. A few cases have also been reported in Belgium, France, West Germany, Ireland, Israel, and France. Cases have also been reported from Greece, Japan, Poland, Italy, Hungary, Mexico, Netherlands, Venezuela, and Argentina.

Several cases of ocular toxocariasis have also had high titers for toxoplasmosis. This is quite understandable as the contamination of the soil with *Toxocara* by the dog can easily be matched with contamination by the cat with the *Toxoplasma* oocyst.

THERAPY

Systemic. A decade ago, 15 mg/kg of diethylcarbamazine[‡] was used in the treatment of toxocariasis on a daily basis for 3 weeks, but thiabendazole has become more commonly used in the United States. Thiabendazole[‡] is administered in daily dosages of 25 to 50 mg/kg in two divided doses for 7 to 10 days. Occasionally, the course has to be repeated a second or a third time. This anthelminthic is used in combination with systemic steroids because it is thought that the reaction to the dead nematode is the factor that is so devastating to the health of the eye. Prednisone in a daily dosage of 2 mg/kg is used orally along with the thiabendazole for 3 weeks to control the vitreitis; in some cases, steroids alone have proved to be successful in clearing the vitreous. Topical steroids are useful if iritis is present. The ocular absorption of thiabendazole is unknown. The most frequent side effects are anorexia, nausea, vomiting, and dizziness. Elevation of SGOT and hyperglycemia with leukopenia and hematuria have been reported, as well as Stevens-Johnson syndrome. Blurring of vision, hypotension, enuresis, and perianal rash have rarely been seen.

Surgical. There are many cases in which various types of surgical treatment are helpful. Peripheral retinal detachment is common, which may develop because of contraction of the vitreous base that produces a peripheral dialysis. A standard scleral buckling procedure alone may be effective; in a few cases, that procedure was all that was necessary for successful results.

In the majority of patients requiring surgery, there is also a significant detachment of the posterior retina that either involves or threatens the macula. This detachment is usually caused by a prominent vitreous band and can be removed only by vitrectomy techniques. A lensectomy is also necessary in some of these patients, either because of cataract formation or in order to remove completely the extreme anterior attachments of the vitreous bands. In addition to the vitrectomy and lensectomy, a scleral buckling procedure may be required.

In rare instances, a vitrectomy can be used simply to remove opaque vitreous; of course, adequate time should be given for the more conservative medical measures.

Using various combinations of these surgical procedures can result in stability or improvement in visual acuity, although reactivation of the uveitis has rarely been reported. Because the natural history and the rate of progression of *T. canis* are not well documented, ophthalmologists should follow these patients very closely and perform surgery whenever a macular detachment occurs or appears eminent or whenever a progressive peripheral detachment should occur.

Some outstanding visual results with surgical treatment have been obtained. Several cases improved from 20/400 or less to 20/40 and 20/30. Of course, if the macula has already been destroyed by a posterior detachment or granuloma, central visual acuity cannot be improved, but stability of peripheral vision can be expected in most cases.

Ocular or Periocular Manifestations

Cornea: Larva; nummular keratitis.
Globe: Diffuse nematode endophthalmitis.
Iris: Granuloma (may be associated with hypopyon).
Lens: Cataract; larva.
Optic Nerve: Granuloma (growing from surface of optic nerve into vitreous); optic neuritis; papillitis.
Retina: Detachment (often confused with retinoblastoma); focal posterior granuloma; peripheral inflammatory granuloma (appearing as a unilateral pars plantis but sometimes also associated with a retinal detachment); retinal fold or vitreous band from the peripheral mass to the optic nerve or posterior pole.
Other: Strabismus.

PRECAUTIONS

Children's sandboxes can be decontaminated by replacing the sand or by steam sterilization. It is estimated that there are between 60 and 80 million dogs in the United States and 30 million cats. Treatment of these animals with piperazine or pyrantel pamoate has been quite effective in managing toxocariasis. Infections in puppies are more common than in the adult dog. A public health awareness of this problem plus a concerted effort to have all dogs and cats dewormed will reduce the incidence of this disease.

COMMENTS

Epidemiologic surveys are being performed to determine the exact incidence and distribution of this disease in the United States. In some areas of Georgia, ELISA titers have been positive in 10 per cent of control groups. In one county of Georgia, 3 per cent of controls tested had positive titers for *Toxocara*. The percentage of dogs with intestinal toxocariasis has been reported to vary from 20 to 86 per cent.

References

Brown DH: Ocular *Toxocara canis*. J Pediatr Ophthalmol 7:182–191, 1970.
Felberg NT, Shields JA, Federman JL: Antibody to *Toxocara canis* in the aqueous humor. Arch Ophthalmol 99:1563–1564, 1981.
Hagler WS, et al: Results of surgery for ocular *Toxocara canis*. Ophthalmology 88:1081–1086, 1981.
Liesegang TJ: Atypical ocular toxocariasis. J Pediatr Ophthalmol 14:349–353, 1977.
Pollard ZF: Long-term follow-up in patients with ocular toxocariasis as measured by ELISA titers. Ann Ophthalmol 19:167–169, 1987.
Pollard ZF, et al: ELISA for diagnosis of ocular toxocariasis. Ophthalmology 86:743–749, 1979.
Rhones JAA, Pratt CB, Johnson WW: Thiabendazole in visceral larva migrans. Am J Dis Child 121:226–229, 1971.

TOXOPLASMOSIS
(Ocular Toxoplasmosis, Toxoplasmic Iridocyclitis, Toxoplasmic Retinochoroiditis)
DANIEL H. SPITZBERG, M.D.
Indianapolis, Indiana

This infection is caused by the protozoal parasite, *Toxoplasma gondii*, which invades and multiplies asexually within the cytoplasm of nucleated host cells. As host immunity develops, multiplication slows, and the parasite develops cysts within cells. These have a predilection for the brain, eye, and muscle. As a result, various symptoms, such as recurrent retinochoroiditis, hydrocephalus, intracerebral calcification, and central nervous system manifestations, may develop. Although ocular toxoplasmosis may not make its first appearance until adulthood, most infections with *T. gondii* are congenital in origin and have a predilection for the nerve fiber layer. Microphthalmos, posterior uveitis, optic atrophy, iritis, strabismus, and nystagmus are the ocular signs most often associated with severe congenital toxoplasmosis and may be well developed at birth. Ophthalmoplegia and nystagmus are usually due to central nervous system involvement. Before toxic systemic medications are prescribed, the ophthalmologist should document the possibility of toxoplasmosis (by a toxoplasmosis titer positive at any level) and should rule out tuberculosis (by performing the tuberculin skin test down to PPD#2) and syphilis (by obtaining a negative FTA-ABS test).

THERAPY

Systemic. *Corticosteroids should not be used without specific antimicrobials.* At one time, it was popular to treat toxoplasmic retinochoroiditis with corticosteroids alone, but occasionally the patients' immunity is not strong enough to prevent the rampant multiplication of the parasite, resulting in serious damage.

Depending on the severity and the location of the retinochoroiditis, one should use up to four drugs: trisulfapyrimidines (sulfadiazine, sulfamethazine, and sulfamerazine), pyrimethamine, clindamycin, and corticosteroids. Since these drugs work in different ways, they may be synergistic; however, synergism has only been demonstrated for pyrimethamine and triple sulfa. Although small peripheral retinal lesions do not demand any medication, patients with large severe ones near the macula or optic disc probably should receive all four drugs. The major defense against *T. gondii* is a cellular response in which immune competent lymphocytes and macrophages participate. In the future, treatment may be directed more toward enhancing the body's immunity than toward the use of antiparasitic drugs.

If only one drug is chosen, trisulfapyrimidines should be the first choice because of their minimal expense, good tolerance, lack of spoilage, and simplicity of use. One must avoid most of the newer sulfonamides because they are less effective. The usual dosage of trisulfapyrimidines is 1 to 1.5 gm given orally four times daily.

The alternate first or second choice would be clindamycin,‡ usually in a dosage of 300 mg every 6 hours. This is an expensive drug and has not yet been approved by the FDA for toxoplasmosis and probably never will be because of the infrequency of toxoplasmosis and the expense of obtaining such approval. A less expensive, but less effective alternative to clindamycin is 500 mg of tetracycline‡ four times daily.

The major problem with pyrimethamine is that it is nauseating and requires two additional steps. One needs to prescribe at least 3 mg of leucovorin a week and obtain a platelet count for depression of the bone marrow at least once a week. A loading dose of 50 mg of pyrimethamine four times a day the first day is followed by 25 mg twice a day thereafter.

Corticosteroids should not be used without the cover of at least one antitoxoplasmic agent, and one must be careful not to use them in an immunosuppressive dosage. Either 100 mg of prednisone every other day after breakfast or periocular injections* every 2 to 3 weeks are recommended.

Ocular. Subtenon injection of steroids* may produce immediate dramatic improvement in patients with ocular toxoplasmosis. Some patients benefit from an oral analgesic sedative approximately 20 minutes before injection. In addition, topical local anesthetics should be applied at least five times over the area to be injected. The head should be tilted so that gravity will pull the anesthetic into the cul-de-sac. An injectable anesthetic is not necessary nor advisable. A 2-ml syringe is used to inject 0.5 ml of the 80 mg/ml concentration of methylprednisolone. The easiest place to make the injection is inferotemporally. The point of the needle should be placed 3 to 4 mm in front of the cul-de-sac and between blood vessels and pushed into the hilt *following the curve* of the sclera. One is helped to follow the curve of the sclera by the use of lateral motion of the needle over an area of 5 mm. This is a most valuable maneuver, since it allows one to hug the sclera as the needle goes in. The barrel of the syringe must be moved a large distance as one goes around the eyeball in order to keep the needle point near the eye. Keeping the needle near the eye with the aperture facing the sclera cuts down on the patient's discomfort and increases the penetration of the steroid because the medication will be closer to the sclera and not out in the orbital tissues. This lateral motion also avoids impaling the eyeball, since the ophthalmologist will immediately be aware that the sclera has been engaged if such a movement is used. By putting the injection far back, the side effects of chemosis and ptosis are decreased and the white material is not visible. If repeated injections are necessary, the superotemporal quadrant is usually varied with the inferotemporal. If a patient develops an allergy to methylprednisolone, the diagnosis should be confirmed by intradermal injection of 0.01 ml and read at 2 days, and the patient should be switched to triamcinolone (40 mg/ml).

Surgical. Freezing the active lesion has been employed in an attempt to kill resistant *T. gondii* and thus to quiet the lesion. This technique should be reserved for unusual cases. The entire lesion may be frozen and thawed three times in one sitting.

Although photocoagulation does kill cysts of *T. gondii*, it also damages normal retina and cannot be relied upon to eradicate all the cysts. Photocoagulation of an active lesion may occasionally be of value in those that have failed to heal after several months of medical treatment or in those patients who cannot tolerate the medication. A controlled study of the prophylactic value of employing photocoagulation around inactive lesions is in order.

Vitrectomy is indicated only for patients with dense membranes and greatly reduced vision. This treatment is not indicated for punctate opacities.

Ocular or Periocular Manifestations

Cornea: Keratic precipitates.
Extraocular Muscles: Esotropia; nystagmus.
Iris: Iritis; synechiae.
Optic Nerve: Atrophy; disc edema; papillitis.
Pupil: Anisocoria; persistent membrane.
Retina: Macular edema; retinitis.
Sclera: Scleritis; thickening.
Vitreous: Cells; exudates; haze; posterior vitreous detachment.
Other: Cataracts; lymphadenopathy; microphthalmos.

PRECAUTIONS

Pseudomembranous colitis may develop with the use of clindamycin; however, this danger is greatly reduced if trisulfapyrimidines are used. If clindamycin is prescribed, patients should be warned to discontinue use of the drug if they have four or more bowel movements a day than is normal for them. In addition, the prescription for clindamycin should be limited to a one-week supply with three refills.

Sometimes a blood picture resembling macrocytic anemia results from administration of pyrimethamine. Platelet counts should be monitored weekly in these patients. This bone marrow depression can be prevented in most patients by oral dosage of leucovorin in any drink without alcohol. This regimen is superior to waiting for thrombocytopenia to develop and then using leucovorin. The use of folic acid, which inactivates the pyrimethamine, should be avoided.

Comments

No method of preventing attacks has been designed at the present time. Patients should be advised to take good care of their general health and to have some medication, such as triple sulfonamides, on hand to take immediately with the first symptoms of a recurrence. It is crucial to start therapy as early as possible, especially before the onset of retinal necrosis if the lesion is near the disc or macula.

Many infants survive acute infection and have no complications or sequelae; however, some have healed scars in the fundus and may develop retinochoroiditis later in life.

References

Dobbie JG: *Toxoplasma* retinochoroiditis. Successful isolation of *Toxoplasma gondii* from the subretinal fluid of the living human eye. Ann Ophthalmol 2:509–513, 1970.
Eyles DE, Coleman N: Synergistic effect of sulfadiazine and Daraprim against experimental toxoplasmosis in mouse. Antibiotics Chemother 3:483–490, 1953.
Fitzgerald CR: Pars plana vitrectomy for vitreous opacity secondary to presumed toxoplasmosis. Arch Ophthalmol 98:321–323, 1980.
Frenkel JK, Hitchings GH: Relative reversal by vitamins (p-aminobenzoic, folic, and folinic acids) of the effects of sulfadiazine and pyrimethamine on *Toxoplasma*, mouse and man. Antibiotics Chemother 7:630–638, 1957.
Ghartey KN, Brockhurst RJ: Photocoagulation of active toxoplasmic retinochoroiditis. Am J Ophthalmol 89:858–864, 1980.
Tabbara KF, O'Connor GR: Treatment of ocular toxoplasmosis with clindamycin and sulfadiazine. Ophthalmology 87:129–134, 1980.
Tessler HH: Quadruple therapy offers rapid, effective results in ocular toxoplasmosis. Ophthalmology Times 5:27, 1979.

TRICHINOSIS
(Trichinellosis)
B.H. KEAN, M.D.
New York, New York

Almost 30 million people throughout the world are infected with *Trichinella spiralis;* most of the cases of trichinosis are in the United States. The disease is acquired by the ingestion of poorly cooked meat, especially pork, or ground beef contaminated by pork in the grinder. Less frequently, the meat of other mammals, such as bear and walrus, is involved.

After meat containing encysted larvae is ingested, the gastric juices release the parasites that develop in the upper portion of the small intestine. The adult females measure 3 to 4 mm by 60 μm, and males are one-third of that size. After 4 days of maturation, the adults produce larvae at the rate of 1000 daily for several weeks while embedded in the mucosa. The larvae disseminate throughout the entire body, but have a predilection for striated muscle, which is invaded and where encystment eventually takes place.

Only a few hundred cases are reported each year because the disease is unrecognized or so mild as to produce few symptoms. Systemic symptoms of trichinosis may include gastrointestinal disturbances, especially diarrhea; fever; generalized muscle pains, sometimes severe; and eosinophilia, often pronounced. The ophthalmologist is often the first to see the patient and has a unique opportunity to suspect the diagnosis. Bilateral edema of the eyelids, barely recognizable or severe enough to shut the eyes, presents as the first symptom of the disease in most patients. There is no consensus regarding the exact mechanism of the edema that may occur from the 6th to the 22nd day of infection, but it certainly is associated with the invasion of the eye muscles and the resulting myositis. Such mistaken diagnoses as kidney disease, mumps, angioneurotic edema, and erysipelas have been made. Other ophthalmic signs of trichinosis may include pain on motion of the eye muscles, pain in one or both eyes, headaches associated with fever, chemosis, and subconjunctival and retinal petechial hemorrhages. Rarer are disturbances in vision, including blurring, strabismus, exophthalmos, nystagmus, photophobia, diplopia, and visual hallucinations. Tiny striated hemorrhages close to the inferior temporal vein have also been reported.

The symptoms and the inevitable eosinophilia make a clinical diagnosis relatively easy. Definitive diagnosis is made by the use of several different serologic tests; the bentonite flocculation test is the most widely used, with a rising titer considered convincing. Muscle biopsy, if positive, is conclusive.

THERAPY

Systemic. If the diagnosis is made early (in the first week), 100 mg of mebendazole[‡] twice a day for 3 to 5 days may be helpful in reducing the intestinal worm load and hence the number of larvae released.

In the muscular stage of severe infection, thiabendazole[‡] is the drug of choice. The usual oral dose is 25 mg/kg, given in divided doses for 3 days and repeated after an interval of 24 to 48 hours. The drug should be taken after meals. In severe cases, corticosteroids should be used in conjunction with thiabendazole.

Some advocate the use of mebendazole and thiabendazole in greater doses and for longer duration than we have recommended. Albendazole is under study as a substitute for mebendazole.

Ocular. Ocular therapy is directed primarily to relief of the severe ocular pain that results from larval invasion of ocular musculature. Topical corticosteroids usually provide significant relief and help reduce swelling. A solution of 0.2 per cent hydrocortisone drops may be used four times daily until symptoms subside. In severe cases, topical corticosteroids may be accompanied by subconjunctival corticosteroid injections; 5 mg/ml of hydrocortisone* is the recommended dosage. Cycloplegics are indicated if anterior uveitis is evident.

Supportive. If the infection is mild and there is no evidence of encephalitis or myocarditis, symptomatic treatment may be sufficient. These patients should be confined to bed and fed high-calorie, protein-rich diets. Ice packs to the eyes, used intermittently, are often welcome. Pain relievers should be used freely, but aspirin should be avoided because it may increase the number and extent of the hemorrhages. Hospitalization is recommended for patients with severe trichinosis.

Ocular or Periocular Manifestations

Conjunctiva: Chemosis; conjunctivitis; diffuse hemorrhages (splinter); petechiae.
Extraocular Muscles: Encysted parasites; paresis or paralysis of sixth nerve.
Eyelids: Edema; erythema.
Globe: Exophthalmos; immobility; proptosis.
Iris: Anterior uveitis.
Optic Nerve: Disc hyperemia; optic neuritis; papilledema.
Pupil: Loss of rapid adaptation to light changes.
Retina: Edema; exudates; hemorrhages.
Other: Decreased accommodation; diplopia; dyschromatopsia; ocular pain; orbital edema; photophobia; scotoma; secondary glaucoma; visual field defects; visual loss.

PRECAUTIONS

Mebendazole, 100 mg twice daily for 4 days, has been replacing thiabendazole because it is better tolerated. Both drugs may produce a hypersensitivity reaction and both are contraindicated in pregnancy. In severe cases 60 mg of prednisone daily should be used in conjunction with one of these anthelminthics.

References

Campbell WC, Denham DA: Chemotherapy. *In* Campbell WC (ed): Trichinella and Trichinosis. New York, Plenum Press, 1983, pp 335–366.

Duke-Elder S (ed): System of Ophthalmology. St. Louis, CV Mosby, 1976, Vol XV, pp 159–160.

Hoskins DW: Trichinellosis (trichinosis). *In* Wyngaarden JB, Smith LH Jr (eds): Textbook of Medicine. 18th ed. Philadelphia, WB Saunders. 1988, pp 1911–1912.

SECTION 3

ENDOCRINE DISORDERS

HYPERPARATHYROIDISM
K.J. MURPHY, F.R.A.C.P.
Woolloongabba, Australia

Hyperparathyroidism is a generalized disorder that results from an increased secretion of parathyroid hormone. The increase may be a primary disorder, or it may be secondary to diseases that cause a low serum calcium. The primary disorder may be caused by adenoma of one of the four parathyroid glands, generalized hyperplasia of all four glands, or carcinoma of one of the glands. Secondary hyperparathyroidism is usually the result of chronic renal failure, with phosphate retention and a resulting low serum calcium. It may be due to other conditions, such as steatorrhea with calcium loss. If the hyperparathyroidism persists after the cause of secondary hyperparathyroidism is removed or corrected, the term "tertiary hyperparathyroidism" is used. Some patients with tertiary hyperparathyroidism have been found to have an adenoma, which presumably results from a prolonged stimulation during the stage of secondary hyperparathyroidism.

Increased parathyroid hormone production can also be caused by drugs, such as lithium. In primary, tertiary, and lithium-induced hyperparathyroidism, the serum calcium is elevated and the serum phosphate is low or normal. In secondary hyperparathyroidism, the serum calcium is low or normal and the serum phosphate is elevated.

The symptoms of hyperparathyroidism are nonspecific. They have been summed up as "stones, bones, abdominal groans, and psychic moans," indicating the possibilities of kidney stones, bone pathology with osteitis fibrosa, either peptic ulcer or pancreatitis, and mental changes (particularly depression). Neurologic changes may include muscle weakness, especially affecting the proximal muscles of the limbs, particularly the lower limbs. Very rarely, even though the serum calcium is raised, there may be status epilepticus.

The most common ocular manifestations of hyperparathyroidism result from metastatic calcification, the likelihood of which is related to the product of calcium times phosphorus in the serum. This product is usually higher in the secondary form than in the primary, because of the relatively greater increase in serum phosphate in the secondary form. The sign most commonly seen is a band keratopathy with deposition of calcium at the corneoscleral junction within the palpebral fissure. However, such calcification can occur in other conditions of hypercalcemia, and it can occur in chronic renal failure without hyperparathyroidism when the product of phosphorus and calcium is high enough. Very rarely, the bones of the skull may be so vascular that a secondary papilledema is produced. This may be followed by optic atrophy. Thus, both hypoparathyroidism and hyperparathyroidism may rarely cause papilledema, and both may cause epilepsy.

The course of primary hyperparathyroidism is unpredictable, but the serum calcium may rise very rapidly to levels that can endanger life. However, most cases of primary hyperparathyroidism are asymptomatic, and the elevated serum calcium is found on a routine biochemical screening.

THERAPY

Systemic. The asymptomatic patient probably requires no treatment. There are no definitive rules regarding surgery in such patients. Patients with such complications as kidney stones, peptic ulcer, or pancreatitis usually require operation for the parathyroid disorder, and patients with markedly elevated serum calcium certainly require treatment.

Systemic treatment is usually aimed at the hypercalcemia. This is best treated by a vigorous diuretic regimen consisting of intravenous infusion of isotonic sodium chloride, up to 1 liter per hour. In addition, furosemide in an oral dose of 40 to 80 mg twice daily is given to maintain urine volume and to promote calcium excretion. Most cases respond to a vigorous diuretic therapy, but occasionally mithramycin may be required in an intravenous dose of 25 to 50 μg/kg in a single daily dose. The oral administration of phosphate in a daily dose of 1 to 2 gm will lower the serum calcium in the short term, but it should not be continued long term because of the risk of further soft tissue calcification. Although the production of parathyroid hormone has been shown to be increased by histamine and beta-adrenergic agents, such as isoproterenol, there have been no convincing responses to either beta blockade with propranolol[‡] or histamine blockade with cimetidine[‡] in established hyperparathyroidism. The lithium-induced increase in parathyroid hormone responds to cessation of the lithium.

Ocular. In patients with band keratopathy, the deposits should first be exposed by mechani-

126 / HYPERPARATHYROIDISM

cal denuding of the corneal epithelium. A solution of 1.85 per cent edetate disodium may then be instilled four to five times hourly for 2 to 3 hours to irrigate the exposed membrane.

Surgical. If a single parathyroid tumor is found, it should be removed surgically. If there is hyperplasia of all glands, the surgeon removes three and a half glands. If the glands in the neck are found to be normal, exploration needs to be extended to the mediastinum. Postoperative hypoparathyroidism requires oral calcium and oral vitamin D or analog. Patients with severe bone disease may start to rapidly recalcify the skeleton in the postoperative period. This can produce severe and sustained hypocalcemia, which requires intravenous infusions of 10 per cent calcium gluconate (up to 200 ml per day). The serum calcium needs to be monitored frequently in such patients.

Ocular or Periocular Manifestations

Conjunctiva: Calcification; glass-like crystals.
Cornea: Band-shaped keratopathy; bleb; opacity.
Optic Nerve: Atrophy; granuloma; papilledema.
Retina: Vascular engorgement accompanying engorgement of the bones of the skull (mainly seen in the secondary form).
Other: Enlarged blind spot; ptosis; scleral thinning; visual loss.

PRECAUTIONS

If the serum calcium rises to dangerous levels, the patient may complain of a nasty metallic taste in the mouth, thirst, possible headache, and drowsiness; stupor and death may result if the serum calcium reaches 20 mg/100 ml. Patients who have been on a stable dose of digitalis preparations may show digitalis toxicity when the serum calcium rises. Successful surgery and the resultant fall in serum calcium may cause tetany or seizures; intravenous calcium may be required.

COMMENTS

Primary hyperparathyroidism may be suspected in patients with recurring bilateral renal calculi, bone disease causing pain or pathologic fracture, pancreatitis (especially if the serum calcium is normal or elevated), recurrent or persistent peptic ulceration, and other evidence of multiple endocrine adenomatosis, particularly if there is a family history. Generally, the symptoms are nonspecific and include fatigue, weakness, headache, thirst, polyuria, skin itching, or muscle weakness. Parathyroid hormone has been shown to exaggerate both hypertension and anemia.

Since the introduction of automated biochemical screening, the majority of cases of primary hyperparathyroidism have been found in asymptomatic patients with hypercalcemia. The diagnosis is confirmed by the finding of a raised level of serum parathyroid hormone on assay in the presence of hypercalcemia. Normally, a raised serum calcium from other causes should depress parathyroid function. The one exception is the syndrome of peptide production by various malignancies; such peptides react in the same way as parathyroid hormones on the assay. Hypercalcemia is usually found in these patients.

Secondary hyperparathyroidism is present in most patients with renal failure from the time they begin to show phosphate retention.

Because it is unusual for an enlarged parathyroid gland to produce a palpable mass in the neck, the most satisfactory localization of the pathology is exploration by an experienced surgeon. If the original exploration is negative and repeat surgery is contemplated, the approximate localization may be shown by cannulation of the draining veins from the separate areas and parathyroid hormone assays on the specimens. Occasionally, ultrasound examination of the neck, barium swallow, or even selective arteriography may demonstrate the affected areas.

In patients with corneal calcification caused by hyperparathyroidism, the calcium salts are deposited extracellularly in the corneal layers and tend to persist unchanged long after serum calcium levels have returned to normal. Deposition of calcium in the conjunctiva of the tarsal plate may lead to continuing irritation.

References

Bilezikian JP: The medical management of primary hyperparathyroidism. Ann Intern Med 96:198–202, 1982.
Cogan DG, Albright F, Bartter FC: Hypercalcemia and band keratopathy. Report of nineteen cases. Arch Ophthalmol 40:624–638, 1948.
Golan A, et al: Band keratopathy due to hyperparathyroidism. Ophthalmologica 171:119–122, 1975.
Mundy GR, Cove DH, Fisken R: Primary hyperparathyroidism: Changes in the pattern of clinical presentation. Lancet 1:1317–1320, 1980.
Sampson MJ, van't Hoff W, Bicknell EJ: The conservative management of primary hyperparathyroidism. Q J Med 65:1009–1014, 1987.
Stevenson JC, Lynn JA: Time to end a conservative treatment for mild hyperparathyroidism. Br Med J (Clin Res) 296:1016–1017, 1988.

HYPOCALCEMIA

MARION H. BROOKS, M.D.
and ANTHONY L. BARBATO, M.D.
Maywood, Illinois

Hypocalcemia may be found in patients with hypoproteinemia, hypoparathyroidism, chronic renal failure, hypomagnesemia, malabsorption syndromes, acute pancreatitis, osteoblastic metastases and other malignant disorders, rickets or osteomalacia, and following administration of anticonvulsants or transfusion of large quantities of citrated blood. A decrease in serum calcium does not always indicate a disturbance of calcium homeostasis. Patients with hypoproteinemia often have a low total but normal ionic serum calcium level. Under these circumstances, there are no symptoms attributable to hypocalcemia, and calcium replacement is unnecessary. In contrast, low levels of ionized serum calcium interfere with cellular function, and treatment is necessary if symptoms, signs, and complications of hypocalcemia are to be avoided or reversed. A decrease in the concentration of ionized calcium in plasma is often associated with an increase in neuromuscular irritability, which is expressed clinically as overt or latent tetany. The patient with tetany may complain of muscle cramps, carpopedal spasms, numbness and tingling of the extremities, palpitations, or fatigue. Physical findings suggestive of hypocalcemia include a positive Chvostek or Trousseau sign, convulsions, laryngeal stridor, alopecia, coarse scaly skin, moniliasis, and hypoplastic teeth. Tetany may also occur in patients with normal serum calcium levels who develop hypokalemia, hypomagnesemia, or alkalosis. Although cataracts are the best-known ocular complication of hypocalcemia, other ocular abnormalities include loss of eyebrows or eyelashes and papilledema.

THERAPY

Systemic. The major therapeutic objective in all forms of hypocalcemia is restoration and maintenance of serum calcium levels in the vicinity of 8.5 to 9.0 mg/100 ml without the development of hypercalciuria. The therapeutic regimen used to achieve this goal depends on the cause of hypocalcemia and the response of the individual patient to therapy.

In chronic hypoparathyroidism, inadequate levels of parathyroid hormone are associated with diminished conversion of vitamin D to its active metabolite, calcitriol, by the kidney. As a consequence, intestinal absorption of calcium and mobilization of calcium from bone are impaired, leading to hypocalcemia. Adequate serum calcium levels can often be maintained in mild hypoparathyroidism with calcium supplements alone, but administration of both vitamin D and calcium are usually required to increase serum calcium levels significantly in patients with hypoparathyroidism. Vitamin D may be administered in the form of ergocalciferol (vitamin D_2), dihydrotachysterol (vitamin D_1), or calcitriol (1α, 25 dihydroxy vitamin D_3). The daily dose of ergocalciferol varies from 25,000 to 200,000 IU, depending upon the patient's response. Some authorities prefer to use dihydrotachysterol in a dose of 0.125 to 5.0 mg per day, since this preparation has a shorter half-life, is three times as potent as ergocalciferol on a weight basis, and does not require 1 alpha-hydroxylation by the kidney to exert its metabolic effects. Despite these theoretical advantages, dihydrotachysterol is more expensive than ergocalciferol and has not been demonstrated to be unequivocally superior to the latter in the treatment of hypoparathyroidism. Treatment with calcitriol is advantageous in that this form of vitamin D is fully active in increasing intestinal calcium absorption. In view of the markedly enhanced potency of calcitriol relative to other preparations of vitamin D, the daily dose is usually in the range of 0.25 to 2.0 μg per day. The dose of any vitamin D preparation must be individualized for each patient. Since the full effect of a given dose may not be apparent for a long period of time, increments in dosage should not be made more often than every 2 to 3 weeks.

In addition to vitamin D, calcium supplements may also be needed to restore serum calcium levels to normal. The most common therapeutic error, which results in persistent hypocalcemia, is failure to appreciate that replacement doses of calcium are expressed in terms of *elemental* calcium, rather than the calcium salt. For example, elemental calcium constitutes only 9.3 percent of the weight of calcium gluconate, 18.4 percent of the weight of calcium lactate, and 40 percent of the weight of calcium carbonate. In view of the relatively low calcium content of calcium gluconate and calcium lactate, it often is necessary to prescribe large numbers of calcium tablets each day to provide the 1 to 3 gm of *elemental* calcium required by patients with hypoparathyroidism. Recent interest in dietary calcium supplements has resulted in widespread availability of several preparations of calcium carbonate that permit the patient to obtain an adequate intake of *elemental* calcium in a smaller number of tablets per day. It should be noted that absorption of calcium from tablets may be unsatisfactory, since some preparations do not dissolve properly unless thoroughly chewed. These considerations may make it desirable to administer calcium supplements to some patients in the form of calcium glubionate syrup or as calcium lactate or calcium carbonate powder dissolved in water or juice. Regardless of the preparation used, the total calcium dose should be divided into equal portions and administered three to four times daily.

Hypocalcemia develops in chronic renal failure because there is inadequate renal parenchyma to convert 25-hydroxyvitamin D to calcitriol despite increased serum parathyroid hormone levels. Administration of calcitriol in a dose of 0.25 to 1.0 μg per day to patients undergoing chronic dialysis often restores serum calcium and parathyroid hormone levels to normal and prevents the development of renal osteodystrophy. In some patients with renal failure, calcium supplements are also required, and it may be necessary to administer aluminum hydroxide orally to reduce serum phosphorus levels by interfering with intestinal phosphorus absorption.

Hypocalcemia due to hypomagnesemia is most often encountered in patients with alcoholic liver disease. In this situation, the secretion of parathyroid hormone and its metabolic effects are impaired as a consequence of magnesium depletion. Restoration of total body magne-

128 / HYPOCALCEMIA

sium stores to normal by administration of magnesium salts is usually associated with an increase in the serum calcium concentration to normal.

The hypocalcemia associated with malabsorption syndromes, rickets, osteomalacia, osteoblastic metastases and other malignant disorders, and administration of anticonvulsants usually responds to treatment of the underlying disease together with administration of vitamin D and calcium supplements in doses similar to those used in the treatment of hypoparathyroidism.

Hypocalcemia that develops in response to parathyroidectomy, acute pancreatitis, or transfusion of large quantities of citrated blood may be associated with the acute onset of tetany and may require intravenous calcium administration for relief of symptoms. Administration of 10 ml of 10 per cent calcium chloride or calcium gluconate may be used; however, since extravasation of calcium solutions into soft tissues elicits a marked inflammatory response, it is preferable to prepare a solution containing 200 mg of elemental calcium in 100 ml of 5 per cent dextrose in water and to administer this solution over a 10-minute period through an indwelling catheter in a large peripheral vein. If symptoms recur, the infusion can be repeated at 6- to 8-hour intervals, or calcium can be administered at a slower rate by constant intravenous infusion.

Dairy products contain calcium but are also rich in phosphate, which can interfere with the absorption of calcium from the intestine and increase serum phosphate levels. For this reason, the intake of dairy products should be limited. Administration of parathyroid hormone has no role in the therapy of chronic hypocalcemia.

Surgical. Since the neuromuscular and metabolic abnormalities associated with hypocalcemia increase the risk of anesthesia and surgery, elective procedures should be postponed until normocalcemia is restored. If cataract extraction is necessary in a normocalcemic patient, standard operative procedures are usually adequate. No special problems are to be anticipated, except for a possible increase in the frequency of postoperative hemorrhage.

If the oral intake of calcium and vitamin D is limited as a consequence of surgery, serum calcium levels must be carefully monitored. If hypocalcemia develops, replacement therapy should be instituted intravenously.

Ocular or Periocular Manifestations

Conjunctiva: Conjunctivitis.
Eyebrows or Eyelids: Blepharitis; blepharospasm; madarosis; pigmentation; ptosis.
Lens: Flake-like, crystalline, punctate, or zonular cataracts.
Optice Nerve: Papilledema.
Other: Decreased visual acuity; diplopia; photophobia; strabismus.

PRECAUTIONS

Hypercalcemia and hypercalciuria leading to renal damage from nephrocalcinosis or nephrolithiasis are potentially serious complications of therapy with calcium and vitamin D. Vitamin D intoxication often develops unexpectedly in patients who have had stable serum calcium levels for prolonged periods. In general, the smallest dose of vitamin D that will provide the desired effects should be used, and patients should be taught to recognize the symptoms of hypercalcemia. The physician should measure serum and urinary calcium levels at weekly intervals during initiation of therapy, at monthly intervals for 6 months when maintenance doses appear to have been reached, and every 3 to 6 months thereafter when serum calcium levels appear to have stabilized at the desired level. If hypercalcemia or hypercalciuria develops, supplemental calcium and vitamin D must be discontinued immediately, and adequate hydration must be ensured with oral or parenteral fluids. Restoration of normal serum calcium and vitamin D levels may not be achieved for several months, since large amounts of vitamin D are stored in adipose tissue and skeletal muscle.

The dose of calcium and vitamin D may need to be increased during pregnancy, lactation, or administration of phenytoin or phenobarbital. Conversely, the requirement for calcium and vitamin D may decrease in patients receiving thiazide diuretics. Care must also be exercised when calcium and vitamin D are administered to patients receiving digitalis preparations, since hypercalcemia can lead to the development of digitalis intoxication and cardiac arrhythmias.

Laboratory evaluation of patients suspected of having hypocalcemia should always include measurements of serum total protein, albumin, urea nitrogen, creatinine, calcium, phosphorus, magnesium, electrolytes, and pH. If the total calcium level is low, the ionized fraction of serum calcium should be measured; additional studies, including serum parathyroid hormone levels, will be necessary to define the cause of hypocalcemia.

COMMENTS

Chronic renal failure with inability to synthesize calcitriol is the most common cause of hypocalcemia. Malabsorption that limits the availability of both calcium and vitamin D is the next leading cause, followed by hypoparathyroidism. Although hypoparathyroidism is usually an iatrogenic disease that develops after thyroid or parathyroid surgery, it may also occur spontaneously in an idiopathic form or as pseudohypoparathyroidism.

Since hypocalcemic cataracts are not reversible, attempts should be made to prevent their development or progression. Careful monitoring of serum calcium levels in all patients for at least 7 days after thyroidectomy, parathyroidectomy, or radical neck dissection is mandatory because the patient may remain asymptomatic despite significant hypocalcemia. The progression of hypocalcemic cataracts is variable in that they may be found as early as 10 days or as late as 22 years after thyroidectomy. The lenticular changes resulting from hypocalcemia are suggestive but not pathognomonic of this disorder and vary from minute, white, punctate opacities to complete opacification of the lens. Despite these variations, there is general agreement that early recognition and vigorous therapy will often prevent the development or halt the progression of cataracts in hypocalcemic patients.

References

Bronsky D et al: Idiopathic hypoparathyroidism and pseudohypoparathyroidism: Case reports and review of the literature. Medicine 37:317–352, 1958.
Brooks MH: Lenticular abnormalities in endocrine dysfunction. In Bellows JG (ed): Cataract and Abnormalities of the Lens. New York, Grune & Stratton, 1975, pp 291–294.
Buckwalter JA, et al: Postoperative hypoparathyroidism. Surg Gynecol Obstet 101:657–666, 1955.
Morris DA: Cataracts and systemic disease. In Duane TD (ed): Clinical Ophthalmology. Hagerstown MD, Harper & Row, 1982, Vol V, pp 41:1–2.
Schneider AB, Sherwood LM: Pathogenesis and management of hypoparathyroidism and other hypocalcemic disorders. Metabolism 24:871–898, 1975.

HYPOPARATHYROIDISM

FELIX O. KOLB, M.D.
San Francisco, California

Hypoparathyroidism is caused by a deficient secretion of parathyroid hormone or, more rarely, resistance to its action due to a receptor defect "pseudohypoparathyroidism". This disorder usually occurs following thyroidectomy, surgery for parathyroid tumor, x-ray irradiation, massive radioactive iodine administration for cancer, or idiopathic conditions. Transient hypoparathyroidism in newborns may result from magnesium deficiency, maternal hypercalcemia, or intake of cow's milk containing large amounts of phosphate. Hypoparathyroidism is characterized by decreased blood calcium and increased serum phosphate in the absence of renal failure. Parathormone levels are low or absent in hypoparathyroidism and elevated in pseudohypoparathyroidism. This disorder may cause tetany, muscle cramps, stridor, carpopedal spasms, and convulsions. Lethargy, personality changes, and mental retardation are evident in chronic cases. Some patients show basal ganglia calcifications best seen on CT scan. The signs of Trousseau and Chvostek may also be present. Idiopathic hypoparathyroidism may be associated with candidiasis, Addison's disease, and thyroiditis due to an autoimmune disorder. The incidence of hypoparathyroidism occurs equally in both sexes and rarely is familial.

The major ocular manifestation in chronic hypoparathyroidism is cataract, characterized by numerous bilateral discrete polychromatic opacities, usually in the cortices and subcapsular zones of the lens. Other ocular complications may include keratoconjunctivitis, blepharospasm, photophobia and diplopia, papilledema, increased intracranial pressure (pseudotumor cerebri), and loss of eyebrows.

THERAPY

Systemic. Acute hypoparathyroidism usually occurs after thyroid surgery and requires immediate treatment. Intravenous infusion of 5 to 10 ml of 10 per cent calcium chloride or 10 to 20 ml of 10 per cent calcium gluconate (preferably dissolved in 500 to 1000 ml of 5 per cent dextrose in water) may be given until tetany ceases. Oral calcium salts and ergocalciferol or its more active analogs should be started as soon as possible to maintain the serum calcium level. Calcium carbonate is the oral calcium salt of choice, and 1 to 2 gm of calcium carbonate two to three times daily are sufficient. Alternatively, 8 gm of calcium gluconate[§] or 4 to 8 gm of calcium lactate[§] powder may be administered orally three times daily. Calcium citrate is better absorbed in most patients. Ergocalciferol may be administered in a daily dosage of 40,000 to 200,000 units (1 to 5 mg). In some patients, up to 7 or 8 mg of ergocalciferol may be needed daily. When a more rapid action is required to control severe hypocalcemia, crystalline dihydrotachysterol (DHT) in a dosage of 0.8 to 2.4 mg may be indicated. After several days, a daily dosage of 0.2 to 1.0 mg will usually maintain blood calcium at a normal level. In addition, daily administration of 10 to 20 ml of oral aluminum hydroxide may be given 1 hour after meals to help lower the serum phosphate level in the initial stage of treatment. In cases refractory to ergocalciferol or DHT, 50 to 100 μg of calcifediol[§] two times daily or preferably 0.25 μg of calcitriol[§] three to four times daily may be needed. Once calcium is normalized, lower doses of calcium, ergocalciferol, or DHT will maintain a normal calcium level. Chlorthalidone[‡] given in a dosage of 50 mg with a low-sodium diet can control mild hypoparathyroidism without the use of ergocalciferol.

Ocular. For ocular keratitis and keratoconjunctivitis, 0.5 or 1 per cent methylcellulose solution may be applied four times daily in combination with 1.5 per cent cortisone ointment every 4 hours to lubricate the eye artificially and to control inflammation.

Supportive. A high-calcium, low-phosphorus diet is important in the treatment of hypoparathyroidism. Patients should omit such foods as milk and cheese during acute hypoparathyroidism.

Surgical. Cataracts may remain stable if hypocalcemia is corrected. If a cataract matures, lens extraction may be performed. There is no apparent increase in postoperative complications compared with other surgery.

Ocular or Periocular Manifestations

Conjunctiva: Conjunctivitis.
Cornea: Epithelial defects; keratitis; nodules; pannus.
Eyebrows: Madarosis.
Eyelids: Blepharospasm; madarosis; ptosis.
Lens: Punctate opacities; subcapsular cataracts.
Optic Nerve: Edema; optic neuritis; papilledema.
Other: Diplopia; myopia; photophobia.

Precautions

Although the treatment of hypoparathyroidism with vitamin D is effective, it is hazardous because the patient's condition may so easily slip over into serious hypercalcemic toxicity. Hypervitaminosis D is a frequent complication of the treatment of hypoparathyroidism, and serum calcium must be monitored frequently and the dosage adjusted accordingly. In severe vitamin D intoxication, corticosteroids may be effective antidotes. Intravenous calcium chloride or calcium gluconate should not be overused to treat tetany or irreversible tissue calcification will occur. Phenothiazine drugs should be administered with caution in hypoparathyroid patients, since they may precipitate dystonic reactions.

Comments

In the prognosis of hypoparathyroidism, some changes may be reversible, but the dental changes, cataracts, and brain calcifications are permanent. Papilledema and increased intracranial pressure disappear with therapy.

The ease of misdiagnosing hypoparathyroidism with convulsion and papilledema as a brain tumor is apparent. The possibility of hypoparathyroidism should be borne in mind when cataracts develop in young children who may have few symptoms, except some mental changes.

References

Along U, Chau JC: Hypocalcemia from deficiency of and resistance to parathyoid hormones. Adv Pediatr 32:439, 1985.
Avioli LV: The therapeutic approach to hypoparathyroidism. Am J Med 57:34–42, 1974.
Bajandas FJ, Smith JL: Optic neuritis in hypoparathyroidism. Neurology 26:451–454, 1976.
Breslau NA, Pak CYC: Hypoparathyroidism. Metabolism 28:1261–1276, 1979.
Camargo CA, Kolb FO: Endocrine disorders. *In* Schroeder SA, et al (eds): Current Medical Diagnosis and Treatment. East Norwalk, CT/San Mateo, CA, Appleton & Lange, 1988, pp 708–711.
Hanno HA, Weiss DI: Hypoparathyroidism, pseudohypoparathyroidism, and pseudo-pseudohypoparathyroidism. Arch Ophthalmol 65:238–242, 1961.
Haussler MR, Cordy PE: Metabolites and analogues of vitamin D. Which for what? JAMA 247:841–844, 1982.
Nusynowitz ML, Frame B, Kolb FO: The spectrum of the hypoparathyroid states: A classification based on physiologic principles. Medicine 55:105–119, 1976.

Okano K, et al: Comparative efficacy of various vitamin D metabolites in the treatment of various types of hypoparathyroidism. J Clin Endocrinol Metab 55:238, 1982.

HYPOTHYROIDISM
(Cretinism, Hypothyroid Goiter, Juvenile Hypothyroidism, Myxedema)
HESKEL M. HADDAD, M.D.
New York, New York

Hypothyroidism is a disease caused by the lack or decrease in systemic thyroid hormones, which results from a deficiency of the thyroid gland or its function. Hypothyroidism may have different causes: 1) primary damage of the thyroid gland (loss of thyroid tissue), which may be congenital as in cretinism, secondary to surgery (thyroidectomy), following treatment with radioactive iodine, after thyroiditis or infectious diseases of the thyroid glands, such as mumps; 2) tumor infiltration of the thyroid gland, either primary or metastatic thyroid carcinoma; 3) or deficiency of iodine in the diet as in endemic goiter. Hypothyroidism could also be secondary to reduced stimulation of the thyroid gland by the pituitary, as in Simmonds' disease or following hypophysectomy, or may be associated with feedback suppression of the thyroid gland through the suppression of TSH (thyroid-stimulating hormones) secretion by the pituitary gland induced by the use of exogenous thyroid hormone. This mechanism is used in the treatment of hypothyroid goiter and occasionally in the management of thyroid nodules.

In infancy and childhood, generalized suppression of the body systems and growth, primarily bone formation, is found. Hypophyseal dysgenesis as recognized radiologically in the newborn is the first clinical sign of cretinism, even before the full-blown picture of the disease develops in the infant. Whereas the retardation of growth reduces weight gain in children, myxedema and swelling of the skin induce a weight gain in adults.

In hypothyroidism, the skin becomes dry and scaly, with yellowish discoloration due to increased carotene in the circulation (carotenemia). The skin is usually pale and cold. In myxedema, the skin appears edematous and thick. The edema may occasionally be localized on the tibia and other bony protuberances. Hair growth may be slowed. There is a retardation in the cuticular growth, especially of the nails and the hair of the armpits and face. This retardation is also manifested by thin brittle hair and alopecia. The mental processes may become dulled and cerebration slow. Mental retardation ensues in infants if the condition is not corrected promptly. The cardiovascular system is affected by bradycardia, hypotension, enlargement of the heart by myxedema, and decreased electrocardiographic parameters with poor circulation, which may further enhance the edema.

Ocular manifestations may include loss of the hair of the eyebrows, especially their temporal third or half. The lids become edematous, but in contrast to endocrine exophthalmos edema, the periorbital myxedema is intradermal with almost bullous formations of the skin. The conjunctiva becomes pale and appears gelatinous, in contrast to the chemosis and hyperemia noted in hyperthyroidism and Graves' disease. The sclera has a very grayish white appearance. There is marked sluggishness of the circulation by funduscopic examination with venostasis. In very rare conditions, an exophthalmos may develop, especially following thyroiditis or Hashimoto's struma. The intraocular pressure tends to be low but with tonography, there is an association of reduction in the outflow facility, as well as the intraocular pressure, which is directly related to the changes in the coefficient of scleral rigidity. There is also a decreased tear secretion resembling keratoconjunctivitis sicca.

THERAPY

Systemic. Management of hypothyroidism is established with thyroid replacement therapy. Although optimal dosage is determined by the patient's clinical response, replacement therapy in an adult can usually be satisfied with 195 mg of thyroglobulin (thyroid extract) daily. Alternatively, levothyroxine may be administered orally in a daily dosage of 0.1 to 0.3 mg or liothyronine in a daily dosage of 25 to 75 μg. Synthetic thyroid hormone derivatives are not recommended as initial therapy nor for use in children.

Ocular: Most of the ocular findings will clear after the systemic disease is treated. Topical ophthalmic lubricants containing methylcellulose or petrolatum may be useful for conjunctival irritation and blepharitis aggravated by lid edema. Carbonic anhydrase inhibitors, such as 125 to 250 mg of acetazolamide or 25 to 50 mg of methazolamide one to four times daily, may be useful to alleviate edema, as the treatment for hypothyroidism is advanced.

PRECAUTIONS

It is imperative that patients treated for myxedema or cretinism be given initial small doses of thyroglobulin to prevent induced cardiac stress and to alleviate the edema of the heart gradually and thus promote better circulation. Otherwise, such patients may develop sudden cardiac failure. Combinations of thyroid products are not recommended because of their higher biologic activity.

In those cases of hypothyroidism caused by failure of the pituitary, attention should be paid to treating the other hormonal deficiencies, particularly adrenal insufficiency. Treatment of the thyroid alone may precipitate severe Addison's disease and may be fatal.

COMMENTS

Usually, the prognosis of hypothyroidism is excellent if recognized and treated early. However, if not recognized and treated promptly in infancy, hypothyroidism can cause permanent mental retardation (cretinism). The association of diabetes with hypothyroidism may create another hazard to the health of the patient, especially if the thyroid is treated without the proper adjustment of diabetic control. The alleged incidence of cataract or glaucoma with hypothyroidism does not appear to be corroborated by current statistics.

References

Brownlie BEW, Newton OAG, Singh SP: Ophthalmopathy associated with primary hypothyroidism. Acta Endocrinol 79:691–699, 1975.

Haddad HM: Tonography and visual fields in endocrine exophthalmos: Report on 29 patients. Am J Ophthalmol 64:63–67, 1967.

Mahto RS: Ocular features of hypothyroidism. Br J Ophthalmol 56:546–549, 1972.

McDougall IR: Treatment of hyper- and hypothyroidism. J Clin Pharmacol 21:365–384, 1981.

Swanson JW, Kelly JJ Jr, McConahey WM: Neurologic aspects of thyroid dysfunction. Mayo Clin Proc 56:504–512, 1981.

Wortsman J, Wavak P: Palpebral redundancy from hypothyroidism. Plast Reconstr Surg 65:1–3, 1980.

SECTION 4

NUTRITIONAL DISORDERS

CROHN'S DISEASE
(Granulomatous Ileocolitis, Regional Enteritis, Terminal Ileitis)

DAVID L. KNOX, M.D.

Baltimore, Maryland

Crohn's disease and ulcerative colitis are the most common inflammatory bowel diseases. Regional enteritis, terminal ileitis, and granulomatous ileocolitis are synonyms that emphasize different features of Crohn's disease. The spotty or regional nature of the disorder affects the enteric canal anywhere from the esophagus to the rectum. It is felt by some that aphthous ulcers of the tongue and buccal mucosa are also a manifestation.

Deep focal ulceration of the mucosa, visualized either by proctosigmoidoscopy or on the surface of excised ileum, is a major feature of Crohn's disease. Some ulcers form fistulas from bowel to bowel, bowel to skin, or bowel to bladder or vagina. Histopathologically, ulcers and thickened gut wall contain acute and chronic inflammatory cells, most characteristically epithelioid and giant cells.

In contrast, ulcerative colitis is characterized by widespread surface ulceration, which may at times become fulminant and lead to perforation. Epithelioid and giant cells are not seen in tissue from patients with ulcerative colitis.

Etiologies have not been proven for either disease. However, Crohn's disease often occurs in siblings or several generations of family members who, like the patient, also have multiple allergies. Many of the patients were not breastfed or had colic and other troubles digesting cow's milk formula.

The initial symptoms are often quite mild, depending on the segment of intestine that is involved. Multiple symptoms of intestinal discomfort, excessive gas, and intermittent diarrhea, mistakenly classified as "irritable bowel syndrome," may precede for months or years an insidious or explosive onset of severe diarrhea, rectal bleeding, fever, malaise, and weight loss in the patient with Crohn's disease. Adolescents may have had an enigmatic failure to grow. The disease can begin at any age, but most cases present between 20 and 40 years of age, with onset in males a little earlier than females. In total, however, males equal females. The disease is protean, highly variable, unpredictable, and with different duration and recurrence patterns. There are some patients whose courses leave the clinician with the nagging feeling that the disease has burned itself out.

Diagnosis depends primarily on histopathology; however, clinical features determined by history, proctocolonoscopy, and radiologic features, such as the "string sign" in the terminal ileum, are the bases of many diagnoses.

Complications can occur with or without the obvious activity associated with Crohn's disease. These complications may also act as indicators of subclinical activity. The systemic complications of Crohn's disease include arthritis, erythema, nodosum, pyoderma gangrenosum, anemia, and amyloidosis. Because malnutrition and weight loss are an obvious result of bowel disease, they are not emphasized, although they are important in consideration of Crohn's disease. Ocular complications occur in about 10 per cent of patients with Crohn's disease and much less frequently in patients with ulcerative colitis.

Ocular complications can be divided into three groups. In the primary group are those complications directly associated with Crohn's disease. These complications occur with a high rate of frequency and respond to systemic therapy, such as corticosteroids, or surgical excision. The next group includes the secondary complications associated with Crohn's disease, and the third group contains the coincidental problems that occur so frequently in normal people that they are considered unrelated to the disease.

Primary ocular complications may include a specific epithelial and anterior stromal keratopathy, limbal corneal infiltrates, episcleritis, scleritis, acute iritis, chronic iridocyclitis, macular edema, papillitis, and orbital inflammation, which can produce proptosis, pain, and limited movement. Optic neuropathy with swelling or loss of vision or both can occur at the optic disc, in the intraorbital or intracranial nerve, and chiasm. Episcleritis is the most common ocular complication of Crohn's disease and represents both a diagnosis point in the differentiation of Crohn's from ulcerative colitis and an indicator of activity of the basic disease.

Secondary ocular complications include cataracts that are caused either by the prolonged use of corticosteroids or by chronic iridocyclitis. Also included in this category are refractive changes that occur when patients start or stop systemic corticosteroids. Exudative retinal detachment, optic disc edema secondary to posterior scleritis, scleromalacia, and *Candida* endophthalmitis from intravenous hyperalimentation have also been seen. Night blindness and dry eyes occur as the result of reduced vegetable intake, which patients follow because it relieves intestinal irritation or because absent or diseased ileum does not allow vitamins to be absorbed.

Coincidental ocular complications include conjunctivitis, recurrent corneal erosion, glaucoma, subconjunctival hemorrhage, and generalized retinal artery narrowing.

THERAPY

Systemic. Systemic corticosteroids are the most commonly used agents because of their standardization, availability, familiarity, and, most importantly, their effectiveness. At first, high doses rapidly reduce abdominal pain, nausea, fever, and diarrhea. Gradual tapering over weeks or months to maintenance doses brings stability to the patient. Sulfasalazine has been shown to be effective in long-term management of ulcerative colitis, and its use has been extended to patients with Crohn's disease. Cytotoxic agents, such as azathioprine‡, are used for patients whose disease does not respond to systemic corticosteroids.

Ocular. Treatment of ocular complications begins with identification of the type of complication. Primary complications require attention to the intestinal disease and clarification of its status. More aggressive treatment, either medically or surgically, may be indicated. The ophthalmologist must work closely with other practitioners. Acute iritis requires topical corticosteroids, cycloplegics, and, at times, systemic corticosteroids. Limbal corneal infiltrates and episcleritis frequently respond to topical steroids.

Chronic iridocyclitis in patients with Crohn's disease is a difficult problem. It is closely associated with active gut disease and has responded to excision of involved intestinal tissue. Systemic corticosteroids given for both disorders help, but are not curative. The characteristic keratopathy does not impair vision, is not painful, and therefore requires no therapy. Macular edema syndromes usually respond to systemic corticosteroids.

Secondary ocular complications first require the recognition of an intervening process. Dry eyes and night blindness are managed by giving the patient either parenteral or oral vitamin A. Exudative retinal detachment requires clarification as to whether it is secondary to scleritis or a remote abscess. Cataracts are managed according to their nature. Early posterior subcapsular opacities often stop progressing when systemic corticosteroids are discontinued. However, activity of the intestinal disease may require continuation of the corticosteroid. In young people, a visually disabling cataract is well managed by extracapsular, irrigation-aspiration techniques through a small limbal incision.

Papillitis from posterior scleritis usually responds to systemic corticosteroids. Endophthalmitis from either bacteria or fungi can be aggressively managed by diagnostic and therapeutic vitrectomy, which provides an organism for culture and removes the mass of infected vitreous. Appropriate antimicrobial therapy depends upon identification and sensitivity studies.

Coincidental ocular disease requires only that the ophthalmologist recognizes it as not being related to the intestinal disorder. Management is the same as for any patient.

Surgical. Surgical intervention is required for intestinal obstruction, abscess from rupture or fistula, large mass of inflamed ileum and adjacent tissue, severe pain, intractable rectal disease, or fistula alone. Some surgeons advise excision of the involved ileum in a patient whom other practitioners might elect to follow medically.

Supportive. General supportive measures, such as a liquid or low roughage diet, pain medication and antispasmodic drugs, give relief.

Precautions

After surgery, many patients do very well. Gut symptoms cease, extraintestinal complications (such as arthritis) subside, and the patients resume entirely normal lives. Other patients will intermittently be afflicted with the disease, requiring occasional medical or surgical management, and a few patients will continue to have relentless attacks of Crohn's disease.

Comments

Treatment of Crohn's disease is difficult, primarily because etiologic mechanisms have not been defined. Family physicians, internists, gastroenterologists, and general surgeons, all with slightly different educations, experiences, and psychologic natures, are the primary and secondary managers of these patients. In their desperation, patients often invoke the care of many different physicians.

An ophthalmologist should not try to manage these patients alone, but should work closely with other experienced practitioners. Management of a patient with an ocular complication of Crohn's disease is difficult and time consuming. Effort must be expended to clarify the status of the intestinal disease and to communicate with the other physicians involved. It is important to utilize the best diagnostic tools. CT scans of the head and abdomen and MRI of the head, orbit, and chiasm are often helpful.

References

Blase WP, Knox DL, Green WR: Granulomatous conjunctivitis in 2 patients with Crohn's disease. Br J Ophthalmol 68:901–903, 1984.

Hopkins DJ, et al: Ocular disorders in a series of 332 patients with Crohn's disease. Br J Ophthalmol 58:732–737, 1974.

Kirsner JB, Shorter RG: Recent developments in "nonspecific" inflammatory bowel disease. (First of two parts). N Engl J Med 306:775–785, 1982.

Kirsner JB, Shorter RG: Recent developments in nonspecific inflammatory bowel disease. (Second of two parts). N Engl J Med 306:837–848, 1982.

Knox DL, Bayless TM: Gastrointestinal and ocular disease. In Mausolf FA (ed): The Eye and Systemic

Disease, 2nd ed. St Lous, CV Mosby, 1980, pp 333–348.

Knox DL, Schachat AP, Mustonen E: Primary, secondary and coincidental ocular complications of Crohn's disease. Ophthalmology 91:163–173, 1984.

Knox DL, Snip RC, Stark WJ: The keratopathy of Crohn's disease. Am J Ophthalmol 90:862–865, 1980.

Macoul KL: Ocular changes in granulomatous ileocolitis. Arch Ophthalmol 84:95–97, 1970.

Schulman MF, Sugar A: Peripheral corneal infiltrates in inflammatory bowel disease. Ann Ophthalmol 13:109–111, 1981.

HYPOVITAMINOSIS A
(Xerophthalmia)

ALFRED SOMMER, M.D., M.H.Sc.

Baltimore, Maryland

Hypovitaminosis A is the presence of depleted tissue stores, usually reflected in low serum levels, of vitamin A. Most often, inadequate dietary intake is the cause. Interference with absorptive, storage, or transport capacities, such as in liver disease, sprue, cystic fibrosis, regional enteritis, and chronic gastroenteritis, can have the same effect. The primary ocular changes indicating vitamin A deficiency are night blindness and xerophthalmia. As a rule, these eye lesions tend to be most serious in the younger age groups, although night blindness is often difficult to substantiate in a small child.

THERAPY

Systemic. The primary treatment for hypovitaminosis A is rapid replenishment of vitamin A stores. In patients with normal absorptive and storage capacities, oral administration of 200,000 IU of vitamin A[§] in oil for 2 successive days, followed by an additional dose 1 to 2 weeks later, is adequate. In patients with severe gastroenteritis, the initial dose might preferably be intramuscular injections of 100,000 IU of vitamin A in water. Patients with severe protein-energy malnutrition require additional large oral doses every 1 to 2 weeks until protein status improves. Patients with persistent underlying malabsorption might be handled by repeated high dosages of oral therapy, with the adequacy determined by periodic serum vitamin A levels. Where this is ineffective, periodic parenteral administration of water-miscible vitamin A may be necessary.

Ocular. Corneal lesions frequently fail to respond to systemic therapy for 2 to 4 days. Although tretinoin is not licensed for use as a topical ophthalmic drug, 0.1 per cent tretinoin[*] in arachis oil applied three times daily will hasten corneal healing during the first critical days of therapy.

Corneal ulcers should be carefully observed and cultured to rule out secondary bacterial infections. Topical broad-spectrum antibiotic ointments may be applied several times daily as prophylaxis until healing is complete. Artificial tears may be used as needed. In children especially, a firm shield should protect ulcerated eyes.

Surgical. Classical vitamin-A-responsive lesions usually improve within 1 week of therapy, and most heal within 2 to 4 weeks. However, Bitot's spots that are not responsive to vitamin A may require simple excision.

Supportive. Adequate food intake, with particular reference to amount and quality of dietary protein and calories, is important.

Ocular or Periocular Manifestations

Conjunctiva: Bitot's spot; xerosis.
Cornea: Edema; erosion; haziness; keratomalacia; opacity; perforation; punctate keratitis; ulcer; xerosis.
Lacrimal System: Loss of tear film wetting action.
Retina: Degeneration; depigmentation; opacity.
Other: Night blindness; scotoma; visual loss.

Precautions

Care is required in the diagnosis of vitamin-A-specific conjunctival epithelial changes. Not every slight degree of dryness or thickening of the conjunctiva should be ascribed to vitamin A depletion. Severe corneal changes, especially ulceration and keratomalacia, often occur in the absence of milder signs of vitamin A deficiency (night blindness, conjunctival xerosis, Bitot's spots). Many patients with corneal involvement have severe generalized malnutrition or systemic diseases (gastroenteritis, tuberculosis) that interfere with vitamin A metabolism and wound healing and require immediate proper attention.

Under no circumstances should oil-miscible vitamin A be used for parenteral therapy. The vitamin is released slowly, if at all, from the injection site.

Use of topical ophthalmic tretinoin can lead to increased scarring and should be reserved for eyes with corneal xerosis, nonaxial ulcers, or for one eye of patients with axial ulcers in both.

Comments

The most sensitive test for vitamin A deficiency is measurement of dark adaptation. Determination of vitamin A concentration in the serum is less reliable, since the serum level may not fall below 0.2 µg/ml until the body's reserves are extensively depleted.

Many of these patients have inadequate aqueous tears, as well as a deficiency of goblet cells and mucus. Tears may be unable to spread over the epithelial surface and maintain a moist protective tear film. The corneal epithelium may be damaged by evaporation and can become susceptible to secondary bacterial infection.

References

Sommer A, Emran N: Topical retinoic acid in the treatment of corneal xerophthalmia. Am J Ophthalmol 86:615–617, 1978.

Sommer A, et al: Vitamin-A-responsive panocular xerophthalmia in a healthy adult. Arch Ophthalmol 96:1630–1634, 1978.

Sommer A, Emran N, Tamba T: Vitamin-A-responsive punctate keratopathy in xerophthalmia. Am J Ophthalmol 87:330–333, 1979.

Sommer A, et al: History of night blindness: A simple tool for xerophthalmia screening. Am J Clin Nutr 33:887–891, 1980.

Sommer A, et al: Oral versus intramuscular vitamin A in the treatment of xerophthalmia. Lancet 1:557–559, 1980.

Sommer A: Nutritional Blindness. New York, Oxford University Press, 1982.

Sommer A, Muhilal T, Tarwotjo I: Protein deficiency and treatment of xerophthalmia. Arch Ophthalmol 100:785–787, 1982.

SECTION 5

DISORDERS OF PROTEIN METABOLISM

CYSTINOSIS

RANDALL V. WONG, M.D.,
and VERNON G. WONG, M.D.
Washington, District of Columbia

Cystinosis is a rare, recessively inherited error of metabolism characterized by increased intracellular (nonprotein) levels of free cystine that appear to be localized within lysosomes. Cystine accumulates within the bone marrow, reticuloendothelial cells, kidneys, cornea, and conjunctiva. Three forms of cystinosis—nephropathic, intermediate, and benign (also known as infantile, adolescent, and adult)—have been described, and in all three forms crystal deposits develop in the cornea and conjunctiva.

The most severe form, nephropathic, becomes symptomatic in the first few years of life and is characterized by polyuria, polydipsia, progressive renal failure (Fanconi's syndrome), rickets, and growth retardation. Late in the course of nephropathic cystinosis, severe hypothyroidism, splenomegaly, and hepatomegaly may be seen at times. The intermediate form has variable renal failure and presents later in life. Death is common within the first decade in nephropathic cystinosis, whereas patients with benign cystinosis, true to its name, appear to have a normal life expectancy.

Ocular symptoms include photophobia and crystal deposits (tinsel-like and glistening) located in the cornea and conjunctiva. An early ocular finding is a peripheral pigmentary retinopathy that will progress to visual impairment.

THERAPY

Systemic. Therapeutic attempts to remove or reduce the cystine load in the cells, thereby reversing or retarding further damage, have been made with penicillamine[‡] and ascorbic acid,[‡] but have been found to be ineffective. Oral mercaptamine[†] at daily doses of 30 to 90 mg/kg appears to be of benefit when instituted early in the disease.

Mercaptamine has been shown to lower cystine levels in vitro and in vivo, and growth can be improved and renal deterioration delayed or prevented.

Ocular. Treatment of the photophobia associated with all forms of this disease is sympto-

matic. Dark glasses and avoidance of bright light are partially effective. Mercaptamine 0.1 per cent eyedrops have been shown to clear corneal crystals in a limited number of children.

Surgical. Treatment of renal failure associated with the nephropathic and intermediate forms has been achieved with renal transplant. The success of this method is sufficient to recommend it when renal failure supervenes.

Successful corneal transplantation has been achieved in one reported case, but recurrent crystal deposition may occur later.

Supportive. Adequate fluid intake, vitamin D supplements, and control of chronic acidosis and hypophosphatemia are important in the nephropathic and later in the intermediate forms of cystinosis. Dietary restriction of cystine and methionine is not effective.

Ocular or Periocular Manifestations

Choroid: Crystal deposits.
Conjunctiva: Crystal deposits.
Cornea: Crystal deposits (initially confined to anterior stroma, but progress to full thickness).
Iris: Crystal deposits.
Retina: Pigment epithelial degeneration (nephropathic form).
Other: Lacrimation; photophobia.

PRECAUTIONS

Mercaptamine therapy has been reported to cause reversible seizures in the higher dosage range of 90 mg/kg.

Long-term follow-up in renal transplant patients demonstrated progression of corneal crystal deposition, as well as progressive retinal pigment degeneration involving the posterior pole and occasionally the macula. Decrease in visual acuity has also been documented. It would appear that, although renal transplant prolongs life, it does not halt progression of the disease.

COMMENTS

The ophthalmologist commonly makes the diagnosis of cystinosis by noting the deposition of crystals in the cornea and conjunctiva, but multiple myeloma may also present a similar appearance. The diagnosis of cystinosis can be confirmed by an assay of cystine content of a conjunctival biopsy specimen, cultured skin fibroblasts, or polymorphonuclear leukocytes. A pulse-label technique can be used with amniotic cells to provide an in utero diagnosis of the homozygote state. The heterozygote state can also be detected, but cystine values may overlap normal values.

References

Gahl WA, et al: Cystinosis: Progress in a prototypic disease. Ann Intern Med 109:557–569, 1988.
Kaiser-Kupfer MI, et al: Removal of corneal crystals by topical cysteamine in nephropathic cystinosis. N Engl J Med 316:775–779, 1987.
Kaiser-Kupfer MI, et al: Clear graft two years later after keratopathy in nephropathic cystinosis. Am J Ophthalmol 105:318–319, 1988.
Katz B, et al: Recurrent crystal deposition after keratopathy in nephropathic cystinosis. Am J Ophthalmol 104:190–191, 1987.
Sanderson PO, et al: Cystinosis: A clinical, histopathologic, and ultrastructural study. Arch Ophthalmol 91:270–274, 1974.
Schneider JA, Schulman JD, Seegmiller JE: Cystinosis and the Fanconi syndrome. In Stanbury JB, Wyngaarden JB, Frederickson DS (eds): The Metabolic Basis of Inherited Disease, 4th ed. New York, McGraw-Hill, 1978, pp 1660–1682.
Wong VG: Ocular manifestations in cystinosis. Birth Defects 12:181–186, 1976.
Wong VG, Lietman PS, Seegmiller JE: Alterations of pigment epithelium in cystinosis. Arch Ophthalmol 77:361–369, 1967.
Yamamoto GK, et al: Long-term ocular changes in cystinosis: Observations in renal transplant recipients. J Pediatr Ophthalmol Strabismus 16:21–25, 1979.

HOMOCYSTINURIA

RAPHAEL S. BLOCH, M.D.
Mount Kisco, New York

Homocystinuria is a genetically determined error of the metabolism of methionine, one of the essential amino acids. The disorder is most commonly caused by the absence or deficiency of cystathionine beta-synthase, an enzyme active in one step of the catabolic pathway through which methionine is ultimately degraded to cysteine. As a consequence of this biochemical defect, there are increased concentrations of methionine and homocyst(e)ine in body fluids and diminished concentrations of cysteine. Elevated tissue levels of homocyst(e)ine are postulated to be responsible for the extensive connective tissue abnormalities observed in this disease. Homocystinuria is inherited by the autosomal recessive mode, but there is considerable heterogeneity in both its biochemical and clinical expressivity. Nearly half of the patients retain a small but measurable amount of beta-synthase activity; this group is less severely affected and more responsive to therapy than those with total absence of the enzyme.

The clinical signs of homocystinuria are not apparent at birth. Beginning in early childhood, however, there is progressive involvement of the eye and nervous, skeletal, and vascular systems. Developmental delays may be detected in the first year, e.g., failure to sit or crawl in the appropriate age range. Mental retardation is evident by mid-childhood in about half of all patients. Subluxation of the lens occurs by the age of 10 in most cases, is usually bilateral, and is often the diagnostic feature of this disease. In later childhood, the patients are typically tall and thin, blond and blue-eyed, with elongated digits, knock-knees, and diffuse osteoporosis on x-ray. The most ominous complication of homocystinuria is the propensity to thromboembolism. This may occur at any age, can involve both the arterial and venous vasculature of any organ, and results in a mortality rate of approximately 25 per cent before age 30.

THERAPY

Systemic. Initially, the only therapy for homocystinuria was nutritional, i.e., restriction of dietary intake of methionine and supplementation with oral cystine. Several low-methionine "medical foods," formulated from both natural and synthetic sources, are commercially available. Such a regimen has been effective in preventing or ameliorating some of the complications of homocystinuria, including the rate of lens dislocation.

At present, pharmacologic doses of pyridoxine,[§] ranging up to 1.2 gm daily, are tired in all cases. Pyridoxine is a co-factor for the deficient enzyme, and its administration results in marked biochemical improvement within several weeks in a significant percentage of patients. Responsiveness to pyridoxine is strongly correlated with detectable residual cystathionine beta-synthase activity. Current studies suggest that, in responsive patients, pyridoxine is effective in reducing the incidence of thromboembolic events, as well as lens dislocation.

For those individuals not responsive to pyridoxine, an alternative approach to management is the use of chemical agents that reverse the catabolic degradation of methionine, thereby preventing the buildup of homocysteine to toxic levels. Betaine,[§] in doses of 6 gm daily, has been successfully employed for this purpose, with substantial biochemical and clinical improvement.

Ocular. Refractive errors should be treated with conventional optical correction for as long as possible. Acute glaucoma caused by incarceration of the ectopic lens in the pupil is an emergency condition and is preferably managed with mydriasis and pressure on the cornea with the patient supine in order to reposition the lens in the posterior chamber. This treatment should be followed by miotic therapy to help retain the lens behind the pupil and a peripheral iridotomy (laser or surgical) to prevent subsequent episodes of pupillary block. In the event that the lens cannot be dislodged, it is advisable to perform the iridotomy and then repeat the repositioning procedure.

Surgical extraction of the dislocated lens is usually a procedure of last resort for impaired vision or pupillary block, as it carries a high risk of vitreous loss and hemorrhage.

Ocular or Periocular Manifestations

Globe: Buphthalmos; posterior staphyloma.
Lens: Subluxation; dislocation; spherophakia; cataract.
Optic Nerve: Atrophy.
Retina: Peripheral cystoid degeneration; peripheral pigmentary degeneration; retinal detachment; retinal artery occlusion.
Uvea: Pigment atrophy of iris and choroid.
Other: Myopia; glaucoma with or without pupillary block; strabismus.

PRECAUTIONS

There is significant morbidity and mortality from thromboembolism following all surgery in homocystinuria, including ophthalmic procedures. The risk is greatest with general anesthesia, which is usually mandatory for young or retarded patients; local anesthesia is also dangerous when it is injected in proximity to important blood vessels. Optimal perioperative management includes adequate hydration, reduction of blood viscosity and platelet adhesiveness with infusion of dextran, and early postoperative ambulation. Conventional anticoagulant therapy is not advisable, but a regimen of dipyridamole or aspirin to inhibit platelet aggregation may be helpful in the postoperative period.

COMMENTS

Early diagnosis and treatment are the keys to effective prevention of the complications of homocystinuria. Mass neonatal screening programs have successfully detected this and several other treatable metabolic diseases. Because of the relatively early appearance of ocular abnormalities, particularly lens subluxation, the ophthalmologist can play a critical role in the diagnosis and management of this sight-threatening and life-threatening disorder.

References

Cross H, Jensen A: Ocular manifestations in the Marfan syndrome and homocystinuria. Am J Ophthalmol 75:405–420, 1973.

Elsas L, Acosta P: Nutrition support of inherited metabolic diseases. In Shils M, Young V (eds): Modern Nutrition in Health and Disease, 7th ed. Philadelphia, Lea & Febiger, 1988, pp 1363–1367.

Mudd S, Levy H: Disorders of transsulfuration. *In* Stanbury J, et al. (eds): The Metabolic Basis of Inherited Disease, 5th ed. New York, McGraw-Hill, 1983, pp 522–559.

Mudd S, et al: The natural history of homocystinuria due to cystathionine beta-synthase deficiency. Am J Hum Genet 37:1–31, 1985.

Parris W, Quimby C: Anesthetic considerations for the patient with homocystinuria. Anesth Analg 61:708–710, 1982.

Wilcken D, et al: Homocystinuria—The effects of betaine in the treatment of patients not responsive to pyridoxine. N Engl J Med 309:448–453, 1983.

MAPLE SYRUP URINE DISEASE
(Branched-Chain Ketoaciduria, MSUD)

LAWRENCE G. TOMASI, M.D., Ph.D.

Loma Linda, California

Maple syrup urine disease (MSUD) is an autosomal recessive disorder characterized by a marked elevation in branched-chain amino acids (leucine, isoleucine, and valine) and their respective ketoacids in the serum. The disease derives its name from the odor similar to maple sugar (burned sugar) in the urine. The enzymatic defect is in the oxidative decarboxylation of these ketoacids by a high-molecular-weight multienzyme complex that involves five closely linked enzymatic reactions and multiple co-factors, including thiamine and lipoic acid. The variability in the symptomatology of the disorder has been correlated with the level of residual enzymatic activity. Currently, the enzymatic abnormalities in MSUD are grouped as follows: 1) classical, 2) intermittent, 3) intermediate, 4) thiamine-responsive, and 5) E_3-deficient phenotypes. These variant groups represent mutations that involve different reactions in the multienzyme complex or, alternatively, may be multiple alleles for a single genetic locus.

The more classical presentations include initial symptoms of poor weight gain, vomiting, lethargy, and seizures that are related to the elevated blood levels of the branched-chain amino acids and their metabolites, particularly leucine. Although leucine-induced hypoglycemia commonly accompanies the metabolic derangement, the mechanisms by which central nervous system injury occurs remain uncertain. Postulated mechanisms include an inhibition of protein synthesis secondary to the disturbed free amino acid pool and/or an inhibition of glutamic acid decarboxylation by the elevated branched-chain ketoacids, leading to altered levels of the putative neurotransmitter gamma-aminobutyric acid (GABA).

Late signs of central nervous system injury include generalized increased muscle tone, opisthotonus, coma, microcephaly, and severe psychomotor delay, with death occurring in untreated patients secondary to an intercurrent infection. In those with classical MSUD, death may occur in the first week of life and almost certainly within the first year.

Neuropathologic studies on patients succumbing during the first month of life demonstrate only a sponginess of the white matter attributed to edema. In those patients who survive well into the first year, a deficiency in myelin and an astrocytosis are noted that are similar to that described in patients with other aminoacidopathies, such as phenylketonuria. These nonspecific alterations within the central nervous system reflect a delay in myelinogenesis, rather than defective synthesis or increased destruction of the myelin. More recently, these neuropathologic findings can be demonstrated antemortem by CT scan or magnetic resonance imaging (MRI). Mild to moderate atrophy with a marked diffuse, low-density attenuation of the white matter has been described in both the cerebellum and the cerebral hemispheres. In addition, abnormalities of the gray matter within the globus pallidus as well as the thalamus are described, a finding that may be unique to MSUD. A reversibility of these abnormalities within the gray matter has been reported after dietary treatment. Status spongiosus, together with dysmyelination, is the pathologic counterpart of the CT and MRI abnormalities.

Increasingly, variants of MSUD have been reported in which intermittent central nervous system dysfunction occurs, rather than the overwhelming illness of the classical disease. Age of onset in these patients is usually in the first decade of life, but has been reported at 40 years of age, with intermittent episodes of lethargy, nystagmus, ataxia, and seizures usually in association with an intercurrent infectious illness. Two recent reports reflect this variability. The mother of a child with intermittent MSUD, and thus an obligatory carrier of the trait, demonstrated neurologic symptoms at 40 years of age that were responsive to dietary therapy. A 15-year follow-up of an infant with thiamine-responsive MSUD reported that the adolescent had a normal social life and attended a regular high school. She exhibited neither epilepsy nor behavioral abnormalities, and her current IQ was 85 on the WISC-R. She had experienced five episodes of metabolic decompensation over this 15-year period with clinical symptomatology of seizures and coma, one of which was of sufficient severity to require peritoneal dialysis.

In such patients, the characteristic elevation in serum and urine branched-chain amino acids and ketoacids is present, although these abnormalities may not be discernible during symptom-free intervals. Confirmation of the diagnosis by direct assay of the branched-chain oxidative decarboxylase activity in either white cells or cultured fibroblasts of patients is possible either during an acute attack or during symptom-free intervals. In general, age of onset and severity of symptoms are related to residual enzymatic activity; classical MSUD patients demonstrating less than 2 per cent of normal activity whereas those with the mildest symptoms have enzymatic activity levels of between 8 and 15 per cent of normal values. Recent studies have precluded a defect in either the transcription of DNA or the processing of RNA in selected cultures of MSUD fibroblasts.

Ocular manifestations have been reported in both classical MSUD and its variants. Their incidence and prevalence, however, are markedly increased in the variant forms perhaps because such signs in classical MSUD are masked by a severe encephalopathy. In contrast to other inborn errors of metabolism in which complex sphingolipids accumulate from conception within the lysosome (i.e., Tay-Sachs disease), these branched-chain amino acids are readily removed from the fetus via the placenta during gestation. Thus, symptoms of MSUD are absent at birth, may become apparent within the first week of life, and fluctuate with both the infant's protein intake and general metabolic status. The commonly noted decreased visual attentiveness on initial presentation is almost certainly due to cerebral cortical rather than ocular dysfunction, with its severity related to the infant's level of consciousness. The optic atrophy described in the older untreated patients has a gray rather than a white hue, reflecting the generalized defect in myelination described throughout the central nervous system, as demonstrated neuropathologically by Franke and co-workers. Disturbances in ocular movements include gaze paresis either upward, combined vertical and horizontal, or adductor. Ptosis and sluggish pupillary light reaction also are commonly reported signs. Nystagmus is a frequently reported finding with the initial clinical symptomatology and also during the recovery phase with treatment. As an initial finding in these patients, it may represent the subtle seizures that are described with the encephalopathy. During recovery, it should not be confused with the progression of the neurologic symptoms. The localization of the dysfunction within the neuro-ophthalmologic pathways is unclear, but diffuse cerebral edema, subtle seizures, and a thiamine-dependent variant should have a greater consideration in the differential diagnosis.

THERAPY

Systemic. Since the branched-chain amino acids cannot be synthesized in animals, therapy of MSUD, as in other aminoacidopathies, is based on dietary control of these essential amino acids. Unlike phenylketonuria, however, such dietary control must be lifelong. In classical MSUD, an amino acid mixture tailored to the patient's weight and growth potential is utilized, whereas patients with the variant form require less stringent dietary control. Frequently, at the time that the diagnosis is initially made, the levels of the branched-chain amino acids and ketoacids are extremely elevated, which produces severe neurologic symptoms and signs that may be life threatening. A similar picture occurs episodically in patients on a prescribed diet or in those with a variant form, usually during an intercurrent illness. As a rule, parenterally administered fluids containing glucose and electrolytes, followed by an amino acid diet in which the branched-chain amino acids are omitted,

140 / MAPLE SYRUP URINE DISEASE

will reverse these findings. Occasionally, this standard regimen is unsatisfactory, and an exchange transfusion or peritoneal dialysis may be lifesaving.

Ocular. Strabismus therapy may require glasses, patching, or surgery. Ptosis surgery may be indicated if warranted by the cosmetic or functional deficit.

Ocular or Periocular Manifestations

Extraocular Muscles: Nystagmus; ophthalmoplegia.
Eyebrows or Eyelids: Elevation; epicanthal folds; ptosis.
Optic Nerve: Atrophy.
Pupil: Decreased or absent reaction to light.
Other: Convergent strabismus; cortical visual inattentiveness.

Precautions

Early diagnosis and dietary treatment are imperative to prevent mental retardation and death. In classical MSUD, generalized systemic symptoms are more prominent that the ocular manifestations. On the other hand, ophthalmoplegia is a relatively uncommon sign in the newborn nursery and has been the initial feature in many infants who become symptomatic during the neonatal period and early infancy. An easily obtainable and rapid screening test for urinary ketoacids utilizing 2,4-dinitrophenylhydrazine is available in most hospitals. Although more specific assays are necessary to establish the diagnosis, this screening test remains useful because of its widespread availability and infrequent false-negative results.

The ophthalmologist is more likely to be confronted with one of the variant forms of MSUD or the patient whose classical MSUD is under treatment but has decompensated with the metabolic stress of an infectious illness. In either case, both the ocular manifestations and biochemical abnormalities will only be present during the period of decompensation. Thus, the screening test for urinary ketoacids will be a useful addition to the diagnostic studies utilized in the evaluation of these ocular manifestations.

Comments

The mean incidence of MSUD from various studies is 1 : 250,000. Although dietary treatment prolongs life and prevents mental retardation, such patients are exceedingly difficult to manage in comparison to those with the more commonly encountered phenylketonuria, which has a disease incidence of 1 : 13,000. In the United States, all 50 states screen for phenylketonuria, whereas 20 states presently are screening for MSUD. Difficulties in management include the necessity to balance three amino acids in the diet, their ubiquitous presence in food from which they cannot be removed, frequent life-threatening decompensations that occur in patients while on treatment, and the apparent need to continue dietary management throughout the life span. Computerized-assisted dietary management plans have been reported for both infants and adults.

Although screening the population for heterozygotes has not proven feasible because of the rarity of this condition, antepartum diagnosis is available to families who are at risk because of an affected child. The enzyme is normally present in fibroblasts grown from amniotic fluid cells, and affected fetuses have been identified in utero.

References

Chabria S, Tomasi LG, Wong PWK: Ophthalmoplegia and bulbar palsy in variant form of maple syrup urine disease. Ann Neurol 6:71–72, 1979.

Ellingsen LI, Haugstad TS, Holm H: Tailoring of the diet for the individual in maple syrup urine disease: Long-term home dietary treatment of an adult patient with MSUD by monitoring of daily intake with a personal computer. A case report. Hum Nutr Appl Nutr 39A:130–136, 1985.

Franke G, et al: Ophthalmologische und histopathologische befunde bei Ahornsirup-Krankheit. Ophthalmology 80:457–459, 1983.

Holmgren G, et al: Intermittent neurological symptoms in a girl with a maple syrup urine disease (MSUD) variant. Neuropediatrics 11:377–383, 1980.

Hu CW, et al: Isolation and sequencing of a cDNA encoding the decarboxylase (E1) alpha precursor of bovine branched-chain alpha-keto acid dehydrogenase complex. Expression of E1 alpha mRNA and subunit in maple-syrup-urine-disease and 3T3-L1 cells. J Biol Chem 263:9007–9014, 1988.

Mantovani JF, et al: MSUD: Presentation with pseudotumor cerebri and CT abnormalities. J Pediatr 96:279–281, 1980.

Naughten ER, et al: Early diagnosis and dietetic management in newborn with maple syrup urine disease. Birth to six weeks. J Inherited Metab Dis 8(Suppl 2):131–132, 1985.

Paul TD, Naylor EW, Guthrie R: Urine screening for metabolic disease in newborn infants. J Pediatr 96:653–656, 1980.

Schriver CR, et al: So-called thiamine-responsive maple syrup urine disease: 15-year follow-up of the original patient. J Pediatr 107:763–765, 1985.

Suzuki S, et al: Cranial computed tomography in a patient with a variant form of maple syrup urine disease. Neuropediatrics 14:102–103, 1983.

Tanaka K, Rosenberg LE: Disorders of branched chain amino acid and organic acid metabolism. *In* Stanbury JB, et al (ed): The Metabolic Basis of Inherited Disease, 5th ed. New York, McGraw-Hill, 1983, pp 440–473.

Taylor D: Ophthalmological features of some human hereditary disorders with demyelination. Bull Soc Belge Ophthalmol 208:405–413, 1983.

Uziel G, Savoiardo M, Nardocci N: CT and MRI in maple syrup urine disease. Neurology 38:486–488, 1988.

OCULOCEREBRORENAL SYNDROME
(Lowe's Syndrome)

ANDREA CIBIS TONGUE, M.D.
Portland, Oregon

Lowe's syndrome is an x-linked recessive metabolic disorder characterized by congenital cataracts, glaucoma, hypotonic facies with frontal bossing and deep-set eyes, mental and motor retardation, muscular hypotonia, areflexia, hyperexcitability, and secondary proximal renal tubular acidosis with proteinuria, aminoaciduria, metabolic acidosis, inability to acidify urine, rickets, and osteomalacia. The disease process can be divided into three stages. Ocular abnormalities and proteinuria may be the only stigmata present during early infancy. Aminoaciduria may not be present until 1 year of age or later. Neurologic abnormalities likewise are often not striking during the first year, but are noted in all affected infants over 1 year of age. Metabolic abnormalities appear during the second stage and can be ameliorated by supportive systemic therapy. During the third stage, metabolic abnormalities may disappear, and systemic therapy may no longer be necessary. Joint dislocation and scoliosis can develop secondary to hypotonia and joint hypermobility. Mental retardation may not be severe, and IQs in the 70s and 80s have been reported.

THERAPY

Systemic. Supportive treatment is aimed at correcting the metabolic abnormalities caused by the proximal renal tubular malfunction. Although the specific biochemical defect has not been elucidated, the finding of undersulfated chondroitin sulfate A in the urine of patients with Lowe's syndrome points to a possible defect in glycosaminoglycan metabolism. Alkali therapy, correction of electrolyte imbalance, and supplements of vitamin D ameliorate the metabolic acidosis, rickets, and osteomalacia.

Surgical. Removal of dense cataracts is indicated in hopes of preventing marked visual impairment. The surgeon should be prepared to perform a posterior capsulotomy and anterior vitrectomy, since the flat discoid lenses are strongly adherent to the anterior vitreous in many patients.

Management of glaucoma is essentially the same as for other types of congenital or infantile glaucomas. The etiology of glaucoma is not clear, but in some patients, it may be secondary to angle anomalies or to pupillary block.

Corneal keloid formation in older children may cause significant visual impairment, initiating an attempt at corneal surgery. Keloids, however, recur and are a most difficult management problem. Exposure and trauma to the epithelium may be contributing factors to the keloid formation, since they are typically in the lower half to two thirds of the cornea. Rarely, they may be seen in the superior cornea, which is covered by the upper lid. Several months after cataract surgery, one patient was observed to develop keloid formation at the entry site of the irrigation cannula in the inferior temporal cornea adjacent to the limbus. Another patient developed keloids after persistent punctate epithelial keratitis of the inferior cornea secondary probably to exposure and recurrent staphylococcal keratitis. This raises the question as to whether corneal incisions should be avoided in these patients.

Spectacle correction of the aphakia may be preferable to contact lens correction because of the need to minimize corneal epithelial trauma. Likewise, efforts should be made to minimize corneal exposure; partial tarsorrhaphy may be helpful.

Ocular or Periocular Manifestations

Anterior Chamber: Embryonic angle.
Cornea: Edema; keloid formation; megalocornea, microcornea (rare); opacity; pannus; thickened Descemet's membrane.
Globe: Buphthalmos; microphthalmos.
Iris or Ciliary Body: Atrophy; hypoplasia and segmental aplasia of dilator pupillae muscle; poorly developed ciliary muscle; posterior synechiae; rudimentary ciliary processes.
Lens: Cataracts, microphakia; posterior lenticonus.
Orbit: Retina: Lange's folds; sclerosis and hyalinization of retinal vessels.
Other: Glaucoma; miosis; nystagmus; strabismus.

PRECAUTIONS

Any male infant with congenital cataracts should be suspected of having Lowe's syndrome. It is important to remember that proteinuria may be the only other early manifestation of the disorder. Typically, the lenticular opacities are flat, discoid, and central. Often, the pupil is miotic and resistant to mydriatics. Glaucoma is not a necessary accompaniment of the disease, but occurs in about 50 per cent of the patients. In older children, degenerative changes of the cornea with vascularization and keloid formation are significant factors in causing further visual impairment.

COMMENTS

Prompt recognition of the disease is necessary for the institution of appropriate systemic therapy and amelioration of the metabolic abnormalities. Genetic counseling with identification of possible carrier females is important. Identification of the carrier females is dependent on thorough pedigree analysis and careful ocular slitlamp examination. Carrier females have increased numbers of cortical fleck opacities (greater than 15 per quadrant) and subcapsular plaques. The lens changes may be progressive and can increase with age. A significant number of carriers also have posterior subcapsular plaques. Some carrier females require relatively early cataract extraction.

Linkage studies have also been shown to be helpful in identifying carrier females in a number of families. The locus for Lowe's syndrome is at Xq25 and is tightly flanked by DXS42 and DXS10. Females at risk for the carrier state of Lowe's syndrome therefore should have slitlamp examinations, preferably after age of 10 and again at age 15 (lens opacities may not be present before then, and linkage studies, especially if the slitlamp examination is negative. Slitlamp examinations in one study were positive in 87 per cent of females identified as carriers by linkage analysis. Positive slitlamp examinations were not present in females who were negative by linkage study. If the slitlamp examination is positive for lens changes of the carrier state, that female is at 50 per cent risk of passing on the gene to each offspring. The risk of producing a carrier female is 1:4 for each pregnancy and 1:2 for each female offspring. The risk of an affected male is 1:4 for each pregnancy, and the risk of being affected is 1:2 for each male offspring. Unaffected males do not carry the gene and will not produce affected offspring.

References

Abbassi V, Lowe C, Calcagno PL: Oculo-cerebro-renal syndrome. A review. Am J Dis Child 115:145–168, 1968.

Brown N, Gardner RJM: Lowe syndrome: Identification of the carrier state. Birth Defects 13:579–595, 1976.

Cibis G, et al: Corneal keloid in Lowe's syndrome. Arch Ophthalmol 100:1795–1799, 1982.

Cibis G, et al: Lenticular opacities in carriers of Lowe's syndrome. Ophthalmology 93:1041–1045, 1986.

Reilly D, et al: Tightly linked flanking markers for the Lowe oculocerebrorenal syndrome, with application to carrier assessment. Am J Hum Genet 42:748–755, 1988.

Tongue A: Lowe's syndrome with particular reference to the carrier state. Trans Pac Coast Otoophthalmol Soc 53:219–227, 1972.

Wappner R: Update: Lowe's syndrome. Compr Ther 13:3–4, 1987.

TYROSINEMIA II
(Pseudodendritic Keratitis, Recessive Keratosis Palmoplantaris, Richner-Hanhart Syndrome, Tyrosinosis)

ROBERT P. BURNS, M.D.

Columbia, Missouri

Tyrosinemia II is an autosomal recessive genetic disease involving distinct metabolic abnormalities, namely, increased tyrosine levels in plasma and urine. It is associated with a charac-

teristic clinical syndrome of eye and skin lesions, which usually occur during the first months of life, although later onset has occurred. Skin lesions, varying from erosions to hyperkeratotic crusted lesions, are almost always limited to the palms and soles, although the knees and elbows may also be involved. These lesions are most prominent on the tips of the fingers, hypothenar eminences, and heels. These lesions may appear and disappear over the course of several days and are invariably painful. Normally, eye and skin lesions are present at the same time. Mental retardation is often present in untreated patients; however, if treatment is given early in the disease, mental retardation may be minimal or absent. Other less common findings in tyrosinemia II may include seizure disorders, multiple congenital anomalies, periodontia, dystrophy of nails, and hypotrichosis.

Common ocular manifestations include corneal erosions, severe keratitis, corneal ulcers, discrete conjunctival plaques and papillary hypertrophy, photophobia, ocular pain, and lacrimation. Neovascularization of the cornea may occur in more advanced lesions; patients with advanced inactive disease have reported nystagmus and subcapsular dots and opacities in the lens. Blindness may occur in untreated patients.

Because of the branching nature of the corneal epithelial lesions caused by tyrosine crystal precipitation in the epithelium with lysosomal enzyme release, herpes simplex dendritic keratitis is most often confused with tyrosinemia II. Bilateralism, early age of onset, and absence of herpes virus aid in making the correct diagnosis.

THERAPY

Systemic. Therapy in tyrosinemia II is primarily dietary. A low tyrosine, low phenylalanine diet (Mead-Johnson 3200 AB diet, containing 80 mg phenylalanine and 40 mg tyrosine/100 gm) usually results in an immediate decrease in the tyrosine level and gradual resolution of skin and eye lesions. After these lesions have been brought under control, the diet can be liberalized somewhat. Maintenance therapy consists of a liberalized 3200 AB diet plus small amounts of regular food; blood tyrosine levels are checked monthly and maintained at three to four times normal levels.

Ocular. Since the primary treatment is dietary, ocular care is symptomatic and protective until the basic underlying metabolic defect can be corrected in part. Topical ocular therapy with corticosteroids or antibiotics has no effect on the corneal lesions. Rarely, conjunctival flaps and electrodesiccation have been used in the management of corneal lesions due to tyrosinemia II. However, the eye lesions usually markedly improve with dietary therapy, and treatment of the corneal lesions is seldom necessary. Polymorphonuclear leukocytes have been implicated as playing a role in the corneal lesions.

Ocular or Periocular Manifestations

Conjunctiva: Discrete plaques; hyperemia; mucous discharge; papillary hypertrophy.
Cornea: Clouding; dendritic erosion; epithelial ridges; haze; keratitis; mucous discharge; plaques; neovascularization.
Lens: Subcapsular opacity.
Other: Nystagmus; ocular pain; photophobia; visual loss.

PRECAUTIONS

Early diagnosis is of paramount importance for effective treatment of tyrosinemia II. Knowledge of the degree of phenotypic variability and the various clinical features of the syndrome is essential for pediatricians, ophthalmologists, and dermatologists, since clinical suspicion is usually necessary before amino acid studies are performed. Without early diagnosis and treatment, severe mental retardation, permanent neurologic damage, and blindness may commonly occur.

COMMENTS

Tyrosinemia I is a rare metabolic defect of recessive inheritance with manifestations of splenomegaly, hepatomegaly, cirrhosis, fever, edema, vomiting, renal glycosuria, gross generalized aminoaciduria, phosphaturia, and rickets. Patients with this disorder do not have the characteristic skin and eye lesions of tyrosinemia II.

References

Burns RP, Gipson IK, Murray MJ: Keratopathy in tyrosinemia. Birth Defects 12:169–180, 1976.
Charlton KH, et al: Pseudodendritic keratitis and systemic tyrosinemia. Ophthalmology 88:355–360, 1981.
Geeraets WJ: Ocular Syndromes, 3rd ed. Philadelphia, Lea & Febiger, 1976, p 212.
Gipson IK, Burns RP, Wolfe-Lande JD: Crystals in corneal epithelial lesions of tyrosine-fed rats. Invest Ophthalmol 14:937–941, 1975.
Goldsmith LA, Reed J: Tyrosine-induced eye and skin lesions. A treatable genetic disease. JAMA 236:382–384, 1976.
Ripple RE, et al: Role of leukocytes in ocular inflammation of tyrosinemia II. Invest Ophthalmol Vis Sci 27:926–931, 1986.

SECTION 6

DISORDERS OF CARBOHYDRATE METABOLISM

DIABETES MELLITUS

SURESH R. CHANDRA, M.D.

Madison, Wisconsin

Diabetes mellitus is a complex disorder of carbohydrate, lipid, and protein metabolism characterized clinically by hyperglycemia and relative or absolute lack of insulin. It is a common disorder that is prevalent worldwide. In the United States, the prevalence of diabetes is 2 per cent of the population. These figures are based on known diabetic patients and do not include the large reservoir of undiagnosed diabetics. The development of diabetes is influenced by multiple factors, both genetic and environmental. The disease may develop in the first and second decades of life (type I) or in middle and late life (type II); more than half of the diabetic individuals above the age of 40 years are overweight. It occurs more commonly in females than males (3 : 2), and a family history of diabetes is positive in 25 per cent of patients. The disease is generally transmitted as a recessive trait without sex linkage.

Although the discovery of insulin has led to increased longevity of diabetics, the longer duration of the disease is associated with an increased incidence of secondary complications, consisting of accelerated atherosclerosis and a triad of retinopathy, nephropathy, and neuropathy.

Diabetic retinopathy is the second leading cause of new blindness and the leading cause of blindness in adults under the age of 65 in the United States. The prevalence of diabetic retinopathy is strongly related to the duration of diabetes. The prevalence of clinically detectable diabetic retinopathy is less than 25 per cent in patients with less than 5 years duration of diabetes, about 50 per cent when diabetes has been present for 5 to 15 years, and exceeds 75 per cent in patients who have had diabetes for more than 15 years. There is evidence to suggest a strong relationship between hyperglycemia and incidence and progression of diabetic retinopathy.

THERAPY

Systemic. Adult-onset diabetic patients whose diabetes cannot be controlled with diet alone or those who are unwilling or unable to adhere to a restrictive diet can be controlled with oral hypoglycemic agents or insulin. Oral hypoglycemic agents are useful only in adult-onset diabetics (type II). Tolbutamide (1.5 gm twice a day), acetohexamide (750 mg twice a day), and chlorpropamide (175 mg twice a day) are some of the commonly used oral hypoglycemic agents.

Most juvenile-onset diabetic patients (type I) and some maturity-onset diabetics (type II) who are uncontrolled with diet and oral hypoglycemic agents require insulin. Single or multiple injections of one or more of various long- and short-acting insulins may be used in combination to control the hyperglycemia. The majority of insulin-dependent diabetics require between 1 and 4 units of insulin per hour or 10 to 20 units for each main meal.

Various pharmacologic agents have been tried to treat diabetic retinopathy. Clofibrate[‡] has been used in an attempt to reduce the amount of hard exudates, and calcium dobesilate[†] has been tried to decrease the capillary fragility and abnormal permeability. However, neither of these drugs is of practical use for diabetic retinopathy in the United States.

It has been suggested that the increased platelet aggregation in diabetic retinopathy may be responsible for its development and progression, perhaps by promoting small vessel obstruction. Theoretically, aspirin, a potent inhibitor of platelet aggregation, might be beneficial in retarding diabetic retinopathy. This possibility is being evaluated by the National Eye Institute-sponsored Early Treatment Diabetic Retinopathy Study (ETDRS).

Surgical. At the present time, photocoagulation is the treatment of choice for proliferative diabetic retinopathy. The beneficial effect of photocoagulation has been demonstrated by the ETDRS. In this study, the beneficial effect of the treatment was observed in both proliferative and severe nonproliferative retinopathy, but was of greater clinical importance in those eyes with the following high-risk characteristics: 1) moderate to severe disc neovascularization, defined as new vessels greater than one fourth to one third the area of the disc and 2) mild disc neovascularization or retinal neovascularization elsewhere, if preretinal or vitreous hemorrhage was present. Although both argon laser and xenon arc photocoagulation were shown to be beneficial, the argon technique was preferred because side effects (decreases in visual acuity and peripheral visual fields) were less frequent.

The treatment technique most commonly used

is called "panretinal" or "scatter" treatment. It consists of application of several hundred 500-micron diameter burns to the midperipheral and peripheral portions of the retina. Treatment extends posteriorly to two disc diameters from the center of the macula in the temporal quadrants and one-half disc diameter nasal to the optic disc. In addition, focal treatment using moderate-intensity confluent burns may be applied to new vessels on the surface of the retina. The total number of burns is usually 1200 to 1600, each with a duration of 0.1 to 0.2 second. Power is adjusted to achieve a moderately white burn. The treatment is applied on an outpatient basis under topical or retrobulbar anesthesia. Focal treatment to new vessels on the optic disc is not necessary.

Regression of disc neovascularization is usually apparent very soon (days to weeks) after treatment, but is not always complete or permanent. When substantial regression of disc neovascularization is not obtained (and maintained), one or more additional scatter treatments over previously untreated retina are often followed by satisfactory regression.

The risk-benefit ratio of photocoagulation in patients with mild to moderate nonproliferative retinopathy is unclear. The ETDRS is evaluating the role of photocoagulation treatment in early nonproliferative retinopathy. The ETDRS recently demonstrated that photocoagulation treatment is beneficial in diabetic macular edema.

Before photocoagulation was widely accepted, pituitary ablation was advocated for patients with rapidly progressive "florid" retinopathy. Because of its attendant mortality and morbidity and because of the effectiveness and safety of photocoagulation, this procedure is rarely used today.

In some cases of traction retinal detachment with or without retinal break, scleral buckling or scleral resection may be useful. In most cases, a pars plana vitrectomy procedure is necessary.

Vitrectomy surgery is used to treat eyes with severe vitreous hemorrhage, tractional retinal detachment, and extensive preretinal membrane formation. In vitrectomy, long-standing vitreous hemorrhage is removed from the eye, and the traction caused by fibrous scar tissue is relieved. The vitreous is replaced with physiologic solution to restore transparency. The National Eye Institute's Diabetic Retinopathy Vitrectomy Study (DRVS) demonstrated that, in patients with nonresolving diabetic vitreous hemorrhage, early vitrectomy is beneficial in type I diabetics but did not provide any advantage in type II diabetics.

In patients with neovascular glaucoma, panretinal photocoagulation is often followed by regression of rubeosis iridis and neovascularization in the anterior chamber angle. In some early cases, photocoagulation plus conventional antiglaucoma medical therapy may be sufficient to control intraocular pressure. Direct photocoagulation of new vessels extending across the chamber angle has also been advocated. When peripheral anterior synechiae are extensive, filtering surgery is required, but the results are often unsatisfactory.

Supportive. The goal of diabetic management should be to educate the patient about diabetes and its complications and to help the patient lead as normal a life as possible. This can be achieved by teaching the patient and family about diabetes and the importance of self-care through regular habits, avoidance of dietary and other excesses and deficiencies, maintenance of normal weight, and finally applied common sense.

Dietary management remains the most important factor in the practical management of diabetes mellitus. The diabetic diet should maintain the prescribed balance between carbohydrates, protein, fat, vitamins, and minerals in order to maintain the patient's ideal body weight.

Ocular or Periocular Manifestations

Ciliary Body: Glycogen deposits in pigment epithelium; thickening of basement membrane.
Cornea: Endothelial pigment deposits; hypesthesia; poor epithelial healing.
Extraocular Muscles: Paralysis of third or sixth nerve.
Iris: Ectropion uveae; glycogen deposits in pigment epithelium; pupillary abnormality; rubeosis iridis.
Lens: Cataracts; pigment deposits on epithelium; premature presbyopia.
Macula: Edema; heterotopia.
Optic Nerve: Atrophy; papillopathy.
Retina: Cotton-wool spots (soft exudates); detachment; dilation and beading of retinal veins; hard exudates; hemorrhages (superficial, deep, and preretinal); intraretinal microvascular abnormalities; microaneurysms; neovascularization and fibrous proliferation; sclerosis of retinal arterioles.
Vitreous: Asteroid hyalosis; detachment; hemorrhages.

PRECAUTIONS

A good control of diabetes may be beneficial in the prevention of diabetic retinopathy. There is some evidence that coexistent hypertension may have an adverse effect on the progression of diabetic retinopathy. Pregnancy carries a high risk of deterioration of retinopathy and significant visual loss in patients with proliferative or severe nonproliferative retinopathy. There is controversy regarding possible increased risk of cardiovascular complications associated with prolonged use of oral hypoglycemic agents.

The most common side effects of panretinal photocoagulation observed in the ETDRS are mild to moderate decrease in visual acuity and constriction of peripheral visual fields. These harmful side effects were more commonly observed with xenon arc than with argon photocoagulation.

Until the results of the DRVS are available, vitrectomy is indicated in long-standing vitreous

146 / DIABETES MELLITUS

hemorrhage and retinal traction involving the macula.

COMMENTS

Diabetic retinopathy poses a major threat of blindness in patients with diabetes mellitus. Treatment with photocoagulation reduces this threat significantly. Careful periodic ophthalmoscopic examinations, preferably through dilated pupils, should be performed on all patients by the physician caring for the diabetic. If the patient develops diabetic retinopathy, its progression should be monitored by an ophthalmologist who can seek specialized care, such as photocoagulation or vitrectomy, at an appropriate time.

References

Blankenship GW, Skyler JS: Diabetic retinopathy: A general survey. Diabetes Care 1:127–137, 1978.
Bresnick GH: Diabetic retinopathy. In Peyman GA, Sanders DR, Goldberg MF (eds): Principles and Practice of Ophthalmology. Philadelphia, WB Saunders, 1980, pp 1205–1276.
Diabetic Retinopathy Study Research Group: Photocoagulation treatment of proliferative diabetic retinopathy. Clinical application of (Diabetic Retinopathy Study) findings: DRS Report Number 8. Ophthalmology 88:583–600, 1981.
Diabetic Retinopathy Vitrectomy Study Research Group: Early vitrectomy for severe vitreous hemorrhage in diabetic retinopathy. Two year results of a randomized trial; Diabetic Retinopathy Vitrectomy Study Report Number 2. Arch Ophthalmol 103:1644–1652, 1985.
Early Treatment Diabetic Retinopathy Study Research Group: Photocoagulation for diabetic macular edema. Early Treatment Diabetic Retinopathy Study Report Number 1. Arch Ophthalmol 103:1796–1806, 1985.
Kahn HA, Bradley RF: Prevalence of diabetic retinopathy. Age, sex, and duration of diabetes. Br J Ophthalmol 59:345–349, 1975.
Kahn HA, Moorhead HB: Statistics on Blindness in a Model Reporting Area, 1969–1970 (DHEW Publication No. NIH 73–427). Washington, DC, Government Printing Office, 1973.
Klein R, Klein B, Davis MD: Wisconsin epidemiologic study of diabetic retinopathy. Prevalence and severity of diabetic retinopathy and its association with risk factors in participants diagnosed to have diabetes mellitus after age 29 years. Preliminary report. Invest Ophthalmol Vis Sci 22(Suppl):68, 1982.

GALACTOSEMIAS

WARREN A. WILSON, M.D.,
(Deceased)
and GEORGE N. DONNELL, M.D.

Los Angeles, California

Galactosemia can result from more than one inborn error of galactose metabolism. The most important source of the sugar is milk, where it is found in the form of the disaccharide lactose. Lactose is hydrolyzed in the intestine to its monosaccharides, glucose and galactose. These are absorbed and used for energy and the synthesis of a number of cell components.

Three major enzymatic reactions are involved in the metabolism of galactose. In the first step of galactose metabolism, galactokinase catalyzes the phosphorylation of galactose. In the second step, the galactose-1-phosphate formed is exchanged with glucose-1-phosphate of uridine diphosphoglucose. This reaction is mediated by the enzyme, galactose-1-phosphate uridyltransferase. The third reaction catalyzed by uridine diphosphogalactose-6-epimerase transforms uridine diphosphogalactose to uridine diphosphoglucose.

Defects in each of these steps have been described. All of the diseases are inherited as autosomal recessive traits; both parents are obligatory heterozygotes and exhibit about half of normal erythrocyte enzyme activity.

In galactokinase deficiency, galactose accumulates in the blood and overflows into the urine. Galactitol is formed in tissues from galactose. Cataracts and pseudotumor cerebri are the only physical findings, and they are thought to result in part from galactitol accumulation in the target organs.

Transferase deficiency results in the accumulation of galactose, intracellular galactose-1-phosphate, and galactitol. Infants with transferase deficiency usually appear normal at birth, but develop vomiting, fever, lethargy, and failure to gain weight within a few days following milk feedings. Additional findings include jaundice, ascites, and hepatomegaly. Severe infections, including septicemia, meningitis, and even osteomyelitis, are common. The mortality rate is high in the untreated infant. Cataracts and mental retardation usually will occur in many of those who survive. Late complications in treated patients have included learning disabilities, speech and language defects, and ovarian failure in the female patients.

The term "oil drop" cataract probably originated with early observers using only an ophthalmoscope for examinations. Slitlamp findings reveal early fetal nuclear involvement of the lens spreading into the posterior third of the cortical area and forming zonular cataracts. Although the central clouding may be dense, these cataracts rarely, if ever, become mature, even in patients undiagnosed at 6 months or more. Originally, it was thought that total regression of the opacities occurred when infants were placed on the proper diet, but some residual punctate opacities are observed with the slitlamp.

Epimerase deficiency is usually benign and confined to the red blood cells. No treatment is required.

THERAPY

Systemic. The management of kinase and transferase deficiencies is identical and requires the immediate withdrawal of all milk and its products. It is essential to maintain strict control during the formative years. This requires cooperation of the parents and the assistance of a nutritionist. The diet should be maintained for life, as it is not believed that tolerance to galactose develops. Early complications of transferase deficiency, such as sepsis or other infections, require appropriate antibiotic treatment, whereas ascites, jaundice, and other systemic conditions usually resolve when the individual is placed on the special diet.

Surgical. Less than half of a large group of patients followed have had cataract changes, even though all of the patients were not diagnosed early. The lens opacities occasionally progress as children grow, even those who are in compliance with the special diet. Some individuals will require surgical intervention because of the increase in the density of the cataracts. The management is the same as for any child with congenital cataracts.

Ocular or Periocular Manifestations

Lens: Nuclear or zonular cataracts.

PRECAUTIONS

Complications related to the disease itself are thought in part to be due to lack of compliance with the diet. Infections and general medical problems are managed by the usual methods. Difficulties associated with cataract surgery are no greater than with similar operations in nongalactosemic patients. Patients with partial cataracts that are not dense enough to need surgery, often have myopia, necessitating spectacles.

COMMENTS

The management of these two diseases is based on dietary control; once instituted, the management is lifelong, and the patients must strictly adhere to this regime. Of 18 female patients between 14 and 29 years of age with galactosemia, 12 had ovarian insufficiency; however, 8 male patients of comparable age had normal male hormones.

References

Donnell GN, Bergren WR: The galactosemias. *In* Raine DN (ed): Treatment of Inherited Metabolic Diseases. New York, American Elsevier, 1974, pp 91–114.
Kaufman FR, et al: Hypergonadotrophic hypogonadism in female patients with galactosemia. N Engl J Med 304:994–998, 1981.
Oberman AE, et al: Galactokinase deficiency cataracts in identical twins. Am J Ophthalmol 74:887–892, 1972.
Wilson WA: Cataracts and galactose metabolism. Trans Am Ophthalmol Soc 65:661–704, 1967.
Wilson WA: Surgery of congenital and childhood cataracts. Trans Pac Coast Otoophthalmol Soc 59:207–219, 1978.
Wilson WA, Donnell GN: Cataracts in galactosemia. Arch Ophthalmol 60:215–222, 1958.
Wilson WA, Donnell GN, Koch R: Galactosemia, a twenty-five year follow-up. *In* XXII Concilium Ophthalmologicum Paris, 1974, Acta Paris, Masson, 1976, Vol I, pp 740–744.

MUCOPOLYSACCHARIDOSIS I-H
(Dysostosis Multiplex, Hurler Syndrome, MPS I-H, Pfaundler-Hurler Syndrome)

T.E. KELLY, M.D., Ph.D.,
Charlottesville, Virginia
and VICTOR A. McKUSICK, M.D.
Baltimore, Maryland

Mucopolysaccharidosis I-H is an autosomal recessive syndrome characterized by deficiency of lysosomal enzyme α-L-iduronidase, which allows the mucopolysaccharides, dermatan sulfate and heparan sulfate, to accumulate in cells throughout the body. The primary manifestations include skeletal abnormalities, enlargement of the spleen and liver, corneal clouding, and mental retardation. Although the child may develop normally for the first few months, typical Hurler manifestations usually begin to appear in the first or second year of life. Clouding of the cornea is present in all patients with this disease. Buphthalmos and megalocornea may also be present. Retinal degeneration occurs in many cases, and optic atrophy is also common. The eyebrows are typically bushy and coarse, and the eyelids are thickened and coarse.

THERAPY

Systemic. Considerable enthusiasm has been generated in England for the use of bone marrow transplantation in the management of inborn errors of metabolism. There have been several reports of successful transplantation in patients with MPS I-H with evidence of enhanced mucopolysaccharide degradation and clinical improvement. This approach is still highly experimental, and there are several major problems: the onset of lysosomal storage diseases is prenatal; the morbidity and mortality of bone marrow transplantation are high; and there is doubt that the changes in viscera observed following a successful transplant will extend to the skeleton and central nervous system, the major organs involved in the mucopolysaccharidoses.

Supportive. The physician should offer the parents sympathetic guidance in dealing with the gross deformities and mental retardation that may develop in these patients. Genetic counseling is also indicated for parents because of the 25 per cent recurrence risk and the availability of prenatal diagnosis.

148 / MUCOPOLYSACCHARIDOSIS I-H

Surgical. Surgical treatment is supportive; it may include repair of hernias and hydroceles, orthopedic surgery for skeletal deformities, or adenoidectomy to provide relief from the persistent upper airway obstruction present in Hurler patients. Penetrating keratoplasty or lamellar corneal graft may be used for corneal clouding. Hydrocephalus and associated papilledema may require shunting or cerebrospinal fluid.

Ocular or Periocular Manifestations

Cornea: Interstitial clouding; megalocornea.
Eyebrows: Bushy; coarse.
Eyelids: Coarse eyelashes; edema; ptosis; tylosis.
Iris: Acid mucopolysaccharide deposits.
Lens: Acid mucopolysaccharide deposits; congenital anterior polar cataract.
Optic Nerve: Atrophy; cupping; disc edema; disc hyperemia.
Orbit: Enlarged optic foramen; hypertelorism; small.
Retina: Detachment; macular edema; pigmentary degeneration.
Sclera: Acid mucopolysaccharide deposits.
Other: Anisocoria; buphthalmos; convergent strabismus; decreased visual acuity; nystagmus.

PRECAUTIONS

Administration of general anesthesia is complicated by the excessive pharyngeal secretions, laryngospasm, cardiac abnormalities, increased frequency of cardiac arrest, hypoxia, and hypotension. Postoperative obstruction or infection may occur in the respiratory tract and require tracheotomy. Many of these complications may be avoided if large doses of atropine are given in the preinduction period and postoperative narcotics are withheld as much as possible.

Plasma infusion is not a practicable means of therapy. Improvement is temporary, if present at all. There are dangers of fluid overload in those patients whose cardiovascular status is compromised.

COMMENTS

The prognosis for the Hurler patient is not encouraging. Mental retardation is invariably present and is especially severe and progressive after the first year, usually reaching a plateau after several years. Deformities of the respiratory tract in this syndrome may cause choking on solid foods or nasal regurgitation of liquids. Some patients may have unexplained spells of cyanosis or even apnea. Death usually occurs in the first decade of life either from cardiac involvement or increased susceptibility to pneumonia and bronchitis.

References

Bloch RS, Henkind P: Ocular manifestations of endocrine and metabolic diseases. *In* Duane TD (ed): Clinical Ophthalmology. Hagerstown, MD, Harper & Row, 1982, Vol V, pp 21:10–12.
Francois J: Ocular manifestations of the mucopolysaccharidoses. Ophthalmologica 169:345–361, 1974.
Hobbs JR: Bone marrow transplantation for inborn errors. Lancet 2:735–739, 1981.
Hobbs JR, et al: Reversal of clinical features of Hurler's disease and biochemical improvement after treatment by bone-marrow transplantation. Lancet 2:709–712, 1981.
Nowaczyk MJ, Clarke JT, Morin JD: Glaucoma as an early complication of Hurler's disease. Arch Dis Child 63:1091–1093, 1988.
McKusick VA: Heritable Disorders of Connective Tissue, 4th ed. St. Louis, CV Mosby, 1972, pp 528–548.

MUCOPOLYSAC-CHARIDOSIS I-H/S
(Hurler/Scheie Syndrome, MPS I-H/S)
T.E. KELLY, M.D., Ph.D.
Charlottesville, Virginia

Mucopolysaccharidosis I-H/S is an autosomal recessive syndrome characterized by deficiency of lysosomal enzyme α-L-iduronidase, which allows the mucopolysaccharides, dermatan sulfate and heparan sulfate, to accumulate in cells throughout the body. The primary manifestations include corneal opacities, cardiac enlargement, umbilical and inguinal hernias, and multiple skeletal changes. Mild mental retardation may be present. Micrognathia and severe acne are features peculiar to this form of mucopolysaccharidosis. Ocular findings also include both diffuse corneal clouding and pigmentary retinopathy. Buphthalmos and megalocornea may also be present. The eyebrows are typically bushy and coarse, and the eyelids are thickened and coarse.

THERAPY

Systemic. Considerable enthusiasm has been generated in England for the use of bone marrow transplantation in the management of inborn errors of metabolism. There have been several reports of successful transplantation in patients with MPS I-H with evidence of enhanced mucopolysaccharide degradation and clinical improvement. This approach is still highly experimental, and there are several major problems: the onset of lysosomal storage diseases is prenatal; the morbidity and mortality of bone marrow transplantation are high; and there is doubt that the changes in viscera observed following a successful transplant will extend to the skeleton and central nervous system, the major organs involved in the mucopolysaccharidoses.

Supportive. The physician should offer the parents guidance in dealing with the gross deformities and mental retardation that may arise in these patients. Life expectancy of these patients is into the twenties, and surgical and medical management of individual problems is appropriate.

Genetic counseling is indicated for parents as a 25 per cent recurrence risk exists. Carrier detection should also be available for other relatives.

Surgical. Surgical treatment is supportive. It may include repair of hernias and hydroceles, orthopedic surgery for skeletal deformities, or adenoidectomy to provide relief from the persistent upper airway obstruction present in these patients. Tympanoplasty and hearing aids may be required to preserve hearing. Penetrating keratoplasty or lamellar corneal graft is the treatment of choice for corneal clouding. Hydrocephalus and associated papilledema may be relieved by shunting of cerebrospinal fluid.

Ocular or Periocular Manifestations

Cornea: Bullous keratopathy; clouding; megalocornea; punctate opacity; thickening.
Eyebrows: Bushy; coarse.
Eyelids: Coarse eyelashes; edema; ptosis; tylosis.
Globe: Buphthalmos; proptosis.
Iris: Acid mucopolysaccharide deposits; distortion; folding; thickening.
Lens: Acid mucopolysaccharide deposits; congenital anterior polar cataract.
Optic Nerve: Atrophy; cupping; disc edema; disc hyperemia.
Orbit: Enlarged optic foramen; hypertelorism; small.
Retina: Detachment; macular edema; pigmentary degeneration; tapetoretinal degeneration.
Sclera: Acid mucopolysaccharide deposits; thickening.
Other: Anisocoria; constriction of visual fields; convergent strabismus; decreased visual acuity; night blindness; secondary glaucoma.

PRECAUTIONS

Plasma infusion is not a practicable means of therapy. Improvement is temporary, if present at all. However, the danger of fluid overload is present in those patients whose cardiovascular status is compromised. Such patients manifest heart disease as cardiomyopathy, conduction defects, and valvular heart disease. Several have died during induction of anesthesia for minor procedures. General anesthesia should be approached with caution.

COMMENTS

The Hurler syndrome and the Scheie syndrome share a common metabolic defect; in both, the enzymatic deficiency is α-L-iduronidase. The mutation in both is presumed to be allelic, and thus it is felt that the inheritance of a Hurler gene and a Scheie gene results in a genetic compound with an intermediate phenotype, the Hurler/Scheie syndrome. This phenotype is distinct, although intermediate in severity between the Hurler and Scheie syndromes. Patients with mucopolysaccharidosis I-H/S usually succumb after protracted cardiac failure. Mental deficiency and dwarfism are less severe than in the Hurler syndrome, although the pattern of radiographic changes is similar. Additional atypical mucopolysaccharidosis patients with the same specific biochemical defect and similar features of Hurler syndrome suggest that several genetically distinct forms of α-L-iduronidase deficiency exist.

References

Chijiiwa T, Inomata H, Yamana Y, Kaibara N: Ocular manifestations of Hurler/Scheie phenotype in two sibs. Jpn J Ophthalmol 27:54–62,1983.
Hobbs JR: Bone marrow transplantation for inborn errors. Lancet 2:735–739, 1981.
Hobbs JR, et al: Reversal of clinical features of Hurler's disease and biochemical improvement after treatment by bone-marrow transplantation. Lancet 2:709–712, 1981.
Kajii T, et al: Hurler/Scheie genetic compound (mucopolysaccharidosis IH/IS) in Japanese brothers. Clin Genet 6:394–400, 1974.
Kelly TE: The mucopolysaccharidoses and mucolipidoses. Clin Orthop 114:116–136, 1976.
Lavery MA, Green WR, Jabs EW, Luckenbach MW, Cox JL: Ocular histopathology and ultrastructure of Sanfilippo's syndrome, type III-B. Arch Ophthalmol 101:1263–1274, 1983.

MUCOPOLYSACCHARIDOSIS I-S
(MPS I-S, Scheie Syndrome)
IRENE H. MAUMENEE, M.D.
Baltimore, Maryland

Mucopolysaccharidosis I-S is an autosomal recessive syndrome characterized by deficiency of the lysosomal enzyme α-L-iduronidase, which allows the mucopolysaccharides dermatan sulfate and heparan sulfate to accumulate intracellularly throughout the body. The primary manifestations include severe progressive corneal clouding and retinal degeneration, joint contractures, facial coarseness, hammer toes, and carpal tunnel syndrome. Glaucoma is a late complication. Aortic regurgitation occurs, but cardiac decompensation at an early age is usually not a major problem. The onset of symptoms in this relatively mild disease usually is after the age of 5 years, although corneal clouding, stiff fingers, and umbilical or inguinal hernias may be detected sooner.

150 / MUCOPOLYSACCHARIDOSIS I-S

THERAPY

Systemic. Several experimental approaches are currently being tried to restore the ability to degrade or clear storage material. Such therapy requires either induction of enzyme synthesis, enhancement of any residual enzyme activity, or replacement therapy with exogenous enzyme.

Surgical. Surgical treatment may include repair of hernias and hydroceles or orthopedic surgery for skeletal deformities. Penetrating keratoplasty is the treatment of choice for corneal clouding. Hydrocephalus and associated papilledema may be relieved by shunting of cerebrospinal fluid.

Supportive. Genetic counseling is indicated for the parents who have a 25 per cent risk of having another similarly affected child. There is no mental involvement, life expectancy is close to normal, and patients may lead fruitful normal lives. The resulting facial coarseness is only mildly debilitating. Chronic care is not needed until very late in the disease, when blindness, cardiac insufficiency, or marked joint stiffness may have occurred.

Ocular or Periocular Manifestations

Cornea: Clouding (more striking in the peripheral than central cornea); punctate opacities; thickening.
Eyebrows: Bushy; coarse.
Eyelids: Coarse eyelashes; edema; tylosis.
Iris: Acid mucopolysaccharide deposits; distortion; folding; thickening.
Optic Nerve: Atrophy; disc edema.
Retina: Macular edema; tapetoretinal degeneration.
Sclera: Acid mucopolysaccharide deposits; thickening.
Other: Anisocoria; cataracts (?); constriction of visual fields; decreased visual acuity; glaucoma (secondary to mucopolysaccharide deposits in trabecular meshwork, also angle-closure attacks); proptosis.

PRECAUTIONS

Administration of general anesthesia is complicated by excessive pharyngeal secretions, laryngospasm, cardiac abnormalities, increased frequency of cardiac arrest, hypoxia, and hypotension. Postoperative obstruction or infection in the respiratory tract may require tracheostomy. Many of these complications may be avoided if large doses of atropine are given in the preinduction period and postoperative narcotics are withheld as much as possible.

Plasma infusion is still not a practicable means of therapy. Improvement is temporary if present at all. The treatment is successful if there is no physical deterioration for a period of time; however, danger of fluid overload is present in those patients whose cardiovascular status is compromised.

COMMENTS

Originally classified as MPS V because of the distinctive phenotype, the Scheie syndrome is currently designated as MPS I-S. Clinically, the patients with MPS I-H and MPS I-S have many similarities (corneal clouding, hepatosplenomegaly, cardiovascular abnormalities, and certain skeletal deformities), but they differ in three important respects. In contrast to patients with MPS I-H, patients with MPS I-S are not dwarfed, are free of neurologic and mental deficits (except for the signs of the carpal tunnel syndrome), and have normal life expectancy.

References

Crocker AC: Present status of treatment of the mucopolysaccharidoses. Birth Defects 10:113–124, 1974.
François J: Ocular manifestations of the mucopolysaccharidoses. Ophthalmologica 169:345–361, 1974.
Hussels IE, et al: Treatment of mucopolysaccharidoses. Birth Defects 10:212–238, 1974.
Kelly TE: The mucopolysaccharidoses and mucolipidoses. Clin Orthop 114:116–136, 1976.
Legum CP, Schorr S, Berman ER: The genetic mucopolysaccharidoses and mucolipidoses. Review and comment. Adv Pediatr 22:305–347, 1976.

MUCOPOLYSACCHAR- IDOSIS II
(Hunter Syndrome, MPS II)
ELAINE R. BERMAN, Ph.D.
Jerusalem, Israel

Mucopolysaccharidosis II is the only known x-linked recessive disorder of mucopolysaccharide metabolism. It is caused by a profound deficiency of iduronate sulfatase, which leads to the intracellular accumulation and excessive urinary excretion of two mucopolysaccharides, dermatan sulfate and heparan sulfate. Mucopolysaccharidosis II is thought to exist in two clinically and genetically distinct forms. In the mild type, intelligence is not impaired, and survival into adulthood and even procreation have been observed. In the severe form, mental retardation and neurologic changes are almost indistinguishable from those found in mucopolysaccharidosis I-H. Other clinical signs in the severe form of MPS II include gargoyle-like facies, dwarfism, hepatosplenomegaly, and early deafness. The corneas remain clear until the fourth decade of life. Papilledema and retinal deterioration are found in most of these patients.

THERAPY

Systemic. Several experimental approaches have been used in an attempt to enhance the degradation of the stored material. Such therapy is based on induction of enzyme, activation of any residual enzyme activity, or replacement therapy with exogenous enzyme. One major modality is plasma therapy, in which perfusions of fresh plasma from a normal donor are administered at regular intervals in order to provide a supply of corrective factor, the particular deficient enzyme. Although plasma infusion can usually do no harm, nevertheless, there is no evidence to date that it causes any improvement by either reversing the severe skeletal changes or contributing to the catabolism of the stored mucopolysaccharides (apart from a transient effect). Fibroblast transplantation therapy is also being investigated and may be of some usefulness in the future.

Supportive. The physician should offer the parents sympathetic guidance in dealing with the gross deformities that characterize both forms of Hunter syndrome. Genetic counseling is indicated for parents at risk (those who already have an affected child).

Surgical. Surgical treatment is supportive; repair of hernias and hydroceles or orthopedic surgery for skeletal deformities may be necessary. Hydrocephalus and associated papilledema, if severe enough to warrant surgical intervention, may be relieved by shunting of cerebrospinal fluid.

Ocular or Periocular Manifestations

Cornea: Acid mucopolysaccharide deposits; stromal haze (late).
Eyebrows or Eyelashes: Bushy; coarse, proptosis.
Eyelids: Edema; ptosis; tylosis.
Iris or Ciliary Body: Acid mucopolysaccharide deposits.
Optic Nerve: Atrophy; cupping; disc hyperemia; papilledema.
Retina: Diminished electroretinogram; pigmentary degeneration.
Sclera: Acid mucopolysaccharide deposits; thickened.

PRECAUTIONS

Administration of a general anesthetic may be complicated by excessive pharyngeal secretions, laryngospasm, cardiac abnormalities, increased frequency of cardiac arrest, hypoxia, or hypotension. Postoperative obstruction or infection may occur in the respiratory tract and may require tracheotomy. Many of these complications may be avoided if large doses of atropine are given in the preinduction period and postoperative narcotics are withheld as much as possible.

COMMENTS

Mucopolysaccharidosis II is an x-linked disorder. Hence, the disease is only transmissible from mother to son. Parents at risk should be informed that there is a 50 per cent chance that their son will be affected and a 50 per cent chance that their daughter will be a carrier. In most cases, the carrier does not manifest any signs of the disease.

Prenatal diagnosis is theoretically possible in any inherited disorder with an established enzymatic defect. In fact, this is the most effective way possible at present to deal with MPS II. Amniocentesis should be performed in pregnancies where the mother has previously given birth to an effected son. The amniotic cells should be cultured and examined for a deficiency of iduronate sulfatase. If such is found, the pregnancy can be interrupted before the seventeenth week of gestation.

References

Beck M, Cole G: Disc oedema in association with Hunter's syndrome: ocular histopathological findings. Br J Ophthalmol 68:590–594, 1984.
Berman ER: Biochemical diagnostic tests in genetic and metabolic eye diseases. *In* Goldberg MF (ed): Genetic and Metabolic Eye Disease. Boston, Little, Brown, 1974, pp 85–92.
Di Natale P, Neufeld EF: Biochemical diagnosis of mucopolysaccharidoses, mucolipidoses and related disorders. Perspect Inherit Metab Dis 2:113–123, 1979.
Gibbs DA, et al: The treatment of lysosomal storage diseases by fibroblast transplantation: Some preliminary observations. Birth Defects 16:457–474, 1980.
Jolly RD, Desnick RJ: Inborn errors of lysosmal catabolism—Principles of heterozygote detection. Am J Med Genet 4:293–307, 1979.
Legum CP, Schorr S, Berman ER: The genetic mucopolysaccharidoses and mucolipidoses: Review and comment. Adv Pediatr 22:305–347, 1976.
McDonnell JM, Green WR, Maumenee IH: Ocular histopathology of systemic mucopolysaccharidosis, type II-A (Hunter syndrome, severe). Ophthalmology 92:1772–1779, 1985.
Sugar A, Podos SM: Ophthalmic aspects of inborn errors of metabolism. *In* Mausolf FA (ed): The Eye and Systemic Disease, 2nd ed. St. Louis, CV Mosby, 1980, pp 48–87.

MUCOPOLYSACCHARIDOSIS III
(MPS III, Sanfilippo Syndrome)

ELAINE R. BERMAN, Ph.D.
Jerusalem, Israel

Mucopolysaccharidosis III is inherited as an autosomal recessive trait and is characterized by excessive tissue storage and urinary excretion of heparan sulfate. There are three subtypes, designated A, B and C, which are indistinguishable clinically. The A form is caused by a deficiency of heparin N-sulfatase, the B form by an α-N-acetylglucosaminidase deficiency, and the C form by a defect in acetyl CoA : α-glucosaminide N-acetyl transferase enzyme. The various forms

152 / MUCOPOLYSACCHARIDOSIS III

of MPS III are nonallelic (the mutations occur at separate genetic loci).

Severe mental retardation and neurologic deterioration are the most prominent clinical signs. Mental and neurologic deficiencies progress to extreme degrees within a few years, and death usually occurs by 10 to 15 years of age. Seizures and aggressive behavior have been noted in most patients. Growth and physical development are within normal limits, and skeletal abnormalities are minimal. The corneas remain clear, but retinal pigmentary degeneration is usual.

THERAPY

Systemic. Several experimental approaches have been used in an attempt to enhance the degradation of the stored material. Such therapy is based on induction of enzyme synthesis, activation of any residual enzyme activity, or replacement therapy with exogenous enzyme. A major modality is plasma therapy, in which perfusions of fresh plasma from a normal donor are administered at regular intervals in order to provide a supply of corrective factor (the particular deficient enzyme). Although plasma infusion can usually do no harm, nevertheless, there is no evidence to date that it causes any improvement by either reversing the severe mental and neurologic changes or contributing to the catabolism of the stored heparan sulfate (apart from a transient effect). Enzyme replacement therapy using HLA-compatible fibroblasts is a promising hope for the future.

Supportive. Genetic counseling is indicated for parents who already have an affected child. They should be informed of the 25 per cent statistical probability of producing affected children in future pregnancies.

There is no surgical or medical treatment available that would contribute to the well-being of the patient.

Ocular or Periocular Manifestations

Cornea: Acid mucopolysaccharide deposits.
Eyebrows: Bushy; coarse.
Iris or Ciliary Body: Acid mucopolysaccharide deposits.
Lens: Acid mucopolysaccharide deposits.
Retina: Pigmentary degeneration.
Sclera: Acid mucopolysaccharide deposits.

PRECAUTIONS

As the physical features of mucopolysaccharidosis III are usually minimal, this disorder may not be included in the differential diagnosis of a child with progressive central nervous system disorder. Urine of suspected patients should be tested for excess mucopolysaccharides, and skin fibroblasts should be cultured and examined for enzyme deficiency. Unless these examinations are undertaken in children who undergo progressive mental deterioration after normal early development, the diagnosis of MPS III may be overlooked.

COMMENTS

Prenatal diagnosis is theoretically possible in any inherited disorder with an established enzymatic defect. In fact, this is the most effective way possible at present to deal with MPS III. Aminocentesis should be performed in pregnancies where the mother has previously given birth to an affected child. The amniotic cells should be cultured and examined for all of the enzymes involved in MPS III. If the enzymes are found to be deficient, pregnancy can be interrupted before the seventeenth week of gestation.

References

Berman ER: Biochemical diagnostic tests in genetic and metabolic eye diseases. *In* Goldberg ME (ed): Genetic and Metabolic Eye Disease. Boston, Little, Brown, 1974, pp 85–92.

Berman ER: Diagnosis of metabolic eye disease by chemical analysis of serum, leukocytes and skin fibroblast tissue culture. Birth Defects *12*:15–51, 1976.

Dean MF, et al: Enzyme replacement therapy by transplantation of HLA-compatible fibroblasts in Sanfilippo A syndrome. Pediatr Res *15*:959–963, 1981.

Del Monte MA, Maumenee IH, Green WR, Kenyon KR: Histopathology of Sanfilippo's syndrome. Arch Ophthalmol *101*:1255–1262, 1983.

Legum CP, Schorr S, Berman ER: The genetic mucopolysaccharidoses and mucolipidoses: Review and comment. Adv Pediatr *22*:305–347, 1976.

McKusick VA: Heritable Disorders of Connective Tissue, 4th ed., St. Louis, CV Mosby, 1972, pp 575–582.

Ricci R, et al: Enzymatic assays of diagnostic value in mucopolysaccharidoses and sphingolipidoses. Perspect Inherited Metab Dis *1*:193, 1979.

MUCOPOLYSACCHARIDOSIS IV
(Chondro-Osteodystrophy, Keratosulfaturia, Morquio-Brailsford Syndrome, Morquio Syndrome, MPS IV)

CYRIL P. LEGUM, M.D.

Tel Aviv, Israel

Mucopolysaccharidosis IV is a progressive autosomal recessive disorder with an enzyme deficiency of N-acetyl-galactosamine-6-sulfate sulfatase that causes keratan sulfate to accumulate in the tissues and be excreted in the urine. By 2 years of age, the clinical and roentgenographic features of mucopolysaccharidosis IV become distinctive, and the disease can be differentiated from the other established mucopolysaccharidoses. In the second or third year of life, gibbus of the thoracolumbar spine, retarded growth, awkward gait, knock-knees, and sternal deformity usually bring the child to medical attention. With advancing age, all these deformities are exaggerated, and growth is severely deficient, coming practically to a standstill by the age of 5 years. Facial features are similar to those of patients with the other mucopolysaccharidoses, with the addition of an early enamel defect of the teeth. Corneal clouding is detectable early by slitlamp examination, but is not grossly apparent until after 8 to 10 years of age. Retinal changes have not been reported, and ocular atrophy is rare.

THERAPY

Systemic. All attempts at enzyme replacement, whether by plasma, lymphocyte infusions, or enzymes packaged in biologic "envelopes," have not influenced the course of the disease in the mucopolysaccharidoses and have ultimately added to its burden.

Supportive. The intelligence of patients with MPS IV is generally normal. With sympathetic guidance, these individuals can usually attend a school for normal children and perhaps even attain college-level training. Institutionalization should generally be avoided. A hearing aid may be of use for hearing loss.

Parents of affected children have a 25 per cent risk of having another affected child with each pregnancy. Intrauterine diagnosis by measurement of the enzyme in cultured amniotic fluid cells and chorionic villi is feasible.

Surgical. Although the Milwaukee brace has been advocated for the prevention of spinal deformity, as has surgery for the correction of genu valgum, neither of these modes of treatment has been shown to be clearly advantageous over no treatment at all. On the other hand, stabilization of the atlanto-occipital joint is firmly recommended to prevent dislocation of this joint, which may cause pressure on or transection of the upper spinal cord. This hazard is especially great when hyperextending the neck for intubation during general anesthesia. Spinal surgery has been performed successfully to relieve pressure on the cord. There is generally no need to resort to keratoplasty for the corneal clouding, as it does not seriously interfere with vision.

Ocular or Periocular Manifestations

Cornea: Clouding.
Eyebrows: Bushy; coarse; splayed.
Optic Nerve: Atrophy.

PRECAUTIONS

At the present time, there is no specific treatment for MPS IV. Hyperextension of the neck should be avoided.

COMMENTS

Although patients with MPS IV may die in childhood or adolescence as the result of pulmonary insufficient (severely reduced lung capacity) or spinal cord complications, adulthood may be attained although severe limitation of mobility may be present.

References

Berman ER: Biochemical diagnostic tests in genetic and metabolic eye diseases. *In* Goldberg MF (ed): Genetic and Metabolic Eye Disease. Boston, Little, Brown, 1974, pp 89–90.
Grossman H: The mucopolysaccharidoses and mucolipidoses. Progr Pediatr Radiol 4:495–544, 1973.
Legum CP, Schorr S, Berman ER: The genetic mucopolysaccharidoses and mucolipidoses: Review and comment. Adv Pediatr 22:305–347, 1976.
Maroteaux P, Lamy M: Hurler's disease, Morquio's disease, and related mucopolysaccharidoses. J Pediatr 67:312–323, 1965.
McKusick VA: Heritable Disorders of Connective Tissue, 4th ed. St. Louis, CV Mosby, 1972, pp 583–611.
Yuen M, Fenson AH: Diagnosis of classical Morquio's disease: N-acetyl-galactosamine-6-sulfate sulfatase activity in cultured fibroblasts, leukocytes, amniotic cells and chorionic villi. J Inherit Metab Dis 8:80–86, 1985.

MUCOPOLYSACCHARIDOSIS VI
(Maroteaux-Lamy Syndrome)
RICHARD G. WELEBER, M.D.,
and JACLYN VIDGOFF, Ph.D.
Portland, Oregon

Mucopolysaccharidosis VI is an autosomal recessive trait with an enzyme deficiency of sulfogalactosamine sulfatase (N-acetyl-galactosamine-4-sulfatase or arylsulfatase B), which causes dermatan sulfate to accumulate within the body. Excessive amounts of dermatan sulfate or chondroitin sulfate B are also present in the urine. There appear to be both mild and severe phenotypes, which may represent different allelic genes. Patients with an intermediate degree of severity have recently been described. The physical findings resemble those of mucopolysaccharidosis I-H with respect to growth retardation, skeletal deformities, and coarse facial features; however, intellectual development is normal. A prominent forehead and sternal protrusion are frequently noted soon after birth. Restriction of joint motion may begin by the first year. Growth retardation is first noted at the age of 2 or 3 years, and skeletal growth may cease entirely after 8 years. By the sixth year, all patients have hepatomegaly, and about half have enlarged spleens. Deafness and inguinal hernias are common. Cardiac involvement is frequent and, with respiratory complications, is the most serious threat to the patients. Generally, the life span is longer than in patients with mucopolysaccharidosis I-H, although, with the severe phenotype, survival past the mid-twenties is rare.

154 / MUCOPOLYSACCHARIDOSIS VI

The significant ocular manifestations of muco-polysaccharidosis VI are corneal clouding, which is moderate in degree and develops early, and optic atrophy. Papilledema has been reported and is thought to be associated with hydrocephalus.

THERAPY

Systemic. Several experimental approaches are currently being tried to restore the ability to degrade or clear the storage material. These include induction of enzyme synthesis, enhancement of any residual enzyme activity, and replacement therapy with exogenous enzyme. Plasma therapy, in which perfusions of fresh plasma are administered in order to provide a corrective factor for the particular enzymatic deficiency, may provide short-term biochemical improvement, but significant difficulties with long-term plasma therapy limit this approach. Another experimental approach is transfusion of lymphocytes. However, at present, no form of therapy has been of lasting benefit.

Supportive. The physician should offer sympathetic guidance in helping the parent deal with the skeletal deformities that arise in these patients. Parents should be informed of available inpatient chronic care facilities. Genetic counseling should be provided to parents and other potential carriers, as well as to patients who reach childbearing age. Both parents of an affected child are carriers of the deficient gene; however, since the gene defect is detectable in amniotic cell cultures, prenatal diagnosis is possible.

Surgical. Surgical treatment is supportive with repair of hernias and hydroceles, orthopedic surgery for skeletal deformities, or adenoidectomy to provide relief from the persistent nasal discharge, as indicated. Penetrating keratoplasy or lamellar corneal graft has been performed for significant corneal clouding. Hydrocephalus and associated papilledema may be relieved by shunting of cerebrospinal fluid.

Ocular or Periocular Manifestations

Choroid: Thinning.
Ciliary Body: Acid mucopolysaccharide deposits.
Cornea: Acid mucopolysaccharide deposits; clouding; opacity; thickening.
Eyebrows: Bushy; coarse.
Optic Nerve: Atrophy; cupping; papilledema.
Retina: Detachment; macular edema; vascular tortuosity.
Sclera: Acid mucopolysaccharide deposits; thickening.
Other: Coarse eyelashes; decreased visual acuity.

PRECAUTIONS

Atlantoaxial subluxation can occur as a result of hypoplasia of the odontoid process. In addition, neurologic deterioration from myelopathy due to thickening of the dura of the cervical spinal cord and consequent cord compression has been reported. Early surgical decompression appears to be beneficial.

COMMENTS

One of the most outstanding features of mucopolysaccharidosis VI is the normal intellectual capacity of the patients. They usually attend regular schools and pass their examinations without difficulties, although visual and physical handicaps eventually will impede their psychomotor performance.

References

Goldberg MF, Scott CI, McKusick VA: Hydrocephalus and papilledema in the Maroteaux-Lamy syndrome (mucopolysaccharidosis type VI). Am J Ophthalmol 69:969–975, 1970.

Kenyon KR, et al: Ocular pathology of the Maroteaux-Lamy syndrome (systemic mucopolysaccharidosis type VI). Histologic and ultrastructural report of two cases. Am J Ophthalmol 73:718–741, 1972.

McKusick VA: Heritable Disorders of Connective Tissue, 4th ed. St. Louis, CV Mosby, 1972, pp 611–627.

McKusick VA, Neufield EF, Kelly TE: The mucopolysaccharide storage diseases. In Stanbury JB, Wyngaarden JB, Fredrickson DS (eds): The Metabolic Basis of Inherited Disease, 4th ed. New York, McGraw-Hill, 1978, pp 1296–1298.

Spranger JW, et al: Mucopolysaccharidosis VI (Maroteaux-Lamy's disease). Helv Paediat Acta 25:337—362, 1970.

Stumpf DA, et al: Mucopolysaccharidosis type VI. (Maroteaux-Lamy syndrome). I. Sulfatase B deficiency in tissues. Am J Dis Child 126:747–755, 1973.

Tamaki N, et al: Myelopathy due to diffuse thickening of the cervical dura mater in Maroteaux-Lamy syndrome: Report of a case. Neurosurgery 21:416–419, 1987.

MUCOPOLYSACCHARIDOSIS VII
(β-Glucuronidase Deficiency, MPS VII)
WILLIAM S. SLY, M.D.
St. Louis, Missouri

Mucopolysaccharidosis VII is a rarely encountered autosomal recessive disorder caused by a deficiency of β-glucuronidase. The enzyme deficiency causes heparan sulfate, dermatan sulfate, and chondroitin-4 or -6-sulfate to accumulate within the body. The disorder is characterized by dwarfism, hepatosplenomegaly, skeletal deformities, mild to moderate mental retardation, hernias, unusual facies, delayed psychomotor development, and frequent symptomatic pulmonary infections. Variable corneal clouding may be present. Phenotypic variation in different pedigrees has been remarkable.

THERAPY

Systemic. Several experimental approaches are currently being tried to restore the ability to degrade or clear the storage material. Such therapy would require induction of enzyme synthesis, enhancement of any residual enzyme activity, or replacement therapy with exogenous enzyme. Other experimental approaches include bone marrow transplantation.

Supportive. The physician should offer the parents sympathetic guidance in dealing with the gross deformities and mental retardation that may arise in these patients. The parents should be informed of any inpatient chronic care facilities that may be available. Genetic counseling is indicated for parents, as the risk of recurrence is 25 per cent in subsequent pregnancies. Prenatal diagnosis is possible from enzyme assays on cells cultured from amniocentesis specimens.

Surgical. Surgical treatment is supportive and might include repair of hernias or orthopedic surgery for skeletal deformities. Penetrating keratoplasty or lamellar corneal graft is the treatment of choice for corneal clouding.

Ocular or Periocular Manifestations

Cornea: Clouding.

PRECAUTIONS

There is no specific treatment for any of the mucopolysaccharidoses. Plasma infusion has occasionally provided temporary improvement, but it is still not a practical means of therapy.

COMMENTS

The phenotypic variability of β-glucuronidase deficiency is quite remarkable and suggests genetic heterogeneity. Recently, several unrelated β-glucuronidase-deficient patients have presented in the newborn period with nonimmune hydrops and have died within the first 12 months. This is the most severe clinical form of the disease; the milder forms resemble the Hunter syndrome phenotype in severity, though symptoms are less progressive in late childhood. Despite considerable variability of β-glucuronidase activity in the plasma and serum of normal individuals, the homozygous-affected patient can readily be diagnosed from serum. For carrier detection, the enzyme should preferably be measured in fibroblast cultures or leukocytes. The relatively simple enzymatic assay on white blood cell lysates provides a means for making or excluding this diagnosis, as well as for determining carrier states. Its application to other patients with mucopolysaccharidoses will help delineate this entity further.

References

Beaudet AL, et al: Variation in the phenotypic expression of β-glucuronidase deficiency. J Pediatr 86:388–394, 1975.

Gitzelmann R, et al: Unusually mild course of β-glucuronidase deficiency in two brothers (mucopolysaccharidosis VII). Helv Paediatr Acta 33:413–428, 1978.

Guibaud P, et al: Mucopolysaccharidosis type VII par deficit en beta-glucuronidase: Etude d'une famille. J Genet Hum 27:29–43, 1979.

Lee JES, Falk RE, Ng WG, Donnell GN: Beta-glucuronidase deficiency; a heterogeneous mucopolysaccharidosis. Am J Dis Child 139:57–59, 1985.

Nelson A, et al: Mucopolysaccharidosis VII (β-glucuronidase deficiency) presenting as nonimmune hydrops fetalis. J Pediatr 101:574–576, 1982.

Sewell AC, Gehler J, Mittermaier G, Mayer E: Mucopolysaccharidosis type VII (beta-glucuronidase deficiency): A report of a new case and a survey of those in the literature. Clin Genet 21:366–373, 1982.

Sly WS, et al: Beta glucuronidase deficiency: Report of clinical, radiologic, and biochemical features of a new mucopolysaccharidosis. J Pediatr 82:249–257, 1973.

SECTION 7

DISORDERS OF LIPID METABOLISM

ANGIOKERATOMA CORPORIS DIFFUSUM UNIVERSALE
(Anderson-Fabry Disease, Fabry's Disease, Glycolipid Lipidosis)

THOMAS A. WEINGEIST, M.D., Ph.D.
Iowa City, Iowa

Angiokeratoma corporis diffusum universale is a rare glycolipid thesaurosis that results from an x-linked recessive inborn error of metabolism. Deficiency of an alpha-galactosidase (formerly called ceramide trihexosidase) has been found to be the major enzymatic defect in this disorder, although recent studies have implicated additional enzymes.

Cutaneous angiokeratomas and a whorl-like corneal dystrophy are the most distinctive physical findings in Fabry's disease. Accumulation of neutral glycosphingolipids in endothelial, perithelial, and smooth muscle cells of the cardiovascular, renal, and cerebrovascular systems results in progressive impairment and premature death. The full-blown manifestations of Fabry's disease occur only in males (hemizygotes). Early in life, affected males frequently have episodic pain, acroparesthesia accompanied by low-grade fever, and an elevated erythrocyte sedimentation rate. Affected males have a reduced alpha-galactosidase level in plasma, serum, leukocytes, tears, and skin fibroblasts. An elevated trihexosyl ceramide level in urine, plasma, and skin fibroblasts can also be demonstrated. Multiple wine-red angiokeratomas involve the trunk, fingers, penis, lips, and tongue. Skin lesions may be distributed in the bathing trunk region in hemizygous adults. Death usually occurs before the fourth or fifth decade from renal or cardiac failure or from cerebrovascular disease. Female carriers (heterozygotes) are involved to a lesser extent and usually develop symptoms at a later age. In heterozygous females, Fabry's disease is usually limited to the eyes; life expectancy is nearly normal, since renal and cerebrovascular involvement is uncommon.

The ocular findings in Fabry's disease are often subtle and seldom interfere with vision. The most characteristic ocular sign is a fine, whorl-like, superficial corneal opacity that occurs in both affected male subjects and female carriers. On slitlamp examination, golden-brown pigmentation is visible in the corneal epithelium. This vortex corneal pattern resembles the corneal changes found after chronic ingestion of chloro-

quine, amiodarone, and other agents that cause a drug-induced lipidosis. The familial corneal dystrophy of Fleischer-Gruber (cornea verticillata), which was once considered a separate entity, has been found to be a manifestation of Fabry's disease. Dilated sausage-shaped conjunctival blood vessels and tortuosity of retinal vessels are common. Two specific types of cataracts occur in Fabry's disease. One type is characterized by granular anterior subcapsular deposits. The other type is an unusual spoke-like posterior subcapsular opacity that is best seen by retroillumination.

In Fabry's disease, decreased visual acuity results primarily from occlusive retinal vascular disease and complications of hypertensive retinopathy. Profound loss of vision from central retinal artery occlusion is sometimes the initial presenting symptom.

Abnormal accumulation of intracytoplasmic lipid occurs throughout endothelial, perithelial, and smooth muscle cells of the eye. Intracellular deposits of lipid also occur in epithelial cells of the conjunctiva, cornea, and lens. Ultrastructural examination of these inclusions reveals that they consist of a single membrane, surrounding concentrically arranged membranous lamellae. These myelin-like structures are not pathognomonic of Fabry's disease.

The histopathologic basis for the whorl-like pattern in the cornea has been the subject of debate. Increasing evidence indicates that it is due to a combination of accumulation of lysosomal granules in the epithelium that have been detected even in the fetus and duplication of the basal lamina of the corneal epithelium.

THERAPY

Systemic. Intravenous administration of purified enzyme (placental alpha-galactosidase)[†] has been investigated but offers little promise. Phlebotomy does not alter plasma or urinary levels of ceramide trihexoside, and plasmapheresis is ineffective in treating the acroparesthesia of Fabry's disease.

Surgical. No satisfactory treatment is currently available. Renal transplantation has been performed for amelioration of chronic uremia. Unfortunately, recurrence of the storage disease is common in the renal allograft. The disproportionately high incidence of sepsis in some patients may be due to deficient immunologic function of lipid-laden leukocytes. Hemodialysis remains an alternative mode of therapy for uremia, but it does not alter the accompanying cerebrovascular disease.

Ocular or Periocular Manifestations

Conjunctiva: Telangiectasia.
Cornea: Cornea verticillata; whorl-like or spoke-like opacity.
Extraocular Muscles: Internuclear ophthalmoplegia.
Eyelids: Edema.
Lens: Anterior and posterior, spoke-like, subcapsular opacity ("Fabry cataract").
Optic Nerve: Disc edema.
Orbit: Periorbital edema.
Retina: Central or branch retinal artery occlusion; hypertensive retinopathy; vascular occlusive disease; vascular tortuosity.

PRECAUTIONS

Genetic counseling and recognition of female carriers are important. The pattern of inheritance is like that of all x-linked recessive disorders. There is absence of father-to-son transmission. All daughters of an affected male will be carriers (heterozygotes). Half the sons of affected daughters will also have Fabry's disease. Identification of all female carriers is difficult, since 25 to 40 per cent of suspected heterozygotes may have normal alpha-galactosidase levels. Recent studies have shown that, with the use of multiple biochemical tests, carriers can now be identified in more than 90 per cent of cases.

Cobra venom‡, cortisone‡, vasoconstrictors‡, vasodilators‡, and antihistamines‡ have been used in the treatment of Fabry's disease, but none has been demonstrated to be effective. Stellate ganglion block and bilateral cervical sympathectomy do not alleviate the pain.

COMMENTS

The diagnosis of Fabry's disease is easily missed, especially in female carriers. The ophthalmologist is in an excellent position to make the diagnosis of Fabry's disease, since corneal changes are the earliest and the most consistent ocular abnormality. Corneal changes occur in about 90 per cent of affected male subjects and may be the only ocular sign in female carriers. The posterior spoke-like cataracts may be pathognomonic. The whorl-like corneal opacities are highly indicative of Fabry's disease, especially if there has been no history of consumption of drugs, such as chloroquine.

References

Beutler E, Westwood B, Dale GL: The effect of phlebotomy as a treatment of Fabry disease. Biochem Med 30:363–368, 1983.
Braine HG, et al: A prospective double-blind study of plasma exchange therapy for the acroparesthesia of Fabry's disease. Transfusion 21:686–689, 1981.
Desnick RJ, et al: Fabry disease: Molecular diagnosis of hemizygotes and heterozygotes. Enzyme 38:54–64, 1987.
Desnick RJ, Grabowski GA: Advances in the treatment of inherited metabolic diseases. Adv Hum Genet 11:281–369, 1981.
Kleijer WJ, et al: Prenatal diagnosis of Fabry's disease by direct analysis of chorionic villi. Prenat. Diagn 7:283–287, 1987.
Mathew TH: Recurrence of disease following renal transplantation. Am J Kidney Dis 12:85–96, 1988.
Riegel EM, et al: Ocular pathology of Fabry's disease in a hemizygous male following renal transplantation. Surv Ophthalmol 26:247–252, 1982.
Rodriguez FH, Hoffmann EO, Ordinario AT: Fabry's disease in a heterozygous woman. Arch Pathol Lab Med 109:89–91, 1985.
Sakuraba H, et al: Effects of vitamin E and ticlopidine on platelet aggregation in Fabry's disease. Clin Genet 31:349–354, 1987.
Tsutsumi A, et al: Corneal findings in a foetus with Fabry's disease. Acta Ophthalmol 62:923–931, 1984.

HYPERLIPOPROTEINEMIA
MALCOLM N. LUXENBERG, M.D.
Augusta, Georgia

Hyperlipoproteinemia is a metabolic disorder characterized by abnormally elevated concentrations of specific lipoprotein particles in the plasma. Hyperlipidemia, which refers to an elevation of the plasma cholesterol and/or triglycerides above the normal range, is present in all these disorders. The hyperlipoproteinemias can be separated into primary and secondary forms, with the secondary form being caused by other diseases, such as diabetes mellitus, pancreatitis, renal disease, or hypothyroidism. The hyperlipoproteinemias can be divided into distinct groups that are determined by the pattern of elevation of the plasma lipoproteins. These groups are not specific diseases, but may represent the final result of various metabolic disorders. Certain ones can be defined as genetically determined, and their mechanisms and modes of inheritance have been determined. The primary groups include chylomicronemia (exogenous or endogenous hyperlipemia), hypercholesterolemia, dysbetalipoproteinemia (hyperlipoproteinemia type 3), hypertriglyceridemia, mixed hyperlipoproteinemia, and combined hyperlipoproteinemia. Clinical manifestations of the hyperlipoproteinemias are caused by deposition of lipids at various sites throughout the body, such as the skin, tendons, vascular system, and eye. Corneal arcus, lipemia retinalis, and xanthelasma are the most common ocular abnormalities.

THERAPY

Systemic. Various drugs, especially those that lower cholesterol and/or triglycerides, may be beneficial in the management of these disorders. Some of the medications used include clofibrate, gemfibrozil, niacin, cholestyramine resin, colestipol, dextrothyroxine, sitosterols, probucol, and some progestational agents. Gemfibrozil, one of the newer drugs, is chemically related to clofibrate and lowers both cholesterol and triglycerides. Because of the possibility of significant side effects and the question as to whether triglycerides are independent risk factors for atherosclerosis, many physicians use drugs to reduce triglyceride levels only when they exceed 500 mg/100 ml. The newest class of HMG Co-A reductase inhibitors (lovastatin) are potent cholesterol-lowering drugs. It is currently recommended that an annual eye examination be done in patients taking these drugs as lens opacities may develop with their use.

Supportive. Diet remains the cornerstone of therapy for hyperlipidemia. Weight reduction is desirable, and saturated fat and cholesterol intake may need to be restricted. Alcohol and estrogens should be avoided in certain types of hyperlipoproteinemias.

Surgical. Ileal bypass surgery and plasmapheresis may be used to lower elevated serum lipids in very selected cases of familial hypercholesterolemia. These forms of therapy should only be used by physicians with experience in this field.

Xanthelasma may be surgically excised, with small defects being primarily closed and large defects requiring skin grafting. Care must be taken to avoid postoperative ectropion. Xanthelasma may also be removed by photocoagulation.

Ocular or Periocular Manifestations

Choroid: Xanthoma (hypercholesterolemia).
Conjunctiva: Lipemia of limbal vessels (dysbetalipoproteinemia); xanthoma (hypercholesterolemia).
Cornea: Arcus (hypercholesterolemia and dysbetalipoproteinemia); lipid keratopathy (chylomicronemia and hypercholesterolemia).
Eyelids: Eruptive xanthoma (chylomicronemia, dysbetalipoproteinemia, and mixed hypertriglyceridemia); xanthelasma (hypercholesterolemia and dysbetalipoproteinemia).
Iris: Xanthoma (chylomicronemia).
Retina: Lipemia retinalis (chylomicronemia and mixed hypertriglyceridemia); xanthoma (chylomicronemia and hypercholesterolemia).

PRECAUTIONS

Hyperlipoproteinemia may be present in children and young adults, and persons with these disorders may develop abnormalities of the vascular system, including ischemic cardiac disease. Therefore, it is important to obtain appropriate medical evaluation, especially in patients under 40 to 45 years of age who have a prominent arcus of the cornea, xanthelasma, or in any patient with lipemia retinalis, in order to establish a diagnosis and initiate therapy when appropriate. Corneal arcus is commonly seen in nor-

mal people, especially in males over the age of 45 years without associated hyperlipidemia. Although xanthelasma may be present without elevation of the serum lipids, about half of the patients have elevated cholesterol levels. Recent studies have demonstrated apolipoprotein abnormalities in patients with xanthelasma, including those with normal cholesterol levels. There may also be an increased prevalence of hyperlipidemia in patients with retinal vein occlusion. In many cases, it is difficult or impossible to determine which patients with these findings have hyperlipidemia, especially when there are no other signs of hyperlipoproteinemia. Therefore, one should consider obtaining serum cholesterol and triglyceride studies in any patient with premature arcus or xanthelasma, as these tests are inexpensive and harmless.

COMMENTS

Measurements of plasma lipid and lipoprotein levels should be performed while the patient is on a regular diet after an overnight fast of 12 to 16 hours. Identification of abnormal lipoprotein patterns can often be made after determining serum cholesterol and triglyceride levels and visual inspection of the plasma sample, which has been stored at 4°C. In some cases, it may be necessary to perform electrophoresis and ultracentrifugation on whole plasma specimens to make a diagnosis.

Lipemia retinalis is caused primarily by elevation of the serum triglycerides, which imparts a milky color to the blood. The changes are usually not seen until the triglyceride level reaches at least 2000 mg per cent and are best observed in the early stages in the peripheral fundus. The vessels initially appear "salmon pink"; as the triglyceride level rises, they assume a whitish appearance. These changes, which begin in the periphery, progress toward the posterior pole as the triglyceride level rises. In severe cases, the vessels are creamy white in color, and it becomes difficult to differentiate arteries from veins. The findings can fluctuate widely from day to day, depending on the triglyceride level. The fundus abnormalities, which improve as the triglycerides return to normal, provide a means of following the patient's course and response to therapy.

Patients suspected or known to have hyperlipoproteinemia should be referred to a physician familiar with these disorders for evaluation and management, as treatment can be difficult, especially regarding selection and use of specific drugs.

References

Bron AJ, Williams HP: Lipaemia of the limbal vessels. Br J Ophthalmol 56:343–346, 1972.
Brunzell JD, Bierman EL: Chylomicronemia syndrome. Interaction of genetic and acquired hypertriglyceridemia. Med Clin North Am 66:455–468, 1982.
Dodson PM, et al: Retinal vein occlusion and the prevalence of lipoprotein abnormalities. Br J Ophthalmol 66:161–164, 1982.

Fredrickson DS, Goldstein JS, Brown MS: The familial hyperlipoproteinemias. *In* Stanbury JB, Wyngaarden JB, Fredrickson DS (eds): The Metabolic Basis of Inherited Disease, 5th ed. New York, McGraw-Hill, 1982, pp 655–671.

Havel RJ, Kane JP: Therapy of hyperlipidemic states. Annu Rev Med 33:417–433, 1982.

Havel RJ, Goldstein JL, Brown MS: Lipoproteins and lipid transport. *In* Bondy PK, Rosenberg LE (eds): Metabolic Control and Disease, 8th ed. Philadelphia, WB Saunders, 1980, pp 393–494.

Kuske TT, Feldman EB: Hyperlipoproteinemia, atherosclerosis risk and dietary management. Arch Intern Med 147:357–360, 1987.

Margolis S: Treatment of hyperlipemia. JAMA 239:2696–2698, 1978.

Rifkind BM: Corneal arcus and hyperlipoproteinemia. Surv Ophthalmol 16:295–304, 1972.

Spaeth GL: Ocular manifestations of the lipodoses. *In* Tasman W (ed): Retinal Diseases in Children. New York, Harper & Row, 1971, pp 127–137.

Vinger PF, Sachs BA: Ocular manifestations of hyperlipoproteinemia. Am J Ophthalmol 70:563–573, 1970.

SECTION 8

OTHER METABOLIC DISORDERS

GOUT
(Hyperuricemia)
SIDNEY LERMAN, M.D.
Atlanta, Georgia

Gout comprises a group of diseases (usually inherited) in which there is an abnormality of purine metabolism or uric acid excretion by the kidneys or both. It is inherited as an autosomal dominant trait, but can have variable expression clinically, ranging from acute gouty arthritis to asymptomatic hyperuricemia. Gouty arthritis is much more prevalent in males than in females (20 to 1 ratio), but simple hyperuricemia appears to occur equally in both sexes. Gouty arthritis is more common in the upper socioeconomic classes, which may be related to dietary habits. In acute gouty arthritis, the feet and ankles are most frequently involved, and the symptomatology consists of acute pain, inflammation, and swelling. However, gouty arthritis can affect any of the extremities, and gouty tophi (accumulation of uric acid deposits) can occur anywhere in the body, although most frequently in joints, bursae, and subcutaneous regions. Tophi in the kidneys can cause severe destruction, resulting in hydronephrosis and/or pyelonephritis. Ocular involvement is relatively rare and generally not severe. Sodium urate deposits occur most frequently in the conjunctiva and episclera, resulting in chronic conjunctivitis and episcleritis. Gouty uveitis is a rather rare ocular manifestation.

THERAPY

Systemic. When therapy is directed against the acute inflammatory condition, colchicine is used to provide relief from an acute attack and also as a prophylactic agent to prevent recurrence. Colchicine appears to act by inhibiting the migration of granulocytic cells to the inflamed area and decreasing lactic acid production, which is commonly associated with phagocytosis. It is thought that this action serves to interrupt the cycle of uric acid crystal deposition and therefore the subsequent inflammatory response. Colchicine is also a well-known antimitotic agent, which may explain its ability to prevent the mobilization of leukocytes during inflammation. It also inhibits histamine release from mast cells. When colchicine is given promptly (within the first few hours of an acute attack of gouty arthritis), it provides dramatic relief in well over 90 per cent of such patients.

This has led to the use of colchicine for diagnostic purposes. The initial dose is 1 mg, followed by 0.5 mg every 2 to 3 hours; therapy is stopped as soon as the pain disappears or gastrointestinal symptoms occur. In most cases, the total dose required to alleviate an attack is approximately 4 to 8 mg. It is important not to repeat colchicine therapy within 3 days because of cumulative toxicity. If necessary, colchicine can be given intravenously in a single dose of approximately 2 mg diluted in 20 ml of 0.9 per cent sodium chloride solution. It is also used as a prophylactic agent during the asymptomatic period for patients with chronic gout and is indicated in patients who are started on chronic allopurinol therapy. Because there is a frequent increase in the incidence of acute attacks during the first few months of therapy with allopurinol or other drugs that increase the renal excretion of uric acid, colchicine therapy is recommended initially in conjunction with allopurinol or uricosuric agent therapy.

Allopurinol is a purine analog that inhibits the terminal steps in the biosynthesis of uric acid. This reduces the plasma concentration and urinary excretion of uric acid and increases the blood levels and renal excretion of the more soluble precursors of uric acid. Allopurinol is rapidly absorbed after oral dosage, and peak plasma concentrations are reached within 2 to 6 hours. It is rapidly cleared from the plasma by conversion to alloxanthine, which in turn is slowly excreted in the urine. Although alloxanthine is a less potent inhibitor of the xanthine oxidase enzyme than allopurinol, it can contribute to the therapeutic effect of allopurinol therapy, since it tends to accumulate with chronic administration of allopurinol. Allopurinol is used to control the hyperuricemia in gout and to maintain the uric acid level in the plasma below 6 mg per cent. It should never be started during an acute attack of gouty arthritis and is generally given initially at low doses to decrease the risk of precipitating and acute attack. Concurrent colchicine therapy is recommended for the first few months of allopurinol therapy. Allopurinol is started with an initial daily dose of 100 mg and increased at 100-mg intervals every week. The usual daily maintenance dose for adults is about 300 mg and can be given as a single dose. In resistant cases, daily doses of 600 to 800 mg may be required. It is important to determine the renal status of the patient, since the dosage must be reduced in patients with renal impairment.

Other drugs that can be used to treat gout are the uricosuric drugs that act by increasing the renal excretion of uric acid and thus reducing the plasma uric acid levels. These include probenecid and sulfinpyrazone.

Ocular. The therapy of the ocular complications of gout includes artificial tears for patients with conjunctivitis and proper lid hygiene. Steroid drops or ointment may be required for patients who develop scleritis and can be given two to three times daily. Topical steroids and cycloplegics are generally very effective for the rare case of gouty uveitis. If band keratopathy develops, a superficial keratectomy can be performed.

Supportive. In addition to drug therapy, attention to dietary intake is an important adjunct, particularly the avoidance of foods that are high in purine content. The obese patient should also be encouraged to lose weight.

Precautions

Allopurinol is contraindicated in patients who have exhibited adverse effects from this form of therapy, such as hypersensitivity reactions involving the skin and the blood. The skin reaction is a pruritic erythematous or maculopapular eruption with fever and malaise. It occurs more frequently in patients with renal impairment. Leukopenia or leukocytosis is rare, but if they occur, allopurinol therapy must be stopped. Allopurinol is also contraindicated in nursing mothers and in children. In addition to these side effects of allopurinol, this agent has also recently been implicated in human cataractogenesis. Allopurinol has been demonstrated in cataractous lenses derived from patients on chronic allopurinol therapy. There is a suggestion that concurrent exposure to ultraviolet radiation may result in the photobinding of this drug to lens proteins, leading to the generation (and permanent retention) of a new photosensitizer within the lens. Such a photosensitizer could exert a cataractogenic influence by enhancing the cumulative photochemical changes already occurring in the ocular lens (as a result of the continuous exposure to ambient ultraviolet radiation). Recent laboratory evidence has demonstrated a relationship between allopurinol, photosensitization, and cataract formation in humans, as well as in experimental animals. If photosensitization plays a role in enhancing allopurinol cataractogenesis, it could be easily prevented by prescribing proper ultraviolet filtering spectacles, which are now available in plastic as well as specially coated glass lenses.

Comments

Since there is no known cure for gout, treatment should be directed toward management of the complications of the disease. The goals of therapy should include rapid termination of the acute attack, prevention of future attacks of gout, lowering the serum uric acid to prevent its accumulation in body tissues, prevention of the formation of uric acid stones, and treatment of disorders accompanying hyperuricemia.

References

Bloch RS, Henkind P: Ocular manifestations of endocrine and metabolic diseases. In Duane TD (ed): Clinical Ophthalmology. Hagerstown, MD, Harper & Row, 1982, Vol V, pp 21:20–21.

Flower RI, Moncada S, Vane JR: Analgesic-antipyretics and anti-inflammatory agents; drugs employed in the treatment of gout. In Gilman AG, Goodman IS, Gilman A (eds): The Pharmacological Basis of Therapeutics, 6th ed. New York, MacMillan, 1980, pp 717–728.

Fraunfelder FT, et al: Cataracts associated with allopurinol therapy. Am J Ophthalmol 94:137–140, 1982.

Lerman S, Megaw JM, Gardner K: Allopurinol therapy and cataractogenesis in humans. Am J Ophthalmol 94:141–146, 1982.

XERODERMA PIGMENTOSUM

JEFFREY FREEDMAN, M.B., B.Ch., Ph.D., F.R.C.S.E.
Brooklyn, New York

Xeroderma pigmentosum is a rare, autosomal recessive disorder characterized by extreme cutaneous photosensitivity to ultraviolet light, early development of cutaneous malignancies of ectodermal and mesodermal origin on ultraviolet light-exposed areas, severe ophthalmologic abnormalities, and, often, early death from malignancy. Neurologic abnormalities are also sometimes present. The range of harmful ultraviolet light is all that up to a wavelength of at least 320 nm and possibly even up to and higher than 340 nm. Consequently, such harmful ultraviolet light from sunlight, germicidal lamps, sunlamps, and even some commonly employed fluorescent light tubes must be avoided.

Symptoms of the disease are usually noted by 3 years of age, but may first become apparent in adult life. Photosensitivity is one of the earliest recognized cutaneous signs, characterized by erythema occurring on exposed areas, especially the face, neck, V area of the chest, forearms, and dorsa of hands. The skin lesions can be divided into six stages: stage 1—Acute sun sensitivity in infancy, and inflammation erythema and bullae; stage 2—Pigmented macules and achromic spots in exposed areas; stage 3—Telangiectasia of exposed areas; stage 4—Atrophy of lids, dryness of conjunctiva, and corneal opacification; stage 5—Benign growths, conjunctival inflammatory masses, symblepharon, and papillomas of lids; stage 6—Neoplasms: epithelioma, basal cell carcinoma, and malignant melanoma.

Corneal involvement may be the most common ocular change occurring with xeroderma pigmentosum. Beginning before 2 years of age, vascularization of the inferior half of the cornea may be followed by vascularization of the upper half of the cornea. The vessels regress, leaving a nonvascularized opaque area so that at 2 years of age the entire cornea is opaque. During the ac-

162 / XERODERMA PIGMENTOSUM

tive stage of vascularization, the patient may experience intensive photophobia and lacrimation. Presumably, the lower half of the cornea is involved early because of its more direct exposure to the sun, the upper half being protected by the lid. Histologically, all layers of the cornea appear to be abnormal, with the most prominent change being a degenerative pannus and irregularity of its superficial corneal stroma. Band-shaped nodular dystrophy, also known as climatic droplet keratopathy, has been noted in a patient with xeroderma pigmentosum. Other ocular lesions may include conjunctival pterygia and pinguecula; benign papillomas and fibromas of the iris occur less frequently. Keratoconus may occur in association with xeroderma pigmentosum; it may be the result of disturbances in the cell differentiation and the function of epithelial cells and keratocytes caused by ultraviolet-light-induced deficient DNA synthesis. The fundus of the eye is not affected in xeroderma pigmentosum.

In a survey of 830 patients with xeroderma pigmentosum, ocular abnormalities were reported in 40 per cent of the patients described and were restricted to tissues exposed to ultraviolet radiation (lid, conjunctiva, and cornea). The abnormalities included ectropion, corneal opacity leading to blindness, and neoplasms. Malignant neoplasms develop in many patients with xeroderma pigmentosa and involve the lids, conjunctiva, or corneoscleral limbus. Conjunctival neoplasms include intraepithelial epithelioma, squamous cell carcinoma, and sarcomas. Corneal tumors may be primary or secondary to invasion from the corneoscleral limbus. Corneal neoplasms include epitheliomas, sarcomas, squamous cell carcinomas, and melanomas. In some patients, the malignancies may invade the orbit.

THERAPY

Systemic. Systemic chemotherapy is used only for patients with known metastasis.

Ocular. Methylcellulose drops or soft contact lenses may be used to keep the cornea moist and to protect against mechanical trauma in patients whose lids are severely deformed. Corneal transplantation can be used to treat patients with corneal opacification due to pannus. If corneal transplantation is undertaken, an anti-rejection regimen must be used. The regimen that has been utilized with some success is a combination of steroids and azathioprine. Prednisolone in a dosage of 200 mg daily is given for 5 days. This is reduced by 10 mg per day to 100 mg. When this level is reached, the dosage is dropped by 10 mg per week to a standing dose of 60 mg daily. Azathioprine is given in a dose of 150 mg daily for 1 month and then dropped to 100 mg daily for a minimum period of 6 months. Weekly blood counts and platelet levels must be performed Azathioprine is stopped if platelets

drop below 150,000 or white cell count below 3000.

Supportive. Since exposure to sunlight results in the skin changes typical of xeroderma pigmentosum, patients must be educated to constantly protect all body surfaces from ultraviolet radiation. In addition to sunlight, ultraviolet exposure may come from germicidal lamps, artificial sunlamps, and to a small extent, the common, unfiltered, cool, white, fluorescent lamps. However, long wavelength ultraviolet radiation from incandescent lamps or sunlight passing through window glass is not known to be harmful. Ultraviolet radiation protection should consist of adopting a life-style to minimize the possibility of ultraviolet radiation exposure; wearing protective clothing, glasses, and hairstyles; and use of sunscreens. When outdoors, patients should wear long-sleeved clothing, long pants, and wide-brimmed hats. Sunglasses or eyeglasses that are completely opaque to ultraviolet radiation should be worn. The glasses should incorporate side shields to protect the eyelids and periorbital skin, as well as the cornea and conjunctiva. Exposed skin should be covered with physical ultraviolet radiation blocking agents, such as zinc oxide ointment, titanium dioxide compounds, or thick makeup. Chemical sunscreens with the highest sun protection factor ratings should be used; these usually contain para-aminobenzoic acid or its derivatives.

Fibroblasts from patients with xeroderma pigmentosum exhibit an abnormally sensitive response to chemical carcinogens, such as benzapyrene derivatives and others. Exposure to such common environmental carcinogens as cigarette smoke should be minimized.

Early detection of cutaneous and ocular lesions is important to permit treatment with minimal morbidity. Patients should be examined weekly by a family member who has been instructed in recognition of cutaneous neoplasms. This examination should include the eyes, scalp, ears, mouth, as well as covered skin areas.

Surgical. Premalignant lesions, such as multiple actinic keratoses, may be treated with superficial freezing with liquid nitrogen or with topical application of fluorouracil. Larger areas have been treated with therapeutic dermatome shaving or dermabrasion. These modalities remove the outer, more damaged epidermal layers. The epidermis is then repopulated by cells from follicles or glands, which by virtue of their deeper location have received less ultraviolet radiation exposure. Each melanoma should be treated as if it were the sole primary melanoma, with the surgical procedure dictated by the histology and location of the lesion. Malignant lesions not amenable to the above modalities can be treated with x-ray.

Neoplasms of the lids, conjunctiva, and cornea are usually treated surgically. All conjunctival surfaces must be examined for malignancies as these can occur in the fornices and may be missed unless looked for.

Ocular or Periocular Manifestations

Conjunctiva: Conjunctivitis; inflammatory nodules; malignancies; pigmentation; symblepharon.
Cornea: Exposure keratitis; malignancies; pannus; perforation; ulcer.
Eyelids: Blepharitis; blepharospasm; ectropion; keratoses; malignancies; pigmentation.
Iris: Anterior uveitis; malignancies.
Other: Photophobia; visual loss.

PRECAUTIONS

Psoralens followed by long wavelength ultraviolet radiation should not be used in xeroderma pigmentosum patients. This treatment results in DNA damage, which is not repaired normally in xeroderma pigmentosum cells, and has been reported to result in an increase in skin cancer in patients with xeroderma pigmentosum and psoriasis. Actinic keratoses have been treated with topical fluorouracil, but patients may eventually become refractory to this treatment.

COMMENTS

In patients in whom systemic chemotherapy must be used, care should be exercised to avoid untoward reactions that might result from the use of a chemotherapeutic drug to which the patient might be abnormally sensitive by virtue of defective DNA repair. The dermatologic changes that occur in patients with xeroderma pigmentosum are due to an inherited deficiency in the repair of DNA damage produced by irradiation with ultraviolet light. DNA damage produced by certain chemicals is also not repaired normally by xeroderma pigmentosum cells. The ocular abnormalities in this disorder probably result both from the intrinsic DNA repair defect in those cells of the eye that are irradiated with sunlight and from impairment of the mechanical protection of the ocular accessory organs.

There is no known prevention for the progressive neurologic abnormalities of xeroderma pigmentosum. However, with early diagnosis, appropriate avoidance of harmful ultraviolet light, and prompt treatment of neoplasms, most xeroderma pigmentosum patients without neurologic abnormalities can now survive well into adulthood and lead productive lives.

References

Blanksma LJ, Donders PC, vanVoorst Vader PC: Xeroderma pigmentosum and keratoconus. Doc Ophthalmol 64:97–103, 1986.
Freedman J: Xeroderma pigmentosum and band-shaped nodular corneal dystrophy. Br J Ophthalmol 61:96–100, 1977.
Freedman J: Corneal transplantation with associated histopathologic description in xeroderma pigmentosum occurring in a black family. Ann Ophthalmol 11:445–448, 1979.
Kraemer KH: Xeroderma pigmentosum. In Demis DJ, Dobson R, McGuire J (eds): Clinical Dermatology. Hagerstown, MD, Harper & Row, 1980.
Kraemer KH, Lee MM, Scotto J: Xeroderma pigmentosum. Cutaneous, ocular and neurologic abnormalities in 830 published cases. Arch Dermatol 123:241–250, 1987.
Newsome DA, Kraemer KH, Robbins JH: Repair of DNA in xeroderma pigmentosum conjunctiva. Arch Ophthalmol 93:660–662, 1975.
Regan JD, et al: Repair of DNA damaged by mutagenic metabolites of benzo(a)pyrene in human cells. Chem Biol Interact 20:279–287, 1978.
Robbins JH: Significance of repair of human DNA: Evidence from studies of xeroderma pigmentosum. J Natl Cancer Inst 61:645–656, 1978.
Robbins, JH, et al: Xeroderma pigmentosum. An inherited disease with sun sensitivity, multiple cutaneous neoplasms, and abnormal DNA repair. Ann Intern Med 80:221–248, 1974.

SECTION 9

HEMATOLOGIC AND CARDIOVASCULAR DISORDERS

ARTERIOVENOUS FISTULA

(Arteriovenous Aneurysm, Arteriovenous Angioma, Arteriovenous Malformation, Cirsoid Aneurysm, Racemose Hemangioma, Varicose Aneurysm)

J. REIMER WOLTER, M.D.

Ann Arbor, Michigan

Arteriovenous fistulas are abnormal communications, single or multiple, between arteries and veins by which arterial blood enters the veins directly without traversing a capillary network. These fistulas can be developmental or acquired. Most acquired arteriovenous fistulas occur secondarily to penetrating injuries or in certain circumstances secondarily to blunt trauma. Malignancy, infection, and arterial aneurysms are also responsible for the development of arteriovenous communications. The congenital arteriovenous fistulas are usually complex structures with many separate or interconnected lesions, most commonly found in the head and neck region. Clinical manifestations may include aching pain, edema, palpitation, substernal pain, and dyspnea. The presence of fistulas in subcutaneous tissue, limb swelling with hypertrophy, visible pulsation with macrofistula communications, and varicose veins in atypical locations are common. The tissue near the fistula may be tender, edematous, and either red or slightly cyanotic. In congenital arteriovenous fistulas, the skin temperature is usually elevated locally but decreased distal to the fistula.

All vascular parts of the eye and its adnexa can be involved by arteriovenous fistulas, which may often be part of more extensive malformations in the eye region, such as Sturge-Weber syndrome. The major outflow of periocular arteriovenous fistulas is the superior ophthalmic veins, which may expand tremendously with engorged orbital and conjunctival veins. These veins become arterialized, producing signs and symptoms of venous congestion. Corneal epithelial edema, flare and cells in the anterior chamber, glaucoma, rubeosis iridis, cataract, retinal venous dilation, and hemorrhages are common manifestations in this condition.

THERAPY

Surgical. Before operating, it is important to obtain complete angiographic studies. The usual clinical studies, including roentgenograms of the skull with laminography are equally important for arteriovenous fistulas of the ocular region.

Single fistulas can be repaired surgically be reestablishing the continuity of the involved artery and vein walls by a variety of procedures, including arteriorrhaphy, end-to-end anastomosis, or grafting. Embolization of feeding arteries using detachable balloons, isobutylcyanoacrylate, or polyvinyl particles has been recorded, but this can lead to complications. Thus, mild cases should be managed conservatively. Multiple fistulas in some cases mainly present as a space-taking problem and can be excised or otherwise obliterated completely.

Eighty-five to 90 percent of all arteriovenous aneurysms are supplied primarily by the carotid circulation. Among the recommended treatments are carotid ligation in the neck and/or intracranial and extracranial internal carotid ligation, with possible additional ligation of the external carotid and ophthalmic arteries. The superior ophthalmic veins may be ligated in the orbit through a superior marginal approach or a resection of the outer orbital wall.

Ocular or Periocular Manifestations

Anterior Chamber: Cells and flare, hemorrhage, shallowing.

Conjunctiva: Chemosis, neovascularization; vascular engorgement, vascular tumor; hemorrhage, necrosis.

Cornea: Bullous keratopathy, clouding, neovascularization.

Eyelids: Edema, vascular tumor, ptosis.

Globe: Exophthalmus, diplopia, glaucoma.

Iris: Atrophy, rubeosis; ectropion uveae.

Optic Nerve: Congestion; vascular tumor; papilledema; atrophy.

Retina: Vascular tumor; congestion; hemorrhage; degeneration; detachment.

Other: Cataract, vitreous hemorrhage; loss of vision; pareses of third or sixth nerves; vascular tumor; congestion of orbit.

CAROTID CAVERNOUS FISTULAS AND CAVERNOUS SINUS ARTERIOVENOUS MALFORMATIONS

BRIAN R. YOUNGE, M.D.
Rochester, Minnesota

Carotid cavernous fistulas (CCFs) are abnormal connections of the carotid arteries directly into the veins of the cavernous sinus; depending on the rate and amount of this shunt, they may produce neuro-ophthalmic manifestations. CCFs are most frequently caused by trauma, although spontaneous fistulas may also occur, particularly in middle-aged and elderly women. A dural sinus arteriovenous malformation (AVM) to the cavernous sinus, in contrast, is an acquired spontaneous shunt, usually of the low-flow type, but it may produce similar ophthalmic manifestations, particularly if the rate of flow is significant. Other predisposing factors include infection, malignancy, aneurysms, carotid dissection, fibromuscular dysplasia, pregnancy, and the Ehlers-Danlos syndrome.

Ocular manifestations (unilateral, bilateral, or even contralateral) include arterialized vessels of the conjunctiva and orbit, proptosis, edema and hyperemia of periorbital structures, papilledema, retinal hemorrhages and macular edema, iritis, iris atrophy, secondary glaucoma, and anterior segment ischemia. Visual loss may supervene from optic nerve compromise or corneal complications and may be accompanied by various extraocular muscle palsies, most commonly third nerve and sixth nerve palsies; aberrant regeneration of the third nerve is common. Bruit audible to the patient is a very annoying symptom and is usually detected by the examiner. Pulsating exophthalmos may also occur in very high-flow shunts. Neither bruit nor exophthalmos is common in clinical AVM. Death from rupture of the cavernous sinus is very rare and occurs most often during pregnancy.

THERAPY

Ocular. Although the treatment may be neurosurgical or interventional by the neuroradiologist, these lesions produce almost exclusively ocular complications, and the ophthalmologist needs to be centrally involved in the decisions about diagnosis and management. Many of the low-flow shunts spontaneously occlude in time. Sometimes, even the investigational procedure of angiography will precipitate cure. Many patients can coexist well with a low-flow shunt and have minimal or no symptoms. Previous carotid occlusive "trapping" procedures rendered the eye even more ischemic and were associated with a significant rate of visual loss and risk of cerebral complications. The one-eyed patient with CCF seldom, if ever, needs surgical treatment because the risk of total blindness is not to

PRECAUTIONS

Even in the absence of untoward effects at the time of operation and soon thereafter, surgical therapy may result in the development of late cerebral signs, such as the comparatively slow onset of hemiplegia with perhaps a fatal termination due to spreading thrombosis. An associated cerebral edema or deterioration of the ocular symptoms, including progressive necrosis and sloughing of the cornea, may also occur.

COMMENTS

The most common traumatic arteriovenous fistula is a rupture of the carotid in the cavernous sinus. Most of these are associated with fractures at the base of the skull, and many involve the body of the sphenoid bone where the artery and veins are intimately apposed.

The majority of spontaneous arteriovenous fistulas occur in women, and 25 per cent occur during pregnancy. The prognosis in this condition is not good. Occasionally, death is sudden and almost immediate, presumably by rupture of the cavernous sinus and cerebral hemorrhage.

References

Brown GC, Shields, JA: Tumors of the optic nerve head. Surv Ophthalmol 29:239–264, 1985.
Coffman JD: Peripheral vascular diseases due to abnormal communications between arteries and veins. Arteriovenous fistula. In Beeson PB, McDermot W (eds): Textbook of Medicine, 14th ed. Philadelphia. WB Saunders, 1975, pp 1082–1083.
Fourman AM: Acute angle closure glaucoma after arteriovenous fistula. Am J Ophthalmol 107:156–159, 1989.
Hanneken AM, Miller NR, Debrun GM, Nauta HJ: Treatment of carotid-cavernous sinus fistulas using a detachable balloon catheter through the superior ophthalmic vein. Arch Ophthalmol 107:87–92, 1989.
Katzen LB, Katzen BT, Katzen MJ: Treatment of carotid-cavernous fistulas with detachable balloon catheter occlusion. Adv Ophthal Plast Reconstr Surg 7:157–165, 1987.
Kupersmith MJ, Berenstein A, Choi IS, Warren F, Flamm E: Management of nontraumatic vascular shunts involving the cavernous sinus. Ophthalmology 95:121–130, 1988.
Mansour AM, Wells CG, Jampol LM, Kalina RE: Ocular complications of arteriovenous communications of the retina. Review article. Arch Ophthalmol 107:232–236, 1989.
Troost BT, Glaser JS: Aneurysms, arteriovenous communications, and related vascular malformations. In Duane TD (ed): Clinical Ophthalmology. Hagerstown, MD, Harper & Row, 1981. Vol. II pp 17:1–30.
Walsh FB, Hoyt WF: Clinical Neuro-Ophthalmology, 3rd ed. Baltimore, Williams & Wilkins, 1969, pp 1714–1735.
Wolter JR: Arteriovenous fistulas of the eye region. Trans Am Ophthalmol Soc 72:253–281, 1974.
Wolter JR: Arteriovenous fistulas involving the eye region. J Pediatr Ophthalmol 12:22–39, 1975.
Wolter JR: Arteriovenous fistula of the eyelid: Secondary to a chalazion. J Pediatr Ophthalmol 14:225–227, 1977.

be taken lightly in a nonlethal disease. Of two such patients described in the literature, one refused treatment of any kind and did well, and the other was subjected to a series of embolization and trapping procedures that resulted in total permanent blindness and a lawsuit against the surgeon. The ophthalmologist must clearly demonstrate to the patient and his or her colleagues the threat to vision, the risks of doing nothing, and the risks of intervention.

In patients with intolerable symptoms or visual compromise, there are now several suitable forms of therapy.

Surgical. CCFs are of two main types: high flow and low flow. The high-flow CCFs are usually direct communications between a rent in the internal carotid artery and the cavernous sinus, and they are most often traumatic in origin. Low-flow CCFs are spontaneous AVMs or dural shunts, although some traumatic CCFs are low flow as well. When treatment is indicated for threatened visual loss or other neuro-ophthalmic complications, the high-flow fistulas are best managed by detachable balloon embolization. Occasionally, they may require direct attack or other arterial occlusion procedures. Low-flow shunts are often managed with either detachable balloon obliteration or embolization of the external carotid artery, depending on the type of shunt. Other approaches to both types have their advocates and have various degrees of success; platinum wire or other materials have been used via percutaneous catheterization of the dilated superior ophthalmic vein, and radiation therapy has been reported to be successful in low-flow shunts.

PRECAUTIONS

Complications can ensue, such as cerebral infarction or death, transient neurologic defects, ophthalmoplegias, pain, and visual loss; late complications can also occur, including recurrence of the fistula and premature deflation of the balloon. Sometimes, late effects of treatment improve the situation by progressive obliteration of the sites of leakage. Abrupt closure of a fistula may in itself produce neurologic deficits, especially in patients with CCFs of long duration, presumably on the basis of the so-called luxury perfusion phenomenon.

References

Barrow DL, et al: Classification and treatment of spontaneous carotid-cavernous sinus fistulas. J Neurosurg 62:248–256, 1985.

Bitoh S, et al: Irradiation of spontaneous carotid-cavernous fistulas. Surg Neurol 17:282–286, 1982.

Debrun GM, et al: Indications for treatment and classification of 132 carotid-cavernous fistulas. Neurosurgery 22:285–289, 1988.

Halbach VV, et al: Normal perfusion pressure breakthrough occurring during treatment of carotid and vertebral fistulas. AJNR 8:751–756, 1987.

Palestine AG, Younge BR, Piepgras DG: Visual prognosis in carotid-cavernous fistula. Arch Ophthalmol 99:1600–1603, 1981.

Sanders MD, Hoyt WF: Hypoxic ocular sequelae of carotid-cavernous fistulae: Study of the causes of visual failure before and after neurosurgical treatment in a series of 25 cases. Br J Ophthalmol 53:82–97, 1969.

Teng MMH, et al: Occlusion of arteriovenous malformations of the cavernous sinus via the superior ophthalmic vein. AJNR 9:539–546, 1988.

CAVERNOUS SINUS THROMBOSIS
MILTON BONIUK, M.D.
Houston, Texas

To many physicians, the term "cavernous sinus thrombosis" implies a severe infectious process of acute onset. The process primarily involves the central nervous system with generalized symptoms and signs of a septic process. The source of infection may be the face, mouth, throat, paranasal sinuses, or ear. The frequency of this disorder has decreased considerably since the introduction of antibiotics.

In addition to the septic variety, an aseptic form of cavernous sinus thrombosis may be seen with crushing fractures through the sphenoid, after surgical treatment of carotid cavernous fistula and tic douloureux, and in association with phlebothrombosis of the orbital veins.

Diagnosis of aseptic thrombosis is difficult, and the condition is most frequently confused with carotid cavernous fistula. The absence of widening of the pulse pressure with tonometry or tonography, the absence of a bruit, and a negative carotid angiogram should make one suspect this diagnosis; the use of orbital venography may also be helpful in confirming a suspected diagnosis. Early recognition of this disorder is obviously important, and perhaps neurosurgeons should institute some prophylactic measures that would help prevent this complication. Suspected cases associated with phlebothrombosis of the orbital veins should have a medical workup to rule out underlying causes or systemic diseases, such as a history of oral contraceptives or evidence of dysproteinemia. If inflammation is present, the possibility of cranial arteritis or some collagen vascular disease should be considered in the differential diagnosis.

The most obvious ocular sign of cavernous sinus thrombosis is proptosis associated with dilation of the episcleral veins. There may be a variable degree of lid and conjunctival edema. If lagophthalmos and exposure keratitis are present, there may be secondary changes, such as staining and ulceration of the cornea. An afferent pupillary defect or dilation of the pupil secondary to an internal ophthalmoplegia may also be seen. The retina may show dilation of the retinal veins with hemorrhages, and in some cases, there may be retinal ischemia and infarction. The optic disc may be swollen or may show signs of an ischemic optic neuritis. Glaucomatous cupping may be seen in some patients with severe secondary open-angle glaucoma. Motility may be restricted as a result of changes in the extraocular muscles or secondary to involvement of the third, fourth, and sixth cranial nerves.

THERAPY

Systemic. Although most cases of *septic cavernous sinus thrombosis* are of bacterial origin, some cases have been reported in association with mucormycosis and *Aspergillus* organisms. It is important therefore to make a precise diagnosis as soon as possible. Doing so requires immediate blood cultures, as well as skull and sinus x-rays and CT or MRI scanning of the head. In some cases, biopsy and cultures from the paranasal sinuses might be necessary to make a diagnosis.

Once the etiologic agent has been identified, treatment with appropriate antibiotics is indicated. Until the specific organism has been isolated, broad-spectrum coverage should include 2 gm of intravenous methicillin every 4 hours or 2 gm of intravenous cephalothin every 4 hours plus up to 5 to 8 mg/kg of gentamicin injected in three equally divided doses.

If a diagnosis of *aseptic cavernous sinus thrombosis* is established in the acute phase, systemic anticoagulants (heparin and/or warfarin) or the combination of 600 mg of aspirin and 150 mg of dipyridamole might be indicated. If there is evidence of inflammation, systemic steroids or other anti-inflammatory agents, such as indomethacin or ibuprofen, might be indicated.

Ocular. In the septic variety, there may be tremendous proptosis, conjunctival chemosis, lagophthalmos, and exposure keratitis. These conditions may require the use of artificial tears, lubricating ointment, taping of the lids, intermarginal sutures, or some type of moisture chamber.

The secondary open-angle glaucoma in both septic and aseptic patients is probably secondary to increased episcleral venous pressure. The glaucoma responds poorly to miotics and other forms of medical therapy. If surgery becomes necessary, a trabeculectomy might be indicated, although the dilated episcleral, iris, and angle vessels might lead to serious operative and postoperative hemorrhage. Cryocyclotherapy, ultrasonic therapy, or use of transcleral YAG laser might be a good alternative to trabeculectomy.

Supportive. The septic patient may require antipyretic and analgesic agents. Intravenous fluids and electrolyte therapy may be required in the nauseated or comatosed patient. Patients with aseptic thrombosis may benefit from elevation of the head, which promotes venous drainage and may relieve some of the symptoms.

Ocular or Periocular Manifestations

Conjunctiva: Chemosis; dilation of episcleral veins.
Cornea: Punctate staining; ulcer.
Extraocular Muscles: Third, fourth, or sixth nerve paralysis.
Eyelids: Edema; ptosis.
Globe: Proptosis.
Pupil: Afferent defect; dilation.
Retina: Hemorrhages; ischemic infarction; venous dilation.
Optic Nerve: Glaucomatous cupping; ischemic neuritis; papilledema.
Other: Glaucoma; orbital cellulitis; visual loss.

PRECAUTIONS

With the septic variety of cavernous sinus thrombosis, prompt diagnosis and early institution of appropriate antibiotic treatment are essential for survival of the patient. It is important to continue systemic antibiotics for several weeks after the acute septic phase has subsided in order to prevent a relapse.

The aseptic variety of cavernous sinus thrombosis is less of an emergency and more difficult to diagnose. If the diagnosis is not established in the acute phase, the use of anticoagulants might be of questionable value.

COMMENTS

In the septic variety of cavernous sinus thrombosis, the mortality rate has dropped dramatically since the introduction of antibiotics. Early aggressive treatment with intravenous antibiotics is necessary in the acute phase, and this must be followed by several weeks of oral antibiotics in order to prevent relapses. Late ocular complications, including glaucoma and corneal or motility problems, require periodic ophthalmologic evaluation and treatment.

In the aseptic variety of cavernous sinus thrombosis, the clinical picture and course of the disease are different. It is difficult to make a diagnosis, and carotid angiography is usually necessary to rule out the possibility of a low-flow carotid cavernous fistula. New techniques that may help in diagnosis include CT scanning and gallium scintigraphy. Although anticoagulants and other drugs, such as aspirin and dipyridamole, may be indicated in the acute phases of the disease, treatment in the later stages is mainly directed toward the secondary glaucoma, which is often difficult to control.

References

Ahmadi J, et al: CT observations pertinent to septic cavernous sinus thrombosis. AJNR 6:755–758, 1985.
Boniuk M: The ocular manifestations of ophthalmic vein and aseptic cavernous sinus thrombosis. Trans Am Acad Ophthalmol Otolaryngol 76:1519–1534, 1972.
Brismar G, Brismar J: Thrombosis of the intraorbital veins and cavernous sinus. Acta Radiol (Diagn) 18:145–153, 1977.
Hasso AN, et al: Venous occlusions of the cavernous area—A complication of crushing fractures of the sphenoid bone. Radiology 132:375–379, 1979.
Palestro CJ, et al: Gallium scintigraphy in a case of septic cavernous sinus thrombosis. Clin Nucl Med 11:636–639, 1986.

Sekhar LN, Dujovny M, Rao GR: Carotid-cavernous sinus thrombosis caused by *Aspergillus fumigatus*. J Neurosurg 52:120–125, 1980.

Yarington CT Jr: Cavernous sinus thrombosis revisited. Proc Roy Soc Med 70:456–459, 1977.

SICKLE CELL DISEASE

STEVEN B. COHEN, M.D.,
LEE M. JAMPOL, M.D.,
and MORTON F. GOLDBERG, M.D.

Chicago, Illinois

Sickle cell disease encompasses a group of genotypes in which hemoglobin S is present. It includes sickle cell anemia (the homozygous state, SS), hemoglobin SC disease (a doubly heterozygous state), and sickle cell betathalassemia (the presence of hemoglobin S plus a defect in synthesis of the beta chain). The mutant gene for hemoglobin S production has become prevalent in parts of the world where malaria is endemic, apparently the result of partial protection from *Plasmodium falciparum* malaria. The sickling hemoglobinopathies are found predominantly, but not exclusively, in blacks. The prevalence of sickle cell trait in American blacks is 8 to 10 per cent, sickle cell anemia 0.5 per cent, and hemoglobin SC disease 0.12 per cent. Sickling of erythrocytes containing hemoglobin S is noted in association with low oxygen tension and acidosis and causes vascular stasis and obstruction. Patients with sickle cell disease may experience aplastic crises and splenic sequestration. Vaso-occlusion may cause painful crises with fever and pain in the arms, legs, or abdomen. Ocular findings, such as retinal neovascularization, are sequelae of intravascular sickling with sluggish blood flow and repetitive vascular occlusions. Hyphema associated with sickling of red cells in the anterior chamber may cause severe secondary glaucoma and loss of vision.

THERAPY

Systemic. In sickle cell crises, the accurate diagnosis and treatment of the precipitating cause are essential. Infections should be promptly treated. If hypoxia is present, oxygen should be administered. Treatment should also include rehydration (using intravenous fluids and electrolytes to correct any abnormality), prompt correction of acidosis, and mild analgesics, such as acetaminophen with or without codeine. Occasionally, stronger analgesic agents are required. It is sometimes useful to add a tranquilizer, such as hydroxyzine. Blood transfusions have been utilized for the therapy of anemic crises, for the termination of severe vaso-occlusive crises, and, in some situations, as a prophylaxis against vaso-occlusion in association with preg-

nancy or surgery or in patients with a past history of stroke. Transfusion reactions and the risk of hepatitis or acquired immunodeficiency syndrome (AIDS) are considerations in these patients.

Other modes of therapy that have been utilized in the past but without proven value include low molecular weight dextran,[‡] carbonic anhydrase inhibitors,[‡] anticoagulants,[‡] urea,[‡] sodium cyanate,[†] zinc,[‡] desmopressin,[‡] and many others. Few controlled clinical trials have been performed.

Ocular. Because of the possibility of vitreous hemorrhage and tractional or rhegmatogenous retinal detachment, attempts at closing retinal neovascularization have been made using diathermy, cryopexy, or xenon arc or argon laser photocoagulation. Photocoagulation of neovascularization has included direct focal ablation, feeder vessel treatment, and panretinal scatter. All appear to be effective under certain circumstances, although complications have been described. Vitrectomy is necessary in patients in whom vitreous hemorrhage does not clear or when vitreous traction leads to detachment of the retina.

Scleral buckling surgery is performed for rhegmatogenous or progressive tractional detachments. Because these patients are at risk of developing anterior segment ischemia after vitrectomy or retinal detachment surgery, such surgery should be preceded by measures that reduce the propensity for sickling. Suggested preoperative management should include use of local anesthesia when possible, pupillary dilation primarily with parasympatholytic drugs, avoidance, if possible, of sympathomimetic agents in local anesthetics and the dilating regimen, and lowering of intraocular pressure. In addition, partial exchange blood transfusion to raise the hemoglobin A to 50 per cent or greater with a final hematocrit of 39 per cent or less should be considered. The status of the fellow eye, surgical risks (including the risks of anesthesia and anterior segment ischemia), and the risk of transfusion reactions, hepatitis, and AIDS must be weighed carefully when deciding upon the use of preoperative exchange transfusion. During surgery, supplemental oxygen should be given; diathermy or heavy cryotherapy should be avoided near the long posterior ciliary vessels, if possible; the rectus muscles should not be detached and traction on these muscles should be minimized; large, tight encircling elements should be avoided; and drainage of subretinal fluid should be performed, whenever feasible. Recommended postoperative measures include supplemental oxygen by face mask for 48 hours and adequate dilation of the pupil.

Supportive. Management of sickle cell disease should include an immunization program for children, including the recently introduced pneumococcal vaccine, maintenance of a good nutritional state, folic acid supplements, and regular check-ups. Patients should be educated about their disease and instructed to avoid known precipitating causes of crises.

Ocular or Periocular Manifestations

Choroid: Acute choroidal ischemia related to occlusion of the ciliary arteries; white wedge-shaped infarcts, which subsequently show hyperpigmentation.
Conjunctiva: Comma signs (apparently isolated, small vascular channels); icterus; pallor.
Iris: Atrophy; neovascularization (rare); vascular occlusion.
Optic Nerve: Atrophy; disc neovascularization (rare); isolated comma-shaped vascular segments.
Retina: Angioid streaks; arteriovenous anastomoses; central retinal artery or macular precapillary arteriolar occlusions; retinal depression signs; chorioretinal scars (black sunbursts); cotton-wool patches; iridescent deposits; macular holes; peripheral arteriolar occlusion with sheathing; peripheral retinal holes; preretinal hemorrhages (salmon patches); retinal detachment; vascular tortuosity.
Vitreous: Hemorrhages; preretinal neovascularization; traction bands.

PRECAUTIONS

Bleeding into the anterior chamber (hyphema) is more deleterious in patients who have sickle cell disease than in normal individuals. Those with sickle cell trait, which is ordinarily a benign condition, are similarly at risk. The anterior chamber environment is particularly noxious for erythrocytes with the propensity for sickling, because of stagnation, hypoxia, and relative acidosis. The cells may therefore readily become sickled and then, in the rigid, elongated, sickled configuration, obstruct the aqueous outflow pathways by creating a logjam in the trabecular meshwork of the anterior chamber angle. Secondary glaucoma may ensue, and only slight to moderate pressure elevations may result in closure of small vessels in the optic nerve and macula. Thus, patients with sickle cell disease or trait and hyphema should have their visual acuity and intraocular pressures carefully observed. Repeated doses of hyperosmotic agents, such as mannitol, and of carbonic anhydrase inhibitors (which constitute the standard medical regimen in hyphema patients who do not have sickle cell disease) are contraindicated because of the dangers of hemoconcentration, acidosis, or both. Early decompression of the anterior chamber by limbal paracentesis is an effective way to lower the intraocular pressure and allow many of the sickled erythrocytes to escape.

COMMENTS

Genetic counseling and family planning are indicated for patients with sickle cell disease. Close medical supervision and periodic ophthalmologic evaluations are essential.

References

Dean J, Schechter AN: Sickle-cell anemia: Molecular and cellular bases of therapeutic approaches (First of three parts). N Engl J Med 299:752–763, 1978.
Dean J, Schechter AN: Sickle-cell anemia: Molecular and cellular bases of therapeutic approaches. (Second of three parts). N Engl J Med 299:804–811, 1978.
Dean J, Schechter AN: Sickle-cell anemia: Molecular and cellular bases of therapeutic approaches. (Third of three parts). N Engl J Med 299:863–870, 1978.
Goldberg MF: Classification and pathogenesis of proliferative sickle retinopathy. Am J Ophthalmol 71:649–665, 1971.
Goldberg MF: Retinal vaso-occlusion in sickling hemoglobinopathies. Birth Defects 12:475–515, 1976.
Goldberg ME: Retinal neovascularization in sickle cell retinopathy. Trans Am Acad Ophthalmol Otolaryngol 83:409–431, 1977.
Goldberg MF, Jampol LM: The treatment of neovascularization, vitreous hemorrhage, and retinal detachment in sickle cell retinopathy. In Symposium on the Retina. St. Louis, CV Mosby, 1983, pp 53–81.
Goldberg MF, et al: Sickled erythrocytes, hyphema, and secondary glaucoma. Ophthalmic Surg 10:17–123, 1979.
Jampol LM: New techniques in treating proliferative sickle cell retinopathy. In Fine SL (ed): Current Concepts in Management of Retinal Vascular and Macular Disease. Baltimore, Williams & Wilkins, 1983.
Jampol LM, Goldbaum MH: Peripheral proliferative retinopathies. Surv Ophthalmol 25:1–14, 1980.
Jampol LM, et al: An update on vitrectomy surgery and retinal detachment repair in sickle cell disease. Arch Ophthalmol 100:591–593, 1982.
Nagpal KC, Goldberg MF, Rabb MF: Ocular manifestation of sickle hemoglobinopathies. Surv Ophthalmol 21:391–411, 1977.
Serjeant GR: The Clinical Features of Sickle Cell Disease. New York, American Elsevier, 1974.

TEMPORAL ARTERITIS
(Giant Cell Arteritis)
NEIL R. MILLER, M.D.
Baltimore, Maryland

Temporal arteritis is a systemic disease characterized by chronic granulomatous inflammation of the wall of large and medium-sized arteries. Affected arteries show fragmentation of the elastic lamina, necrosis of smooth muscle cells, and infiltration with lymphocytes, epithelial cells, and giant cells. The process has a predilection for the extradural cranial arteries, including the ophthalmic and posterior ciliary arteries, but it may affect the large arteries of the head and neck, the coronary arteries, the renal arteries, and the peripheral arteries as well. The cause of temporal arteritis is unknown, but studies demonstrating immunoglobulin deposition in affected vessels suggest that there may be an underlying immunologic defect.

Temporal arteritis occurs almost exclusively in patients over 50 years of age. Its prevalence increases with advancing age, such that 1 per cent of patients 80 years of age or older will develop the disease. Males and females are equally affected.

Most patients with temporal arteritis have constitutional symptoms and signs, including intermittent fever, malaise, anorexia, migratory arthralgia (polymyalgia rheumatica), and weight loss. They may complain of severe temple pain, scalp tenderness, jaw pain or claudication, or ear pain. They often have exquisite tenderness in the region of the superficial temporal artery on one or both sides. One or both arteries may be prominent but nonpulsatile. Many patients with temporal arteritis develop visual symptoms as the initial manifestation of the disease. In others, visual symptoms predominate, but a careful history will elicit the constitutional symptoms described earlier.

Systemic sequelae of temporal arteritis include stroke, heart attack, kidney failure, and arterial insufficiency of the upper and lower extremities. Ocular complications occur in about 50 per cent of patients. The most common ocular disturbance is visual loss, which may affect one or both eyes and which may be partial or complete. The visual loss may result from retinal or choroidal ischemia, central retinal artery occlusion, anterior or posterior ischemic optic neuropathy, or cerebral ischemia. Homonymous visual field defects may result from occlusion of one of the posterior cerebral arteries or its branches. Diplopia may also occur in patients with temporal arteritis. It results from oculomotor nerve paresis, usually abducens nerve paresis or pupil-sparing oculomotor nerve paresis, and from extraocular muscle ischemia. Some patients develop complete ocular ischemia from occlusion of the ipsilateral internal carotid or ophthalmic arteries.

The diagnosis of temporal arteritis is a *clinical* one. Temporal arteritis should be considered in any elderly patient with acute visual loss, and a careful history should be obtained with respect to the various constitutional symptoms described earlier. Once the diagnosis is suspected, an emergency erythrocyte sedimentation rate (ESR) should be obtained. The most popular procedure used to perform an ESR is the Westergren method, which is extremely accurate for high ESRs; however, other procedures, such as the Wintrobe and Zeta methods, are also used in some laboratories. If the ESR is elevated or if the ESR is normal but the patient is thought to have a clinical picture compatible with temporal arteritis, therapy should be initiated immediately, and a temporal artery biopsy should be performed within 8 days. The biopsy initially may be performed on one side only. The specimen obtained should be at least 2 cm long. It should be fixed in formalin, embedded on end, and serially sectioned until the tissue is exhausted. The slides should be examined by a pathologist acquainted with the pathologic appearance of temporal arteritis. If the biopsy specimen is negative but it is thought that temporal arteritis is a likely diagnosis, the opposite temporal artery should be biopsied. If this biopsy specimen is also negative, the physician should search for another cause of the patient's symptoms, such as an occult malignancy. It is important to obtain a temporal artery biopsy in all patients with suspected temporal arteritis, even if the clinical picture is thought to be pathognomonic of the disease, because of the potential side effects of systemic corticosteroid therapy.

THERAPY

Systemic. Corticosteroid therapy is the only effective treatment for temporal arteritis. It should therefore be instituted as soon as the diagnosis of temporal arteritis is suspected and blood has been drawn for an ESR. The usual dose is 1.5 to 2.0 mg/kg of prednisone or prednisolone daily in single or divided doses taken orally. Some authors advocate intravenous corticosteroid therapy for those patients with acute visual loss from anterior or retrobulbar ischemic optic neuropathy. Such patients are given 0.5 to 1.0 gm of methylprednisolone intravenously every 12 hours for 3 to 5 days, after which time the patient is switched to an oral corticosteroid in the dose described above.

Most patients experience relief of systemic symptoms within 24 hours after starting corticosteroid therapy, although vision, once lost, almost never returns and the ESR may take 2 to 14 days to decrease. Even if symptoms abate immediately and the ESR becomes normal, patients should be maintained on a stable dose of corticosteroid for about 2 to 3 weeks. The dose should then be reduced at the rate of no more than 5 to 10 mg/week, and the patient's symptoms and ESR should be monitored on a weekly basis. As long as the patient remains free of symptoms and the ESR remains normal, the corticosteroid dose may be lowered. If symptoms return, the ESR begins to increase, or both, the steroid dose should be increased and kept stable until symptoms once again abate and the ESR normalizes. Alternate-day corticosteroid therapy does not suppress the inflammatory response on the day on which no steroids are taken. It is therefore thought that there is a risk of visual loss in patients placed on this regimen.

It must be remembered that temporal arteritis is often a *chronic* disease that may last for 6 to 18 months and often longer. Patients may therefore require corticosteroid therapy for many months, and attempts to wean them from therapy too fast may result in catastrophic visual or systemic complications from the persistent disease.

Ocular or Periocular Manifestations

Choroid: Infarction.
Extraocular Muscles: Diplopia, ophthalmoplegia; abducens nerve paresis; pupil-sparing oculomotor nerve paresis; trochlear nerve paresis.
Eyelid: Ptosis.
Optic Nerve: Ischemic optic neuropathy (anterior and retrobulbar).
Pupil: Relative afferent defect; tonic pupil.

Retina: Central retinal artery occlusion; ischemic retinopathy; cotton-wool spots; hemorrhage.
Other: Cortical blindness; homonymous visual field defects.

PRECAUTIONS

Systemic corticosteroid therapy is associated with well-described systemic side effects, especially increased incidence of bacterial and fungal infections. All patients taking systemic corticosteroids for temporal arteritis should be monitored carefully by an internist, general practitioner, or gerontologist familiar with temporal arteritis and with the systemic side effects of corticosteroid therapy.

COMMENTS

The major problems in dealing with patients who have temporal arteritis are that, too often, it is not until vision is lost that the diagnosis is considered, and that the treatment for this condition is often as bad as the disease. It is to be hoped that a better treatment for this condition can be found in the future.

References

Beevers DG, et al: Giant cell arteritis: The need for prolonged treatment. J Chronic Dis 26:571–584, 1973.
Caselli RJ, et al: Neurologic disease in biopsy-proven giant cell (temporal) arteritis. Neurology 38:352–359, 1988.
Clark AE, Victor WH: An unusual presentation of temporal arteritis. Ann Ophthalmol 19:343–346, 1987.
Cullen JF, Coleiro JA: Ophthalmic complications of giant cell arteritis. Surv Ophthalmol 20:247–260, 1976.
Eshaghian J: Controversies regarding giant cell (temporal, cranial) arteritis. Doc Ophthalmol 47:43–67, 1979.
Hunder GG, et al: Daily and alternate-day corticosteroid regimens in treatment of giant cell arteritis. Ann Intern Med 82:613–618, 1975.
Machado EBV, et al: Temporal arteritis: Clinical and epidemiological features from a community-based study, 1950 to 1985. Ann Neurol 22:148, 1987.
McDonnell PJ, et al: Temporal arteritis. Ophthalmology 93:518–530, 1986.
Mehler ME, Rabinowich L: The neuro-ophthalmological spectrum of temporal arteritis. Ann Neurol 22:147–148, 1987.
Nevyas JY, Nevyas HJ: Giant cell arteritis with normal erythrocyte sedimentation rate: A management dilemma. Metab Pediatr System Ophthalmol 10:18–21, 1987.
Rosenfeld SI, et al: Treatment of temporal arteritis with ocular involvement. Am J Med 80:143–145, 1986.
Wong RL, Korn JH: Temporal arteritis without an elevated erythrocyte sedimentation rate. Am J Med 80:959–964, 1986.

THALASSEMIA
STEPHEN S. FEMAN, M.D.
Nashville, Tennessee

Thalassemia is a group of hereditary disorders characterized by decreased rates of synthesis of hemoglobin polypeptide chains. In the past, these disorders had a variety of names (Cooley's anemia, thalassemia major, thalassemia minor, etc.); now, a more inclusive nomenclature based on the involved polypeptide chain is in common use (alpha-thalassemia, beta-thalassemia, etc.). The clinical feature most characteristic of thalassemia is the development of a hypochromic microcystic anemia. In some varieties, however, the thalassemic change represents such a small fraction of total globin synthesis that this feature is difficult to measure with standard techniques.

In general, when a patient has one thalassemia gene and one normal gene, the disorder is thalassemia trait (thalassemia minor in the older literature) and relatively mild anemia is present. When two similar genes are present, there is a severe impairment of hemoglobin synthesis (or thalassemia major). However, thalassemia can be subdivided just as well by identifying the rate of synthesis of polypeptide chains. On that basis, one can describe various degrees of hemoglobin synthesis impairment; this results in the more clinically relevant descriptions of severe, mild, and silent forms of thalassemia.

The most common type of thalassemia, which was described by Cooley and Lee in 1925, is a defect in the rate of synthesis of the beta-polypeptide chain of hemoglobin A. This defect causes a relative increase in the levels of hemoglobin A2 and hemoglobin F, along with microcystic hypochromic anemia. In addition, splenomegaly, hepatomegaly, and discoloration of the skin and sclera occur. It was thought that this disorder had a specific geographic distribution that extended from the Mediterranean through the Middle East, India, and Southeast Asia, it is now found worldwide.

THERAPY

Systemic. Transfusions to prevent the symptoms of anemia have been the standard of treatment for many years. In time, such therapy will result in an iron overload and hemosiderosis; this complication had been the most common cause of death in these patients. However, with the use of iron chelators, such as deferoxamine, this danger is lessened. Splenomegaly becomes a major problem for such patients and can be resolved with splenectomy when needed.

Ocular: The most serious threats to vision occur in patients with thalassemia and sickle cell trait. Such patients develop peripheral retinal neovascularizations that result in vitreous hemorrhages. The vessels feeding and draining the neovascular growth can be identified by fluorescein angiography. Photocoagulation to occlude

172 / THALASSEMIA

the feeding and draining vessels can close the neovascular growth and prevent such hemorrhages. The surrounding area of ischemic retina can be treated then with a scatter photocoagulation pattern to reduce the stimulus for recurrent neovascularization and prevent recurring problems in that retinal region.

Ocular or Periocular Manifestations

Conjunctiva: Focal regions of dilated and tortuous vessels.

Retina: Vascular tortuosity; pigmented chorioretinal scars (black sunburst pattern); iridescent intraretinal deposits; focal arterial occlusions; neovascularizations; hemorrhages; angioid streaks.

Vitreous: Hemorrhages.

PRECAUTIONS

Ocular complications usually indicate that the patient has a combination of thalassemia and some other hemoglobin abnormality. The treatment of the ocular manifestations of the other hemoglobin abnormality offers the greatest visual benefit to the patient.

COMMENTS

Intraocular hemorrhages without neovascularization and visual field defects have been reported in thalassemia patients; treatment of the underlying systemic disorder can prevent additional changes of this type. When retinal neovascular changes are identified, one must search for additional hemoglobin abnormalities. When such features are found, the treatment should be directed to the ocular and systemic manifestations of the other co-existing hemoglobinopathy in order to prevent additional visual loss.

References

Comings DE: Thalassemia. *In* Williams WJ, et al (eds): Hematology, New York, McGraw-Hill, 1972, pp 328–345.

Condon PI, Serjeant GR: Ocular findings in sickle cell thalassemia in Jamaica. Am J Ophthalmol 74:1105–1109, 1972.

Cooley TB, Lee P: A series of cases of splenomegaly in children with anemia and peculiar bone changes. Trans Am Pediatr Soc 37:29–35, 1925.

Feman SS, Westrich DJ: Macular arteriolar occlusions in sickle cell beta-thalassemia. Am J Ophthalmol 101:739–740, 1986.

Goldberg MF, Charache S, Acacio I: Ophthalmologic manifestations of sickle cell thalassemia. Arch Intern Med 128:33–39, 1971.

Magli A, et al: Ocular manifestations in thalassemia minor. Ophthalmologica 184:139–146, 1982.

WEGENER'S GRANULOMATOSIS

JAMES L. KINYOUN, M.D.
Seattle, Washington

Wegener's granulomatosis is a necrotizing, granulomatous vasculitis of the sinuses (upper respiratory tract), lungs (lower respiratory tract), and kidneys. A limited form of the disease exists in which renal lesions are not present. All age groups can be affected, and symptoms include rhinorrhea, sinus pain, cough, malaise, and weight loss. There is no sexual or racial predilection. Although the etiology remains unknown, available evidence (deposition of immune complexes) indicates that immunopathogenic mechanisms are responsible. Histopathology shows a necrotizing granulomatous vasculitis with infiltrate of neutrophils, lymphocytes, plasma cells, histiocytes, and giant cells. The most common ophthalmic manifestation of this disease is proptosis due to orbital involvement via extension from adjacent sinuses.

THERAPY

Systemic. Cytotoxic drugs have greatly improved the prognosis for patients with Wegener's granulomatosis. Cyclophosphamide‡ in a daily oral dosage of 2 mg/kg is a successful treatment for most patients, whereas the 2-year mortality rate before this drug was over 90 per cent. Treatment should be continued for 1 year after all signs of active disease have subsided. Erythrocyte sedimentation rate is a useful laboratory test to monitor disease activity.

Systemic corticosteroids (e.g., oral prednisone 60 to 80 mg daily) are recommended to control inflammation during the first 2 weeks of induction therapy with cyclophosphamide. After 2 weeks, the steroids can usually be tapered and discontinued.

Ocular. Specific ocular therapy is not usually necessary because appropriate systemic treatment alleviates associated ocular disease.

Surgical. Orbital decompression procedures should be considered in patients with optic nerve compression that is unresponsive to medical treatment. Grafts may be necessary to treat severe corneal and scleral ulceration.

Topical. Surface lubricants, such as petrolatum ointment every 30 minutes to 4 hours, may be necessary for corneal drying caused by proptosis. Topical antibiotic solution or ointment (e.g., tobramycin every 3 to 4 hours) is recommended for patients with corneal ulceration to prevent and treat superinfections. Topical ophthalmic corticosteroid drops, such as 1 per cent prednisolone every 3 to 4 hours, are useful in controlling superficial ocular inflammation (conjunctivitis, episcleritis, and scleritis) and anterior uveitis. Ciliary spasm associated with uveitis can be treated with topical 1 per cent cyclopentolate every 4 hours.

Supportive. Affected patients require a minimum of 1 year of drug treatment in addition to possible hospitalizations and surgical procedures, such as biopsies of lung or sinuses. Therefore, considerable health care expenditures are required. Financial assistance for those patients in need will be necessary.

Counseling. Affected patients need to understand the chronicity of this disease, its unknown etiology, the relatively optimistic outlook for most cases, and possible treatment complications. Of primary concern to patients considering parenthood or more offspring is that treatment can cause sterility. Sperm banking may be desired before beginning treatment in male patients. Females should use safe contraceptive methods during treatment because cytotoxic drugs are known to be teratogenic. Normal reproductive functions resume in some, but not all, patients after cytotoxic drug treatment is discontinued.

Irradiation. Irradiation of affected tissues has been attempted to control disease, but is of questionable efficacy and no longer recommended.

Ocular or Periocular Manifestations

Conjunctiva: Conjunctivitis.
Cornea: Peripheral and central ulcers.
Eyelids: Edema.
Lacrimal System: Obstruction of nasolacrimal duct.
Optic Nerve: Optic neuritis; papilledema.
Orbit: Proptosis.
Retina: Central retinal artery occlusion; vasculitis.
Sclera: Episcleritis; scleritis.
Uvea: Choriocapillaritis; uveitis.

Precautions

Complications of treatment with cyclophosphamide include bone marrow suppression, hemorrhagic cystitis, azoospermia, bladder carcinoma, nausea, vomiting, and hair loss. The leukocyte count should be followed closely during therapy (initially every other day and weekly during maintenance therapy) and should not decrease below 3000 cells/cubic millimeter. Granulocyte count below 1500 cells/cubic millimeter increases the risk of infection. Dosages must be decreased at the first signs of bone marrow suppression because the full effect of the present dosage will not be manifest in the white count until one week later. Hemorrhagic cystitis can be minimized by adequate hydration to avoid concentrated urine. Fortunately, hair regrows in most patients who experience hair loss while taking cyclophosphamide.

Complications of systemic corticosteroids include fluid retention, weight gain, "moon" facies, hyperglycemia, osteoporosis, bone fractures, psychological disturbances, peptic ulcer, and infection. Side effects can be minimized by switching to every other day treatment and discontinuing steroids as soon as inflammation is controlled.

Accurate diagnosis depends on clinical findings (sinus and lung involvement with or without renal disease) and histopathology (granulomatous inflammation with necrotizing vasculitis). Detection of autoantibodies against cytoplasmic components of neutrophil granulocytes (ACPA) reportedly is useful in the diagnosis and estimation of disease activity. A closely related disease with a poorer prognosis is lymphomatoid granulomatosis, which can be differentiated histopathologically by demonstrating angiocentric infiltration of atypical lymphoid cells. Other similar diseases include the Churg-Strauss syndrome and necrotizing sarcoid granulomatosis.

Comments

Because ophthalmic symptoms can be the initial manifestation of Wegener's granulomatosis, ophthalmologists should be aware of this disorder. Prompt referral to an internist and early treatment with cytotoxic and immunosuppressive drugs may not only save life but also preserve useful vision. Affected patients will need to be followed by internists and ophthalmologists to monitor treatment effectiveness and side effects of cytotoxic and immunosuppressive drugs. Depending on disease activity, follow-up examinations daily or at several month intervals are appropriate.

References

Biglan AW, et al: Corneal perforation in Wegener's granulomatosis treated with corneal transplantation: Case report. Ann Ophthalmol 9:799–801, 1977.

Bullen CL, et al: Ocular complications of Wegener's granulomatosis. Ophthalmology 90:279–290, 1983.

Cupps TR, Fauci AS: The vasculitides. *In* Smith LH Jr: Major Problems in Internal Medicine. Philadelphia, WB Saunders, 1981, Vol XXI, pp 155–173.

Fauci AS, Wolff SM: Wegener's granulomatosis: Studies in eighteen patients and a review of the literature. Medicine 52:535–561, 1973.

Fauci AS, Haynes BF, Katz P: The spectrum of vasculitis: Clinical, pathologic, immunologic, and therapeutic considerations. Ann Intern Med 89:660–671, 1978.

Haynes BF, et al: The ocular manifestations of Wegener's granulomatosis. Am J Med 63:131–141, 1977.

Kinyoun JL, Kalina RE, Klein ML: Choroidal involvement in systemic necrotizing vasculitis. Arch Ophthalmol 105:939–942, 1987.

Leavitt RY, Fauci AS: Pulmonary vasculitis. Am Rev Respir Dis 134:149–166, 1986.

Robin JB, et al: Ocular involvement in the respiratory vasculities. Surv Ophthalmol 30:127–140, 1985.

van der Woude FJ, et al: Autoantibodies against neutrophils and monocytes: Tool for diagnosis and marker of disease activity in Wegener's granulomatosis. Lancet I:425–429, 1985.

SECTION 10

DERMATOLOGIC DISORDERS

ACRODERMATITIS ENTEROPATHICA

J. DOUGLAS CAMERON, M.D.,
and DONALD J. DOUGHMAN, M.D.
Minneapolis, Minnesota

Acrodermatitis enteropathica is a rare hereditary disease characterized by skin lesions, alopecia, failure to thrive, diarrhea, and impaired immune function with frequent infections. A variety of ocular lesions also may occur. Involvement in siblings, but not in parents, and a history of familial occurrence in 65 per cent of patients suggest an autosomal recessive mode of inheritance. The disease usually manifests itself early in infancy, often just after weaning from human breast milk. Children with this disorder tend to be listless, apathetic, and anorectic and develop psychomotor retardation. Acrodermatitis enteropathica is characterized by a fluctuating course with severe exacerbations. If untreated, the disease is fatal; however, mild cases may improve at puberty and require no further therapy.

The dermatitis consists of vesiculobullous cutaneous eruptions distributed symmetrically, periorificially, and acrally. The areas about the eyes, occiput, elbows, hands, knees, feet, and especially the paronychial areas of the fingers and toes are involved. The skin lesions crust quickly and become psoriasiform; secondary infections, especially with *Candida*, are common. Alopecia involving the scalp, eyebrows, and eyelashes usually follows the dermatitis. Nonspecific conjunctivitis associated with photophobia frequently accompanies the dermatitis. Linear subepithelial corneal opacities are occasionally found during exacerbations of the dermatitis. Punctal stenosis, cataracts, and optic atrophy have also been reported in patients with acrodermatitis enteropathica.

THERAPY

Systemic. Oral zinc therapy (10 to 50 mg of zinc base as zinc sulfate or zinc gluconate per day) produces complete remission in acrodermatitis enteropathica, allowing normal growth with cessation of diarrhea, correction of immune deficiency, and disappearance of skin lesions. In most cases, zinc supplementation must be continued throughout the life span.

Ocular. The development of ocular lesions is generally prevented by oral zinc supplementation. Occasionally, supportive measures, such as artificial tears or dark glasses, may be necessary. Punctal dilation may be required in those cases with punctal stenosis.

Ocular or Periocular Manifestations

Cornea: Anterior corneal scarring; epithelial thinning; linear subepithelial opacities.
Eyebrows or Eyelids: Madarosis; nonspecific blepharitis; vesiculobullous eruptions.
Other: Abnormalities of dark adaptation; lacrimal punctal stenosis; nonspecific conjunctivitis; photophobia.

PRECAUTIONS

There are no recognized untoward effects of supplemental zinc therapy. Some patients have now lived long enough to complete normal pregnancies without teratologic complications. Occasionally, a single dose may cause transient emesis. Iodoquinol is no longer used in the treatment of acrodermatitis enteropathica.

COMMENTS

It was noted initially that feeding with human breast milk would improve the complications of acrodermatitis enteropathica. In the early 1950s, it was found that treatment with the antifungal agent, iodoquinol, improved the signs of acrodermatitis. In 1973, Barnes and Moynahan made the fortuitous discovery that oral zinc therapy produces dramatic improvements in this disease process. Indeed, the beneficial results from iodoquinol therapy were subsequently found to be due to increased zinc absorption caused by this drug. It is now generally accepted that the signs and symptoms of acrodermatitis enteropathica are caused by zinc deficiency and are identical to those seen in animals made zinc deficient by dietary means or with hereditary zinc malabsorption. The mechanism for this disease currently is thought to be depressed intestinal zinc absorption, probably through a failure in the production of a low molecular weight zinc-binding ligand that facilitates zinc absorption.

Severe zinc deficiency is found in a variety of more common processes, such as chronic alcoholism, sickle cell anemia, regional enteritis, short bowel syndrome, and total parenteral nutrition, to name only a few. Ocular abnormalities may complicate these states of acquired zinc deficiency just as in the hereditary disease of abnormal zinc metabolism, acrodermatitis entero pathica. Studies in zinc-deficient animals have recently confirmed the essential role of zinc in normal ocular function.

References

Barnes PM, Moynahan EJ: Zinc deficiency in acrodermatitis enteropathica: Multiple dietary intolerance treated with synthetic diet. Proc Roy Soc Med 66:327–329, 1973.
Cameron JD, McClain CJ: Ocular histopathology of acrodermatitis enteropathica. Br J Ophthalmol 70:662–667, 1986.
Leure-duPree AE: Electron-opaque inclusions in the rat retinal pigment epithelium after treatment with chelators of zinc. Invest Ophthalmol Vis Sci 21:1–9, 1981.
Matta CS, Felker GV, Ide CH: Eye manifestations in acrodermatitis enteropathica. Arch Ophthalmol 93:140–142, 1975.
Racz P, et al: Bilateral cataract in acrodermatitis enteropathica. J Pediatr Ophthalmol Strabismus 16:180–182, 1979.
Sunderman FW Jr: Current status of zinc deficiency in the pathogenesis of neurological, dermatological and musculoskeletal disorders. Ann Clin Lab Sci 5:132–145, 1975.
Warshawsky RS, et al: Acrodermatitis enteropathica. Corneal involvement with histochemical and electron micrographic studies. Arch Ophthalmol 93:194–197, 1975.
Wirsching L Jr: Eye symptoms in acrodermatitis enteropathica. A description of a brother and sister, with corneal changes. Acta Ophthalmol 40:567–574, 1962.

ATOPIC DERMATITIS
(Atopic Eczema, Besnier's Prurigo)
MITCHELL H. FRIEDLAENDER, M.D.
La Jolla, California

Atopic dermatitis is one of the eczematous skin eruptions. It often occurs in childhood, but may be seen in adolescents and adults as well. The incidence in children under 5 years of age is estimated at 3 per cent. Frequently, patients with atopic dermatitis have a history of respiratory allergy or allergic reactions to certain foods. Although immunologic abnormalities have been noted in atopic dermatitis, this condition also seems to represent an abnormal reactivity of the skin to various stimuli. This abnormal skin reactivity may be genetically determined, and it is considered by some to represent a metabolic or biochemical defect. Although patients with atopic dermatitis undergo extensive allergic testing, it is frequently impossible to find a relationship between this condition and a known allergy.

Serum IgE concentrations are generally elevated in patients with atopic dermatitis. Recent evidence indicates that a deficiency of cellular immunity may also exist. Cutaneous delayed hypersensitivity responses to ubiquitous antigens, such as *Candida* and streptokinase-streptodornase, may be poor. A deficiency of T-suppressor cells may be responsible for the failure to terminate IgE antibody responses to certain antigens in atopic dermatitis. IgE binds to mast cells in the skin, initiating the release of histamine and chemical mediators during antigenic stimulation. The overly reactive skin of atopic patients may respond excessively to the effects of histamine and other chemical mediators.

THERAPY

Topical. Topical steroids may be used for the skin lesions. A fluorinated corticosteroid in a water-soluble base, such as triamcinolone or betamethasone, may be applied three times a day to localized skin lesions. For exudative lesions, wet saline dressings may be applied several times a day. For thick and lichenified lesions, 1 per cent crude coal tar in Lassar's paste or cold cream may be effective. Coal tar derivatives, however, can sensitize the skin to strong sunlight.

Systemic. If the skin lesions are widespread and not controlled by topical therapy, oral corticosteroids may be added. As little as 5 to 10 mg of prednisone a day combined with a full regimen of topical treatment may keep a patient relatively free of dermatitis. For acute involvement of large areas of skin, a high dose of prednisone may be given and tapered slowly until skin lesions improve. Long-term use of corticosteroids should be avoided, especially in children, because of the tendency of these drugs to suppress growth.

Antihistamines, such as hydroxyzine, may be given in doses of 5 to 25 mg as often as four times a day to help control itching.

Ocular. If an inciting antigen can be identified in atopic keratoconjunctivitis, it should be eliminated. Topical corticosteroids may be used for short periods of time; however, their long-term usage should be avoided. In general, the lowest dose of corticosteroid required to control the patient's symptoms should be administered as infrequently as possible. Cold compresses and topical vasoconstrictor/antihistamine eyedrops may be all that are necessary to maintain comfort. Some recent success has been obtained with the use of 2 to 4 per cent cromolyn eyedrops. This medication stabilizes mast cells and prevents the release of their mediators.

Surgical. Surgery of atopic cataracts should not be undertaken lightly. Several investigators have reported such complications as severe hemorrhage, retinal detachment, iridocyclitis, and corneal edema. A relatively high incidence of pre- and postoperative retinal detachment has been reported. In patients with keratoconus associated with atopic eczema, penetrating keratoplasty may be carried out with a high degree of success.

Counseling. The skin of atopic dermatitis patients is easily irritated. Therefore, these patients should take care to avoid these factors—

176 / ATOPIC DERMATITIS

bathing too frequently, excessive sweating, chapping in cold weather, scratching, emotional stress, such irritating fabrics as wool and nylon, and nonspecific irritants, such as harsh soaps and detergents.

Ocular or Periocular Manifestations

Conjunctiva: Chemosis; filamentary discharge; giant papillary hypertrophy; hyperemia; linear or stellate scarring; shrinkage of the fornices; Trantas' dots.
Cornea: Cicatrization; keratoconus; punctate staining; vascularization.
Eyelids: Erythema; exudates; scaling and crusting; secondary staphylococcal blepharitis.
Lens: Cataracts.
Retina: Detachment.

PRECAUTIONS

Patients with active atopic dermatitis should not be vaccinated for smallpox because of the danger of developing a disseminated vaccinia infection. Corticosteroids should be used with restraint for ocular and skin manifestations. Cataracts, glaucoma, and secondary infections are known to develop in atopic patients treated excessively with corticosteroids. Surgery of atopic cataracts has been associated with complications, including hemorrhage, retinal detachment, iridocyclitis, and corneal edema.

COMMENTS

Atopic dermatitis is a chronic disease, and manifestations vary depending on the patient's age. A dermatologist should manage the patient's dermatitis. Ocular findings occur in a small percentage of atopic dermatitis patients; however, they can be the most severe aspect of the condition. Supportive treatment with cold compresses and topical vasoconstrictor/antihistamine eyedrops may be all that is required. Topical corticosteroids may be necessary, but should be used with restraint because they may eventually induce cataract formation and other problems. Cromolyn shows great promise in the treatment of this condition, and other antiallergic drugs are also being developed. Since atopic patients are prone to secondary infections, these should be looked for and treated appropriately.

References

Amemiya T, Matsuda H, Uehara M: Ocular findings in atopic dermatitis with special reference to the clinical features of atopic cataract. Ophthalmologica *180*:129–132, 1980.
Christiansen SC: Evaluation and treatment of the allergic patient. Int Ophthalmol Clin 28:282–293, 1988.
Donshik PC: Allergic conjunctivitis. Int Ophthalmol Clin 28:294–302, 1988.
Friedlaender MH: Allergy and Immunology of the Eye. Hagerstown, Md, Harper & Row, 1979, pp 76–79.

Hanifin JM, Lobitz WC Jr: Newer concepts of atopic dermatitis. Arch Dermatol *113*:663–670, 1977.
Hogan MJ: Atopic keratoconjunctivitis. Am J Ophthalmol 36:937–947, 1953.
McGeady SJ, Buckley RH: Depression of cell-mediated immunity in atopic eczema. J Allergy Clin Immunol 56:393–406, 1975.
Uehara M, Ofuji S: Atopic dermatitis: A discussion of theories concerning its pathogenesis. J Dermatol 7:231–238, 1980.

CONTACT DERMATITIS
(Dermatitis Venenata)
MITCHELL H. FRIEDLAENDER, M.D.
La Jolla, California

Contact dermatitis is probably the most common immunologic disease encountered by dermatologists. It results from the exposure of the skin to a wide variety of substances commonly found in the environment, including drugs, dyes, plant resins, preservatives, cosmetics, and metals. There are two varieties of contact dermatitis: 1) irritant, the more common form, and 2) allergic. Irritant contact dermatitis is caused by excessive moisture or by acids, alkalis, resins, or chemicals capable of injuring any person's skin if persistent contact is allowed. Allergy or hypersensitivity plays no role in irritant contact dermatitis. Allergic contact dermatitis, unlike the irritant variety, only occurs in sensitized individuals and involves the mechanism of cell-mediated immunity. In allergic contact dermatitis, an individual becomes sensitized to a given chemical or other sensitizing substance, and upon re-exposure to the same chemical, an erythematous delayed skin reaction is elicited.

Irritant dermatitis is provoked by substances with primary irritant properties or by frequent defatting of the skin caused by excessive moisture. With repeated exposure, edema, erythema, vesication, and scaling of the skin develop. In allergic contact dermatitis, the sensitizing substances are generally haptens of small molecular weight, which bind to dermal proteins forming complete antigens. Initial exposure to the hapten results in sensitization of T lymphocytes. A second application elicits an inflammatory response.

THERAPY

Systemic. The only form of contact dermatitis that may require systemic corticosteroids is widespread, severe poison ivy dermatitis. A 10- to 14-day course of prednisone may be used in this situation, since it may lessen the intensity of the disease, as well as the loss of time from work or school. Desensitization treatment by the oral and parenteral routes has been tried with poison ivy; however, the efficacy of this mode of therapy is still in dispute.

Ocular. The eye is a frequent site of involvement in contact dermatitis. Such drugs as neomycin, atropine and its derivatives, chloramphenicol, and penicillin and its related compounds may all act as sensitizers. The basis of treatment in contact dermatitis is the removal of the allergen or irritant from the patient's environment. When the allergen is identified, use of the compound containing it should be discontinued and avoided in the future. For conjunctivitis or keratoconjunctivitis associated with drugs that are primary irritant substances or contact allergens, the best treatment is withdrawal of the drug and substitution of an appropriate, nonirritating medication.

Topical. In acute skin lesions, cool saline compresses should be applied. Topical fluorinated corticosteroid lotions, such as triamcinolone or betamethasone, may be used. In chronic lesions, steroid lotions or ointments are also of use.

Supportive. It may be difficult or impractical to remove the allergen or irritant from the patient's environment due to economic or occupational factors. If continued exposure to an allergen is necessary, well-designed clothing may offer suitable protection.

Ocular or Periocular Manifestations

Conjunctiva: Chemosis; papillary reaction; vasodilation; watery discharge.

Cornea: Fine, epithelial, punctate keratitis; small, yellow, necrotic limbal opacity.

Eyelids: Crusting; eczema; edema; erythematous blepharitis; exudates; lichenification; scaling; vesicles.

PRECAUTIONS

Rubbing the eyes after handling soaps, detergents, or chemicals may provoke a contact dermatitis reaction. Allergic reactions to cosmetics affect primarily the eyebrows and upper lids because of the method of application. Mascara, eyebrow pencil, and face creams may also act as allergens. Nail polish can cause sensitization around the eye by accidental touching of the area. Lip gloss and eye gloss cosmetics contain lanolin fractions that may also act as sensitizers.

Parabens are used in a great many lotions, creams, and cosmetics because they are excellent antimicrobial agents that prevent spoilage from bacterial and fungal growth. Paraben allergy is one of the leading causes of contact dermatitis at the present time. Nickel sulfate is a common sensitizer found in jewelry and undergarments. Chromates used in costume jewelry, leather products, bleaches, and fabrics are also common offenders.

Many ocular medications are excellent contact sensitizers. Neomycin is perhaps the most common. Other antibiotics, anesthetics, and dilating agents, as well as preservatives, can cause similar problems. Development of a red eye while on chronic eyedrops should alert the ophthalmologist to the possibility of contact sensitivity. Patch testing by the dermatologist or simply discontinuation of the medication will generally make the diagnosis apparent.

COMMENTS

Contact sensitivity is a common problem in ophthalmology because of the everyday exposure to chemicals. The best form of treatment is discontinuation of the offending substance. Steroid therapy can reduce symptoms, but is not recommended on a long-term basis. Patch testing can be very helpful in determining the cause of contact dermatitis and in selecting alternative drugs to which the patient is not sensitive.

References

Claman HN, et al: Control of experimental contact sensitivity. Adv Immunol 30:121–157, 1980.

Friedlaender MH: Allergy and Immunology of the Eye. Hagerstown MD, Harper & Row, 1979, pp 79–81.

Friedlaender MH, Cyr RJ: Contact sensitivity in the guinea pig eye. Curr Eye Res 1:403–407, 1981.

Friedlaender MH: Contact allergy and toxicity in the eye. Int Ophthalmol Clin 28:317–320, 1988.

Mathias CGT, et al: Allergic contact dermatitis to echothiophate iodide and phenylephrine. Arch Ophthalmol 97:286–287, 1979.

Mathias CGT, et al: Delayed hypersensitivity to retrobulbar injections of methylprednisolone acetate. Am J Ophthalmol 86:816–819, 1978.

ERYTHEMA MULTIFORME
(Erythema Multiforme Exudativum, Stevens-Johnson Syndrome)

GEORGE M. HOWARD, M.D.
New York, New York

Erythema multiforme is an acute inflammatory polymorphic skin disease of multiple or undetermined origins. Drugs and x-ray therapy are usually implicated in adults, and infectious causes, such as herpes simplex, coxsackie and echoviruses, *Mycoplasma pneumoniae*, psittacosis, and histoplasmosis, are found in children and young adults. Incidence is highest in the first three decades, and males are more commonly affected. Erythema multiforme may begin abruptly with fever and malaise, followed within a few days by an eruptive maculopapular disorder. Vesicles and bullae appear, and an ulcerative stomatitis and conjunctivitis may ensue. Erythema multiforme exudativum is a term reserved for severe forms of erythema multiforme that usually, but not always, involve the eye. The term "Stevens-Johnson syndrome" definitely

178 / ERYTHEMA MULTIFORME

implies ocular disease; acute ocular manifestations usually consist of bilateral catarrhal, purulent, or pseudomembranous conjunctivitis. In severe cases, corneal ulcers, perforations, and panophthalmitis may occur.

THERAPY

Systemic. Although systemic corticosteroids have little specific anti-inflammatory effects on the eye, they have produced good recovery from systemic illness in several cases. Pediatric supervision of corticosteroid dosage is advisable.

Antibiotics should be used to combat secondary bacterial infection. Oral tetracycline may be given in a 250 mg dose four times daily. Sulfisoxazole may be given orally in a dosage of 0.5 gm four times daily when other measures fail. Pediatric consultation is advisable whenever systemic antibiotics are prescribed.

Recently, systemic chemotherapy with immunosuppressive agents[‡] has been used in treatment of certain dry eye syndromes. Originally developed for therapy of severe ocular cicatricial pemphigoid, immunosuppressive agents have been found useful in the management of chronic complications of Stevens-Johnson syndrome. It need hardly be mentioned that consultation with a knowledgeable and competent specialist in internal medicine is necessary during the administration of all systemic immunosuppressive agents.

Ocular. *Staphylococcus aureus* superinfection is common, and topical antibiotics known to be effective against this bacterium should be used until cultures are returned. Topical ophthalmic bacitracin, gentamicin, or tobramycin solution or ointment should be applied every 2 to 3 hours. Treatment should be continued for at least 48 hours after the eye appears healed.

Topical corticosteroids may be used to control ocular inflammation. Conjunctival irrigation with prednisolone solution in conjunction with topical ophthalmic antibiotics may be used every few hours. Severe ocular discomfort may be partially relieved by warm moist compresses or warm saline irrigations every 2 to 3 hours. Conjunctival discharge should be removed with sterile moist cotton swabs. Once or twice a day under topical anesthesia, the fornices may need to be swept gently with a glass rod to separate fresh adhesions between the conjunctival surfaces. Scleral shells, if tolerated by the patient, may help maintain the fornices.

All eyes that are clinically dry or photophobic should be treated continuously with methylcellulose drops or other tear substitutes, which are administered as often as every half-hour. Tight-fitting moisture chambers may be indicated for patients with chronic ocular involvement. Dark glasses may be helpful for photophobia.

Persistent anterior uveitis may require the use of 1 per cent atropine instilled into the eye one to two times a day.

Surgical. Early canthotomy may be considered in patients with severe swelling of the lids that prevents adequate irrigation of the cul-de-sacs.

To prevent impending blindness or greatly reduced visual acuity, tarsorrhaphy should be performed before the deep vessels start to invade the cornea if lacrimal insufficiency is established. Tarsorrhaphy only arrests corneal opacification, but such arrest may be beneficial in patients with severe corneal drying. However, if the central opening is too large in tarsorrhaphy, the patient may still experience discomfort and develop corneal ulcers. Punctal occlusion is very helpful in tear deficiency syndromes and should be performed before determining the need for tarsorrhaphy.

Cryosurgery, diathermic epilation, or appropriate plastic procedures are indicated to relieve trichiasis. If the trichiasis is due to entropion, a transverse blepharotomy and marginal rotation are recommended.

For incurable keratitis sicca, transposition of the parotid duct to the conjunctival cul-de-sac has been attempted, but rarely relieves dry eye symptoms or improves vision. Even then, subsequent surgery may be necessary to relieve excess salivary secretion.

Supportive. Bedrest and good nursing care are indicated when fever is present. Causative factors, such as chronic systemic infections, focal infections, or sensitizing drugs, should be treated, eliminated, or avoided. Simple erythema often requires no treatment. Vesicles and bullous lesions can be treated with intermittent tap water compresses.

Ocular or Periocular Manifestations

Conjunctiva: Adhesions; catarrhal, pseudomembranous, or purulent conjunctivitis; chemosis; collagen degeneration; cysts; hyperemia; subconjunctival hemorrhages; symblepharon; vesicles; widespread fibrinoid necrosis of arterioles and venules.

Cornea: Cicatrization; dense opacity; infiltration; keratoconjunctivitis sicca; neovascularization; pannus; perforation; punctate keratitis; ulcer.

Eyelids: Blepharitis; blepharospasm; cicatrization; edema; entropion; trichiasis; ulcer.

Globe: Endophthalmitis; immobility; panophthalmitis; phthisis bulbi; rupture.

Lacrimal System: Decreased tear secretion; occlusion of the lacrimal puncta.

Other: Anterior uveitis; cataract; episcleral nodules; miosis; optic neuritis.

PRECAUTIONS

In most cases, topical corticosteroids are of little value in the treatment of ocular complications. They are recommended only in small doses when the eyes are inflamed, and topical therapy with them should be closely monitored because a bacterial or fungal corneal ulcer could develop and perforate rapidly.

After the acute stage of conjunctival inflammation has passed, extended-wear soft contact lenses may be of some help in the treatment of the dry eye syndrome. In this respect, the ultra-thin soft contact lenses may be employed as a bandage lens.

Antihistamine drugs have been used in the treatment of erythema multiforme; however, conclusive evidence for the efficacy of these drugs is wanting.

COMMENTS

At the onset of the disease, the eyes frequently require immediate attention to prevent secondary infection. Topical ophthalmic antibiotics are generally indicated, especially in the presence of purulent conjunctivitis and conjunctival ulceration. The role of systemic and local corticosteroids is less clear; however, most ophthalmologists use local corticosteroids in combination with topical ophthalmic antibiotics.

In mild and moderate cases, complete recovery without systemic or ophthalmic complications is to be expected. However, in severe cases with pseudomembranous formation, scarring of the conjunctiva and cornea may progress for many years after original recovery.

References

Anderson RL, Harvey JT: Lid splitting and posterior lamella cryosurgery for congenital and acquired distichiasis. Arch Ophthalmol 99:631–634, 1981.
Beyer CK: The management of special problems associated with Stevens-Johnson syndrome and ocular pemphigoid. Trans Am Acad Ophthalmol Otolaryngol 83:701–707, 1977.
Citron J, Dyer JA: The use of therapeutic soft contact lenses in corneal disease. Mayo Clin Proc 50:443–452, 1975.
Foster CS, et al: Episodic conjunctival inflammation after Stevens-Johnson syndrome. Ophthalmology 95:453–462, 1988.
Foster CS, et al: Recurrent Stevens-Johnson syndrome of the conjunctiva. Ophthalmology 94(suppl):83, 1987.
Maumenee AE: Keratinization of the conjunctiva. Trans Am Ophthalmol Soc 77:133–143, 1979.
Omerod LD, Fong LP, Foster CS: Corneal infection in mucosal scarring disorders and Sjögren's syndrome. Am J Ophthalmol 105:512–518, 1988.
Tuberville AW, Frederick WR, Wood TO: Punctal occlusion in tear deficiency syndromes. Ophthalmology 89:1170–1172, 1982.
Wright P, Collin JR: The ocular complications of erythema multiforme (Stevens-Johnson syndrome) and their management. Trans Ophthalmol Soc UK 103:338–341, 1983.

HYPERTRICHOSIS
(Hirsutism)

DAVID T. TSE, M.D., F.A.C.S.,
Fort Lauderdale, Florida

and RICHARD L. ANDERSON, M.D., F.A.C.S.
Salt Lake City, Utah

There is some overlap between the terms "hirsutism" and "hypertrichosis." Hirsutism is conventionally defined as a disease of women and children in which there is excessive growth of body hair in response to androgens, resulting in a male distribution of hair growth. Hypertrichosis has meant that congenital or acquired presence of excessive hair growth of vellus or lanugo hair in areas not usually hairy. Lanugo is a fine, short hair covering the entire body of the developing fetus; it usually completes its growth cycle before birth. Vellus hair is similar to the fetal lanugo hair, but makes its appearance in postnatal life; it is generally unpigmented. Excessive accumulation of vellus hair may give a "peach fuzz" appearance, particularly when localized in the facial region. Generalized hypertrichosis may affect any part of the body, with the exceptions of palms and soles. It has been reported in association with the following: congenital hypertrichosis lanuginosa, acquired hypertrichosis lanuginosa, anorexia nervosa and malnutrition, central nervous system disorders, hereditary disorders, endocrine disturbances, drug-induced abnormalities, and dermatomyositis. In congenital hypertrichosis lanuginosa, the lanugo hair follicles of the fetus persist as lanugo hair follicles into adult life; often these patients exhibit a covering of fine hair over the lids, with the eyebrows participating in the abundant hair growth. Likewise, the hair follicles in acquired hypertrichosis lanuginosa revert to production of the fetal lanugo hair. In these patients, the disorder is often related to an underlying malignancy. In some, the hypertrichosis may precede the presentation of the neoplasm by up to 2 years; but in the majority, disseminated malignancy is present when the increased hair was first noted.

Localized hypertrichosis sometimes results from chronic localized low-grade physical or chemical trauma or hormonal stimulation. It may also be associated with nevi, particularly congenital nevi, and is often seen with porphyria. Topical corticosteroids that are used in patients for the therapy of chronic diseases, such as eczema, psoriasis, and disseminated lupus erythematosus, sometimes stimulate hair growth. This has been seen primarily in adults who have used potent fluorinated corticosteroids with or without plastic film occlusion.

Congenital ocular hypertrichosis may manifest itself as an increase in the length or the number of eyelashes or eyebrows. Synophrys (fusion of eyebrows across the midline), trichomegaly (an increase in the length of cilia), and polytrichia (an increase in number) are common in this condition. Ectropic cilia, reduplication of the ciliary

180 / HYPERTRICHOSIS

follicles, and cilium inversum are rare hypertrichotic anomalies. Duplication supercilia, in which two rows of eyebrows are present, has also been described.

Hirsutism may be caused by physiologic states (precocious puberty, menopause) or endocrinologic states (Cushing's syndrome, malignancies).

THERAPY

Systemic. In patients whose hirsutism presents a problem beyond that which can be handled by local physical means, various drug regimens have been used on an empiric basis. New growth of unwanted hair associated with primary adrenal androgenic hyperfunction can often be inhibited by long-term low-dose corticosteroids; a dosage of 5 to 10 mg of oral prednisone daily may be effective. Measurement of plasma and/or urinary parameters after several weeks of glucocorticoids may be of some predictive use. If androgen parameters are lowered by the corticosteroids, the physician is encouraged to pursue long-term management with this agent, providing that secondary side effects are kept at a minimum. Excessive hair growth associated with primary ovarian hyperfunction sometimes may be controlled by a combined progestogen-estrogen combination, usually in the form of oral contraceptives. Again, measurement of androgen parameters after one or more cycles of suppression may encourage the continuation of this therapy. Many difficulties are associated with these forms of treatment, not least of which is their poor effectiveness. In the case of an androgen-secreting tumor, removal of the lesion is occasionally followed by partial or, more rarely, complete regression of the hirsutism. Physicians should thus be cautioned against making overly optimistic predictions as to outcome.

Recently, the realization that androgenic receptors are present in the hair follicles, combined with the availability of several compounds with anti-androgenic properties, has afforded new approaches to the treatment of hirsutism. Spironolactone,[‡] an aldosterone antagonist, appears to be remarkably effective for the treatment of hirsutism. In one small series, spironolactone at a dose of 200 mg a day was administered to two groups of patients with hirsutism: 1) those with polycystic ovary disease with excessive ovarian androgen production and 2) those with normal androgen levels and idiopathic hirsutism. Treatment with spironolactone resulted in improvement of hirsutism in 19 of 20 patients, with regression in terms of diameter, density, and the rate of facial hair growth within 2 months. Although these results are encouraging, spironolactone is not an entirely benign medication. Until additional data are available from a larger number of patients, spironolactone cannot be recommended as an entirely benign and effective treatment for hirsutism.

The oral administration of the powerful anti-androgen, cyproterone acetate,[‡] alone or in combination with ethinyl estradiol[‡] has been found to be successful in several European trials. These progestin-like agents may have several sites of action, including suppression of testosterone production and direct anti-androgen action at one or more target organ sites. This treatment is presently at the investigational stage. Cimetidine[‡] has recently been found to have anti-androgenic activity, and preliminary clinical results suggest that this drug may be a safe, effective treatment of androgen-dependent hirsutism.

Supportive. Attempts should be made to determine the cause of the hypertrichosis or hirsutism. If the cause is not physiologic, therapy should be directed to correction of the underlying condition. In the great majority of cases, the hirsutism represents a genetically based normal variation, and the patient can be reassured that the excess hair has no pathologic significance. However, many patients will insist on treatment for cosmetic reasons. In these cases, the least irritating methods should be applied. Cutting or shaving the hair is not likely to irritate the skin. However, there is often a certain resistance to shaving because of the myth that it stimulates hair to grow faster or more coarsely. A simple solution is to bleach the hair with hydrogen peroxide, thus rendering it less conspicuous. Alternatively, application of a depilatory cream or wax or removal with tweezers may also be beneficial. However, epilating creams and waxes are generally too irritating to use around the eye, and none of these methods permanently remove the overgrowth of hair.

Surgical. Electrolysis is usually a successful method for permanent hair removal, particularly if there are relatively few hairs; it can also be an effective adjunct with a medication regimen in more severe cases. Properly performed, electrolysis can be a safe and effective method of hair removal. However, it is a time-consuming, expensive, and moderately uncomfortable procedure. It is generally suitable for only small areas, such as the face and eyelids. Minimal puncture scarring may result. Expertise in this field can be quite variable, since commercial electrolysis is an unlicensed field in many areas of the country. Care should thus be exercised in selecting an electrolysist.

The management of polytrichosis of the eyelids is discussed in detail in the section on distichiasis.

Ocular or Periocular Manifestations

Cornea: Irritative keratitis.
Eyebrows: Excessive cilia; synophrys.
Eyelids: Ectropic cilia; monilethrix; pili torti; polytrichosis; reduplication of ciliary follicles; trichomegaly.

PRECAUTIONS

If there is a diffuse coarsening of hairs, especially in the area of the upper lid, electrolysis may produce poor results. Electrolysis is a tedious procedure that usually requires multiple treatment sessions. A history of keloid formation is an important medical contraindication to electrolysis. Too vigorous electrolysis treatment can produce perceptible cutaneous scarring.

Under no circumstances should radiotherapy be employed in the treatment of hypertrichosis. Permanent depilation can be achieved only at the expense of eventual radiodermatitis, which is both disfiguring and dangerous.

Topical application of depilation waxes or lotions containing barium sulfide or thioglycollates may produce contact dermatitis. Troublesome folliculitis is a frequent complication unless the procedure is carried out under skilled supervision. For this reason, such applications are generally not recommended in the periocular area.

COMMENTS

In at least 90 per cent of women who consider themselves hirsute, the hirsutism is genetically determined and must be considered physiologic. In the small percentage of patients in whom hirsutism is a manifestation of a defined and reversible medical disorder, it is important that an accurate diagnosis be made at an early stage.

Most cases of acquired hypertrichosis are reversible, assuming that the underlying cause is recognized and can be treated. Careful planned investigation by an endocrinologist to identify the etiology is advisable for all such patients, particularly if hormonal abnormalities are suggested.

References

Anderson JAR: An assessment of (1) cyproterone acetate and (2) ethinyl oestradiol and lynoestrenol (Minilyn) in the treatment of idiopathic hirsutism. Br J Dermatol 99:545–552, 1978.
Cumming DC, et al: Treatment of hirsutism with spironolactone. JAMA 247:1295–1298, 1982.
Duke-Elder S (ed): System of Ophthalmology. St. Louis, CV Mosby, 1963, Vol III, pp 873–881.
Maguire HC: Diseases of the hair. *In* Moschella SL, Pillsbury DM, Hurley HJ Jr (eds): Dermatology. Philadelphia, WB Saunders, 1975, pp 1215–1221.
Muller SA: Hirsutism. Am J Med 46:803–817, 1969.
Vigersky RA, et al: Treatment of hirsute women with cimetidine. A preliminary report. N Engl J Med 303:1042, 1980.

ICHTHYOSIS
(Epidermolytic Hyperkeratosis, Ichthyosis Vulgaris, Lamellar Ichthyosis, X-Linked Ichthyosis)

RAYMOND J. SEVER, M.D.

Temple Terrace, Florida

The ichthyosiform dermatoses are a relatively uncommon group of disorders characterized by fish-like scaling of the skin. Ichthyosis vulgaris is by far the most common and is inherited as an autosomal dominant trait. In this disorder, dry skin and follicular accentuation (keratosis pilaris) usually appear at puberty. Scaling is most prominent over the trunk, abdomen, buttocks, and legs. The flexural areas, such as the antecubital fossa, are spared.

X-linked ichthyosis is a more severe disorder affecting males. Generalized scaling is present at or shortly after birth. This scaling is most prominent over the extremities, neck, trunk, and buttocks. The flexural creases, palms, and soles are spared. Irregular deep corneal opacities are found in the male patients with x-linked ichthyosis and may be used to distinguish this form of ichthyosis from all others. Female carriers may have minor corneal opacities. The corneal opacities are not known to affect visual acuity. Recent studies have shown deficient steroid-sulfatase in fibroblasts grown from the skin and in leukocytes from patients with x-linked ichthyosis.

Lamellar ichthyosis, a more severe form of dermatosis, is an autosomal recessive trait. Children who are born with lamellar ichthyosis are called "collodion babies" and are covered at birth by a thickened membrane that is subsequently shed. The scaling of the skin involves the whole body with no sparing of the flexural creases. Ectropion may be produced by drying and tautness of the facial skin. Secondary conjunctival and corneal changes may ensue from the exposure.

Epidermolytic hyperkeratosis is an autosomal dominant disorder. At birth, the skin is moist, red, and tender. Thick verrucous scaling occurs within a few days.

The ichthyoses differ in their cellular kinetics. The epidermal turnover of ichthyosis vulgaris and x-linked ichthyosis is normal. Lamellar ichthyosis and epidermolytic hyperkeratosis show a significantly increased transit rate.

THERAPY

Systemic. In epidermolytic hyperkeratosis, recurrent and chronic bacterial infections of the skin require frequent systemic antibiotics.

Ocular. In patients with lamellar ichthyosis, care must be taken to avoid ectropion. Treatment is a two-step process. The first step, hydration, is accomplished with petrolatum jelly and urea. The jelly is used on the lower lid when the skin is moist after a bath. Urea in a 10 per cent cream is effective when applied several times daily. The second step, the slowing of the epidermal turnover rate, is accomplished with a daily application of 0.1 per cent tretinoin cream. If exposure keratitis occurs, artificial tears or occlusive therapy may be needed.

Supportive. All treatments for ichthyosis are aimed at three principal goals: hydration of the stratum corneum, removal of the scale, and slowing of the epidermal turnover rate when increased cellular proliferation occurs. Overall care is a dermatologic problem.

182 / ICHTHYOSIS

Ocular or Periocular Manifestations

Conjunctiva: Keratinization and thickening secondary to ectropion (in lamellar ichthyosis).
Cornea: Exposure keratitis secondary to ectropion (in lamellar ichthyosis); opacities (in x-linked ichthyosis).
Eyelids: Ectropion (in lamellar ichthyosis).

PRECAUTIONS

Tretinoin may be very irritating to the skin if used frequently and should not be allowed to penetrate the conjunctival sac.

COMMENTS

Other than the diagnostic help that the ophthalmologist can give in x-linked ichthyosis, he or she has no real function in the treatment of x-linked ichthyosis or ichthyosis vulgaris.

References

Frost P: Disorders of cornification. *In* Moschella SL, Pillsbury DM, Hurley HJ Jr (eds): Dermatology. Philadelphia, WB Saunders, 1975, pp 1056–1084.
Grekin JL, Basler RS: New treatments for ichthyosis. Cutis 25:432–434, 1980.
Orth DH, Fretzin DF, Abramson V: Collodion baby with transient bilateral upper lid ectropion. Review of ocular manifestations in ichthyosis. Arch Ophthalmol 91:206–207, 1974.
Sever RJ, Frost P, Weinstein G: Eye changes in ichthyosis. JAMA 206:2283–2286, 1968.
Shapiro LJ, et al: X-linked ichthyosis due to steroid-sulphatase deficiency. Lancet 1:70–72, 1978.

IMPETIGO

ALAN SUGAR, M.D.

Ann Arbor, Michigan

Impetigo is a superficial infection of the skin caused by group A streptococcus or *Staphylococcus aureus* or both. It occurs primarily in newborns and young children. The more common form is caused by streptococci (streptococcal pyoderma), although staphylococci may also be cultured later from the same lesions. Impetigo secondary to streptococcus, often called impetigo contagiosa, is easily transmitted among young people. The initial lesions are tiny vesicles in the superficial epidermis that develop into larger pustules. Initially, there is very little underlying erythema. The lesions become covered by a thin crust that thickens to a honey-colored purulent crust and appears to be "tacked on" to the skin. An erythematous base and regional lymphadenopathy may develop, although there are no systemic symptoms. Deeper skin ulceration (ecthyma) may follow. The lesions occur in exposed areas, particularly the face and arms, and are especially common in late summer and following minor skin trauma. An important systemic sequela is the development of glomerulonephritis when nephrogenic streptococcal strains are involved (about a 1 per cent incidence). Bullous impetigo is caused by staphylococci and begins with the development of large bullae, which rupture leaving a thin clear crust. Ocular involvement in impetigo is secondary to periocular skin involvement.

THERAPY

Systemic. Untreated impetigo may become a chronic skin disease and lead to acute glomerulonephritis. Systemic antibiotic therapy is the most effective treatment, either alone or in combination with topical therapy, and results in a higher cure rate than topical therapy alone. Penicillins are rapidly effective. A 10-day course of 250,000 to 500,000 units of oral penicillin V three to four times daily is an adequate regimen. Intramuscular benzathine penicillin G in a single 0.6 to 1.2 million unit injection is effective when compliance is a problem. In penicillin-allergic patients, a 10-day course of 20 to 40 mg/kg of erythromycin may be given in four divided doses. Penicillin-resistant staphylococci in bullous impetigo may be treated with 25 to 50 mg/kg of cloxacillin[§] or dicloxacillin[§] four times a day. Benzathine penicillin G injection is effective prophylactically to prevent infection of family members.

Topical. Traditionally, impetigo has been treated with cleansing of the crusts and scrubbing with bacteriostatic soaps, followed by application of bacitracin or neomycin ointment. Recent studies, however, have shown that scrubbing may delay healing. Topical 2 per cent mupirocin ointment is as effective as oral erythromycin. Systemic antibiotics may be more effective than topical ointments in prevention of nephritis from nephrogenic streptococci.

Ocular or Periocular Manifestations

Conjunctiva: Acute bacterial conjunctivitis.
Cornea: Bacterial ulcer (rare).
Eyelids: Blepharitis; cicatricial ankyloblepharon (rare); local skin lesions.

PRECAUTIONS

Isolation and skin wound precautions should be observed to prevent spread of infection to family members or to other patients. Prophylactic treatment of family members, especially young children, can be effective.

COMMENTS

Systemic antibiotic treatment is the most effective form of therapy. Topical treatment is probably ineffective.

References

Eels LD, Mertz PM, Piovanetti Y, et al: Topical antibiotic treatment of impetigo with mupirocin. Arch Dermatol 122:1273–1276, 1986.

Ferrieri P, Dajani AS, Wannamaker LW: A controlled study of penicillin prophylaxis against streptococcal impetigo. J Infect Dis 129:429–438, 1974.

Margolis HS, et al: Acute glomerulonephritis and streptococcal skin lesions in Eskimo children. Am J Dis Child 134:681–685, 1980.

Mupirocin—A new topical antibiotic. Med Lett Drug Ther 30:55–56, 1988.

Peter G, Smith AL: Group A streptococcal infections of the skin and pharynx. (First of two parts). N Engl J Med 297:311–317, 1977.

NEURODERMATITIS
(Lichen Simplex Chronicus)

WESLEY KING GALEN, M.D.

New Orleans, Louisiana

Neurodermatitis is a condition in which the skin becomes altered because of the effects of chronic rubbing or scratching. The chronic trauma may result in erythema, excoriations, and erosions, but commonly, lichenification (thickening of the skin), hyperpigmentation, or hypopigmentation result. Pruritus is the major presenting symptom, and the multitude of precipitating causes may include atopic dermatitis, seborrheic dermatitis, allergic contact dermatitis, or even seasonal allergic conjunctivitis. As the patient responds to this symptom by rubbing, the skin becomes damaged, thickened, and more sensitive. Thus, a vicious itch-scratch cycle is set up, which may be further exacerbated by numerous environmental or psychogenic factors. Neurodermatitis may be generalized and involve many areas of the skin, including the eyelids, or it may be localized. Common sites for localized involvement include the neck, lower extremities, scalp, or genital or perianal area. It may also be localized just to the eyelids. Whatever the underlying cause, ocular manifestations of neurodermatitis primarily involve the lids, which present with edema, changes in pigmentation, and lichenification that is sometimes dramatic. Other associated ocular problems include atopic cataracts, keratoconus, and keratoconjunctivitis.

THERAPY

Supportive. The physician should explain the role that chronic rubbing and scratching play in the formation of lesions and encourage the patient to restrain when possible. Reassurance is helpful. Teaching the patient to avoid precipitating causes, such as contact allergens, is also important. Rarely, psychiatric counseling may be necessary if psychogenic causes are dominant and all other possible underlying causes have been ruled out or treated.

Cool compresses with clear water or very dilute boric acid solution may provide symptomatic relief for affected areas. Antihistamines may be very useful, both for their sedative properties and for their antihistaminic effects. An oral dosage of 25 to 50 mg of either diphenhydramine or hydroxyzine every 4 to 6 hours may be given. Terfadine 60 mg may be given every 12 hours for less sedation.

Topical corticosteroid creams or ointments applied to affected skin for short periods of time (1 to 3 weeks) or intermittently may be very helpful. Generally, sterile ointments acceptable for ocular use are preferred as the medication may possibly spread into the eye. Topical ophthalmic 1.5 per cent hydrocortisone or 0.05 per cent dexamethasone ointment is recommended. Strong fluorinated corticosteroids should probably be avoided, especially for chronic use. However, it may be necessary to use intermediate-potency corticosteroids, such as 0.05 per cent desonide or 0.1 per cent triamcinolone, on very difficult cases that are unresponsive to more traditional therapy. Occasionally, occlusion with a porous plastic wrap (Handiwrap) may be required for short courses of therapy, such as preparing a patient for cataract surgery.

Rarely, plaques due to neurodermatitis do not respond to topical treatment and may require intralesional injection of corticosteroids, although the author has never had to resort to this method. The very rare occasions when the physician feels that intralesional corticosteroids are indicated, an extremely dilute form of corticosteroid should be used. The first injection should not exceed 1.0 mg/ml of triamcinolone. If well tolerated, this dose may be increased to 2.0 to 2.5 mg/ml. Although intralesional corticosteroid injections are used with confidence in other areas of the body, they should be avoided if possible around the eye, owing to the danger of significant atrophy and telangiectasia and consequently poor cosmetic results.

Ocular. Patients with eyelid involvement should be treated with topical ophthalmic corticosteroid ointments as described earlier. In addition, most patients with keratoconjunctivitis can be managed with the administration of artificial tears.

PRECAUTIONS

Topical corticosteroid therapy should be carefully monitored in these patients. A number of cases of corticosteroid-induced glaucoma have been reported as a result of periocular corticosteroid application. They are probably caused by melting of the ointment, which inadvertently allows the medication to penetrate the tear film by gravity.

Atrophy, telangiectasia, and stria formation may develop after prolonged use of topical corticosteroid ointments. If intralesional injection of corticosteroids proves to be unavoidable, the physician should advise the patient that transient or permanent localized atrophy or pigmentary changes may occur.

Patients with atopic dermatitis should be informed of their increased potential to develop cataracts at an early age, prior to the use of corticosteroids. The use of topical anesthetics, topical antihistamines, and complex mixtures of antibiotics and corticosteroids should be avoided in the treatment of neurodermatitis because of the sensitizing tendencies of these agents. The superimposition of a contact dermatitis upon the neurodermatitis lesions would be disastrous, and any associated secondary infection should be treated concurrently.

COMMENTS

Manipulating, rubbing, and scratching the face and, in some, the periocular area is a common habitual tic. It can also occur in some patients postoperatively who cannot seem to keep their fingers away from their lids. This activity, in part, can be aggravated by the drying of ocular medication on the eyelid. Although this is rare, it can give rise to well-demarcated neurodermatitis of the eyelids.

References

Arndt KA: Manual of Dermatologic Therapeutics, with Essentials of Diagnosis, 2nd ed. Boston, Little, Brown, and Co, 1978, pp 55–57.
Duke-Elder S (ed): System of Ophthalmology. St. Louis, CV Mosby, 1976, Vol XV, p 108.
Galen WK: Neurodermatitis. In Conn HF (ed): Current Therapy, Philadelphia, WB Saunders, 1978, p 601.
Pillsbury DM: Principles of clinical diagnosis. In Moschella SL, Pillsbury DM, Hurley HJ Jr (eds): Dermatology. Philadelphia, WB Saunders, 1975, pp 131, 147, 151.

OCULAR ROSACEA

JOSEPH FRUCHT, M.D.,
and STUART I. BROWN, M.D.

San Diego, California

Rosacea is a common chronic skin disorder of unknown etiology. It is more prevalent in females and is usually manifested between the ages of 30 to 50 years. Characteristically, the facial flush areas (forehead, nose, and cheeks) and the V of the neck are involved. The presence of telangiectasia pustules and rhinophyma is diagnostic of rosacea, and supporting findings include erythema, hypertrophic sebaceous glands, and papules. Intermittent exacerbation and remissions are common.

Ocular manifestations of rosacea mainly involve the lids, conjunctiva, and cornea. Diffusely hyperemic conjunctiva, blepharitis, meibomianitis or styes are common, and episcleritis may also occur. Corneal involvement includes punctate epithelial erosions, peripheral vascularization, and subepithelial infiltrates with thinning central to vascularization. Corneal perforation may ensue secondary to the infiltrate and thinning. Patients usually complain of burning and tearing and general irritation.

THERAPY

Systemic. Treatment with oral tetracyclines[‡] is necessary to alleviate the symptoms and signs of ocular rosacea. Recent experience shows that doxycycline, a semisynthetic tetracycline, can alleviate the ocular symptoms as efficiently as tetracycline and is better tolerated. The dose of 100 mg of doxycycline is given once a day for 6 weeks. If the patient's symptoms have responded, the dose is tapered to 50 mg daily for one month, then 50 mg every other day, and finally stopped. However, if the symptoms remain unchanged, the doxycycline is discontinued, 250 mg of tetracycline is given four times a day, and the dose is slowly tapered according to the patient's symptoms and response.

Improvement is expected within the first 3 weeks; irritation is usually diminished before the signs resolve. Most of the treated patients require some daily medication indefinitely. Abrupt tapering may cause recurrence of the disease, which may be very difficult to treat with full doses of tetracycline, and some of these cases become unresponsive to these drugs.

Ocular. Topical antibiotics are ineffective in ocular rosacea. Topical steroids may be useful to treat subepithelial corneal infiltrates or episcleritis; however, these drugs should always be applied in addition to oral tetracyclines. Associated blepharitis will respond to systemic doxycycline or tetracycline.

Surgical. Small corneal perforations, especially peripheral, may be treated with application of cyanoacrylate adhesive and a bandage soft contact lens or by lamellar patch graft. In patients with large central perforations or with visual disability from scarred and vascularized corneas, a penetrating keratoplasty may be done. Concurrent treatment with tetracycline or doxycycline is crucial during these surgical maneuvers.

Topical. Facial lesions respond to treatment with tetracycline. Patients rarely require topical corticosteroid preparations to decrease signs of the disorder.

Ocular or Periocular Manifestations

Conjunctiva: Hyperemia.
Cornea: Pannus; perforation; punctate erosion (recurrent); subepithelial infiltration; superficial or deep wedge-shaped neovascularization; thinning.
Eyelids: Chalazion; chronic blepharoconjunctivitis; erythema of lid margins; hordeolum; increased meibomian secretions; thickening.
Sclera: Nodular episcleritis.

Other: Burning; decreased visual acuity; foreign body sensation; irritation; pain.

PRECAUTIONS

Tetracycline or doxycycline should not be used in children under the age of 8 years or until enamel deposition on the maturing teeth is completed. Likewise, it should not be given to pregnant or lactating women. Vaginal yeast superinfection may occur and can be treated by gradual tapering of the tetracycline doses or with local antifungal agents. Tetracycline should be administered on an empty stomach, and concurrent administration of antacids, dairy products, or iron preparations is not recommended because gastrointestinal absorption of the drug is diminished by these agents. Doxycycline can be used at any time. Although milk products insignificantly affect the absorption of doxycycline, concurrent antacids or milk products are not recommended with its use.

COMMENTS

The diagnosis of ocular rosacea is often missed. All examinations for external eye disorders should be performed with good illumination and removal of facial makeup if present to enable the discovery of subtle signs. Ocular signs and symptoms may be unilateral, and rosacea patients may present with a unilateral red eye. It is important to counsel patients, since this disease may be chronic and some signs of meibomianitis or blepharitis may persist after most symptoms are relieved.

References

Brown SI, Shahinian L Jr: Diagnosis and treatment of ocular rosacea. Ophthalmology 85:779–786, 1978.
Jenkins MS, et al: Ocular rosacea. Am J Ophthalmol 88:618–622, 1979.
Lempert SL, Jenkins MS, Brown SI: Chalazia and rosacea. Arch Ophthalmol 97:1652–1653, 1979.
Marmion VJ: Tetracyclines in the treatment of ocular rosacea. Proc Roy Soc Med 62:11–12, 1969.
Sneddon IB: A clinical trial of tetracycline in rosacea. Br J Dermatol 78:649–652, 1966.
Tolman EL: Acne and acneiform dermatoses. *In* Moschella SL, Pillsbury DM, Harley HJ Jr (eds): Dermatology. Philadelphia, WB Saunders, 1975, pp 1139–1142.

PHOTOSENSITIVITY AND SUNBURN

JOHN A. PARRISH, M.D.,
and BARRY S. PAUL, M.D.

Boston, Massachusetts

Photosensitivity is an enhanced responsiveness to natural or artificial nonionizing electromagnetic radiation. Direct symptomatic reactions of the skin may result from absorption of the middle wavelength ultraviolet (UVB, 290 to 320 nm). An acute sunburn reaction that is characterized by erythema with tenderness, pain, edema, and sometimes vesiculation is an example of a direct symptomatic reaction. The severity of the reaction depends upon the incident exposure dose and host defenses, such as the melanin content of the skin or the thickness of the stratum corneum. Severe cases of sunburn may be accompanied by systemic signs, such as fever, nausea, chills, and delirium. Chronic exposure to sunlight results in cumulative skin damage that may be seen as erythema, irregular pigmentation, telangiectasia, atrophy or hyperplasia, dyskeratosis, or the anaplasia of actinic keratosis or squamous cell carcinomas.

Chemical phototoxicity is caused by the presence of some absorber that enhances reaction to radiation. It may be of exogenous origin from drugs or other chemicals or endogenous origin from underlying systemic or genetic disorders. Most such reactions require exposure to long wavelength ultraviolet (UVA, 320 to 400 nm) or to visible light. Clinical manifestations of chemical phototoxicity vary depending upon the particular offending agent or systemic disease.

The most common ocular abnormality caused directly by ultraviolet radiation is photokeratoconjunctivitis, which results from absorption of short (UVC, 200 to 290 nm) and middle (UVB, 290 to 320 nm) wavelength ultraviolet radiation by the outer viable cell layers of the cornea and conjunctiva. The clinical picture of photokeratitis follows a characteristic course. After exposure, a period of latency varies somewhat inversely with the exposure dose, being as short as 30 minutes to as long as 24 hours. Conjunctivitis, often accompanied by erythema of the periorbital skin, is associated with a foreign body sensation, varying degrees of photophobia, lacrimation, and blepharospasm. Corneal pain can be very severe. The individual is usually incapacitated for 6 to 24 hours, but all discomfort usually disappears within 48 hours. Very rarely does exposure result in permanent damage. Unlike the skin, the ocular system does not develop tolerance to repeated exposure.

Ocular manifestations of chemical photosensitivity are becoming increasingly important with the widespread use of psoralen plus UVA (PUVA) photochemotherapy in the treatment of psoriasis, as well as other dermatologic diseases. Methoxsalen (8-MOP), a psoralen, is ingested orally 2 hours before exposure with a high-intensity UVA source. The 8-MOP serves as a chromophore upon which absorbing UVA produces photoproducts with proteins and DNA cross-links that interfere with DNA replication and hence cellular proliferation. It has been shown that 8-MOP enters the lens and can be found in the cortex, nucleus, and epithelial cells. If kept in the dark for 12 hours, the free 8-MOP will diffuse out of the lens. However, if exposed to UVA (which is abundantly present in sunlight), it will bind to lens proteins and DNA. Because the lens is completely encapsulated and never sheds any

186 / PHOTOSENSITIVITY AND SUNBURN

cells, bound 8-MOP may accumulate with repeated exposures. This may result in enhanced photo-oxidation reactions and eventually be cataractogenic. In young children whose lenses transmit UVA and in aphakic patients, PUVA may potentially result in damage to the retina.

THERAPY

Systemic. Severe generalized photosensitivity reactions may require systemic corticosteroids to afford symptomatic relief; however, these drugs do not reduce the erythema. An oral dosage of 40 to 60 mg of prednisone should be tapered gradually over 10 to 14 days.

Some patients with polymorphous light eruptions (PMLE) may be treated with topical sunscreens; however, in many patients, systemic therapy is required. A short course of 200 mg of hydorxychloroquine[‡] once or twice daily or oral prednisone beginning 2 to 3 days before sun exposure may prevent an episode of PMLE. A patient with PMLE may also undergo the induction of tolerance with a 3-week course of either PUVA or UVB before sun exposure.

Ocular. Symptomatic relief of photosensitivity of the eyelids may be obtained with cold compresses of isotonic saline, Burow's solution 1 : 40, or plain tap water. Cold compresses reduce the blepharospasm and the accompanying paroxymal pain. Topical fluorinated corticosteroids, such as 0.2 per cent betamethasone, may be applied three to four times daily to reduce erythema, pruritus, and edema.

Symptomatic relief from acute solar conjunctivitis may be obtained by bandaging the eyes. Broad-spectrum antibiotic ointments applied three to four times daily may help prevent infection that could prolong the symptoms. In severe cases, homatropine eyedrops may help relieve the ciliary spasm and extreme miosis.

Clinical and subclinical solar keratosis of the eyelids may be removed with topical cream containing 5 per cent fluorouracil. This must be applied twice a day for 2 to 3 weeks with extreme caution and care as it results in an inflammatory response that may be quite vigorous. Cryosurgery using liquid nitrogen that creates a freeze lasting 10 to 20 seconds and surgical excision or curettage followed by light electrodesiccation will remove any clinically evident actinic keratosis. Care must be taken not to affect the orbital contents when treating the lid with liquid nitrogen.

Supportive. The best therapy for all photosensitivity disorders is avoidance of exposure to ultraviolet radiation. For those for whom this is not possible, prophylaxis with sunscreening lotions is essential. Effective sunscreens against middle wavelength ultraviolet are 5 per cent aminobenzoic acid in alcohol, esters of aminobenzoic acid, and certain benzophenone-containing combination products. For those who re-quire protection from the long wavelength ultraviolet, additional protection may be obtained with benzophenones alone or in combination with 5 per cent aminobenzoic acid.

PRECAUTIONS

The use of hydroxychloroquine to treat patients affected by PMLE is not listed in the manufacturer's official directive. This drug should not be used for prolonged periods, as it may lead to irreversible retinal change. Ocular examinations once or twice yearly are advisable. Sunglasses or other eyewear with appropriate ultraviolet-absorbing properties may prevent photokeratitis and reduce the long-term risks associated with certain systemically administered photosensitizers, such as psoralens or chlorpromazine. Because of epidemiologic evidence linking solar ultraviolet with the incidence of brunescent cataracts, it may be appropriate for persons chronically exposed to bright sunlight to wear appropriate sunglasses.

All patients receiving PUVA therapy should wear protective sunglasses for at least 12 hours after ingestion of methoxsalen. The sunglasses must be opaque to UVA; examples of such are Noir, Foster Grant, and Cool Ray. It should be remembered that UVA passes through window glass, so that the sunglasses must be worn when riding in an automobile during the daytime.

COMMENTS

Endogenous photosensitivity is clinically apparent as cutaneous manifestations of systemic diseases or abnormalities, such as porphyria, amino aciduria, lupus erythematosus, solar urticaria, polymorphous light eruption, xeroderma pigmentosum, and Cockayne's syndrome. These clinical manifestations will vary with the underlying cause. Management, therefore, should be directed toward the underlying cause and supplemented with avoidance of natural or artificial ultraviolet radiation and the use of appropriate sunscreens. Unfortunately, the etiology of some photodermatoses, such as polymorphous light eruption and solar urticaria, remains obscure.

References

Duke-Elder S (ed): System of Ophthalmology. St. Louis, CV Mosby, 1965, Vol VIII, pp 512–515; 1974, Vol XIII, pp 78–79, 349, 404–406; 1972, Vol XIV, pp 888–893, 921–928, 930–932, 1294–1297.

Lerman S: Radiant Energy and the Eye. New York, Macmillan, 1980.

Parrish JA: Photosensitivity and sunburn, *In* Conn HF (ed): Current Therapy. Philadelphia, WB Saunders, 1979, pp 607–608.

Taylor HR, West SK, Rosenthal FS, et al: Effect of ultraviolet radiation on cataract formation. N Engl J Med *319*:1429–1433, 1988

Willis I: Photosensitivity. *In* Moschella SL, Pillsbury DM, Hurley HJ Jr (eds): Dermatology. Philadelphia, WB Saunders, 1975, pp 324–349.

POISON IVY, OAK, OR SUMAC DERMATITIS
(Rhus Dermatitis)

WILLIAM L. EPSTEIN, M.D.

San Francisco, California

Several plants in the *Rhus* genus are capable of producing contact dermatitis. Poison ivy (*Rhus radicans*) dermatitis is by far the most common, but poison oak (*R. toxicodendron*) and poison sumac (*R. vernix*) dermatitis may also occur. The most characteristic lesion is a linear one, appearing on an extremity that has brushed past an offending plant. The rash is initially red and very itchy; it rapidly becomes vesicular and may spread from the patient's extremities to face or genitals. In severe cases, the patient is acutely uncomfortable, due to the oozing, crusting, itching, and smarting that occur during the active stages of infection. Resolution of *Rhus* dermatitis usually occurs in 2 to 3 weeks. Ocular involvement almost always results from transmission of the irritant to the ocular adnexae by the hands. The lids become edematous and hyperemic, vesiculation occurs, and a secondary pyoderma may lead to pustulation. In severe cases, a chemotic conjunctival reaction may be present. The cornea may be involved, causing pain, photophobia, and blepharospasm.

THERAPY

Systemic. If edema becomes noticeable or the dermatitis is severe, systemic corticosteroids may be employed. A repository corticotropin injection of 80 units may be given intramuscularly on the patient's first visit. Repeat injections given on the third and fifth days often provide sufficient relief. However, the dose and frequency of injection depend upon the patient's response. The same degree of control requires an initial dose of 400 to 600 mg of hydrocortisone or its equivalent (80 to 100 mg of triamcinolone or methylprednisolone).

Ocular. Ocular therapy is symptomatic. Cool compresses may provide relief for itching and burning. In the earliest stages before marked vesiculation has occurred, topical corticosteroids, such as 0.2 per cent betamethasone cream, may be applied three times daily to the eyelids for a few days. If conjunctival or corneal involvement occurs, topical ophthalmic corticosteroids, such as 0.05 per cent dexamethasone ointment, may be used four times daily. If an anterior uveitis is present, 5 per cent homatropine one to four times daily may be used.

Supportive. Before vesiculation occurs and during the healing stage, topical corticosteroids may be applied to the affected area. High-potency corticosteroids in a gel base or an optimized vehicle are preferred for skin lesions, whereas topical ophthalmic ointments are necessary for use around the eye. Topical 0.05 to 0.5 per cent fluocinolone, fluocinonide, or betamethasone may be used three times daily.

After vesication occurs, conventional therapy relies on the use of cold soaks (Burow's solution 1:40), tepid baths (starch and soda, Aveeno oatmeal), and lotions (calamine without additives). However, drying and cracking of the skin from overzealous bathing should be avoided, as this tends to increase pruritus. Care must be taken not to allow these materials to touch the eye.

Sedatives or antihistamines may help alleviate pruritus. Aspirin may be given in a dosage of 0.6 gm every 3 to 4 hours. Occasionally, 0.5 to 2.0 gm of chloral hydrate at bedtime may be necessary.

Ocular or Periocular Manifestations

Conjunctiva: Chemosis.
Cornea: Infiltration; keratitis.
Eyelids: Blepharospasm; edema; hyperemia; pustules; vesicles.
Other: Ocular pain; photophobia.

Precautions

The effectiveness of topical corticosteroids is greatly reduced after vesiculation has begun. Because of the high potency of recommended topical corticosteroids, they should not be used for long periods of time or over large areas of the body. Prolonged use of topical corticosteroids near the periocular area should be avoided because of the potential danger of glaucoma. If systemic corticosteroids are used, the value of a very large initial dose cannot be overemphasized; most failures in this form of therapy are caused by hesitation to use a therapeutic dose of corticosteroid. Flare-ups may occur if the dosage of corticosteroids is reduced too rapidly. Local subcutaneous injections of corticosteroids can cause atrophic changes.

Administration of poison ivy extract is contraindicated in the management of acute cases. It usually produces no effect, and occasionally the dermatitis is aggravated by this therapeutic measure.

Comments

The *Rhus* plants produce a dermatitis by means of a group of antigens common to all three plants. The same group of antigens may also be found in the shell of the cashew nut, the mango rind, Japanese lacquer, Indian marking nut, the ginkgo tree, and several other exotic plants and trees from South America and Southeast Asia. The dermatitis caused by these antigens is more likely to be vesicular and bullous than many other common forms of contact dermatitis.

Rhus dermatitis occurs most commonly in children during spring and summer and in those whose occupations bring them into contact with the species. Poison ivy dermatitis is very com-

188 / POISON IVY, OAK, OR SUMAC DERMATITIS

mon and constitutes a significant source of disability.

References

Duke-Elder S (ed): System of Ophthalmology. St. Louis, CV Mosby, 1974, Vol XIII, p 60.

Epstein WL: Allergic contact dermatitis. *In* Fitzpatrick TB et al (eds): Dermatology in General Medicine, 3rd ed. New York, McGraw-Hill, 1987, pp 1373–1383.

Epstein WL: The poison ivy picker of pennypack park. J Invest Dermatol 88:7s–11s, 1987.

Grant WM: Toxicology of the Eye, 3rd ed. Springfield, IL, Charles C Thomas, 1986, pp 749–750.

PRURITUS

JAMES D. HOGAN, M.D.

La Crosse, Wisconsin

Pruritus is an unpleasant sensation perceived in the skin that elicits the response of scratching. Pruritus may be sharp and well localized (epicritic), diffuse (protopathic), scattered with multiple distant foci of itching after primary focal itch, or referred itch within the same dermatome of primary focal itch. It may result from physiologic or pathologic causes, as a generalized hyperresponsiveness of itchy skin, such as in urticaria with dermatographism, and, more recently, central neural itch as mediated by the central nervous system without primary cutaneous changes.

Itch receptors' free nerve endings and networks pass through a rich milieu in the dermis of blood vessels, mast cells, and connective tissue, forming a plexus of receptor sites at the dermalepidermal junction. Itch and pain are separate sensations, though increasing itch stimulus can result in pain. Removal of the epidermis and upper dermis abolishes itch but not pain sensation. Both pain and itch are transmitted to the spinal cord by small diameter fibers and are probably integrated at a common site in the dorsal horn of each spinal segment. Impulse conduction is then transmitted to the contralateral anterolateral spinothalamic tracts of the spinal cord to secondary neuronal relay centers in the thalamus. However, evidence of tertiary cortical itch receptors in the sensory cortex is inferential.

The best-known mediator of itch is histamine. Histamine is known to be present in mast cells surrounding dermal vessels. Serotonin is present in activated platelets; however, serotonin is not found primarily in skin. Epidermal proteases or peptidases obtained from inflamed skin will provoke itch, leading to the conclusion that products obtained from keratinocytes or leukocytes during inflammation may directly activate itch receptors. Additionally, kinin peptides, vasoactive intestinal polypeptides, enkephalin, substance P, and neurotensin all can either modulate itch

directly or the sensation of itch. These peptides appear to modulate itch through release of histamine, as well as having a direct effect upon the itch receptor. Prostaglandin E_1 potentiates histamine-induced itching and may have a direct pruritogenic action on nerve endings. Histamine may provoke itch by a direct action in H_1 receptors and perhaps an indirect action due to secondary release of other mediators. H_2 receptors do not appear to be involved in histamine-induced itch, although H_2 blockers, such as cimetidine, may be beneficial in idiopathic chronic urticaria. Central itch may be mediated by the neuropeptides, endorphins, as naloxone may either inhibit or potentiate central perception of itch depending on the direction of placebo response, i.e., it may abolish the placebo response or stimulate the placebo response. Direct pathologic itch may be mediated by pruritogenic dihydroxy bile salts as in primary biliary cirrhosis; however, poor correlation is observed between depletion of the suspected mediator and symptomatic benefit. Additionally, the mediator in uremic pruritus is unknown, although systemic benefit is provided by phototherapy with ultraviolet B (290 to 320 nm) treatment.

Pruritus may be subdivided into generalized sensation of pruritus without skin changes; pruritus with primary skin lesions, such as macular erythema, papules, vesicles, urticaria, and eczematization; and pruritus with secondary skin lesions of excoriations, secondary infection, or lichenification.

Systemic diseases with focal or generalized itching include the following: *CNS disease* (senile pruritus, multiple sclerosis, psychosis with delusions of parasitosis), *liver disease* (hepatitis, primary biliary cirrhosis, extrahepatic biliary obstruction, drug-induced intrahepatic cholestasis, pruritus gravidarum), *renal disease* (uremic pruritus, secondary hyperparathyroidism), *metabolic disease* (hyperthyroidism; hypothyroidism; hypoglycemia; diabetes; cutaneous paresthesias as numbness, tingling, crawling sensations accompanying peripheral neuropathy; pruritus ani), *hematopoietic disorder* (iron-deficiency anemia, polycythemia vera, paraproteinemia, hypereosinophilic syndrome), and *malignancy* (Hodgkin's disease, carcinoid syndrome, myeloid metaplasia, mycosis fungoides, adenocarcinomas including adenocarcinoma colon with iron-deficiency anemia or hepatic metastases, nasal pruritus with brain tumor, lymphoma, multiple myeloma). Subclinical *drug reactions* (angiotension-converting enzyme inhibitors; beta-blockers; thiazide diuretics; antiarrhythmics, such as quinidine, procainamide; tocainide, encainide, and amiodarone; warfarin; phenothiazines; antidepressants; cocaine; morphine; codeine; aspirin; nonsteroidal anti-inflammatory agents; vitamin B complex) as well as *miscellaneous causes* (excessive bathing, harsh soaps usually advertised as antibacterial that leave no soapy films) may also be responsible for pruritus. Other factors that may induce pruritus include *contact urticaria* to enzymes or fragrances in liquid detergents, fragrance in fabric softeners, optical brighteners in powdered detergents, or fiberglass and *solar exposure*, which causes a type of polymorphous light eruption. Rarely, brachial-radial pruritus, dermatomal pruritus from nerve compression, hereditary pruritus localized to the midback or scapular tip, caffeine-induced pruritus, premenstrual pruritus, aspartame-induced pruritus or frank urticaria, nasal pruritus of atypical angina, autoimmune progesterone dermatitis, mastocytosis, and aquagenic pruritus may occur.

Pruritus may present with the primary cutaneous lesion of urticaria. If present less than 4 weeks, urticaria is classified as *acute* and most often is the result of 1) drug exposure; 2) preceding or intercurrent viral, bacterial, or parasitic infection; 3) immediate, intermediate, or delayed phase food reaction; 4) inhalation allergy, as an intrinsic or extrinsic seasonal or nonseasonal activation of the atopic state; 5) local or systematized *Hymenoptera* or insect venom reaction; or 6) local or systematized contact urticaria to chemicals, cosmetics, etc. *Chronic* urticaria is diagnosed when hives have been present for 4 to 6 weeks or more. Generally, if the individual hive persists for greater than 24 hours, a skin biopsy is indicated to rule out urticarial vasculitis of an idiopathic nature, either associated with hypocomplementemia with or without nephritis or presenting as systemic lupus erythematosus. Pruritus may accompany individual lesions of Henoch-Schönlein purpura and ordinary leukocytoblastic vasculitis. Physical urticaria, such as solar, pressure, aquagenic, vibratory, dermographism, and cholinergic (induced by exercise, heat, stress, or cold) urticaria, should be excluded by history and appropriate testing. Cholinergic urticaria, a common chronic physical urticarial problem, can be diagnosed by observing typical 1- to 3-mm wheals with a surrounding 0.5- to 3-cm zone of erythema. A rare variety of diffuse erythema can also signify cholinergic urticaria. Exercise- or cold-induced cholinergic urticaria may trigger systemic anaphylaxis, and testing must be performed under controlled conditions. Other rare forms of urticaria include adrenergic urticaria, hereditary or acquired angioneurotic edema caused by C1-esterase inhibitor deficiency, functional protein abnormality, or atypical serum protein as in the acquired form. Life-threatening airway swelling may occur with angioneurotic edema. The acquired form requires a search for associated malignancy. Generally, most chronic urticaria does not have an identifiable etiology and seems to reflect feedback instability in the mast cell population itself.

THERAPY

Supportive. An attempt should be made to determine if pruritus is a manifestation of internal disease, a reaction to drugs, associated with primary skin disease elsewhere, or a contact urticarial, irritant, or contact allergic reaction limited to the periorbital region. Therapy should be directed to correcting or avoiding the underlying cause where possible. If all such determinable causes can be excluded, then symptomatic treatment may be directed to the pruritus.

The patient should be advised to avoid scratching the area as doing so lowers the itch threshold and reinforces the itch-scratch cycle. Nails should be trimmed to avoid excoriations. Cultures for bacteria should be obtained as indicated, since altered skin integrity may allow pathogenic staphylococcal or streptococcal colonization that can contribute to pruritogenic stimulus by release of keratinocyte peptidases and cytotoxic antibody production. The patient should avoid fatigue, strain, alcohol, and caffeine as these may lower the itch threshold. A constant climate and avoidance of excessive moisture or dryness are preferable.

Topical. In the active, wet, vesiculated, or exudative phase with secondary infected areas, open compresses with cool tap water or Burow's solution should be applied for 10 to 20 minutes three or four times daily. The compresses should then be removed and the skin allowed to air dry. Calamine lotion may also be applied to enhance drying, if desired. This routine should be repeated until this phase has been converted into a drier state, usually in 3 to 5 days.

If the skin is fissured with eczematization, the skin should again be hydrated with tap water compresses, but then immediately covered with a bland soothing moisturizing lotion, such as Vaseline brand Dermatology Formula Lotion. If redness and itching persist after rehydration, the skin may be covered with a weak steroid cream or ointment, such as 0.025 per cent triamcinolone. If more moisture needs to be retained without promoting maceration, an ointment rather than a cream base should be used. The steroid cream or ointment should be given until symptoms have abated, usually in 5 to 7 days.

In the dry state with lichenification with thickening, hydration compresses with tap water should be applied three to four times daily. Direct application of a weak 1 per cent hydrocortisone ointment may be used until redness and pruritus abate, followed by daily application with plain USP white petrolatum.

Acceptable topical corticosteroids for initial control of inflammation include 2.5 per cent hydrocortisone, 0.025 per cent triamcinolone cream or ointment, or 0.2 per cent hydrocortisone valerate cream. After the initial period necessary to control the inflammation, which is usually 5 to 7 days, 1 per cent hydrocortisone should be used to maintain the symptom-free skin until a bland emollient base, such as plain USP white petrolatum, Complex 15 moisturizing cream or lotion, or Vaseline Dermatology Formula Lotion, can be applied. The importance of not using stronger steroids in the periocular region cannot be overemphasized because of the need to avoid topical steroid side effects to the thin skin in this area and as not to potentiate ocular absorption of steroid that can lead to elevated ocular pressure and precipitate acute angle-closure glaucoma.

Systemic. If systemic therapy is needed to augment topical anti-inflammatory measures, antihistamines may be useful. Initial side effects can be minimized by beginning treatment at night before bedtime and then increasing the dose as the body develops tolerance to the drug. Often, significant antipruritic effect is not established because the full 24-hour dose of the antihistamine is not employed. In children, it is important to establish the full 24-hour dose on a mg/kg scale and then employ the medication in appropriate divided doses. Hydroxyzine has been shown to be a superior antipruritic agent in several studies; however, many comparison trials have not been conducted on an equivalent potency basis, and therefore, a clear choice of the best antihistamine for the individual patient rests on the patient's response to a full dose of what is often an empiric choice. If antipruritic effects are not beneficial, one should then choose another antihistamine H_1 blocker from a different class of parent compound. Ethanolamine derivatives (diphenhydramine), alkylamine derivatives (chlorpheniramine), ethylenediamine derivatives (tripelennamine), piperazine derivatives (hydroxyzine), phenothiazine derivatives (trimeprazine), or cyproheptadine are examples of other antihistamines from which to choose. Treatment might begin in adults with hydroxyzine at bedtime and an increase to 25 mg five times daily. If this fails to relieve symptoms, the oral dose may be increased to a maximum of 100 mg four times daily. In children, the elixir is useful with a maximum daily dose of 2 mg/kg in divided doses. Tranquilizers, such as 2 to 5 mg of diazepam or 5 to 10 mg of chlordiazepoxide three to four times per day, may be beneficial in allaying anxiety associated with pruritus in some patients. In senile pruritus, doxepin may be useful in the absence of organic causes for itch.

Newer nonsedating H_1 blockers include 60 mg of terfenadine once or twice daily and the most recent introduction, 10 mg of astemizole[†] administered as a single daily dose. Double blind crossover trials show astemzole effective as a single agent compared to placebo. The main side effects of these newer drugs were increased appetite and mild weight gain. Mild sedation was also noted, but a high frequency of remission after cessation of the drug is encouraging. If necessary, a minimally sedating adjunct regimen would include either 1 mg of azatadine twice daily or 4 mg of chlorpheniramine two or three times daily. For early morning break-through, the addition of 25 mg of hydroxyzine every night has been helpful. For cold-induced urticaria, 10 mg of doxepin three times daily appears superior to cyproheptadine. In the elderly, doxepin and other sedating antihistamines should be used with caution, especially at full doses, because of the increased risk of unsteadiness, falls, and injury. Doxepin and other antihistamines with anticholinergic activity are contraindicated in narrow-angle glaucoma and in patients with a tendency toward urinary retention.

Severe allergic contact dermatitis may necessitate systemic steroids. Prednisone beginning at 40 to 60 mg initially, then tapered over 10 to 14 days, will control the immunologically mediated reaction and prevent flare break-through. Other methods that may help include the H_2 blocker cimetidine,[‡] especially in some cases of chronic urticaria. Administration of 300 mg of cimetidine may be given twice daily and titrated to threshold suppression, with special concern for its side effects and problems with long-term usage.

PRECAUTIONS

When more potent steroid creams or ointments are applied, they should be used for as brief a period as possible and in as low a potency as is efficacious. It is now known that repeated applications of topical steroids enhance their potency, and what has little effect initially will become more potent with continued usage. Another factor that enhances potency is frequent application, and twice-daily application is sufficient initially, with subsequent daily application to begin after the symptomatic period has ended. Additionally, absorption through dermatitic skin where the stratum corneum barrier has been broken will increase steroid absorption. This factor along with the extreme thinness of the eyelid skin can dramatically increase potency over one hundred times. It is also known that the absence of fluorinated steroid application is not a guarantee of long-term safety and that steroid-induced toxicity can occur with 1 per cent hydrocortisone alone.

COMMENTS

Other medications in mastocytosis that have proven useful include oral cromolyn sodium[‡] for gastrointestinal mastocytosis. Newer agents include ketotifen,[†] which can inhibit mast cell release of mediators without needing blocking action as do the classic H_1 blockers. Except for some cases of mastocytosis, prostaglandin inhibitors have not been studied for their antipruritic effect, and aspirin[‡] may increase or decrease the itch threshold in different patients. Topical cromolyn* has not been shown to have antipruritic action over placebo. Newer studies have shown topical doxepin* to have histamine-induced pruritus blocking effect, although large-scale studies have not been done. Naloxone[‡] has been tested for central itch block, but results are not conclusive to recommend its use for regular antipruritic therapy. For pruritus associated with cholestasis, removal of any cholestatic drug is indicated where possible, and the use of activated charcoal plasma exchange or oral charcoal is helpful. For uremic pruritus, phototherapy with UVB is also helpful in many patients.

References

Bernard JD: Clinical aspects of pruritus. *In* Fitzpatrick TB, et al (eds): Dermatology in General Medicine. New York, McGraw-Hill, 1987, pp 78–90.

Bircher AJ: Aquagenic pruritus. Arch Dermatol *124*:84–89, 1988.

Bleehan SS, et al: Cimetidine and chlorpheniramine in the treatment of chronic idiopathic urticaria: A multi-

centre randomized double blind study. Br J Dermatol 117:81–88, 1987.
Denman ST: A review of pruritus. J Am Acad Dermatol 14:375–392, 1986.
Fox RW, et al: The treatment of mild to severe chronic idiopathic urticaria with astemazole: Double blind and open trials. J Allergy Clin Immunol 78:1159–1166, 1986.
Goldsobel AB, et al: Efficacy of doxepin in the treatment of chronic idiopathic urticaria. J Allergy Clin Immunol 78:867–873, 1986.
Hirschmann JV, et al: Cholinergic urticaria: A clinical and histologic study. Arch Dermatol 123:462–467, 1987.
Monroe EW: Chronic urticaria: Review of nonsedating H_1 antihistamines in treatment. J Am Acad Dermatol 19:842–846, 1988.
Papadopoulas NM: Electrophoretic differentiation of acquired angioedema from hereditary angioedema. Clin Chim Acta 163:231–234, 1987.
Pola J, et al: Urticaria caused by caffeine. Ann Allergy 60:207–208, 1988.
Shelley WB, Shelley ED: Adrenergic urticaria: A new form of stress induced hives. Lancet 2:1031–1033, 1985.
Wanderer AA: Clinical characteristics of cold-induced systemic reactions in acquired cold urticaria syndromes. J Allergy Clin Immunol 78:417–429, 1986.

PSORIASIS
WILLIAM B. GLEW, M.D.,
and THOMAS P. NIGRA, M.D.
Washington, District of Columbia

Psoriasis vulgaris is a chronic skin disease of unknown etiology affecting 1 to 4 per cent of the population. It is characterized by sharply circumscribed, elevated, thick red plaques of skin covered with coarse, dry, silvery scales. The epidermal cells in patches of psoriasis have lost regulatory control and turn over several times more rapidly than normal epidermal cells. Most patients have minimal amounts of psoriasis limited to such areas as elbows, knees, scalp, and gluteal cleft; approximately 15 per cent of the psoriatic population have severe generalized psoriasis.

Removal of the silvery scale produces minute bleeding points (Auspitz sign). In an active case of psoriasis, stroking of normal skin with a blunt instrument will result in the development of typical papules a few weeks later in the area of trauma (Köbner phenomenon). This probably accounts for the frequency of psoriasis seen on elbows and knees, since there is constant trauma to these areas.

Psoriasis infrequently affects the skin of the eyelids, but plaques may extend to the conjunctiva where they can cause irritation. Marginal keratitis and uveitis are also uncommon, but may occur more frequently in psoriatics than in the general population. Psoriasis is a capricious disease that can appear at any age. It is characterized by flares sometimes associated with streptococcal infection and stress, and there can be spontaneous remission of the lesions.

THERAPY

Systemic. Chemotherapy for psoriasis is based on drugs that interfere with reproduction of epidermal cells. Methotrexate is the only systemic drug approved for use in severe psoriasis. The usual dosage range of methotrexate is 2.5 to 5.0 mg at 12-hour intervals for three doses each week. Monitoring of renal, liver, and bone marrow functions is essential. Other drugs, such as hydroxyurea[‡] and aminopterin,[†] have been used to treat psoriasis. In addition, the use of aromatic retinoid etretinate has been shown to be very effective, particularly in association with ultraviolet therapy. For unresponsive cases, cyclosporine[‡] has been helpful.

Perhaps the greatest advances in the treatment of psoriasis have come in the areas of phototherapy. Since the 1920s when patients were hospitalized on an average of 21 days and treated intensively (Goeckerman regimen), tar and ultraviolet light therapy have been used to clear psoriasis. This modality has proven safe and effective for psoriasis, although it is time consuming and costly and does not have any effect on prevention of recurrences.

In 1974, a new form of photochemotherapy known as PUVA was developed. This therapy employs the systemic use of psoralen, methoxsalen, which sensitizes the skin to long wave ultraviolet light in the 320 to 400 nm range (UVA). The skin is irradiated with UVA in a carefully monitored chamber 2 hours after ingestion of methoxsalen, resulting in a controlled phototoxic response that is therapeutic. On the average, 90 per cent of patients treated with this modality at intervals of two to three times weekly clear in 21 treatments. They are then maintained in a clearing phase with follow-up treatments every 1 to 4 weeks. After a clearing and short maintenance phase, approximately 60 per cent remain clear for greater than 1 year. This modality has recently been approved by the FDA and must be done under strict protocol only on severe disabling psoriasis. It has a long-term risk of skin carcinogenesis and cataracts.

Since the development of PUVA, there has been a resurgence of ultraviolet light therapy in general for psoriasis. Today, intense sunburn spectrum 280 to 320 nm (UVA) light therapy given in association with topical application of tar or anthralin derivatives is very effective on an outpatient basis for treating generalized psoriasis. Maintenance and slow tapering of the therapy subsequent to clearing (average 30 treatments) result in a longer remission than the Goeckerman regimen. If patients respond to this therapy and maintain a good remission, PUVA is not necessarily indicated.

Ocular. Keratoconjunctivitis, which may be associated with psoriasis even in the absence of facial lesions, responds to ocular steroid drops four times daily and ointment during the night.

Uveitis usually responds to 30 mg of oral prednisone daily. Keratitis sicca, trichiasis, cicatrization, symblepharon, and ectropion are rare secondary findings for which a variety of tear replacements and ocular lubricants can be helpful.

Topical. Topical therapy is indicated for minimal psoriasis. The potent fluorinated steroids, such as halcinonide, fluocinonide, betamethasone, and triamcinolone, as well as hydrocortisone, are the most commonly used preparations. In the past, occlusive dressings were needed to potentiate the corticosteroid effectiveness. Currently, application of halcinonide two times a day is very effective in most cases. Other modalities of delivering corticosteroids to the skin include the use of impregnated tape or direct injection of 5 mg/ml of triamcinolone in saline into the dermal area of a lesion by raising a wheal.

It is important also to treat the normal skin of psoriatics, since dry skin serves as a locus for the Köbner phenomenon that may result in more extensive psoriasis. Patients should use various preparations of bath oils and topical emollients, such as lotions and creams, to keep their skin healthy and well lubricated.

Finally, coal tar has been effective in treatment and can be used in association with fluorinated steroids in derivative form or by itself in a 5 per cent concentration in white petrolatum in association with ultraviolet light. For the scalp, coal tar shampoos containing sulfur and salicylic acid or in association with fluorinated steroid solutions are very effective.

PRECAUTIONS

Systemic corticosteroids should not be used in the treatment of psoriasis because of the high doses necessary and the severe exacerbations that often occur after the steroids are stopped.

Methotrexate should be used very carefully. It has the potential risk of hepatic cirrhosis when high cumulative doses have been used or in association with alcohol ingestion. Hematologic function also needs to be monitored for suppression of marrow components.

Phototherapy has been reported to produce skin cancer, as does sunlight. To prevent the development of cataracts associated with phototherapy, adequate ocular photoprotection can be achieved by wearing goggles and spectacles that are tested and confirmed as *opaque to ultraviolet light*. Goggles must be worn during irradiation; wraparound spectacles should be worn after ingestion of photosensitizers and for the 24-hour period of potential photosensitization following each drug dose. Ordinary sunglasses are not adequate.

COMMENTS

The combination of psoralens and UVA in the treatment of psoriasis is now established as a successful mode of therapy for severe generalized psoriasis, but the increased incidence of skin carcinomas and potential for cataractogenesis mandate continued caution in the administration of this innovative therapy.

References

Current status of oral PUVA therapy for psoriasis: Eye protection revisions. J Am Acad Dermatol 6:851–855, 1982.

Eustace P, Pierse D: Ocular psoriasis. Br J Ophthalmol 54:810–813, 1970.

Fritsch PO, et al: Augmentation of oral methoxsalen-photochemotherapy with an oral retinoic acid derivative. J Invest Dermatol 70:178–182, 1978.

Glew WB, et al: Photochemotherapy and the eye: Photoprotective factors. Trans Am Ophthalmol Soc 78:243–254, 1980.

Knox DL: Psoriasis and intraocular inflammation. Trans Am Ophthalmol Soc 77:210–224, 1979.

Lerman S, Megaw J, Willis I: Potential ocular complications from PUVA therapy and their prevention. J Invest Dermatol 74:197–199, 1980.

Melski JW, et al: Oral methoxsalen photochemotherapy for the treatment of psoriasis: A cooperative clinical trial. J Invest Dermatol 68:328–335, 1977.

Parrish JA, et al: Photochemotherapy of psoriasis with oral methoxsalen and longwave ultraviolet light. N Engl J Med 291:1207–1211, 1974.

Roenigk HH Jr, et al: Methotrexate guidelines—revised. J Am Acad Dermatol 6:145–155, 1982.

Sandvig K, Westerberg P: Ocular findings in psoriatics. Acta Ophthalmol 33:463–467, 1955.

URTICARIA AND HEREDITARY ANGIOEDEMA
(Angioneurotic Edema, Giant Edema, Giant Urticaria, Hives, Nettle Rash, Quincke's Disease)

MITCHELL H. FRIEDLAENDER, M.D.

La Jolla, California

Urticaria is a cutaneous eruption with multiple pathogenic mechanisms that may be immunologic or nonimmunologic. Its prevalence in the general population is high and is estimated to be between 10 and 25 per cent. No specific cause can be found in 70 per cent of patients with chronic urticaria; in others, psychogenic, allergic, and physical factors may play a role.

The skin lesions of urticaria are sharply circumscribed, elevated areas of edema. If the swelling is extensive and involves the subcutaneous tissues, the term "angioedema" is used. Urticaria may be divided into acute and chronic forms. Acute urticaria is often associated with immunologic mechanisms. Chronic urticaria, which lasts more than 8 weeks, frequently has no identifiable cause. At times, emotional or allergic factors may be implicated.

The immunologic mechanisms involved in urticaria are not well understood. The clinical signs of urticaria may be simulated by injection of histamine into the skin. Presumably, histamine and other vasoactive mediators are released from mast cells by immunologic or nonimmunologic means in urticaria.

Hereditary angioedema is characterized by repeated attacks of epithelial edema involving the skin, respiratory tract, and gastrointestinal tract. Urticaria does not occur in this condition, although the skin may be well demarcated. Although hereditary angioedema was first recognized by Osler in 1888, it was only recently discovered that a biochemical abnormality in the complement system exists in this entity. Patients with hereditary angioedema have an inherited deficiency of C1-esterase inhibitor, a protein that inhibits activation of the first component of complement. The deficiency leads to uncontrolled activation of the complement pathway and generation of a kinin-like substance. Repeated episodes of angioedema involving the skin and respiratory tract may lead to death from pharyngeal edema and asphyxiation. About 85 per cent of patients' kindreds have markedly deficient or absent C1-esterase inhibitor. In the remaining 15 per cent, the inhibitor is present in normal amounts, but is functionally inactive.

THERAPY

Systemic. Antihistamines are frequently effective in control of urticaria and may be effective for angioedema, particularly if administered soon after the onset of symptoms. Daily administration of 30 to 100 mg of hydroxyzine in divided doses has become increasingly popular for the treatment of urticaria, regardless of cause. Beta-adrenergic drugs, such as ephedrine and terbutaline, are now being used as adjuncts to antihistamines for therapy of urticaria. These drugs elevate intracellular cyclic AMP levels and, in turn, suppress mediator release from mast cells. Systemic corticosteroids may be required for control of severe cases of acute urticaria or angioedema, but in general, they have no place in the regular therapy of chronic urticaria. Aqueous epinephrine may be given subcutaneously for temporary relief of acute urticaria.

In patients with hereditary angioedema, three groups of medications are useful: antifibrinolytic agents, anabolic steroids and impeded androgens, and fresh-frozen plasma. The antifibrinolytic agent aminocaproic acid[‡] has been used successfully to prevent attacks of hereditary angioedema. The effective dose in adults is 18 gm daily in divided doses. Tranexamic acid[‡] is a newer, more potent antifibrinolytic agent that markedly reduces the frequency of attacks of hereditary angioedema at a dose of 3 gm daily. Methyltestosterone[‡] (an anabolic steroid) and danazol or oxymetholone[‡] (impeded androgens) have been shown to prevent attacks of hereditary angioedema. These drugs induce synthesis of C1 inhibitor. In acute attacks, administration of fresh-frozen plasma as the source of C1 inhibitor provides a rapid method to terminate attacks.

Ocular. Systemic therapy will generally control ocular as well as other systemic manifestations of these two diseases. However, subcutaneous injection or application of cotton pads soaked in 1:1000 epinephrine[‡] may be used for treatment of severe conjunctival edema.

Surgical. If orbital edema develops to such an extent that the globe or optic nerve is threatened, relief from pressure should be provided. The most effective method to remove pressure appears to be an osteoplastic decompression of the lateral orbital wall. This should rarely be necessary.

Supportive. A specific etiologic agent may sometimes be identified in urticaria. In food allergy, the suspected food may be eliminated from the diet for several weeks and subsequently tried again to determine its relation to the urticaria. Drug allergy requires a careful history and elimination of the suspected drug.

In hereditary angioedema, prevention of airway obstruction is essential.

Counseling. Cholinergic urticaria may be associated with exercise, emotional stress, and overheating. Sunlight, trauma, and sudden changes of temperature may also precipitate urticaria due to physical allergy. Sunscreen lotions or topical antipruritic medications, such as calamine lotion, may also be of value in prophylaxis.

Hereditary angioedema may be precipitated by trauma, dental extractions, wearing of tight garments, physical exertion, infections, heat or cold, emotional stress, and menstruation.

Ocular or Periocular Manifestations

Conjunctiva: Chemosis.
Eyelids: Edema; hyperemia.
Optic Nerve: Optic neuritis; papilledema.
Other: Central serous retinopathy; exophthalmos; nystagmus; orbital edema; secondary glaucoma; uveitis; visual field defects.

PRECAUTIONS

Pharyngeal edema is a life-threatening situation that must be treated immediately. Some patients present with abdominal attacks that mimic intra-abdominal crises, and not infrequently patients are subjected to laparotomies. Approximately 50 per cent of cases present before the age of 6 years.

If the eye is not threatened, overenthusiastic treatment is not encouraged, since the edema will usually resolve in a few days. Corticosteroids should not be considered a substitute for epinephrine in the emergency treatment of severe cases.

Antihistamines may cause drowsiness, and patients taking them should be warned not to drive or operate machinery.

COMMENTS

Urticaria has numerous causes, and its pathogenesis is poorly understood. Basically, it is associated with uncontrolled mast cell degranulation and release of mediators. Therapy is designed to prevent mast cell release or inhibit the mediators of inflammation.

Hereditary angioedema is an inherited deficiency of C1-esterase inhibitor and represents a chronic condition that is life threatening. Patients must be counseled intensively, and emergency therapy must be available to them.

References

Ballogh Z, Whaley K: Hereditary angio-oedema: Its pathogenesis and management. Scott Med J 25:187–195, 1980.

Casale TB, Sampson HA, Hanifin J, et al: Guide to physical urticarias. J Allergy Clin Immunol 82:758–763, 1988.

Christiansen SC: Evaluation and treatment of the allergic patient. Int Ophthalmol Clin 28:282–293,1988.

Friedlaender MH: Allergy and Immunology of the Eye. Hagerstown, Md, Harper & Row, 1979, pp 81–85.

Kaplan AP: The pathogenic basis of urticaria and angioedema: Recent advances. Am J Med 70:755–758, 1981.

Mathews KP: Management of urticaria and angioedema. J Allergy Clin Immunol 66:347–357, 1980.

VITILIGO

FRANK PARKER, M.D.

Portland, Oregon

Vitiligo is a patchy depigmentary disorder of the skin that is generally progressive over many years and occurs in 1 to 2 per cent of the general population. The depigmentation is due to a destruction of melanocytes in the involved skin. Nearly 40 per cent of patients have a positive family history, with an autosomal dominant inheritance pattern. The depigmentation may appear anywhere on the skin surface, although the lesions most often are symmetrically distributed bilaterally on the backs of the hands, on the forearms, face and neck, around body orifices, and over bony prominences. In over 50 per cent of patients, vitiligo first develops before the age of 20 years. Early lesions may show only patchy loss of melanin pigment; however, total loss of pigment in the involved area is almost invariable as time passes. The borders of the enlarging depigmented areas are sharply delineated and may display mild inflammation, as well as hyperpigmentation. The extent of the disease varies from a few small patches to universal loss of pigment. Hairs in the patches usually lose their pigment. The lesions of vitiligo are benign and asymptomatic. However, the areas are subject to painful sunburn.

Vitiligo frequently begins with rapid loss of pigment, which may be followed by a lengthy period when the skin color does not change. Later, pigment loss may begin anew. The loss of color may continue until, for unknown reasons, the process stops. Cycles of pigment loss, followed by periods of stability, may continue indefinitely. It is rare for any patient with vitiligo to repigment or regain significant skin color spontaneously.

Vitiligo can take several other forms, such as halo nevi, segmental vitiligo (involving a region supplied by peripheral nerves), veloce vitiligo (rapid graying hair and sudden appearance of extensive vitiligo after an episode of acute emotional or physical trauma), or chemical vitiligo (depigmentation seen on the hands of people working with germicidal detergents or rubber containing monobenzone). Once the process of chemical vitiligo is set in motion locally, loss of pigment cells can occur in parts of the body remote from sites of actual contact.

No matter how extensive vitiligo is, the color of the eyes under ordinary examination does not change. However, 3 of 51 patients with vitiligo studied with a slitlamp biomicroscope were found to have a focal loss of pigment in the irides. Most common are lesions in the ocular fundus suggestive of chorioretinitis or atrophy of the pigment layers of the eyes. It is likely that destruction of melanocytes in the eye may be an important factor in the pathogenesis of certain types of uveitis. This process could also play an initiating role in sympathetic ophthalmia.

Vitiligo may occur in association with hyper- or hypothyroidism, thyroiditis, alopecia areata, pernicious anemia, juvenile and adult diabetes, and Addison's disease. In addition, vitiligo may be associated with ocular syndromes, such as Vogt-Koyanagi syndrome and sympathetic ophthalmia. Vitiligo may precede the clinical appearance of these conditions by several years and occurs in 8 to 20 per cent of people with these disorders.

The presence of thyroid, adrenal, and gastric parietal cell antibodies in many patients with both vitiligo and endocrine disease suggests a common, perhaps autoimmune origin. The autoimmune theory of vitiligo is further strengthened by the increased prevalence of organ-specific autoantibodies in several, but not all large series of patients with vitiligo. Recently, the presence of a circulating complement-fixing antibody that binds melanocytes of human skin and nevus cells in two patients with vitiligo and multiple endocrine insufficiencies has provided further evidence regarding the autoimmune nature of vitiligo. Presumably, such IgG antibodies play some role in the destruction of the melanocytes in the vitiliginous skin. Other theories regarding the etiology of vitiligo are that 1) abnormal functioning nerve cells may injure nearby pigment cells and 2) the malanocytic cells may be self-destructive (autotoxic).

THERAPY

Supportive. Complete spontaneous cure is unusual. Some temporary and partial repigmentation is detectable in about 50 per cent of patients during the summer months. The treatment of vitiligo is usually unsatisfactory, and in most cases, it is best to advise patients to seek effective cosmetic camouflage.

Topical. Especially in darker-skinned persons, treatment of vitiligo often consists of the application of cosmetic cover creams to the involved areas. Opaque formulations containing zinc oxide are the most favorable camouflaging agents as they combine a broad-spectrum sunscreen agent with a water-resistant opaque base. These preparations come in various shades, imparting a natural look.

The depigmented patches may also be painted with dihydroxyacetone. Cosmetic cover-up lotions containing dihydroxyacetone and certain analine dyes impart fairly natural color to amelanotic areas. Reapplication is required after washing as these compounds are water soluble. Protection from the sun by a benzophene or an aminobenzoic acid sunscreen cream is advisable. Patients with skin types I or II (light skin with little melanin pigmentation who sunburn readily) benefit from artificial suntan formulations containing 5 per cent dihydroxyacetone, which often gives satisfactory skin color. Care should be taken with these preparations as they impart a greenish color to the skin after the formulation is 6 to 9 months old.

In patients whose vitiliginous lesions are limited to a small area, topical application of psoralens followed by ultraviolet light (PUVA therapy) is indicated. Methoxsalen lotion or 0.1 per cent methoxsalen in hydrophilic ointment may be applied to the affected area. After 45 minutes to an hour, the area is exposed to long wavelength ultraviolet light. The first exposure should last 15 seconds; subsequent exposures, every other day, are increased by 15-second increments until a visible erythema has appeared in the affected area. Subsequent exposures are given or slightly increased at this time level until pigment fills in from the normally pigmented skin borders and the perifollicular melanocytes. The distance of the light source to the skin should be kept constant for each exposure.

Steroid preparation may promote repigmentation in vitiligo lesions. Topical betamethasone[‡] and clobetasol[‡] have been used with variable results. Local injections of corticosteroids[‡] have also been used, with 60 per cent of patients' vitiligo responding to a variable degree in one series. Care must be used with such injections, as skin atrophy is a common and unwelcome complication.

Tattooing ferrous oxide[†] pigment into the dermis of vitiliginous areas, if they are of limited extent, may also be of some benefit.

A small group of patients with widespread vitiligo who have not responded to psoralens and UV light or who do not want to commit to 100 to 300 sessions of photochemotherapy and who desire complete depigmentation can be given a trial of 20 per cent monobenzone. This medication is applied to the normal pigmented areas twice daily and decreases pigment in the normal areas within 2 to 3 months. Full depigmentation is achieved in 4 to 12 months in 50 to 60 per cent of patients. Complications from the monobenzone include burning, itching, erythema, dryness, and contact dermatitis.

Systemic. Occasionally, oral psoralen treatment is worth trying, especially when the vitiligo is widespread and the patient highly motivated. Two hours before exposure to natural sunlight or long wavelength ultraviolet light (UVA 320 to 380 nm), a psoralen preparation is given (trioxsalen or methoxsalen). Oral trioxsalen is the preferred drug when sunlight is used because it is less phototoxic than methoxsalen. The patient using trioxsalen should begin with a one-minute exposure to sunlight, and the times are gradually increased every other day 2 hours after taking the trioxsalen, until visible erythema occurs in the affected areas. If artificial UVA light booths are used, 20 to 40 mg of methoxsalen is given 1 to 2 hours before light exposure. The treatment continues every other day at the time or energy exposure that gives erythema, until repigmentation occurs. This often takes months, and if repigmentation is not seen, increasing the methoxsalen dosage to 60 mg has been advocated. Perifollicular macules of repigmentation in the depigmented areas first appear after 15 to 30 treatments. Complete repigmentation usually requires 200 to 300 treatments. Some repigmentation may be achieved in 15 to 20 per cent of patients. Certain areas of the body are more responsive than the others. The face, especially the periorbital area, responds quite well, followed by the neck and trunk. Vitiliginous areas over bony prominences, hands, feet, and mucosa are the most resistant. Young patients often respond more rapidly than older individuals.

Phenylalanine[‡] and UVA light have also been used for treating generalized vitiligo. A success rate of 95 per cent repigmentation has been reported with this method, as well as less sun sensitivity of affected areas after therapy.

Ocular. There is no treatment for uveal or retinal depigmentation.

Ocular or Periocular Manifestations

Choroid: Posterior uveitis.
Eyebrows or Eyelids: Depigmentation of skin and lashes.
Iris: Depigmentation.
Retina: Atrophy; depigmentation.

PRECAUTIONS

In laboratory studies liver toxicity has developed in animals following the use of oral psoralens. However, there appears to be no evidence that such an effect occurs in humans receiving oral psoralens. Patients sometimes experience nausea after receiving oral methoxsalen; however, taking the drug after a glass of milk or a sandwich usually allays the sensation of nausea. Presently, there is some concern that long-term therapy with high-dose oral psoralens plus UVA therapy may result in ocular damage and skin cancers. It is advisable to have the patient undergo a baseline ophthalmologic examination before instituting oral psoralen therapy and have periodic subsequent examinations.

While on PUVA treatments, special protective glasses are recommended on the days the psoralen is taken. After a patient has used either topical or oral psoralens, the skin is also sensitive to ultraviolet light for at least 24 hours. Sunscreens or cover-ups should be used if the patient must be exposed to sunlight for longer periods of time than the therapeutic exposure period. Care should also be taken with topical psoralens, as they may cause intense dermatitis reactions with vesiculation and blistering.

COMMENTS

The etiology of vitiligo remains obscure. Among the various hypotheses that have been proposed to explain the pathogenesis of the disease, autoimmune mechanisms have been prominent. Recent research suggests that a nondermatomal vitiligo may be due to an autoimmune mechanism, whereas a dermatomally distributed vitiligo derives from a disturbance in the sympathetic nerves of the affected area.

References

Albert DM, Nordlund JJ, Lerner AB: Ocular abnormalities occurring with vitiligo. Ophthalmology 86:1145–1158, 1979.

Benmaman O, Sanchez SL: Treatment and camouflaging of pigmentary disorders. Clin Dermatol 6:50–61, 1988.

Cormane RH, et al: Phenylalanine and UV-A light for the treatment of vitiligo. Arch Dermatol Res 277:126–130, 1985.

Duke-Elder S (ed): System of Ophthalmology. St. Louis, CV Mosby, 1974, Vol XIII, pp 369–371.

Koga M: Vitiligo: A new classification and therapy. Br J Dermatol 97:255–261, 1977.

Lerner AB, Nordlund JJ: Vitiligo. What is it? Is it important? JAMA 239:1183–1187, 1978.

Lorincz AL: Disturbances of melanin pigmentation. In Moschella SL, Pillsbury DM, Hurley JJ Jr (eds): Dermatology. Philadelphia, WB Saunders, 1975, pp 1096–1128.

Lowe D: Pigmentary disturbances. In Conn HF (ed): Current Therapy. Philadelphia, WB Saunders, 1982, pp 673–677.

SECTION 11

CONNECTIVE TISSUE DISORDERS

JUVENILE RHEUMATOID ARTHRITIS
(JA, JRA, Juvenile Arthritis, Still's Disease)

JERRY C. JACOBS, M.D.,
and HAROLD F. SPALTER, M.D.
New York, New York

Juvenile rheumatoid arthritis has been the diagnostic label applied to all forms of persistent arthritis of childhood onset. During the past decade, it has become apparent that currently accepted diagnostic criteria identify a consortium of different disorders with different genetic susceptibility determinants, environmental offsets, pathology, prognoses, and clinical patterns. It has also become apparent that all forms of both "childhood" and "adult" arthritis may begin at any age.

The eyes are frequently affected in two different forms of childhood arthritis: pauciarticular arthritis and spondyloarthritis. Subacute or chronic iridocyclitis occurs primarily in association with pauciarticular arthritis (four or fewer affected joints). Girls are predominantly afflicted (9:1), and the median age of onset is 2 years of age. In 50 per cent of cases, arthritis is limited to the knee at the time of onset, and 74 per cent of cases are monarticular; 40 per cent of girls in this subset develop uveitis, and half of these patients have a positive test for antinuclear antibody (ANA). The eye inflammation is usually silent and only discovered by routine slitlamp screening examination, which should be performed every 3 months in this subset. In one series, 92 per cent of these patients possessed human leukocyte antigen (HLA)-DRw5. Those who develop iridocyclitis most frequently do so within the first year after onset of arthritis, but uveitis may first occur at any time and may recur many years later.

Acute iridocyclitis occurs primarily in patients with spondyloarthritis, a form of arthritis related pathologically and genetically to the prototypic disorders, ankylosing spondylitis and Reiter's syndrome. Most patients present with pauciarticular arthritis of the lower extremities. Boys are more frequently afflicted, and the median age of onset is 10 years of age. In one series, 8 per cent of children with this form of arthritis developed uveitis during childhood, but the lifetime risk is probably about 25 per cent. The ANA test is usually negative, but occasionally may be transiently positive at the onset of arthritis. Most patients possess HLA-B27, and a family history of similar arthritis and/or uveitis may frequently be established in these patients. Subacute or chronic iritis is less frequent in this subset, but does occur. Chronic blepharitis and conjunctivitis are also associated with spondyloarthritis.

Iridocyclitis is not known to occur in childhood-onset rheumatoid-factor positive adult rheumatoid arthritis and is rare in polyarticular and systemic-onset (Still's disease) forms of childhood arthritis. However, all forms of arthritis lack precise definition and tend to be confused with each other. Therefore, all children with arthritis require regular slitlamp examinations for detection of silent uveitis. In the past, 2 per cent of all children with arthritis lost all vision, and the risk of total blindness was much higher in the highly susceptible subsets.

THERAPY

Systemic. Aspirin and other nonsteroidal anti-inflammatory agents are the drugs of choice in all forms of childhood arthritis. "Slow-acting" agents, such as gold salts, penicillamine, and hydroxychloroquine, may be required by some patients. Immunosuppressive agents, such as azathioprine and methotrexate,[‡] are used in a few selected cases. All patients and their parents are taught a physical medicine regimen to maintain the functional range of motion of the affected joints.

Ocular. Unless the inflammation is so severe that vision is threatened, all patients are initially treated with mydriatics and topical steroid drops administered at frequent intervals. If vision is threatened or a prompt response is not obtained, 1 to 2 mg/kg of oral prednisone daily in divided doses may be used until the inflammation is completely controlled (usually a few weeks). The dosage should then be changed to an alternate-day regimen (2 to 5 mg/kg, with a daily maximum of 150 mg). Provided the inflammation remains controlled, the dose is gradually reduced with careful monitoring of the eyes.

Surgical. If bilateral complicated cataracts occur at any age and residual vision is unacceptable or if there is no vision in a single eye at an age where amblyopia ex anopsia may result, surgical removal of the cataract may be required. Experience suggests that the optimal surgical technique is phacoemulsification with preservation of the posterior capsule. To control inflammation completely, corticosteroid coverage should be provided beginning the day before surgery, with a sufficient daily dose provided on the day of surgery and throughout the postoperative period. Intraocular steroids are administered by subtenon injection* during the surgery and again, if necessary, during the postoperative period. As soon as the surgical result is assured, the steroids are changed to an alternate-day regimen as detailed earlier. In appropriate cases, such as when the lens is also dislocated or severe vitreitis is present, lensectomy with vitrectomy is an alternative procedure. Conventional surgical techniques for complicated cataracts have historically yielded extraordinarily poor results and should no longer be used in these children with chronic uveitis.

Secondary glaucoma must be controlled both before and after surgery; this can usually be accomplished with appropriate drug therapy, but standard surgical techniques may also be used if required. Successful restoration of vision following surgery for complicated cataract is dependent upon restoring vision to an eye that is not also blinded by inadequately treated glaucoma or amblyopia ex anopsia.

Band keratopathy may be treated with curettage and chelating agents, such as edetate disodium.*

Ocular or Periocular Manifestations

Anterior Chamber: Cells; protein flare.
Cornea: Keratitic precipitates.
Iris or Ciliary Body: Ciliary flush (rare); iris bombé; synechiae.
Other: Decreased visual acuity; glaucoma; ocular pain (rare); papillitis; photophobia; macular edema; vitreous cells.

PRECAUTIONS

Topical ocular steroids can induce cataract and glaucoma; systemic steroids can also cause these and many other adverse effects, including avascular necrosis of bone, but these risks are acceptable to most patients in an effort to prevent blindness. Aspirin toxicity may produce gastrointestinal, auditory, and metabolic disturbances and increases the risk of Reye's syndrome. Nonsteroidal anti-inflammatory agents are not known to increase the risk of Reye's syndrome, but otherwise have similar risks as aspirin and greater risks of renal complications. A high incidence of serious side effects, including changes in macular retinal pigment epithelium, has discouraged long-term use of hydroxychloroquine in the treatment of juvenile rheumatoid arthritis. Gold and penicillamine are high-risk agents of uncertain efficacy; azathioprine and methotrexate pose an even higher risk.

COMMENTS

Obsessive screening with early diagnosis and aggressive corticosteroid treatment of uveitis in arthritic children are capable of preventing visual disability in most children. Recognition of ANA, HLA-DRw5, HLA-B27, and pauciarticular disease as risk factors warranting even more frequent screening and vigilance has also improved the visual prognosis. For children whose vision is compromised as a result of complicated cataracts, newer surgical techniques and improved management have transformed what was an essentially hopeless situation into practically 100 per cent restoration of adequate vision. These newer surgical techniques, including phacoemulsification, lensectomy, and vitrectomy, are supported by dynamic corticosteroid control of postoperative inflammation and by careful attention to glaucoma and to the potential for amblyopia ex anopsia. These goals have been primarily achieved in large clinics specializing in the care of eye complications of arthritic children, but may now be extended to other settings where both pediatric rheumatologic support and informed ophthalmologic medical and surgical care are available.

References

Chylack LT Jr, Dueker DK, Pihlaja DJ: Ocular manifestations of juvenile rheumatoid arthritis: Pathology, fluorescein iris angiography, and patient care patterns. *In* Miller JJ III (ed): Juvenile Rheumatoid Arthritis. Littleton, MA, Publishing Sciences Group, 1979, pp 149–163.

Diamond JG, Kaplan HJ: Lensectomy and vitrectomy for complicated cataract secondary to uveitis. Arch Ophthalmol 96:1798–1804, 1978.

Jacobs JC: Pediatric Rheumatology for the Practitioner. New York, Springer-Verlag, 1982.

Jacobs JC, Berdon WE, Johnston AD: HLA-B27-associated spondyloarthritis and enthesopathy in childhood: Clinical, pathologic, and radiologic observations in 58 patients. J Pediatr 100:521–528, 1982.

Kanski JJ: Anterior uveitis in juvenile rheumatoid arthritis. Arch Ophthalmol 95:1794–1797, 1977.

Kanski JJ, Crick MDP: Lensectomy. Trans Ophthalmol Soc UK 97:52–57, 1977.

Kanski JJ: Care of children with anterior uveitis. Trans Ophthalmol Soc UK 101:387–390, 1981.

Kanski JJ, Shun-Shin GA: Systemic uveitis syndromes in childhood: An analysis of 340 cases. J Ophthalmol 91:1247–1252, 1984.

Petty RE: Current knowledge of the etiology and pathogenesis of chronic uveitis accompanying juvenile rheumatoid arthritis. Rheum Dis Clin North Am 13:19–36, 1987.

Praeger DL, et al: Kelman procedure in the treatment of complicated cataract of the uveitis of Still's disease. Trans Ophthalmol Soc UK 96:168–172, 1976.

Spalter HF: The visual prognosis in juvenile rheumatoid arthritis. Trans Am Ophthalmol Soc 73:554–570, 1975.

Suciu-Foca N, et al: HLA-DR5 in juvenile rheumatoid arthritis confined to few joints. Lancet 2:40, 1980.

POLYARTERITIS NODOSA
(Necrotizing Angiitis, PAN, Periarteritis Nodosa)

JOHN J. WEITER, M.D., Ph.D.,
and JOHN A. MILLS, M.D.

Boston, Massachusetts

Polyarteritis nodosa is a widespread inflammatory and necrotizing vasculitis that usually affects small- and medium-sized muscular arteries, although venous involvement may occur. The lesions are typically focal or segmental, are often in different stages of development, and have a predilection for branch points and bifurcations of vessels. The pathologic hallmark of the disease is acute necrotizing inflammation of the arterial media, with fibrinoid necrosis and extensive inflammatory cell infiltration of all vessel coats and surrounding tissue. Aneurysmal dilations and rupture may occur, and thrombosis and fibrosis may lead to occlusion of the lumen. Such vascular lesions may involve virtually every organ of the body, with characteristic involvement of renal and visceral arteries and sparing of the pulmonary circulation. The cause of polyarteritis is unknown. It is usually grouped with the so-called collagen diseases and may be mediated by deposition of immune complexes. Polyarteritis nodosa has been reported to occur in patients of all ages, although the usual age of onset is between 20 and 50 years. Males are affected more commonly in a ratio of 2.5 : 1. In a variant of this entity called cutaneous polyarteritis nodosa, the lesions are restricted to the small muscular arteries of the subcutaneous tissue. This localized disease spares visceral arteries and is therefore not a true systemic vasculitis syndrome. The relationship between this disorder and true periarteritis seems analogous to the relationship between discoid and systemic lupus erythematosus.

Clinical manifestations of polyarteritis nodosa are protean and variable, reflecting the widespread vascular involvement, the degree of ischemia, and the resulting necrosis. The clincal onset may be abrupt, with chills, fever, and tachycardia, or insidious, with low-grade fever, myalgia, arthralgia, anorexia, weight loss, and nonspecific weakness and fatigue. Hypertension occurs in 50 per cent of patients and renal involvement in 75 per cent. Mucous membrane lesions and a wide variety of cutaneous abnormalities develop, including purpura, petechiae, urticaria, subcutaneous nodules, and skin ulceration. Involvement of the gastrointestinal and both central and peripheral nervous systems is common. Ocular involvement may result as lesions in the cerebral vasculature affect the visual or oculomotor pathways. The retinal and choroidal vasculatures may be affected directly by local lesions or through secondary changes, resulting from nephrogenic hypertension. The external eye and anterior segment of the eye rarely may have inflammatory and ischemic lesions.

THERAPY

Systemic. The 5-year survival rate for untreated patients with polyarteritis nodosa is approximately 10 per cent. This high mortality justifies an aggressive therapeutic approach. The use of corticosteroids has improved the 5-year survival to approximately 50 per cent. Prednisone should be used at a level of 1 to 2 mg/kg and adjusted upward if necessary. Efficacy of therapy should be assessed on the basis of symptom control and degree of organ involvement while the erythrocyte sedimentation rate and white blood cell count are followed. The episodic course of periarteritis nodosa makes the effects of therapy difficult to follow. When the disease appears to be controlled, a slow, cautious, stepwise reduction of corticosteroid dosage may be undertaken at 1- to 2-week intervals. If long-term therapy is required, an alternate-day regimen may be attempted. Although a remission may occur during therapy with corticosteroids, these drugs frequently mask inflammatory activity while the disease progresses.

Cytotoxic agents are gaining greater acceptance in the therapy for polyarteritis nodosa. The combination of corticosteroids and immunosuppressive agents has resulted in an increased survival rate. The most commonly used immunosuppressive agents are azathioprine[‡] and cyclophosphamide.[‡] Cyclophosphamide has induced clinical remission in patients with severe necrotizing vasculitis that had been refractory to other therapeutic modalities. Oral administration of 2 mg/kg of cyclophosphamide daily should be started together with 1 to 2 mg/kg of prednisone daily. If symptoms are controlled after 2 weeks, the prednisone dosage is slowly tapered to an alternate-day regimen, and the cyclophosphamide dosage is adjusted to maintain a white blood cell count of 3000/cubic millimeter.

Ocular. Ocular treatment is generally symptomatic. Early systemic control of the disease with corticosteroids and immunosuppressive agents tends to lessen the ocular symptoms. Inflammation of the anterior segment should be treated with topical corticosteroids and mydriatics. Control of systemic hypertension decreases retinal vascular disease. Retrobulbar injection[*] of vasodilators may be tried for their antispasmodic effects, but they are often found to be ineffective.

Supportive. Management of complications consists largely of support in the event of organ failure or intervention in the event of hemorrhage or organ infarction. Systemic hypertension should be carefully controlled, since sustained hypertension will add further insult to kidneys already damaged by vasculitis or glomerulonephritis. Furthermore, systemic hypertension is a major contributor to late complications, such as stroke and myocardial infarction. Physical therapy may be employed to sustain muscular tone and arterial function in patients with musculoskeletal involvement, and splints are useful to prevent contractures. Analgesics, such as aspirin, are useful adjuncts for treating myalgias and arthralgias.

Ocular or Periocular Manifestations

Conjunctiva: Edema; hyperemia; subconjunctival hemorrhages; ulcer.
Cornea: Keratoconjunctivitis sicca; marginal ulcer; necrotizing sclerokeratitis.

Extraocular Muscles: Nystagmus; paralysis; tenonitis.

Eyelids: Edema; ptosis.

Globe: Proptosis or pseudotumor (rarely, in contradistinction to Wegener's granulomatosis).

Optic Nerve: Atrophy; disc edema.

Retina or Choroid: Central retinal artery occlusion; cotton-wool spots; edema; exudates; hemorrhages; hypertensive retinopathy; nonrhegmatogenous (exudative) retinal detachment; vasculitis of specific retinal and choroidal arteries.

Sclera: Necrotizing nodular scleritis; nodular episcleritis; sclero-uveitis.

Other: Anterior uveitis; Argyll Robertson pupil; cataracts; cortical blindness; hemianopsia.

PRECAUTIONS

Both of the therapeutic agents recommended earlier, corticosteroids and cytotoxic drugs, have significant adverse side effects of which the physician should be aware. The multitude of side effects related to corticosteroid therapy have been reviewed in detail; they include suppression of the hypothalamic-pituitary axis, cataracts, and osteonecrosis. These adverse effects are predictable and related directly to dosage and duration of therapy; dosage should therefore be tapered, when possible, to an alternate-day regimen, and the minimal efficacious dose should be determined.

Immediate and long-term complications have been reported with the use of cyclophosphamide. Cyclophosphamide directly suppresses the bone marrow, and this effect should be monitored through peripheral leukocyte counts. Other complications include lower urinary tract problems, such as hemorrhagic cystitis and bladder fibrosis. Finally, any patient undergoing immunosuppressive therapy should be carefully observed for signs of infection, particularly by such opportunistic organisms as cytomegalovirus, *Candida*, and *Toxoplasma gondii*.

COMMENTS

The treatment strategy described earlier is designed to modulate or suppress the immune mechanisms underlying the vasculitis. Other modalities less commonly employed to alter the host immune response are antilymphocyte serum and lymphoplasmapheresis. Plasmapheresis has been used in an attempt to remove immune complexes. This approach is based upon the yet unproven supposition that periarteritis nodosa is an immune complex disease.

Even with treatment, the prognosis is poor. Renal failure, ruptured aneurysms, strokes, and cardiovascular disease are the major causes of death. The cutaneous variant, cutaneous polyarteritis nodosa, runs a chronic course with a good long-term prognosis.

References

Axelrod L: Glucocorticoid therapy. Medicine 55:39–65, 1976.

Cupps TR, Fauci AS: The vasculitides. Major Probl Intern Med 21:1–211, 1981.

Diaz-Perez JL, Winkelmann RK: Cutaneous periarteritis nodosa. Arch Dermatol 110:407–414, 1974.

Frohnert PP, Sheps SG: Long-term follow-up study of periarteritis nodosa. Am J Med 43:8–14, 1967.

Leib ES, Restivo C, Paulus HE: Immunosuppressive and corticosteroid therapy of polyarteritis nodosa. Am J Med 67:941–947, 1979.

Schein PS, Winokur SH: Immunosuppressive and cytotoxic chemotherapy: Long-term complications. Ann Intern Med 82:84–95, 1975.

Steinberg AD et al: Cytotoxic drugs in treatment of nonmalignant diseases. Ann Intern Med 76:619–642, 1972.

PSEUDOXANTHOMA ELASTICUM
(Grönblad-Strandberg Syndrome, PXE)

DAVID S. HULL, M.D.

Augusta, Georgia

Pseudoxanthoma elasticum is an inherited connective tissue disorder characterized by redundant folds of soft, wrinkled, and lax skin typically located on the neck, lower abdomen, or perineum and in the flexures of the arms, popliteal fossae, axillary, and groin areas. It is transmitted as either an autosomal dominant or an autosomal recessive trait. It usually appears by age 30, although it may appear in childhood or in old age. Although it may affect the elastic tissue of the skin, eyes, or cardiovascular system, the primary defect appears to be premature degeneration and calcium deposition in the dermal elastic fibers. The xanthomatous eruptions are perfectly symmetric, small (1 to 3 mm in diameter), yellow nodules that have a plucked-chicken appearance. The skin is loose but not hyperelastic. Cardiovascular complications may accompany the disorder, and patients may exhibit hypertension, coronary insufficiency, arterial insufficiency in the extremities, dilation of the aorta, vascular aneurysms, and gastrointestinal or cerebral hemorrhages.

Similar changes occur in the elastic lamina of Bruch's membrane, resulting in the formation of angioid streaks in the fundi of approximately 85 per cent of patients. This form of the disease is known as Grönblad-Strandberg syndrome. It is complicated by disciform macular degeneration and loss of central vision as a result of macular hemorrhage. Angioid streaks usually occur bilaterally, develop in the second or third decades, and gradually increase over several years. They may not be visible ophthalmoscopically; however, they can be clearly seen on fluorescein angiography. The angioid streaks that occur in the fundus have been well described as resembling cracks in old oil paintings. They tend to radiate from the disc and lie deep to the retinal vessels. They are gray or brown, and there may be small white borders on either side of the stria. They are not connected with the retinal vessels.

Diffuse mottling or peau d'orange, often associated with widespread drusen-like spots, may be the earliest fundus changes in this disease. These disturbances may be present with or without angioid streaks.

THERAPY

Systemic. Treatment is conservative and symptomatic. Hypertension may occur frequently in patients with pseudoxanthoma elasticum and may require treatment. Patients with ischemic symptoms may require arteriography. The cosmetic appearance of the skin may be improved by plastic surgery.
Ocular. Patients with angioid streaks of the fundus and neovascular membranes should be considered for fluorescein angiography. Laser photocoagulation can be employed to abolish or limit choroidal neovascularization at angioid streaks and reduce the occurrence or extent of subretinal hemorrhage or edema.
Counseling. Genetic counseling is especially important in view of the newly detected autosomal dominant variants of pseudoxanthoma elasticum where the risk of transmission is increased to 50 per cent.

Ocular or Periocular Manifestations

Choroid or Retina: Angioid streaks; detachment; macular hemorrhages; mottling; prominent choroidal vessels; scarring; vascular sclerosis.
Cornea: Descemet's wrinkles; keratoconus; opacity.
Lens: Cataracts; subluxation.
Other: Blue scleral coloration; exophthalmos (orbital hematoma); optic atrophy; paralysis of extraocular muscles (secondary to vascular lesions of central nervous system); visual field defects; visual loss; vitreal hemorrhages.

PRECAUTIONS

Patients with pseudoxanthoma elasticum may be at increased risk during anesthesia. Coronary artery insufficiency may predispose the patient to arrhythmias and sudden death. Accurate blood pressure readings and electrocardiogram monitoring are essential. A nasogastric tube should be avoided because of the tendency for gastric bleeding. Since even minor trauma can cause retinal hemorrhage, contact sports should be avoided.

COMMENTS

The underlying defect in pseudoxanthoma elasticum is the abnormal presence of stainable polyanion in the dermal elastic fibers. These polyanions play a role in the subsequent calcification of the affected fibers. The calcium content of skin lesions increases with the severity of the lesions, and the lesions do not occur without deposited calcium. The changes of Bruch's membrane are caused by tears, which later result in angioid streaks. These may subsequently be followed by pigment epithelial degeneration and fibrovascular tissue proliferation. Focal retinal degeneration and visual loss seem more related to repeated hemorrhages in the region of reaction to angioid streaks than to the angioid streaks themselves. The retinal vessels appear normal, and hemorrhages originate from choroidal vessels or their offshoots for reasons that are not yet understood.

References

Archer DB, Logan WC: Angioid streaks. In Krill AE (ed): Hereditary Retinal and Choroidal Diseases. Hagerstown, MD, Harper & Row, Vol II, 1977, pp 851–909.
Eddy DD, Farber EM: Pseudoxanthoma elasticum. Internal manifestations: A report of cases and a statistical review of the literature. Arch Dermatol 86:729–740, 1962.
Francois J, et al: Neovascularization after argon laser photocoagulation of macular lesions. Am J Ophthalmol 79:206–210, 1975.
Hull DS, Aaberg TM: Fluorescein study of a family with angioid streaks and pseudoxanthoma elasticum. Br J Ophthalmol 58:738–745, 1974.
Kadri W, Rosen E, Harcourt B: Intraretinal changes in the Grönblad-Strandberg syndrome. Br J Ophthalmol 57:588–592, 1973.
Kaplan EN, Henjyoji EY: Pseudoxanthoma elasticum: A dermal elastosis with surgical implications. Plast Reconstr Surg 58:595–600, 1976.
Krechel SLW, Ramirez-Inawat RC, Fabian LW: Anesthetic considerations in pseudoxanthoma elasticum. Anesth Analg 60:344–347, 1981.
Martinez-Hernandez A, Huffer WE: Pseudoxanthoma elasticum: Dermal polyanions and the mineralization of elastic fibers. Lab Invest 31:181–186, 1974.
Meislik J, et al: Laser treatment in maculopathy of pseudoxanthoma elasticum. Can J Ophthalmol 13:210–212, 1978.
Pope FM: Autosomal dominant pseudoxanthoma elasticum. J Med Genet 11:152–157, 1974.
Pope FM: Two types of autosomal recessive pseudoxanthoma elasticum. Arch Dermatol 110:209–212, 1974.

RELAPSING POLYCHONDRITIS

PETER G. WATSON, M.A., M.B., B.Chir., F.R.C.S., D.O.
Cambridge, England

EAMON P. O'DONOGHUE, M.B., B.Ch., B.A.O., F.R.C.S. (Ed.)
London, England

Relapsing polychondritis causes inflammation of cartilaginous structures throughout the body, but most commonly affects the nasal, tracheal and auricular cartilage. The characteristic features of the disease are destruction of cartilage

202 / RELAPSING POLYCHONDRITIS

and eventual replacement with connective tissue. Migratory oligo- or polyarthritis is frequently the earliest sign and is generally progressive. The chondritis typically is of sudden onset and very painful. If the costal, tracheal, and laryngeal cartilage also become involved, the trachea may collapse and death may result from acute bronchial obstruction.

Diagnostic criteria were described by McAdam in 1976 and consist of three or more of the following: 1, recurrent chondritis of both auricles; 2, nonerosive inflammatory polyarthritis; 3, chondritis of nasal cartilage; 4, inflammation of ocular structures; 5, laryngotracheal chondritis; or 6, Vestibular or cochlear inflammation. This was modified further by Damiani in 1979 to include histopathologic evidence for the disease. The 5 and 10 year survival rates are 74 percent and 55 percent respectively, with death due mainly to infection, vasculitis and malignancy. Anemia at diagnosis is a poor prognostic indicator at any age, as well as saddle nose deformity and systemic vasculitis in patients under 51 years. Myocardial, aortic and cardiac valvular involvement in addition to renal and liver dysfunction have also been observed. Ocular involvement occurs in 50 to 65 per cent of patients. The most frequent ocular signs are episcleritis and scleritis and less commonly keratoconjunctivitis sicca, iritis, retinopathy, and cataract.

THERAPY

Systemic. This is a notoriously difficult disease to treat. Treatment is by suppression of the inflammation in the sclera, cartilage, and connective tissue by corticosteroids that are also especially effective against laryngotracheobronchial and external ear manifestations. Prednisone is usually started in a dosage of 60 mg daily, or an equivalent dose of another corticosteroid preparation may be used. In exceptionally severe acute disease, it is sometimes necessary to suppress the inflammation by the use of 500 mg of methylprednisolone, given intravenously in an infusion over a period of at least 1 hour. This may need to be repeated after 2 days. (Perioperative pulsed intravenous methylprednisolone should also be considered when planning surgery to vulnerable tissues.) If this fails to control the condition or there is evidence of raised circulating immune complexes, 500 mg of cyclophosphamide‡ given intravenously will probably induce a remission of the disease. A second dose may need to be given intravenously after a week, and all therapy may need to be continued. Patients on cyclophosphamide must be well hydrated so that if the drug is given by intravenous infusion it should be followed for 24 hours with intravenous fluids. Most patients can be maintained on low doses of oral steroid alone, although some will require addition of the immunosuppressive drugs, such as cyclophosphamide‡ or azathioprine.‡

Ocular. Topical ophthalmic corticosteroids are sometimes helpful for recurrent ocular problems. Prednisolone eyedrops or ointment may be applied on an hourly basis for acute episodes and then tapered. One per cent atropine applied one to three times daily may be of value in controlling the uveitis.

Supportive. Any sign of respiratory distress with tracheal inflammation should be observed closely and treated early by intubation. If perichondrial inflammatory masses narrow the airway, surgical removal of the masses and reconstruction of the airway may be indicated.

Since collapse of the nasal cartilage or development of nasal tip deformity usually worsens after surgery, cosmetic surgery is not recommended. In extreme cases of cardiac vascular involvement, valvular replacement with prosthetic valves or aortic aneurysm resection may become necessary symptomatic treatment.

Ocular or Periocular Manifestations

Conjunctiva: Chemosis; conjunctivitis; infiltration.
Cornea: Edema; keratoconjunctivitis sicca; opacity; perforation; stromal infiltration; thinning; ulcer.
Globe: Exophthalmos; phthisis bulbi; proptosis.
Optic Nerve: Edema; hemorrhages; optic neuritis; papilledema.
Retina: Exudative detachment; retinal artery thrombosis; striae.
Sclera: Blue coloration; episcleritis; scleritis; thinning.
Vitreous: Opacity; syneresis.
Other: Cataracts; decreased visual acuity; diplopia; nystagmus; ocular pain; paresis of third or sixth nerve; photophobia; scotoma; secondary glaucoma; uveitis; dacryocystitis; lid edema, tarsitis.

PRECAUTIONS

Relapsing polychondritis should be considered not only in patients presenting with scleral disease but also in those who develop diffuse joint disease. When the diagnosis has been established, corticosteroid therapy must be started as early as possible. However, it must be remembered that corticosteroids neither stop the disease progression in the more aggressive cases nor the development of potential lethal organ system involvement. There is some evidence that cyclophosphamide may induce a prolonged remission. The use of subconjunctival corticosteroids should be avoided, as diseased sclera may be lost at the site of the injection.

Though there are no specific serological markers for relapsing polychondritis, the anticytoplasmic autoantibody, which is highly specific for Wegeners granulomatosis, will help discriminate these two conditions in equivocal cases.

Careful radiological evaluation of major airways and joints are of paramount importance for diagnostic, prognostic and management purposes. Computed tomography is useful in assessing extent of disease.

The major airways are affected in over 50 percent of cases. Hughes et al (1973) estimated that

44 percent of deaths in relapsing polychondritis related to respiratory involvement; more recently, however, Michet et al (1986) has reported that fatality rate due to respiratory problems is closer to 10 per cent.

If elective surgical procedures are considered, they should be undertaken only during periods of remission and with immunosuppression. These patients tolerate anesthesia poorly, especially if tracheobronchial involvement is present and active and expert anesthesia care is required.

Comments

Although relapsing polychondritis is more commonly a chronic, low-grade, episodic disease, it may be a fulminant disease with a rapid downhill course. The critical organ system involved in relapsing polychondritis is the respiratory tract. However, death from ruptured abdominal aneurysms or progressive heart failure secondary to aortic regurgitation has also occurred. Because of the variation in severity and the episodic nature of the disease, careful prolonged follow-up and individualized therapy are the keys to optimal treatment. Aggressive therapy may be necessary during an acute attack.

References

Arkin CR, Masi AT: Relapsing polychondritis: Review of current status and case report. Sem Arthritis Rheum 5:41–62, 1975.
Booth A, Dieppe PA, Goddard PL, Watt I: The radiological manifestations of relapsing polychondritis. Clin Radiol 40:147–149, 1989.
Damian JM, Levine HL: Relapsing polychondritis—Report of ten cases. Laryngoscope 89:929–944, 1979.
Hayward AW, Al-Shaikh B, Relapsing polychondritis and the anaesthetist. Anaesthesia, 43:573–577, 1988.
Isaak BL, Liesgang TJ, Michet CJ: Ocular and systemic findings in relapsing polychondritis. Ophthalmology 93:681–689, 1986.
McAdam LP, et al: Relapsing polychondritis: Prospective study of 23 patients and a review of the literature. Medicine 55:193–215, 1976.
McKay DAR, Watson PG, Lyne AJ: Relapsing polychondritis and eye disease. Br J Ophthalmol 58:600–605, 1974.
Mendelson DS, et al: Relapsing polychondritis studied by computerized tomography, Radiology, 157:489–490, 1985.
Michet CJ, et al: Relapsing polychondritis: Survival and predictive role of early disease manifestations. Ann Intern Med 104:74–78, 1986.
Specks U, et al: Anticytoplasmic autoantibodies in diagnosis and follow-up of Wegeners granulomatosis. Mayo Clin Proc 64:28–36, 1989.

RHEUMATOID ARTHRITIS
JAMES T. ROSENBAUM, M.D.
Portland, Oregon

Rheumatoid arthritis is a systemic, immune-mediated disease that primarily affects females with an onset during middle age. Approximately 80 per cent of patients with rheumatoid arthritis have a positive test for rheumatoid factor, which indicates an IgM type immunoglobulin that binds to an IgG. In general, the arthritis characteristic of rheumatoid arthritis is symmetric. Joints most likely to be affected include the proximal interphalangeal joints of the hands and feet, the metacarpal-phalangeal joints, the metatarsal-phalangeal joints, wrists, ankles, knees, hips, shoulders, and temporomandibular joints. The extra-articular manifestations of rheumatoid arthritis include subcutaneous nodules, vasculitis, pleuropericarditis, leukopenia and anemia as in Felty's syndrome, and interstitial lung disease. The arthritis characteristic of rheumatoid arthritis is generally clinically and radiographically distinct from such other causes of arthritis as systemic-onset juvenile rheumatoid arthritis, ankylosing spondylitis, Reiter's syndrome, and gout.

Keratoconjunctivitis sicca is an extremely common complication of rheumatoid arthritis. In autopsy studies, nearly all patients with rheumatoid arthritis have a lymphocytic infiltration of salivary glands, as is characteristic of Sjögren's syndrome. Patients with rheumatoid arthritis frequently have abnormal Schirmer's tests, abnormal rose bengal staining of the conjunctiva, and complaints related to ocular dryness. Treatment of rheumatoid arthritis does not generally alter keratoconjunctivitis. Symptomatic therapy for Sjögren's syndrome secondary to rheumatoid arthritis should therefore not differ from treatment for Sjögren's syndrome that is primary, i.e., unassociated with another connective tissue syndrome.

Other ocular manifestations of rheumatoid arthritis include scleritis, episcleritis, peripheral corneal infiltrates (Wesseley rings), and marginal corneal thinning (corneal melts). In rheumatoid arthritis, rarely a tendonitis of the sheath of the superior oblique muscle can impair the function of that muscle, resulting in Brown's syndrome. Complications from anterior scleritis include glaucoma and iritis. Although posterior scleritis is a less frequent manifestation of rheumatoid arthritis, it does occur and may be associated with such complications as retinal detachment and disc edema. In contrast to ankylosing spondylitis and some subsets of juvenile rheumatoid arthritis, iritis is not a manifestation of rheumatoid arthritis, unless it occurs secondarily to scleritis or vasculitis.

Scleritis develops most commonly in patients with rheumatoid arthritis who have other extra-articular manifestations of the disease, such as vasculitis and nodules. These patients ordinarily have strongly positive tests for rheumatoid factor. Rheumatoid arthritis is the most common systemic disease associated with scleritis. A painful, necrotizing scleritis should be distinguished from the more indolent condition, scleromalacia perforans. Approximately 50 per cent of all patients with scleromalacia perforans have rheumatoid arthritis, usually in association with subcutaneous nodules. The therapy for either a scleritis or a corneal melt in the setting of rheumatoid arthritis is optimized if the underlying joint disease is well controlled.

THERAPY

Systemic. The therapy for rheumatoid arthritis includes nonsteroidal anti-inflammatory drugs, more potent medications that are generally considered to be disease-modifying agents, and adjunctive measures, such as physical therapy, rest, and joint protection. The nonsteroidal anti-inflammatory drugs include aspirin, indomethacin, ibuprofen, phenylbutazone, naproxen, piroxicam, and tolmetin, among others. These medications work in part by inhibiting the synthesis of prostaglandins. If tolerated, one of these agents should always be included in the therapy for scleritis. Most published reports on scleritis discuss experience with either 25 to 50 mg of indomethacin administered orally three to four times daily or 100 mg of phenylbutazone administered orally three to four times daily. The author's preference is to begin with indomethacin and to consider phenylbutazone if an adequate therapeutic response is not achieved in 2 weeks.

Disease-modifying drugs for rheumatoid arthritis include antimalarials, injectable and oral gold salts, penicillamine, and immunosuppressants, including methotrexate,[‡] azathioprine, and cyclophosphamide.[‡] The antimalarials (200 mg of oral hydroxychloroquine two times daily or 250 mg of oral chloroquine once daily) are the least toxic disease-modifying agents. Unfortunately, only about 40 per cent of patients respond to this class of medication, and the onset of benefit is frequently as long as 12 weeks after initiating therapy.

Intramuscular gold injection is the first choice of many rheumatologists when selecting a disease-modifying drug. Either aurothioglucose or gold sodium thiomalate is given by injection as frequently as every week up to a dose of 50 mg. After a total dose of 1 gm, the frequency of injections is generally reduced. The complete blood count and urinalysis must be monitored frequently while either of these drugs is given. About 70 per cent of patients with rheumatoid arthritis will have sustained improvement from gold injections. The onset of benefit may be delayed as long as 3 months after the initiation of treatment. Gold may also be taken orally as auranofin, usually at a dose of 3 mg two times daily. While efficacious, most rheumatologists do not consider oral gold to be as potent as intramuscular gold. The mechanism of action of the orally administered drug may differ from that of the intramuscular drug.

Penicillamine is an alternative to intramuscular gold as a disease-modifying drug. Penicillamine is given orally at daily doses as high as 0.75 to 1.5 gm. The drug is usually begun at a daily dose of 125 mg, and the dosage is increased by 125 mg/day every 2 weeks. As with gold, the complete blood count and urinalysis must be monitored carefully, and 3 months or more may be required before therapeutic benefit is achieved. Toxicity may include loss of taste, thrombocytopenia, nephrotic syndrome, and a variety of presumably immune-mediated side effects.

Sulfasalazine[‡] (2 to 3 gm daily in divided doses) appears to be effective for rheumatoid arthritis, especially if the disease is of recent onset. Its role in severe disease or in the arrest of the progression of erosive bone changes has not been established.

Immunosuppressant drugs are also effective for rheumatoid arthritis. Azathioprine at an oral dose of 1 to 2 mg/kg daily has been approved by the Food and Drug Administration for rheumatoid arthritis. Oral or intramuscular methotrexate,[‡] usually at a dose from 5 to 15 mg weekly, has become extremely popular as a treatment for rheumatoid arthritis. Its unique virtues include a low likelihood of leukopenia at the recommended dose (if the baseline renal function is normal) and a rapid onset of action, such that patients generally benefit within 2 to 3 weeks after initiating therapy. Although methotrexate is an excellent drug for the articular manifestations of rheumatoid arthritis, its role in treating rheumatoid nodules or vasculitis is less established. Since scleritis and corneal melts tend to correlate with these aspects of rheumatoid disease, the role of methotrexate for ocular complications of rheumatoid arthritis has not been established. Cyclophosphamide[‡] (usually 1 to 2 mg/kg daily) is one of the most potent cytotoxic drugs available. It is an excellent choice for a complication of rheumatoid arthritis, such as a corneal melt, if other less toxic modalities of therapy have failed.

Corticosteroids, either orally or injected locally, can provide prompt, but transient, improvement in rheumatoid arthritis. In general, a corticosteroid dose greater than what is comparable to 10 mg of prednisone should be used only as a temporary measure in rheumatoid arthritis. An acute ocular complication, such as a scleritis or a corneal melt, might be an indication for a limited course of oral corticosteroids. The long-term safety of prednisone at a daily dose of less than 10 mg is still debated.

The role of cyclosporine,[‡] drug combinations, pulse methylprednisolone, total lymphoid irradiation, and lymphoplasmapheresis is less well established in rheumatoid disease. Recent reports suggest a role for oral cyclosporine in the treatment of a corneal melt.

Ocular or Periocular Manifestations

Cornea: Keratoconjunctivitis sicca; marginal corneal thinning or keratolysis; peripheral corneal infiltrates.

Extraocular: Tendonitis affecting the superior oblique muscle sheath.

Sclera: Anterior or posterior scleritis; episcleritis; scleromalacia perforans.

Other: Complications of scleritis including iritis, glaucoma, exudative choroiditis, disc edema. Complications from medications including chrysiasis from gold; retinal pigment changes or corneal opacities from antimalarials; blurry vision from nonsteroidal antiinflammatory drugs; posterior subcapsular cataracts and glaucoma from corticosteroids.

PRECAUTIONS

Potential toxicities from nonsteroidal anti-inflammatory drugs include gastrointestinal bleeding, such central nervous system effects as mood swings or headache, reduction in glomerular filtration rate and fluid retention, and reduced platelet function. Reversible blurring of vision can also occur with nonsteroidal anti-inflammatory drugs. Optic neuritis may be a rare complication from this class of medications. Phenylbutazone has rarely been associated with a fatal aplastic anemia.

Retinal toxicity should be monitored closely on antimalarial therapy, although it is rare if the recommended doses are not exceeded. Reversible corneal deposits can also induce visual halos in patients receiving antimalarial therapy.

Potential toxicities of gold salts include anemia, leukopenia, thrombocytopenia, rash, stomatitis, flushing, and renal disease. The deposition of gold in the cornea or chrysiasis occurs in 75 percent of patients who receive a cumulative intramuscular dose greater than 1.5 gm; however, this accumulation is rarely clinically significant.

The long-term use of corticosteroids may be associated with numerous toxicities. Some of these adverse effects, such as osteopenia and a reduced response to infection, are especially troublesome in patients with rheumatoid arthritis.

COMMENTS

Rheumatoid arthritis should be distinguished from other causes of joint inflammation such as osteoarthritis and Reiter's syndrome. Most patients with rheumatoid arthritis have positive tests for rheumatoid factor and a polyarticular, symmetric arthritis. Only a minority of patients with juvenile rheumatoid arthritis have a disease which resembles that seen in adults.

Keratoconjunctivitis is a frequent manifestation of rheumatoid arthritis. Scleritis affects only a small percentage of patients with rheumatoid arthritis, but rheumatoid arthritis is the systemic disease most commonly associated with scleritis. Patients with scleritis often have other extraarticular manifestations of rheumatoid disease. Optimal treatment for scleritis associated with rheumatoid arthritis includes therapy for the systemic disease, but therapy of the arthritis does not alter ocular dryness.

Many of the medications used to treat rheumatoid arthritis have potential ocular toxicities.

References

Brown SI, Grayson M: Marginal furrows: A characteristic corneal lesion of rheumatoid arthritis. Arch Ophthalmol 79:563–567, 1968.
Foster CS, Forstot SL, Wilson LA: Mortality rate in rheumatoid arthritis patients developing necrotizing scleritis or peripheral ulcerative keratitis. Effects of systemic immunosuppression. Ophthalmology 91:1253–1262, 1984.
Jayson MIV, Jones DEP: Scleritis and rheumatoid arthritis. Ann Rheum Dis 30:343–347, 1971.
Lyne AJ, Pitkeathley DA: Episcleritis and scleritis. Association with connective tissue disease. Arch Ophthalmol 80:171–176, 1968.
McGavin DD, et al: Episcleritis and scleritis: A study of their clinical manifestations and association with rheumatoid arthritis. Br J Ophthalmol 60:192–226, 1976.
Watson PG, Hayreh SS: Scleritis and episcleritis. Br J Ophthalmol 60:163–191, 1976.

SJÖGREN'S SYNDROME
(Gougerot-Sjögren's Syndrome)
MICHAEL A. LEMP, M.D.
Washington, District of Columbia

Sjögren's syndrome is an autoimmunogenic disease characterized by the triad of dry eyes (keratoconjunctivitis sicca), dry mouth (xerostomia), and a connective tissue disease. The majority of patients presenting with keratoconjunctivitis sicca do not have overt evidence of systemic disease. However, those patients with collagen vascular disorders, particularly rheumatoid arthritis, have an unusually high incidence of keratoconjunctivitis sicca. There is chronic lymphocytic infiltration of the main and accessory lacrimal glands in this disorder, and the evidence supporting an autoimmune pathogenesis is strong. Sjögren's syndrome has been associated with rheumatoid arthritis, lupus erythematosus, Wegener's granulomatosis, lymphoproliferative diseases, paraproteinemias, and even drug reactions.

Sjögren's syndrome has been associated with a significantly higher incidence of the HLA-B8 antigen, and it is thought that this antigen is genetically linked to immune response genes that predispose the individual to autoimmune phenomena. Other diseases associated with Sjögren's syndrome include scleroderma, polymyositis, Hashimoto's thyroiditis, panarteritis, and interstitial pulmonary fibrosis.

The onset of this condition is gradual. In patients presenting with signs and symptoms of keratoconjunctivitis sicca, questioning might reveal the presence of dry mouth, arthritic complaints, and/or other symptoms.

THERAPY

Systemic. Attention to inflammatory diseases of an autoimmune nature accompanying Sjögren's syndrome is of paramount importance. Systemic corticosteroids play a major role in the management of many of these conditions. Systemic antimetabolite therapy is also useful and occasionally lifesaving in the management of these conditions.

Ocular. The use of artificial tear supplements remains the mainstay in the treatment of keratoconjunctivitis sicca (see page 206). The frequent instillation of artificial tears of low viscosity with

206 / SJÖGREN'S SYNDROME

an adsorptive polymer will manage most cases. The use of nightly ointments can also be quite useful. Sustained-release polymeric rods of hydroxypropyl cellulose that dissolve over a 6- to 12-hour period can be very useful in most severe cases. In the most severe cases, the use of moist chambers or punctal occlusion or both can be quite helpful.

In a subgroup of patients with keratoconjunctivitis sicca, the irritative symptoms are secondary to a marked increase in viscosity of the ocular mucin. The use of a 10 or 20 per cent solution of acetylcysteine* to decrease the viscosity of tears is very useful.

Soft bandage contact lenses have a significant place in the treatment of filamentary keratitis and severe cases of sicca. They must, however, be used in conjunction with artificial tears, and they present a very real danger of infection. The use of prophylactic antibiotics does not entirely remove the danger of infection. The use of bandage lenses should be limited to those cases that cannot be managed adequately otherwise.

Ocular or Periocular Manifestations

Conjunctiva: Chemosis; hyperemia; lusterless appearance.
Cornea: Mucous plaques; perforation; superficial punctate erosions; thinning; ulcer.
Eyelids: Blepharitis; chalazion; hordeolum; meibomianitis.
Lacrimal System: Decreased tear film stability (rapid break-up time); increased debris in the tear film; increased tear film viscosity.

PRECAUTIONS

Patients with Sjögren's syndrome have decreased ocular surface defense mechanisms associated with keratoconjunctivitis sicca, thereby making them more prone to infections. Moreover, because of the autoimmune nature of their disease, they are more likely to sustain sterile necrotic ulcerations secondary to vasculitis. This combination of susceptibilities makes marginal corneal ulceration, and even perforation, a possibility. Corticosteroids therefore should be used with great care in the management of these conditions. The management of the systemic manifestations of Sjögren's syndrome should be coordinated with an internist because of the frequent monitoring necessary in anticipation of the side effects of drug therapy.

COMMENTS

One point should be emphasized. The majority of people presenting with keratoconjunctivitis sicca do not have and will not develop discernible systemic disease. Those people, however, who do have evidence of systemic disease conforming to the criteria for Sjögren's syndrome can be reassured that the majority of patients can be successfully managed throughout life without the loss of vision.

References

Ericson S, Sundmark E: Studies on the sicca syndrome in patients with rheumatoid arthritis. Acta Rheum Scand 16:60–80, 1970.
Gudas PP Jr, et al: Corneal perforations in Sjögren's syndrome. Arch Ophthalmol 90:470–472, 1973.
Holly FJ, Lemp MA: Tear physiology and dry eyes. Surv Ophthalmol 22:69–87, 1977.
Lemp MA: Dry eye. In Spaeth GL, Katz LJ, Parker KW (eds): Current Therapy in Ophthalmic Surgery. Toronto, B.C. Decker Inc., 1989, pp 96–99.
Tabbara KF, et al: Sjögren's syndrome. Trans Am Acad Ophthalmol Otolaryngol 77:820–821, 1973.
Tuberville AW, Frederick WR, Wood TO: Punctal occlusion in tear deficiency syndromes. Ophthalmology 89:1170–1172, 1982.

SYSTEMIC LUPUS ERYTHEMATOSUS
JAMES T. ROSENBAUM, M.D.
Portland, Oregon

Systemic lupus erythematosus (SLE) is an immunologically mediated disease of uncertain etiology that has the potential to affect virtually any organ system. The American College of Rheumatology has suggested 11 diagnostic criteria for SLE. Patients are considered to have lupus if they meet four of the following criteria and have no alternate diagnostic explanation for the abnormalities: 1) malar rash; 2) discoid rash; 3) photosensitive rash; 4) oral ulcers; 5) nonerosive arthritis in two or more joints; 6) pleuritis or pericarditis; 7) glomerulonephritis or proteinuria; 8) seizures or psychosis; 9) hemolytic anemia, leukopenia, lymphopenia, or thrombocytopenia; 10) immunologic laboratory abnormality, such as antibodies to double-stranded DNA or the SM antigen, or a false-positive serologic test for syphilis; and 11) a positive antinuclear antibody test that is not caused by a medication. SLE is much more common in females than males. The prognosis depends largely on the organ system involved.

Keratoconjunctivitis sicca is the most common ocular manifestation of SLE. Cotton-wool spots are seen in as many as 28 per cent of patients with SLE. Some authorities believe that the presence of cotton-wool spots correlates with the likelihood of central nervous system disease. Other potential ocular manifestations of SLE include conjunctivitis, retinal vasculitis or retinal vascular occlusion, optic neuritis, scleritis, episcleritis, marginal corneal ulcer, eyelid rash, central nervous system disease affecting vision or extraocular muscles, and iritis. Papilledema may be present in association with pseudotumor cerebri.

As many as 50 to 60 per cent of patients with SLE have antibodies to a phospholipid known as cardiolipin. These antibodies may prolong the partial thromboplastin time. Because of this laboratory property, antibodies to cardiolipin are sometimes referred to as the lupus anticoagulant, although they are rarely associated with clinical bleeding. In fact, paradoxically, antiphospholipid antibodies are frequently associated with thrombosis. Antibodies to phospholipid may be responsible for false-positive serologic tests for syphilis. Antibodies to cardiolipin may be present without any manifestation of either systemic lupus or other autoimmune disease.

Antibodies to cardiolipin are strongly associated with thrombosis, including deep venous thrombosis, pulmonary embolism, nonbacterial thrombotic endocarditis, and central nervous system infarction. These antibodies may be causally related to spontaneous abortion. Antibodies to cardiolipin have been detected in association with an occlusive retinal vasculitis.

THERAPY

The treatment for SLE depends largely on the organ system that is involved and the severity of that involvement.

Systemic. Arthritis and pleuropericarditis are generally improved by nonsteroidal anti-inflammatory drugs, such as aspirin or indomethacin (75 to 200 mg daily). Antimalarials, including hydroxychloroquine[‡] (200 mg twice daily) and chloroquine[‡] (250 mg once daily), are particularly effective for discoid rash and the serositis. Anticoagulation may be indicated for thrombosis secondary to antiphospholipid antibodies.

Immunosuppressive therapy is indicated for SLE when the disease involves a critical organ, such as the kidney. Oral corticosteroids are generally the drug of first choice. The dosage depends on the activity of the disease. An initial dose comparable to 60 mg of prednisone is appropriate for active nephritis. A cytotoxic drug, such as azathioprine or cyclophosphamide,[‡] may be added if the corticosteroid alone is inadequate. Either of these cytotoxic drugs is generally administered at a daily dose of 1 to 2 mg/kg. The dose is adjusted based on toxicity, especially leukopenia. A monthly intravenous bolus of cyclophosphamide appears to be highly effective and perhaps safer than a daily oral regimen. Intravenous cyclophosphamide is generally begun at 500 mg/square meter. The dose may be increased, depending largely on hematologic toxicity. Pulse therapy with intravenous methylprednisolone, plasmapheresis, and total lymphoid irradiation are additional forms of immunosuppression that have been tried when more conventional therapy is not efficacious.

The section on rheumatoid arthritis (see page 203) contains additional discussion of therapy with nonsteroidal anti-inflammatory drugs, antimalarials, and cytotoxics.

Ocular. The treatment for sicca is described in the section of Sjögren's syndrome (see page 205). No form of immunosuppressive therapy has been found to increase tear formation.

Topical. Dermatologic manifestations of lupus are usually treated by topical corticosteroid preparations.

Ocular or Periocular Manifestations

Conjunctiva: Conjunctivitis.
Cornea: Keratoconjunctivitis sicca; peripheral corneal infiltrates; marginal corneal ulcer or keratolysis.
Eyelids: Erythematous, hyperkeratotic rash; telangiectasia.
Retina: Cotton wool spots or cytoid bodies; retinal vasculitis; retinal vasoocculusive disease including central or branch retinal artery or vein occlusions; secondary hypertensive retinopathy.
Optic nerve: Optic neuritis; ischemia; optic atrophy; papilledema; pseudotumor cerebri.
Sclera: Scleritis; episcleritis.
Other: Iritis; changes secondary to central nervous system infarction including cranial nerve palsies, homonymous hemianopsia, nystagmus, and intranuclear ophthalmoplegia.

PRECAUTIONS

The section on uveitis (see page 47) contains a more complete discussion of the adverse effects of corticosteroids.

COMMENTS

Systemic lupus erythematosus is a multisystem disease that may involve the eye. Although antinuclear antibodies are characteristic of this disease, a positive test for antinuclear antibodies does not establish a diagnosis in the absence of clinical findings.

The two most common ocular manifestations of systemic lupus are dry eyes and cotton wool spots.

Patients with lupus who have retinal ischemic events have a greater likelihood to have central nervous system disease. The lupus anticoagulant or antiphospholipid antibodies such as those to cardiolipin may be causally related to some instances of retinal vascular occlusion. The treatment for retinal vasculitis may differ from the treatment for anticardiolipin-mediated retinal occlusive disease.

References

Austin HA, et al: Therapy of lupus nephritis. Controlled trial of prednisone and cytotoxic drugs. N Engl J Med 314:614–619, 1986.
Boey ML, et al: Thrombosis in systemic lupus erythematosus: Striking association with the presence of circulating lupus anticoagulant. Br Med J 287:1021–1023, 1983.
Gold DM, Morris DA, Henkind P: Ocular findings in systemic lupus erythematosus. Br J Ophthalmol 56:800–804, 1972.
Jabs DA, et al: Severe retinal vaso-occlusive disease in systemic lupus erythematosus. Arch Ophthalmol 104:558–563, 1986.
Levine SR, et al: Visual symptoms associated with the presence of a lupus anticoagulant. Ophthalmology 95:686–692, 1988.
Tan EM, et al: The 1982 revised criteria for the classification of systemic lupus erythematosus (SLE). Arthritis Rheum 25:1271–1277, 1982.

SYSTEMIC SCLEROSIS
(Scleroderma)

DOUGLAS A. JABS, M.D.
Baltimore, Maryland

Progressive systemic sclerosis is a generalized disorder of connective tissue of unknown etiology, characterized by fibrous and degenerative changes in the skin and viscera, vascular insufficiency, and vasospasm. It usually affects patients between the ages of 30 and 50 years, and females are affected four times more frequently than males. The skin changes consist of thickening, tightening, and induration, leading to loss of normal mobility and to contracture (scleroderma). These changes are usually preceded by an edematous phase, lasting weeks to months. The fingers (sclerodactyly), arms, and face are usually affected early, but the process may spread to involve the entire body. Raynaud's phenomenon occurs in more than 95 per cent of patients with progressive systemic sclerosis.

Visceral involvement includes esophageal dysfunction with gastroesophageal reflux, pulmonary fibrosis, cardiac abnormalities (such as pulmonary hypertension and arrhythmias), gastrointestinal hypomotility, and renal disease (scleroderma kidney). Renal failure is a major cause of mortality in progressive systemic sclerosis, and it is often associated with the onset of malignant hypertension. Other manifestations include digital ulcers, telangiectasia, polyarthralgias, polyarticular arthritis (occasionally), and myositis.

Progressive systemic sclerosis has a clinical spectrum ranging from the relatively benign, slowly progressive CREST syndrome (*c*alcinosis, *R*aynaud's phenomenon, *e*sophageal dysfunction, *s*clerodactyly, and *t*elangiectasia) to a more severe course with rapidly progressive visceral involvement and death. "Overlap" syndromes occur with other connective tissue diseases, such as sclerodermatomyositis and mixed connective tissue disease. The latter is characterized by high titers of antibody to ribonucleoprotein and a combination of features of systemic lupus erythematosus, progressive systemic sclerosis, and polymyositis. Localized benign forms of scleroderma without vascular or visceral disease also occur.

Ocular complications of progressive systemic sclerosis usually result from involvement of the facial skin and lacrimal glands. Involvement of the eyelids leads to tightness of the lids, lagophthalmos, blepharophimosis, and ptosis. Telangiectasia may be present on the lids, and the conjunctival fornices are shortened. Exposure keratitis may occur, but it is not common. Tear secretion is often decreased, which may lead to keratoconjunctivitis sicca. Abnormalities of the conjunctival vessels, including venous dilation, varicosities, vascular sludging, and telangiectasia, are common. Grade IV hypertensive retinopathy with hemorrhages, cotton-wool spots, and papilledema is usually present during scleroderma-renal crises. Ocular myositis has been described in a patient with systemic myositis.

THERAPY

Systemic. No specific agent or agents have been found that halt the progression of scleroderma. In recent years, penicillamine,[‡] a compound that interferes with the intermolecular cross-linking of collagen, has been used experimentally in treating progressive systemic sclerosis. Results of penicillamine therapy have thus far been equivocal; even in the most encouraging study, long-term therapy (average 2.3 years) was required for improvement. Therapy is, therefore, mainly directed toward management of the various complications of the disease.

Ocular. When keratoconjunctivitis sicca or exposure keratitis problems are present, tear substitutes containing cellulose derivatives or polyvinyl alcohol should be used at frequent intervals. Bland lubricating ointments should be used at night.

Supportive. Skin care is essential. Special soaps, creams, and lotions are used to relieve dryness and increase pliability. Ulcerations should be kept clean to avoid secondary infections. Articular complaints may be helped by aspirin or nonsteroidal anti-inflammatory drugs. Avoiding cold exposure and use of warm protective clothing help protect against Raynaud's phenomenon. Previous experience with vasodilator therapy to treat Raynaud's phenomenon has been disappointing. However, newer vasodilators, such as prazosin and nifedipine, may prove useful. Systemic corticosteroids are used to treat the myositis; 40 to 60 mg of prednisone may be needed daily. In a few cases, aggressive antihypertensive therapy has been shown to reverse renal failure in the scleroderma-renal crisis.

Ocular or Periocular Manifestations

Choroid: Patchy choroidal nonperfusion.
Conjunctiva: Chemosis; shortened fornices; telangiectasia; varicosities; vascular sludging; venous dilation.
Cornea: Exposure keratitis; keratoconjunctivitis sicca.
Eyelids: Blepharophimosis; lagophthalmos; ptosis; tightness.
Orbit: Periorbital edema.
Retina: Cotton-wool spots; hemorrhages; papilledema; venous thrombosis.
Other: Decreased tear secretion; ocular myositis; paralysis of extraocular muscles; Sjögren's syndrome.

PRECAUTIONS

Because of the high frequency of abnormalities of tear secretion in these patients, tear production should be evaluated. If tear replacement therapy is necessary, it should be started.

If extraocular muscle involvement caused by myositis is observed, it should be brought to the attention of the patient's internist or rheumatologist because it suggests a generalized inflammatory process that may be treatable with anti-inflammatory agents. Early recognition of this ocular complication may reveal treatable systemic components of this disease and thereby prevent unnecessary morbidity.

COMMENTS

The main ocular manifestations of progressive systemic sclerosis are eyelid involvement (about 65 per cent of cases), decreased tear production (40 to 50 per cent), keratoconjunctivitis sicca (30 per cent), shallow conjunctival fornices (20 per cent), and conjunctival vascular abnormalities (70 per cent). Visual impairment is seldom a problem unless severe corneal damage occurs as a result of dry eyes.

The retinal lesions in progressive systemic sclerosis are clinically and histopathologically indistinguishable from those of malignant hypertension. However, they have been described in one normotensive scleroderma patient and in scleroderma patients with blood pressures lower than expected compared to the severity of fundus changes. This finding suggests an underlying abnormality of the retinal vasculature. One study utilizing fluorescein angiography has demonstrated patchy choroidal nonperfusion in half of the patients. This change was unrelated to hypertension and seemed to have no effect on retinal function. Lastly, results of lid biopsies have suggested that lacrimal and salivary gland involvement may be due to either inflammatory lesions (Sjögren's syndrome) or to glandular fibrosis.

References

Cipoletti JF, et al: Sjögren's syndrome in progressive systemic sclerosis. Ann Intern Med 87:535–541, 1977.
Grennan DM, Forrester J: Involvement of the eye in SLE and scleroderma. A study using fluorescein angiography in addition to clinical ophthalmic assessment. Ann Rheum Dis 36:152–156, 1977.
Horan EC: Ophthalmic manifestations of progressive systemic sclerosis. Br J Ophthalmol 53:388–392, 1969.
Jabs DA: The rheumatic diseases. In Ryan SJ (ed): Retina. Volume II, St. Louis, CV Mosby Company, 1989, pp 457–480.
MacLean H, Guthrie W: Retinopathy in scleroderma. Trans Ophthalmol Soc UK 89:209–220, 1969.
Michels RG: Ocular manifestations in connective tissue disorders (CTD). In Ryan SJ Jr, Smith RE (eds): Selected topics on the Eye in Systemic Disease. New York, Grune & Stratton, 1974, pp 310–312.
Seibold JR: Scleroderma. In Kelley WN, Harris ED, Jr, Ruddy S, Sledge, CB (eds): Textbook of Rheumatology. 3rd ed. Philadelphia, WB Saunders Company, 1989, pp 1215–1244.
West RH, Barnett AJ: Ocular involvement in scleroderma. Br J Ophthalmol 63:845–847, 1979.

WEILL-MARCHESANI SYNDROME
DAVID S. WALTON, M.D.
Boston, Massachusetts

The Weill-Marchesani syndrome is an hereditary cause of ectopia lentis and secondary glaucoma. The usual mode of inheritance is autosomal recessive, and affected persons demonstrate microspherophakia, short stature, stubby hands and feet, and brachycephaly. The affected lenses possess an abnormally small equatorial diameter, can be thickened in the anterior-posterior diameter, and become subluxated. The lens capsule and zonules are abnormal when viewed microscopically. Lens movement usually occurs inferiorly or anteriorly. The abnormal shape of the lens and anterior displacement predispose the eye to the development of pupillary-block glaucoma, which may be acute or chronic and may begin in childhood.

THERAPY

Ocular. Lenticular myopia is a constant finding in this syndrome and often is progressive. Appropriate spectacle or contact lens correction is indicated. Astigmatism secondary to subluxation in the coronal plane cannot be corrected by contact lenses and requires spectacle correction.

Visual loss may occur at a young age secondary to glaucoma. Regular anterior segment examinations are indicated to recognize the presence or development of anterior chamber shallowing and increased lens-iris contact, which predispose to pupillary-block glaucoma. The finding of peripheral anterior synechia is certain evidence of past episodes of pupillary block and secondary angle closure. Acute glaucoma in this syndrome should be initially managed medically, utilizing osmotic agents, carbonic anhydrase inhibitors, and topical cycloplegic-mydriatic agents. Relief of the pupillary block can be induced by instillation of 1 per cent cyclopentolate or 2.5 per cent phenylephrine; however, these cycloplegic-mydriatics can predispose the eye to lens subluxation further into the anterior chamber. Manual posterior displacement of the lens using a muscle hook against the cornea may also be helpful if relief of the pupillary blockage does not occur in 1 to 2 hours.

When first seen in adolescence or adult years, patients with this syndrome may have chronic glaucoma secondary to permanent angle-closure glaucoma. Iridectomy, of course, does not reverse this condition, but only prevents further blockage of the trabecular meshwork associated with the continued occurrence of angle closure in the untreated eye. Medical treatment with timolol, carbonic anhydrase inhibitors, and epinephrine agents is indicated for the chronic glaucoma.

Surgical. When the eye is at risk for pupillary-block glaucoma as indicated by the iris-lens

210 / WEILL-MARCHESANI SYNDROME

configuration on gonioscopy or when there is evidence of past or present pupillary block, laser iridotomy is indicated to prevent repeated attacks and the development of further permanent angle closure. It should be remembered that this development is a frequent and early complication in this syndrome, and prophylactic surgery must be considered for the fellow eye. The more affected eye will often possess a shallower anterior chamber. Laser iridotomy is probably safer than surgical iridectomy. The opening should be placed as peripherally as possible to prevent blockage of the opening by the lens. Miotics may be safely used in this syndrome after iridotomy or iridotomy to induce miosis and hold the lens behind the iris.

When there is inadequate control of medical treatment for chronic glaucoma, external filtration surgery will be necessary. The considerations relevant to such procedures performed with aphakia must be considered, especially in respect to the potential for vitreous entry into the anterior chamber and filter site.

Supportive: Careful screening of the relatives of patients with this syndrome is indicated. Children with threatening anterior segment findings may be asymptomatic and require prophylactic treatment. Other relatives may possess normal eyes and only the systemic features of this syndrome. Appropriate genetic counseling is indicated for all family members.

Ocular or Periocular Manifestations

Anterior Chamber: Abnormally shallow.

Ciliary Body: Prominence of the uveal meshwork in the ciliary body band region (infrequent).

Cornea: Megalocornea; microcornea; opacities related to lenticulocorneal contact.

Lens: Anterior displacement; inferior displacement; microspherophakia; punctate cortical opacities.

Optic Nerve: Glaucomatous cupping.

Other: Convex iris; lenticular myopia; pupillary-block glaucoma.

Precautions

Miotics increase the severity of the pupillary block mechanism in this syndrome. Increased iris-lens contact may develop secondary to the miosis and relaxation of the lens zonules. As a provocative test in this syndrome, this maneuver is of undetermined value. Angle-closure glaucoma also may be initiated by cycloplegia and pupillary dilation.

Surgical iridectomy may be complicated by vitreous loss more readily in the presence of compromised zonules. Subluxation of the lens into the anterior chamber may occur and is not prevented by iridectomy.

Comments

The poor visual prognosis in this disease is probably due in part to the fact that the frequently asymptomatic glaucoma and secondary field loss occur in children. Earlier surgical intervention would be beneficial, but the absence of a family history is this usually recessively inherited disorder makes early detection difficult. Certainly all siblings of affected individuals should be thoroughly evaluated and appropriately treated as early as possible. The high frequency of visual loss occurring prior to surgery, the fact that delay of surgery permits irreversible angle damage, and the favorable postoperative intraocular tension control emphasize the need for early diagnosis and surgical intervention in microspherophakic eyes with glaucoma.

References

Gorlin RJ, L'Heureux PR, Shapiro I: Weill-Marchesani syndrome of two generations: Genetic heterogeneity or pseudodominance? J Pediatr Ophthalmol 11:139-144, 1974.

Jensen AD, Cross HE, Paton D: Ocular complications in the Weill-Marchesani syndrome. Am J Ophthalmol 77:261-269, 1974.

Willi M, Kut L, Cotlier E: Pupillary-block glaucoma in the Marchesani syndrome. Arch Ophthalmol 90:504-508, 1973.

Wright KW, Chrousos GA: Weill-Marchesani syndrome with bilateral angle-closure glaucoma. J Pediatr Ophthalmol Strabismus 22:129-132, 1985.

SECTION 12

SKELETAL DISORDERS

Craniostenosis

CROUZON'S DISEASE
(Craniofacial Dysostosis, Dysostosis Craniofacialis)

PAUL TESSIER, M.D.
Paris, France

Crouzon's disease is usually a dominantly inherited syndrome involving cranial and facial bones. It is characterized by the premature fusion of several cranial sutures and probably by the premature closure of facial bones to the cranial base. The disease is manifested by exophthalmos, retrusion of the maxilla, which gives an appearance of mandibular prognathism, occasionally enlargement of the interorbital distance, and bony abnormalities in the region of the superior longitudinal sinus and bregma. The anomaly is present at birth, but becomes more conspicuous during the first year of life when the head grows rapidly. Increased intracranial pressure may be present at birth or may develop later. If it persists for a longer period of time, it will cause headaches, convulsions, mental deterioration, optic atrophy, lack of nasal breathing, and sometimes secondary deformities of the mandible. The changes in the eyes are secondary to the orbital anomalies. The interpupillary distance is sometimes widened (hypertelorism), and the shortened orbits produce exophthalmos that may be so extreme that luxation of the eyelids may occur behind the globe. Obliquity of the palpebral fissure with the outer canthus slanting downward may occur, although this is more frequent in Apert's syndrome. The optic atrophy is usually of the secondary type and is preceded by papilledema. Strabismus, usually exotropia and hypotropia, is often present, although nystagmus may also sometimes occur. Congenital absence of the superior recti has been reported.

THERAPY

Surgical. A total osteotomy of the face, to achieve a posterior-anterior movement of the whole facial mass, should be considered in anyone over 12 years of age, and earlier if the ocular problem is particularly acute. The procedure has three aims: to establish normal dental occlusion, to develop the nasopharynx, and to increase orbital capacity by developing the depth of these short orbital cavities.

The main incision is a bitemporal one, followed by two infraorbital incisions and a vestibular incision inside the mouth. The principal osteotomies are frontomalar and frontonaso-orbital. Through the oral incision, an interpterygomaxillary disjunction is performed with a 10-mm curved chisel. By the temporal route, the three lines of the malar steps are marked out with an oscillating saw from the infraorbital fissure to the medial wall. The osteotomy of the frontomalar area is cut in the shape of a spur, and then a vertical cut from the upper lateral angle to the infraorbital fissure is made through the lateral orbital wall. In the frontonasal area 10 mm behind the posterior lacrimal crest, a vertical osteotomy is made of the medial wall to the floor by means of a chisel. Then an intercraniofacial "V-shaped" osteotomy (under the cribriform plate) is performed. A transverse cut is made approximately 10 to 15 mm deep, slightly above the frontonasal angle, to bring the frontal process within the lower section. Its exact level and depth will depend upon the x-ray indications. On each side, the osteotomy is undertaken, beginning near the roof in the upper medial angle. These osteotomies converge toward the frontonasal angle, which they reach in the depth. The slope of the saw is regulated so that it will be parallel to the slope of the anterior cranial base, and its depth is regulated according to the size of the latter. At this time, the mobility of the facial mass is tested. The vomer is the last obstacle. A long curved chisel is introduced into the interfrontonasal osteotomy in the direction of the posterior nasal spine, and the midface is separated from the skull.

Disjunction and projection can be done either by levers introduced into the interpterygomaxillary section of the Rowe disimpacting forceps. The facial mass is disimpacted and freed by progressive powerful tractions, applied either on the maxillary arch or behind the maxilla. A 10-mm overprojection must be attempted to overcome residual resistance. The posterior and lateral defects made by the midface advancement are finally filled with bone grafts taken from the ilium and ribs.

Ocular or Periocular Manifestations

Cornea: Dystrophy; exposure keratitis.
Eyelids: Canthal displacement; ptosis.
Optic Nerve: Atrophy; papilledema.
Orbit: Exophthalmos; hypertelorism; shallow orbital cavity.
Other: Blue sclera; cataract; divergent strabismus; nystagmus; visual field defects; visual loss.

PRECAUTIONS

Surgery should aim at simultaneous correction of all critical deformations. The frontofacial advancement is best undertaken through compound extracranial and intracranial methods. The extracranial approach alone does not radically change the shape of the forehead or completely correct severe exophthalmos. To divide the surgery into several stages is not only wrong in attitude but is also doomed to failure. The maxillary problems must not be separated from the orbital or nasal problems. The frontofacial advancement allows a fixation of the upper jaw to the cranium without any dependence on the mandible. This is an incomparable advantage when operating on children with deciduous teeth. The absence of intermaxillary fixation also gives more safety after surgery. The intracranial approach also allows additional expansion of the cranial cavity, an increase in the depth of the orbital cavity, an enlargement of the nasopharynx, improvement of the dental malocclusion, and correction of the proportions and appearance of the forehead and midface, all while recontouring the cranial vault.

The greatest surgical risk is on and around the cribriform plate. Possible sloping of the anterior cranial base, prolapse of the olfactory grooves, and nasal meningoencephalocele should be considered. Scraping the periosteum from the bone around the lacrimal sac below the trochlea and inferior oblique muscle is the only way to protect these structures from injury. This should be done before exploring the medial wall of the orbit and before cutting deeply into the lower medial orbital angle. The movement necessary for disimpaction tends to break the maxillomalar suture where the weak infraorbital rim is thin and hypoplastic.

COMMENTS

Craniofacial dysostosis is a syndrome involving both Crouzon's disease and Apert's syndrome. Crouzon's disease is the main feature of craniofacial dysostosis, its hallmarks being coronal synostosis and faciostenosis with extreme eye proptosis. Apart from the syndactylism of Apert's syndrome, nothing specific differentiates the two diseases. Craniostenosis is rare, affecting 1 child out of 1000. Boys are affected two to four times more frequently than girls. There is no variation of incidence with race. There is a facial element in about 5 per cent of the total number of patients showing craniostenosis.

References

Apert E: De l'acrocéphalosyndactylie. Bull Soc Med Hop Paris 23:1310–1330, 1906.
Blodi FC: Developmental anomalies of the skull affecting the eye. Arch Ophthalmol 57:593–610, 1957.
Crouzon O: Dysostose cranio-faciale héréditaire. Bull Soc Med Hop Paris 33:545–555, 1912.
Tessier P: Relationship of craniostenoses to craniofacial dysostoses, and to faciostenoses. A study with therapeutic implications. Plast Reconstr Surg 48:224–237, 1971.
Tessier P: The definitive plastic surgical treatment of the severe facial deformities of craniofacial dysostosis. Crouzon's and Apert's diseases. Plast Reconstr Surg 48:419–442, 1971.

ENGELMANN'S DISEASE
(Camurati-Engelmann's Disease, Diaphyseal Dysplasia, Hereditary Diaphyseal Dysplasia, Hereditary Multiple Diaphyseal Sclerosis, Hyperostosis Corticalis Generalisata Familiaris, Juvenile Paget's Disease, Osteopathia Hyperostotica Sclerotisans Multiplex Infantilis, Progressive Hyperostosis)

PETER H. MORSE, M.D., F.A.C.S.,
and COLETTA M. MILLER, D.D.S.
Chicago, Illinois

Engelmann's disease is a rare, usually progressive bone dystrophy of unknown etiology that is included in a spectrum of disorders known as the craniotubular (osteosclerotic) dysplasias. Uncertainty in the diagnosis exists in some of the reported cases, and several diseases having similar manifestations may have been described under this eponym. Radiographs demonstrate a symmetric, spindle-shaped, sclerotic, cortical thickening of the intermediate segment of the shaft of the long tubular bones. With progression, the osteosclerosis extends proximally and distally. The base of the skull, calvarium, mandible, cervical vertebrae, clavicles, and bones of the pelvis are often involved. The scapulae, ribs, and bones of the hands and feet are rarely affected.

The various clinical symptoms and signs are pain in the limbs, easy fatigability, delayed ambulation, generalized neuromuscular weakness, inability to run, broad-based waddling gait, thin legs, poor musculature and disproportionately long limbs, bowing of the tibiae, abnormal deep tendon reflexes, hepatosplenomegaly, failure to thrive, delayed puberty, hypogonadism, delay of secondary sex characteristics after apparent early sexual precocity, dry skin, absence of subcutaneous fat, delayed dentition, hypoplasia of the enamel of the upper front teeth, carious teeth, exophthalmos, papilledema, optic atrophy, and deafness.

The age of patients ranges from 3 months to 57 years with a mean age of 19.2 years. There is a slightly greater prevalence of males than females, and the disease is predominantly seen in

Caucasians. Hereditary transmission is not definitely established and may be variable. Several families with an autosomal dominant pattern have been reported. The penetrance and expressivity, the spectrum of manifestations, the severity of the disease, and the rate of progression may vary. The severe form in older age may resemble myelosclerosis, chronic sclerosing osteitis, tertiary syphilis, or osteoblastic carcinomatosis.

THERAPY

Systemic. The progression and degree of activity of the disease should be determined by clinical, radiologic, and laboratory examination before any therapy is begun. Treatment should be directed toward the demonstrated activity or a dynamic process. Corticosteroids have been used in an attempt to suppress bone formation and increase resorption with a calciuric effect. The dosage is 0.5 to 2.0 mg/kg of oral prednisone daily. If there is evidence of abnormal phosphate metabolism, aluminum hydroxide or probenecid might be useful. In the absence of hypocalcemia, a diet low in calcium with cellulose phosphate may be tried. The rapid regrowth of bones may be controlled with diphosphonates. The use of calcitonin and etidronate disodium (EHDP) seems illogical unless the specific medication is used with respect to bone formation activity.

Ocular. Secondary glaucoma may be treated with antiglaucomatous medications. One must be aware of the possibility of induced secondary glaucoma in patients undergoing corticosteroid therapy. If the glaucoma is caused by an increased pressure on the globe secondary to bony overgrowth that creates decreased orbital volume, a surgical decompression may be necessary.

Surgical. Luxation of the globe may require surgery. Lysis of the lateral canthal tendon and resection of Müller's muscle may prevent exposure of the cornea. With progression of the disease, these procedures may not be permanently effective. Orbital decompression may be necessary to counteract secondary glaucoma, and unroofing of the optic canal has been used to alleviate disc edema. However, the rapid regrowth of bone renders this surgical therapy only temporarily successful.

Ocular or Periocular Manifestations

Extraocular Muscles: Convergence insufficiency; diplopia; palsy of lateral rectus muscle.
Eyelids: Lagophthalmos; ptosis; skin atrophy.
Globe: Luxation.
Optic Nerve: Disc edema; pallor or atrophy; vascular tortuosity.
Orbit: Exophthalmos; proptosis; secondary hypertelorism.
Other: Cataracts; decreased visual acuity; epiphora; irritation; secondary glaucoma.

PRECAUTIONS

No specific etiology or effective therapy exists for Engelmann's disease. Patients being treated with systemic corticosteroids must always be observed for the potential complications of glaucoma or cataract.

COMMENTS

Despite the fact that the underlying metabolic defect in Engelmann's disease is unknown, most of the clinical signs and symptoms are a result of the osteosclerotic process and bony overgrowth. This is particularly true of the ocular manifestations, which are the consequence of the physical limitation of the size of the orbit and compression of the nerves.

References

Brodrick JD: Luxation of the globe in Engelmann's disease. Am J Ophthalmol 83:870–873, 1977.
Hundley JD, Wilson FC: Progressive diaphyseal dysplasia. Review of the literature and report of seven cases in one family. J Bone Joint Surg 55-A:461–474, 1973.
Krohel GB, Wirth CR: Engelmann's disease. Am J Ophthalmol 84:520–525, 1977.
Kumar B, Murphy WA, Whyte MP: Progressive diaphyseal dysplasia (Englemann disease): Scintigraphic-radiographic-clinical correlations. Radiology 140: 87–92, 1981.
Morse PH, Walsh FB, McCormick JR: Ocular findings in hereditary diaphyseal dysplasia (Engelmann's disease). Am J Ophthalmol 68:100–104, 1969.
Ramon Y, Buchner A: Camurati-Engelmann's disease affecting the jaws. Oral Surg 22:592–599, 1966.
Smith R, et al: Clinical and biochemical studies in Engelmann's disease (Progressive diaphyseal dysplasia). Q J Med 46:273–294, 1977.
Yoshioka H, et al: Muscular changes in Engelmann's disease. Arch Dis Child 55:716–719, 1980.

ORBITAL HYPERTELORISM
(Greig's Syndrome)
LOIS A. LLOYD, M.D., F.R.C.S.(C),
and RAYMOND BUNCIC, M.D.,
F.R.C.S.(C)
Toronto, Ontario

Orbital hypertelorism is an abnormally increased distance between the orbits. It is an indicator of craniofacial anomaly and produces a significant cosmetic facial defect. Orbital hypertelorism can be classified on the basis of unilateral or bilateral orbital displacement, its severity of deformity, or axial rotation. Tessier has ranked the severity of deformity according to the interorbital distance: first degree, 30 to 34 mm; second degree, 34 to 40 mm; and third degree, greater than 40 mm. However, these distances

214 / ORBITAL HYPERTELORISM

are only applicable to adults and must be scaled downward for children and infants. The orbital displacement may be uniaxial in the lateral plane, but it is more frequently polyaxial with the lateral orbital wall rotated posteriorly. There may also be vertical rotation or displacement causing three-dimensional malposition of the orbit.

Orbital hypertelorism has been ascribed to arrested development of the first branchial arch. This produces a deficiency in the midline that allows the brain to herniate anteroinferior and to intrude between the orbits, preventing their forward growth during embryonic and fetal life. A facial cleft may also be present.

Hypertelorism seldom exists alone. Associated cranial anomalies include encephaloceles that deform the malar, sphenoidal, and frontal bones; brachycephaly that stretches the supraorbital arch and flattens the supraorbital rims; or gigantic frontal bone pneumatization and widened ethmoidal cells that displace the orbits laterally. Orbital hypertelorism may be associated with craniostenosis in which the volume of the cranial vault is decreased and intracranial pressure is occasionally increased. Crouzon's disease, Apert's syndrome, Englemann's disease, and Aarskrog's syndrome may manifest hypertelorism secondary to craniostenosis. Rarely, hypertelorism is secondary to fibrous dysplasia or trauma.

THERAPY

Surgical. Clinical measurements alone are inadequate criteria for recommending surgery. Roentgenographic methods of measuring hypertelorism are difficult if the dacryon is masked by ethmoidal air cells or basal tomograms are not available. Similarly, magnified photographs fail to demonstrate the facial midline accurately, making photographic intercanthal measurements unreliable. The real indications for cosmetic surgery are the relationship between the interorbital distance and width of the skull—that is, the general proportions of the child's head and face—the patient's social acceptance by others, as well as his or her success in maintaining binocular vision.

The clinical assessment and management of patients with hypertelorism should be done by a craniofacial reconstruction team consisting of the following: plastic surgeon, neurosurgeon, neuro-ophthalmologist, neuro-otologist, dentist, radiologist, psychiatrist, psychologist, geneticist, anthropologist, medical photographer, speech therapist, social worker, and cosmetologist. A medical illustrator projects possible changes by imposing an overlay on a photograph of the patient. A Styrofoam model of the patient's face outlines contours from the stereophotographs of the face, which are transferred to a terraced model done to actual scale. The model can be cut in all dimensions and the parts moved to correct the facial deformity. Once plans are complete and the social and psychologic factors are considered, correction is undertaken surgically by a team of neurosurgeon and plastic surgeon.

The operation is usually performed at the age of 2 years. In children younger than 2 years, the cranium is too small to produce successful results. The entire operation is done without external scars on the nose or cheeks. It is performed under hypotensive anesthesia in approximately 5 hours. The scalp incision is made from ear to ear, and skin is turned forward over the face. A frontal bone flap is raised by the neurosurgeon so that the frontal lobes can be retracted from the orbital roofs. The bony forehead can then be advanced or recessed as necessary. The plastic surgeon separates the orbital soft tissues from the bony orbits by subperiosteal dissection, using an incision through the lower fornices and proceeding as far back as the superior orbital fissures. The apex of the orbits and the orbital nerves remain untouched. The incisions through the bony orbital walls anterior to the superior orbital fissures allow displacement of the orbits as a bony box-like unit in any direction—medially, upward, downward, or obliquely.

The U-shaped osteotomy is used for minor corrections up to 15 mm. It mobilizes the lateral orbital wall, the inferior orbital rim and floor, and the medial orbital wall as a single block. Medial orbital wall migration can be augmented by medial movement of the lateral orbital wall or by insertion of a bone graft to the lateral orbital wall. The extracranial technique can be used only if there is no prolapse of the cribriform plate between the medial orbital walls. The intracranial technique of Tessier and Converse mobilizes the majority of the orbit as a box.

The predetermined width of the nasal bone and ethmoidal cells is removed. A glabellar part of the frontal bone and the anterior cranial fossa anterior to the cribriform plate are left intact. The reconstructed bony walls are wired together through the supraorbital ridges and to the frontal bone. Bone chips from the patient's own iliac crest fill any bony gaps in the orbital walls. The medial canthal ligaments are wired to each other by drilling through the anterior lacrimal crests, and the soft tissues are similarly wired. It is important to identify the medial canthal ligaments and perform transnasal canthoplasty after orbital depositioning by fixing the ligaments at the dacryon with a transnasal wire. Excess skin and tissue over the roof of the nose and glabellar areas are resected, and the upper canthal fold is corrected if necessary.

In patients with a recessed midface, the entire midfacial skeletal block may be freed, advanced, and rotated downward to repair maxillary malocclusion. The dentist wires the mandibular arch to the frontal bone to maintain the condyle in the glenoid fossa.

Ocular surgery to correct muscle imbalance follows in about 6 months if necessary.

Ocular. Primary therapeutic measures by the ophthalmologist include care of strabismus, treatment of lagophthalmos with tarsorrhaphy and medication, and both pre- and postoperative assessment and treatment of tearing, ptosis, and visual loss.

Ocular or Periocular Manifestations

Cornea: Microcornea.
Extraocular Muscles: Strabismus; vertical muscle imbalance; V-pattern exotropia.
Eyelids: Coloboma; ptosis.
Globe: Microphthalmos.
Optic Nerve: Atrophy; papilledema.
Orbit: Exophthalmos; lateral displacement of the eyes; misalignment.
Other: Dyschromatopsia; retinal anomalies (congenital); visual field defects; visual loss.

Precautions

Telecanthus is a lateral displacement of the inner canthi seen in Waardenburg's syndrome. It is not true orbital hypertelorism.

The surgical excision of the bone in the midline produces an eso-movement of the globes, thereby improving any preoperative exotropia or producing a frank esotropia. The esotropia is caused by abduction difficulties secondary to medial movement of the anterior two thirds of the orbits. The surgery is also associated with marked overaction of the inferior oblique muscles, underaction of the superior rectus muscles, and underaction of the superior oblique muscles.

Binocularity preoperatively may result in diplopia postoperatively. It is helped by alternate patching of the eyes. Narrowing of the palpebral fissure, lateral ptosis from eyelid tension, and incorrect alignment of the canthal regions are complications that are often difficult to avoid.

Advancement of the orbital bony rim ideally corrects any lagophthalmos, but overcorrection may produce lack of apposition of the ocular globe to the inner lid surface and occasionally tightness of the lid margins due to lateral tension, with resultant tearing.

Following orbital dissection, an intraorbital hematoma occurring during the procedure may produce acute visual loss by optic nerve compression and ischemia. Once the visual loss is recognized, this uncommon complication responds to prompt evacuation of the hematoma before the child leaves the operating room.

Comments

Pure cases of idiopathic orbital hypertelorism are rare. The condition may be inherited as an autosomal dominant or recessive condition, has an unknown sex ratio, and is usually detected early in life. Familial cases are not frequent.

Hypertelorism is one of the most difficult craniofacial problems to correct completely. These patients should be treated by experienced surgical teams located in only a few centers in the world. The risks include death, brain damage, blindness, and infection with osteomyelitis.

References

Buncic R, Lloyd LA: Treatment of craniofacial anomalies in pediatric ophthalmology. *In* Crawford JS, Morin JD (eds): The Eye in Childhood. New York, Grune & Stratton, 1983.
Converse JM, et al: Ocular hypertelorism and pseudohypertelorism. Advances in surgical treatment. Plast Reconstr Surg 45:1–13, 1970.
Lloyd LA: Craniofacial reconstruction: Ocular management of orbital hypertelorism. Trans Am Ophthalmol Soc 73:123–140, 1975.
Mullihen JB, et al: Facial skeletal changes following hypertelorism correction. J Plast Reconstr Surg 77:7–16, 1986.
Munro IR: Orbito-cranio-facial surgery: The team approach. Plast Reconstr Surg 55:170–176, 1975.
Munro IR, Das SK: Improving results in orbital hypertelorism correction. Ann Plast Surg 2:499–507, 1979.
Tessier P: Orbital hypertelorism. I. Successive surgical attempts. Materials and methods. Causes and mechanisms. Scand J Plast Reconstr Surg 6:135–155, 1972.
Tessier P, Guiot G, Derome P: Orbital hypertelorism. II. Definite treatment of orbital hypertelorism (OR.H.) by craniofacial or by extracranial osteotomies. Scand J Plast Reconstr Surg 7:39–58, 1973.
Whitaker LA, et al: Orbital reconstruction in hypertelorism. Otolaryngol Clin North Am 21:199–214, 1988.

Dwarfism

COCKAYNE'S SYNDROME
WILLIAM H. COLES, M.D., M.S.
Buffalo, New York

Children with Cockayne's syndrome have a normal birth and normal development for the first year of life. Then in the second year, their growth is retarded, and the full syndrome becomes apparent. Dwarfism, with disproportionately large hands and feet, is the predominant feature; beak-like noses, sunken eyes, and the prominent jaws of prognathism with associated dental malocclusion and carious teeth are common manifestations. The head is microcephalic, and progressive retardation develops. Additional signs that are not present in all patients include photosensitivity, hypertension, and emphysema. By the second decade, these children appear severely aged. They rarely live beyond 20 years. Pneumonia is a common cause of death.

Although the condition is rare, reported cases have established an autosomal recessive inheritance from the following characteristics: frequent occurrence in siblings, an equal sex distribution, and not infrequent history of parent consanguinity of affected children. Examination of amniotic cells from the uterus of a high-risk

COCKAYNE'S SYNDROME

mother may help in establishing a prenatal diagnosis of Cockayne's syndrome of the fetus. Cockayne's syndrome should not be confused with progeria (premature aging) or Seckel (bird-headed) dwarfism.

THERAPY

Ocular. If corneal changes occur that may be due to corneal drying, artificial tears or mild ophthalmic ointments are indicated.

Surgical. Both acquired and congenital cataracts of severe enough density to require surgery have been reported. No corneal transplant has been required for corneal changes. Cosmetic surgery is not indicated.

Supportive. Guidance and support help parents deal with the progressive retardation. The children usually have a pleasant and very social nature, and they can frequently be cared for at home until the very late stages of their disease, despite their retardation. Genetic counseling is also indicated if parents are planning to have other children.

Ocular or Periocular Manifestations

Cornea: Keratoconjunctivitis sicca; opacity.
Lens: Nuclear, zonular, and fleck cataracts.
Optic Nerve: Atrophy; pallor.
Retina: Attenuation of vessels; spotty "peppered," pigmentary degeneration of the posterior pole.
Other: Enophthalmos; exotropia; nystagmus (usually pendular).

PRECAUTIONS

Cataract extraction in the late stages of the disease should be considered carefully. Frequently, retinal and optic nerve changes contribute more to visual loss than do cataracts. In many of these patients, cataract removal has a very poor visual prognosis. The emphysema and hypertension that occur in these patients make them poor anesthesia risks, especially in the second decade of life.

COMMENTS

Cultured skin fibroblasts from patients with Cockayne's syndrome show a change in the postultraviolet colony-forming ability, a feature shared with xeroderma pigmentosa. However, other features of cultured cells (fibroblasts and lymphocytes) differ between the two diseases; in Cockayne's syndrome patients, there is no increase in carcinogenesis, as is seen in xeroderma pigmentosa patients.

The pathology in the central nervous system is patchy tigroid demyelination similar to Pelizaeus-Merzbacher disease; however, there are few clinical similarities between these two conditions. Enlarged ventricles are also a feature of Cockayne's syndrome, but the clinical changes are not caused by hydrocephalus.

In Cockayne's syndrome, calcifications may be found in the basal ganglion, cerebellum, and cerebrum. Also, tapering of the thoracic vertebral bodies and a steepening of the iliac crest in the small pelvis are seen as the disease progresses.

References

Cheng WS, et al: Ultraviolet light-induced sister chromatid exchanges in xeroderma pigmentosum and in Cockayne's syndrome lymphocyte cells lines. Cancer Res 38:1601–1609, 1978.
Coles WH: Ocular manifestations of Cockayne's syndrome. Am J Ophthalmol 67:762–764, 1969.
Lambert WC: Genetic diseases associated with DNA and chromosomal instability. Dermatol Clin 5:85–105, 1987.
Lehmann AR: Prenatal diagnosis of Cockayne's syndrome. Lancet 1:486–488, 1985.
Moossy J: The neuropathology of Cockayne's syndrome. J Neuropathol Exp Neurol 26:654–660, 1967.
Pearce WG: Ocular and genetic features of Cockayne's syndrome. Can J Ophthalmol 7:435–444, 1972.
Riggs W Jr, Seibert J: Cockayne's syndrome. Roentgen findings. Am J Roentgenol 116:623–633, 1972.
Schmickel RD, et al: Cockayne syndrome: A cellular sensitivity to ultraviolet light. Pediatrics 60:135–139, 1977.
Soffer D, et al: Cockayne syndrome: Unusual neuropathological findings and review of the literature. Ann Neurol 6:340–348, 1979.
Timme TL, Moses RE: Review: Diseases with DNA damage-processing defects. Am J Med Sci 295:40–48, 1988.
Tanaka K, et al: Genetic complementation groups in Cockayne syndrome. Somatic Cell Genet 7:445–455, 1981.

DOWN'S SYNDROME
(**Mongolism, Trisomy 21**)

EDWARD A. JAEGER, M.D.
Philadelphia, Pennsylvania

Down in 1866 first ascribed the term "mongolism" to those with short stature, mental deficiency, and mongolian features. It was the first multisystem disease syndrome to be related to abnormal chromosome numbers. Several chromosome patterns are found in Down's syndrome. The most common is tripling of chromosome 21 found in 95 per cent of those with mongolism; hence, the more appropriate title, trisomy 21. A total chromosome number of 47 is present in all cells, rather than the normal 46. A second pattern, termed "translocation," occurs when the extra chromosome 21 becomes attached to another chromosome. In this case, the total number of chromosomes is 46. A third pattern results if the failure in chromosome separation occurs in a cell division after fertilization. Some cells then contain the normal 46 chromosomes, whereas others contain 47. These individuals are termed "mosaics." There are no significant clinical differences, including the eye findings, among these chromosomal patterns.

The physical appearance of those with Down's syndrome is easily recognizable and characteristic. Nonophthalmologic physical features include an anteriorly and posteriorly flattened head, fissured and protruding tongue, short broad neck, dry skin, shortened extremities and phalanges, simian palmar crease, cardiac disorders, and a wide variation in the degree of mental retardation (an I.Q. below 60 to 70).

The ocular findings in Down's syndrome include epicanthus, upward and outward slanting of palpebral fissures, external infections, keratoconus, Brushfield's spots, strabismus, high refractive errors, nystagmus, lacrimal obstruction, cataracts, and an increase in the number of small retinal vessels radiating from the disc. Ocular abnormalities due to self-inflicted trauma may also be seen.

THERAPY

Ocular. The commonly encountered external ocular problems of blepharitis, styes, chalazions, and conjunctivitis are treated in the standard manner. In the therapy of these conditions, it is important to remember that the use of corticosteroids can contribute to the development of a herpes simplex keratitis in patients with Down's syndrome.

Surgical. Although surgical corrections of ocular manifestations of Down's syndrome may result in a more productive life for these individuals, there is no specific therapy.

Those with keratoconus must be watched for the development of hydrops and corneal perforation. Corneal transplant is indicated in impending perforation. Traumatic ocular injuries should be treated in the usual manner.

High refractive errors, such as myopia, hyperopia, and astigmatism, are common, but high myopia appears to be predominant. There is some evidence that early correction of high refractive errors leads to a better visual and neurosensory environmental adjustment.

Full hypermetropic correction should be tried in those cases of accommodative esotropia. The surgical correction of nonaccommodative estropia is indicated in selected cases. However, bifoveal fixation is seldom achieved after surgery. Patching for amblyopia is difficult, but may be attempted in those patients with a strongly supportive environment. Fortunately, profound amblyopia secondary to strabismus is less frequent than might be anticipated in those with Down's syndrome.

Lacrimal surgery must be approached with caution as excess bleeding in the immediate postoperative phase may be encountered.

The development of senile cataracts presents special problems in patients with trisomy 21. These patients appear to age more rapidly, and lens opacification is another manifestation of this process. Better general medical care, along with improved family and institutional awareness, has increased the life expectancy of many persons with Down's syndrome; hence, a greater incidence of cataracts in this group.

Cataract extraction is indicated when vision has deteriorated to the point that self-care and general function are significantly impaired. Since family members or attendants are often in the best position to evaluate visual function, the ophthalmologist should rely heavily on their input. The standard extracapsular extraction is the procedure of choice, and the implantation of a posterior chamber lens does not appear to present undue risk. However, if posterior capsule opacification develops, YAG laser capsulotomy may be difficult. The use of anterior chamber lenses presents some additional concern. If the posterior capsule is not intact or an intraoperative complication has occurred, it may be best not to implant an intraocular lens. Many patients with Down's syndrome do well as aphakes, even without correction. Since general anesthesia is required, the presence of a close family member or familiar attendant is absolutely necessary for a reasonably calm pre- and postoperative period. Returning the patient to familiar surroundings, preferably the same day, is also helpful; likewise, a well-sutured wound provides for surgeon tranquility. It is surprising how well some of these patients tolerate the procedure. Careful planning is imperative, however.

Supportive. Those with Down's syndrome are susceptible to respiratory infections and cardiac problems and have a higher incidence of leukemia. The trend in management of multiple handicapped individuals is to return as many systems as possible to normal early in life. This philosophy holds true for those with Down's syndrome, although it must be judiciously applied to the individual.

The ophthalmologist often is asked to examine patients with Down's syndrome early in life because of manifest or pseudo strabismus. An awareness of the ocular and systemic problems is helpful in further counseling of parents.

There is some evidence that those persons with Down's syndrome who are raised in an understanding and supportive environment achieve a greater degree of adjustment and advancement than institutionalized persons. Day schools and work centers have also been quite successful in contributing to the development and social adjustment of these individuals.

Ocular or Periocular Manifestations

Cornea: Keratoconus.
Extraocular Muscles: Accommodative or nonaccommodative esotropia; nystagmus.
Eyelids: Blepharitis; chalazion; epicanthus; hordeolum; lateral upward slope of palpebral fissures.
Iris: Brushfield's spots; hypoplasia.
Lacrimal System: Obstruction of nasolacrimal duct or canaliculi.
Lens: Cataracts.

218 / DOWN'S SYNDROME

Retina: Detachment; vascular proliferation (radiating in spoke-like fashion from the disc).

Other: Astigmatism; conjunctivitis; hyperopia; myopia.

PRECAUTIONS

Persons with Down's syndrome have been thought to be unusually sensitive to atropine, which produces a rapid heart rate. However, this has not been found in controlled studies involving systemic and topically administered atropine. The possibility of unreported ocular trauma must be kept in mind. When ocular surgery is performed on patients with Down's syndrome, every contingency must be anticipated in the immediate pre- and postoperative periods. Familiar surroundings and attendants are the best precautions.

COMMENTS

Down's syndrome occurs once in every 600 to 700 live births; however, because of increased life span, the percentage of the population with Down's syndrome has increased. It has been associated with increased maternal age; in one study, the maternal age for Down's births was found to be 34.43 years compared to 28.17 years for normal births.

Improved techniques in prenatal genetic testing have made it possible to diagnose Down's syndrome early in pregnancy. Amniocentesis and chorionic villus biopsy utilizing DNA analysis have resulted in safe and increasingly accurate diagnoses in a wide variety of genetic disorders and should be discussed with those mothers at significant risk of bearing a mongoloid child.

References

Clarke CM, Edwards JH, Smallpiece V: 21-Trisomy/normal mosaicism in an intelligent child with some mongoloid characters. Lancet *1*:1028–1030, 1961.

Down JL: Observations on the ethnic classification of idiots. London Hosp Rep *3*:259–262, 1866.

Hiles DA, Hoyme SH, McFarlane F: Down's syndrome and strabismus. Am Orthopt J *24*:63–68, 1974.

Jaeger EA: Ocular findings in Down's syndrome. Trans Am Ophthalmol Soc 78:808–845, 1980.

Lejeune J, Gauthier M, Turpin R: Les chromosomes humains en culture de tissus. CR Acad Sci *248*:602–603, 1959.

Mir GH, Cumming GR: Response to atropine in Down's syndrome. Arch Dis Child *46*:61–65, 1971.

Nelson LB, Jackson LG: Techniques in prenatal genetic diagnoses. *In* Duane TD, Jaeger EA (ed): Biomedical Foundations of Ophthalmology, Vol 3. Philadelphia, JB Lippincott, 1988.

Smith GF, Berg JM: Down's Anomaly, Edinburgh, Churchill Livingstone, 1976, pp 1–13, 246–263.

Ullman S, Nelson LB, Jackson LG: Prenatal diagnostic techniques. Chorionic villus sampling. Sur Ophthal *30*:33–40, 1985.

Williams EJ, McCormick AQ, Tischler B: Retinal vessels in Down's syndrome. Arch Ophthalmol 89:269–271, 1973.

WERNER'S SYNDROME

JOHN D. BULLOCK, M.D., M.S., F.A.C.S.
Dayton, Ohio

and STUART H. GOLDBERG, M.D.
Hershey, Pennsylvania

Werner's syndrome is a rare multisystem disorder described as either a partial phenocopy of aging or one of a group of chromosome instability syndromes. It is an autosomal recessive condition that becomes manifest in the second or third decade of life. Cardinal characteristics include short stature, premature graying and baldness, atrophic changes of the skin with loss of underlying connective tissue and muscle, bilateral cataracts, trophic ulcers of the legs, and hypogonadism. The general picture is that of a prematurely aged, short patient with thin extremities, stocky trunk, and markedly atrophic skin. The characteristic facies—a "beaked" nose, thin lips, and sunken orbits—results from taut, adherent facial skin. Other features include Mönckeberg-type vascular calcification, which leads to diffuse arteriosclerosis, adult-onset diabetes mellitus, osteoporosis, increased consanguinity rates among affected families, and an increased incidence of neoplasia. Although the disease has been likened to premature aging, it is more likely a condition that merely displays features of normal aging.

The constant ocular manifestation is the development of bilateral cataracts early in the clinical course. These cataracts mature rapidly and are generally characterized by posterior subcapsular opacities that may appear striated or homogeneous. Another common finding is apparent proptosis secondary to atrophy of circumorbital tissue. The incidence of retinopathy appears to be no greater and possibly less frequent in Werner's syndrome patients with diabetes mellitus compared with the general diabetic population.

THERAPY

Systemic. Diabetes mellitus in Werner's syndrome can generally be controlled by diet; however, insulin or oral hypoglycemic agents may be required. Insulin resistance is common, but ketoacidosis is rare. Diffuse arteriosclerosis may lead to development of a variety of problems (hypertension, coronary artery disease, and nephropathy), necessitating appropriate medical therapy.

Surgical. Good visual results can be achieved with cataract extraction. Ulcerations of the legs and feet may benefit from treatment with skin grafting.

Supportive. No curative therapy for Werner's syndrome exists. Individual problems are treated palliatively. Genetic counseling should be offered to patients and their relatives. Management by dermatologic and orthopedic specialists is required for the treatment of the crippling ulcerations of the lower extremities.

Ocular or Periocular Manifestations

Cornea: Arcus senilis; keratoconjunctivitis.
Eyelids or Eyebrows: Madarosis; poliosis.
Globe: Apparent proptosis.
Iris: Telangiectasia.
Lens: Cataracts (usually posterior subcapsular).
Retina: Chorioretinitis; macular degeneration; pigmented retinal dystrophy.
Other: Blue scleral coloration; decreased accommodation; decreased tear secretion.

PRECAUTIONS

A high incidence of postoperative complications following cataract extraction in patients with Werner's syndrome has been reported by several authors. Corneal endothelial decompensation, corneal ulceration, wound dehiscence, iris prolapse, and secondary glaucoma have occurred. The surgical approach should be individualized; technique and management should anticipate poor wound healing and aim to minimize endothelial cell damage.

COMMENTS

Ophthalmologic and dermatologic manifestations are the major sources of morbidity early in the course of the disease. Diffuse arteriosclerosis is the major cause of organ failure and mortality. Patients usually die of malignancy or myocardial or cerebrovascular accidents in the fourth or fifth decade.

The relationship of the pathologic process in Werner's syndrome to natural aging has prompted considerable research and debate. Recent cytogenetic and clinical observations in Werner's syndrome have led some to include this disorder in the category of autosomal recessive genetic diseases with chromosome instability and increased incidence of neoplasia. These genetic diseases are ataxia telangiectasia, Fanconi's anemia, Bloom's syndrome, and xeroderma pigmentosum. Patients with Werner's syndrome have been found to have hyaluronic aciduria; their abnormal connective tissue may be due to aberrations of collagen and/or proteoglycans. Fibroblast abnormalities are the subject of a large volume of current research.

References

Bullock JD, Howard RO: Werner syndrome. Arch Ophthalmol 90:53–56, 1973.
Epstein CJ: Werner's syndrome and aging: A reappraisal. Adv Exp Med Biol 190:219–228, 1985.
Epstein CJ et al: Werner's syndrome: A review of its symptomatology, natural history, pathologic features, genetics and relationship to the natural aging process. Medicine 45:177–221, 1966.
Jonas JB, et al: Ophthalmic surgical complications in Werner's syndrome: Report on 18 eyes of nine patients. Ophthalmic Surg 18:760–764, 1987.
Petrohelos MA: Werner's syndrome. A survey of three cases, with review of the literature. Am J Ophthalmol 56:941–953, 1963.
Salk D: Werner's syndrome: A review of recent research with an analysis of connective tissue metabolism, growth control of cultured cells, and chromosomal aberrations. Hum Genet 62:1–15, 1982.

Fragile Bone Disease

ANKYLOSING SPONDYLITIS
(Marie-Strumpell Disease)

DOUGLAS A. JABS, M.D.
Baltimore, Maryland

Ankylosing spondylitis is a chronic inflammatory disorder characterized by involvement of the cartilaginous joints of the axial skeleton. It is typically a disease of young people, with onset usually between 16 and 40 years of age. Males are affected more frequently than females, with a sex ratio of 7:3. Ankylosing spondylitis has a strong association with the histocompatibility of antigen HLA-B27.

The susceptible joints in ankylosing spondylitis are the sacroiliac joints, the intervertebral spaces, and the apophyseal and costovertebral articulations. The most frequent manifestation is chronic low back pain. If the disease is persistent and untreated, it may progress during several years and cause loss of motion and fusion of the involved joints. This may result in a fixed forward flexion of the spine and hips. Peripheral joints, particularly the shoulders, hips, and knees, can also be involved. A potentially severe manifestation of ankylosing spondylitis is cardiac involvement, which can result in heart block or hemodynamically significant aortic insufficiency.

The characteristic ocular manifestation of ankylosing spondylitis is recurrent acute iridocyclitis. Bouts of anterior segment inflammation usually involve only one eye at a time, and they often recur after a lapse of months to years. Both eyes may eventually be involved. In some patients, the repeated attacks of iridocyclitis are mild; in others, the attacks may be severe. Some patients develop a severe fibrinous exudate ("plastic iritis") or hypopyon. Posterior synechiae, band keratopathy, and rarely even phthisis bulbi can occur. Scleritis has been reported rarely in patients with ankylosing spondylitis.

THERAPY

Systemic. Systemic anti-inflammatory drugs are important in the treatment of ankylosing spondylitis. The two most frequently used agents are phenylbutazone, at a dosage of 100 to 200 mg two times daily, and indomethacin, at a dosage of 25 to 50 mg three times a day. A good therapeutic response to aspirin is unusual. Other nonsteroidal antiinflammatory agents, such as ibuprofen,‡ naproxen,‡ fenoprofen,‡ and tolmetin,‡ are now being evaluated in ankylosing spondylitis. There is no evidence that systemic corticosteroids are effective.

Ocular. The treatment of iridocyclitis associated with ankylosing spondylitis consists of local cycloplegics and topical corticosteroids. Cycloplegics are used to relieve ocular pain and to minimize formation of posterior synechiae. Either 1 per cent atropine or 5 per cent homatropine ophthalmic solution, given two to four times daily, may be used. Topical corticosteroids are used to control inflammation. Although combined preparations of various steroid agents are available, 1 per cent prednisolone is preferred. One or two drops should be instilled in the affected eye as frequently as necessary to suppress the inflammation; this may vary from hourly applications to use of the drops every other day.

Supportive. A daily exercise program designed to maintain chest expansibility, maximal spinal mobility, and a full range of motion of the proximal joints is the cornerstone of managing ankylosing spondylitis. Education of the patients and lifelong cooperative effort on their part are essential to successful therapy.

Ocular or Periocular Manifestations

Anterior Chamber: Aqueous flare and cells; hypopyon.

Cornea: Band keratopathy; keratic precipitates.

Iris: Anterior uveitis ("plastic iritis"); synechiae.

Other: Ocular pain; photophobia; scleritis; visual loss.

PRECAUTIONS

Topical steroids used to treat ocular inflammation should be tapered and withdrawn as soon as the anterior chamber reaction clears and should be given again only if the inflammation recurs. Long-term topical corticosteroid therapy should be avoided because of possible complications, including glaucoma and cataract formation.

Systemic drugs used to treat ankylosing spondylitis have various, sometimes severe side effects. These drugs should be prescribed by an internist or rheumatologist. Side effects secondary to phenylbutazone include the Stevens-Johnson syndrome and bone marrow suppression, in addition to gastric intolerance that may also occur secondary to indomethacin. Various ocular complications of drug therapy have also been described, although it is not always clear that a causal relation exists. However, in the event of an ocular reaction of a sort not usually associated with uveitis, a drug-induced effect should be considered.

COMMENTS

A strong genetic component is present in the pathogenesis of ankylosing spondylitis, as is demonstrated by the association of this condition with the antigen HLA-B27. Approximately 90 per cent of Caucasian patients and 50 per cent of black patients with ankylosing spondylitis are HLA-B27 positive, as compared to a 4 to 8 per cent prevalence of this gene in control populations. A similar relation with HLA-B27 antigen has been demonstrated for other spondylarthropathies, such as Reiter's syndrome and psoriatic spondylitis.

There is no clear evidence that systemic antiinflammatory drugs alter the natural history of the disease; their major role is in the relief of pain and stiffness, thus allowing the patient to pursue an exercise program and maintain a normal life-style. For this reason, such drugs are valuable.

Iridocyclitis occurs in about 25 per cent of patients with ankylosing spondylitis. Furthermore, studies of patients with "idiopathic" acute non-granulomatous iridocyclitis demonstrate a high frequency (over 50 per cent) with subtle clinical, radiographic or scintigraphic evidence of spondylarthropathy or the presence of HLA-B27 (about 50 per cent). Therefore, the possibility of ankylosing spondylitis should be considered in any young person presenting with acute iridocyclitis, and appropriate clinical and radiologic investigations should be obtained.

References

Calina R: Ankylosing spondylitis. *In* Kelley WN, Harris ED Jr, Ruddy S, Sledge CB (eds): Textbook of Rheumatology. 3rd ed. Philadelphia, WB Saunders Company, 1989, pp 1021–1037.

Jabs DA: The rheumatic diseases. *In* Ryan SJ (ed): Retina. Volume II, St. Louis, CV Mosby Company, 1989, pp 457–480.

Kimura SJ, et al: Uveitis and joint diseases: A review of 191 cases. Trans Am Ophthalmol Soc 64:291–310, 1966

Michels RG: Ocular manifestations in arthritis. *In* Ryan SJ Jr, Smith RE (eds): Selected Topics on the Eye in Systemic Disease. New York, Grune & Stratton, 1974, pp 372–373.

Russell AS, et al: Scintigraphy of sacroiliac joints in acute anterior uveitis. A study of thirty patients. Ann Intern Med 85:606–608, 1976.

Watson PG, Hazleman BL: The Sclera and Systemic Disorders. Philadelphia, WB Saunders, 1976, pp 246–252.

OSTEOPETROSIS

(Albers-Schönberg Disease, Marble Bone Disease, Osteosclerosis Congenita Diffusa, Osteosclerosis Fragilis Generalista)

JONATHAN D. WIRTSCHAFTER, M.D.
Minneapolis, Minnesota

Osteopetrosis describes a group of at least eight inherited disorders of reduced osteoclast function that results in failure of bone resorption and a generalized increase in bone density. In some of these disorders, there is an abnormality in bone marrow stem cells that affects osteoclasts and macrophages. Abnormalities of macrophages and neutrophil activation partially explain the high susceptibility to infection. In some of these disorders, abnormal osteoclast function may result from local environmental products that influence cellular differentiation or regulation.

Anemia, hepatosplenomegaly, and extramedullary hematopoiesis result from the reduced marrow space and replacement of its normal contents by chondro-osseous tissue in the sclerotic bones. Pathologic fractures limit mobility. Juvenile-onset osteopetrosis has been subdivided into malignant (formerly "lethal"), nonlethal, carbonic anhydrase II (CAII) deficiencies, and inactive parathyroid hormone types. Most children presenting with osteopetrosis in infancy have the autosomal recessively inherited "infantile" or "malignant" form of the disease. These children have limited longevity because of hematologic and neurologic involvement. The most common form of the disease (osteopetrosis tarda) is an autosomal dominantly inherited form and usually presents in childhood, but may not be symptomatic until after the seventh decade. Some obligate carriers of the dominant type have no phenotypic features.

The radiographic examination of patients with the dominant forms may show pronounced sclerosis of the cranial vault (type 1) or of the cranial base, vertebrae, and pelvis (type 2). Serial roentgencephalometry documents craniofacial abnormalities, including narrowed optic canals, orbital hypertelorism, defective growth of the middle and lower face, decreased intracranial volume, and calcified secondary cartilage. Cerebral calcifications are seen in the CAII disorder.

Visual loss may occur as a result of several mechanisms: compressive optic atrophy, hydrocephalus, papilledema, or an infantile amaurosis (simulating Leber's congenital amaurosis) characterized by a markedly abnormal electroretinogram (ERG) at the first examination and associated with degeneration of all layers of the neural retina. Assessment of visual function is frequently difficult in affected children because of deafness and impaired communication skills. These problems and the effects of anticonvulsive medications compound structural causes of impaired mental function. Serial visual evoked potential (VEP) examinations may be the only objective measure of visual deterioration or improvement.

THERAPY

Systemic. Bone marrow transplantation is the only definitive therapy for the previously lethal infantile or malignant form of the disease. The success rate is approaching 50 per cent. After successful transplantation, magnetic resonance (MR) of the spine shows that material of high signal intensity fills in the marrow cavity of the vertebrae where once there was a complete signal void. However, successful transplantation may not reverse optic canal compression in a timely manner or at all. Therefore, bone marrow transplantation may not greatly affect the indications for optic canal decompression nor for shunting patients with hydrocephalus.

Ocular. Bony decompression of the superior half of the optic canal (with or without widening of the canal) may be indicated in those children where there is computed tomographic evidence (2 mm or thinner sections and bone window display) of narrowing of the optic canals, a normal ERG, and subjective and objective evidence, such as progressive abnormality on serial VEP examination, of decreased optic nerve function. The VEP may show further deterioration in the first weeks after surgery and then improve. Intraoperative VEP monitoring is probably not indicated. Surgery was performed at the age of 8 months in the youngest reported case with a successful visual result. That patient had a mild systemic disease and did not require bone marrow transplantation. Bilateral decompression at a single sitting amounts essentially to sequential operations using the pterional approach and is not recommended for infants. Optic canal decompression is probably of no value for those patients whose osteopetrosis is associated with an extinguished ERG.

Surgical. Decompression of the facial and vestibular nerves is sometimes indicated.

Supportive. Although the adult patient may require little or no support other than the treatment of an occasional fracture, the management of deafness, and the treatment of dental caries, the child may require extreme measures to maintain normal blood cell populations (splenectomy, corticosteroids, transfusions), to control infections (antibiotics and surgical drainage), to maintain weight gain, and to encourage normal psychologic development. There have been reports of hematologic improvement after the use of high-dose intravenous methylprednisolone or prednisolone, and a low-calcium, high-phosphate diet in juvenile osteopetrosis.

Ocular or Periocular Manifestations

Extraocular Muscles: Paralysis of the third, fourth, or sixth cranial nerves.
Eyelids: Ptosis; weakness due to facial nerve paralysis.
Globe: Proptosis.
Lens: Congenital cataracts.
Optic Nerve: Ischemic swelling of the nerve head; optic atrophy may be primary and associated with retinal degeneration or secondary to compression, increased intracranial pressure, meningitis, or other infections; papilledema.
Orbit: Hypertelorism.
Pupil: Anisocoria.
Retina: Primary degeneration; vascular dilation.
Other: Nystagmus; strabismus; trigeminal neuralgia; visual field constriction.

PRECAUTIONS

The ophthalmic surgeon should be aware that the sclerotic bone encroaches on many structures and may cause unforeseen complications, such as hypopituitarism, sleep apnea, and foraminal occlusion of an internal jugular vein with dural sinus thrombosis. Other problems include intracranial hemorrhage and seizures.

COMMENTS

In addition to bone marrow transplantation, other more specific therapies will be advocated when more is known about the mechanisms of this heterogeneous group of disorders, particularly for those forms of the disease where abnormal osteoclast function may result from local environmental products that influence cellular differentiation or regulation. The indications for optic canal decompression are still uncertain, but surgical intervention seems to be useful for selected patients within the first decade of life. Optic canal decompressions may be indicated shortly before or soon after bone marrow transplantation in infants with what was once a uniformly lethal disease.

References

Al-Mefty O, et al: Optic nerve decompression in osteopetrosis. J Neurosurg 68:80–84, 1988.

Coccia PF, et al: Successful bone marrow transplantation for infantile malignant osteopetrosis. N Engl J Med 302:701–708, 1980.

Ellis PP, Jackson E: Osteopetrosis: A clinical study of optic nerve involvement. Am J Ophthalmol 53:943–953, 1962.

Haines SJ, Erickson DL, Wirtschafter JD: Optic nerve decompression for osteopetrosis in early childhood. Neurosurg 23:470–475, 1988.

Hoyt CS, Billson FD: Visual loss in osteopetrosis. Am J Dis Child 133:955–958, 1979.

Key L, et al: Treatment of congenital osteopetrosis with high-dose calcitriol. N Engl J Med 310:409–415, 1984.

Kieth CG: Retinal atrophy of osteopetrosis. Arch Ophthalmol 79:234–241, 1968.

Marks SC: Osteopetrosis—Multiple pathways for the interception of osteoclast function. Appl Pathol 5:172–183, 1987.

Merin S, Harwood-Nash DC, Crawford JS: Axial tomography of optic canals in diagnosis of children's eye and optic nerve defects. Am J Ophthalmol 72:1122–1129, 1971.

Yarington CT Jr, Sprinkle PM: Facial palsy in osteopetrosis. Relief by endotemporal decompression. JAMA 202:549, 1967.

Mandibulofacial Dysostosis

HALLERMANN-STREIFF-FRANCOIS SYNDROME

(Francois-Hallermann-Streiff Syndrome, Francois Syndrome, Hallermann-Streiff Syndrome, Mandibulo-Oculofacial Dyscephaly, Mandibulo-Oculofacial Dysmorphia)

DAVID J. HOPKINS, M.B., F.R.C.S., D.O.

Bradford, England

The Hallermann-Streiff-Francois syndrome is a complex of congenital skeletal and ocular anomalies. The principle features are dyscephaly or bird face; dental anomalies; proportionate dwarfism; atrophy of the skin, head, and nose; sparse thin hair; and ocular abnormalities. Spontaneous absorption of the cataract is a common ocular feature. This is believed to lead to hypersensitivity to the lens substance and loss of vision from chronic uveitis and refractory secondary glaucoma. Many other frequently encountered ocular features of the syndrome have been described. There is no definite chromosomal abnormality in this disease, and family occurrence is infrequent; the presence of a single gene mutation seems likely.

THERAPY

Ocular. Treatment of glaucoma in these patients is a difficult therapeutic problem. Local miotics beta blockers, and systemic carbonic anhydrase inhibitors are the most advantageous medications. The addition of topical ophthalmic 1 per cent epinephrine may be useful; this solution may be applied twice daily.

Surgical. Early bilateral lensectomy is recommended to reduce the risk of loss of vision from uveitis and secondary glaucoma and also to avoid suppression amblyopia. Surgical treatment of established glaucoma is unlikely to be successful. Airway management may present difficulties for the anesthesiologist.

Supportive. Patients who have had cataracts removed require frequent, regular follow-up examinations to ensure that, if intraocular inflammation occurs, it will be diagnosed and treated properly. Spectacle correction of aphakia should be carried out as soon as possible after surgery, and orthoptic support is necessary to optimize visual acuity.

Ocular or Periocular Manifestations

Choroid: Coloboma; peripapillary choroidal atrophy.

Cornea: Keratoglobus; microcornea, sclerocornea.

Eyebrows or Eyelids: Antimongoloid slant; madarosis.

Iris: Atrophy; coloboma; granulomatous anterior uveitis; synechiae.

Orbit: Reduced intraorbital distance; small.
Retina: Folds; subretinal pigmentary band.
Other: Abnormal anterior chamber angle; decreased visual acuity; optic disc coloboma; secondary glaucoma.

Precautions

The ophthalmic surgeon should not delay intervention in the hope that spontaneous cataract absorption will occur in these patients, because the attendant chronic uveitis and secondary glaucoma will lead to irreversible loss of sight.

Comments

In many cases, the condition is discovered in older children or adults, and it appears that these individuals may have a normal life span. Pulmonary insufficiency is the main cause of death in children with the syndrome. Appropriate investigation and treatment should therefore be carried out.

Glaucoma in the Hallermann-Streiff-Francois syndrome mainly results from intraocular inflammation. The inflammation may represent a hypersensitivity reaction to the lens, since a granulomatous anterior uveitis occurs most often where there has been surgical or spontaneous release of the lens matter into the anterior chamber. Less frequently, the glaucoma may be the result of the developmental anomalies of the anterior chamber.

References

Francois J: Les nanismes essentiels. J Fr Ophthalmol 4:511–524, 1981.

Francois J: Francois dyscephalic syndrome. Birth defects. Original article series 18:595–619, 1982.

Hopkins DJ, Horan EC: Glaucoma in the Hallermann-Streiff syndrome. Br J Ophthalmol 54:416–422, 1970.

Sataloff RT, Roberts B-R: Airway management in Hallermann-Streiff syndrome. Am J Otolaryngol 5:64–67, 1984.

Schanzlin DJ, Goldberg DB, Brown SI: Hallermann-Streiff syndrome associated with sclerocornea, Aniridia and a chromosal abnormality. Am J Ophthalmol 90:411–415, 1980.

Solomon LM, Esterly NB: The Skin and the Eye. In Goldberg MF (ed): Genetic and Metabolic Eye Disease. Boston, Little, Brown and Co, 1974, pp 505–506.

Sugar A, Bigger JF, Podos SM: Hallermann-Streiff-Francois syndrome. J Pediatr Ophthalmol 8:234–238, 1971.

MANDIBULOFACIAL DYSOSTOSIS
(Berry Syndrome, Franceschetti Syndrome, Treacher Collins Syndrome)

TREVOR H. KIRKHAM, M.D., F.R.C.S.
Montreal, Quebec

Mandibulofacial dysostosis is a congenital anomaly caused by the effects of an incompletely penetrant dominant autosomal gene with pleiotropic manifestations. The major effects of the gene are to retard fusion of the embryonic facial clefts and to inhibit development of the facial bones derived from the first branchial arch. The syndrome is characterized by hypoplasia of the maxilla and mandible, malformation of the pinnae, and a beaked nose. There is a marked antimongoloid obliquity of the palpebral fissures, characteristically with a pronounced coloboma of the outer third of the lower lids. The mouth appears wide and fishlike. The hairline projects prominently in front of the ears onto the cheeks. A high arched palate and dental abnormalities may be present. There are sometimes blind fistulas on the cheeks between the ears and the angles of the mouth. Conductive deafness resulting from malformation of the ossicular chain may be present. Less commonly, other skeletal anomalies occur. The ophthalmic problem is usually cosmetic. Recognition of the syndrome is clinical, and there are no reported biochemical or chromosomal abnormalities.

THERAPY

Surgical. A team approach of orbitocraniofacial surgery may produce dramatic cosmetic improvement in the facial appearance. Detailed preoperative ophthalmic examination, particularly of ocular alignment and the lacrimal system, is a medicolegal safeguard. Otolaryngologic reconstruction of the ossicular chain may be possible. The eyelid defects may be repaired at an early stage, sometimes after initial build-up of the hypoplastic maxilla by cartilage or other tissue. Various methods have been suggested for the repair of colobomas, including full-thickness skin grafts and transposition of flaps. Early repair for extensive colobomas is recommended to obviate corneal damage. Sometimes, the antimongoloid slant of the palpebral fissures may be lifted.

Supportive. The unusual facial appearance and possible deafness may lead to a mistaken diagnosis of mental retardation. Early evaluation of hearing is necessary; if there appears to be a speech problem, speech therapy is essential. Psychiatric help and genetic counseling are recommended for the patients and their families.

Ocular or Periocular Manifestations

Extraocular Muscles: Strabismus; underdeveloped orbicularis oculi muscle.
Eyelids: Antimongoloid slant; coloboma of temporal third of lower lid.
Lens: Cataract; ectopia.

Precautions

Early recognition of the syndrome is important, since children born into affected families should be examined for deafness at an early age. A series of reconstructive procedures must usually be undertaken, some during infancy and

224 / MANDIBULOFACIAL DYSOSTOSIS

childhood and others deferred until adolescence or adult life.

COMMENTS

Many incomplete forms of the syndrome have been described, and patients displaying all the manifestations of the syndrome are rare.

References

Kirkham TH: Mandibulofacial dysostosis with ectopia lentis. Am J Ophthalmol 70:947–949, 1970.
Rogers BO: The surgical treatment of mandibulofacial dysostosis (Berry syndrome; Treacher Collins syndrome; Franceschetti-Zwahlen-Klein syndrome). Clin Plast Surg 3:653–666, 1976.

OCULOAURICULO-VERTEBRAL DYSPLASIA
(Goldenhar's Syndrome)

CHARLES R. LEONE, JR., M.D.

San Antonio, Texas

Goldenhar's syndrome is a disorder characterized by a triad of anomalies: epibulbar dermoids or dermolipomas, deformity of the ears, and vertebral skeletal defects. The syndrome does not appear to be inherited as most cases have been sporadic, with males being affected in 60 per cent of cases. The disease is usually unilateral, although the epibulbar dermoids may occur bilaterally in 25 per cent of patients. The epibulbar dermoids are typically located in the lower temporal limbal area and are present in 75 per cent of cases. The dermolipomas are less frequent, occupy the upper lateral fornix, and are usually unilateral. Upper eyelid colobomas are present in 25 per cent of cases, are unilateral, and occur in the medial aspect of the upper lid. There is also a significant incidence of lacrimal obstruction on the affected side, usually in the nasolacrimal duct.

The ear deformity consists of preauricular appendages, misshapen ears due to hypoplasia of the pinna, and absent external auditory meati. There may also be a suggestion of hemifacial microsomia. Cervical vertebral anomalies consisting of fusion of the vertebrae, hemivertebrae, and occipitalization of the atlas may be present.

THERAPY

Ocular. Rarely, decreased corneal sensitivity may require ocular lubricants to moisten and lubricate the eyes. Either 0.5 per cent methylcellulose solution or petrolatum ointment may be applied several times daily.

Surgical. If the limbal epibulbar dermoids are producing visual disturbance or an obvious cosmetic blemish, they can be excised. It is important to keep in mind that limbal dermoids may involve the entire thickness of the cornea.

Therefore, it is advisable to remove only the part elevated from the cornea, followed by the diamond burr to smooth the surface flush with the normal cornea. If a large area of cornea is involved, it may be necessary to do a lamellar transplant.

Dermolipomas that bulge between the lids temporally should be removed with caution. If there is a pilosebaceous area with cilia present, it can be removed along with the lipomatous mass underlying the conjunctiva. Large excisions of the epidermalized conjunctiva should be avoided, as should excision of fat beyond the anterior orbit.

Repair of the upper eyelid coloboma is dependent on the size and degree of corneal exposure. Small colobomas are better left alone. If the defect involves the entire tarsus but the cornea is protected, the repair can be done when the child is a good anesthetic risk. If the cornea shows signs of mechanical injury or exposure keratopathy despite lubricants, repair should be undertaken. It is necessary to freshen the edges of the coloboma vertically to prevent notching and possibly to use stay sutures across the incision to prevent separation.

A lacrimal obstruction is usually not amenable to probing, and dacryocystorhinotomy is usually necessary.

Supportive. Parents should be aware that only 10 per cent of those affected with oculoauriculovertebral dysplasia may be retarded.

Ocular or Periocular Manifestations

Choroid: Coloboma.
Conjunctiva: Dermolipoma; epibulbar dermoid.
Cornea: Dermoid; hypesthesia; keratoconus; microcornea.
Extraocular Muscles: Duane's retraction syndrome; strabismus.
Eyelids: Coloboma (upper eyelid); ptosis.
Globe: Anophthalmos; exophthalmos; microphthalmia.
Iris: Atrophy; coloboma.
Lacrimal System: Dacryocystitis; obstruction of nasolacrimal duct; punctal or canalicular atresia or absence.
Orbit: Dermolipoma; hypoplasia.
Other: Amblyopia, astigmatism; cataract; persistent pupillary membrane.

PRECAUTIONS

Because of cervical vertebral abnormalities, the neck may not extend sufficiently, making intubation for general anesthesia very difficult. Tracheostomy may be necessary in these cases.

Care must be exercised in approaching limbal dermoids; since many of them involve full-thickness cornea, corneal perforation may result from attempting complete removal. It is far better to remove only the part that protrudes from the corneal surface. In some cases following surgery, there can be conjunctival overgrowth resembling a pterygium.

Radical excision of a dermolipoma could result in foreshortening of the lateral fornix, inadvertent removal of the palpebral portion of the lacrimal gland, or injury to the levator or lateral rectus muscles. Therefore, removal of only the part that is visible between the eyelids is recommended.

Although most colobomas will not produce exposure keratopathy, large colobomas must be watched closely for signs of exposure, especially those that are close to the midline. After repairing a coloboma, there is usually tethering of the upper eyelid, resulting in a ptosis that may require correction in the future.

COMMENTS

Corneal dermoids cause a disturbance of vision by encroachment on the visual axis or distortion by the induced astigmatism. Despite removal, strabismus and amblyopia may follow and require further therapy.

The diagnosis of Goldenhar's syndrome should lead to complete examination for associated systemic abnormalities, especially cardiovascular, renal, genitourinary, and gastrointestinal defects.

References

Bowen DI, Collum LMT, Rees DO: Clinical aspects of oculo-auriculo-vertebral dysplasia. Br J Ophthalmol 55:145–154, 1971.

Geeraets WJ: Ocular Syndromes, 3rd ed. Philadelphia, Lea & Febiger, 1976, p 194.

Mortada A: Orbital dermo-lipoma with Goldenhar's syndrome and exophthalmos. Br J Ophthalmol 53:786–788, 1969.

Peyman GA, Sanders DR, Goldberg MF (eds): Principles and Practice of Ophthalmology. Philadelphia, WB Saunders, 1980, pp 2235, 2409.

Sargent RA, Ousterhout DK: Ocular manifestations of skeletal diseases. *In* Harley RD: Pediatric Ophthalmology, 2nd ed. Philadelphia, WB Saunders, 1983, pp 1041–1044.

Zion VM, Billet E: Musculoskeletal disorders. *In* Duane TD (ed): Clinical Ophthalmology. Hagerstown, MD, Harper & Row, 1982, Vol V, pp 29:1–20.

ROBIN SEQUENCE
(Pierre Robin Syndrome, Robin Anomalad)

G. FRANK JUDISCH, M.D.

Iowa City, Iowa

Robin sequence is a disorder characterized by the triad of micrognathia (mandibular hypoplasia), glossoptosis (posterior and inferior displacement of the tongue), and usually, though not invariably, some degree of posterior clefting of the secondary palate. It is currently thought that the most probable initiating event is the development of mandibular hypoplasia before 9 weeks in utero. This shifts the tongue posteriorly, interposing it between the merging palatine shelves and precluding their normal fusion. The palatal defect in these patients is usually U-shaped, conforming to the contour of the posteriorly placed tongue, as opposed to the inverted V-shape of the cleft palates caused by intrinsic abnormalities in the palatine shelves. This difference in cleft shapes is considered strong evidence in support of the mandible-tongue pathogenesis in Robin clefts.

Although once considered a specific syndrome, it is now known that many individuals with the Robin sequence are otherwise entirely normal. However, about 25 per cent of Robin patients also have definitive syndromes for which specific but varying genetic counseling is indicated, whereas about 35 per cent have one or more additional abnormalities that fail to constitute a recognized syndrome. Of the syndromes known to be associated with the Robin sequence, the Stickler syndrome is the most common. The Robin sequence is also a common finding in the camptomelic syndrome, the cerebrocostomandibular syndrome, and persistent left superior vena cava syndrome. Rarely, it is seen with the Beckwith-Wiedemann syndrome, fetal alcohol syndrome, fetal hydantoin syndrome, diastrophic dwarfism, congenital myotonic dystrophy, and congenital spondyloepiphyseal dysplasia.

Abnormalities associated with the Robin sequence as a part of a broader pattern of malformation include, in decreasing order of frequency, positional limb deformities; cardiovascular defects; microcephaly; dental, ear, genital, and thoracic anomalies; short neck; renal dysplasia; and pyloric stenosis.

Respiratory and feeding difficulties, which may be present at birth or may develop over the first few weeks, are the most serious symptoms. The glossoptosis permits the tongue to act like a ball valve, blocking inspiration while permitting expiration. Depending on the severity of the obstruction, cyanosis, acidosis, failure to thrive, and cor pulmonale may develop. The respiratory problems are compounded by feeding difficulties and choking fits that are ascribed to malposition of the tongue, in addition to the palatal defect.

Only 10 to 20 per cent of Robin sequence patients also have one or more ocular anomalies. Congenital glaucoma is usually of the open-angle type. Several ocular lesions have been reported with the Robin sequence that do not represent a specific entity; strabismus is the most common of these. Some of the earlier reported eye abnormalities in Robin sequence seem to be examples of unrecognized Stickler syndrome.

THERAPY

Ocular. The eye abnormalities seen with the Robin sequence are not therapeutically unique and are treated as if they were isolated findings. The glaucoma is typical of congenital glaucoma and is responsive to the usual surgical proce-

226 / ROBIN SEQUENCE

dures for congenital glaucoma. This is further discussed in the section on infantile glaucoma.

Surgical. Infrequently, a surgical procedure, such as some variant of the Douglas procedure or a Kirshner wire, may be necessary to fix the tongue anteriorly. A tracheostomy is the last resort in those patients unresponsive to everything else.

Supportive. Most Robin sequence patients can be effectively managed by strict attention to proper placement in an absolutely prone position. The respiratory and feeding problems usually become progressively less marked as the child develops. By 4 to 6 months of age, jaw growth and neuromuscular development in the area usually eliminate further obstruction and swallowing difficulties. Palate surgery may, in some cases, be delayed until 3 to 4 years of age, as long as the palatine shelves continue to develop toward the midline. Continued growth of the mandible usually produces an essentially normal profile by 4 to 6 years of age.

Ocular or Periocular Manifestations

(R) refers to Robin sequence; (S) indicates Stickler syndrome.
Globe: Microphthalmos (R).
Iris: Coloboma (R).
Retina: Detachment (S); perivascular pigmentary retinopathy (S).
Other: Cataract (R, S); congenital glaucoma, usually open-angle glaucoma (R, S); high myopia (S); strabismus (R); vitreoretinal degeneration (S).

PRECAUTIONS

The Stickler syndrome should be one of the first considerations for the ophthalmologist evaluating a Robin sequence patient because of its serious and prominent ocular features. It is one of the most common autosomal dominant connective tissue disorders among those of predominantly North European ancestry. As soon as permissible, a complete eye examination should be performed, using sedation or general anesthesia, if necessary; particular attention should be used in the evaluation for glaucoma, myopia, and retinopathy. With early recognition of the Stickler syndrome, blindness may be prevented by glaucoma treatment or prophylactic treatment of the retinopathy. If a diagnosis of the Stickler syndrome is made, the need for close ocular follow-up as well as appropriate genetic counseling cannot be overemphasized.

COMMENTS

Although the reported incidence of Robin sequence is about 1/30,000 live births, it is probably more common. A relatively recent study reported, a 26 per cent mortality; all of the deaths occurred within the first 3 months. Obviously, any mortality figure will be greatly influenced by the severity of the Robin sequence in the patients studied. If they survive infancy, the prognosis for these patients is good, although as many as 20 per cent may exhibit major mental retardation, depending on the severity of Robin sequence and the presence of additional anomalies.

Interdisciplinary systemic evaluation for an associated syndrome or concomitant anomalies should be strongly encouraged. This helps ensure an accurate diagnosis, which is mandatory for appropriate treatment and counseling.

References

Blair NP, et al: Hereditary progressive arthro-ophthalmopathy of Stickler. Am J Ophthalmol 88:876–888, 1979.
Bush PG, Williams AJ: Incidence of the Robin anomalad (Pierre Robin syndrome). Br J Plast Surg 36:434–437, 1983.
Cohen MM Jr: The Robin anomalad—its nonspecificity and associated syndromes. J Oral Surg 34:587–593, 1976.
Cosman B, Keyser JJ: Eye abnormalities and skeletal deformities in the Pierre Robin syndrome: A balanced evaluation. Cleft Palate J 11:404–411, 1974.
Edwards JRG, Newall DR: The Pierre Robin syndrome reassessed in the light of recent research. Br J Plast Surg 38:339–342, 1985.
Hanson JW, Smith DW: U-shaped palatal defect in the Robin anomalad: Developmental and clinical relevance. J Pediatr 87:30–33, 1975.
Lewis MB, Pashayan HM: Management of infants with Robin anomaly. Clin Pediatr 19:519–528, 1980.
Pasyayan HM, Lewis MB: Clinical experience with the Robin sequence. Cleft Palate J 21:270–276, 1984.
Smith JD: Treatment of airway obstruction in Pierre Robin syndrome. A modified lip-tongue adhesion. Arch Otolaryngol 107:419–421, 1981.
Smith JL, Stowe FR: The Pierre Robin syndrome (glossoptosis, micrognathia, cleft palate). A review of 39 cases with emphasis on associated ocular lesions. Pediatrics 27:128–133, 1961.
Smith JL, Cavanaugh JJA, Stowe FC: Ocular manifestations of the Pierre Robin syndrome. Arch Ophthalmol 63:984–992, 1960.
Spranger J et al: Errors of morphogenesis: Concepts and terms. J Pediatr 100:160–165, 1982.
Williams AJ et al: The Robin anomalad (Pierre Robin syndrome)—a follow up study. Arch Dis Child 56:663–668, 1981.

WAARDENBURG'S SYNDROME
(Klein-Waardenburg Syndrome)
ANGELO M. DIGEORGE, M.D.
Philadelphia, Pennsylvania

Waardenburg's syndrome is a rare genetic disorder involving the pigmentary, auditory, and ocular systems. Three subtypes have been delineated; all are inherited in an autosomal dominant fashion. Hirschsprung's disease (aganglionic megacolon) has been reported in association with Waardenburg's syndrome in several dozen patients (both type I and type II). A few instances of atretic lesions of the gastrointestinal tract and one of atresia of the vagina have also been associated.

Type I is characterized by lateral displacement of the medial canthi (dystopia canthorum) and of the inferior lacrimal punctae. This leads to shortening of the palpebral fissures (blepharophimosis) and reduced visibility of the medial parts of the sclera, giving the mistaken impression of strabismus. The distance between the medial canthi is increased, but the distances between the pupils and between the lateral canthi are normal.

Other characteristics include partial or total heterochromia of the irides, a white forelock or premature graying of the hair, congenital sensorineural deafness, prominence of the nasal root, hyperplasia of the medial portions of the eyebrows, hypoplasia of the alae nasi, and full lips. Penetrance of the components of the syndrome varies. The laterally displaced medial canthus is present in virtually all patients who carry the gene for the type I disorder; whereas, the manifestations of heterochromia iridum, white forelock, and deafness each occur in only about one third of affected patients. Ptosis has been noted in six patients; in two instances, it was related to the Horner syndrome, and in two others, it was of the Marcus Gunn type.

Type II is characterized by the pigmentary disorder and the deafness, but lateral displacement of the medial canthi is absent. The prominence of the nasal root and synophrys occur less often, but the white forelock and heterochromia iridum develop in about the same percentage of patients as in type I. Deafness occurs in slightly over 50 per cent of affected patients and is usually bilateral.

Type III has been reported in only a few patients and consists of the type I syndrome in association with hypoplastic upper limb anomalies.

All the congenital anomalies in this syndrome, as well as associated disorders, such as aganglionic megacolon, are thought to be related to a primary defect in migration of cells of the anterior neural crest.

THERAPY

Supportive. All individuals with the Waardenburg syndrome should be subjected to careful audiometric studies. Unilateral or partial hearing loss may be easily overlooked in the absence of testing.

Other family members should be examined for evidence of the syndrome, and genetic counseling should be provided, particularly in regard to the risk of recurrence of deafness.

Surgical. The lateral displacement of the inferior lacrimal punctae occasionally leads to chronic dacryocystitis. Nasal transposition of the lacrimal punctae and medial canthi may be indicated to remedy this defect.

Ocular or Periocular Manifestations

Choroid or Retina: Hypopigmentation; hypoplasia.
Cornea: Cornea plana; microcornea.
Eyebrows: Hyperplasia of medial portion; poliosis; synophrys.
Eyelids: Blepharophimosis; caruncle hypoplasia; epicanthus; lateral displacement of medial canthi.
Lacrimal System: Lateral displacement of inferior punctae; lengthening of lacrimal canaliculi.
Lens: Lenticonus; microphakia.
Other: Heterochromia (partial or total).

PRECAUTIONS

One should be aware of the rare associations such as Hirschsprung megacolon or genital anomalies.

COMMENTS

The type I disorder has been reported twice as frequently as type II. The laterally displaced canthi (in type I) are critical clues in the detection of affected infants who may not manifest heterochromia or the other pigmentary changes. Detection of this condition can lead to early recognition of deafness.

References

Curri ABM, et al: Associated developmental abnormalities of the anterior end of the neural crest: Hirschsprung's disease-Waardenburg syndrome. J Pediatr Surg 21:248–250, 1986.
DiGeorge AM, Olmsted RW, Harley RD: Waardenburg's syndrome. A syndrome of heterochromia of the irides, lateral displacement of the medial canthi and lacrimal puncta, congenital deafness, and other characteristic associated defects. J Pediatr 57:649–669, 1960.
Goldberg ME: Waardenburg's syndrome with fundus and other anomalies. Arch Ophthalmol 76:797–810, 1966.
Goodman RM, et al: Absence of a vagina and right sided adnexa uteri in the Waardenburg syndrome: A possible clue to the embryological defect. J Med Genet 25:355–357, 1988.
Hageman MJ, Delleman JW: Heterogeneity in Waardenburg syndrome. Am J Hum Genet 29:468–485, 1977.
Klein D: Historical background and evidence for dominant inheritance of the Klein-Waardenburg syndrome (Type III). Am J Med Genet 14:231–239, 1983.
Meire F, et al: Waardenburg syndrome, Hirschsprung megacolon, and Marcus Gunn ptosis. Am J Med Genet 27:683–686, 1987.
Waardenburg PJ: A new syndrome combining developmental anomalies of the eyelids, eyebrows and nose root with pigmentary defects of the iris and head hair and with congenital deafness. Am J Hum Genet 3:195–253, 1951.

SECTION 13

PHAKOMATOSES

ANGIOMATOSIS RETINAE
(Angiomatosis of the Retina and Central
Nervous System, Retinal and Optic Disc
Capillary Hemangiomas, Retinal Capillary
Hamartoma, Retinal Hemangioblastoma, von
Hippel-Lindau Disease, von Hippel's Disease)

JOHN J. WEITER, M.D., Ph.D.
Boston, Massachusetts

Angiomatosis retinae is characterized by congenital capillary angiomatous hamartomas of the retina and optic nerve. If there are associated central nervous system and visceral angiomas, the condition is called von Hippel-Lindau disease. The retinal angiomas are usually diagnosed when the patient is between 10 and 30 years old. Central nervous system and visceral tumors are frequently noted after the ocular symptoms become manifest. The mode of transmission of these angiomas is autosomal dominant with incomplete penetrance and variable expressivity. There is no well-established predilection for sex or race. The retinal tumors are often multiple and are bilateral in more than 50 per cent of the cases. Approximately 20 per cent of patients with retinal angiomas develop central nervous system tumors.

These ocular angiomas may develop in the retina, optic nerve head or peripapillary retina, or the retrobulbar portion of the optic nerve. The retinal angiomas usually arise from the inner (endophytic) layers of the retina and are discrete angiomas, whereas the peripapillary angiomas frequently arise from the outer (exophytic) retinal layers and are diffuse.

These angiomas consist of masses of capillaries that tend to exhibit an embryonic appearance (hemangioblastoma) and often have abnormal fenestrations. Glial proliferation (astrocytes) separates the vascular channels and frequently contain large lipid-filled vacuoles, most likely representing astrocytic phagocytosis of leaking plasma. The retinal tumors are usually located at the equator or in the peripheral retina and have a propensity for the temporal side. The tumor characteristically remains stable or grows very slowly. With the gradual growth of these tumors, arteriovenous shunting usually occurs within the tumor, resulting in an increasingly dilated, tortuous, feeding artery and draining vein. With time, subretinal fluid and yellow exudate begin to accumulate around the lesion. There is also a tendency for the exudate to accumulate in the macular region as the tumor enlarges. (The visual change from this macular accumulation of exuda-

tion from a peripheral tumor is frequently the presenting sign). The endophytic tumors are frequently associated with vitreous traction that can lead to vitreous hemorrhage and a tractional retinal detachment that may be either rhegmatogenous or nonrhegmatogenous. The peripapillary angiomas tend to be endophytic and relatively flat, without feeding and draining vessels. Their clinical appearance is similar to outer retinal telangiectasia. Hemangiomas of the optic disc often clinically simulate papilledema or disc edema. Untreated retinal angiomatosis frequently leads to vitreous hemorrhage, total retinal detachment, secondary glaucoma, and phthisis bulbi.

THERAPY

Surgical. Since angiomatosis retinae is usually a progressive disease, therapy should be initiated as soon as the diagnosis is made. The treatment selected should depend upon the size and location of the tumor, the clarity of the ocular media, and the associated ocular complications. Argon laser photocoagulation or xenon arc photocoagulation has proven to be effective in the treatment of smaller tumors with a clear media. Treatment should consist of large spot size, low-intensity, and long-duration burns directed at the angioma itself. Multiple treatment sessions should be planned for all but the smallest tumors. The end point should be based on obliteration of the tumor by both clinical observation and fluorescein angiography. Once the tumor becomes yellowish in appearance secondary to gliosis and lipid ingestion, photocoagulation of the tumor becomes difficult because of poor penetrance of the laser light.

Anterior angiomas and larger posterior angiomas may be successfully treated by cryotherapy, using a repetitive freeze-thaw technique. Only two to three freeze-thaw cycles should be used at each therapy session in order to minimize the risk of hemorrhage. Multiple treatment sessions are usually required. Eradication of the tumor by either photocoagulation or cryotherapy usually results in resolution of the macular edema and improved visual acuity.

For large angiomas, angiomas not responding to photocoagulation or cryotherapy, and angiomas associated with retinal detachment, penetrating diathermy under a lamellar scleral bed has proven effective. If there is extensive subretinal exudation, the fluid should be drained and a scleral buckling procedure considered.

Frequently, large tumors develop surface membranes and vitreous traction that can lead to vitreous hemorrhage and/or rhegmatogenous retinal detachments. These complications may be amenable to treatment using vitreous surgery techniques, endodiathermy, or scleral buckling procedures.

The peripapillary and optic disc angiomas are difficult to treat without destroying useful central vision. Diffuse exophytic peripapillary hemangiomas with associated visual loss may be considered for laser photocoagulation, using a wavelength that spares the inner retina and is absorbed well by blood. Treatment should be conservative and aimed at the foci of greatest leakage.

Ocular or Periocular Manifestations

Globe: Phthisis bulbi.
Optic Nerve: Angioma; disc edema; hard exudates.
Retina: Angioma; circinate exudative retinopathy; dilated tortuous vessels; epiretinal membranes; exudate; hemorrhages; macular star exudation; retinal detachment.
Vitreous: Hemorrhage; proliferative vitreoretinopathy.
Other: Secondary glaucoma; visual loss.

PRECAUTIONS

Since these tumors are highly vascular, any form of treatment may cause further leakage or hemorrhage before the vascular channels are obliterated. This may result in further loss of vision from macular exudation, vitreous hemorrhage, and retinal detachment. Proliferative vitreoretinopathy frequently occurs after treatment of large tumors. Most of these complications are only an exacerbation of the normal course of the disease process. Many complications can be avoided by treatment of the angioma in multiple sessions, rather than an aggressive single-session treatment.

Treatment is best accomplished when the tumor is small. The visual prognosis is related to the size, location, and associated complications at the time that therapy is initiated. Early detection of a peripheral tumor results in a good prognosis, whereas large tumors with an associated retinal detachment or angiomas of the optic nerve have a less favorable prognosis. Since these tumors tend to be multiple and/or bilateral, it is important to have close follow-up once a tumor is diagnosed. Furthermore, since there is a familial tendency, other family members should be evaluated.

COMMENTS

Multiple tumors tend to occur frequently in the same quadrant of the retina. The earliest endophytic tumors tend to be in the peripheral retina. Subsequent tumors often occur proximally in the same quadrant, having the same feeding and draining vessels. Fluorescein angiography shows evidence of arteriovenous shunting of blood through the tumor with an associated relative hypoperfusion of the retina peripheral to the tumor, suggestive of a vascular steal syndrome. Although not proven, the subsequent, more proximal angiomas may very well represent a "neovascular angiomatous" reaction in a susceptible vascular bed.

Since approximately 20 per cent of patients presenting with retinal angiomas develop multiple systemic involvement including central nervous system tumors (von Hippel-Lindau syndrome), patients with angiomatosis retinae should have a thorough systemic evaluation. The cerebellar hemangioma is the typical central nervous system tumor in the von Hippel-Lindau syndrome and tends to occur somewhat later than the retinal angioma. The cerebellar tumor is similar to the retinal angioma in having large feeding and draining blood vessels and in histologic appearance. In the von Hippel-Lindau syndrome angiomas may also be found in the medulla oblongata, spinal cord, liver, or kidney. Cysts of the liver, pancreas, kidney, and epididymus are occasionally found, as well as a higher incidence of pheochromocytoma and renal cell carcinoma.

References

Annesley WJ Jr, et al: Fifteen-year review of treated cases of retinal angiomatosis. Trans Am Acad Ophthalmol Otolaryngol 83:446–453, 1977.
Font RL, Ferry AP: The phakomatosis. Int Ophthalmol Clin 12:1–50, 1972.
Machmichael IM: von Hippel-Lindau's disease of the optic disc. Trans Ophthalmol Soc UK 90:877–885, 1970.
Nicholson DH, Green WR, Kenyon KR: Light and electron microscopic study of early lesions in angiomatosis retinae. Am J Ophthalmol 82:193–204, 1976.
Shields JA: Diagnosis and Management of Intraocular Tumors. St. Louis, CV Mosby, 1983, pp 534–556.
Welch RB: von Hippel-Lindau disease: The recognition and treatment of early angiomatosis retinae and the use of cryosurgery as an adjunct to therapy. Trans Am Ophthalmol Soc 68:367–424, 1970.

NEUROFIBROMATOSIS
(von Recklinghausen Disease, NF-1)
RICHARD A. LEWIS, M.D., M.S.
Houston, Texas

Characterized as a distinct entity in 1882 by von Recklinghausen, classical neurofibromatosis, now designated NF-1, is among the most common inherited disorders in humans, with an estimated frequency of approximately 1 per 3000. About half of the affected individuals clearly inherit the disease from a parent as an autosomal dominant trait, whereas the disease in the other half of affected individuals results from a new genetic mutation, which once having occurred will also be transmitted in that same autosomal dominant fashion. For those afflicted individuals with a negative antecedent family history, about half give a history of advanced paternal age at the time of the index case's birth. The NF-1 gene has recently been localized to the pericentromeric region of chromosome 17. Linkages are not yet sufficient for accurate prenatal diagnosis.

The defining features of von Recklinghausen neurofibromatosis are 1) the presence of six or more hyperpigmented skin macules over 5 mm in greatest diameter in prepubertal individuals and over 15 mm in postpubertal individuals, usually described as café-au-lait spots; 2) two or more cutaneous neurofibromata or one plexiform neurofibroma; 3) and melanocytic hamartomata of the iris, eponymically termed Lisch nodules. Other characteristic features include axillary freckling (and freckling of other skin-apposed areas, such as the inframammary, inguinal, or gluteal creases), areolar neurofibromata (in 85 per cent of postpubertal females), neural crest tumors (meningiomas, pheochromocytomas, neurofibrosarcomas, and malignant schwannomas), cervicothoracic kyphoscoliosis, and distinctive osseous lesions, such as sphenoid dysplasia, thinning of the long bone cortex, or pseudoarthrosis. Both short stature and either relative or absolute (>97 percentile) macrocephaly may occur, as well as seizure disorders, overt mental retardation, learning disabilities, and school behavior problems in children and adolescents.

Usually, only café-au-lait spots are present from birth into the first year of life, although they may become darker and more numerous with age. Congenital plexiform neurofibromata may appear anywhere on the body, but have significance if they occur across the midline, especially if they have an overlying "pancake" zone of hyperpigmentation or if the tumor involves the orbit. Cutaneous and deep neurofibromata may be undetectable or minimal until puberty ensues. They may be punctiform or nodular on the eyelids and face or enlarge on the torso to be sessile or even pedunculated. Exacerbation of tumor growth also occurs in both puberty and pregnancy.

Ophthalmic features of von Recklinghausen neurofibromatosis may involve all tissues of the eyelid, orbit, and globe, except the crystalline lens. Extensive plexiform neurofibroma involving the lid and orbit may be associated with ipsilateral facial hemihypertrophy or asymmetric enlargement of orbital volume. Exophthalmos may occur either with diffuse orbital neurofibromatosis; with a tumor of specific tissue in the orbit, such as glioma of optic nerve or chiasm, meningioma, and astrocytoma; or with an occasionally pulsatile herniation of intracranial contents (meningocele, brain) into the orbit through a defect in the bony wall, most often involving a dysplasia of the sphenoid bone. Rarely, either pulsatile or nonpulsatile enophthalmos may occur.

Eyelids may show small café-au-lait spots or punctiform neurofibromata in about one third of cases. Although thickening of the upper lid margin by plexiform neurofibroma with S-shaped configuration of the upper outer one third is highly characteristic, it probably occurs in only 5 per cent of patients. Even though the association of congenital glaucoma with neurofibromatosis is well established, its occurrence in the absence of orbital or upper lid involvement is extremely rare.

THERAPY

Surgical. Close follow-up for early recognition of surgically amenable complications and surgical intervention at the earliest possible time are the only ways to minimize serious problems. Even then, surgery may not resolve the problem entirely, and at times surgery is not possible. Surgical removal of cutaneous neurofibromas should be reserved for those that are especially disfiguring or functionally compromising or both. In general, these tumors are progressive and radioresistant. The removal of orbital tumors may mandate optic nerve section and a definitive sacrifice of vision. The management of intracranial tumors is more problematic. Many anterior optic gliomas identified on routine scanning may not progress.

Supportive. Once the diagnosis of von Recklinghausen disease is made, genetic counseling explains that recurrence of the trait follows the classical pattern for autosomal dominant transmission with 100 per cent penetrance of the phenotype. However, the patient must be advised of the markedly variable expressivity, with the risk that at least 25 per cent of affected individuals will have moderate or severe disease.

For a patient's first-degree relative (parent, sibling, offspring) who is postpubertal and has no café-au-lait spots, neurofibromas, or Lisch nodules, counseling is also uncomplicated. It is unlikely that the individual is afflicted, and therefore his or her risk of producing affected children is essentially that of the general population.

Problematic individuals should be studied carefully for both defining and other characteristic features and followed as necessary for evolving problems. That evaluation may include 1) a detailed history of cognitive or psychomotor deficiencies, constipation, pain, and vision problems; 2) a family history of at least two antecedent generations; 3) physical examination evaluating systemic hypertension, scoliosis, macrocephaly, proptosis, iris Lisch nodules, short stature, precocious puberty or hypogonadism, café-au-lait macules, and cutaneous neurofibromas; and 4) contrast CT scan or paramagnetic contrast-enhanced MRI scans.

Ocular or Periocular Manifestations

Choroid: Melanocytic hamartomas ("nevi") (melanoma is reported, but the relative frequency compared to the general population is not established); neurofibroma.

Conjunctiva or Episclera: Neurofibroma.
Cornea: Prominent corneal nerves.
Eyelids: Café-au-lait spots or lentigines; plexiform neurofibroma; ptosis; punctate or nodular neurofibroma.
Globe: Buphthalmos (usually associated with orbital plexiform neurofibromas); intermittent or pulsatile exophthalmos or enophthalmos.
Iris or Ciliary Body: Ectropion uveae; Lisch nodules; melanoma (rare); neurofibroma (rare).
Optic Nerve: Glioma; meningioma.
Orbit: Bony asymmetry (orbital neurofibroma); dysplasia of orbital bones (sphenoid); enlarged optic foramen (optic nerve glioma).
Retina: Astrocytic hamartoma (extremely rare); a purported association with congenital myelinated nerve fibers has not been substantiated.

Precautions

No laboratory feature uniquely diagnoses von Recklinghausen NF-1, including histopathologic details of the primary lesions. Single gene molecular DNA probes are not yet available. In light of the defining features listed earlier, all persons afflicted with or at risk for neurofibromatosis should undergo a meticulous evaluation to define the diagnosis, to identify complications, and to monitor progression. That evaluation may include cranial CT scanning with or without contrast or paramagnetic contrast-enhanced MRI scanning, including the orbits and the optic chiasm; ophthalmologic consultation with emphasis on biomicroscopy and indirect stereo-ophthalmoscopy; electroencephalography; audiometry; and psychometric testing. The ophthalmologist must respect not only the problems and complications within his or her purview but also must recognize a 6 per cent lifelong risk for development of malignancy associated with this disorder. However, significant and progressive disfigurement and a heavy psychosocial burden are the most significant long-term complications.

Comments

Although von Recklinghausen NF-1 is the most recognized variant, several other entities can be confused with it. Bilateral acoustic neurofibromatosis, designated NF-2, is characterized by bilateral eighth nerve masses seen with appropriate imaging techniques; or a first-degree relative with NF-2 and either unilateral eighth nerve mass or two of the following: neurofibroma, meningioma, glioma, schwannoma, or juvenile posterior cortical lenticular opacities. NF-2 is also an autosomal dominant disease with a relative paucity of café-au-lait spots and cutaneous neurofibromas and has no other ocular signs except in the lens. NF-2 has been assigned to chromosome 22q2. Segmental neurofibromatosis, in which café-au-lait spots and neurofibromas are restricted to a single body segment and do not cross the midline, presumably occurs as a somatic (nonheritable) mutation. Multiple café-au-lait spots may occur as an autosomal dominant variant with no other systemic features. In addition, there is an "adult" neurofibromatosis, an apparently nonheritable variant, with neurofibromas, lipomas, and other tumefactions and no ocular features. This entity is as yet poorly understood and reported.

References

Barker D, et al: Gene for von Recklinghausen neurofibromatosis is in the pericentromeric region of chromosome 7. Science 236:1100–1102, 1987.
Holt JF: Neurofibromatosis in children. Am J Roentgenol 130:615–639, 1978.
Imes RK, Hoyt WF: Childhood chiasmal gliomas: Update on the fate of patients in the 1969 San Francisco study. Br J Ophthalmol 70:179–182, 1986.
Lewis RA, Riccardi VM: von Recklinghausen neurofibromatosis. Incidence of iris hamartomata. Ophthalmology 88:348–354, 1981.
Lewis RA, Gerson LP, Axelson KA, Riccardi VM, Whitford RP: von Recklinghausen neurofibromatosis II: Incidence of optic gliomata. Ophthalmology 91:929–935, 1984.
Martuza RL, Eldridge R: Neurofibromatosis 2 (bilateral acoustic neurofibromatosis). N Engl J Med 318:684–688, 1988.
Miller RM, Sparkes RS: Segmental neurofibromatosis. Arch Dermatol 113:837–838, 1977.
National Institutes of Health Consensus Development Conference: Neurofibromatosis: Conference Statement. Arch Neurol 45:575–578, 1988.
Riccardi VM: von Recklinghausen neurofibromatosis. N Engl J Med 305:1617–1627, 1981.
Seiff SR, et al: Orbital optic glioma in neurofibromatosis: Magnetic resonance diagnosis of perineural arachnoidal gliomatosis. Arch Ophthalmol 105:1689–1692, 1987.
Wright JE, McDonald WI, Call NB: Management of optic nerve gliomas. Br J Ophthalmol 64:545–552, 1980.

STURGE-WEBER SYNDROME
(Encephalotrigeminal Syndrome)

F. HAMPTON ROY, M.D.
Little Rock, Arkansas

The Sturge-Weber syndrome is a congenital malformation that is characterized by angiomatosis that involves the central nervous system, skin, and eye. The complete syndrome includes intracranial and facial hemangiomas with an ipsilateral choroidal hemangioma and often glaucoma. Along with epilepsy, hemiplegia, hemianopsia, and mental deterioration, meningeal angiomatosis must be also considered in this disorder. The port-wine nevus or nevus flammeus is generally distributed over the branches of the trigeminal nerve and is usually unilateral. The ocular significance of Sturge-Weber syndrome is its frequent association with glaucoma and cho-

232 / STURGE-WEBER SYNDROME

roidal hemangioma. Glaucoma is caused by high episcleral venous pressure, which results in arteriovenous shunting in episcleral and intrascleral hemangiomas.

THERAPY

Ocular. Because the high intraocular pressure is caused by high episcleral venous pressure, medical treatment to reduce aqueous formation or to improve aqueous outflow is not very effective. It can narrow the gap between the intraocular pressure and episcleral venous pressure, but cannot lower intraocular pressure below the episcleral venous pressure.

One per cent epinephrine twice daily or 4 percent pilocarpine four times a day can improve aqueous outflow. Reduction of aqueous formation can be accomplished with a beta blocker, such as 0.5 per cent timolol twice daily. Oral administration of 5 mg/kg of acetazolamide four times daily in infants or young children or up to 1 gm daily in older children and adults may be indicated if topical ophthalmic therapy is inadequate.

Surgical. Goniotomy and trabeculotomy are usually ineffective. Trabeculotomy, however, is the treatment of choice when medical therapy of glaucoma proves inadequate and the optic disc is becoming damaged by the elevated intraocular pressure. A large choroidal effusion may form during surgery. This can be anticipated and treated by a posterior sclerotomy over the ciliary body for drainage before entering the anterior chamber. If trabeculotomy fails, cryotherapy may be used as a last resort.

Supportive. Cosmetics are helpful to camouflage the facial blemishes as skin lesions are usually too extensive to be treated surgically. Anticonvulsant medications are indicated for epilepsy, but the seizures may be difficult to control.

Ocular or Periocular Manifestations

Anterior Chamber: Blood reflux in Schlemm's canal; wide angle.

Choroid: Hemangioma.
Conjunctiva: Episcleral and conjunctival hemangioma; increased vascularity.
Eyelids: Port-wine stain.
Globe: Buphthalmos.
Optic Nerve: Cupping.
Other: Anisometropia; facial port-wine stain; hemianopsia; increased corneal diameter; increased intraocular pressure; retinal detachment; visual loss.

PRECAUTIONS

The age of onset of glaucoma is unpredictable and seldom symptomatic. Therefore, frequent examinations are essential.

Port-wine nevus has no propensity to regress. Although cryosurgery is useful in treating some hemangiomas, it has proved inadequate for producing regression of the port-wine nevus.

COMMENTS

Early diagnosis and treatment of elevated intraocular pressures are essential and, if instituted early, can lower intraocular pressure to prevent visual loss. When the facial area supplied by both the ophthalmic and maxillary division of the trigeminal nerve is involved, there is a 15 per cent chance of glaucoma and a 30 per cent chance of the patient being a glaucoma suspect and having elevated intraocular pressure. Patients with only mandibular involvement seldom have glaucoma.

References

Cibis GW, Tripathi RC, Tripathi BJ: Glaucoma in Sturge-Weber syndrome. Ophthalmology 91:1061–1071, 1984.
Phelps CD: The pathogenesis of glaucoma in Sturge-Weber syndrome. Ophthalmology 85:276–286, 1978.
Shihab ZM, Kristan RW: Recurrent intraoperative choroidal effusion in Sturge-Weber syndrome. J Pediatr Ophthalmol Strabismus 20:250–252, 1983.

SECTION 14

NEUROLOGIC DISORDERS

ACUTE IDIOPATHIC POLYNEURITIS
(Acute Febrile Polyneuritis, Acute Infectious Polyneuritis, Fisher's Syndrome, Guillain-Barré Syndrome, Inflammatory Polyradiculoneuropathy, Landry-Guillain-Barré-Strohl Syndrome, Landry's Paralysis, Postinfectious Polyneuritis)

KAY-UWE HAMANN, M.D.
Hamburg, Germany

The nosology of acute idiopathic polyneuritis remains obscure. It is a reversible paralytic disease of unknown etiology and pathogenesis, usually starting with complaints of symmetric bilateral weakness involving the extremities, most likely the legs, and emerging into an ascending type of paralysis involving the respiratory muscles and eventually causing bulbar paralysis. In about 35 per cent of all patients, a previous harmless viral infection can be traced, though this disease may follow a variety of other disorders. An inflammatory infiltration of the nerve roots suggesting a lymphocyte-mediated autoimmune reaction probably against the myelin of the peripheral nerve has been reported. On cerebrospinal fluid examination, a high protein level with poor cellular response confirms the diagnosis. However this finding is not a prerequisite to establish the diagnosis, though certain features of the syndrome are closely linked to the albuminocellular dissociation.

The ocular findings in the bulbar variant include a painless, rapidly progressive ophthalmoplegia with bilateral symmetric involvement, mimicking a supra- or internuclear disorder of ocular motility. The lid elevators are affected only to a lesser degree. The autonomic nervous system serving pupillary function, accommodation, and lacrimal secretion may or may not be spared, and corneal sensation may be reduced. The appearance of papilledema in inflammatory polyneuritis is rare. The different evolution of impairment of ocular motility in both eyes renders the diagnosis more difficult; however, the presence of facial diplegia virtually precludes other disorders. Fisher's syndrome comprises the ophthalmoplegic variant of acute idiopathic polyneuritis, including oculomotor palsies, areflexia, and ataxia.

THERAPY

Systemic. The vague knowledge of this syndrome makes an assessment of therapeutic trials difficult. The treatment that is most widely employed consists of corticosteroids in full doses with low-salt diets and precautions against peptic ulcerations. Although beneficial effects following steroid medication have been reported, oral administration of 45 to 60 mg of prednisone[‡] daily is still a matter of controversy, since controlled studies revealed the inefficacy of this drug, as well as detrimental side effects. Immunosuppressive drugs[‡] are used sparsely, but no affirmative report on this medication is available.

Ocular. In the patient with facial and trigeminal involvement, the cornea is threatened by the development of exposure and neuroparalytic keratitis. Lack of lacrimal secretion compounds the problem. To prevent ulceration of the cornea and epidermalization of the conjunctiva, precautions to moisten the cornea by using artificial tears, to shield the eye by producing a moist chamber, or to employ permanent or temporary tarsorrhaphies should be taken. Paresis or paralysis of one of the oculomotor nerves is treated by patching as soon as diplopia ensues. Strabismus surgery is not considered until the stability of the deviation is proven and prism balance is tolerated. Correction of the ptosis and the extraocular muscles should not be performed in one procedure. Decreased accommodation may require reading glasses employing convergence prisms. Papilledema resolves spontaneously.

Supportive. If the vital capacity declines below 800 to 1000 ml, mechanical respiratory assistance and tracheostomy are required to maintain oxygen supply with minimal positive-pressure breathing during mechanical ventilation. Secretions from the tracheobronchial tree are removed and pulmonary infections combatted. The support of blood pressure in the face of hypotension completes the therapeutic regimen. The best results are obtained in an intensive care unit under the surveillance of a skilled staff. Under these circumstances, the mortality rate can be reduced from 20 to 5 per cent. Physiotherapy and orthopedic procedures should be initiated for the long-term permanent muscle weakness and contractures.

Ocular or Periocular Manifestations

Cornea: Exposure keratitis; keratoconjunctivitis sicca; neuroparalytic keratitis.

Extraocular Muscles: Gaze paresis (in symmetric involvement); internuclear ophthalmoplegia of abduction; paresis or paralysis of the third, fourth, or sixth nerve.

234 / ACUTE IDIOPATHIC POLYNEURITIS

Eyelids: Ectropion; lagophthalmos; ptosis.
Optic Nerve: Hemorrhages; papilledema.
Pupil: Anisocoria; dilation lag.
Other: Decreased accommodation; dyschromatopsia; photophobia; scotoma.

PRECAUTIONS

Patients with the tentative diagnosis of acute idiopathic neuropathy require prompt attention and surveillance. It is an anxiety-laden experience for the patient and the next of kin alike, and the approach to this patient should be thoughtful. The physician should not hesitate to admit the patient to an intensive care unit if the vital capacity drops. The clinical course is variable, and permanent paralysis ensues in 5 to 10 per cent of all patients. Children have a greater tendency for residual weakness; skeletal deformity before skeletal maturity is achieved presents a further hazard.

COMMENTS

Acute idiopathic polyneuritis causes long-term disability secondary to paresis and paralysis of various muscles. The various specialists—the neurologist, the plastic and orthopedic surgeons, and the ophthalmologist—should be consulted to elicit functional impairment, to initiate proper therapeutic procedures, and to mitigate permanent disability.

References

Asbury AK, Arnason BG, Adams RD: The inflammatory lesion in idiopathic polyneuritis. Its role in pathogenesis. Medicine *48*:173–215, 1969.
Ashworth B: Ophthalmoplegia in the Guillain-Barré syndrome. Trans Ophthalmol Soc UK *93*:207–211, 1973.
Banerji NK, Millar JHD: Guillain-Barré syndrome in children, with special reference to serial nerve conduction studies. Dev Med Child Neurol *14*:56–63, 1972.
Behan PO, Geschwind N: The ophthalmoplegic form of the Guillain-Barré syndrome: An immunologic study. Acta Ophthalmol *51*:529–542, 1973.
Grunnet ML, Lubow M: Ascending polyneuritis and ophthalmoplegia. Am J Ophthalmol *74*:1155–1160, 1972.
Hamann K-U: Die dissoziierte Ophthalmoplegie der Abduktion; hintere "internukleäre" Ophthalmoplegia im Rahmen eines Fisher-Syndroms. Ophthalmologica *178*:365–372, 1979.
Hughes RAC, et al: Controlled trial of prednisolone in acute polyneuropathy. Lancet *2*:750–753, 1978.
Morley JB, Reynolds EH: Papilledema and the Landry-Guillain-Barré syndrome. Brain *89*:205–222, 1966.
Pollard JD, McLoad JG, Gatenby P, Kronenberg H: Prediction of response to plasma exchange in chronic relapsing polyneuropathy. J Neurol Sci *58*:269–287, 1983.
Ravin H: The Landry-Guillain-Barré syndrome. A survey and a clinical report of 127 cases. Acta Neurol Scand *43*:(Suppl) 9–64, 1967.
Sherman WH, Olarte MR, McKiermann G, Sweeney K, Latov N, Hays AP: Plasma exchange treatment of peripheral neuropathy associated with plasma cell dyscrasia. J Neurol Neurosurg Psychiat *47*:813–819, 1984.

BELL'S PALSY
(Idiopathic Facial Paralysis)

THOMAS R. HEDGES, JR., M.D.,
Philadelphia, Pennsylvania

and THOMAS R. HEDGES, III, M.D.
Boston, Massachusetts

Bell's palsy is a unilateral facial nerve paralysis of sudden onset and gradual recovery that involves the nerve as it runs through the Fallopian canal. The cause is unknown, although ischemic (vascular), autoimmune, and viral theories of etiology are currently popular. Definable causes of a facial paralysis must be ruled out by a thorough examination of the ears, nose, throat, and cranial nerves. If there are any doubts about the clinical findings, computerized tomographic scanning with special attention to the temporal bones should be considered.

Early ipsilateral symptoms of Bell's palsy include aching in the ear or mastoid, tingling or numbness of the cheek or mouth, alteration of taste, hyperacusis, epiphora, ocular burning, blurred vision, and facial weakness. Ocular complications are caused by lagophthalmos, ectropion of the lower lid, and decreased tear output; increased evaporation and poor tear distribution further compound the problem. Corneal erosion, infection, and ulceration may also occur.

Late ocular manifestations are caused by permanent damage and aberrant regeneration of the facial nerve. These include motor synkinesis (reverse jaw winking), which is characterized by contracture of the facial muscle (a twitch of the corner of the mouth or a dimpling of the chin that occurs simultaneously with every blink); facial contracture, with an ipsilaterally deepened nasolabial fold; and autonomic synkinesis (crocodile tears), where tearing occurs with meals. Several months after Bell's palsy, there may be mild generalized (mass) contracture of the facial muscles, rendering the affected palpebral fissure more narrow than the opposite one.

In addition to Bell's palsy, facial paralysis may be caused by pontine lesions (stroke, multiple sclerosis, tumor); cerebellopontine angle disorders (tumor, sarcoidosis, meningitis); geniculate ganglion infection (herpes zoster oticus); otitis media, parotid gland disease (tumor, inflammation); congenital malformation, and trauma.

THERAPY

Systemic. A short course of high-dose steroids may dramatically relieve pain when it is present and may decrease the incidence of late complications, such as aberrant regeneration of the facial nerve, in cases of severe paralysis. A daily dosage of 60 mg of prednisone for the first 7 to 10 days with rapid tapering thereafter is recommended.

Histamine,[‡] niacin,[‡] diphenhydramine,[‡] and cromolyn[‡] are of no proven benefit.

Ocular. In most cases of Bell's palsy, topical

ocular therapy is sufficient to prevent the complications of corneal exposure. An artificial tear preparation instilled frequently during the day, with a bland ophthalmic ointment containing petrolatum used at bedtime, works well. Occasionally, ointment must be instilled around the clock on a three-times-a-day basis. Although ointment blurs the patient's vision, makes the lids sticky, and is messy, it is usually well tolerated for a few weeks. If an associated conjunctivitis should occur, an antibiotic ointment should be used.

Hydrophilic soft contact lens in conjunction with lubricating drops shows real promise in preventing corneal exposure. The old problem of keeping a contact lens in position on the cornea in the presence of lagophthalmos appears to be much easier to manage with this lens.

Lid taping with clear plastic tape or applying a pressure patch can be used for 1 or 2 days to help heal corneal erosions. Upper lid closure can also be accomplished with a lid suture placed in mattress fashion through the skin of the upper lid, taping the ends firmly to the upper cheek to close the eyelid. Because of the danger of infection, the lid suture should only be used as a temporary measure when recovery is imminent. A final method uses clear plastic wrap, 8 by 10 cm, applied with generous amounts of ointment as a nighttime occlusive bandage.

Moisture chambers are bulky affairs and are seldom necessary. Wraparound sunglasses are useful for the patient who is comfortable indoors, but suffers outdoors because of wind exposure.

Lower lid ectropion or droop can be temporarily helped by tape applied below the lid margin in the center of the lower lid, pulling the lid laterally and upward to anchor on the orbital rim.

Surgical. Surgery for Bell's palsy is done for three reasons: to decompress the facial nerve, to correct lid abnormalities, and to restore dynamic lid closure.

Surgery to decompress the facial nerve is controversial, based on experimental evidence that immediate facial nerve decompression prevents nerve degeneration. It is used in complete Bell's palsy patients who have not responded to medical therapy and who show evidence of facial nerve degeneration by electrodiagnostic testing. More than 1 week after the onset of the palsy, surgery is probably of no benefit.

Surgery to correct lower lid droop and ectropion includes tarsorrhaphy, lid shortening, tarsoconjunctival ellipse, and canthoplasty. Lateral tarsorrhaphy is very useful in patients with mild orbicularis oculi palsy and lagophthalmos. It decreases horizontal lid opening and allows an effective blink, better support of the precorneal lake of tears, and better coverage of the eye during sleep. Horizontal lid wedge shortening accomplishes these same objectives, but is not reversible, unlike lateral tarsorrhaphy. In severe permanent palsy, these procedures are not useful by themselves because lid laxity will recur.

Epiphora due to punctal eversion with mild laxity of the lower lid can be treated by excising a horizontal tarsoconjunctival ellipse of tissue inferior to the lower lid punctum (protecting the canaliculus with a probe) and suturing the edges of the ellipse together. Punctal eversion associated with severe lid laxity requires medial canthoplasty combined with horizontal shortening of the lower lid and tarsoconjunctival ellipse. Severe lid laxity of a permanent nature often requires lateral canthoplasty that supports the lower lid from the lateral orbital rim.

A host of ingenuous devices have been invented to restore dynamic lid closure in cases of severe symptomatic lagophthalmos. All overcome the elevator action of the levator palpebrae superioris muscle. A weight-adjustable magnet, palpebral spring, or silicone-encircling band can be inserted into the lids. These devices require frequent patient examination for adjustment and are subject to infection, breakage, and extrusion of the mechanism.

Finally, temporal muscle transplant, or reinnervation of the facial nerve through cross-facial nerve grafting or hypoglossal-facial nerve anastomosis, can be used in cases of significant permanent paralysis to help restore relatively normal function to the orbicularis oculi muscle or eyelids.

Ocular or Periocular Manifestations

Cornea: Erosion; infection; ulcer.
Extraocular Muscles: Paresis or paralysis of orbicularis oculi muscles.
Eyelids: Ectropion; lagophthalmos; paralysis; ptosis.
Lacrimal System: Epiphora.
Other: Decreased visual acuity; diplopia; ocular irritation.

PRECAUTIONS

A careful examination looking for possible causes of facial paralysis must be performed. Bell's palsy rarely occurs with other cranial nerve palsies or brainstem signs. Facial palsy in children may be caused by pontine glioma; whereas in young and middle-aged adults, facial palsy can be the early sign of a cerebellopontine tumor.

Aberrant regeneration of the facial nerve must be differentiated from spastic paretic facial contracture, spastic facial contracture and myokymia associated with multiple sclerosis, and hemifacial spasm. Aberrant regeneration of the facial nerve is recognized by the abnormal contraction of the facial muscles, usually a twitch at the corner of the mouth, that occurs only and simultaneously with every blink. Even if the history and physical findings are characteristic of aberrant regeneration of the facial nerve, a brainstem mass lesion must be ruled out by neuroradiologic evaluation if associated brainstem signs are present.

Lid taping and application of a loose pressure patch should be avoided in obtunded patients or those with pre-existing corneal hypesthesia. Even with the most diligent nursing, the loose patch or tape will often move out of position and

236 / BELL'S PALSY

expose or even erode into the cornea. A firm-splinted, properly applied pressure dressing with lids firmly closed is an excellent temporary procedure, however.

COMMENTS

Bell's palsy is more common in adults, diabetics, and predisposed families. It recurs in 3 to 10 per cent of patients either on the same or opposite side. Prognosis for complete recovery of mild cases is almost universally good and occurs in a few days to weeks. In severe paralysis, recovery may be prolonged for several months, especially in the elderly patient; in 15 to 25 per cent of these cases, permanent facial weakness and aberrant regeneration of the facial nerve may result. The treatment of Bell's palsy should be conservative, guided by the severity and probable prognosis in each particular case. Electrodiagnostic tests can help improve accuracy of prognosis in problem cases. Topical ocular therapy is successful in all but severe or prolonged cases. In these cases, the best procedure is a lateral tarsorrhaphy. This procedure eliminates the necessity of constant drops and ointments, improves cosmesis by eliminating lid sag while preserving vision on the affected side, and can be taken down wholly or in part whenever recovery occurs.

References

Fisch U: Surgery for Bell's palsy. Arch Otolaryngol 107:1–11, 1981.

Jelks GW, Smith B, Bosniak S: The evaluation and management of the eye in facial palsy. Clin Plast Surg 6:397–419, 1979.

Katusic SK, et al: Incidence, clinical features, and prognosis in Bell's palsy, Rochester, Minnesota, 1968–1982. Ann Neurol 20:622–627, 1986.

Levine RE: Management of the eye in facial paralysis. Otolaryngol Clin North Am 7:531–544, 1974.

Mitchell JM, Smith JL: Spastic paretic facial contracture. In Smith JL: Neuro-Ophthalmology Update. New York, Masson, 1982, pp 239–246.

Wepman B, Baum JL: Ocular findings in Bell's palsy. Ophthalmology 86:1943–1946, 1979.

Wolf SM, et al: Treatment of Bell palsy with prednisone: A prospective randomized study. Neurology 28:158–161, 1978.

BENIGN INTRACRANIAL HYPERTENSION AND PSEUDOTUMOR CEREBRI

SATOSHI KASHII, M.D.,
WILLIAM L. BASUK, M.D.,
and RONALD M. BURDE, M.D.

Bronx, New York

The term "pseudotumor cerebri" (PTC) is commonly used to describe a condition charac-

terized by raised intracranial pressure (ICP), with normal cerebrospinal fluid (CSF) constituents and bilateral papilledema, in the absence of hydrocephalus or space-occupying lesions. ICP, when measured, is usually elevated, but may vary from normal to very high. The term "benign intracranial hypertension" (BIH) was introduced by Foley to describe such patients without known cause. Over time, the two terms have been used interchangeably. This article uses the term "idiopathic intracranial hypertension" (IIH) for that form of the disease for which no cause is known, thus eliminating the implication of the term "benign." Four criteria are proposed for diagnosis of IIH: 1) elevated CSF pressure (>200 mm Hg), 2) normal CSF composition (CSF protein concentration may be low, <20 mg/dl), 3) symptoms and signs restricted to those of elevated ICP, and 4) normal neuroimaging studies, excluding nonspecific findings of increased ICP (CT scans may demonstrate small, slit-like ventricles).

The use of some medications and certain disease conditions have induced or been associated with a disese state that mimics IIH. Since there is a hint of causality, the authors prefer to call this condition secondary IIH. Therapeutic use of drugs producing secondary IIH include systemic corticosteroids (use and withdrawal), nalidixic acid, nitrofurantoin, and tetracycline in children. Hypervitaminosis A produced by the use of vitamin A or its congener, retinoic acid, used for treating various skin disorders consistently produces secondary IIH. Systemic conditions, such as hypoparathyroidism, iron-deficiency anemia, systemic lupus erythematosis (SLE), periarteritis nodosa, and sarcoidosis, may produce secondary IIH. In addition, dural sinus thrombosis following such entities as middle ear infection, the use of oral contraceptives, pregnancy, and SLE with circulating cardiolipins can produce secondary IIH.

The peak incidence of IIH occurs during the third decade, and there is a significant predominance in females. The ratio of females to males ranges from approximately 2:1 to 10:1. Obesity is a common finding (44 to 90 per cent). Thus, the typical patient is a young obese female. Although the literature indicates that the condition is self-limited to 3 to 9 months in most patients, IIH is now considered by many to be a chronic disease that requires careful follow-up. Recurrence rate has been low, usually less than 10 per cent; but a recrudescence may occur many years later.

The mechanisms underlying increased ICP in IIH is unknown. Using the compartmental model of Foley; there are four possible mechanisms that could lead to elevated intracranial pressure: 1) increased blood volume, 2) increased CSF production, 3) decreased absorption, or 4) parenchymal brain edema. At the present time, decreased absorption of CSF is the most-often invoked theory. It is postulated that in IIH there is a relative obstruction to CSF absorption across the arachnoid villi. Decreased absorption could be caused by increased resistance within the villi themselves or by an increase in the draining venous system. In the latter case, there is a reversed normal gradient between the sinus and subarachnoid space. Increased resistance to CSF outflow (absorption block) has been demonstrated by studies utilizing intrathecal saline infusion and radioisotope cisternography. Thus, it would appear that IIH is somewhat analogous to primary open-angle glaucoma.

Similarly, it is believed that the secondary IIH associated with hypovitaminosis A and acute systemic corticosteroid withdrawal are caused by an increase in arachnoidal resistance.

It can be argued that the finding of smaller-than-normal ventricles on CT scanning in primary or secondary IIH excludes an increase in resistance to CSF absorption as a possible mechanism. In fact, it has been shown that the normalization of the CSF pressure is associated with an increase in ventricular volume into normal range. This suggests that parenchymal edema may be the underlying pathogenetic mechanism.

The supposition that parenchymal edema is the cause of IIH has been supported by altered cerebrovascular reactivity at the capillary-venule level, and it has been postulated that changes in vascular permeability result in parenchymal edema. However, a CSF absorption block could also result in cerebral interstitial edema. Elevated CSF pressure could produce an increase of transependymal transport of CSF fluid from ventricular spaces into brain tissues. Although a 33 per cent increase in cerebral blood volume was noted in one series, it was pointed out that this would produce a 1 per cent increase in intracranial contents, far less than needed to sustain an elevation in ICP. Some compensatory increase in cerebral blood volume would be expected as an autoregulatory response of the cerebral vasculature to elevated ICP. Evidence to support the theory that hypersecretion of CSF is the cause of IIH is contradictory. Therefore, individual patients may have different underlying causative mechanisms in primary and secondary IIH.

Headache is the initial symptom in 99 per cent of the patients seen by neurologists, but in only 80 to 85 per cent of those who initially see an ophthalmologist. The headache is usually generalized in nature, is worse early in the morning, and is exacerbated by anything that produces a Valsalva maneuver and in some by head turning.

Other symptoms of IIH are related to the visual system. Transient visual obscurations (TVOs) are a presenting symptom in 46 to 72 per cent of patients. TVOs usually last between 1 and 5 seconds and rarely more than 30 seconds. It is postulated that the increased ICP produces a relative decrease in perfusion of the prelaminar disc, leading to further compromise of capillary perfusion. This failure of perfusion is secondary to an increase in the intrinsic tissue pressure in the optic nerve. Superimposed upon this, a transient alteration of the perfusion pressure to the nerve head by suddenly standing up, bending over, or a transient increase in the intraocular pressure by rubbing of the eyes will produce TVOs.

The only serious complications of this condition are loss of visual field or loss of central vision. The characteristic visual field abnormalities in IIH are disc related and mimic those defects associated with glaucoma. Thus, if one single test is to be used to follow patients with this disease process, it would be a quantitative visual field, either kinetic or static. Enlarged blind spots are found in virtually all patients with papilledema. These have been attributed to displacement and detachment of the peripapillary retina by the swollen axons, but recently this blind spot enlargement has been demonstrated to be refractive in nature. In addition, in patients with papilledema there are often peripapillary choroidal folds or striae that can increase the size of the blind spot and remain enlarged long after the papilledema has disappeared. Initially, peripheral nerve fiber involvement causes constriction of the visual field, progressing to nasal depression and steps and then overt arcuate defects. When sufficient nerve fiber loss occurs, visual acuity is reduced. One study noted that 21 per cent of patients with IIH sustained loss of visual acuity (8 per cent—less than 20/40), as well as severe field loss.

Occasionally, patients with papilledema may experience acute visual loss. Mechanical distortion of the peripapillary tissues can cause a break in Bruch's membrane, allowing the formation of subretinal neovascular capillary net. Transudation or overt bleeding from this membrane can spread to the macular area. Central retinal vein occlusion has also been reported to cause acute visual loss in these patients. Superimposed anterior ischemic optic neuropathy with acute field defects has been reported to occur in patients with IIH. Whether this is a fortuitous occurrence or is pathogenetically associated is not known.

Diplopia, when present, is almost always horizontal and is a unilateral or bilateral sixth nerve palsy. This is a nonspecific effect of increased pressure on the abducens nerves as they course through the subarachnoid space. Rare reports of skew deviation, III, and fourth nerve palsies are to be found. In addition, paralysis of the seventh nerve has also been reported. How these findings relate to the disease process is not clear. Such findings should place the diagnosis of primary IIH in question.

Patients may experience dizziness, nausea, vomiting and other nonspecific symptoms. None of these symptoms correlates well with recorded CSF pressure, appearance of the papilledema, or the ultimate prognosis.

If a patient presents with signs and symptoms of IIH and neuroimaging technique has excluded the presence of an intracranial mass lesion, a spinal tap is indicated to measure the ICP and to assess the constituents of the CSF. If the pressure is not elevated on one or two successive taps, 24-hour monitoring of the ICP is indicated. In IIH, there is free communication of spinal subarachnoid with intracranial subarachnoid space. ICP can be readily and simply monitored

BENIGN INTRACRANIAL HYPERTENSION AND PSEUDOTUMOR CEREBRI

by inserting a catheter into the lumbar subarachnoid space and connecting it to a transducer. Interestingly, patients with IIH and florid papilledema frequently have a normal ICP during the day, whereas during rapid eye movement (REM) sleep, their ICP reaches heights of systemic arteriolar pressure. Thus, in patients suspected to have IIH whose ICP on spinal tap is normal, a baseline must be obtained over a 24-hour period, including REM sleep. Repeated CSF taps late in the course of the disease are only indicated in the face of progressive visual dysfunction despite appropriate intervention.

As mentioned previously, continuous monitoring of visual fields and measurement of visual acuity, as well as sequential fundus photographs, are fundamental in the follow-up care of patients with IIH. Because therapy for IIH is determined by the degree and progression of visual dysfunction, it has been suggested by some that specific visual field strategies should be employed. Because of the similarity of visual field loss in IIH and glaucoma, kinetic perimetry utilizing the modified Armaly-Drance strategy has been recommended for routine examinations. Automated threshold static perimetry (e.g., Octopus program 32 or Humphrey 30-1) has been advocated by others who feel that it may be a more sensitive methodology for detecting visual field change. Visual function testing should be carried out at regular intervals, the length of which should be determined by the patient's clinical condition. Slitlamp examination with measurement of intraocular pressure is necessary at regular intervals if systemic corticosteroids are used.

THERAPY

Systemic. Severe and intractable headaches and evidence of optic neuropathy (i.e., visual dysfunction) are the primary reasons for initiating treatment. Visual loss when present at the time of the first examination is considered by some to be an indication for intensive therapy.

No prospective randomized study comparing various treatments has been done. Although there are claims of a high spontaneous remission rate for IIH, there are no controlled data on the natural history of untreated IIH. Some patients only briefly experience symptoms of IIH that may disappear after the initial diagnostic tap, and it is difficult to know whether reported improvements are the result of treatment or simply represent the natural course of the disease.

The first line of therapy in the treatment of IIH is the systemic use of carbonic anhydrase inhibitors (CAIs). CAIs have been shown to decrease CSF secretion in humans following intravenous bolus injections of 1 gm of acetazolamide.[§] CSF production is inhibited for approximately 2 hours after such an injection. Daily doses of 60 mg/kg (2 to 4 gm) of acetazolamide[§] in its sustained release form in divided doses effectively lower ICP, even in patients with mass lesions. The side effects from the use of acetazolamide are for the most part dose related and may be bothersome at a dose as little as 500 mg daily. These side effects include drowsiness; tingling of the fingers, toes, and circumoral region; metalic taste; nausea; and anorexia. The use of the drug is associated with a metabolic acidosis accompanied by an alkalization of the urine, reducing the solubility of oxylate and predisposing susceptible individuals to the development of calcium oxylate stones. Unfortunately, it has been shown that lower daily doses as acetazolamide (0.5 to 2.5 gm) are ineffective in lowering ICP or relieving symptoms. It is known that methazolamide more readily penetrates the blood-brain barrier, and it has been postulated to be effective in relatively lower doses, thus reducing some side effects but not the drowsiness. Although the use of CAIs reduces the serum concentration of potassium, total intracellular stores are not affected. The metabolic acidosis remains relatively constant.

CAIs are sulfonamides and therefore can produce an idiosyncratic agranulocytopenia or aplastic anemia; thus, a baseline complete blood count is indicated. In addition, the sulfonamides have been reported to be teratogenic and should be used with caution during pregnancy.

In spite of apocryphal statements to the contrary, there is little evidence available demonstrating the efficacy of thiazide diuretics, furosemide,[‡] or ethacrynic acid[‡] in treating IIH. In an uncontrolled study, chlorthalidone,[‡] a long-acting thiazide, has been reported to be effective in treating IIH.

Oral hyperosmotic agents can acutely lower ICP. A single dose of 1 gm/kg of glycerol will raise serum osmolality from 295 to 320 mosm/l in 90 minutes and concomitantly reduce CSF pressure for 3 to 5 hours. Obviously, treatment would be required every 4 hours. Glycerin is extraordinarily fattening and can produce either ketoacidosis or nonketotic hyperosmolar coma. The taste of glycerin is terribly sweet and often so nauseates patients that they cannot swallow; it can be made more tolerable by diluting it with orange juice and serving it over ice. A reversed osmotic gradient and a rebound increase in ICP can occur. In addition, glycerin is metabolized and can have an adverse effect on serum glucose concentration. Isosorbide, which is not metabolized, can be substituted for glycerin at a dose level of 2 cc/kg. The use of hyperosmotics in IIH should be limited to a few days in an attempt to "break" the cycle.

Cardiac glycosides[‡] have been reported to reduce CSF production, but the efficacy of such therapy has never been substantiated.

If CAIs do not relieve the symptoms or a patient cannot tolerate their side effects, a 2-week course of oral corticosteroids (60 mg of prednisone daily) may be instituted. If remission occurs, it is noted usually within 4 days of the start of prednisone therapy. If there is no response by the end of the first week, the corticosteroids should be discontinued. Prednisone treatment can be discontinued after 2 weeks of therapy without a recrudescence of the disorder. It is curious that both the use of and the withdrawal of systemic corticosteroids have been associated with the onset of IIH.

It is well known that long-term use of systemic corticosteroids can raise intraocular pressure and cause posterior subcapsular cataracts, but such side effects are unlikely to occur with a short course. On the other hand, the increase in intraocular pressure caused by the use of orally administered corticosteroids for an injudicious amount of time may act as the final insult to produce ischemic damage of the optic nerve head. The systemic side effects are of greater importance. The immediate effects of systemic corticosteroids include aggravation of underlying hypertension and disturbance in control of serum glucose in susceptible individuals. They also have a profound effect on mentation, causing insomnia, a hyperactive state, or depression. The long-term effects of variably induced Cushing's syndrome are well known.

Surgical. Because no single drug or combination of medications has proven to be effective or tolerated in patients with IIH, surgical intervention should be contemplated before serious visual loss has developed. Most physicians choose to demonstrate progressive visual field loss before recommending surgery, but the finding of significant visual field loss at the time of the initial examination may itself prove to be an indication for intervention.

Multiple or repeated spinal punctures are mentioned only for historical interest. A lumbar puncture has a short-lived effect on CSF pressure. The CSF pressure returns to pretap levels within 60 to 90 minutes, unless an inadvertent nip is made in the meninges at the time of the tap. Most patients find the experience of a spinal tap so unpleasant that the suggestion of multiple taps causes them either not to seek help (thus, taking the chance of developing visual dysfunction) or seeking help elsewhere.

Subtemporal decompression has been generally abandoned because of significant morbidity and mortality. It has been replaced by CSF shunting procedures. Lumboperitoneal shunts are preferable to ventricular shunts; because the ventricles are by definition normal or small in size in patients with IIH, access is technically difficult. A lumbar cisternogram is usually done before shunting to ensure patency of the subarachnoid space. The major problem associated with lumboperitoneal shunts are 1) testing their patency because of the surrounding adipose tissue as these patients are usually obese and 2) the high rate of shunt failure caused by obstruction. Cervical-peritoneal shunting was proposed to solve this problem, but no large series has been forthcoming.

Optic nerve sheath decompression is considered by many to be the procedure of choice in preventing the visual dysfunction associated with chronic papilledema. Technically, there are two ways to approach the optic nerve: with or without orbitotomy. However, using the operative microscope, the medial approach has become standard for most surgeons. This approach has a low operative morbidity, and by operating on the medial aspect of the optic nerve, the critical foveomacular projection is avoided. This approach is also a relatively safe method of access to the retrobulbar optic nerve in order to obtain tissue and fluid for chemical and cytologic analysis.

Under local anesthesia, a peritomy is made, and the medial rectus muscle is detached from the globe. The globe is retracted laterally to expose the optic nerve. A window is cut in the optic nerve dural sheath nasally, just posterior to the globe, utilizing an operating microscope to avoid the myriad of vessels in the region where the nerve arises from the globe. Some prefer to make multiple longitudinal slits. Improvement in disc edema may not occur for weeks, but visual function ordinarily begins to improve within days. The presence of preoperative disc pallor (early optic atrophy) does not necessarily indicate a poor prognosis. This procedure does not affect the ICP and rarely relieves contralateral papilledema. Therefore, optic nerve sheath decompression is thought to affect and improve local factors contributing to intravaginal fluid accumulation and disc edema, usually without alteration of ICP.

There is substantial evidence both clinically and experimentally that unilateral optic nerve sheath decompression effectively produces a bilateral defervescence of papilledema. The variable results with respect to the contralateral side are thought to be caused by variations in the meshwork of the subarachnoid space at the optic canal that connects intracranial meningeal space to intraorbital meningeal space. In addition, whether the meninges collapse around the nerve, thereby sealing the subarachnoid space, or whether the fenetration procedure remains patent affects the results. The meshwork appears to play an important role in determining the extent to which the entire subarachnoid space is decompressed by a unilateral or bilateral optic nerve decompression.

This procedure is extraordinarily effective in preventing further deterioration of visual function, but has a variable effect on the headache. Complications include transient asymmetry of the pupils, probably from trauma to posterior ciliary nerves, horizontal motility disturbances from disinsertion of the medial rectus muscle, and recurrence of papilledema. Early failure is usually due to orbital tissue plugging the fenestration site, and late failure is due to inadequate decompression of the multiple meshwork channels.

Ocular or Periocular Manifestations

Extraocular Muscles: Abducens nerve palsy.
Optic Nerve: Papilledema, optic nerve atrophy, opticocilliary shunt vessels.
Retina: Choroidal folds, subretinal neovascular membrane.
Other: Visual field defect—enlargement of the blind spot and generalized constriction, nasal (especially inferonasal) loss, central, paracen-

tral and cecocentral scotomas, and altitudinal patterns of loss.

PRECAUTIONS

The single most important risk factor associated with visual loss in a patient with IIH is systemic hypertension. Rapid lowering of an elevated blood pressure may contribute to ischemic damage of the optic disc in the presence of papilledema with compromised perfusion of the prelaminar nerve. This is especially true in patients with secondary IIH undergoing hemodialysis for chronic renal failure, in whom hypotensive episodes are more common.

Obese hypertensive females seem to be at greatest risk for visual field defects. Weight reduction by diet has been advocated as a treatment of IIH. Others have suggested surgically induced weight loss by gastric exclusion to stabilize the visual function. The relationship of obesity to the pathogenesis of IIH is uncertain. It has been postulated that estrone produced exclusively by adipocyte (via the aromatization of circulating androstenedione) could increase the rate of CSF production. In obese females, who have a reduced absorptive capacity of CSF, this combination of factors could result in IIH. It has been the experience of most physicians dealing with this patient population that dieting and weight loss are unachievable goals, thus leaving only the options of medical or surgical intervention.

COMMENTS

IIH may be benign from the standpoint that it is not life threatening, but it should not be considered benign in the functional sense because it can produce devastating visual loss. Permanent visual loss in adults with IIH occurs in from 6 to 25 per cent of patients. Moreover, permanent visual impairment can occur in children as well. Hypothalamic-hypophyseal dysfunction has been attributed to increased ICP. It is postulated that long-standing intracranial hypertension may weaken the diaphragm sellae and through uncertain mechanisms allow the pituitary gland to be flattened against the floor of the sella turcica, producing a so-called empty sella syndrome. Rare cases of chiasmal herniation into the sellae with concomitant visual field loss have been reported. Even when the pituitary gland is flattened against the floor of the sella, endocrine function appears to remain normal, although it is suggested that pituitary dysfunction may eventually develop.

Supported in part by an unrestricted grant from RPB, New York.

References

Amaral JF, et al: Reversal of benign intracranial hypertension by surgically induced weight loss. Arch Surg 122:946–949, 1987.

Beatty R: Cervical peritoneal shunt in the treatment of pseudotumor cerebri. J Neurosurg 57:853–855, 1982.

Brourman ND, Spoor TC, Ramocki JM: Optic nerve sheath decompression for pseudotumor cerebri. Arch Ophthalmol 106:1378–1383, 1988.

Corbett JJ: Problems in the diagnosis and treatment of pseudo-tumor cerebri. Can J Neurol Sci 10:221–229, 1983.

Corbett JJ, et al: Results of optic nerve sheath fenestration for pseudotumor cerebri. Arch Ophthalmol 106:1391–1397, 1988.

Foley J: Benign forms of intracranial hypertension— "toxic" and "otitic" hydrocephalis. Brain 18:1–41, 1955.

Hupp SL, Glaser JS, Frazier-Byrne S: Optic nerve sheath decompression. Arch Ophthalmol 105:386–389, 1987.

Kaye AH, Galbraith JEK, King J: Intracranial pressure following optic nerve decompression for benign intracranial hypertension. J Neurosurg 55:453–456, 1981.

Keltner JL: Optic nerve sheath decompression. Arch Ophthalmol 106:1365–1369, 1988.

Kilpatrick CJ, et al: Optic nerve decompression in benign intracranial hypertension. Clin Exp Neurol 18:161–168, 1981.

Sergott RC, Savino PJ, Bosley TM: Modified optic nerve sheath decompression provides long-term visual improvement for pseudotumor cerebri. Arch Ophthalmol 106:1384–1390, 1988.

Tse DT, et al: Optic nerve sheath fenestration in pseudotumor cerebri. Arch Ophthalmol 106:1458–1462, 1988.

BLINDNESS

ROBERT L. BERRY, M.D.

Little Rock, Arkansas

Blindness is defined as correctable distant visual acuity of 20/200 or poorer in the better eye or a visual field of less than 20° in its widest diameter. There are an estimated 15 million totally blind people in the world today. The leading causes of blindness in the world are trachoma, cataract, onchocerciasis, and xerophthalmia.

Within the United States, approximately 0.5 million people are considered legally blind. Of these, 53 per cent are 65 years of age or older. In order of decreasing frequency, the causes of legal blindness in the United States are glaucoma, macular degeneration, senile cataract, optic nerve atrophy, diabetic retinopathy, and retinitis pigmentosa. In total, these diagnoses account for 51 per cent of the blind persons. Trauma accounts for only 4 per cent of blindness in the United States, whereas hereditary or congenital conditions account for some 20 per cent. Of these, the most widespread hereditary condition is retinitis pigmentosa, followed by prenatal cataract, congenital glaucoma, albinism, and congenital optic nerve atrophy. Genetic counseling is resulting in a gradual decrease in new hereditary cases of blindness.

THERAPY

Supportive. The major role of the ophthalmologist in treatment of the newly blinded person is to offer psychologic support. When the blinded patient is psychologically ready, the ophthalmologist should speak plainly yet compassionately and advise him or her of the inevitable need for personal adjustment. The physician should make proper referrals to the appropriate rehabilitative services as soon as the patient has begun to accept the disability. The quicker the patient can return to the mainstream of life, the fewer psychologic problems will be encountered. Sometimes, the blind patient becomes severely depressed and may require the services of a psychiatrist. It is important that the legally blind person be evaluated by a low-vision professional to ensure that all of his or her full vision potential is being used. Genetic counseling is necessary when the cause of blindness is hereditary. This counseling service should be provided to help families live more comfortably with the disease that affects them and to help with family planning decisions.

PRECAUTIONS

The psychologic reaction to blindness is often overwhelming, particularly if it has occurred suddenly. These patients are members of a psychiatrically high-risk population. Anxiety, low self-esteem, and depression may result in suicidal tendencies. An open and supportive relationship between physician and patient is essential for the promotion of good mental health. It is important that the physician not offer false hope to the patient or the family. It is also important that the physician ensure the patient and family that a blind person can live a full and productive life. Ophthalmologists may have unfounded feelings of guilt and consequently are uncomfortable when dealing with blind patients. It is essential that physicians accept that they cannot cure all blindness and that they learn to be more comfortable and communicate with their blind patients.

COMMENTS

The number of visually impaired or partially sighted persons in the United States is estimated to be 11 million. Of these, 3.4 million are monocularly blind, and a small proportion have a defective but not blind second eye. Because these individuals have the potential for improved vision, low-vision clinics and optical aids should be recommended by ophthalmologists.

New devices are being developed every day to help blind persons live more normal and productive lives. Electronic devices, including talking calculators and watches, sonar sensor canes, and auditory aids are now available; however, these aids may not be affordable by the majority of the blind.

References

Hatfield EM: Estimates of blindness in the United States. Sight-Saving Rev 43:69–80, 1973.
Hiatt RL: World blindness. J Tenn Med Assoc 80:403–406, 1987.
National Society to Prevent Blindness: Vision Problems in the U.S. New York, National Society, 1980.
Perry EC, Roy FH: Light in the Shadows: Feelings about Blindness. Little Rock, World Eye Foundation, 1982.

CEREBRAL PALSY
(Brain Damage Syndrome, Perinatal Encephalopathy)

PETER BLACK, B.Sc., M.B., F.R.C.S., D.O.
Gorleston, England

Cerebral palsy is a group of conditions of widely differing etiologies caused by brain damage that is produced either before, during, or after birth. These disorders have broadly similar and fairly characteristic clinical pictures. They are nonprogressive, but not unchanging, and are dominated by the motor abnormality, with which convulsions, emotional instability, mental subnormality, speech defects, and abnormalities of hearing and vision are commonly associated. The brain damage may occur in utero secondary to infections with rubella or cytomegalovirus and placental insufficiency. It may occur during birth or in the immediate perinatal period and may be related to prematurity, intracranial hemorrhage, hypoxia, hypoglycemia, hyperbilirubinemia, or accidents during labor and delivery. The brain damage may also occur after the perinatal period from such causes as accidental and nonaccidental injury, meningitis, cerebral abscess, and intracranial hemorrhage. Some 10 per cent of affected children have cerebral palsy for no known reason, and a very small number have familial cerebral palsy. In any unselected population of children with these disorders, there are a few with well-defined, recognizable clinical syndromes.

Cerebral palsy is usually classified according to the motor abnormality and its topography. Spastic, athetoid, and ataxic forms are the most common, with mixed forms also being found. With the exception of purely athetoid cerebral palsy, it is rarely possible to localize the sites of the intracerebral lesions. The widely differing nature of the disabilities is a reflection of the diffuse nature of the lesions. This is supported by postmortem studies.

Abnormalities of the visual apparatus are common; the incidence of ocular changes has been reported between 50 and 80 per cent. The range

242 / CEREBRAL PALSY

of disorders is wide, with refractive errors, squint, amblyopia, visual field defects, nystagmus, and optic atrophy being particularly common. Spastic types of cerebral palsy are most likely to have associated ocular abnormalities, and athetoid types the least. There is evidence that the incidence of ocular abnormalities increases with the degree of mental subnormality. The problems caused by the ocular abnormalities are compounded by visual-spatial and perceptual difficulties.

THERAPY

Ocular. Refractive errors should be fully corrected after the instillation of a cytoplegic. Depending on the age of the child, 1 per cent atropine or 1 per cent cyclopentolate may be used. For older children with any degree of mental subnormality or abnormal head movements, a subjective refraction is rarely possible and a cycloplegic refraction is necessary. At the same time, the fundus can be examined by indirect ophthalmoscopy. Anisometropia of sufficient degree to cause amblyopia must be detected at an early enough age to allow conventional treatment with occlusion of the "good" eye and visual stimulation of the amblyopic eye to be carried out.

Strabismus is detected in the usual manner. Full correction of refractive error based on cycloplegic refraction must be given, followed by occlusion of the squinting eye and orthoptic treatment, if necessary. Rarely, this treatment may entail the use of appropriate prisms. The aim is to give the child binocularity or at least good vision in both eyes before surgery, if indicated.

There is some evidence that successful treatment of squint may improve the coordination in such children. Defects of retina and optic nerve associated with squint must be identified to prevent treatment in eyes in which there is no hope of improving vision.

Surgical. For nonaccommodative esotropia and exotropia, recession and resection of the appropriate muscles are usually adequate. The degree to which the horizontal muscles are weakened or strengthened must be determined by repeated observations because of the variable angles often found in squints in these children. Particularly when squints present a purely cosmetic problem and one eye has a very poor vision that cannot be improved, the aim should be to undercorrect the deviation because overcorrections are common. Vertical deviations are fairly common, most of which are manifest as overaction of the inferior oblique muscles. There are several causes for this deviation. In these cases, simple recession of the inferior oblique muscles is satisfactory.

In children with bilateral cataract, lens aspiration or lensectomy/vitrectomy may be carried out. Surgery for unilateral cataract is not advised. Rarely, other abnormalities amenable to surgical treatment, such as congenital glaucoma, may be seen and should be treated along standard lines.

Supportive. The aim of examination is to identify at an early age those ocular defects that are treatable and to undertake such treatment as if the child were otherwise normal. Of equal importance is to identify those children with severe visual handicap that is not amenable to therapy. The ophthalmologist is then in a position to counsel the parents on the placement of the child in the correct educational environment. As well as the parents, those responsible for assessing the child's intellectual ability and those who will educate the child need to know of the child's visual status. Teachers, in particular, need to know the visual acuity, the size of the visual field, and the child's ability to match colors. Many of these children are deaf, and their education relies heavily on visual stimulation. The ophthalmologic findings cannot be taken in isolation. Assessment and treatment must be coordinated with other disciplines, and to this end, the ophthalmologist should be part of a team including psychologists, teachers, and other physicians concerned with the other disabilities. There is a continual need for reassessment as the child grows. Parents and teachers need constant reassurance. The aim of the ophthalmologist is to help provide the child with the best possible chance of attaining independence or minimizing the amount of institutional care required when the child leaves the shelter of school.

Ocular or Periocular Manifestations

Extraocular Muscles: Esophoria; esotropia; exophoria; exotropia; hypertropia; paralysis of the third, fourth, or sixth nerve.
Eyelids: Epicanthus; ptosis.
Iris: Coloboma; heterochromia.
Lens: Cataracts.
Optic Nerve: Atrophy; coloboma; hypoplasia.
Retina: Choroidoretinal scars; coloboma; pigmentary changes; retinopathy of prematurity.
Other: Amblyopia; astigmatism; gaze palsies; hypermetropia; leukoma; microphthalmos; myopia; nystagmus; visual field defect.

PRECAUTIONS

Examination of these children is often difficult, particularly those with mental subnormality. Subjective tests, such as those for visual acuity, are unreliable, and the examination may need to be repeated on several occasions before the ophthalmologist can be sure of the findings. It is easy to underestimate a child's visual performance, particularly in those with gross disturbances of motility, such as athetosis, and in those with hemianopic field defects. Young and severely handicapped children should be examined in familiar surroundings, if possible, with someone they know and trust alongside them. Doing so allays their fears and, in some cases, is necessary because children with speech disorders and deafness may need to have their responses interpreted. Topical drugs with known systemic side effects should be used with caution, since these children seem to be unusually prone to adverse reactions. This caution particularly applies to anticholinesterase drugs, such as echothiophate, since they may have an adverse effect on the child's behavior. For this reason, use of these drugs in accommodative esotropia is not recommended.

It is important that surgical therapy, usually for squint, be planned in conjunction with the other disciplines concerned with the medical care of the child, since these children are often submitted to multiple surgical procedures, particularly for musculoskeletal problems. Few guidelines exist on the management of squint in these children. The information available suggests that squints should be treated as if the child were otherwise normal.

Comments

It is apparent from the literature that visual problems in children with cerebral palsy are either overlooked or ignored because they are overshadowed by the more dramatic musculoskeletal and intellectual problems. The diagnosis of cerebral palsy has usually been made by the time that such a child attains 18 months of age. The initial ophthalmologic examination should also be made by then. At that time, treatment for probable amblyopia can be started or planned. Continued reassessment is necessary, particularly before the child starts his or her education and during schooling, so that appropriate decisions regarding training can be made at the earliest opportunity. The overall aim of the medical care and training is to enable the child to become independent. This aim will not be feasible in those who are severely handicapped, but this may not be apparent until the child reaches the second decade of life. All the help possible will be required by the child before then. To this end, all treatable defects should be identified at a sufficiently early age to enable appropriate measures to be carried out.

References

Black PD: Visual disorders associated with cerebral palsy. Br J Ophthalmol 66:46–52, 1982.
Douglas AA: The eyes in vision and infantile cerebral palsy. Trans Ophthalmol Soc UK 80:311–325, 1960.
Fantl EW, Perlstein MA: Refractive errors in cerebral palsy. Am J Ophthalmol 63:857–863, 1967.
Harcourt B: Strabismus affecting children with multiple handicaps. Br J Ophthalmol 58:272–280, 1974.
Hiles DA, Wallar PH, McFarlane F: Current concepts in the management of strabismus in children with cerebral palsy. Ann Ophthalmol 7:789–798, 1975.
O'Malley J, et al: An ophthalmic review of cerebral palsy in Queensland, 1980. Aust J Ophthalmol 9:91–95, 1981.

CHRONIC PROGRESSIVE EXTERNAL OPHTHALMOPLEGIA

(Abiotrophic Ophthalmoplegia, Chronic Progressive External Ophthalmoplegia with Ragged Red Fibers, Chronic Progressive Muscular Dystrophy, Kearns-Sayre-Daroff Syndrome, Kearns-Sayre Syndrome, Kearns-Shy Syndrome, Ocular Myopathy, Oculocraniosomatic Neuromuscular Disease, Oculopharyngeal Muscular Dystrophy Syndrome, Oculoskeletal Myopathy, Ophthalmoplegia Plus, Progressive Dystrophy of the Extraocular Muscles)

JOSEPH ESHAGIAN, M.D.
Los Angeles, California

Chronic progressive external ophthalmoplegia encompasses a conglomeration of diseases causing bilaterally impaired extraocular motility and blepharoptosis. It is called "external" ophthalmoplegia because the iris and ciliary body muscles are not affected. The onset of the disease may occur at any age, and about half of the cases are familial. These patients present with diplopia, blepharoptosis, poor vision, weakness, syncopal episodes, dysphagia and weight loss, or symptoms of exposure keratopathy. Chronic progressive external ophthalmoplegia usually has a slow, gradual onset with an insidious course. At the end stage, the eyes may be totally immobile, and there may be no levator action. Almost any of the body's skeletal muscles may be weak. When the face is involved, a myopathic or Hutchinson facies occurs.

The multitude of associated neurodegenerative disorders that may occur with chronic progressive external ophthalmoplegia include dysthyroid ophthalmopathy, myasthenia gravis, myotonic dystrophy, hereditary oculopharyngeal dystrophy, Bassen Kornzweig syndrome, Refsum's syndrome, progressive supranuclear palsy, symptomatic focal (neurogenic) ophthalmoplegia, abiotrophic ophthalmoplegia externa, muscular dystrophy, retinal pigmentary degeneration, retinitis pigmentosa with spastic quadraplegia or heart block, spongiform encephalopathy, and a generalized disorder of the nervous system, skeletal muscle, and heart resembling Refsum's disease and Hurler's syndrome (Shy).

Kearns and Sayre described the triad of retinitis pigmentosa, chronic progressive external ophthalmoplegia, and complete heart block. Daroff emphasized the spongiform encephalopathic aspect of this syndrome. Childhood onset, high cerebrospinal fluid proteins, abnormal muscle mitochondria, and ragged red fibers are associated with the Kearns-Sayre syndrome. Ragged red fibers are muscle fibers containing abnormal mitochondria and excessive amounts of subsarcolemmal and intermyofibrillar lipid droplets that stain red with the modified trichrome stain. However, no ragged red fibers were found in ophthalmoplegia patients with myasthenia

244 / CHRONIC PROGRESSIVE EXTERNAL OPHTHALMOPLEGIA

gravis, myotonic dystrophy, thyrotoxicosis, or Möbius syndrome. Therefore, it appears the chronic progressive external ophthalmoplegia with ragged red fibers and no positive family history represented a distinct entity, namely oculocraniosomatic neuromuscular (Olson's) disease, which may be differentiated histologically and clinically from the oculopharyngeal syndrome. Oculopharyngeal muscular dystrophy syndrome consists of progressive dysphagia, symmetric ptosis (usually of late onset, after the fourth decade), either sporadic or familial (autosomal dominant), and insidious onset with slow progression. The oculopharyngeal syndrome usually has rimmed vacuoles (on muscle biopsy) and does not have ragged red fibers. Unlike the Kearns-Sayre syndrome, oculopharyngeal "dystrophy" does not have central nervous system, retinal, or cardiac abnormalities.

THERAPY

Ocular. Certain ocular features of chronic progressive external ophthalmoplegia are remediable. The blepharoptosis may be treated with lid crutches, adhesive (Scotch) tape, or surgical repair. Lid crutches may prevent the eyelid from closing and may cause exposure keratopathy. Scotch tape usually does not keep the eyelid up because moisture causes the tape to slip. Therefore, most patients soon become unhappy with lid crutches and Scotch tape for treatment of the blepharoptosis.

Surgical repair of the blepharoptosis, with either a fascial sling brow suspension or levator surgery, is usually the most satisfactory treatment in properly chosen patients. In patients with more than 5 mm of levator function, resection, tucking, or advancement of the levator aponeurosis usually yields excellent results. When levator function is less than 5 mm, levatory surgery sufficient to lift the upper eyelid above the pupil may cause an inability of the eyelid to close fully; hence, exposure keratopathy may occur.

Exposure keratopathy may be aggravated at night, as many of these patients have poor Bell's phenomenon and some have dry eyes. Although these patients usually have weak orbicularis oculi muscles, they often have strong frontalis or brow muscles. It is presently generally felt that the best sling material for a suspension operation is autogenous fascia, which may be either obtained from the limb or from the temporalis. The usual measures of treating exposure keratopathy are advisable for chronic progressive external ophthalmoplegia and may include the use of artificial tears, bland ophthalmic ointment, humidification of the air, patching the eyes, swimmer's or protective goggles, closure of the lacrimal puncta, and pyridostigmine.

Base-down reading prisms may be helpful if voluntary downward gaze is severely limited. These patients usually see better with two pairs of glasses (one for near and the other for distance), rather than with bifocals.

Supportive. The dysphagia and aspiration (usually associated with the oculopharyngeal form of chronic progressive external ophthalmoplegia) may be treated with cricopharyngeal myotomy. For heart block and Stokes-Adams attacks, which may be fatal, a pacemaker may be lifesaving. Genetic counseling should also be offered.

Ocular or Periocular Manifestations

Choroid: Atrophy.

Cornea: Exposure keratopathy; filamentary keratitis; keratoconjunctivitis sicca; scarring.

Extraocular Muscles: Esotropia; exotropia; gaze paresis or paralysis; low amplitude to no opticokinetic nystagmus; low amplitude or no response to caloric stimulation; ragged red fibers (mitochondrial abnormalities).

Eyelids: Incomplete eyelid closure; levator paresis or paralysis; ptosis; weak orbicularis oculi muscles.

Lens: Posterior subcapsular opacity (rare).

Optic Nerve: Pallor or even atrophy.

Retina: Atypical pigmentary retinopathy (tapetoretinal degeneration).

Other: Constriction of visual fields; diplopia.

Precautions

Properly establishing the diagnosis of chronic progressive external ophthalmoplegia is critical for management. A complete workup of chronic progressive external ophthalmoplegia requires a number of clinical and laboratory tests that would delineate the amount of "ophthalmoplegia plus" and would rule out diseases that mimic the idiopathic form of chronic progressive external ophthalmoplegia. A workup of such patients should include a complete family history with examination of photographs of family members for blepharoptosis and strabismus and a physical examination with review of systems, particularly neurologic and ophthalmic systems. A dilated funduscopic examination should be done to check for pigmentary retinopathy. Yearly electrocardiograms would rule out cardiac conduction defects, cardiomyopathy, and the need for a pacemaker. Electromyography, nerve conduction velocities, and repetitive stimulation tests may reveal a myopathy, neuropathy, neuromyopathy, myasthenia, or myotonia. Electroencephalography might reveal abnormalities not suspected clinically. The cerebrospinal fluid could be examined for an elevated protein as commonly seen in the Kearns-Sayre syndrome. Muscle enzymes (aldolase, CPK), lactic acid, or pyruvic acid levels may be elevated. The dysphagia, which may be remediable, may be elucidated by a barium swallow or cinemography. Abetalipoproteinemia should be ruled out (lipoprotein electrophoresis, peripheral smear for acanthocytes). Refsum's disease should be ruled out (phytanic acid if motor nerve conduction velocities are slow). Dysthyroidism and myasthenia should be ruled out. Myasthenia gravis may be difficult to differentiate from chronic progressive external ophthalmoplegia (without myasthenia), since some patients with chronic progressive external ophthalmoplegia are supersensitive to edrophonium and curariform agents. Such hypersensitivity in some patients with chronic progressive external ophthalmoplegia requires administration of curare with great caution. Some patients with chronic progressive external ophthalmoplegia have been misdiagnosed for years as having myasthenia gravis or dysthyroidism. A limb muscle biopsy is helpful in better categorizing the type of chronic progressive external ophthalmoplegia. Ragged red fibers are usually found in the oculocraniosomatic neuromuscular (Olson) disease, whereas rimmed vacuoles are usually found in the oculopharyngeal syndrome.

Comments

An ongoing controversy has raged over the basic nature of chronic progressive external ophthalmoplegia. The pendulum has swung back and forth between authorities supporting the nuclear-neuropathic, myopathic, and myo-neuropathic schools. Later, slow viruses were proposed as the etiologic agent, and then biochemical defects in pyruvate-lactate metabolism were postulated to be responsible for the marked proliferation of abnormal mitochondria. Hyman felt that abnormal mitochondria in chronic progressive external ophthalmoplegia were morphologic reflections of the metabolic defect. One cannot be certain that the syndromes described in the older literature are the same as those in the modern literature because of the different histochemical stains available. Drachman found so-called "myopathic" changes in patients with the chronic denervation of poliomyelitis and subsequently confirmed this finding experimentally. Alvarado found that denervation of a cat's rectus muscle led to so-called myopathic changes and ragged red fibers. Drachman concluded that electromyographic and histologic criteria to distinguish myopathic and neuropathic lesions in limb muscles do not apply to ocular muscles. Moreover, Rowland questioned whether the so-called muscular dystrophies are neurogenic. A myopathic hypothesis of chronic progressive external ophthalmoplegia does not explain abnormalities in liver functions and cerebrospinal fluid enzymes. The vacuolation and ataxia of chronic progressive external ophthalmoplegia are similar to those of the spongiform encephalopathies of slow viral diseases.

Melmed infused uncouplers of oxidate phosphorylation into rats and caused lactic acidosis. Muscle histochemistry showed "ragged red" fibers. Electron microscopy showed abnormal mitochondria. Reske-Neilson performed light and electron microscopy and found abnormal mitochondria and degeneration of muscle and nerve in patients with chronic progressive external ophthalmoplegia who had abnormal pyruvate or lactate levels. They therefore suggested that a biochemical defect in pyruvate-lactate metabolism could cause a proliferation of abnormal mitochondria.

In summary, the etiology of chronic progressive external ophthalmoplegia is disputed. It has been postulated to be a nuclear, neuropathic, myopathic, supranuclear, viral, metabolic, and/or autoimmune disease by different authorities.

References

Anderson RL, Dixon RS: Neuromycopathic ptosis. A new surgical approach. Arch Ophthalmol 97:1129–1131, 1979.

Carroll JE, et al: Depressed ventilatory response in oculocraniosomatic neuromuscular disease. Neurology 26:140–146, 1976.

Drachman DA: Ophthalmoplegia plus: A classification of the disorders associated with progressive external ophthalmoplegia. *In* Vinken PJ, Bruyn GW (eds): Handbook of Clinical Neurology. New York, American Elsevier, 1975, Vol 22, pp 203–216.

Drachman DB, et al: "Myopathic" changes in chronically denervated muscle. Arch Neurol 16:14–24, 1967.

Drachman DA, et al: Experimental denervation of ocular muscles: A critique of the concept of "ocular myopathy." Arch Neurol 21:170–183, 1969.

Eshaghian J, et al: Orbicularis oculi muscle in chronic progressive external ophthalmoplegia. Arch Ophthalmol 98:1070–1073, 1980.

Hyman BN, Patten BM, Dodson RF: Mitochondrial abnormalities in progressive external ophthalmoplegia. Am J Ophthalmol 83:362–371, 1977.

Johnson CC, Kuwabara T: Oculopharyngeal muscular dystrophy. Am J Ophthalmol 77:872–879, 1974.

Kearns TP, Sayre GP: Retinitis pigmentosa, external ophthalmoplegia, and complete heart block: Unusual syndrome with histologic study in one of two cases. Arch Ophthalmol 60:280–289, 1958.

Melmed C, Karpati G, Carpenter S: Experimental mitochondrial myopathy produced by *in vivo* uncoupling of oxidative phosphorylation. J Neurol Sci 26:305–318, 1975.

Olson W, et al: Oculocraniosomatic neuromuscular disease with "ragged-red" fibers. Histochemical and ultrastructural changes in limb muscles of a group of patients with idiopathic progressive external ophthalmoplegia. Arch Neurol 26:193–211, 1972.

Rowland LP: Trophic functions of the neuron. IV. Clinical disorders of trophic function: Muscular dystrophy? Are the muscular dystrophies neurogenic? Ann NY Acad Sci 228:244–260, 1974.

Shy GM, et al: A generalized disorder of nervous system, skeletal muscle and heart resembling Refsum's disease and Hurler's syndrome. I. Clinical, pathologic and biochemical characteristics. Am J Med 42:163–168, 1967.

248 / CREUTZFELDT-JAKOB DISEASE

developed Creutzfeldt-Jakob disease after operation in the same neurosurgical unit. Creutzfeldt-Jakob disease has been reported in patients receiving pooled human growth hormone and dura mater grafts. Since 15 per cent of Creutzfeldt-Jakob disease is familial, it has been suggested that blood and organ donations should be avoided in family members of patients with Creutzfeldt-Jakob disease.

An association with intraocular pressure testing performed within 2 years of onset of Creutzfeldt-Jakob disease has been reported. Concern about the risk of applanation tonometry as a means of transmitting Creutzfeldt-Jakob agent and a suggestion that all patients with dementia should have their intraocular pressure taken with a sterile disposable tonometer or with a cover on the corneal surface of the tonometer have also been expressed.

Creutzfeldt-Jakob disease has been transmitted to laboratory animals by intracerebral, subcutaneous, intraperitoneal, intramuscular, or intravenous injection. Creutzfeldt-Jakob-like disease has been reported among primates after exposure to animals infected with Creutzfeldt-Jakob disease.

Any tissue being discarded from patients should be incinerated because its infectivity is not destroyed by storage either in formalin, glutaraldehyde, ethylene oxide, or alcohol. Care should be taken with electroencephalography, electromyography, or tonometry. No tissue should be used for transplantation.

Fully effective sterilization procedures for Creutzfeldt-Jakob disease tissues and contaminated materials are steam autoclaving for 1 hour at 132° C and immersion in 1N sodium hydroxide for 1 hour at room temperature. Partially effective procedures include steam autoclaving at either 121° or 132° C for 15 to 30 minutes, immersion in 1N sodium hydroxide for 15 minutes or lower concentrations (less than 0.5N) for 1 hour, and immersion in hypochlorite (undiluted, or up to 1:10 dilution) for 1 hour. Ineffective procedures include boiling, ultraviolet irradiation, ethylene oxide sterilization, and immersion in ethanol, formaldehyde solution, B-propiolactone, detergents, quaternary ammonium compounds, Lysol, alcoholic iodine, acetone, and potassium permanganate.

COMMENTS

Creutzfeldt-Jakob disease is found worldwide with a risk of about one per million. It may be caused by a prion, which is a small proteinaceous particle that resists inactivation by procedures modifying nucleic acid. Characteristically, the infection has a long incubation period, noninflammatory response, no recovery, no inclusion body, no interferon sensitivity, degenerative histopathology, and no change with immunosuppression or immunopotentiation. It has been shown that scrapie, another spongiform encephalopathy, may also be caused by a prion. A cellular isoform of the scrapie prion protein (PRP) has been identified. An immunologic re-

sponse to purified Creutzfeldt-Jakob disease prion proteins has been demonstrated in mice and humans.

Evidence that a prion is not the infectious agent responsible for Creutzfeldt-Jakob disease has been presented. Creutzfeldt-Jakob disease is also thought to be caused by an undefined agent consisting of protein and nucleic acid.

References

Austin JH: Precautions in Creutzfeldt-Jakob disease. Ann Neurol 20:748, 1986.
Centers for Disease Control: Human-to-human transmission of rabies via a corneal transplant—France. MMWR 29:25–26, 1980.
Committee on Health Care Issues, American Neurological Association: Precautions in handling tissues, fluids, and other contaminated materials from patients with documented or suspected Creutzfeldt-Jakob disease. Ann Neurol 19:75–77, 1986.
Davanipour Z, et al: Possible modes of transmission of Creutzfeldt-Jakob disease. N Engl J Med 311:1582–1583, 1984.
Davanipour Z, et al: Creutzfeldt-Jakob disease: Possible medical risk factors. Neurology 35:1483–1486, 1985.
Rizzo M, Corbett JJ, Thompson HS: Is applanation tonometry a risk factor for transmission of Creutzfeldt-Jakob disease? Arch Ophthalmol 105:314, 1987.
Taylor DM: Decontamination of Creutzfeldt-Jakob disease agent. Ann Neurol 20:749–750, 1986.
Traub RD: Pathogenesis of Creutzfeldt-Jakob disease. Neurology 37:1821, 1987.

DYSLEXIA

MARSHALL P. KEYS, M.D.
Rockville, Maryland

Dyslexia, primary or specific reading disability, strephosymbolia, and congenital word blindness are just a few of the terms used in describing children or adults with a primary defect in their ability to read. In spite of intact senses, normal intelligence, and proper motivation, these individuals demonstrate various degrees of inability to interpret written symbols. A family history of reading problems is common. In general, the label "dyslexia" excludes all those learning disorders considered secondary to other recognizable entities, such as seizure states, emotional disorders, mental retardation, environmental deprivation, poor teaching, and physical handicaps (including eye and ear defects).

Boder's classification of dyslexia is based on three reading-spelling patterns and is helpful in understanding and planning remedial therapy. Children with dysphonetic dyslexia are unable to decipher a word phonetically. They lack word analysis skills and avoid interpreting words that are not part of their sight memorized vocabulary. The second group labeled dyseidetic or gestalt-blind dyslexia demonstrates poor memory for whole words (gestalts) and has difficulty in discriminating similar letters. These children read by phonetic analysis and have a limited sight memory vocabulary. Spelling mistakes are frequently phonetic, such as "laf" for "laugh." The third group is a mixture of the first two and is therefore the most difficult group to approach through usual remedial reading techniques.

In a broader sense, it is important to realize that children with dyslexia usually fit into a syndrome with a variety of confusing labels. Minimal brain dysfunction syndrome (MBDS) or attention deficit disorder (ADD) consists of three main areas of concern: 1) learning disability possibly affecting visual or auditory perception, sequencing ability, right/left orientation, memory, language, or motor skills; 2) hyperactivity, distractibility, or short attention span (occurs in about 40 per cent of children with MBDS); 3) secondary emotional problems, which can be expected in a child with normal intelligence who is aware of school failures and peer pressures.

Ocular or Periocular Manifestations

During routine ophthalmologic examination, a history of school difficulties, speech problems, defective memory, or poor coordination is common. Poor attention span and distractibility may be obvious. The afflicted child may have difficulty labeling letters on a vision chart yet be able to accurately trace them in the air.

Right/left disorientation may be exemplified by reading chart lines backward. During "E"-game testing, a weaker score on horizontal as compared to vertical characters may also reflect a right/left conflict. Attempts at reading graded paragraphs (Gilmore, Gray) can be quite revealing and should be part of routine near vision testing for elementary school students.

Although strabismus, amblyopia, and refractive errors may occur simultaneously with dyslexia, a cause-and-effect relationship should not be assumed.

THERAPY

Systemic. Medication, including psychostimulants, tranquilizers, and antidepressants, is used in therapy of hyperactivity and should only be prescribed by physicians familiar with their effects. These drugs are used in specific cases to enhance attention so that acceptable *educational* techniques may be instituted.

There are many other types of therapy that lack adequate study. These controversial therapies include visual training, neurologic reorganization, megavitamins, and motion sickness medication.

Supportive. A general examination to rule out underlying disease and neurologic disorders should especially screen for visual and auditory deficiencies. Neurologic or psychiatric consultation may be indicated. A more specific educational workup is usually available through learning disability specialists within the school system. Outside authorities are also frequently helpful.

Precautions

Regardless of the method of treating learning disability, there are some children and adults who have almost no capacity for reading. These individuals can benefit from tape recorders and equipment used for the visually handicapped, such as "talking books for the blind."

Obviously, coexistent ocular disorders require customary treatment. However, parents must be warned that glasses or strabismus therapy will not correct deficiencies in right/left orientation, vision memory, and symbol interpretation. These concepts are emphasized in the recently revised statement on dyslexia available from the American Academy of Ophthalmology.

Comments

Above all, it is the physician's responsibility to provide adequate counseling so that families do not fall prey to the many cults offering quick cures. Specific referral to educational specialists using appropriate therapeutic programs is an acceptable and positive approach. In addition to testing and tutoring, experienced educational professionals can fulfill an advocacy role to ensure support for the child in the school system and provide counseling in preparation for college or vocational training.

References

American Academy of Ophthalmology: Policy Statement: Learning Disabilities, Dyslexia and Vision. San Francisco, American Academy of Ophthalmology, 1982.

Boder E: Developmental dyslexia: A diagnostic approach based on three atypical reading-spelling patterns. Dev Med Child Neurol 15:663–687, 1973.

Duane D, Rawson M (ed): Reading, Perception and Language. Papers from the World Congress on Dyslexia. Baltimore, York Press, 1975.

Gilmore JV: Oral Reading Test. Chicago, World Book, 1971.

Hartstein J (ed): Current Concepts in Dyslexia. St. Louis, CV Mosby, 1971.

Keys MP: Dyslexia and reading disorders. *In* Kelly VC (ed): Practice of Pediatrics. Hagerstown, MD, Harper & Row, Vol IV, 1977, Chapter 57A, pp 1–10.

Levine, MD: Reading disability: Do the eyes have it? Pediatrics 73:869–870, 1984.

Metzger RL, Werner DB: Use of visual training for reading disabilities: A review. Pediatrics 73:824–829, 1984.

Silver LB: The minimal brain dysfunction syndrome. *In* Noshpitz JD (ed): Basic Handbook of Child Psychiatry. New York, Basic Books, Vol II, 1979, pp 416–439.

Silver LB: The Misunderstood Child. A Parents' Guide to Raising Their Child or Adolescent with Learning Disabilities. New York, McGraw-Hill, 1984.

Silver LB: Controversial approaches to treating learning disabilities and attention deficit disorder, Am J Dis Child 140:1045, 1986.

Vellutino, F: Dyslexia. Sci Am 256:34, 1987.

FUNCTIONAL AMBLYOPIA

RONALD V. KEECH, M.D.
Iowa City, Iowa

Amblyopia is a decrease in vision in one or both eyes with no apparent organic abnormality that would account for the visual loss. The etiology is thought to be formed vision deprivation, competitive binocular interaction, or both of these factors. Some precipitating clinical conditions include strabismus, hypermetropia, anisometropia, cataracts, corneal opacities, and complete blepharoptosis. Amblyopia begins in early childhood and is most successfully treated soon after its onset. The incidence is between 2 and 4 per cent of the general population.

THERAPY

Ocular. Although many therapeutic approaches for amblyopia have been suggested, the most effective treatment is occlusion of the dominant eye. Constant occlusion during waking hours is preferable and is accomplished best with commercially available patches applied to the skin. An occluder placed over glasses should be avoided, since it requires more patient cooperation and is generally less effective. An opaque contact lens may be a useful alternative to a patch, especially if the patient is already wearing contact lenses for aphakia or anisometropia.

During occlusion therapy, the frequency of follow-up visits will vary depending on the patient's age. The rule of thumb is no more than 1 week of constant patching between examinations for every year of the patient's age. This is especially important with children under 2 years of age, when occlusion amblyopia is most likely to occur. With older children, the patching interval is less critical and generally varies between 3 to 6 weeks, depending on the severity of amblyopia and the speed of improvement.

If for any reason the interval between examinations must be longer than suggested or the patient has previously demonstrated occlusion amblyopia, patching may be alternated between the dominant and the nondominant eye. The ratio of alternate patching will vary depending on the patient's age, follow-up interval, and level of amblyopia, usually a 2 : 1 to a 6 : 1 day ratio is used. Treatment is continued until significant improvement is noted after 3 months of full-time occlusion. Once the best possible vision has been attained, patching may be discontinued or instituted on a part-time basis, depending on the patient's age and response to therapy.

An alternative form of therapy for amblyopia is penalization. This technique uses cycloplegics, long-acting miotics, and glasses in various combinations to alter accommodation. The purpose is to blur the dominant eye, thereby enhancing the use of the amblyopic eye. The best results are attained in moderate to high hypermetropes with mild amblyopia. Atropine is administered to the undercorrected dominant eye while the amblyopic eye is given a full optical correction. Penalization is most useful when occlusion therapy is not tolerated, as with skin allergies, and in patients requiring maintenance therapy following successful occlusion.

Anisometropic amblyopia may require occlusion therapy, as well as correction of the refractive error. If the amblyopia is mild, glasses alone may, in time, restore vision to normal. With dense amblyopia, patching and glasses are begun simultaneously. After the vision improves, a contact lens may be tried if the patient is symptomatic or has poor fusion due to aniseikonia.

Surgical. If deprivational amblyopia is a result of remedial ocular opacity, such as a cataract, persistent hyperplastic primary vitreous, or corneal opacity, surgical intervention should be considered. There is good evidence that very early surgery, optical correction, and aggressive amblyopia therapy can produce excellent visual results in selected cases.

Strabismus surgery is usually performed only after the amblyopia is resolved. Once this has been attained, the correction of any strabismus may aid in maintaining vision if fusion is present. Amblyopia, however, frequently recurs despite strabismus surgery.

Supportive. Home exercises with graded sizes of letters and objects in combination with occlusion may offer psychologic support, as well as providing a real benefit. Treatment with pleoptics, prisms, and red filters is controversial. At present, these approaches are not commonly used.

Ocular or Periocular Manifestations

Cornea: Opacities.
Extraocular Muscles: Nystagmus; strabismus.
Eyelids: Hemangioma, ptosis.
Lens: Developmental or traumatic cataracts.
Vitreous: Persistent hyperplastic primary vitreous.
Other: Anisometropia; high hypermetropia.

PRECAUTIONS

Most of the problems with amblyopia therapy can usually be averted with careful management. The most serious complication is occlusion amblyopia. Children under 2 years of age and those with mild amblyopia are most susceptible. Although uncommon, it may be irreversible and may result in eccentric fixation. Accurate assessment of visual acuity at frequent intervals is the best prevention.

If the amblyopia is slow to respond to treatment, an organic abnormality must be considered. A repeat refraction and ophthalmoscopy are indicated. Attempts to improve an organic abnormality with occlusion therapy are frustrating for the child, parent, and physician.

Another potential problem is the development of a new strabismus or the deterioration of a pre-existent strabismus as a result of patching. Parents should be made aware of this possibility at the onset of treatment.

Skin irritation from a patch can be an obstacle to successful occlusion therapy. Tincture of benzoin applied to the involved areas will help prevent this problem. Another approach is to rub cold cream into the skin and allow it to dry before applying the patch. This will decrease the adherence of the patch and prevent skin breakdown.

Comments

Long-term follow-up is critical for the proper management of amblyopia. The response to therapy and the tendency for a recurrence differ for each individual. Special care must be taken with strabismus patients after surgery; they may attain good alignment and some fusion, yet still develop amblyopia.

The treatment of amblyopia requires a considerable amount of patient and parent cooperation. This can best be elicited with a thorough explanation of the problem and the rationale for treatment. Parent participation by observing the child's fixation pattern when the patch is removed and involvement in visual games can also enhance the results. Another useful measure is to write a "prescription" indicating the eye to be patched, the duration and frequency of patching, and the date for a reassessment of vision.

References

Beller R, et al: Good visual function after neonatal surgery for congenital monocular cataracts. Am J Ophthalmol 91:559–565, 1981.
Boyd BF: Highlights of Ophthalmology, 25th ed. Panama, Highlights of Ophthalmology, 1981, pp 413–416.
Greenwald MJ, Parks MM: Treatment of amblyopia. In Duane TD, Jaeger EA (eds): Clinical Ophthalmology. Philadelphia, JB Lippincott, 1988, pp 11:1–9.
Swan KC: Esotropia precipitated by occlusion. Am Orthop J 30:49–55, 1980.
von Noorden GK: Application of basic research data to clinical amblyopia. Ophthalmology 85:496–504, 1978.
von Noorden GK: Binocular Vision and Ocular Motility, 3rd ed. St. Louis, CV Mosby, 1985, pp 210–239.

HEADACHE

THOMAS R. HEDGES, JR., M.D.
Philadelphia, Pennsylvania

Migraine is commonly misdiagnosed by the ophthalmologist mainly because the examiner does not listen carefully to the patient's symptoms and does not ask pertinent questions. Ophthalmologists tend not to be familiar with the subject and consider it to be beyond their capabilities in management.

It is of primary importance to identify the type of *vascular headache* by taking a careful history, including the chief complaint and past history of headache, which are of equal importance. The most important characteristic identifying migraine or one of its equivalents is periodicity. Migraine occurs as a major or minor attack of cephalalgia depending on its severity, in contrast to tension headache, which does not follow such a pattern. The next major identifying feature is a preceding aura (usually visual), which is present in classic migraine but absent in common migraine. The aftermath of a migraine attack of any severity is lassitude or a feeling of being "washed out." A family history is of great help in diagnosing migraine headache. The age of the patient is very important. Pediatric, ophthalmoplegic, and basilar migraine occur in children and adolescents. Classic and common migraine are most common in adults between 20 and 40 years of age, and isolated ophthalmic migraine occurs mostly in older patients. Once one has identified the type of vascular headache, treatment or management can be pursued appropriately.

Classic migraine occurs in young and in middle-aged adults. It is easy to diagnose when it presents as a periodic episode characterized by a visual aura and a throbbing unilateral or generalized headache of variable duration and severity. The more severe the headache, the more it is accompanied by nausea and vomiting, postheadache lassitude, or complete exhaustion. Obtaining a family history is of great importance. One must above all emphasize any family history of significant headache often labeled "sinus headache" or "nerves."

A wide spectrum of symptoms may occur, which may vary in both severity and duration. A typical fortification scotoma of 20 minutes duration or any unformed visual hallucinations precede or overlap the onset of headache, which typically is a pounding hemicrania that builds to a peak, often becoming generalized.

The pathophysiology of this important entity is classically explained by vasoconstriction during the aura, which typically causes fortification scotoma or more rarely aphasia, numbness, or motor weakness. This lasts 10 to 30 minutes and either totally precedes or overlaps the vasodilative phase, which creates the headache.

Patients with classic migraine are most commonly seen by the ophthalmologist because of the visual episode that precedes or accompanies the headache. Therefore, it is the examiner's duty to inquire about all the symptoms stated earlier in order to make a proper diagnosis and direct the patient toward the best mode of treatment. The ophthalmologist may manage the patient him- or herself or refer the patient to an internist or headache specialist, depending on the severity of the headache problem.

Common migraine does not have an aura or vasocontrictive prodrome. It begins with a build-up of headache and rises to a peak of pain. It is highly variable in severity, but is the most frequently encountered migraine syndrome, often beginning in the teens and lasting through the menopause in females. Its hallmarks are periodicity and postheadache fatigue. The severity of the headache dictates the amount of accompanying nausea, vomiting, and prostration. All migraine patients want to be alone or in a dark room.

Isolated ophthalmic migraine is commonly encountered in ophthalmic practice because of the alarming and often disabling attack of visual obscuration. The terms "isolated ophthalmic migraine," "migraine accompaniments," and "acephalgic migraine" have been used to describe these attacks. They occur in older patients with an average age of 55 years, but can occur in patients from 20 through 70 years of age. These patients usually have not had migraine headaches in the past.

In isolated ophthalmic migraine, the visual attack comes on suddenly as a typical fortification scotoma lasting 15 to 20 minutes. It appears much the same as the aura of classic migraine, but is not accompanied or followed by headache or other symptoms; thus, the appellation, isolated ophthalmic migraine. If the attacks are typically hemianopic with jagged lines of prisms of light, the origin is related to posterior cerebral-calcarine vascular insufficiency. Retinal migraine has been described as a unilateral attack of blurred vision lasting 10 to 30 minutes. It should not be confused with amaurosis fugax (lasting from seconds to 1 to 2 minutes). Even if monocularity is claimed by alternately covering the eyes, the author feels these are most commonly homonymous attacks in which the patient notices only the large temporal field affected, neglecting the smaller nasal field deficit on the other side. These attacks occur infrequently, but are very frightening. They are probably due to sludging or dysautoregulation in the terminal posterior cerebral or calcarine arteries, but the exact cause is unknown.

Pediatric migraine occurs in children usually between 6 and 14 years of age. Complaints of headache and blurred vision are ill defined, and one must take a very specific history to obtain the story of an episodic, often poorly defined headache. The headache is periodic. Head pain is accompanied by an atypical fuzzy vision and is therefore referred to by the term "fragmented" in comparison to adult migraine. Typically, the child comes home from school with a headache, may or may not have vague descriptions of unformed visual hallucinations, and then refuses supper because of mild nausea and goes to bed and sleeps. Thus, the classic combinations of episodic headache, blurred vision, nausea, and lassitude that are the hallmarks of the migraine syndrome are still present, but are more ill defined. Obtaining a family history of headache is most important in helping establish the diagnosis. Such questions as "Is anyone in the family headachy?" and "Did you or your spouse ever have headaches as a child?" are helpful. Many people forget that they had headache or were told they were nervous or had sinus problems as children. Females who have had headache at the time of their menstrual period do not realize that migraine commonly presents this way.

Ophthalmoplegic migraine is a very rare form of complicated migraine. Most of these patients are under 10 years of age. The patient first complains of lingering severe headache followed by ptosis and extraocular muscle paralysis; the pupil is usually involved as part of a third nerve paresis. This entity then emerges with the syndrome of painful ophthalmoplegia, which responds dramatically to oral steroids. The headaches preceding or accompanying the paresis in complicated migraine attacks are more severe and prolonged than usual. They may respond to ergotamine initially, but provoke concern regarding the differential diagnosis of aneurysms of the internal carotid-posterior communicating artery.

Cluster headache has been labeled as sphenopalatine, vidian and other neuralgias, and histamine cephalgia. Presently, it is most probably considered a migraine variant of vascular origin. It occurs more in males than females in contrast to true migraine, tends to be seasonal, and occurs in a series of episodes (clusters). Conversely, these attacks can often be quite isolated and infrequent. Cluster headache has no familial or constitutional background and is less responsive to routine migraine therapy.

These patients suffer from severe unilateral, periorbital headache with an onset in the early morning hours; it often awakens them from sleep. In contrast to migraineurs, these patients want to be active. In its extreme phase of severity, the pain generally lasts 20 to 30 minutes. The attack gradually subsides, but leaves the patient with pain in the eyeball or in and around the orbit. The eyeball usually remains white and quiet. Rhinorrhea and suffusions occur with severe attacks. A careful evaluation of the eye, including the cornea, the anterior chamber and its angle, the pupil, and intraocular tension, is vitally important in all cases. Horner's syndrome occurs infrequently in this entity. Chronic narrow-angle glaucoma must be ruled out.

Headache and *transient blurred vision* are so commonly seen in general ophthalmic practice that one cannot discuss one without the other. Even though at first one may wonder why migraine has anything to do with vascular disease of the carotid-ophthalmic or vertebral-basilar-posterior cerebral arteries, with experience one realizes that the visual prodroma of migraine and transient binocular attacks experienced without headache are so much alike they cannot be separated.

The term "transient blurred vision" covers a wide spectrum of conditions from short-lived unilateral transient ischemic attacks or transient monocular blur (TMB) to cerebral hemianopic episodes of transient binocular blur (TBB) of 20 to 30 minutes duration. Researchers have stated that any patient over 40 years of age with classic migraine should be considered a potential victim of vaso-occlusive disease. The author's personal clinical experience shows that patients over 40 years can have headaches of a classic migraine type and very rarely have a vaso-occlusive disease.

Any patient complaining of visual blurring should be asked the following questions: 1) Is the blur in one eye or to one side? (it should be remembered that patients tend to neglect the blurring in the small nasal field of the eye contralateral to the homonymous field loss), 2) How long does it last?, 3) Is there an association with any other vasomotor problems, such as hypertension or hematopoietic disorders (polycythemia, anemia, lipidemias, or platelet coagulability)?, 4) Are there cervical orthopedic problems, such as spondylitis?, and 5) Is there any association with stress?

Wavy vision is described as a homonymous hemianopic "spectral march" or fortification scotoma with or without lights and altitudinal "heat wave" type of blurring. It is a common complaint in middle-aged and older individuals. Although it may occur at any age, in the author's experience, the average age is about 52 years. These symptoms resemble in every way the aura or prodroma of migraine, but little or no headache accompanies this often frightening phenomenon. The more typical attacks vary in length from 10 minutes to as long as 2 hours, whereas the true fortification scotoma averages 20 minutes in duration. These patients may be reassured after a physical examination and other appropriate studies to rule out sludging phenomenon due to hematopoietic disorders. It is particularly important to rule out hypertension and/or atherosclerotic disease, which must be treated accordingly.

Transient ischemic attacks occurring in one eye (amaurosis fugax) are very fleeting, lasting seconds to minutes. These patients readily identify the attacks as monocular, even when they do not cover one eye. They are most commonly caused by emboli from extracranial carotid atheromata.

Monocular attacks of long duration (i.e., several hours or days) are often associated with hypertension, diabetes, or hematopoietic disorders. Prolonged monocular blindness should be differentiated from transient visual obscurations that last only seconds and are seen in chronic papilledema usually caused by pseudotumor cerebri and anterior ischemic neuropathy or amaurosis fugax.

Transient blurred vision in young people may be due to the prolonged use of oral contraceptive pills, emboli from a prolapsed mitral valve (Barlow's syndrome), other cardiac abnormalities, or postoperative complications of surgery to correct these defects.

Tension headache is probably the most common headache encountered in clinical practice. It rarely occurs in the very young or very elderly. It is described typically as a band-like or pressure sensation in the frontal region, nuchal area, or top of the head. It follows no pattern, does not have periodicity as its hallmark, but when severe may simulate migraine because of the accompanying physical fatigue that is augmented by the emotional state of the patient. Tension headache occurs with migraine, even in young people, and is commonly concurrent in 60 to 70 per cent of migraineurs. These patients often cannot verbalize, recognize, or accept a cause for the tension state.

The ophthalmologist rarely sees patients with *cranial neuralgias* initially, but must be aware of trigeminal neuralgias. This unilateral, excruciating facial pain in the first, second, and third division of the fifth nerve is usually present in middle-aged patients and presents characteristically as acute lancinating pain of brief duration. It is triggered by stimulation of the skin and is repetitive over a period of minutes.

The most serious cause of secondary trigeminal neuralgia is herpes zoster ophthalmicus, which begins acutely with unilateral head pain. It can be a tricky diagnostic problem because erythema and vesicle formation may not appear for days. Ocular involvement may have a sudden onset, especially if the nasociliary branch is involved.

Multiple sclerosis and internal carotid artery occlusion can also produce unilateral neuralgic-type head pain.

Intracranial neoplasms and vascular lesions, such as aneurysms and arteriovenous malformations, often must be ruled out when unilateral facial pain is persistent, especially when accompanied by sixth nerve palsy, nasopharyngeal carcinoma, chordoma, or aspergillosis. For all of these conditions, appropriate studies must be pursued. MRI is most helpful in making the diagnosis, its value far exceeding that of any other study.

THERAPY

Systemic. Ergotamine and ergot-like drugs remain the cornerstone of migraine therapy. Treatment of common migraine depends on the severity of the attacks, the age of the patient, and any complicating medical or psychiatric problem. Each patient and each attack must be approached individually. Thus, patients often complain of failure when therapy has not been tailored to the type of attack and its severity. Sublingual ergotamine is good therapy for on-the-spot treatment of common migraine attacks. It is vital that the patient take the medication at the onset of the attack to cause vasoconstriction and to abort the vasodilative headache.

"Spot" treatment of classic migraine consists of ergotamine/belladonna/caffeine/pentobarbital combination administered at the onset of the visual aura, thus giving this oral medication sufficient time to cause vasoconstriction and to prevent the onset of the headache caused by vasodilation. Synthetic sympathomimetic drugs, such as isometheptene/dichloralphenazone combinations, can be used if the patient is sensi-

254 / HEADACHE

tive to ergotamine. These medications are also valuable in treating migraine-tension headache. It must be remembered that 70 per cent of migraine sufferers also have tension headache.

Prophylactic treatment of classic migraine involves the use of a beta-blocker. It should be used when migraine attacks occur frequently (i.e., four to six times a month) and they become incapacitating. Prevention of classic migraine by digital massage of the superficial temporal arteries recently has been re-emphasized.

Carbon dioxide inhalation has also been used for many years to abort the visual attack of classic and isolated ophthalmic migraine, with a 50 to 60 per cent success rate in the latter. A small plastic sandwich bag should be available at *all* times. The patient should remain seated while rebreathing in the bag, and the opening of the plastic bag should be held over the mouth only. The patient should be instructed to exhale *fully* into the bag to fill it and then inhale and exhale deeply, rebreathing the air in the bag. This should be continued for 1.5 to 3 minutes at the most or until the visual disturbance begins to disappear. This procedure is to be performed as soon as possible after the onset of visual disturbance, not after 10 to 15 minutes have elapsed and definitely not after the onset of headache.

Recently, isoproterenol‡ inhalation has been used successfully to abort the visual attack. Sublingual nitroglycerin‡ also has been used with limited success.

Aspirin rarely helps an individual attack of common migraine, but it has been helpful in prophylaxis. Aspirin/caffeine/butalbital combinations are often helpful when stress is prominent. Isometheptene/dichloralphenazone contains a sympathomimetic plus a tranquilizer and is quite effective in prophylaxis of common migraine in many patients.

Patients with isolated ophthalmic migraines need careful ophthalmologic evaluation and medical referral when deemed necessary. Angiography is unnecessary, unless other neurologic signs are present. The administration of aspirin and carbon dioxide inhalation aborts isolated ophthalmic migraine in approximately 60 per cent of these patients. Monocular attacks of transient visual loss of variable duration deserve much more concern. Carotid bruits, significant difference in ophthalmodynametric readings greater than 20 per cent, and ophthalmoscopic evidence of atheromatous embolic disease (Hollenhorst plaques) must be searched for diligently.

Treatment of pediatric migraine is usually unnecessary. Aspirin is usually sufficient, since the syndrome is so fragmented and mild. However, there are rare instances in which ergotamine is indicated in common or classic migraine in children. A careful eye examination is important to rule out refractive errors and muscle imbalance; although these conditions have little or nothing to do with the headache, they must be treated if present. The parents should be advised that any prescription for glasses may have no effect on the headache problem and if beneficial is only a dividend. Asthenopic or eye fatigue headaches should be clinically evident after a refraction is done.

Steroid therapy given at the onset of symptoms should be considered in all patients with ophthalmoplegic migraine, unless other neurologic signs indicate the presence of an aneurysm, in which case angiography should be done immediately. However, it would be most unusual to have an aneurysm in most patients with ophthalmoplegic migraine because of the young age group.

Cluster headache responds best to sublingual ergotamine used at the onset of the attack. It can be a serious, recurrent, incapacitating headache, which can be extremely difficult to control if severe. Prophylactic or interim headache treatment may require the use of steroids, as well as ergotamine therapy. Oxygen therapy at home or referral to a headache specialist may also be necessary.

Aspirin or dipyridamole therapy is indicated for all patients with transient blurred vision complaints. The use of carbon dioxide inhalation may also be a source of reassurance, but does not rule out other more serious causes of cerebral hypoxia. The inspiration of 1 per cent isoproterenol‡ via a nebulizer in conjunction with aspirin treatment at the onset of visual symptoms may not only abort the visual attack but also prevent permanent visual loss that can occur in these patients. Patients with amaurosis fugax should be examined for carotid bruits, retinal emboli, and coronary, femoral, or aortic atheromatous disease. Ophthalmologists should perform ophthalmodynamometry and take blood pressure readings on all patients with these symptoms, in addition to ordering blood studies and a medical vascular workup. These patients should also have arterial digital subtraction angiography. If carotid artery stenosis is discovered, endarterectomy should be considered. Despite current controversy, this operation has definite value, as seen by each patient being judged after all data and arteriography results are studied individually. If negative, further investigation is necessary, especially regarding the heart.

Treatment of tension headache should start with aspirin and progress to a combination of aspirin/caffeine/butalbital or any adjunctive or psychiatric treatment when deemed necessary.

As in many other facial neuralgias, treatment with carbamazepine‡ can be successful in patients with cranial neuralgias, but often surgery of the fifth nerve, its ganglia, or tract is necessary for relief. Secondary trigeminal neuralgia due to herpes zoster ophthalmicus may be treated with 600 to 800 mg of acyclovir administered four times daily for 2 weeks in conjunction with 100 mg of prednisone daily, unless the patient is diabetic. Prophylactic cimetidine should also be used with the above regimen to prevent stomach ulcers. This is the most effective way of avoiding the dreaded ocular complications and postherpetic neuralgia. Steroids have also been successful in treating cranial oculomotor nerve palsies and uveitis, the common ocular complications of herpes zoster.

Comments

The initial procedure for headache problems should be to listen carefully to the patient's symptoms, discern any headache or visual obscuration problems, and then put these in a diagnostic category to enable proper management by the ophthalmologist or referring physician. When this is not done, the patient may be misdiagnosed and poorly managed. When diagnosis is pursued in a knowledgeable, systematic fashion, the patient obtains the necessary relief and psychologic support. Patients appreciate the ophthalmologist's interest in their headache and hearing an explanation of the type of headache they have with some indication of the treatment or studies necessary. At this point, the physician can decide whether primary management or referral is the best course to follow. This decision is made depending on the personnel and facilities available. If no headache specialist is available, the primary care must of necessity be given by the ophthalmologist. Otherwise, a referring letter to the patient's general physician, internist, or neurologist will enable that physician to take over the procedures and treatment indicated. Indeed, the interested ophthalmologist can be the deciding factor in starting the headache patient on his or her course to treatment and long-term management.

References

Buci ER, Herlot CP, Rufflieux C: Oral acyclovir in the treatment of acute herpes zoster opthalmicus. Am J Ophthalmol 102:531–532, 1986.
Cruciger HH: Ophthalmoplegic migraine. Am J Ophthalmol 86:414–417, 1978.
Fisher CM: Late life migraine accompaniments as a cause of unexplained transient ischemic attacks. Can J Neurol Sci 7:9–17, 1980.
Fisher CM: Late life migraine accompaniments—Further experience. Stroke 17:1033–1042, 1986.
Hachinski EH: Pediatric migraine. Neurology 23:570–579, 1973.
Hedges TR Jr: Terminology of transient visual loss due to vascular insufficiency. Stroke 15:907–908, 1984.
Hedges TR Jr, Lackman RD: Isolated ophthalmic migraine in the differential diagnosis of cerebro-ocular ischemia. Stroke 7:4, 1976.
Kupersmith MA, Hass WK, Chase NE: Isoproterenol treatment of visual symptoms in migraine. Stroke 10:299–305, 1979.
Kupersmith MA, Warren FA, Hass WK: The non-benign aspect of migraine. Neuro-Ophthalmol. 7:1–10, 1987.
Lipton SA: Prevention of classic migraine headache by digital massage of the superficial temporal arteries during visual aura. Ann Neurol 19:515–516, 1986.
Prensky AL, Sommer D: Diagnosis and treatment of migraine in children. Neurology 29:506–510, 1979.

HYSTERIA, MALINGERING, AND ANXIETY STATES

AUGUST L. READER, III, M.D., F.A.C.S.
Los Angeles, California

Medical practitioners are often faced with patients whose ocular examination does not correlate with their complaints. These patients may be feigning ocular disease for psychologic or physical gain. Occasionally, organic disease can develop secondary to the stress accompanying a constant or periodically recurring emotional state.

Malingering may be defined as the willful exaggeration or simulation of symptoms of an illness, usually to obtain some physical gain (financial, evasion of military service). Occasionally, dissimulation occurs where the patient claims to be normal when disease or disability is present in order to obtain a goal, such as to qualify for a specific occupation (pilots, truck drivers). Hysteria is the feigning of disease or injury on an unconscious level in order to satisfy certain unconscious psychologic needs. There are three main groups of hysteric symptoms: conversion symptoms (aphonia, blindness, deafness, paralysis of a limb, hemiplegia), dissociative state (fugues, multiple personality), and somatic symptoms. Both hysteria and malingering may arise from and be complicated by a state of anxiety, characterized by a subjective feeling of fear and uneasy anticipation. These anxiety states may present separately from hysteria and malingering, with organic disease manifested periocularly from emotional stress (angioneurotic edema, rosacea). Certain psychosomatic symptoms are commonly associated with anxiety states and include irritability, fearfulness, disorientation, insomnia, tachycardia, shortness of breath, fatigue, vertigo, pains in the chest, and blurred vision. These symptoms may lead the patient to present to a physician with fears of a serious physical disorder.

THERAPY

Systemic. In acute anxiety states, temporary relief is usually obtained with benzodiazepines, such as diazepam, given orally in doses of 5 to 10 mg three times daily. Patients liable to sudden attacks of panic gain security from carrying capsules of a rapidly acting anxiolytic, such as 50 mg of amobarbital. In patients with depression or a sleep disorder associated with their disability, 25 to 75 mg of amitriptyline at bedtime can be of help. Patients with organic disease secondary to anxiety (blepharospasm) may be helped by biofeedback therapy. In all cases where the chronic use of any medication is indicated, evaluation and treatment should be under the direction of an internist, neurologist, or psychiatrist.

256 / HYSTERIA, MALINGERING, AND ANXIETY STATES

Supportive. A short discussion with the patient and family about the findings of the examination in a very frank and open manner is usually well accepted by patients who appear to have chronic complaints of a hysterical nature. In patients whose hysteria is mild, simple autosuggestion or pointing out inconsistencies in complaints may produce a normal examination. Hysterics are suggestible and may improve with placebo therapy.

Removal of a patient from an anxiety-producing situation may alleviate anxiety-based complaints. Discussing the possible causes for the complaints may be the only therapy necessary. Reassurance is very important and therapeutic for these patients. If the anxiety state is severe and long standing, psychiatric help should be sought.

Ocular or Periocular Manifestations

Choroid or Retina: Anxiety-induced angiospastic or central serous retinopathy; anxiety-induced or aggravated posterior uveitis.
Conjunctiva: Conjunctivitis (self-induced); hyperemia.
Cornea: Epithelial erosions (traumatic); hypesthesia; phlyctenular keratitis; recurrent herpetic keratitis.
Eyelids: Angioneurotic edema; blepharospasm; chronic blepharitis; contact dermatitis; eczema; hordeola and chalazia; loss of cilia; ptosis; recurrent herpetic vesicles; rosacea.
Pupil: Anisocoria; hippus; peculiar pupillary reflexes.
Other: Accommodative spasm; amaurosis fugax; anxiety-induced optic neuritis; disturbance of conjugate movement; dyschromatopsia; facial tic; hypersecretion glaucoma; increased or decreased tear secretion; night blindness; nystagmus; photophobia; strabismus; visual loss.

PRECAUTIONS

Moralizing about hysterical illness or exhortations to stop imagining symptoms should be avoided. Direct discussion of the nature and causation of the symptoms should be done carefully, stating unequivocally that physical illness has been excluded. Medical examination in patients with presumed hysteria should be conducted and brought to an end quickly. In patients who are felt to be malingering, the examination should be extended or resumed another day to allow the patient to "maintain face." Ambitious medical or surgical intervention is contraindicated, since such measures tend to reinforce the patient's invalidism. Drugs have a limited role in the treatment of hysteria; if they are used, they should be kept under strict supervision, confined to a transitional period, and terminated within a few weeks.

In unmasking conscious or unconscious ocular fraud, the ophthalmologist should remember that hysterics will have positive tests, just as malingerers. Cases of the greatest difficulty to detect are patients with ocular diseases that cause anxiety and induce additional symptoms.

COMMENTS

In both hysteria and malingering, well-documented records and a complete examination to rule out disease are essential. Malpractice litigation in cases of feigned disease are difficult to defend unless the records explain the discrepancy between the complaints and the examination. Anxiety-induced ocular disease can respond to routine therapy, but will recur if the underlying stress is not treated.

References

Catalano RA, Simon JW, Krohel GB, et al: Functional visual loss in children. Ophthalmol 93:385–390, 1986.
Kettner JL, May WN, Johnson CA, et al: The California syndrome: Functional visual complaints with potential economic impact. Ophthalmol 92:427–435, 1985.
Kramer KK, La Piana FG, Appleton B: Ocular malingering and hysteria: Diagnosis and management. Surv Ophthalmol 24:89–96, 1979.
Miller BW: A review of practical tests for ocular malingering and hysteria. Surv Ophthalmol 17:241–246, 1973.
Smith CH, Beck RW, Mills RP: Functional disease in neuro-ophthalmology. Neurol Clin 1:955–971, 1983.
Thompson HS: Functional visual loss. Am J Ophthalmol 100:209–213, 1985.

LOW VISION

THOMAS E. TALBOT, M.D.,
and K. NOLEN TANNER, M.D., Ph.D.
Portland, Oregon

With a progressively aging population, ophthalmologists are seeing older patients in greater numbers. It was estimated there were over 2 million partially sighted Americans in 1984. Of this number, about one-half million were legally blind. Reduced visual function, whether present at birth or appearing later in life, has a profound influence on one's self-esteem and life-style. Patients with low vision that cannot be improved by medical or surgical therapy must be given the opportunity to take advantage of low-vision aids and alternative methods to resolve the problems of sight loss. Of the visually handicapped elderly, 75 per cent are in need of help for household chores and cooking in order to maintain independence. Twenty-five per cent of all seriously visually impaired elderly reside in nursing homes.

Of the diseases that reduce corrected visual acuity to stressful levels, the macular degenerations are most prevalent. Diabetic retinopathy, glaucoma and other optic nerve disease are relatively frequent causes, as well as corneal diseases, including keratopathy from pseudophakia complications. In general, congenital and developmental visual defects respond best to low-vision aids, whereas chronic, progressive degenerative adult-onset diseases are less responsive. The elderly are the largest group with serious vision loss, with 65 per cent of persons with low vision over 65 years of age.

Diagnosis is established with a comprehensive eye examination with only minor embellishments but always including a careful refraction. An assessment of the patient's desires for employment, leisure-time activities, and problems in home management and travel enables one to choose the most useful aids. Visual acuity levels below 20/80 are recorded on more precise intervals, i.e., a patient with 20/140 is more promising than one with 20/200 and needs less magnification. Finger counting as a measure of visual acuity should be avoided as it implies hopeless vision and discourages the patient. Visual acuity charts with finely graded levels above 20/80 are available (Lighthouse, Keeler, Sloan, Bailey-Lovey, etc.). Good illumination often improves acuity by three or four lines. Near test cards generally designed for use at 40 cm (Lighthouse) or 25 cm (Keeler) have graded-sized letters on a logarithmic scale for the lower levels of acuity. Cross cylinders of 0.50 to 1.00 diopter make axis and power changes much easier to see for the patient. Contrast sensitivity testing, although not imperative, may be helpful in predicting the patient's reading ability. Phorias and tropias are often present with occasional diplopia or amblyopic histories. Visual fields are helpful. Amsler grid fields can be quickly done, and fixation may be enhanced by adding lines through the center in the form of an X from corner to corner. Watching the patient's eyes as he or she reads single letters may disclose eccentric fixation. Color testing may suggest the severity of macular involvement, optic nerve disorder, or hereditary dysfunctions.

THERAPY

Supportive. Medical and surgical treatment, including contact lenses, should be considered when indicated, but magnification is the cornerstone of low-vision treatment. Magnifying devices come in the form of head-borne, high-power spectacles and spectacle adds, hand-held and stand magnifiers, telescopes, and closed circuit television (CCTV). CCTV, although capable of 40 to 60 times magnification, is expensive and beyond the budget of most elderly patients. With a practical maximum of 10 to 15 power, spectacles or hand-lenses are relatively inexpensive and are very portable. The ophthalmologist should be familiar with a variety of good-quality inexpensive hand-lenses and high-power microscopic spectacles. These magnifiers may be available from opticians, local shops, or from catalogs from national nonprofit institutions for the visually handicapped, such as the American Foundation for the Blind, the National Association for the Visually Handicapped, and the New York Lighthouse, and from commercial optical firms.

Magnification must be used with care when the peripheral field is impaired, as in retinitis pigmentosa or advanced glaucoma, since the object of regard may be magnified out of sight; phrases become words and words become isolated letters with resulting severe impairment of reading speed.

An intraocular lens implant will retain a better field image relationship after cataract surgery than leaving the patient aphakic. In addition, an aphakic patient will require a very large plus power in a low-vision aid, which causes serious aberration problems.

Binocular vision is often better than monocular vision, especially with macular degeneration, so it should be used when possible. The short working distance with high plus reading adds, however, taxes the convergence. This is relieved by using base in prism in the reading aid. A good rule of thumb is to use one prism diopter for each diopter of sphere power in each lens, i.e. plus 10 spheres have 10 diopters each of base in prism. Trial frames can be used for testing the patient's response to high-power lenses with base in prism, but it is often best done by using the finished product. Half-eye spectacles up to plus 12 diopters with corresponding prisms are available from several sources. Powers higher than 12 diopters (3×) can be tried, but more often than not, the patient reverts to monocular reading. If there is a large disparity in acuity or refractive error between the two eyes, patients almost invariably use monocular vision. Hand-held monocular and binocular telescopes from 2.5 to 8 power that focus for both distance and near, sometimes with clip-on reading lenses, are catalog items. Binocular Galileian telescopes have a longer working distance when used for reading with no need for base in prism. Binoculars or telescopes above 8 power require a fixed mount to avoid a blurred image from hand-held movement. A patient with a tremor may be limited to a 3 power or less telescope or opera glass.

CCTV can provide magnification of printed material of 40 times or more and may allow a patient to read when no other device is satisfactory. Its expense may be justified for students, teachers, or businesspersons, or to maintain secretarial employment. It is often available for public use through the local libraries and at times is loaned to needy patients from local government commissions for the visually impaired.

In general, to maximize reading speed, the lowest magnification necessary to read the print at hand should be used. Newsprint, for example, can be rapidly read at the 20/50 level of acuity. To read newsprint, a patient with 20/100 acuity requires 2× magnification, whereas one with 20/200 acuity needs 4×. The needed magnification for newsprint is therefore the ratio of 20/50 to the patient's measured best acuity. Print with smaller or larger Snellen equivalent may be used as the numerator when required.

Low-vision patients are best refracted at 10 feet (3 meters), which is the distance used by

258 / LOW VISION

most low-vision acuity charts (Keeler, Sloan, etc.); however, these charts can be used at other distances with suitable adjustment of acuity. Near acuity is generally remarkably consistent with distance acuity. Near acuity is measured, with suitable add, at a standard reference distance that is 25 cm (Keeler) or 40 cm (Sloan & others). The near acuity charts for the specific reference distance usually list the power and the equivalent dioptric needed to read newsprint. For 25-cm reference distance, the dioptric multiplier is 4; that is, 3× magnification is obtained by +12 diopters. For 40-cm reference distance, the multiplier is 2.5; i.e., 2× magnification requires +5 diopters. It is important to remember that magnification can be achieved by bringing the object of regard closer; halving the distance doubles the angular subtend. An appropriate add must be used to keep it in focus. On the other hand, an enlarged, erect, virtual image at an increased distance is created by a hand lens held just short of the focal length from the print to be read. Such a lens produces the same magnification when used either way. A +10 diopter lens yields the same magnification used as a hand lens on the lap or as a reading add with the print held at 10 cm from the eye.

Although acuity testing usually yields the magnification and dioptric needed to resolve an object, such as newsprint, the ability to use this resolution for effective and rapid reading varies markedly from patient to patient and depends on previous reading experience, adaptability, motivation, comprehension, and on the particular pathology involved.

Control of lighting is extremely important. Increased illumination is best achieved with an adjustable light source, such as a gooseneck lamp. A 60-watt bulb at 10 inches from the page is much brighter than a 300-watt bulb in a ceiling reflector lamp. A simple typoscope, which consists of a horizontal slot in black paper that eliminates all but one or two lines of print on the page, may reduce glare, improve contrast, and greatly improve the reading ability of patients with glare-inducing disease, such as early cataracts. In such conditions as achromotopsia, for example, the patient may require reduced illumination. Dark glasses may be essential to allow a patient to see in daylight. However, filtering out blue light scatter with a yellow or amber lens may improve contrast and acuity, but block out the color of traffic lights. Very high absorptive lenses may reduce acuity so trial before purchase is wise. The television picture is best resolved simply by moving closer to the set, which is usually more practical than buying a larger screen or telescopic viewing devices. Reducing the viewing distance by half doubles the image size; however, some patients may prefer sports spectacles for television.

Large-print books and magazines, such as *Readers Digest*, are available from private sources or free from the Library of Congress, and many patients prefer such material to optically magnified print. A specially designed computer with large type that is easily scrolled is available for the visually handicapped. Large-print playing cards and nonoptical devices, such as needle threaders, large numeral cooking timers, and measuring tapes, may enhance the low-vision patient's way of life. Talking clocks, watches, calculators, and computers, as well as talking books, are available.

Tactile markers, such as High Marks and Braille print markers, may be of great help. High Marks is a quick-drying plastic that makes small bumps that one can feel to identify stove dials and other hard-to-see items. Reading machines are in the early stages of development and expensive, but hold future promise.

PRECAUTIONS

The patient's depression and shock at the sudden or rapid loss of vision and his or her inability to cope may nullify the potential help of a low-vision aid. Therefore, providing encouragement and time in training the patient to use the aid and one or more return visits to assess progress are essential. Loaned devices reduce the anxiety of what may seem like a large economic outlay. Retraining with a different device may be necessary. If no return appointment is given, the patient may infer that nothing more can be done. Telephone contact with the patient after an initial visit for a low-vision aid may often answer questions and boost morale. A sympathetic, trained technician can greatly improve patient relationships in a practice.

COMMENTS

Referral for rehabilitation should be in the early states of progressive sight loss as patients will fail to return for follow-up when they think or are told nothing more can be done. The chance and hope for rehabilitation may be lost as disease progression is accompanied by fear, depression, and hopelessness.

Rehabilitation in the form of home help in daily living may be provided through social service agencies, such as state departments of rehabilitation and services to the blind. These services may allow patients to stay in their own homes and maintain their independence. Travel and new employment training, special education, psychosocial counseling, financial assistance, and support group help are available in most states and many communities. Peer groups and volunteer services are very helpful in supporting the visually handicapped. Many patients live alone and have no family to reinforce continued learning with a low-vision aid. Groups at senior centers can often arrange classes, lectures, and social gatherings of great value to these patients. The federally funded Talking Books program through the Library of Congress, rehabilitation, orientation, mobility instruction, and in-the-home counseling by trained personnel to solve daily living problems are all services many communities provide.

Unfortunately, providing rehabilitation information to the ophthalmologist and staff has been and continues to hold a low priority in ophthalmic journals, meetings, and conferences. To widen one's knowledge of low-vision management, much literature and many textbooks are available. Monthly journals, such as the *Journal of Visual Rehabilitation* and the *Journal of Visual Impairment and Blindness,* are also available. Other sources of information include American Academy of Ophthalmology courses. Also, some low-vision aid centers, such as the Lighthouse of New York and Pacific Presbyterian Medical Center in San Francisco, offer short courses and fellowships. The Pennsylvania College of Optometry also offers courses in low-vision aids.

Most ophthalmology residency training programs now require training in low-vision aids, but they give little attention to rehabilitation of the visually impaired or blind. As our aging population increases in longevity, the percentage of patients with visual impairments will increase. One must remember to never close the door on these patients and to avoid telling them that nothing more can be done. Low-vision training and rehabilitation can give these patients new capabilities and help them adjust to their visual deprivation.

References

Faye EE: Clinical Low Vision. Boston, Little, Brown and Co, 1976.
Fonda G: Management of Patients with Subnormal Vision. St. Louis, CV Mosby, 1970.
Jose RT: Understanding Low Vision. New York, American Foundation for the Blind, 1983.
Mehr EB, Fried AN: Low Vision Care. Chicago, Professional Press, 1975.
Rosenblum AA, Morgan MW (eds): Vision and Aging. General and Clinical Perspectives. New York, Professional Press, 1986.
Sloan LL: Recommended Aids for the Partially Sighted. New York, American Foundation for the Blind, 1971.

MULTIPLE SCLEROSIS
ROBERT S. HEPLER, M.D.
Los Angeles, California

Multiple sclerosis is a complex, poorly understood disorder of the brain affecting primarily young individuals between the ages of 10 and 40 years. It is characterized by multifocal dysfunction of white matter (demyelination). The optic nerves and the medial longitudinal fasciculi are often involved; hence, the significance of this disorder to ophthalmologists. Optic neuritis is the most common manifestation requiring ophthalmologic evaluation and possible treatment.

The cause of multiple sclerosis is not known. Epidemiologic and immunologic data suggest the possible influence of early viral infection of individuals who later acquire clinical multiple sclerosis or possible altered immune states as significant causative factors.

THERAPY

Ocular. The most commonly applied treatments are corticosteroid therapy, using such agents as prednisone,[‡] and corticotropin.[‡] Such treatment is unproven and controversial, yet it is frequently administered. Either corticotropin or corticosteroid therapy will probably decrease the retrobulbar pain associated with the onset of optic neuritis and may shorten the time of severe visual impairment slightly, but beneficial effect upon the ultimate visual outcome is unproven. Whether to use corticotropin or corticosteroid therapy appears to depend upon regional preferences. Although some have used orbital injections of corticosteroids[*], this technique adds the risks of such injections to the unproven efficacy of treatment.

Evaluation of the effects of treatment is exceedingly difficult because of the strong tendency toward spontaneous improvement from the episodes of demyelination that is characteristic of this disorder. For instance, a youthful patient with hand motion visual acuity may be given prednisone, and 6 weeks later vision in the involved eye is 20/30. This patient would very likely have had the same ultimate visual acuity without corticosteroids!

In approaching the dilemma of whether to treat or not, one logical approach is to use the concept of informed consent. One may provide the patient or the patient's family with a discussion of the pros and cons of steroid therapy. Circumstances in which the patient may be encouraged to decline therapy include the presence of known medical or psychiatric contraindications, such as significant affective disorder, peptic ulcer disease, tuberculosis, or diabetes mellitus; history of previous similar optic neuritis that recovered well without steroid therapy; or history suggesting that spontaneous improvement has already begun. Circumstances in which the patient may be encouraged to request corticosteroid or corticotropin therapy include optic neuritis in an only remaining, sighted eye; history of previous episodes that recovered well during or after corticosteroid therapy; particularly severe loss of vision, such as loss of all light perception; or bilateral simultaneous involvement of both optic nerves.

Most patients with optic neuritis do not need treatment. Those who are treated should receive clearance from their general physician before starting the following regimen: 80 mg of oral prednisone for 3 days, followed by 60 mg for 3 days, and then 40 mg for 7 days before discontinuation of the drug. A more gradual tapering dosage is not required if treatment is limited to 2 weeks. Routinely, the patients are given 1 ml of liquid antacid 2 hours after each meal and at bedtime. The patients are also encouraged to supplement their usual dietary potassium intake (tomatoes, citrus fruits, bananas) and are instructed to report immediately any troublesome side effects, such as gastric distress.

Occasionally, a patient may be disabled by prolonged optic neuritis despite use of corticosteroids. In such a case, one may wish to engage the assistance of research groups who are working with newer modalities, such as antimetabolites,‡ lymphocytopheresis,‡ and interferon.‡ Such modes of treatment of multiple sclerosis are unproven and experimental and therefore only to be considered under exceptional circumstances.

Ocular or Periocular Manifestations

Extraocular Muscles: Internuclear ophthalmoplegia, nystagmus.
Optic Nerve: Optic neuritis.
Pupil: Afferent pupillary defect.
Other: Central scotoma, dyschromatopsia; retrobulbar pain; visual loss (sudden onset).

Precautions

Correct clinical diagnosis is exceptionally important in multiple sclerosis. The disorder cannot be proven by biopsy or confirmatory biochemical or radiologic means; therefore, one must understand the clinical presentation to distinguish the signs and symptoms from those caused, for instance, by compressive tumors. The clinician must constantly assess whether the mode of onset, course, associated symptoms (if any), and examination findings in cases of optic nerve disease are consistent with multiple sclerosis. Since tumors missed by failure to understand and apply such criteria are better treated early than late, the patient suffers from delayed diagnosis.

What has been termed steroid-responsive optic neuritis is usually a treacherous occurrence of optic nerve compression by tumor that shrinks under the influence of systemic steroid and thereby simulates optic neuritis. It is seldom correct to apply the term "optic neuritis" to acute visual loss in persons over 45 years of age; such cases usually are examples of ischemic optic neuropathy as can be suspected by the age of onset, lack of associated pain, and presence of characteristic fundus and visual field findings.

Patients with presumed optic neuritis deserve a careful review of their history and neuro-ophthalmologic examination, including assessment of the visual field in the uninvolved eye. This can be performed by any well-trained general ophthalmologist. If the history and findings fit the diagnosis of optic neuritis perfectly, little laboratory and neuro-radiologic evaluation may be indicated. However, even in what appears to be clear-cut optic neuritis, it is appropriate to consider obtaining a general physical examination, complete blood count, Westergren erythrocyte sedimentation rate, antinuclear antibody, LE prep, and FTA-Abs and then to follow the patient closely for the characteristic confirmatory improvement in vision in about 2 months. This improvement in vision helps confirm the diagnosis of optic neuritis, and without it further evaluation is clearly indicated. Some neuro-ophthalmologists recommend obtaining CT or MR scanning even in typical optic neuritis patients, whereas others are content to reserve such studies for atypical cases. It should be noted that MR scanning frequently shows multiple white intracerebral lesions that are *not* necessarily diagnostic of multiple sclerosis, as was one time thought to be the case. The prime reason for performing a CT or MR scan is to rule out occult tumor compressing an optic nerve. It is appropriate to request neurologic consultation in atypical cases. The consulting neurologist may wish to perform spinal fluid analysis for gamma globulin abnormalities, which may support a diagnosis of demyelinating disease. In any case, it is important to see the patient again roughly 6 to 8 weeks after onset to determine whether he or she is showing the characteristic improvement in vision that helps confirm the diagnosis of optic neuritis.

Precise figures indicating the risk of development of multiple sclerosis associated with a single episode of optic neuritis vary from one publication to the next. However, the risk is probably greater than was believed to be the case in the past and, over the course of 10 years, may approach an incidence of 90 per cent in females and somewhat lower risk in males. Since the etiology of multiple sclerosis is unknown and there are no proven treatments or significant recommendations to avoid further episodes, it is debatable whether to raise the possibility of multiple sclerosis in the patient who is having his or first episode of optic neuritis. If there is a second episode, it is wise for the patient to have a general neurologic examination by a sensitive neurologist who can consider how much to tell and how to inform the patient in a manner that is constructive and supportive. The ophthalmologist is not the appropriate specialist to discuss this general neurologic disorder and to answer such questions as recommendations for exercise limitation, avoidance of heat, utilization of support groups, and family planning.

Comments

The National Eye Institute has established a collaborative, multi-center study to determine statistically whether or not there is benefit associated with the treatment of optic neuritis by systemic corticosteroids. Physicians who manage multiple sclerosis patients might wish to become aware of participating medical centers in their region, for referral of patients, and all such physicians will want to watch for the results of this study which will be published by 1990.

References

Beck RW: The optic neuritis treatment trial. Arch Ophthalmol 106:1051–1053, 1988.

Breen LA, et al: The VER: A status report. J Clin Neuro-Ophthalmol 1:277–278, 1981.

Burde RM, et al: Clinical Decisions in Neuro-Ophthalmology. St. Louis, CV Mosby, 1985, p 37.

Ellison GW, Myers LW: Multiple sclerosis. *In* Conn HE (ed): Current Therapy. Philadelphia, WB Saunders, 1982, pp 749–753.

Francis DA, et al: A reassessment of the risk of multiple sclerosis developing in patients with optic neuritis after extended follow-up. J Neurol Neurosurg Psychiatr 50:758–765, 1987.

Hepler RS: Management of optic neuritis. Surv Ophthalmol 20:350–357, 1976.

Jacobs L et al: Intrathecal interferon reduces exacerbations of multiple sclerosis. Science 214:1026–1028, 1981.

Jacobs L, et al: Silent brain lesions in patients with isolated idiopathic optic neuritis. Arch Neurol 45:452–455, 1986.

Miller DH, et al: Magnetic resonance imaging of the optic nerve in optic neuritis. Neurology 38:175–179, 1988.

Miller NR: Optic neuritis. *In* Walsh and Hoyt's Clinical Neuro-Ophthalmology, Vol 1, Baltimore, Williams & Wilkins, 1982, pp 227–248.

Rose AS: Multiple sclerosis: An overview. Adv Neurol 31:3–9, 1981.

MYASTHENIA GRAVIS
NEIL R. MILLER, M.D.,
and ALAN PESTRONK, M.D.
Baltimore, Maryland

Myasthenia gravis is a disorder of muscles characterized by weakness and fatigability. Ptosis and diplopia are typical presenting symptoms because the extraocular muscles and elevators of the eyelids are frequently affected early in this disease. When the bulbar musculature is affected, there may be impairment of speech, chewing, swallowing, and facial expression. More generalized disease may affect muscles of the trunk and limbs. If the muscles of respiration or swallowing are affected, necessitating respiratory or nutritional assistance, the patient is said to be in "crisis." Symptoms are often least prominent in the morning and after rest, but tend to worsen later in the day or after exercise.

Myasthenia gravis may begin at any age, but reaches a peak incidence in the third decade in females and in the fifth to sixth decades in males. A family history of myasthenia gravis is present in about 5 per cent of cases.

The basic abnormality in myasthenia gravis is a deficiency of acetylcholine receptors at neuromuscular junctions caused by an antibody-mediated autoimmune process. The deficiency of acetylcholine receptors results in muscle weakness and fatigue on repeated activity because of impaired neuromuscular transmission. The factors that trigger the production of autoantibodies in myasthenia gravis are not known, but the complex relationship of the thymus gland to myasthenia suggests that this organ may play a role in the pathogenesis of myasthenia.

THERAPY

Systemic. Although the basic autoimmune disorder is systemic, clinical weakness may remain confined to the extraocular muscles in up to 40 per cent of patients. If the symptoms are mild or intermittent, one might consider no therapy whatsoever. Such patients may be forced to patch one eye occasionally, and many prefer to do so, rather than to take medication.

Anticholinesterase agents continue to be used as the first line of treatment for most patients with myasthenia gravis. Pyridostigmine is the most widely used oral anticholinesterase drug; its effect begins within 10 to 30 minutes, reaches a peak at 1 to 2 hours, and declines at 3 to 4 hours. The correct dosage must be determined empirically. The timing of doses should be adjusted to avoid fluctuations in symptoms and to anticipate periods of greatest need or weakness. The usual starting dose is 60 mg every 4 to 6 hours during the day. The dosage is then adjusted on the basis of an individual's requirements. It is unusual for a patient to benefit from more than 120 mg of pyridostigmine every 3 hours. Sustained-release preparations are available, but should be used only at bedtime. It is important to note that ocular symptoms of myasthenia are usually more refractory to anticholinesterase treatment than are systemic symptoms.

Immunosuppression may be considered for any myasthenic patient whose weakness is not satisfactorily controlled by anticholinesterase medication and/or thymectomy. Adrenal corticosteroids are the immunosuppressive agents most widely used in the treatment of myasthenia gravis. The ocular symptoms as well as systemic symptoms of myasthenia gravis often respond dramatically to alternate-day prednisone therapy, especially when combined with optimum doses of anticholinesterase medication. Older patients are considered good candidates for steroid treatment, since they respond particularly well to this mode of therapy. Before beginning steroid therapy, patients should be told of the serious side effects that may occur, including cataracts, osteoporosis, reduced resistance to infection, ulcer disease, hypertension, exacerbation of diabetes, and salt and fluid retention. Relative contraindications to prednisone treatment include pre-existing diabetes, hypertension, and ulcer disease, although these problems can usually be controlled. Patients who are unable or unwilling to be followed medically should never be treated with steroids.

When treatment is begun with high doses of steroids, such as prednisone, a proportion of patients will experience exacerbation of myasthenic weakness within the first weeks of treatment. A gradually increasing dosage schedule (sometimes with observation in the hospital) usually avoids this problem. When the daily goal of 50 mg of oral prednisone is reached or when a satisfactory dosage has been achieved at a lower dosage level, administration of prednisone is then gradually shifted toward an alternate-day treatment schedule. Prednisone is then tapered

262 / MYASTHENIA GRAVIS

to establish the *minimum* dose required by the individual patient.

Other immunosuppressive drugs, such as azathioprine[‡] and cyclophosphamide,[‡] have been used in the treatment of myasthenia gravis. However, the beneficial effects of these drugs may take from several months to a year to appear, and the toxicity of these agents limits their use to severely affected patients cared for in institutions with special expertise.

Plasmapheresis has proven of temporary benefit in some cases of myasthenia, but is usually not needed. In general, this method of treatment is useful in improving the clinical condition quickly and getting the patient through such difficult periods as a myasthenic crisis, preparation for thymectomy, or the initiation of immunosuppressive therapy.

Ocular. Although attempts have been made to treat purely ocular myasthenic patients with prisms and/or ptosis crutches, these are generally ineffective. The incomitance of the strabismus often precludes successful therapy, and ptosis crutches often cause severe exposure keratopathy.

Surgical. If no adequate response is obtained within a reasonable period of time, a decision must be made about an alternative therapy. Thymectomy is rarely used to treat purely ocular myasthenia gravis. However, it is the treatment of choice in myasthenia gravis to remove a tumor of the thymus or to produce improvement in generalized myasthenic weakness. Thymectomy is recommended in postpubertal patients under the age of 45 to 50 years with generalized myasthenia gravis that is not satisfactorily controlled by anticholinesterase drugs. Thymectomy should only be carried out at centers that have experience with this procedure. Under such circumstances, the mortality rate is close to zero. The maximum benefits of thymectomy are realized on a delayed time scale, 1 to 2 years after surgery. In the meantime, other therapeutic measures may be needed.

Ocular or Periocular Manifestations

Extraocular Muscles: Accommodative insufficiency (rare); generalized limitation of ocular motility; pseudogaze palsy; pseudo-internuclear ophthalmoplegia.

Eyelids: Cogan's lid twitch; orbicularis oculi weakness; paradoxical lid retraction; ptosis.

Other: Diplopia; nystagmus.

PRECAUTIONS

If surgery is needed, oral medication may have to be discontinued. Anticholinesterase medication may be given by intravenous infusion pump. The full equivalent dose of 60 mg of oral pyridostigmine is 1 to 2 mg of intravenous neostigmine. If prednisone has been used prior to surgery, parenteral hydrocortisone and methylprednisolone should be maintained in a daily dose equivalent to the "on" day dose of oral prednisone.

Curare forms of drugs should never be used during surgery. Certain other drugs are also contraindicated in myasthenic patients because they increase weakness. These include quinine, quinidine, and procainamide. Aminoglycoside antibiotics may increase weakness, but should be used when necessary.

Myasthenic patients should be allowed to regulate their own activity levels. The effects of overexertion are reversible, and the patient will learn his or her own limitations. These patients should be instructed to contact their physicians immediately if infections of any sort develop. Overdosage of anticholinesterase compounds can cause symptoms similar to worsening of myasthenia gravis but rarely result in worsening of eye movement.

COMMENTS

Before initiating or modifying treatment in the myasthenic patient, it is necessary to establish the diagnosis unequivocally, to document the severity of myasthenia gravis, and to evaluate the possibility of related or unrelated intercurrent conditions. The diagnosis of myasthenia gravis may be suspected from atypical history of fluctuating symptoms that become worse with fatigue. On physical examination, the strength of the orbicularis oculi should be tested, since this is the most consistently involved muscle. Quantitative movements of ocular motility and eyelid function with evaluation of fatigue are also useful. Observation of Cogan's lid twitch may help confirm the diagnosis. The time at which ptosis develops on upward gaze is a useful objective measurement that may be used to evaluate the success of later treatment. Other quantitative tests of systemic muscle function and fatigue, such as the arm abduction time and the vital capacity, are also useful.

Once myasthenia is suspected, several diagnostic maneuvers may be carried out to confirm the diagnosis. Pharmacologic testing using edrophonium or neostigmine is often performed. These tests are most reliable when an alternative placebo treatment is also given, evaluation of the patient is carried out by a blinded observer, and quantitative measurements of the patient's function are carried out before and after each medication. Other diagnostic tests on such individuals may include repetitive nerve stimulation and measurements of anti-acetylcholine receptor antibodies. Conditions that may exacerbate myasthenia gravis and should be searched for in every patient include intercurrent infection, thyroid disease, and thymoma. Most patients should also be screened for the presence of other autoimmune diseases, and a careful drug history should be taken.

References

Drachman DB: The biology of myasthenia gravis. Annu Rev Neurosci 4:195–225, 1981.
Drachman DB: Myasthenia gravis. *In* Conn HF (ed):

Current Therapy. Philadelphia, WB Saunders, 1982, pp 754–758.
Drachman DB: Present and future treatment of myasthenia gravis. N Engl J Med 316:743–745, 1987.
Grob D: Myasthenia gravis: Pathophysiology and management. Ann NY Acad Sci 377:1–898, 1981.
Miller NR: Walsh and Hoyt's Clinical Neuro-Ophthalmology, 4th ed. Baltimore, Williams & Wilkins, 1985, Vol 2, pp 841–866.
Walton J (ed): Disorders of Voluntary Muscle, 4th ed. New York, Churchill Livingstone, 1981.

PARKINSON'S DISEASE
STEVEN GANCHER, M.D.
Portland, Oregon

Parkinson's disease (PD) is a slowly progressive, degenerative neurologic illness. It most typically affects middle-aged or elderly individuals, although it may occur in young adults. It usually starts insidiously and progresses at a variable rate. Typical symptoms are resting tremor, rigidity, a flexed posture, retropulsion, and bradykinesia. The latter symptom, which produces difficulty in initiating and maintaining movement, can be the most disabling yet least obvious aspect of the disease. The most severe neuropharmacologic deficit is a deficiency of dopamine in the basal ganglia caused by loss of pigmented, nigrostriatal neurons in the substantia nigra, although other neurotransmitter systems, such as serotonin and norepinephrine, are also affected.

There is considerable overlap with other, related degenerative disorders that cause bradykinesia, and early in its course, it may be difficult to separate these other disorders from idiopathic PD. The most common related illness, progressive supranuclear palsy (PSP), may present with very similar symptoms initially before the supranuclear vertical ophthalmoplegia becomes apparent.

A variety of ocular abnormalities, chiefly involving the eyelids and eye movements, may be observed in PD and related conditions. Common to PD, PSP, and other disorders causing bradykinesia are a loss of facial expression and infrequency of blinking, giving rise to the typical "parkinsonian stare." Blepharoclonus, tremor of the eyelids with gentle eye closure, is also common, especially if there is associated head or chin tremor, and apraxia of eye opening may occasionally occur. Myerson's sign, an inability to suppress blinking following tapping on the nasion, is also very common. Seborrhea is also common in PD and may lead to recurrent hordeola and blepharitis.

A variety of eye movement disturbances also occur in PD. An increase in saccadic latency, hypometric saccades, a mild degree of saccadic slowing, and a breakdown in smooth pursuit are the most common abnormalities. A mild degree of limitation in upgaze also occurs but is also common with "normal" aging. Other eye movement disturbances, such as nystagmus, horizontal or marked vertical ophthalmoplegia, or apraxia of eye opening, may occur, but are uncommon and should suggest an alternative diagnosis. Oculogyric crises do not occur in idiopathic PD, but are common in postencephalitic parkinsonism and also occur as an acute dystonic reaction to neuroleptics.

Other abnormalities in the visual pathway, including visual neglect, prolonged latency of visual evoked response, and elevated threshold in foveal contrast sensitivity, may also occur.

THERAPY

Systemic. Drug treatment of Parkinson's disease is symptomatic as there is currently no treatment that affects the natural course of the illness. Levodopa replacement (usually combined with a peripheral decarboxylase inhibitor, such as carbidopa) is initially very effective, but diurnal fluctuations in motor state and drug-induced choreoathetosis or dystonia commonly emerge with chronic treatment, especially in younger patients. Thus, levodopa is usually reserved for those patients who are refractory to other medications or have moderately severe disease at presentation. For patients with predominant tremor, anticholinergics may be effective, but are limited by accommodative paralysis, miosis, dry mouth, and memory loss. Other useful medications include amantadine, bromocriptine, propranolol,[‡] and antidepressants.[‡] Unfortunately, some degree of residual parkinsonism is nearly always present, despite the above treatments.

Ocular. Infrequent blinking may necessitate the use of artificial tears. Ocular secretions tend to be greasy and may lead to blepharitis and hordeola, which may be avoided by good lid hygiene.

Supportive. Psychologic support, with reassurance, encouragement, and supportive counseling, is very useful in managing the major symptoms of parkinsonism. Patient support groups may provide considerable practical advice, as well as emotional support for the patient and caregiver. Adult day care may also be very helpful to avoid caregiver "burnout."

Ocular or Periocular Manifestations

Extraocular Muscles: Decreased convergence; hypometric saccades; limited upgaze (especially in PSP); oculogyric crises (postencephalitic); saccadic pursuit.

Eyelids: Blepharoplegia; blepharospasm; hordeolum; infrequent blinking; seborrheic blepharitis.

Other: Abnormal visual evoked responses; increased foveal threshold; visual neglect.

PRECAUTIONS

Confusion with PSP is a common problem, even in clinics specializing in Parkinson's disease. Early recognition of this disease, which has a worse prognosis, will avoid presenting an incorrect prognosis to the patient and family. Avoidance of anticholinergics in the patient with memory impairment is also crucial. Other side effects seen with anticholinergics, including decreased accommodative ability and miosis, are important to recognize. Drug-induced dyskinesias may also interfere with treatment.

COMMENTS

Ophthalmic evaluation and treatment, such as slitlamp examination or surgery, may be difficult either because of parkinsonian tremor or head and neck dyskinesias, and evaluation of the patient both before and after a dose of levodopa may be needed. Narcotics or benzodiazepines typically do not markedly affect the tremor, although deep sedation with any drug usually suppresses tremor or dyskinesia. Intravenous diphenhydramine, administered in 25-mg increments, has been found to be useful. Before general anesthesia, it is best to avoid levodopa for at least 4 to 6 hours, as the risk of cardiac arrhythmias may be increased with increased plasma dopamine levels due to incomplete inhibition of levodopa decarboxylase.

References

Bodis-Wollner I, Onofrj M: The visual system in Parkinson's disease. Adv Neurol 45:323–327, 1986.
Kupersmith MJ, et al: Visual system abnormalities in patients with Parkinson's disease. Arch Neurol 39:284–286, 1982.
Lesser RP, et al: Analysis of the clinical problems in parkinsonism and the complications of long-term levodopa therapy. Neurology 29:1253–1260, 1979.
Stone DJ, DiFazio CA: Sedation for patients with Parkinson's disease undergoing ophthalmologic surgery. Anesthesiology 68:821, 1988.
Villardita C, Smirni P, Zappala G: Visual neglect in Parkinson's disease. Arch Neurol 40:737–739, 1983.
White OB, et al: Ocular motor defects in Parkinson's disease. II. Control of the saccadic and smooth pursuit systems. Brain 106:571–588, 1983.

TOLOSA-HUNT SYNDROME
(Painful Ophthalmoplegia)
WILLIAM E. HUNT, M.D.
and SUSAN C. BENES, M.D.
Columbus, Ohio

The Tolosa-Hunt syndrome is a painful ophthalmoplegia caused by a nonspecific steroid-sensitive granuloma in the cavernous sinus. A steady pain, frequently described as "gnawing" or "boring," may precede the ophthalmoplegia by days or even weeks or may not appear until cranial nerve deficit is seen. The third, fourth, or sixth nerves and the ophthalmic or, rarely, maxillary divisions of the fifth nerve may be involved. There may be balanced or unbalanced loss of the parasympathetic and sympathetic pupillomotor fibers. Symptoms may last for weeks or months. Spontaneous remission may occur, sometimes with residual neurologic deficits. Recurrences are found at intervals of months to years. Rarely, the syndrome may alternate sides, or a single attack may have bilateral but asymmetric findings.

Diagnosis of the Tolosa-Hunt syndrome is made by exclusion after other causes of subacute painful ophthalmoplegia have been thoroughly ruled out. This requires CT scanning of the orbits and the cavernous and paranasal sinuses. Cerebral angiography is necessary to rule out aneurysms, arteriovenous malformations, and carotid cavernous fistulas. Infrequently, orbital venography may be deemed necessary to show stenosis of the third segment of the superior orbital vein. Bloodwork for systemic infections, inflammations, or hematologic malignancies should be done, including complete blood counts, erythrocyte sedimentation rates, protein studies, and vasculitis markers (ANA, rheumatoid factor, angiotensin-converting enzyme). The causes of the Tolosa-Hunt syndrome are still unknown, but probably include dysfunction of the delayed cell-mediated immunity system.

THERAPY

Systemic. After excluding other disorders, corticosteroids are the treatment of choice for the Tolosa-Hunt syndrome, and an immediate response is expected when large doses are prescribed. The usual oral adult dose is 80 to 100 mg of prednisone daily. Although there may be a rapid initial response to therapy (within hours), recurrences do not respond as well and require larger doses. Therefore, corticosteroids should be tapered to a maintenance level and gradually discontinued when the pain has abated. The ophthalmoplegia may not resolve for some weeks after clearing of the painful inflammation if severe nerve damage has occurred.

If treatment is prolonged, steroid dependency may be a problem, accompanied by all the Cushingoid side effects. This complication is usually avoided by the practice of tapering medication within a week of the subsidence of pain. If response is poor, reinvestigation to rule out neoplasm should be undertaken. Immunosuppression with 1 to 3 mg/kg of oral cyclophosphamide[‡] daily may be used to diminish the steroid requirements.

Ocular or Periocular Manifestations

Extraocular Muscles: Paralysis of third, fourth, or sixth nerve.
Eyelids: Ptosis.

Globe: Proptosis (rare).
Pupil: Anisocoria; Marcus Gunn pupil; sympathetic and/or parasympathetic paralysis.
Other: Decreased visual acuity; diplopia; ocular and periocular pain; orbital inflammatory signs (rare); scotoma.

PRECAUTIONS

Prompt relapse may follow corticosteroid withdrawal in some patients. Patients treated with corticosteroids for any length of time should be appropriately evaluated before therapy and carefully followed for the complications of this treatment. Cyclophosphamide in childbearing women should be avoided. Careful monitoring for hepatotoxicity and hematopoietic toxicity is necessary.

COMMENTS

Prednisone may produce its effect by reducing edema and inflammation of the granulomatous tissue in the cavernous sinus, thereby relieving pressure on the adjacent cranial nerves. This generally requires a 3-week or longer course. Although rapid improvement following corticosteroid therapy may be highly suggestive of the Tolosa-Hunt syndrome, it must be remembered that temporary remission may also be seen when the pain and ophthalmoplegia are of neoplastic origin or are caused by aneurysms in a growth or leak phase, cavernous sinus fistulas, or other such steroid-sensitive processes as granulomatous infections, Wegener's granulomatosis, lymphoma, and infiltrative leukemias.

The Tolosa-Hunt syndrome and orbital pseudotumor (idiopathic, noncaseating, granulomatous inflammation of the orbit) may be the same disease process on two sides of the superior ophthalmic fissure.

References

Glaser JS: Infranuclear disorders of eye movements. *In* Duane TD (ed): Clinical Ophthalmology. Hagerstown, MD, Harper & Row, 1982, Vol II, pp 12:18–19.
Hoes MJAJM, Bruyn GW, Vielvoye GJ: The Tolosa-Hunt syndrome—literature review: Seven new cases and a hypothesis. Cephalalgia 1:181–194, 1981.
Hunt WE: Tolosa-Hunt syndrome: One cause of painful ophthalmoplegia. J Neurosurg 44:544–549, 1976.
Hunt WE et al: Painful ophthalmoplegia. Its relation to indolent inflammation of the cavernous sinus. Neurology 11:56–62, 1961.
Roca PD: Painful ophthalmoplegia: The Tolosa-Hunt syndrome. Ann Ophthalmol 7:828–834, 1975.
Schatz NJ, Farmer P: Tolosa-Hunt syndrome: The pathology of painful ophthalmoplegia. *In* Smith JL (ed): Neuro-Ophthalmology. St. Louis, CV Mosby, 1972, Vol VI, pp 102–112.
Smith JL, Taxdal DSR: Painful ophthalmoplegia. The Tolosa-Hunt syndrome. Am J Ophthalmol 61:1466–1472, 1966.
Tolosa E: Periarteritic lesions of the carotid siphon with the clinical features of a carotid infraclinoidal aneurysm. J Neurol Neurosurg Psychiatry 17:300–302, 1954.

TRIGEMINAL NEURALGIA
(Tic Douloureux)
BAIRD S. GRIMSON, M.D.
Chapel Hill, North Carolina

Trigeminal neuralgia is a brief, sharp, unilateral facial pain that usually occurs in the middle or lower face within the distribution of the second or third division of the trigeminal nerve. Occasionally, the first division of the trigeminal nerve is involved with the cephalgia occurring in or around the eye. The "stabbing," "searing," "lightning-like," or "electrical" pain most often occurs in patients over 40 years of age and is experienced more frequently by females than males. The right side of the face is involved more often than the left. Characteristically, this memorable pain is precipitated by mechanical stimulation of trigger zones within the ipsilateral face or mouth during such activities as chewing, swallowing, laughing, brushing teeth, combing one's hair, or shaving. Each attack of trigeminal neuralgia usually lasts for only several seconds or minutes, often presenting intermittently at first, but can increase to many episodes per day. Spontaneous exacerbations and remissions of tic douloureux are not uncommon and can complicate judgments on the efficacy of therapeutic measures for controlling the pain. If the pain presents bilaterally, the rare occurrence of multiple sclerosis as an underlying etiology of trigeminal neuralgia should be suspected.

THERAPY

Systemic. Carbamazepine or phenytoin[‡] is particularly useful when started shortly after the onset of tic douloureux. Although carbamazepine usually proves more effective, prolonged use of either of these drugs is limited because of their side effects and the tendency for trigeminal neuralgia to become refractory to medical management. Balcofen[‡] is also useful in the management of trigeminal neuralgia.

Carbamazepine is initiated in dosages of 100 mg orally twice a day following meals, with subsequent increments of 100 mg every 12 hours until the pain is relieved or toxic side effects are observed. The total daily dose of carbamazepine usually ranges between 400 and 800 mg, but should never exceed 1.2 gm. Between 300 and 700 mg of phenytoin are required daily for adequate relief from trigeminal neuralgia. Balcofen should be started at 5 mg orally three times a day for 3 days, then increased to 10 mg three times a day for 3 days, and then 20 mg three times a day. The total daily dosage should not exceed 80 mg of balcofen.

Surgical. Surgical intervention for tic douloureux is reserved for those patients who have become refractory to medical management. Numerous surgical procedures have been tried in the past, but radiofrequency trigeminal gangliolysis and microsurgical decompression of the trigeminal nerve rootlet are the current procedures of choice, as they provide the best chance for permanent relief of pain while producing minimal postoperative complications. Thermal trigeminal gangliolysis is performed by the percutaneous insertion of the radiofrequency needle through the foramen ovale directly into the trigeminal nerve rootlet. After radiofrequency stimulation locates the rootlets responsible for the trigeminal pain, the needle tip is heated for thermocoagulation. This procedure does not require a craniotomy, but occasionally produces disagreeable subjective sensations within the trigeminal nerve distribution and sometimes objective trigeminal involvement (hypalgesia, neuroparalytic keratitis, weakness of the jaw muscles). A significant recurrence rate of the trigeminal neuralgia does occur over time, but radiofrequency thermocoagulation can then be repeated without difficulty. Microsurgical decompression of the trigeminal nerve root near the brainstem does require a suboccipital craniotomy, but this has proved to be a relatively safe procedure associated with a low incidence of postoperative trigeminal nerve dysfunction and rare return of pain in the postoperative period.

Ocular or Periocular Manifestations

Conjunctiva: Ipsilateral hyperemia accompanying the pain.
Lacrimal System: Ipsilateral lacrimation during the pain.
Other: Periorbital pain.

PRECAUTIONS

Among the common side effects of carbamazepine therapy are lightheadedness, drowsiness, and lethargy. Ataxia, nausea and vomiting, and skin rashes can also occur. Cardiac arrhythmias and congestive heart failure may develop, and carbamazepine should be used with caution in patients with heart disease. A rare, but serious drug reaction is the development of leukopenia, thrombocytopenia, or aplastic anemia. A complete blood and platelet count is recommended before starting carbamazepine, every week or two after its initiation for several months, and then every 3 or 4 months during maintenance therapy.

Side effects of phenytoin include nystagmus, ataxia, slurred speech, dizziness, nausea, vomiting, and epigastric pain. Gingival hyperplasia, peripheral neuropathy, hirsutism, skin rashes, and a generalized lymphadenopathy may also develop. Liver dysfunction occasionally occurs, and rarely leukopenia, agranulocytopenia, thrombocytopenia, or pancytopenia has been observed.

Balcofen is usually well tolerated, but can cause drowsiness, weakness, fatigue, headache, dizziness, nausea, and hypotension.

Although carbamazepine, phenytoin, and balcofen are very successful at first in controlling the pain, the trigeminal neuralgia often becomes refractory to systemic treatment over several years.

COMMENTS

If objective trigeminal nerve involvement is detected on the initial evaluation or if other parasellar cranial nerve palsies (third, fourth, or sixth) are found, the diagnosis of trigeminal neuralgia is in question, and an investigation for a parasellar mass lesion, including CT, MRI, and possible carotid arteriography, should be initiated. However, if these ipsilateral parasellar cranial nerve palsies are documented soon after surgery for trigeminal neuralgia, no further investigation is indicated as these findings most likely represent postoperative sequelae.

References

Fromm GH, Terrence CF, Chattha AS: Baclofen in the treatment of trigeminal neuralgia: Double-blind study and long-term follow-up. Ann Neurol 15:240–244, 1984.

Grimson BS, Boone SC: Six nerve palsy complicating percutaneous thermal ablation of the trigeminal nerve rootlet. Am J Ophthalmol 92:225–229, 1981.

Hart RG, Easton, JD: Carbamazepine and hematological monitoring. Ann Neurol 11:309–312, 1982.

Jannetta PJ, Sweet, WH: Trigeminal neuralgia. In Wilson CB, Hoff JT (eds): Current Surgical Management of Neurologic Disease. New York, Churchill Livingstone, 1980, pp 279–299.

Voorhies R, Patterson RH: Management of trigeminal neuralgia (tic douloureux). JAMA 245:2521–2523, 1981.

SECTION 15

NEOPLASMS

Benign

ACTINIC AND SEBORRHEIC KERATOSIS

RONALD R. LUBRITZ, M.D.
New Orleans, Louisiana

Actinic keratosis (solar keratoma) is a precancerous lesion that appears as an erythematous, scaly excrescence and occurs most commonly on sunlight-exposed areas of the skin, such as the face, neck, and dorsa of the hands. It may occur in young children, but is more common in middle-aged or older individuals. It is pre-eminently noted in fair-complexioned individuals.

Seborrheic keratosis is a benign epithelial tumor that appears predominantly on the trunk and head. It is rare in children, but very common in adults over 40 years of age.

Seborrheic keratoses can occur both on the eyebrows and eyelids. The upper lids are more often involved than the lower. When on the lids, seborrheic keratoses can occasionally be somewhat pedunculated. Actinic keratoses most often involve the eyebrows. Although they can occur on the eyelids, this is uncommon because the eyelids, especially the upper eyelids, are usually protected from sunlight.

THERAPY

Surgical. Cryosurgery is a natural choice as a primary method of therapy for keratoses. These lesions are superficial and as such do not have to be treated deeply for eradication. Although utilization of a cotton-tipped applicator saturated with liquid nitrogen may possibly be indicated for certain areas of the skin, it is not indicated for treatment around the eyes because of potential drip problems. For single or multiple lesions of actinic keratosis, freezing with a portable liquid nitrogen spray unit is effective for clinical cure of these growths. No local anesthetic is necessary. When treating multiple lesions, it is sometimes advisable to mark those for therapy; because of the short freeze and thaw times, edema and erythema occasionally cannot be relied on to flag the treated sites. For most lesions, the spray tip is placed at the center of the target site and then carried in an ever-widening circle or spiral pattern until the entire lesion is covered. The keratoses should be frozen just outside the border. Timing the thaw period is an effective means of judging the adequacy of the freeze. The thaw time is defined as the elapsed time from the last application of the spray or probe until the entire lesion is thawed. This end point is detected by the disappearance of the white frosted appearance of the surface or disappearance of any hard area on palpation. A thaw time of 20 to 30 seconds is usually sufficient. Within a few days, the lesion will undergo a vesicular crusted stage; and by the tenth to fourteenth day, the eschar will usually slough off, leaving a residual smooth cutaneous surface.

Flat seborrheic keratoses may be treated in a manner similar to that for actinic keratoses. However, raised lesions do not respond adequately to simple freezing. For these, a light spray is employed first. While the lesion is still superficially frozen, a sharp curette is then used to remove the raised tumor level with the skin. If the seborrheic keratosis is raised and on loose periorbital skin, the above two methods may not be able to be utilized. Instead, local anesthetic injection is used followed by light electrodessication and curettage. If the lesion is somewhat pedunculated, a small curved iris scissors may be used to remove the tumor mass from the skin, rather than a curette. Hemostasis is effected with Gelfoam or a similar dressing. A bandage can then be applied if the area permits.

Periocular Manifestations

Seborrheic keratoses are usually asymptomatic but can become large enough to interfere with vision. They usually occur as brownish or black, somewhat verrucous excrescences. In the periocular area they are usually somewhat small, being only several millimeters to a centimeter in size. They can be somewhat larger around the eyebrow and outer canthi.

Actinic keratoses, on the other hand, are usually flatter, more red or reddish brown in color and usually present with some degree of hyperkeratosis or scaling. Although most are asymptomatic, some can become inflamed or irritated and then cause burning or stinging. They will become more noticeable if the patient is exposed to heavy sunlight.

CAPILLARY HEMANGIOMA

(Angioblastic Hemangioma, Benign Hemangio-Endothelioma, Hemangioblastoma, Strawberry Hemangioma)

BARRETT G. HAIK, M.D.
New Orleans, Louisiana

Capillary hemangiomas are among the most common orbital tumors in the pediatric population. These are not true neoplasms, but appear to be hamartomatous proliferations of primitive vasoformative tissues. This tumor consists of anastomosing blood-filled endothelial-lined channels and typically has an infiltrative growth pattern with no true encapsulation. With rare exception, these tumors present in the first 6 months of life, and one third are clinically obvious at birth. These tumors follow a characteristic clinical course with a period of rapid hypertrophy for 3 to 12 months, followed by a period of stabilization and then involution. The major degree of involution takes place by 5 years of age; however, smaller degrees of tumor regression may be noted until the end of the first decade. Involution is complete with no significant cosmetic sequelae in the majority of cases. However, in some larger lesions, especially those with a combined subcutaneous superficial component, it is not uncommon to observe cosmetically disturbing defects. Additionally, ocular complications, primarily in the form of amblyopia, have been noted in 50 to 75 per cent of cases with orbital and adnexal hemangiomas. Rarer dermatologic and systemic complications may occur secondary to this vascular mass.

THERAPY

Supportive. The great majority of capillary hemangiomas undergo significant spontaneous regression. Although it is well established that therapy can speed regression of these tumors, it will not significantly affect the final amount of tumor involution and the cosmetic result. Therefore, unless there are specific ocular, dermatologic, or systemic indications for rapid resolution, treatment should be withheld, since all of the available therapeutic modalities have significant real or theoretic risks. It is generally of great value to discuss the natural history of the tumor with the family and explain the advantages and disadvantages of administering or withholding therapy in any particular case. Likewise, parents of these patients often find it advantageous to study photographs of children who have undergone spontaneous regression and to speak with parents of children who have reached the stage of maximal tumor regression.

Systemic. Corticosteroids have been shown to be effective in significantly speeding natural tumor involution. Details of their inhibitory effects are not definitely known, but appear related to a vasoconstrictor effect. The typical oral administration of corticosteroids is either 2 mg/kg of prednisone daily or 4 mg/kg on an alternate-day basis. Most patients show a significant decrease of tumor size within 1 week after administration. Unfortunately, this involution does not persist in many cases when the steroid level is discontinued or significantly reduced. Because of this rebound growth, it can therefore be difficult to taper corticosteroids in these patients, and corticosteroid complications are a threat after extended use in this infantile population. Recently, the use of intralesional corticosteroid injections has been suggested and appears to be a promising method of maximizing steroid effect in the area of the tumor mass while minimizing systemic absorption levels. It is suggested that a combination of both the rapidly acting betamethasone and the prolonged-acting triamcinolone be injected with a 27-gauge needle into the tumor mass, often at several different sites to distribute the medication throughout the tumor.

Radiation. Radiation has been shown to be effective in creating microembolic episodes in these vascular tumors and leading to hemangioma regression. Superficial or ortho-voltage radiotherapy may be administered in a single treatment of 200 rads, with appropriate shielding of the globe and adjacent uninvolved tissues. The involuntionary response usually is noted in 1 to 2 weeks, and these treatments may be repeated up to two times, if necessary.

Surgical. Various surgical modalities exist that attempt to reduce tumor size through compromise of the major arterial feeding vessels, constriction and sclerosing of the smaller vascular channels, or primary surgical excision of the mass. Ligation of afferent vessels surgically or through intra-arterial embolization can be an effective means of decreasing blood flow to the tumor mass, therefore stimulating further involution or decreasing vascularity before excisional surgery. Such treatments require accurate radiographic visualization of the major vascular channels supplying the tumor to enable selective interference with the tumor's vascular supply. This is often difficult because of the complex configurations and anastomoses assumed by major feeding vessels to such tumors. Attempts to stimulate the natural involutionary process by destroying smaller vascular channels and stimulating thrombosis include cryotherapy, diathermy, and injections of sclerosing solutions or boiling water. These certainly can speed tumor involution, but often lead to more significant cosmetic and functional deformities than would have occurred with natural involution or alternative forms of therapy.

Primary surgical excision of tumors has limited value because of the diffusely infiltrative nature of these masses, lack of encapsulation, and the resultant difficulty in differentiating them from adjacent or infiltrative critical orbital structures. When surgery is necessary for diagnosis or therapy, it is strongly recommended that one obtain an arteriogram or digital intravenous angiogram before surgery so that the major vascular channels of the tumor are delineated. When surgery is performed, hypotensive anesthesia is recommended to aid in minimizing the volume of blood loss from these infants and permitting more accurate visualization of orbital structures during surgery.

Ocular or Periocular Manifestations

Conjunctiva: Hemangioma.
Eyelids: Hemangioma; ptosis.
Globe: Displacement; proptosis.
Lacrimal System: Hemangioma of lacrimal gland or sac.
Optic Nerve: Secondary optic atrophy.
Other: Amblyopia (refractive, occlusive, strabismus); anisometropia (astigmatism or relative myopia in affected eye); diplopia; exposure keratitis; strabismus.

PRECAUTIONS

Potential complications of prolonged administration of systemic corticosteroids in infants include delayed growth, iatrogenic Cushing's syndrome, and adrenal suppression. Ocular and systemic complications from corticosteroid usage generally follow relatively high-dose, long-term use, but should not accompany "pulse" treatment of several weeks. Complications reported from intralesional corticosteroid injections at this time have been insignificant and include mild pigmentary disturbances in the overlying skin, especially in darkly pigmented children, and the persistence of solid corticosteroid and carrier complexes beneath the skin for several months after injection. All children receiving systemic or intralesional corticosteroids should avoid routine pediatric immunizations with live attenuated viruses during and for 2 weeks before and after administration of corticosteroids.

Radiation precautions include shielding of radiation-sensitive ocular structures, such as the lens, uninvolved adjacent tissues, and the thyroid gland, even if the tumor extends to the neck area. There is a real risk of radiation oncogenesis when the thyroid is inadvertently exposed to low levels of radiation and a theoretic but unproven risk of radiation oncogenesis in the orbital area after low-dose irradiation. Radiation, however, should not be excluded from the treatment regimen, since it is highly effective and there are no known reported cases of radiation oncogenesis in the orbital region with modern low-level techniques (despite the theoretic risk).

Because surgical embolization and ligation techniques can be associated with damage to adjacent crucial structures secondary to inadvertent ischemia following occlusion, they should be reserved for masses causing significant functional complications that are resistant to other forms of therapy.

Destructive techniques, such as diathermy, cryotherapy, and the injection of sclerosing solutions, often cause significant scarring and deformity of the treated area and are rarely, if ever, indicated in the orbital region. Surgical excision of hemangiomatous tissue is rarely indicated because it often involves sacrificing critical orbital structures infiltrated with hemangiomatous tissue that are impossible to surgically distinguish or separate. Surgery is occasionally effective in small, relatively localized adnexal hemangiomas and for excision of fibrovascular remnants after regression. Complications of surgery include the inevitable creation of surgical scars and excision of critical vascular, muscular, and neurogenic components of the orbit.

COMMENTS

Clinically, these tumors may be detected in the orbit and periocular area in three ways. Most commonly, a bluish-purple subcutaneous mass with normal overlying skin is noted in the anterior orbit. Second, approximately one third of the patients have an obvious superficial component consisting of an overlying strawberry hemangioma, and lastly, 5 per cent of patients present with a deep orbital mass and have no signs suggesting the diagnosis. This last group of patients is by far the most clinically perplexing and diagnostically important, since the differential diagnosis of deep orbital tumors in a young infant includes such malignancies as rhabdomyosarcoma and metastatic neuroblastoma. Fortunately, the diagnosis of capillary hemangioma can usually be made on clinical grounds alone, and biopsy will not be necessary.

Although clinical examination of the cutaneous and subcutaneous lesions usually leads to the diagnosis, several associated clinical findings can be supportive in establishing a secure diagnosis. Approximately one third of all patients have obvious hemangiomatous involvement of the palpebral or forniceal conjunctiva or lacrimal gland. One fourth of patients have superficial strawberry hemangiomas on other portions of the body. It is also quite common to observe an increase in the size of a subcutaneous hemangiomatous tumor when the child undergoes a Valsalva maneuver, such as crying.

There are many ancillary tests available to aid in the diagnosis, treatment plan, and subsequent management of this condition. Plain radiographs and computed tomography reveal diffuse enlargement of the orbit without evidence of bony erosion. CT studies with contrast, angiography, and digital intravenous angiography reveal the existence and the extent of the diffusely infiltrating vascular tumor, as well as outline the major feeding vessels supplying this tumor. Ultrasonographic studies are valuable in determining the presence and extent of orbital involvement and permit a safe noninvasive method of monitoring tumor growth and regression.

The most important factors governing the management of capillary hemangiomas are treatment indications. Children afflicted with this condition may not ultimately be helped cosmetically by treatment and may indeed be cosmetically disfigured by surgical scars or may develop systemic or local complications from corticosteroids or radiotherapy. Therefore, treatment should be reserved for those patients in whom the rapidity of tumor regression will significantly influence the clinical outcome. Ocular indications for treatment include threatened amblyopia from mechanical occlusion of the palpebral aperture and, more rarely, exposure keratitis or optic nerve compression from the expanding orbital mass. Although it is known that a high degree of myopia and astigmatism is noted in the globe of the affected orbit, there is no definite evidence that treatment of these masses reduces or alters the final refractive error of the globe. Systemic indications for treatment include oral or nasopharyngeal obstruction from extensive hemangiomatous tissue, high output congestive heart failure caused by the multiple vascular shunts in extensive masses, thrombocytopenia, hemolytic anemia, and disseminating intravascular coagulation. All forms of treatment must include periodic evaluation of refractive errors and amblyopia therapy, when indicated.

References

de Venecia G, Lobeck CC: Successful treatment of eyelid hemangioma with prednisone. Arch Ophthalmol 84:98–102, 1970.

Haik BC: Vascular tumors of the orbit. *In* Hornblass A (ed): Ophthalmic and Orbital Plastic and Reconstructive Surgery. Baltimore, Williams & Wilkins, 1989.

Haik BG, et al: Capillary hemangioma of the lids and orbit: An analysis of the clinical features and therapeutic results in 101 cases. Ophthalmology 86:760–789, 1979.

Kushner BJ: Infantile adnexal hemangioma: Eyelid and orbital. *In* Smith BC, Lisman RD (eds): Ophthalmic Plastic and Reconstructive Surgery. St. Louis, CV Mosby 1987, Vol 2, pp 846–852.

Kushner BJ: Intralesional corticosteroid injection for infantile adnexal hemangioma. Am J Ophthalmol 93:496–506, 1982.

Richards RD: Congenital hemangioma of the orbit and lid. South Med J 67:489–500, 1974.

Robb RM: Refractive errors associated with hemangiomas of the eyelids and orbit in infancy. Am J Ophthalmol 83:52–58, 1977.

Stigmar G et al: Ophthalmic sequelae of infantile hemangiomas of the eyelids and orbit. Am J Ophthalmol 85:806–813, 1978.

CAVERNOUS HEMANGIOMA

BARRETT G. HAIK, M.D.
New Orleans, Louisiana

Cavernous hemangiomas are among the most common orbital tumors of adults. They are benign vascular hamartomas that occur more commonly in females and usually present in the third to fifth decade of life. Although multiple tumors have been reported simultaneously or sequentially separated by long intervals, the majority of cavernous hemangiomas are single lesions and are unassociated with vascular lesions in the eye or elsewhere in the body. These masses can occur in any portion of the orbit, but usually develop in the muscle cone; they are usually round or oval in shape with a slightly nodular surface and a purplish-red color. The tumor is typically circumscribed and contained within a firm fibrous capsule with only small vessels penetrating the tumor surface. Microscopically, cavernous hemangiomas are composed of large blood-filled vascular channels that are lined by flattened endothelial cells and are often separated by multiple fibrous septae.

A characteristic clinical course of slow progressive enlargement typically occurs and may be associated with ophthalmologic findings related to compression or displacement of ocular or orbital structures.

THERAPY

Surgical. The primary treatment modality available is surgical excision. Nonsurgical means of treatment, such as radiation or pharmacologic therapy, have been ineffective. Surgical therapy optimally consists of total excision of the tumor mass through whichever standard orbital approach is dictated by tumor location. In certain cases where the tumor abuts the optic nerve or other critical structures in the orbital apex, incomplete excision may be acceptable in order to avoid damage to these structures. Cavernous hemangiomas have not been reported to recur even after incomplete excision, and it is generally assumed that the residual mass of incompletely excised tumor is obliterated by postsurgical fibrosis.

Ocular or Periocular Manifestations

Choroid: Striae.
Conjunctiva: Subconjunctival hemorrhages.
Globe: Displacement; proptosis.
Optic Nerve: Secondary edema or atrophy.
Other: Anisometropia (astigmatism or relative hyperopia in affected eye); diplopia; exposure keratitis; strabismus.

PRECAUTIONS

In the rare cases where a secure clinical diagnosis can be established without surgery and the tumor is adjacent to critical orbital structures, observation alone may be indicated. In these cases, even subtotal excision may present a significant risk of visual complications, thus outweighing the benefit of surgery. This period of observation should include not only clinical examination but also serial computed tomograms, ultrasonograms, and visual fields to dictate if and when surgical intervention should take place.

COMMENTS

The clinical symptoms and signs at the time of diagnosis are generally proptosis of the affected eye. This is usually axial proptosis, but occasionally can present with associated horizontal or vertical displacement. Additionally, the tumor can exert pressure on the posterior sclera sufficient to cause hyperopia and choroidal folds. Restriction of extraocular motility may be present, as well as diplopia in extreme positions of gaze. There are rare reports in which headaches have existed on the side of the orbital tumor, as well as recurrent subconjunctival hemorrhages in the affected eye.

A number of ancillary diagnostic tests may aid in differentiating cavernous hemangiomas from other benign and malignant orbital conditions. Plain orbital x-rays may show an increase in soft tissue density and, more rarely, phlebolith formation. Additionally, orbital asymmetry secondary to diffuse orbital enlargement, local fossa formation, or hyperostosis may be detected following chronic pressure on the orbital bone. A- and B-scan ultrasonography can reveal the presence and location of a circumscribed mass in the orbit. Sound transmission through the tumor is usually good with a high degree of internal reflectivity produced by the blood septae interfaces of these vascularized lesions. On CT scan, a discrete circumscribed orbital mass may be detected and localized. The rounded or oval contour of this mass is well portrayed. When the mass is adjacent to the optic nerve, distinct separation may not be possible. Internal heterogeneity and loculation of the mass are often noted. Enhancement of the tumor mass following intravenous contrast injection is usually present, but can be totally absent in some cases. Magnetic resonance studies of a limited patient population reveal a well-circumscribed mass that is hypointense on T1-weighted sequences and hyperintense on T2-weighted sequences.

References

Coleman DJ, Jack RL, Franzen LA: II. Hemangiomas of the orbit. Arch Ophthalmol 88:368–374, 1972.
Haik BG: Vascular tumors of the orbit. *In* Hornblass A (ed): Ophthalmic and Orbital Plastic and Reconstructive Surgery. Baltimore, Williams & Wilkins, 1989.
Harnett AN, et al: Cavernous hemangioma presenting as an orbital mass after enucleation for a choroidal melanoma: Case report. Br J Ophthalmol 72:618–620, 1988.
Harris GJ, Jakobiec FA: Cavernous hemangioma of the orbit: A clinicopathologic analysis of sixty-six cases. *In* Jakobiec FA (ed): Ocular and Adnexal Tumors. Birmingham, Aesculapius, 1978, pp 741–781.
Henderson JW: Orbital Tumors, 2nd ed. New York, Brian C Decker, 1980, pp 128–133.
Moss HM: Expanding lesions of the orbit. A clinical study of 230 consecutive cases. Am J Ophthalmol 54:761–770, 1962.
Ohbayashi M, et al: Multiple cavernous hemangiomas of the orbits. Surg Neurol 29:32–34, 1988.
Reese AB: Tumors of the Eye, 3rd ed. Hagerstown, MD, Harper & Row, 1976, p 272.

CRANIOPHARYNGIOMA
HAROLD J. HOFFMAN, M.D.,
B.Sc. (Med), F.R.C.S.(C)
Toronto, Ontario

Craniopharyngiomas are benign congenital tumors arising from epithelial remnants of Rathke's pouch. They are the most common nonglial intracranial tumor in childhood. These slowly growing tumors of squamous epithelium arise in the pituitary stalk and infundibulum and encroach and compress adjacent structures. In general, they compress the optic chiasm in front, the diaphragm and pituitary gland below, and the cavity of the third ventricle above, which frequently results in hydrocephalus. In most cases, cysts form in the center of the tumor. The tumor may project extensively enough to cause varied pituitary and hypothalamic constitutional symptoms, including infantilism, diabetes insipidus, and abnormal sexual development.

Craniopharyngiomas can be divided into three anatomic subtypes. The sellar tumors are relatively small tumors that enlarge the sella tursica and encroach on the pituitary gland. Patients with sellar tumors therefore present with endocrine deficiency symptoms and headache. The prechiasmatic tumors protrude forward between the two optic nerves. These tumors push back on chiasm, producing severe visual loss and usually affecting one optic nerve more than the other. The patients with prechiasmatic tumors rarely have raised intracranial pressure, but do have headaches and frequently have endocrine symptomatology. The retrochiasmatic tumors protrude upward into the third ventricle and push the chiasm forward. As they fill the third ventricle, they produce hydrocephalus and thus raised intracranial pressure. These patients present with papilledema, may have endocrine problems, but rarely do they have visual symptomatology other than papilledema. About 5 per cent of craniopharyngiomas are sellar in location, 35 per cent are prechiasmatic, and 60 per cent are retrochiasmatic.

THERAPY

Surgical. Surgical removal of a craniopharyngioma was regarded as a discouraging proposition in the past owing to the nature of the surrounding structures and its anatomically remote location. In recent years, sophisticated endocrinologic management, the new imaging facilities of CT and MRI scanning that enable earlier diagnosis, the development of the operating microscope and its accompanying armamentarium of elaborate surgical instrumentation, and the development of surgically destructive tools, such as the cavitron and the laser beam, that can deal with solid tumors in delicate locations, have evolved. The availability of these tremendous clinical and technologic advances has greatly reduced operative morbidity and permitted a much higher incidence of complete excision of tumor.

When a tumor has reached a size where it has obliterated the foramen of Monro and has produced significant hydrocephalus with grossly raised intracranial pressure (typically a retrochiasmatic tumor), a bypass diversionary shunt may be necessary as an initial step before removal of the tumor. However, if the hydrocephalus is not particularly severe, the tumor removal will usually resolve the disturbed cerebrospinal fluid dynamics.

Irradiation. Radiotherapy appears to have some destructive influence on craniopharyngioma epithelium. However, unlike conventional radiosensitive tumors, craniopharyn-

giomas never completely resorb after radiation. Furthermore, radiotherapy is not completely benign. There are numerous reports of parenchymal damage to the brain, as well as damage to brain vasculature, caused by radiotherapy. There is also a risk of a radiation-induced tumor, the most common of which is a sarcoma. For these reasons, radiation is used only when surgery has failed to control the tumor.

Supportive. Since more than half of the patients with craniopharyngiomas present with endocrine deficiency, a preoperative endocrine workup should be done, and specific endocrine deficiencies, particularly those of corticosteroids and electrolyte abnormalities, should be corrected.

Dexamethasone in a dosage of 1 to 4 mg every 6 hours should be started immediately preoperatively and continued postoperatively for 48 to 72 hours, at which point maintenance doses of cortisone (25 mg/square meter) are substituted. Eventually, the cortisone should be reduced to the lowest effective level, with a warning to the patient that an increase in dosage may be necessary to avoid possible addisonian crisis during periods of stress or infection.

Total removal of a craniopharyngioma almost invariably results in diabetes insipidus, a condition that usually is manifested during the first 24 to 48 hours postoperatively. Treatment with desmopressin administered by nasal instillation in doses of 5 to 20 μg every 12 to 24 hours is now available for management of this disorder.

Because of surgical retraction of the frontal lobe during surgery, prophylactic doses of 5 to 7 mg/kg of phenytoin should be administered daily for a period of 7 to 10 days postoperatively.

Ocular or Periocular Manifestations

Extraocular Muscles: Paresis of third or sixth nerve.
Optic Nerve: Atrophy; optic neuritis; pallor; papilledema.
Pupil: Abnormal response to light; dilation.
Other: Diplopia; hemianopsia; nystagmus; ocular pain; scotoma; visual field defects; visual loss.

PRECAUTIONS

Any episode of sudden blindness in otherwise healthy individuals, especially children, should be suspected of being caused by craniopharyngioma. Plain skull x-rays show calcification of craniopharyngioma in 26 per cent of the cases, but the CT scan is a far more definitive investigative tool. Angiography has largely been replaced by the MRI scan, which provides an accurate picture of the relationship between tumor and cerebral vessels.

Physicians should be aware of the difficulties associated with total removal of the tumor, particularly when it is adherent to the internal carotid arteries. If part of the tumor is left behind, careful follow-up becomes necessary. However, CT scanning has made this follow-up a matter of relative ease.

Comments

The unusual feature of craniopharyngiomas in children, and particularly in adults, is the frequency of finding normal optic discs when there may be extensive loss of visual fields and sometimes visual acuity. A retained pupillary response in the presence of total blindness may also occur, suggesting that only pupillomotor fibers have remained functional. After surgical removal of the tumor, an almost blind eye may recover a remarkable amount of vision.

Although craniopharyngiomas are benign, they will recur in a significant proportion of patients if any portion of tumor is left behind. Late diagnosis may not preclude total removal of the tumor, but can certainly lead to more advanced compression of the optic apparatus and a poor visual prognosis. In the era before corticosteroid replacement therapy, the mortality rate of patients with craniopharyngiomas was extremely high. The present availability of replacement endocrine medication, the use of CT and MRI scanning for early diagnosis, and the development of better neurosurgical instruments have led to far better management of these tumors and a tremendously improved outlook for patients with this disorder.

References

Adams RD, Hochberg F, Webster H deF: Neoplastic disease of the brain. In Isselbacher KJ et al (eds): Harrison's Principles of Internal Medicine, 9th ed. New York, McGraw-Hill, 1980, p 1957.

Amacher AL: Craniopharyngioma: The controversy regarding radiotherapy. Child's Brain 6:57–64, 1980

Hoffman HJ: Craniopharyngioma in children. In Ransohoff J (ed): Modern Technics in Surgery: Neurosurgery. Mt. Kisco, NY. Futura, 1979, pp 5:1–6.

Hoffman HJ, Buncic JR: Craniopharyngioma in children. In Smith JL: Neuro-Ophthalmology Update. New York, Masson, 1977, pp 241–252.

Hoffman HJ, et al: Management of craniopharyngioma in children. J Neurosurg 47:218–227, 1977.

Matson DD, Crigler JF Jr: Management of craniopharyngioma in childhood. J Neurosurg 30:377–390, 1969.

Ross HS, Rosenberg S, Friedman AH: Delayed radiation necrosis of the optic nerve. Am J Ophthalmol 76:683–686, 1973.

Sweet WH: Radical surgical treatment of craniopharyngioma. Clin Neurosurg 23:52–79, 1975.

Waga S, Handa H: Radiation-induced meningioma: With review of literature. Surg Neurol 5:212–219, 1976.

Walsh FB, Hoyt WF: Clinical Neuro-Ophthalmology, 3rd ed. Baltimore, Williams & Wilkins, 1969, pp 2157–2162.

Waltz TA, Brownell B: Sarcoma: A possible late result of effective radiation therapy for pituitary adenoma. Report of two cases. J Neurosurg 24:901–907, 1966.

DERMOID
(Dermoid Choristoma, Dermoid Cyst, Dermolipoma, Lipodermoid)

ARTHUR S. GROVE, JR., M.D.
Boston, Massachusetts

Dermoids are benign tumors that are usually considered to be choristomas, rather than neoplasms. A choristoma is a growth that arises during embryologic development from tissue elements that are not normally present in the location of the lesion. Most dermoids are cystic and are believed to be caused by developmental sequestrations of surface epidermis, frequently adjacent to bony suture lines around the orbit. Some dermoids are chiefly solid with large quantities of fatty tissue, in which case they are described as dermolipomas or lipodermoids.

Histologically, dermoids are composed of epidermal tissue together with one or more dermal adnexal structures and skin appendages, such as hair follicles, sebaceous glands, and sweat glands. The cystic component is lined by keratinizing epidermis and may be filled with keratin, hairs, and fatty material. If these contents are released into the orbit either spontaneously or during surgery, an inflammatory reaction may result. Dermolipomas are usually found beneath the conjunctiva over the surface of the globe. Hairs may arise from these solid tumors and irritate the eye.

Anatomically, dermoids can be classified into three groups: superficial subcutaneous dermoids, deep orbital dermoids, and subconjunctival dermoids. Superficial dermoids are usually found during childhood, when they appear as painless subcutaneous nodules that often occur beneath the lateral brow. Deep orbital dermoids may not be discovered until maturity, since a long period of slow growth may precede displacement of the eye and exophthalmos. Subconjunctival dermoids are frequently dermolipomas, which are usually located on the temporal surface of the globe and may extend far into the posterior orbit.

Orbital x-rays are usually normal in patients with superficial subcutaneous dermoids and subconjunctival dermoids or dermolipomas. However, deep orbital dermoids often displace the orbital walls or cause sharply marginated defects in the orbital bones adjacent to the lesion. Ultrasonography and CT scanning usually demonstrate a cyst, and sometimes an adjacent solid component may be seen as well.

THERAPY

Surgical. Superficial subcutaneous dermoids can usually be removed through a skin incision directly over the lesion. The deep surface of the tumor is nearly always adherent to periosteum, from which it must be sharply divided. The diagnosis of these lesions can commonly be made from their clinical appearance, and excision may be delayed when the abnormality is discovered in young children.

Deep orbital dermoids are often located in areas that cannot be adequately visualized without removing the lateral orbital rim. If the lesion is located in the upper orbit, a superolateral approach similar to that described for removal of lacrimal gland tumors may be used. Deep dermoid cysts located in the lower orbit may be removed using an inferolateral approach. Excision is sometimes made easier by careful removal of the contents before dissection of the cyst wall. Some deep orbital dermoids extend through the orbital bones and involve the intracranial space, in which case they should usually be removed through a neurosurgical approach.

Subconjunctival dermoids or dermolipomas can also be recognized by their location and appearance in most instances. These lesions are usually located adjacent to the temporal surface of the globe and are commonly yellow or white. Hairs may project from the surface of the tumor and irritate the eye. Solid epibulbar dermoids may occur in Goldenhar's syndrome together with eyelid colobomas and auricular appendages. Subconjunctival dermoids may have deep orbital extensions that lie near the levator and extraocular muscles. Excision of these tumors may be complicated by damage to the eye, decreased lacrimal secretion, restricted eye movement, and ptosis. Because of the potential for complications, excision of subconjunctival dermoids or dermolipomas should usually be avoided if possible. If excision is necessary because of enlargement, cosmetic deformity, or irritation, surgery should be performed with great care.

Ocular or Periocular Manifestations

Conjunctiva: Dermoid.
Cornea: Dermoid; exposure keratitis (secondary to dermolipoma surgery).
Extraocular Muscles: Paresis or paralysis.
Eyebrows or Eyelids: Dermoid; ptosis.
Orbit: Exophthalmos.
Other: Astigmatism (caused by pressure against the cornea); visual loss (rare).

PRECAUTIONS

Cystic dermoids should be removed with care to avoid spilling their potentially irritating contents into the orbit or beneath the skin. If some spillage occurs, it is usually adequate to irrigate the area thoroughly to remove debris. Solid dermoids and dermolipomas are often located near the levator and extraocular muscles. Excision of these tumors should either be avoided or performed with great care to avoid such damage to the eye as ptosis or restricted extraocular muscle movement.

COMMENTS

The diagnosis and localization of dermoids can usually be made on the basis of clinical findings and CT scanning. X-rays and ultrasonography may contribute to the evaluation of these lesions. Since dermoids are benign, the benefits of surgery should be balanced against the risks of operation. Cystic dermoids commonly enlarge progressively and therefore should usually be completely removed, if possible. Solid dermoids (most often subconjunctival dermolipomas) may remain relatively stable in size. Therefore, dermolipomas are frequently observed without surgery, since excision may be complicated by damage to surrounding tissues.

References

Grove AS Jr: Giant dermoid cysts of the orbit. Ophthalmology 86:1513–1520, 1979.
Grove AS Jr: Surgery of the orbit. *In* Spaeth GL (ed): Ophthalmic Surgery: Principles and Practice. Philadelphia, WB Saunders, 1982, pp 431–546.
Henderson JW: Orbital Tumors, 2nd ed. New York, Brian C Decker, 1980, pp 75–114.
Paris GL, Beard C: Blepharoptosis following dermolipoma surgery. Ann Ophthalmol 5:697–699, 1973.

JUVENILE XANTHOGRANULOMA
(JXG, Nevoxanthoendothelioma)

PAUL E. ROMANO, M.D., M.S.O.
and LYN A. SEDWICK, M.D.
Gainesville, Florida

Juvenile xanthogranuloma is a disease of infancy and childhood of unknown etiology characterized by multiple benign tumors. The skin is most frequently involved, with yellow, elevated, papular, sharply demarcated lesions singly or in groups that have a predilection for the head or neck. These lesions spontaneously regress over several years.

Ocular and adnexal juvenile xanthogranuloma has been recognized since 1949 and may occur independently of concurrent skin lesions. The iris or ciliary body is commonly affected, and typical presentation in an infant is a salmon or darkly pigmented solitary iris lesion with spontaneous unilateral hyphema. Orbital, corneal, epibulbar, and lid lesions as well as bilateral iris involvement have been described. Although most eye lesions manifest in infancy (85 per cent at age less than 1 year, 64 per cent at age less than 7 months), adult cases have also been reported.

THERAPY

Supportive. The natural course of juvenile xanthogranuloma of the iris and ciliary body in infancy is spontaneous regression punctuated by one or more episodes of spontaneous bleeding. Whether juvenile xanthogranuloma iris lesions occur without bleeding is currently unknown, as eye involvement is usually recognized only after spontaneous hyphema. Such hyphemas may progress to secondary glaucoma. Therefore, prophylactic therapy may be advisable. Experience with other ocular lesions is very limited, but suggests self-limited disease, if not spontaneous regression. The following treatment modalities have been used or advocated by numerous authors; none has had the benefit of controlled studies.

Systemic. Topical or usually both topical and systemic corticosteroids should be given to promote involution of the ocular lesions. Oral prednisone‡ in a daily dosage of 2 mg/kg may be given in divided doses for no more than 4 to 6 weeks. In patients with corneal or intraocular lesions, one drop of topical ophthalmic 1 per cent prednisolone‡ solution may be applied several times daily. However, such therapy should not be administered for more than a few weeks. Orbital disease responds well, but steroids alone may not stabilize intraocular lesions.

Irradiation. Many authors consider radiation therapy to be the most effective treatment modality. Though even smaller doses are advocated, most authors report regression of lesions with a total dose of between 250 and 500 rads, given in divided doses of 150 to 200 rads to minimize cataractogenic effects. Cataract has not to date been reported following such dosage.

Surgical. Iridectomy and iridocyclectomy have been used for both diagnosis and therapy. However, the location of the lesions, their friability, and the propensity to bleed make such procedures technically difficult, and some authors caution against surgical intervention. Large incisions in infantile eyes are hazardous, and refractive and other changes following surgery may cause a functional amblyopia, with a poor visual prognosis akin to a unilateral infantile cataract.

Ocular or Periocular Manifestations

Conjunctiva: Epibulbar mass (very rare).
Cornea: Blood stained (from hyphema); edema (from glaucoma).
Eyelids: Yellow to brown papules or nodules.
Iris or Ciliary Body: Heterochromia; salmon-colored lesion; uveitis.
Pupil: Oval and/or eccentric.
Other: Proptosis (rare); spontaneous hyphema (common).

Precautions

Prolonged use of either topical or systemic corticosteroids may cause glaucoma, cataract, or iatrogenic Cushing's syndrome. Fluorinated corticosteroids should not be used in children.

Comments

When ocular juvenile xanthogranuloma occurs with typical skin lesions, diagnosis can be confirmed by skin biopsy. In about 50 per cent of cases, however, ocular juvenile xanthogranuloma presents without such lesions. Iris lesions may present as unilateral glaucoma, spontaneous hyphema, uveitis, or heterochromia. In such cases, ultrasonic echography or examination under anesthesia or both are indicated to rule out retinoblastoma. Anterior chamber tap for cytology may be useful, though not without some hazard. When glaucoma secondary to hyphema does occur, standard medical and surgical therapy may not control progression to a blind, painful eye. Thus, steroid and radiation therapy is especially important early in the disease process to accelerate natural involution and regression.

References

Hadden OB: Bilateral juvenile xanthogranuloma of the iris. Br J Ophthalmol 59:699–702, 1975.
Harley RD, Romayananda N, Chan GH: Juvenile xanthogranuloma. J Pediatr Ophthalmol Strabismus 19:33–39, 1982.
Sanders TE: Infantile xanthogranuloma of the orbit. A report of three cases. Am J Ophthalmol 61:1299–1306, 1966.
Schwartz LW, Rodrigues MM, Hallett JW: Juvenile xanthogranuloma diagnosed by paracentesis. Am J Ophthalmol 77:243–246, 1974.
Smith JLS, Ingram RM: Juvenile oculodermal xanthogranuloma. Br J Ophthalmol 52:696–703, 1968.
Zimmerman LE: Ocular lesions of juvenile xanthogranuloma. Nevoxanthoendothelioma. Am J Ophthalmol 60:1011–1035, 1965.

KERATOACANTHOMA
J. BROOKS CRAWFORD, M.D.
San Francisco, California

Keratoacanthoma is a benign epithelial tumor on sun-exposed Caucasian skin in patients of middle or old age. Most are solitary. The majority of these occur on the face (including the eyelids and rarely the conjunctiva), where they may be unusually aggressive, and on the hands. Multiple keratoacanthomas are rare and sometimes occur in families. An eruptive form of the disease (thousands of small keratoacanthomas over the whole body) is very rare. Keratoacanthomas may occur in patients with xeroderma pigmentosum, in immunologically compromised patients (such as recipients of renal transplants, patients with metastatic cancer, and patients with leukemia and lymphoma), and as part of the Muir-Torre syndrome (multiple internal malignancies with cutaneous sebaceous proliferations and keratoacanthomas). The lesions are raised, dome-shaped tumors with rolled lateral borders and a central keratin core. They are characterized by an abrupt onset and rapid growth. Most reach a maximum size of 1 to 2 cm in 6 to 8 weeks and then spontaneously involute over a period of months. Some lesions, particularly those on the face, may grow larger and regress more slowly. In most patients, the presence of a rapidly growing lump is the main symptom, but occasionally pain, discomfort, or irritation may occur.

THERAPY

Surgical. Despite the tendency for these tumors to involute spontaneously, surgery is usually the treatment of choice. Small lesions can be completely excised; larger lesions can be biopsied after which they often undergo an accelerated rate of involution.

There are several reasons why surgery is generally preferred over observation. Keratoacanthomas are benign, but may closely resemble squamous cell carcinomas, which are malignant and can metastasize. Lesions on the face are usually disfiguring, and many patients prefer not to wait the time required for spontaneous involution. Small lesions can be removed before they enlarge and produce destruction of cosmetically and functionally important areas. Basal cell carcinomas and squamous cell carcinomas may occur at the base or edges of a true keratoacanthoma. Some keratoacanthomas never regress.

All the methods used to treat the two common skin cancers, basal and squamous cell carcinoma, have been used successfully to treat keratoacanthomas. In addition to excision, other surgical measures include cryotherapy and curettage with electrocoagulation. Nonsurgical treatments include radiation therapy and the use of fluorouracil, which can be injected into the lesion* or applied as a cream or ointment. Synthetic retinoids‡ have successfully been used for a few cases of multiple keratoacanthomas that failed to resolve or recurred after conventional surgery or the use of fluorouracil. In patients who refuse surgery or for whom surgery is contraindicated, these alternative modalities may be effective. However, if the lesions do not regress as expected with these methods, a biopsy should be performed to be certain that the lesion is not a basal or squamous cell carcinoma.

Ocular or Periocular Manifestations

Conjunctiva: Nodules.
Eyelids: Nodules.
Other: Irritation; ocular pain.

Precautions

An adequate biopsy is essential in order to rule out the possibility of squamous cell carcinoma, which keratoacanthoma closely resembles. Oc-

casional progression and malignant change of keratoacanthomas, especially in immunosuppressed patients, have been documented. However, most reports of these benign tumors that later undergo malignant change and metastasize are probably cases of carcinomas that are not recognized initially, either because of an inadequate biopsy or because it is occasionally impossible to differentiate a keratoacanthoma from a squamous cell carcinoma on histologic evaluation alone. The biopsy should include a spindle-shaped portion across the entire lesion including the center, subcutaneous tissue beneath the lesion, and normal tissue at both edges of the lesion. Many large tumors undergo an accelerated rate of spontaneous involution after such a biopsy. Recurrences of keratoacanthomas are rare, but occasionally occur; some keratoacanthomas, particularly those on the eyelids and face, have an especially aggressive behavior.

Comments

The etiology of keratoacanthomas is unknown. Since most occur on sun-exposed areas of light-skinned individuals and may occur in patients with xeroderma pigmentosum, ultraviolet radiation has been implicated. Exposure to tar and oil products has also been suspected in the etiology. Immunologic depression may play a role in some patients. Multiple keratoacanthomas occasionally have a hereditary component.

References

Boniuk M, Zimmerman LE: Eyelid tumors with reference to lesions confused with squamous cell carcinoma. III. Keratoacanthoma. Arch Ophthalmol 77:29–40, 1967.

Boynton JR, Searl SS, Caldwell EH: Large periocular keratoacanthoma: The case for definitive treatment. Ophthalmic Surg 17:565–569, 1986.

Font RL: Eyelids and lacrimal drainage system. *In* Spencer WH (ed): Ophthalmic Pathology. Philadelphia, WB Saunders, 1986, Vol 3, pp 2151–2155.

Haydey RP, Reed ML, Dzubow LM, Shipack JL: Treatment of keratoacanthomas with oral 13-cis retinoic acid. N Engl J Med 303:500–502, 1980.

Lever WF, Schaumberg-Lever G: Histopathology of the Skin, 5th ed. Philadelphia, JB Lippincott, 1975, pp 483–486.

Parker CM, Hanke CW: Large keratoacanthomas in difficult locations treated with intralesional 5-fluorouracil. J Am Acad Dermatol 14:770–777, 1986.

Poleksic S, Yeung KY: Rapid development of keratoacanthoma and accelerated transformation into squamous cell carcinoma of the skin. Cancer 41:12–16, 1978.

Popkin GL et al: A technique of biopsy recommended for keratoacanthomas. Arch Dermatol 94:191–193, 1966.

Rook A, Whimster I: Keratoacanthoma—a thirty year retrospect. Br J Dermatol 100:41–47, 1979.

Schwartz RA: The keratoacanthoma: A review. J Surg Oncol 12:305–317, 1979.

Shaw JC, White CR Jr: Treatment of multiple keratoacanthomas with oral isotretinoin. J Am Acad Dermatol 15:1079, 1082, 1986.

LEIOMYOMA
DAVID SEVEL, M.D., Ph.D., F.A.C.S.
La Jolla, California

Leiomyoma is a rare, benign tumor that arises from smooth muscle; it comprises only 2 to 14 per cent of all primary iris tumors. It may be located in the iris, the ciliary body, or the orbit and originates in these structures from the sphincter or dilator pupillae muscle, the ciliary muscle, and Müller's or capsulopalpebral muscle, respectively.

Leiomyoma of the iris is reported most frequently in white female subjects and occurs in a wide age group, ranging from 10 to 80 years of age. This white or pink tumor commonly involves the inferior temporal iris and is well circumscribed and elevated. A presenting feature may be a distorted pupil, ectropion uveae, or hyphema. Vision is not affected unless there is a complication of glaucoma or cataract. Clinically, a leiomyoma of the iris cannot be differentiated from an amelanotic malignant melanoma.

Leiomyoma of the ciliary body usually presents as a pigmented mass of the ciliary body that slowly increases in size and may distort the iris, compress the lens, or locally occlude the filtration angle. Clinically, it cannot be differentiated from a malignant melanoma of the ciliary body.

A leiomyoma of the orbit is an extremely rare, well-encapsulated, vascular tumor that is usually located in an extraconal position. Irrespective of the primary site of the tumor, the diagnosis of leiomyoma is only made on histologic examination. Although local recurrences may occur if the tumor is incompletely removed, distant metastases have not been described.

THERAPY

Supportive. Leiomyomas of the iris and ciliary body are only excised if the tumors increase in size, bleed, or cause complications, such as glaucoma or cataract. Repeated frequent examinations (every 6 months) should include photography of the tumor to aid in the assessment of the size, gonioscopy, and fluorescein iridography.

Surgical. The tumor should be removed in toto, as local recurrences may occur if the tumor is incompletely excised. Fluorescein iridography helps determine the actual tumor size, which may extend beyond that noted on clinical observation. In addition, the blood supply of the tumor may be ascertained preoperatively. Radioactive phosphorus uptake may be done preoperatively to help assess the vascularity of the tumor. Perhaps of greater importance, the extension of the tumor in the filtration angle can be determined, helping one decide whether or not an iridectomy or iridocyclectomy is required. A tumor of the ciliary body is treated by an iridocyclectomy, which can involve up to a quarter of the ciliary body circumference. A leiomyoma of the orbit is well encapsulated and is easily removed.

Ocular or Periocular Manifestations

(C) refers to ciliary body leiomyoma; (I) indicates iris leiomyoma; (O) refers to orbital leiomyoma.
Anterior Chamber: Hyphema (I); shallow angle (C).
Ciliary Body: Pigmented tumor (C).
Globe: Proptosis (O).
Iris: Distorted pupil (I); ectropion uveae (I); pale tumor (I).
Other: Glaucoma (C,I); localized cataract (C,I).

PRECAUTIONS

An iris or ciliary body leiomyoma cannot be differentiated clinically from a malignant melanoma and is diagnosed on histologic examination. The tumor must be totally removed; otherwise, recurrences are inevitable.

Orbital leiomyoma is localized and well encapsulated and usually shells out without difficulty. The tumor is removed in toto. Patients may experience intermittent episodes of pain, a feature not common with other benign orbital growths. This symptomatology may be related to the vascularity of the tumor.

COMMENTS

Leiomyoma has a propensity for slow growth. Although degeneration may occur within its substance, resulting in hemorrhage and local necrosis, spread by continuity, contiguity, or metastases has not been recorded.

Histologically, a leiomyoma is composed of interlacing, tightly arranged spindle-shaped cells with oval nuclei and blunted ends. There is only a moderate amount of eosinophilic cytoplasm. Longitudinal fibrils are noted within the cells and are best seen with phosphotungstic acid hematoxylin stain. With light microscopy, a leiomyoma can be difficult to differentiate from a neurofibroma, an amelanotic spindle-shaped malignant melanoma, or a neurilemoma, especially as phosphotungstic acid hematoxylin stain does not differentiate myofibrils from neurofibrils. Electron microscopy may be the only means of differentiating these tumors from a leiomyoma.

It has also been suggested that oxytalan fiber demonstration can differentiate between a leiomyoma and a spindle-cell malignant melanoma of the iris. However, in the diagnosis of leiomyoma of the ciliary body, oxytalan fiber demonstration is not of use because these fibers are normally present in the ciliary body.

References

de Buen S, Olivares ML, Charlin VC: Leiomyoma of the iris. Report of a case. Br J Ophthalmol 55:353–356, 1971.

Henderson JW, Harrison EG Jr: Vascular leiomyoma of the orbit: Report of a case. Trans Am Acad Ophthalmol Otolaryngol 74:970–974, 1970.

Meyer SL, et al: Leiomyoma of the ciliary body. Electron microscopic verification. Am J Ophthalmol 66:1061–1068, 1968.

Sevel D, Tobias B: The value of fluorescein iridography with leiomyoma of the iris. Am J Ophthalmol 74:475–478, 1972.

Sunba MSN, et al: Tumours of the anterior uvea. III. Oxytalan fibers in the differential diagnosis of leiomyoma and malignant melanoma of the iris. Br J Ophthalmol 64:867–874, 1980.

LYMPHANGIOMA

IRA SNOW JONES, M.D.,
and HILARY J. RONNER, M.D.
New York, New York

Lymphangiomas are congenital, benign, slow-growing tumors of the lymphatic system. They can arise in various parts of the body, but are found most frequently on the neck, face and scalp and within the lids, conjunctiva, and orbit. A rich vascular supply is often present within the lesions. Some dispute has arisen as to whether orbital lymphangiomas are distinct entities or variants of venous malformations. This latter speculation is the result of venographic studies that revealed abnormal and dilated venous channels in close proximity to orbital lymphangiomas. Presently, it is held, however, that lymphangiomas are distinct and true entities within the orbit. A fluctuating clinical course is typical with an orbital lymphangioma. Hemorrhage into the lesion with or without trauma is a characteristic complication, with resulting chocolate cyst formation and fulminant proptosis. This proptosis often leads to the recognition of these otherwise occult lesions. Lymphangiomas, unlike infantile hemangiomas, do not undergo spontaneous regression.

THERAPY

Supportive. Orbital lymphangiomas frequently have several active lymph follicles within them, and younger patients often exhibit exacerbation of their proptosis during or after an upper respiratory infection. Topical steroids may be of some benefit in these cases. For very deep lesions, systemic steroids may be utilized.

Surgical. The surgical management of orbital lymphangiomas carries considerable risk. Because of their infiltrative growth pattern with diffuse borders, it is surgically very difficult to create a cleavage plane that permits total removal without damaging other vital orbital structures. Because of this lesion's slow growth pattern, partial excisions and plastic repairs may be spread over a long period of time. Repeated small excisions of tumor seem to give the best results. With the introduction of the carbon dioxide laser into ophthalmic surgery, bulky lesions may be excised with hemostasis achieved simultaneously. Radical surgery, such as exenteration of the orbit, is only indicated in a blind eye with a severe cosmetic deformity. Superficial, localized lymphangiomas of the lids and conjunctiva may be excised, and chocolate cysts of the orbit should be drained, with repeated procedures often being necessary.

Ocular or Periocular Manifestations

Conjunctiva: Hemorrhages; hyperemia; lymphangioma.
Eyelids: Cellulitis; hemorrhages; lymphangioma; ptosis.
Globe: Exophthalmos (episodic, stationary, variable).
Orbit: Asymmetry (on x-ray); blood cysts; lymphangioma.
Other: Amblyopia secondary to induced astigmatism; extraocular muscle imbalance; facial lymphangioma; nasopharyngeal lymphangioma; optic disc edema; retinal and choroidal striae.

PRECAUTIONS

Treatment of orbital lymphangioma is indicated when the lesion interferes with use of the eye or when severe cosmetic deformity is present. Because lymphangiomas are not radiosensitive, therapy therefore consists of surgical excision. Recurrences of the lesion are often a problem.

COMMENTS

The growth rate of lymphangiomas of the orbit is comparable to that of the rest of the body. A stationary point of growth of a lymphangioma is commonly reached in early adulthood. They have the tendency to grow during or subsequent to an upper respiratory infection. It is very important to keep in mind, however, that an orbital rhabdomyosarcoma may also enlarge during a viral illness of the upper respiratory tract, although much more rarely.

Spontaneous hemorrhages play an important role in the diagnosis and treatment of orbital lymphangiomas. Orbital and lid lesions may remain occult until there is a sudden orbital or eyelid hemorrhage with resultant proptosis of the eye. If the hemorrhage is superficial, it may appear almost black in color as a result of static, nonaerated blood and hemosiderin and may also be mistaken for a melanoma.

References

Iliff WJ, Green WR: Orbital tumors in children. In Jakobiec FA (ed): Ocular and Adnexal Tumors. Birmingham, Aesculapius, 1978, pp 677–678.

Iliff WJ, Green WR: Orbital lymphangiomas. Ophthalmology 86:914–929, 1979.

Jakobiec FA, Font RL: Orbit. In Spencer WH (ed): Ophthalmic Pathology. Philadelphia, WB Saunders, 1986, Vol 3, pp 2533–2538.

Jones IS: Lymphangiomas of the ocular adnexa: An analysis of 62 cases. Trans Am Ophthalmol Soc 57:602–665, 1959.

Reese AB: Expanding lesions of the orbit. Trans Ophthalmol Soc UK 91:85–104, 1971.

Reese AB: Tumors of the Eye, 3rd ed. Hagerstown, MD, Harper & Row, 1976, pp 290–293.

Reese AB, Howard GM: Unusual manifestations of ocular lymphangioma and lymphangiectasis. Surv Ophthalmol 18:226–231, 1973.

Wright JE: Orbital vascular anomalies. Trans Am Acad Ophthalmol Otolaryngol 78:606–616, 1974.

MEDULLOEPITHELIOMA
(Diktyoma)

LEONARD APT, M.D.

Los Angeles, California

Medulloepithelioma is a rare congenital tumor that arises from the primitive, nonpigmented medullary epithelium of the ciliary body before differentiation into its various derivatives (sixth week of gestation). Occasionally, the tumor originates in the iris, the retina, and the optic nerve. Medulloepithelioma commonly is called "diktyoma" (from the Greek diktyon, meaning net) because, at times, it has a lace- or net-like appearance.

These tumors are classified into nonteratoid and teratoid types, and each is further divided into benign and malignant varieties. Nonteratoid medulloepitheliomas contain tissue resembling medullary epithelium, but may also contain tissue derived from secondary optic vesicle, such as retinal pigment epithelium, ciliary epithelium, vitreous, and neuroglia. The teratoid group exhibits heteroplasia; that is, it contains tissues not normally present in the eye, such as cartilage, brain tissue, and striated muscle. The teratoid types are more likely than the nonteratoid to be malignant. Criteria for malignancy in these tumors include 1) local invasion of other ocular tissues with or without extraocular extension, 2) many poorly differentiated neuroblastic cells that may resemble retinoblastoma, 3) increased pleomorphism or mitotic activity, and 4) appearance of sarcomatous areas. Medulloepitheliomas are locally destructive, but also may metastasize. They should be considered potentially malignant tumors.

Medulloepitheliomas tend to affect children in the first decade of life, commonly between 2 and 4 years of age. The tumor, however, has been observed in young infants and occasionally in adults, the oldest being in a 79-year-old individual. In one large series of cases, the first clinical manifestation was noted at an average age of 3.8 years, and the average time of final diagnosis by enucleation was 5 years of age. Medulloepitheliomas almost always are unilateral, with no laterality preference, and exhibit no hereditary, racial, or sexual predilection. These tumors occur spontaneously and are not related to any predisposing condition such as trauma or inflammation.

The clinical course of medulloepitheliomas is not uniform; most often they grow as a localized, relatively benign tumor in the ciliary body and iris, proceed to cover the lens surface and posterior surface of the iris, and then may fill the anterior chamber or even extend posteriorly to detach the retina. More often, the lesion is recognized inferiorly. Medulloepitheliomas may occur as a solid or cystic tumor or as a net-like mass that extends into adjacent cavities. Although these tumors are slow growing, they may crowd the anterior chamber angle and cause secondary glaucoma.

Ocular or Periocular Manifestations

Anterior Chamber: Shallow; hyphema; medulloepithelioma (rare).
Conjunctiva: Hyperemia.
Cornea: Breaks in Descemet's membrane; tumor infiltration.
Globe: Exophthalmos; buphthalmos (infants, young children).
Iris or Ciliary Body: Heterochromia; medulloepithelioma (solid or cystic); iritis; rubeosis iridis; synechiae.
Lens: Cataract; colombomatous in tumor area.
Optic Nerve: Medulloepithelioma (rare).
Orbit: Medulloepithelioma extension.
Pupil: Fixed or deformed; abnormal reflexes; leukocoria.
Retina: Detachment; medulloepithelioma (rare).
Vitreous: Retrolental membrane with dilated blood vessels; net-like strands; hemorrhage.
Other: Visual loss; pain; strabismus; secondary glaucoma.

The color of the tumor varies, appearing as white, gray, yellow, pigmented or brown in the center, or fleshy pink. In some cases, cysts dislodge from the tumor and float freely in the anterior chamber or enter the vitreous cavity. If the lens appears colobomatous inferiorly as a result of partial absorption in the area of the tumor and there is neovascular glaucoma and rubeosis iridis but no uveal coloboma or retinal abnormality, the diagnosis of medulloepithelioma may be considered.

Differential diagnosis includes retinoblastoma, persistent hyperplastic primary vitreous (occasionally coexists with medulloepithelioma), peripheral uveitis (pars planitis, cyclitis), nematode granuloma (usually *Toxocara canis*), iris cyst, nevus, amelanotic and melanotic melanoma, leiomyoma, neurofibroma of the iris or ciliary body, juvenile xanthogranuloma, and primary tumors of the pigmented or nonpigmented ciliary epithelium, e.g., adenoma and adenocarcinoma.

The clinical diagnosis of medulloepithelioma usually is based on 1) the tumor's appearance on indirect ophthalmoscopy and slitlamp biomicroscopy and 2) familiarity with the tumor's growth pattern. Correct clinical diagnosis before microscopic tissue study, however, has been infrequent. Fluorescein angiography, ultrasonography, and computed tomography have not been diagnostic. Because of the cystic component of some medulloepitheliomas, ultrasonography possibly could be of some diagnostic assistance if the globe is so positioned as to permit proper placement of the instrument's probe. Studies using magnetic resonance imaging have yet to be reported. Definitive diagnosis of medulloepithelioma is made by light and electron microscopy examination of material obtained on aspiration, biopsy, or excision.

THERAPY

Surgical. Treatment of medulloepitheliomas is based on early recognition and surgical management. If the tumor is confined to the iris and growth is documented, excisional biopsy (iridectomy) is indicated. If the tumor is small, well circumscribed, and confined to the ciliary body, cyclectomy or iridocyclectomy is recommended; unfortunately, tumors in the ciliary body usually are large before clinical manifestations lead to their detection. Enucleation generally is required for most medulloepitheliomas because of one or more of the following reasons: tumor size, location, encroachment on or destruction of adjacent ocular tissues, pain, secondary glaucoma, incomplete excision or local recurrence of tumor, malignant changes observed in an excised histopathologic specimen, or failure to exclude an intraocular malignancy such as retinoblastoma.

Precautions

Since medulloepithelioma is slow growing, early enucleation generally results in a high survival rate. Spread may lead to fatality, however, since the tumor then grows into the orbital bones and brain and may metastasize to the regional lymph nodes and lungs. Following enucleation, the patient should be observed closely for local recurrences or metastases. If extraocular extension has occurred, exenteration of the orbit is necessary. The rare optic nerve medulloepithelioma, because of its location and invasive tendency, requires enucleation with long section of the optic nerve or exenteration; removal of the intracanalicular and intracranial portions of the optic nerve may also be necessary.

Comments

Treatment of medulloepithelioma with radiotherapy or chemotherapy has been used too infrequently to judge its true value. Medulloepitheliomas are likely to be radiosensitive as are most embryonic tumors, such as retinoblastoma and neuroblastoma. The actual radiation response of ocular medulloepithelioma, however, is unknown because of the lack of experience with this method of treatment. The probable radiation dose for tumor ablation by conventional external beam techniques might produce serious ocular complications. Whether newer approaches, such as radioisotope applicators or particle beams, could eliminate the tumor without undue morbidity remains unanswered. In cases with local recurrence of tumor or metastasis to distant organs, the use of irradiation and chemotherapy should be considered.

References

Anderson SR: Intraocular epithelial tumors and cysts. *In* Garner A, Klintworth GK (eds): Pathology of Ocular Disease. A Dynamic Approach. New York, Marcel Dekker, 1982, pp 635–650.

Apt L, et al: Diktyoma (embryonal medulloepithelioma). Recent review and case report. J Pediatr Ophthalmol 10:30–38, 1973.

Broughton WL, Zimmerman LE: A clinicopathologic study of 56 cases of intraocular medulloepitheliomas. Am J Ophthalmol 85:407–418, 1978.

Canning CR, McCartney ACE, Hungerford J: Medulloepithelioma (diktyoma). Br J Ophthalmol 72:764–767, 1988.

Floyd BB: Intraocular medulloepithelioma in a 79-year-old man. Ophthalmology 89:1088–1094, 1982.

Green WR, Iliff WJ, Trotter RR: Malignant teratoid medulloepithelioma of the optic nerve. Arch Ophthalmol 91:451–454, 1974.

Jakobiec FA, et al: Electron microscopic diagnosis of medulloepithelioma. Am J Ophthalmol 79:321–329, 1975.

Reese AB: Tumors of the Eye, 3rd ed. Hagerstown, MD, Harper & Row, 1976, pp 66–72.

Shields JA: Diagnosis and Management of Intraocular Tumors. St. Louis, CV Mosby Co., 1983, pp 329–359.

MENINGIOMA

DUNCAN P. ANDERSON, M.D.C.M., F.R.C.S.(C)

Montreal, Quebec

Meningiomas are generally benign, slow-growing tumors that arise from the arachnoid matter, the middle layer of meninges that lies inside the dura mater, and outside the pia mater. They comprise about 15 per cent of adult intracranial tumors and 2 per cent of pediatric intracranial tumors. They are three times more common in females than males and reach a peak incidence in the seventh decade of life.

Meningiomas are seldom invasive. They produce signs and symptoms by compressing adjacent structures; these signs and symptoms obviously depend on the site of origin of the tumor. Because of the characteristic slow tumor growth, the clinical findings have usually been present for a long time before correct diagnosis is made. It is important to recognize these signs and symptoms because surgery performed early in the course of the tumor generally has good results, whereas surgery performed late is fraught with complications.

Approximately half of all meningiomas occur parasagittally or over the convexity of the cerebral hemispheres. Those tumors that arise anteriorly present with a long history of headache, mental change, and chronic papilledema, as a result of long-standing increased intracranial pressure. Those that arise posteriorly present more acutely with seizures, hemiplegia, or homonymous hemianopsia from compression of motor and sensory cortical areas.

Approximately one third of meningiomas arise from the arachnoid over the sphenoid bone. Those arising from the inner one third of the sphenoid wing produce early symptoms due to involvement of cranial nerves II, III, IV, V, and VI, resulting in slowly progressive visual loss, decreased corneal reflex, and disorders of ocular motility. Middle third sphenoid wing meningiomas present later with signs of increased intracranial pressure (headache, vomiting, papilledema) and few cranial nerve signs. Lateral third sphenoid wing meningiomas are usually of the en plaque type and produce slowly progressive, painless exophthalmos and fullness in the temporal fossa, with relative preservation of vision and ocular motility.

Meningiomas that arise from the tuberculum sellae of the sphenoid bone (anterior wall of sella turcica) produce early and isolated visual symptoms because the optic nerves and chiasm are immediately above and behind this structure. These patients present with vague monocular field defects that slowly progress to involve central vision. If the diagnosis is delayed, the second eye is eventually involved. Associated neurologic signs and symptoms are invariably absent.

Meningiomas arising slightly more anteriorly from the planum sphenoidale and olfactory groove (floor of anterior fossa) present late with anosmia, mental changes, and papilledema. If they grow posteriorly, visual changes may result from direct compression.

Sphenoid meningiomas may also arise from or invade the optic canal and spread down the optic nerve sheath into the orbit, causing optic atrophy, opticociliary shunt vessels, and proptosis.

Less than 1 per cent of meningiomas arise primarily, from the arachnoid of the optic nerve sheath, but these patients present exclusively with visual complaints. Those that arise anteriorly in the orbit present with decreased vision, proptosis, mechanical restriction of ocular motility, and choroidal folds. Those arising in the apex of the orbit or in the optic canal develop visual loss early because minimal growth of a very small tumor compresses the optic nerve against unyielding bony structures. These patients have no other neurologic or ophthalmologic findings apart from failing vision, optic atrophy, and occasional opticociliary shunt vessels.

THERAPY

Surgical. Since most meningiomas are encapsulated and noninvasive early in their course, surgical excision at this time is usually curative. As the tumor grows, it surrounds vital neural and vascular structures and grows down the foramina, so that in the late stages a surgical cure is almost impossible. When diagnosed late, partial removal of the tumor and adjacent bony structures in an effort to decompress the anterior visual system will usually give many years of useful visual function. Attempted complete excision of a large tumor surrounding the optic nerve or chiasm usually has devastating visual results because removal of the tumor is invariably accompanied by removal of most of the blood supply of these vital structures.

In general, meningioma surgery is the domain of the neurosurgeon. Even in primary optic nerve sheath meningioma, a combined intracranial-orbital approach is preferred as many of these tumors extend into the orbital apex and optic canal. The ophthalmologist's main role is in early diagnosis and rapid referral to the neurosurgeon so that he or she may operate early while the tumor is still resectable.

Supportive. Elderly meningioma patients with unilateral, slowly progressive visual symptoms may be better left alone. Tarsorrhaphy or orbital decompression may be necessary to save the globe in advanced cases.

Irradiation. Apart from preoperative reduction of tumor vascularity, irradiation has little convincing long-term therapeutic effect on meningiomas. A few recent articles suggest that irradiation reduces the recurrence rate in incompletely resected meningiomas.

Ocular or Periocular Manifestations

Cornea: Exposure keratopathy; hypesthesia (fifth nerve).
Extraocular Muscles: Imbalance or paralysis (third, fourth, or sixth nerve).
Globe: Proptosis.
Optic Nerve: Atrophy; opticociliary shunts; papilledema.
Other: Afferent pupil defect (second nerve); choroidal folds; hyperopia; ocular and facial pain (fifth nerve); visual field defect; visual loss (second nerve).

PRECAUTIONS

The signs and symptoms of meningiomas occasionally improve with systemic steroids; one must not misdiagnose these cases as optic neuritis or multiple sclerosis. Pregnancy occasionally results in worsening of these signs and symptoms. Chemotherapy has not been shown to be of any value in the treatment of meningiomas.

COMMENTS

Early diagnosis and rapid referral are of upmost importance so that the neurosurgeon may excise the meningioma before it has compromised vital neural and vascular structures. Careful and repeated patient evaluation with appropriately directed neuroradiologic investigations (hypocycloidal polytomography, fine matrix CT scanning, and magnetic resonance imaging), will usually demonstrate the tumor. Selective internal and external carotid angiography should be performed preoperatively. Once patients have undergone partial or total excision of the tumor, they should be carefully watched for signs and symptoms of recurrence and followed for life with repeated evaluations of visual acuity, color vision, visual fields, exophthalmometry, corneal sensation, and ocular motility. Periodic repeat radiologic investigations should also be performed.

References

Anderson DP: *In* Miller N (ed): Walsh and Hoyt's Clinical Neuro-Ophthalmology, 4th ed., vol. 3, pp. 1325–1379. Baltimore, Williams & Wilkins, 1988.

Anderson D, Khalil M: Meningioma and the ophthalmologist. A review of 80 cases. Ophthalmology 88:1004–1009, 1981.

Barbaro NM, Gutin PH, Wilson CB, et al: Radiation therapy in the treatment of partially resected meningiomas. Neurosurgery 20:525–528, 1987.

Finn JE, Mount LA: Meningiomas of the tuberculum sellae and planum sphenoidale. A review of 83 cases. Arch Ophthalmol 92:23–27, 1974.

Jane JA, McKissock W: Importance of failing vision in early diagnosis of suprasellar meningiomas. Br Med J 2:5–7, 1962.

Knight CL, Hoyt WF, Wilson CB: Syndrome of incipient prechiasmal optic nerve compression. Progress toward early diagnosis and surgical management. Arch Ophthalmol 87:1–11, 1972.

Kupersmith MJ, Warren FA, Newall J, Ransohoff J: Irradiation of meningiomas of the intracranial anterior visual pathway: Ann Neurol 21:131–137, 1987.

Newell FW, Beaman TC: Ocular signs of meningioma. Am J Ophthalmol 45:30–40, 1958.

Wilson WB: Meningiomas of the anterior visual system. Surv Ophthalmol 26:109–127, 1981.

MUCOCELE
(Pyocele)

IRA A. ABRAHAMSON, M.D.

Cincinnati, Ohio

Mucocele is an accumulation and retention of mucoid material within the sinus as a result of continuous or periodic obstruction of the sinus osteum. X-ray studies may show the frontal sinus completely obliterated by bone density with no bone erosion or destruction. The occurrence of mucocele involving the paranasal sinuses is not as rare a condition as previously reported. The literature reveals many reports of mucoceles involving the various paranasal sinuses.

A gradual onset of headaches, orbital or forehead pain unilateral proptosis, and limited ocular motility should make the physician suspicious of a paranasal sinus mucocele. The patient may also complain of decreased or blurred vision or diplopia, which may be the presenting symptom.

The frontal and ethmoid sinuses are the two most common locations of the mucocele. The least common location is in the maxillary sinus, where the mucocele produces bulging of the turbinates with subsequent occlusion of the nasal passages, loosening of the teeth, erosion of the orbital floor, and compression of the orbital fissure. Proptosis, diplopia, and even blindness may result on the involved side.

In the frontal sinus, erosion of the anterior wall results in a tender fluctuant mass beneath the periosteum of the frontal bone, commonly known as a Pott's puffy tumor or a subcutaneous abscess, which requires local drainage or exenteration of the sinus. Erosion of the posterior sinus wall may produce an epidural abscess, subdural empyema, meningitis, or brain abscess.

Ethmoid sinus mucoceles encroach upon the medial wall of the orbit and the orbital fissure, producing proptosis and ocular motility disturbances.

Mucocele of the sphenoid sinus is less frequent than those of the frontal and ethmoid sinuses and can produce variable clinical pictures. It must be differentiated from retrobulbar neuritis, pituitary tumors, and ophthalmoplegic migraine.

THERAPY

Surgical. A team approach to complete surgical drainage and removal of the tumor and diseased mucous membrane should be utilized. An osteoplastic anterior wall approach to the frontal sinus is performed with obliteration of the sinus cavity by abdominal wall fat. Under general anesthesia, both the face and abdominal wall are prepared. Bilateral eyebrow butterfly-type incisions are made, and the superior flap is elevated. The periosteum is left attached to the cranium. A previously sterilized precut template of the Caldwell view of the frontal sinus is outlined on the periosteum over the sinus. A Stryker saw is used to cut the bone after incising the periosteum, and flap bone is hinged inferiorly upon entering the frontal sinus. After aspirating the contents of the sinus cavity and the cyst and removing the sinus mucosa, the inside of the sinus wall is drilled with a cutting burr of the Jordan Day drill until all the inner periosteum is removed. A tantalum mesh is fashioned to replace the deficient orbital roof. The frontal sinus cavity is then obliterated with the fat obtained from the abdominal wall. The bone flap is then repositioned, and the periosteum is closed. The skin flap is laid back and closed in layers, and a pressure-type dressing may be applied.

Ocular or Periocular Manifestations

Extraocular Muscles: Paralysis.
Globe: Exophthalmos; proptosis.
Lacrimal System: Lacrimation.
Orbit: Erosion of bony walls; mucocele.
Other: Decreased visual acuity; diplopia.

PRECAUTIONS

The diagnosis of a frontal sinus mucocele is established by laminographic radiography. However, this clinical picture may also be caused by several other conditions. Included in a differential diagnosis are thyroid disease, retrobulbar tumor, retrobulbar neuritis, pseudotumor, temporal arteritis, acute or chronic sinusitis, and sinus, nasal, or pharyngeal tumors. Tomography is essential in investigating this lesion and establishing a diagnosis.

COMMENTS

The diagnosis and management of mucoceles have much improved over the past few years. The use of laminograms have greatly aided the diagnosis. However, a team approach (ophthalmologist, radiologist, otorhinolaryngologist, and neurosurgeon) is essential for an accurate diagnosis and therapeutic approach to this problem. A precut template from the Caldwell projection is a very useful device to outline the contours of the frontal sinus during surgery. The not-so-frequent use of abdominal fat to fill the frontal sinus cavity has been utilized with no apparent postoperative fat necrosis.

References

Abrahamson IA Jr, et al: Frontal sinus mucocele. Ann Ophthalmol 11:173–178, 1979.
Evans C: Aetiology and treatment of fronto-ethmoidal mucocele. J Laryngol Otol 95:361–375, 1981.
Feldman M, Lowry LD, Rao VM, et al: Mucoceles of the paranasal sinuses. Trans PA Acad Ophthalmol 39:614–617, 1987.
Gillespie RP, Marshall A, Ludlow P: Use of the CUSA in removal of a recurrent intraorbital mucocele. Otolaryngol Head Neck Surg 99:71–72, 1988.
Jones JL, Kaufman PW: Mucopyocele of the maxillary sinus. J Oral Surg 39:948–950, 1981.
Kaufman SJ: Orbital mucopyoceles. Two cases and a review. Surv Ophthalmol 25:253–262, 1981.
Lund VJ: Anatomical considerations in the aetiology of fronto-ethmoidal mucoceles. Rhinology 25:83–88, 1987.
Schaefer SD, Anderson RG, Carder HM: Epidural mucopyocele: Diagnosis and management. Otolaryngol Head Neck Surg 89:523–527, 1981.
Stankiewicz JA: The endoscopic approach to the sphenoid sinus. Laryngoscope 99:218–221, 1989.
Weinstein GS, Biglan AW, Patterson JH: Congenital lacrimal sac mucoceles. Am J Ophthalmol 94:106–110, 1982.

NEURILEMOMA
(Neurinoma, Schwannoma)
NORMAN S. LEVY, M.D., Ph.D., F.A.C.S.
Gainesville, Florida

Neurilemoma is a slow-growing encapsulated neoplasm arising from the Schwann cells of nerves. Some of these are malignant. These tumors have been found diffusely in both the sensory and motor nerves, but their frequency in sensory nerves is several hundred-fold greater than in motor nerves. They account for 2 per cent of orbital tumors. They have also been reported within the uveal tissues of the eye.

Involvement of any branches of the trigeminal nerve is the most common periocular presentation. Retro-orbital headaches, facial numbness, progressive proptosis, lid swelling, intermittent pain, numbness or paresthesias in the distribution of the appropriate sensory nerve branch, or atypical trigeminal neuralgia have been described as initial signs. The presenting findings in neurilemomas of the third, fourth, and sixth cranial nerves include diplopia or blurring of vision. The proximity of the optic nerve to the expanding tumor within the orbit has occasionally resulted in loss of vision.

CT scanning of the suspected tumor can be extremely helpful in characterizing its size and extent. Magnetic resonance imaging (MRI) has high sensitivity in defining the nature and invasiveness of the tumor.

THERAPY

Surgical. The tumor should be anatomically defined by appropriate radiographic studies. Complete surgical excision is the therapy of choice. Tumors are not highly vascular so that bleeding is rarely a problem. Dissection of the tumor from the adjacent tissues is facilitated by preoperative CT and MRI radiography and microscopic surgical control. Occasionally, the extent and location of the tumor prevent complete excision or cause damage to the nerve and adjacent tissues. In such cases, incomplete excision may be required. If growth continues, repeated excision, radiation, or chemotherapy are indicated.

Irradiation. When histologic examination of the tissue confirms malignancy or radiographic recurrence has been documented, focal application of up to 6000 rads of 10 MeV photons may be employed for local treatment.

Systemic. Intravenous combination chemotherapy consisting of 2 mg of vincristine,[‡] 100 mg of doxorubicin,[‡] 1 gm of cyclophosphamide,[‡] and 500 mg of dacarbazine[‡] has been employed. This therapy should be undertaken over a 5-day intensive course, followed by weekly administration of vincristine. Recurrent courses may be required based upon clinical response to therapy. Such chemotherapy should only be undertaken by a physician trained in these procedures.

Ocular or Periocular Manifestations

Conjunctiva: Localized swelling or mass.
Cornea: Discrete mass.
Extraocular Muscles: Diplopia or blurring.
Eyelids: Horner's syndrome; localized mass; ptosis.
Globe: Proptosis.
Uvea: Discrete mass.
Other: Visual loss.

PRECAUTIONS

Accurate diagnosis of the tumor is only achieved histologically, although radiographic studies can be suggestive. The histologic evaluation must be done by a pathologist who is extremely familiar with this type of tumor. Studies indicate that the morphology and histology of the collagen of such tumors can be useful in their differentiation. Electron microscopy is often useful when standard histologic techniques are not definitive. Human glia-specific proteins, S100 and GFA, have been useful in characterizing the malignancy of these tumors.

The importance of a surgically aggressive approach to patients with malignant neurilemomas cannot be overemphasized. The 5-year survival in one study was 48 per cent. Even tumors initially classified as low grade histologically often eventually metastasize and cause death.

Young patients with von Recklinghausen's disease may develop neurilemomas, which tend to be multiple in location. If these neurilemomas are malignant, the 5-year survival is less than that for patients with solitary malignant neurilemomas.

COMMENTS

The increased incidence of malignant neurilemomas in sites of prior irradiation and in patients with von Recklinghausen's disease must be recognized. Prognosis of any lesion is dependent upon its location, size, the adequacy of excision, and the malignant potential of that particular neurilemoma.

References

Bojen-Miller M, Myhre-Jensen D: A consecutive series of 30 malignant schwannomas. Survival in relation to clinico-pathological parameters and treatment. Acta Pathol Microbiol Immunol Scand 92:147–155, 1984.
Ho KL: Schwannoma of the trochlear nerve. Case report. J Neurosurg 55:132–135, 1981.
Jacque, CM, et al: GFA and S100 protein levels as an index for malignancy in human gliomas and neurinomas. J Natl Cancer Inst 62:479–483, 1979.
Mafee MF, et al: Orbital space-occupying lesions: Role of computed tomography and magnetic resonance imaging. An analysis of 145 cases. Radiol Clin North Am 25:529–559, 1987.
Sayed AK, et al: Heterochromia iridis and Horner's syndrome due to paravertebral neurilemmoma. J Surg Oncol 22:15–16, 1983.
Shields JA, et al: Benign peripheral nerve tumor of the choroid: A clinicopathologic correlation and review

of the literature. Ophthalmology 88:1322–1329, 1981.
Smith PA, et al: Anterior uveal neurilemmoma; a rare neoplasm simulating malignant melanoma. Br J Ophthalmol 71:34–40, 1987.
Sordillo PP, et al: Malignant schwannoma—Clinical characteristics, survival, and response to therapy. Cancer 47:2503–2509, 1981.
Taxy JB, et al: Electron microscopy in the diagnosis of malignant schwannoma. Cancer 48:1381–1391, 1981.

OPTIC GLIOMAS

BRIAN R. YOUNGE, M.D.
Rochester, Minnesota

Optic gliomas are intrinsic tumors of the optic nerve, chiasm, or tract that may involve any or all of these structures and extend beyond into the hypothalamus and ventricles. They are generally low-grade astrocytomas, usually are apparent within the first two decades of life, and grow slowly, permitting survival for many years. There are, however, many exceptions, and these have stirred controversy for nearly 100 years, both in terms of their nature and the best treatment. Clearly, the patient with a unilateral tumor of a single optic nerve has the best chance of survival with surgical resection. Conversely, an untreated glioma of either the nerve or chiasm carries a much poorer prognosis, but again survival can be long.

There remain several questions today as to the nature and management of these tumors: are these tumors hamartomas and do they grow along the optic pathways; what is the natural history of these tumors; what is more useful for following patients: computed tomography (CT) or magnetic resonance imaging (MRI); what treatment is best in unilateral cases: radiation or surgery; does radiation help in chiasmal cases; and finally, does chemotherapy help? These and other questions will probably continue to haunt clinicians for years because each new case encountered by any one individual is likely to be unique and unpredictable.

There is no way to conduct a randomized treatment protocol for this disease because there are so few cases and very long follow-up is needed, in the order of 20 years or more. Nonetheless, some basic facts from the literature have emerged, and the author has drawn from this as well as from his fairly extensive experience. It is convenient to divide the location of these tumors into two main groups: 1) unilateral optic nerve and 2) all the others, which are called chiasmal gliomas, with the realization that there may be multiple sites and extensive involvement of neighboring structures.

Optic nerve gliomas present most often within the first few years of life with unilateral proptosis. The proptosis often has been present for some time, ranging from a month to a year. There is little evidence of visual loss until later in the evolution of the tumor, not only because of the child's age but also because vision persists at fairly good levels for a long time. Strabismus may ensue, but more often the globe is axially displaced forward in the orbit without other deviation until later. Retropulsion of the globe is met with resistance, but the tumor itself is usually not palpable externally. Motility is often good, becoming limited with the further protrusion. Often, there is a relative afferent pupil defect, and if testable, color vision is mildly reduced (as with the Ishihara plates). The optic nerve head may be moderately pale, with some evidence of swelling, and occasionally there are shunt vessels similar to those typical of optic nerve meningioma. Choroidal folds are not typical, despite the obvious displacement of the eye forward.

In contrast to unilateral optic nerve gliomas, *chiasmal gliomas* present at a later age, and visual loss is the key symptom. Because of the obscure and slowly progressive nature of the visual loss, it is often several months to a year or more before the diagnosis is established. Behavioral changes, seizures, headaches, or even a fortuitous detection of pale optic nerve heads during routine examination of the fundi may be the first clue to the abnormality. Optic atrophy is often pronounced by the time the symptoms become manifest, and it is not accompanied by disc swelling. Field defects, when plottable, are of the chiasmal type, but are rarely of a classic nature. Symptoms of obstructive hydrocephalus may ensue if the tumor involves the hypothalamus and third ventricle. Other developmental delays may result from involvement of contiguous hypothalamic structures.

Multicentric origin of these tumors is suggested by the rare occurrence of bilateral optic nerve tumors and by tumors of the orbit and chiasm together. That one is the extension of another is a more likely explanation, even to the nerve of the other side. The optic tract may be involved primarily, as may the optic radiations by extension. Recent studies of patients with type I neurofibromatosis offer some evidence that other tumors may be more common elsewhere in the brain, along with optic gliomas, but it should be emphasized that acoustic neuroma and optic glioma do not coexist because they are manifestations of two different types of neurofibromatosis.

It is of value to inspect the skin for patches of brownish pigmentation (café-au-lait spots) and to examine the pupil for pigmented nodules (Lisch nodules) because many affected children have neurofibromatosis. Other skin manifestations of this disorder include cutaneous tumors, subcutaneous neurofibromas, plexiform neuromas, and axillary freckling, which is quite characteristic.

Even before the advent of modern CT and MRI scanning, there were sophisticated means of examining the area of the optic canal and chiasmal region. Plain skull films and optic canal views were the simplest means of study, and they showed an abnormality in more than half of the patients studied. Hypocycloidal axial polytomography of the optic canals became a most sensitive means for detecting minor bony changes along the canals and into the chiasmal region. When CT became available, these tumors suddenly became visible to the neuroradiologist, and a whole new era of diagnostic imaging changed our approach to these tumors, along with our ability to find other lesions, characterize changes over time, and tailor therapy to individual cases. MRI has added the latest dimension to studying these tumors and has suggested other abnormal findings not seen on CT. The role of gadolinium-enhanced MRI has not yet been determined. Positron emission tomography also promises to be helpful for delineating newer aspects of these lesions, but it may have limited application because of the cost factors.

THERAPY

Surgical. Unilateral optic nerve gliomas are best treated by complete excision. However, if there is useful vision, not much proptosis, no evidence of extension into the intracranial area, and opportunity for adequate follow-up of the patient, a period of careful follow-up may be indicated. The child with unilateral proptosis whose vision is compromised and who has a tumor of the optic nerve should have complete excision of the tumor. Although many approaches to the tumor have been advocated, it is important to obtain free margins of optic nerve behind the tumor. In many cases, this goal requires unroofing of the optic canal and excision of the nerve just anterior to the chiasm. In a few cases in which orbitotomy has been the primary approach, incomplete excision has resulted, and recurrence intracranially has ensued. In only one case has "pathologically proven" complete excision resulted in death, whereas incompletely excised tumors have sometimes recurred and been the cause of death.

Bilateral tumors of each optic nerve invariably involve the optic chiasm and may extend into the tract as well. These and frank chiasmal gliomas are not amenable to complete excision, and surgery is palliative for relief of obstructive hydrocephalus and tumor compression of nearby vital structures. Radiation therapy has proved in many cases to be of value, even to the point of improving vision and fields, at least for a time. Because of the slow growth of these tumors, long survival is possible even in the absence of any treatment; most experts agree that radiation does prolong useful vision and life in chiasmal glioma. No useful data link any form of chemotherapy to improvement of either visual function or prognosis for life.

References

Alvord EC Jr, Lofton S: Gliomas of the optic nerve or chiasm: Outcome by patients' age, tumor site, and treatment. J Neurosurg 68:85–98, 1988.
Glaser JS, Hoyt WF, Corbett J: Visual morbidity with chiasmal glioma: Long-term studies of visual fields

OPTIC GLIOMAS

in untreated and irradiated cases. Arch Ophthalmol 85:3–12, 1971.

Hoyt WF, Baghdassarian SA: Optic glioma of childhood: Natural history and rationale for conservative management. Br J Ophthalmol 53:793–798, 1969.

Lloyd LA: Gliomas of the optic nerve and chiasm in childhood. Trans Am Ophthalmol Soc 71:488–535, 1973.

Miller NR, Iliff WJ, Green WR: Evaluation and management of gliomas of the anterior visual pathways. Brain 97:743–754, 1974.

Packer RJ, et al: Chiasmatic gliomas of childhood: A reappraisal of natural history and effectiveness of cranial irradiation. Child's Brain 10:393–403, 1983.

Riccardi VM: Neurofibromatosis. In Gomez MR (ed): Neurocutaneous Diseases: A Practical Approach. Boston, Butterworths, 1987, pp 11–29.

Rush JA, et al: Optic glioma: Long-term follow-up of 85 histopathologically verified cases. Ophthalmology 89:1213–1219, 1982.

Wilson WB, et al: Malignant evolution of childhood chiasmal pilocytic astrocytoma. Neurology 26:322–325, 1976.

Wilson WB, et al: Tumor spread in unilateral optic glioma—I. Neuro-Ophthalmol 7:179–184, 1987.

Wilson WB, et al: Tumor spread in unilateral optic glioma—II. Neuro-Ophthalmol (In press).

PAPILLOMA
(Verruca, Wart)

FRED M. WILSON II, M.D.
Indianapolis, Indiana

A papilloma is a cutaneous or mucosal tumor that consists of a cluster of finger-like projections of proliferating epithelial and fibrovascular tissues. Each projection is composed of hypertrophic (and sometimes hyperkeratotic) epithelium, subepithelial connective tissue stroma and a central vascular core. A papilloma is recognized clinically by its mulberry-like or cauliflower-like appearance on the cutaneous or mucosal surface. Mucosal papillomas may be sufficiently translucent that their frond-like vascular cores are visible.

Papillomas may be of viral etiology, caused by the human papilloma (wart) virus, or of a noninfectious etiology, representing primary squamous neoplasia. Papillomas of viral origin include verrucae (common cutaneous warts), condylomata acuminata (anogenital warts), and laryngeal papillomas. Noninfectious papillomas include all cutaneous and mucosal squamous neoplasms, whether benign or malignant, that happen to have papillomatous configurations.

Papillomas can be encountered on the eyelids, conjunctiva, cornea, or mucosa of the lacrimal system. Common infectious warts occur most commonly on the palpebral conjunctiva and the eyelids. Viral papillomas are usually asymptomatic, but low-grade chronic papillary conjunctivitis or punctate epithelial keratitis may result. Noninfectious papillomas may involve the eyelids, bulbar conjunctiva, limbus, or cornea. They are usually encountered in older adults and are not multiple or associated with cutaneous warts. They may be benign, premalignant, or malignant. Papillomas of the lacrimal mucosa, whether viral or noninfectious, can cause bleeding from the puncta.

THERAPY

Supportive. Conservative treatment is advised for viral papillomas because they are likely to disappear spontaneously, usually within a period of 2 years or less. Every effort should be made to await these spontaneous cures because the attempted excision or ablation of a single lesion may result in the subsequent appearance of several lesions.

The successes of "wart charmers" have been touted for generations. Whether these successes relate only to coincidental spontaneous regressions or to some obscure psychogenic effect on the body's immune system is unclear. In any case, warts (viral papillomas) may disappear following such apparently worthless efforts as the reciting of chants or the performance of rituals.

Surgical. Excisional biopsy is currently the mainstay of treatment for noninfectious papillomas. Excisional biopsy of either kind of papilloma provides a histopathologic diagnosis and a good chance for elimination of the lesion, although recurrences are possible. Excision should be sufficiently wide as to include some normal tissue. A viral papilloma should not be removed by cutting across its stalk; the head of the lesion, the stalk, and some normal tissue surrounding the base of the stalk should be excised.

Cryotherapy is useful as an adjunct to excision of viral papillomas. However, when cryotherapy is used as the sole method of treatment, there is always the danger that incomplete destruction of virus or proliferating cells will result in recurrence. Cryotherapy with a cryoprobe or cryospray following excisional biopsy is probably of value for reducing the likelihood of recurrence. A viral papilloma of the eyelid or conjunctiva may be treated with application of a cryoprobe at $-70°$ to $-100°$C for 30 to 60 seconds. The lesion can be expected to disappear in 10 to 30 days if cryoablation has been successful. Despite extensive dermatologic experience with liquid nitrogen spray in the treatment of cutaneous papillomas, it probably should be regarded only as an experimental method for treating viral papillomas of the conjunctiva. Cryotherapy for *noninfectious* papillomas of the eyelid or eye must presently be considered to be only in the experimental stages of development, but it may very well reduce the probability of recurrence when it is used immediately following surgical excision.

After excision of either a viral or noninfectious papilloma, the remaining cut edges of conjunctiva and the tissues underlying the site of the tumor (sclera, limbus, cornea, or tarsus) may be treated with contiguous or slightly overlapping, superficial, 1- to 2-second applications of a cryoprobe. A double freeze-thaw technique (two consecutive applications of the cryotherapy) might be more efficacious than a single treatment.

Electrodesiccation is essentially equal in efficacy to cryotherapy. It is used mainly for the treatment of verrucae of the eyelids, although it could be used cautiously for treating viral papillomas of the conjunctiva. Following local anesthesia, the electric needle is inserted into the lesion and kept in place until the tissue begins to bubble. The wart is then curetted away. Care must be taken to minimize scarring by not inserting the needle too deeply. As is the case with cryotherapy, electrodesiccation can be followed by recurrence. Electrodesiccation should not be used for noninfectious papillomas.

Although not widely available to ophthalmologists, the carbon dioxide (CO_2) laser seems to be very effective for treating viral papillomas of the eye and other sites, with or without surgical excision and cryotherapy, even when all other current methods of treatment have been unsuccessful. The emission wavelength of the laser corresponds to the absorption band of water, so water-containing tissue can be vaporized, rapidly, as well as carbonized and coagulated. The causative virus seems also to be readily destroyed, thus helping greatly to protect against recurrence. Low energy levels and short exposure times are advised for treating ocular lesions, e.g., 5 watts of energy for 0.2 seconds in a spot size of 2 mm.

Irradiation. Radiotherapy is rarely, if ever, indicated as primary treatment for viral papillomas. It might possibly be considered when there is extensive involvement of the eyelid or conjunctiva or when there have been multiple recurrences after surgery. Even in these trying circumstances, however, consideration should probably be given first to CO_2 laser therapy, cryotherapy, or immunotherapy.

However, beta irradiation can be utilized rather safely in difficult cases as an adjunct to surgical excision. After excision of a wart of the eyelid, 1000 to 2500 rads of beta radiation may be applied in the hope of reducing the likelihood of recurrence. A dosage of 1000 to 2000 rads may be used following excision of a viral papilloma of the conjunctiva. Especially recalcitrant viral papillomas of the eyelids or conjunctiva may be treated with a combination of excision, cryotherapy, and beta irradiation. Beta rays may also be used after excision of a neoplastic papilloma of the eyelid or conjunctiva, but they should not be relied upon as a primary means of therapy.

Topical. Immunotherapy is a promising, but still experimental method of therapy. Dinitrochlorobenzene[†] has been used successfully to eradicate multiple and recurrent papillomatous squamous tumors of the conjunctiva and lacrimal mucosa that had previously resisted all conventional forms of therapy. It was unclear whether these lesions were infectious or noninfectious papillomas. By applying dinitrochlorobenzene repeatedly to the skin, the patient is made sensitive ("allergic") to this agent, which is a potent contact sensitizer. The chemical is then given topically to the ocular tumor, whereupon a type IV (thymus-derived, lymphocyte-mediated) hypersensitivity reaction occurs and destroys the tumors.

Ocular or Periocular Manifestations

Conjunctiva: Follicular or papillary conjunctivitis; hemorrhages; hyperemia; keratinization; papilloma (noninfectious, viral); pseudopterygium.
Cornea: Infiltration; keratinization; opacity; papilloma (noninfectious); pseudopterygium; punctate epithelial keratitis; vascularization.
Eyelids: Hemorrhages; papilloma (noninfectious, viral); ulcer.
Lacrimal System: Hemorrhages; obstruction; papilloma (noninfectious, viral).

PRECAUTIONS

Papillomas are fundamentally epithelial lesions; subepithelial fibrovascular proliferation probably occurs only because the proliferating epithelium requires a vascular supply. To minimize the chance of recurrence, it is necessary only to remove the epithelial component of the lesion. It is quite permissible for the surgical plane in the conjunctiva to extend down to the level of Tenon's capsule or even to sclera because these tissues heal rapidly with relatively little scarring and it is difficult to remove only the epithelial layer of the conjunctiva. However, surgical planes in the eyelid or cornea should be superficial so as to avoid unnecessary scarring and loss of tissue. Corneal papillomas, in fact, should merely be scraped gently from the corneal surface, leaving Bowman's layer intact except in the rare instance in which a frankly carcinomatous papilloma has invaded the deeper layers.

Care must be taken when using cryotherapy not to freeze too deeply. It is mainly the epithelial layer of the conjunctiva that should be frozen, although no harm is done by allowing the freeze to enter Tenon's layer. Overzealous freezing of sclera, however, can occasionally cause scleral thinning. Inadvertent freezing of the ciliary body and processes can cause uveitis and hypotony. Freezing of the corneal endothelium can cause endothelial dysfunction and corneal edema. Excessive freezing of the eyelid may cause necrosis, scarring, notching, and trichiasis.

Intact human papilloma virus DNA can be liberated into the air during CO_2 laser treatment. Practitioners should realize that the liberated smoke and vapor might be infectious and should take precautions to avoid being infected themselves by these emissions by using gloves, masks, goggles, and proper suctioning apparatus.

COMMENTS

Viral papillomas tend to occur mainly in children and young adults and are transmissible by direct or indirect contact and autoinoculation.

These lesions may be multiple and are self-limited. They undergo malignant transformation very rarely, if ever. Whether, after apparent resolution, these lesions might years later lead to squamous dysplasia or carcinoma is unknown, but the DNA of human papilloma virus types 6, 11, 16, 18, and 31 has been found both in papillomas and squamous neoplasms of the genital tract. Types 6, 11, and 13 have been associated with mild or moderate dysplasia in the cervix, vulva, penis, and anus, whereas types 16 and 18 have been associated with severe dysplasia and with in situ and invasive carcinoma. The time between infection and malignant transformation seems to be about 30 years. Altogether, 32 distinct types of human papilloma virus have been differentiated by DNA molecular hybridization techniques. Types 6 and 11, both of which seem to be able to cause dysplasia in the genital tract, have so far been found in conjunctival papillomas.

Noninfectious papillomas have a predilection for older individuals and are neither transmissible nor multiple. They are not self-limited and frequently undergo malignant transformation.

References

Dunlap EA (ed): Gordon's Medical Management of Ocular Disease, 2nd ed. Hagerstown, MD, Harper & Row, 1976, pp 126, 165–166.

Ferry AP, Meltzer MA, Taub RN: Immunotherapy with dinitrochlorbenzene (DNCB) for recurrent squamous cell tumor of conjunctiva. Trans Am Ophthalmol Soc 74:154–171, 1977.

Gal AA, Meyer PR, Taylor CR: Papillomavirus antigens in anorectal condyloma and carcinoma in homosexual men. JAMA 257:337–340, 1987.

Garden JM, et al: Papillomavirus in the vapor of carbon dioxide laser-treated verrucae. JAMA 259:1199–1202, 1988.

Holmes KK: Infectious diseases. JAMA 254:2254–2257, 1985.

Jackson WB, Beraja R, Codere F: Laser therapy of conjunctival papillomas. Can J Ophthalmol 22:45–47, 1987.

Nelson JH Jr, Averette HE, Richart RM: Dysplasia, carcinoma in situ, and early invasive cervical carcinoma. Ca-A Cancer J Clinicians 34:306–327, 1984.

Pearce WB, et al: Conjunctival papillomas in northern Canadian natives. Can Med J 112:1423–1426, 1975.

Reese AB: Tumors of the Eye, 3rd ed. Hagerstown, MD, Harper & Row, 1976, pp 54–56.

Schachat A, Iliff WJ, Kashima HK: Carbon dioxide laser therapy of recurrent squamous papilloma of the conjunctiva. Ophthalmic Surg 13:916–918, 1982.

Malignant

BASAL CELL CARCINOMA

JOHN L. WOBIG, M.D.
Portland, Oregon

Basal cell carcinoma is the most common malignant neoplasm of the eyelids. The lesion is locally infiltrative and only rarely metastasizes. Basal cell carcinoma may be classified as nodular, ulcerative, syringoid, adenoid, basosquamous, multicentric, recurrent, morpheaform, or sclerosing. Nodular basal cell carcinomas are generally easy to treat, whereas sclerosing and morpheaform basal cell carcinomas are difficult to cure.

Clinically, approximately 90 per cent of the malignant neoplasms of the eyelid are basal cell carcinomas. The lesion is primarily found in the lower lid and medial canthus, with less frequent occurrence in the lateral canthus and upper lid. Variation is typical in the clinical course of a basal cell carcinoma. Initially, the lesion is usually a discrete nodule with or without ulceration and distinct margins. Eventually, the central area becomes ulcerated with rolled waxy borders.

Histologically, the tumor is composed of solid masses of uniform cells with basophilic nuclei and scanty cytoplasm. Palisading of the peripheral cells of tumor lobules is characteristic. Squamoid differentiation can be present in basal cell carcinomas.

THERAPY

Irradiation. Irradiation should be used with caution in the medial canthus, since permanent scarring of the canalicular system can result. If irradiation is used, silicone intubation should be placed in the lacrimal excretory system before any such therapy. Radiotherapy is effective only in the early stages of basal cell carcinoma; however, it makes surgical repair more difficult in the reconstructive phase.

Surgical. Mohs' fresh tissue, microscopically controlled surgery gives the highest success rate for cure. The tumor removal can be done as an outpatient under local anesthesia with surgical reconstruction following. The excised tumor mass is based on clinical margins. The base and sides remaining are cut into 2-mm strips and divided into portions that are placed on a glass slide. All edges are marked with different colored dyes. Frozen sections are made, and residual tumor is marked on a map. Residual tumor is then resected until the lesion is tumor-free, proven microscopically.

Electrodesiccation and curettage are occasionally used for removal of basal cell carcinomas. All the tumor is curetted away, and the base and sides are electrodesiccated. Since only the medial canthus tends to heal by granulation without significant scarring, this method is not used for most eyelid lesions.

Cryosurgery for the management of basal cell carcinomas of the eyelids has had increasing use, probably more so in dermatology than in ophthalmology. Both in cure rates and cosmetic results, carefully performed cryosurgery by an experienced physician is probably equally effective compared to other modalities, especially for lesions less than 1 cm in diameter. However, other forms of therapy should be considered for lesions larger than this size and for those without raised margins, which make it difficult to ascertain the extent of the edge of the tumor. After outlining 3 to 4 mm of normal tissue around the suspected tumor edge, equal parts of bupivacaine and lidocaine are injected around the involved area. The edge of the tumor can be seen best under a slitlamp by pulling on the skin adjacent to the tumor. If any of the skin's stress lines are distorted, then the tumor probably involves that area. A thermocouple needle is placed within 1 to 2 mm inside of the black felt pen outline, and the tumor is frozen to −25° C. It is allowed to completely thaw to 30° C, and then this is repeated. Whenever the tumor is located near the eye, a bone plate should be inserted in the cul-de-sac to protect the globe.

PRECAUTIONS

It appears that larger lesions are best treated by Mohs' technique. Nodular lesions, which are small, can be controlled by almost any technique. Sclerosing lesions need careful monitoring because it is impossible to determine clinically the free margins.

Complications of cryosurgery and irradiation include the difficulty of late repair to tissue treated by those methods. Extreme care must be taken in the medial canthus to preserve the canalicular system. This may include silicone intubation prior to the above treatment. Pigmentary changes and loss of eyelashes with occasional tissue loss are also complications that must be considered.

The low cost of cryotherapy is certainly an advantage. However, it is important not to use cryotherapy without a thermocouple to monitor the tissue temperatures. The tissue does not need to be frozen beyond −25° C. Also, the freezing of lid tissue must be observed, since defense against infection of the lid is reduced in the initial healing period.

The reconstructive surgery must be well conceived because occasionally more tissue than anticipated is removed. The lid surgery repair may include rebuilding a total lid and canthus, and a physician experienced in this procedure should be available.

COMMENTS

Basal cell carcinoma is a malignant tumor that needs to be treated accordingly. Local infiltration in the periorbital region can extend to the globe, bone, and surrounding sinuses. The reconstruction of the lids and lacrimal apparatus is important in the functional as well as the cosmetic result. For recurrences, the best approach is Mohs' microscopically controlled excision. These patients should especially be examined for tumors of the skin and other regions, as well as for recurrence in the eyelids. Any lid lesion that does not heal should arouse suspicion of a tumor.

References

Domonkos AN: Treatment of eyelid carcinoma. Arch Dermatol 91:364–371, 1965.
Fraunfelder FT, et al: The role of cryosurgery in external ocular and periocular disease. Trans Am Acad Ophthalmol Otolaryngol 83:713–724, 1977.
Jones LT, Wobig JL: Surgery of the Eyelids and Lacrimal System. Birmingham, Aesculapius, 1976.
Older JJ, Quickert MH, Beard C: Surgical removal of basal cell carcinoma of the eyelids utilizing frozen section control. Trans Am Acad Ophthalmol Otolaryngol 79:658–663, 1975.
Payne JW, et al: Basal cell carcinoma of the eyelids. A long-term follow-up study. Arch Ophthalmol 81:553–558, 1969.

CONJUNCTIVAL OR CORNEAL INTRAEPITHELIAL NEOPLASIA (CIN) AND SQUAMOUS CELL CARCINOMA
(Invasive Neoplasm)

F.T. FRAUNFELDER, M.D.
Portland, Oregon

Conjunctival or corneal intraepithelial neoplasms are not uncommon tumors that include all dysplastic lesions of the conjunctival and corneal epithelium, regardless of their severity. Clinical and laboratory investigations have led to a simple classification of the intraepithelial process, ranging from mild dysplasia (partial-thickness intraepithelial neoplasia) to severe dysplasia (full-thickness intraepithelial neoplasia). If the dysplastic process breaks through the basement membrane, the end stage of this process is invasive neoplasia or squamous cell carcinoma. This terminology replaces such previously used terms as Bowen's disease of the eye, carcinoma in situ (CIS), intraepithelial epithelioma, intraepithelioma, and intraepithelial dysplasia.

Conjunctival or corneal intraepithelial neoplasia (CIN) has a distinctive clinical course, which is characterized by slow growth and relatively low malignancy potential. The most common cell types comprising dysplastic processes of the conjunctiva and cornea are elongated spindle cells with a monotonous appearance and epidermoid cells; these atypical cells grow upward from an initial basal location. The clinical appearance of the lesions is that of an elevated, gelatinous, leukoplakic, or papilliform limbal mass. The lesions are almost always unilateral

290 / CIN AND SQUAMOUS CELL CARCINOMA

and generally unifocal; they are primarily located at the nasal or temporal limbus, although some may involve the cornea only or conjunctiva only. CIN more often affects males than females and is predominantly a disease of the sixth and seventh decades. Intraocular extension and metastatic disease may occur secondary to developing squamous cell carcinoma.

THERAPY

Surgical. Local surgical excision of CIN lesions combined with cryotherapy utilizing a double-cycle freeze-thaw-refreeze technique has been found to have the lowest recurrence rate. Since the margins of the tumor are indistinct because of the root-like subepithelial extension, lesions may not always stain with rose bengal; individual or multiple conjunctival scrapings with Papanicolaou stain can often aid in outlining the area to be excised. Topical ocular anesthetics, such as proparacaine or cocaine, are instilled, and the conjunctiva under and around the lesion is elevated with subconjunctival injection of 1 per cent lidocaine with epinephrine. The conjunctiva will elevate easily in cases not previously treated; if the conjunctiva does not elevate in these eyes, the diagnosis of squamous cell carcinoma may be suspected. Multiple conjunctival cautery applications 1.5 to 2 mm from the suspected tumor margin are used to outline the area to be excised. An incision is then made through these marks down to bare sclera. The conjunctival and episcleral tissues are then surgically dissected to the limbus. In areas where the conjunctiva is adherent to the episcleral area, a superficial sclerectomy may be necessary. The area of corneal involvement must be outlined by retroillumination before surgery. Multiple applications of a local anesthetic are then used to soften the corneal epithelium. Using a No. 64 Beaver blade, 1 mm of normal epithelium and the involved corneal epithelium are removed by simply "bulldozing" the epithelium to the limbus. A superficial limbal keratectomy is not usually performed because a pannus may form postoperatively, although areas with prior surgical keratectomies or suspected tumor invasion may require a superficial keratectomy.

A Brymill CryAc unit with either a 2- or 4-mm liquid nitrogen cryoprobe tip is used to freeze the limbal area. The most important area to obtain adequate freezing is at the limbus, since this is the site of most recurrences. The end point of the freeze is a 1-second application that, upon removal of the probe, causes a white circular imprint of the probe tip on the eye. Multiple overlapping imprints are done to cover the entire surgical limbus twice. If a scleral or limbal area of inadequate dissection is suspected, a triple freeze-thaw technique should be performed; however, an attempt should be made not to freeze more than 1 mm of peripheral clear cornea. No suturing is necessary. A topical antibiotic-corticosteroid preparation may be given three times daily for 3 days.

Squamous cell carcinoma is treated in the same manner, but more aggressive cryotherapy (triple freeze-thaw) with wider margins around the tumor and deeper sclerectomy and keratectomy is recommended. Deep invasion of the sclera and cornea requires full eye wall resection. Lamellar transplants are seldom used, since they cover the signs of an early recurrence. Small intraocular extension can be treated with iridocyclectomy, whereas larger intraocular extensions may require enucleation.

PRECAUTIONS

Although deep cryotherapy may result in severe iritis, posterior synechiae, and corneal scarring, the complications of superficial cryosurgery are minimal, even when the cornea is treated. To avoid adherence of the cryoprobe, it is of utmost importance to have the probe completely frozen before ocular application. If the probe is applied warm and then frozen, it will cause a tight ocular adherence that is not easily removed without a sterile liquid and may result in excessive freezing.

Squamous cell carcinoma of the conjunctiva with regional or distant metastasis may be life threatening if it is not treated. Biopsy of the excised tissue is essential, with special attention paid to the surgical margins and base of the tumor. Careful clinical follow-up examination after resection of such lesions is further recommended for the detection of early signs of recurrence.

COMMENTS

An obvious advantage of cryosurgery over other modalities for CIN is that "root tips" missed by surgery alone, especially at the limbus, can be treated. This procedure results in a higher cure rate and avoids grafting and symblepharon formation. To date, surgical excision combined with cryotherapy has almost tripled previous cure rates with surgery alone.

Despite the low virulence of CIN, it can be difficult to cure. CIN recurrence has been found to be dependent on the status of the surgical bed and margins and not on the clinical appearance, presence of invasion, degree of dysplasia, or cell types. However, not all incompletely excised lesions recur, and some may revert to normal. Recurrence most often develops in the first 2 years postoperatively; thus, close follow-up is suggested. The histopathologic features of the recurrence may or may not show the same cell pattern.

References

Campbell RJ, Bourne WM: Unilateral central corneal epithelial dysplasia. Ophthalmology 88:1231–1238, 1981.

Divine RD, Anderson RL: Nitrous oxide cryotherapy for intraepithelial epithelioma of the conjunctiva. Arch Ophthalmol 101:782–786, 1983.

Dutton JJ, Anderson RL, Tse DT: Combined surgery and cryotherapy for scleral invasion of epithelial malignancies. Ophthalmic Surg 15:289–294, 1984.

Erie JC, Campbell RJ, Liesegang TJ: Conjunctival and corneal intraepithelial and invasive neoplasia. Ophthalmology 93:176–183, 1986.

Fraunfelder FT, Wingfield D: Management of intraepithelial conjunctival tumors and squamous cell carcinomas. Am J Ophthalmol 95:359–363, 1983.

Geggel HS, Friend J, Boruchoff SA: Corneal epithelial dysplasia. Ann Ophthalmol 17:27–31, 1985.

Tabbara KF, et al: Metastatic squamous cell carcinoma of the conjunctiva. Ophthalmology 95:318–321, 1988.

Waring GO III, Roth AM, Ekins MB: Clinical and pathologic description of 17 cases of corneal intraepithelial neoplasia. Am J Ophthalmol 97:547–559, 1984.

EWING'S SARCOMA

F.T. FRAUNFELDER, M.D.
Portland, Oregon

Ewing's sarcoma is a highly metastatic round cell tumor of bone. The primary lesion may involve any bone, but most commonly arises in the femur, pelvis, tibia, fibula, humerus, scapula, or ribs. Tumor metastases are common and often involve adjacent soft tissues. Ewing's sarcoma is most often a disease of the second decade of life. It is more common in males than females and is extremely rare in blacks. The major presenting symptoms are pain or a mass or both. Primary involvement of the orbit is quite rare; however, metastatic involvement can occur. Signs of orbital involvement include a rapidly developing unilateral proptosis and visual loss, with orbital hemorrhages and necrosis.

THERAPY

Systemic. Before receiving definite local control with radiotherapy or surgery or both, the patient should receive two 9-week cycles of a four-drug combination chemotherapy regimen. During the first 3 weeks, a single intravenous infusion of 1200 mg/square meter of cyclophosphamide[‡] and 1.5 mg/square meter of vincristine[‡] in combination with a daily intravenous dosage of 30 mg/square meter of doxorubicin for 2 days should be administered. During the second 3-week period, daily dosages of 400 mg/square meter of cyclophosphamide and 0.5 mg/square meter of dactinomycin are given for 3 days. During the final 3-week period, a single intravenous infusion of 1200 mg/square meter of cyclophosphamide in combination with daily intravenous dosages of 30 mg/square meter of doxorubicin for 2 days is given. Carmustine,[‡] ifosfamide,[†] and etoposide[‡] have also been shown to be effective in the treatment of Ewing's sarcoma. Each drug retreatment period is separated by approximately 2 weeks to allow time for hematologic recovery from the drugs. After radiation or surgery, chemotherapy is continued for two additional 9-week cycles, for a total of four courses of chemotherapy given over approximately 10 months.

Irradiation. Radiation therapy combined with multiple drug chemotherapy may afford the best chance for cure. Local radiotherapy of 4000 to 4500 rads to the entire diseased bone with a booster of 1500 rads to a small field of primary tumor is effective in controlling local disease. The suggested therapy for orbital Ewing's sarcoma is high-dose radiation therapy to orbital bone, delivered over a 5- to 6-week period.

Surgical. Radical surgery removing the whole tumor-bearing compartment is usually limited to amputation. Centrally located tumors may be treated with incomplete surgical resection followed by a moderate dose of radiation administered to the remainder of the tumor-bearing compartment and the surgical field after resection.

Ocular or Periocular Manifestations

Globe: Exophthalmos; proptosis.
Orbit: Ewing's sarcoma; hemorrhages; necrosis.

PRECAUTIONS

Because of the poor prognosis and the tendency for the lesions to be multicentric, wide surgical excision is generally discouraged. Widespread metastases follow both aggressive surgery and irradiation.

High-dose irradiation of an epiphyseal plate arrests bone growth and may produce ankylosis when administered to the full width of a joint. Therefore, careful irradiation technique is required to minimize bone and joint deformity and to avoid irradiation to the entire width of an extremity with the subsequent production of lymphatic obstruction. Prophylactic pulmonary irradiation is of doubtful value, since the disease metastasizes as frequently to other bones as to the lungs. Radiation therapy in combination with chemotherapy can cause lethal pulmonary fibrosis, and irradiation of the lungs should be limited to 1400 rads, delivered in 100-rad fractions. Irradiation of large volumes of bone marrow should be avoided because it may compromise the value of chemotherapy.

COMMENTS

Surgery and radiotherapy appear to be equally effective for small lesions; however, a trend toward a better prognosis has been seen in surgically treated patients with large lesions. The failure rate is higher in patients undergoing irradiation alone. The majority of relapses occur within the first year of diagnosis, and recurrence after 3 years of disease-free interval is unlikely.

Disease-free survival rates have improved dramatically with aggressive combinations of radiation therapy and multiple chemotherapy with or without surgery. Although the cure rates for localized Ewing's sarcoma of a distal extremity are quite respectable, the prognosis for other groups of patients remains poor. Among concepts being explored to improve these results are aggressive induction chemotherapy, irradiation to the bulky site of disease, and surgical resection of persistent pulmonary nodules. Another approach includes total body irradiation with possible autologous bone marrow reconstitution as part of the therapy.

References

Halperin EC: Pediatric radiation oncology. Invest Radiol 21:429–436, 1986.

Jakobiec FA, Rootman J, Jones IS: Secondary and metastatic tumors of the orbit. In Duane TD (ed): Clinical Ophthalmology. Hagerstown, MD, Harper & Row, 1982, Vol II, pp 46:51–52.

Jurgens H, et al: Multidisciplinary treatment of primary Ewing's sarcoma of bone. A 6-year experience of a European Cooperative Trial. Cancer 61:23–32, 1988.

Rosen G: The current management of malignant bone tumours: Where do we go from here? Med J Aust 148:373–377, 1988.

Sauer R, et al: Prognostic factors in the treatment of Ewing's sarcoma. The Ewing's Sarcoma Study Group of the German Society of Paediatric Oncology CESS 81. Radiother Oncol 10:101–110, 1987.

Woodruff G, Thorner P, Skarf B: Primary Ewing's sarcoma of the orbit presenting with visual loss. Br J Ophthalmol 72:786–792, 1988.

FIBROSARCOMA

F. HAMPTON ROY, M.D.

Little Rock, Arkansas

Fibrosarcoma is a malignant tumor that is most common in adults aged 30 to 70 years. Most tumors arise in the soft tissue of extremities, but some arise in the bone. Those that arise in the bone are more likely to involve the knee region and may be the delayed result of radiation exposure. The usual symptoms of fibrosarcoma include the presence of a mass with gradually progressive pain and variable swelling.

Primary fibrosarcoma of the orbit is unusual, but most often occurs secondary to invasion from nearby paranasal sinuses or adjacent bones. Another source of fibrosarcoma includes irradiation of sarcomas following extensive radiotherapy for prior malignancies of the eye or adnexa, which are most commonly retinoblastoma. The most common age of onset for primary orbital fibrosarcoma is 55 to 60 years, but 30 to 50 years would be the expected age of onset of a secondary orbital fibrosarcoma. When a mass is found in the soft tissue of the orbit or the area of the lacrimal sac, primary fibrosarcoma should be strongly considered. It can, however, occur on the eyelid, sclera, or conjunctiva.

THERAPY

Surgical. Complete excision is the only hope for survival. Total removal may be possible without undue sacrifice of tissue in those rare cases where the tumor is located on or near the surface of the eyelid, eyeball, or in the area of the lacrimal sac. The complete removal of those growths primary in the orbital cavity is more difficult. In these situations, surgical manipulations affecting the integrity of ocular functions and the psychologic impact of visual loss on the patient are subtle barriers to adequate excision. In addition, some fibrosarcomas in this area are partially circumscribed, rather than grossly infiltrative. This feature provides an easier anatomic plane for surgical dissection and may lull the surgeon into the mistaken belief that the neoplasm has been completely removed. Nevertheless, the patient should still be advised to undergo an orbital exenteration. Most complex is the surgical eradication of the secondary fibrosarcomas from the maxilla, nasal cavity, or paranasal sinuses. These neoplasms are infiltrative. Widespread excision of affected soft tissues and bold sacrifice of underlying bone are recommended. Although the recurrence rate of these secondary tumors is high, repeated radical surgery may result in the rare survival of an affected patient. Surgical management of those fibrosarcomas induced by prior irradiation or of those located in the deeper recesses of the face and orbit adjacent to the intracranial foramina is almost hopeless. Chemotherapy and radiotherapy are ineffective, except as palliative or psychologically directed measures.

Ocular or Periocular Manifestations

Extraocular Muscles: Paralysis.
Eyelids: Fibrosarcoma.
Globe: Proptosis.
Lacrimal Sac: Fibrosarcoma.
Orbit: Edema; erosion of bony walls; fibrosarcoma; increased intraorbital pressure.
Sclera: Fibrosarcoma.

PRECAUTIONS

Once the diagnosis is established by incisional or excisional biopsy, the patient should be informed of the malignant nature of the neoplasm, and plans should be made for a more radical removal, such as maxillectomy or exenteration. The longer the duration of symptoms or the greater the interval before definitive surgery, the greater is the chance of a fatal outcome. When radical surgery is undertaken, it should be done in a facility with expertise in frozen-tissue examination to provide on-the-spot information of the extent of neoplastic cells in the periphery of the surgical specimen.

COMMENTS

Although orbital fibrosarcomas develop at a slower rate and the interval between recurrences is longer than in many other sarcomas, they should not be regarded as benign on the basis of this less aggressive behavior. Recurrences, metastases, or intracranial extensions of the neoplasm usually develop within 6 to 8 years from the time of definitive surgery, but it is unwise to consider a cure until 10 to 12 years have passed from the last operation.

The histologic diagnosis of fibrosarcoma is not as easy as once believed. The examiner should be aware of the capabilities of the malignant fibrocyte to merge with or develop into one of the other related tumors of supportive tissue, such as may arise from Schwann cells, histiocytes, lipoblasts, and rhabdomyoblasts. Also, care should be taken to differentiate these tumors from an aggressive type of tumor that is classified as a fibromatosis, rather than a sarcoma. When in doubt, electron microscopy of the tissue specimen may be helpful. With this medium, the true fibroblast has a highly developed, rough-surfaced endoplasmic reticulum, a prominent Golgi apparatus, poorly developed desmosomes, and no basement membrane formation.

References

Fraunfelder FT, et al: The role of cryosurgery in external ocular and periocular disease. Trans Am Acad Ophthalmol Otolaryngol 83:713–724, 1977.
Jakobiec FA: Ocular and Adnexal Tumors. Birmingham, Aesculapius, 1978.
Jones LT, Wobig JL: Surgery of the Eyelids and Lacrimal System. Birmingham, Aesculapius, 1976.

HODGKIN'S DISEASE
STUART A. GROSSMAN, M.D.,
and NEIL R. MILLER, M.D.
Baltimore, Maryland

Hodgkin's disease is a malignant lymphoma of unknown cause that generally arises in the lymph nodes. The clinical course of this disease is quite variable. It may present with relatively localized infiltration of cervical, supraclavicular, or mediastinal lymph nodes; however, all lymph node areas may eventually become affected by disease. Extension beyond the lymph nodes to the liver, spleen, bones, bone marrow, orbit, and brain may also occur. In the early stages of Hodgkin's disease, the patient is often asymptomatic, but systemic symptoms, including fever, night sweats, and weight loss, develop in more advanced cases.

The ocular manifestations of Hodgkin's disease result from damage to the eye, the orbit, and the intracranial visual sensory and oculomotor systems. Infiltration of orbital and intracranial structures usually occurs after systemic evidence of the disease is already present. In rare instances, however, a discrete orbital or subconjunctival mass or loss of vision from infiltration or compression of the optic nerves or chiasm may be the initial manifestation of the disease. Central and peripheral nervous system damage in Hodgkin's disease may result in neuro-ophthalmologic abnormalities, including papilledema from increased intracranial pressure, optic neuropathy, optic atrophy, visual field defects, cortical blindness, and oculomotor nerve paresis. Horner's syndrome may result when the cervical lymph nodes are affected. Motor, sensory, and autonomic peripheral neuropathies may occur in patients with Hodgkin's disease. They are usually caused by infiltration of peripheral nerves by the tumor, but in extremely rare cases, the peripheral neuropathy, as well as optic neuropathy and other central nervous system dysfunction including generalized encephalopathy and cerebellar degeneration, may be part of a paraneoplastic syndrome associated with Hodgkin's disease. In general, damage to the central nervous system in Hodgkin's disease occurs late in the course of the disorder, but cases of primary intracranial Hodgkin's disease occasionally occur.

THERAPY

Irradiation. Radiation therapy with megavoltage equipment is the major form of treatment for early stages of Hodgkin's disease. Radiation therapy is most commonly delivered not only to affected nodes but also to adjacent draining node groups and to areas of potential node involvement. Doses of 4000 to 4500 rads are usually required to eradicate permanently any site of infiltration. Radiation therapy of this potentially curable neoplasm should be administered at centers that have substantial experience in treating the disease.

Systemic. Combination chemotherapy is the treatment of choice for advanced Hodgkin's disease. The introduction of combination chemotherapy with MOPP (mechlorethamine, Oncovin (vincristine), procarbazine, prednisone) in 1964 was a breakthrough in the therapy of Hodgkin's disease. Complete remission rates of 80 per cent have been described with MOPP and similar combination chemotherapy regimens, and a cure can be expected in over 50 per cent of patients with advanced disease. Approaches that include chemotherapy in patients with less advanced disease, the combined use of radiation therapy and chemotherapy, alternating non-cross-resistant chemotherapy regimens, and aggressive salvage protocols have the potential to improve upon these results.

Ocular or Periocular Manifestations

Anterior Chamber: Uveitis.
Choroid: Infiltration.
Conjunctiva: Infiltration.
Cornea: Keratitis.

294 / HODGKIN'S DISEASE

Extraocular Muscle: Infiltration.
Iris: Posterior synechiae.
Lacrimal Gland: Infiltration.
Lens: Cataract.
Optic Nerve: Infiltration; papilledema; paraneoplastic optic neuropathy.
Orbit: Infiltration; tumor mass.
Retina: Exudates; hemorrhages; ischemia; perivascular sheathing; vasculitis.
Sclera: Episcleritis.
Other: Cortical blindness; Horner's syndrome; oculomotor nerve paresis; visual field defects.

PRECAUTIONS

Because of the cytotoxic effects of antineoplastic agents on normal hematopoiesis, the immune system, the gastrointestinal tract, and the cardiorespiratory system, considerable experience is required in order to use these agents properly and safely. Patients vary greatly in their tolerance of antineoplastic agents and should be evaluated frequently for clinical manifestations of drug toxicity. Chronic drug toxicity, such as secondary cancers, sterility, and the side effects of systemic corticosteroids, are of as much importance as acute drug toxicity. Patients receiving antineoplastic drugs are also more likely to develop systemic infections from opportunistic organisms during the course of their therapy. Finally, patients who receive radiation therapy to the mediastinum may become hypothyroid from the effects of the radiation.

COMMENTS

Advances in the use of combination chemotherapy and radiation therapy in Hodgkin's disease have increased the importance of accurate pathologic subclassification and staging of the extent of the disease. Staging procedures include a meticulous history (particularly looking for such predisposing factors as acquired immunodeficiency syndrome) and physical examination, a complete blood count, and tests of renal and hepatic function, including uric acid determination. Computed tomographic scanning of the chest and abdomen, lymphangiography, and bone marrow aspiration and biopsy are also important. In some patients, magnetic resonance imaging, nuclear medicine scanning, or a staging laparotomy and splenectomy are helpful in accurately assessing the extent of disease.

The optimum therapy for Hodgkin's disease is continuously changing and is an area of extensive research. Advances in diagnostic and therapeutic techniques have resulted in an increasingly improved prognosis. Cure is attainable for most patients with early stages of Hodgkin's disease, and even patients with advanced and recurrent disease have a significant chance of cure or long-term disease-free survival. Treatment of these patients is best performed at a center where surgeons, medical oncologists, radiation therapists, and pathologists work closely together as a team.

References

Appelbaum FR, et al: Treatment of malignant lymphoma in 100 patients with chemotherapy, total body irradiation, and marrow transplantation. J Clin Oncol 5:1340–1347, 1987.

Behrens BC, Young RC, DeVita VT Jr: Current management of Hodgkin's disease. Drugs 30:355–367, 1985.

Bonadonna G: Chemotherapy of malignant lymphomas. Sem Oncol 12(Suppl 6):1–14, 1985.

Bonadonna G, Valagussa P, Santoro A: Alternating non-cross-resistant combination chemotherapy or MOPP in stage IV Hodgkin's disease: A report of 8-year results. Ann Intern Med 104:739–746, 1986.

DeVita VT Jr, Hellman S, Rosenberg SA: Hodgkin's disease and the non-Hodgkin's lymphomas. *In* DeVita VT Jr, Hellman S (eds): Cancer: Principles and Practice of Oncology, 2nd ed. Philadelphia, JB Lippincott, 1985, pp 1623–1709.

Fratkin JD, Shammas HF, Miller SD: Disseminated Hodkin's disease with bilateral orbital involvement. Arch Ophthalmol 96:102–104, 1978.

Kielar RA: Orbital granuloma in Hodgkin's disease. Ann Ophthalmol 13:1197–1199, 1981.

Miller NR: Clinical Neuro-Ophthalmology, 4th ed., Baltimore, Williams & Wilkins, 1988, Vol 3, pp 1588–1596.

Miller NR, Iliff, WJ: Visual loss as the initial symptom of Hodgkin disease. Arch Ophthalmol 93:1158–1161, 1975.

Rowland KM Jr, Murthy A: Hodgkin's disease: Long-term effects of therapy. Med Pediatr Oncol 14:88–96, 1986.

van Rijswijk REN et al: Five-year survival in Hodgkin's disease: The prospective value of immune status at diagnosis. Cancer 57:1489–1496, 1986.

Wessel K et al: Paraneoplastic cerebellar degeneration associated with Hodgkin's disease. J Neurol 235:122–124, 1987.

KAPOSI'S SARCOMA
(Idiopathic Multiple Pigmented Sarcoma)
BIJAN SAFAI, M.D., D.S.C.
New York, New York

Kaposi's sarcoma is a multicentric disease that generally presents as red-purple macules, plaques, or nodules on the lower extremities, but may appear anywhere in skin, mucous membrane, lymph nodes, or internal organs. The disease is primarily seen in males (15 : 1) and is rare except in certain endemic pockets, including Eastern Europe, Italy, Equatorial Africa, and North America. The course of the disease ranges from slow and indolent to rapid and fulminant, with average survival time in American series ranging from 8 to 13 years. In Africa, a lymphadenopathic form of the disease, which is highly fatal, is seen in children. Furthermore, a more aggressive form of Kaposi's sarcoma has been observed in kidney transplant recipients and in patients with a variety of immunologic disorders who have been on immunosuppressive therapy. Kaposi's sarcoma has been seen more frequently among individuals who are infected with human immunodeficiency virus (HIV), specifically among homosexual and bisexual men. More than 6,000 cases of AIDS-associated Kaposi's sarcoma have been reported since the beginning of the epidemic. The victims of this epidemic have been shown to suffer from a profound cellular immune deficiency and usually succumb to death from opportunistic infections. Kaposi's sarcoma in these patients appears to have an aggressive course involving skin, gastrointestinal tract and lymph nodes, with occasional dissemination causing death. An increased incidence of second primary malignancies, especially that of lymphoma, has been observed in patients with Kaposi's sarcoma. Some recent data indicate a close association of Kaposi's sarcoma and cytomegalovirus. In addition, endothelial cells have been suspected to be the cell of origin of Kaposi's sarcoma.

Kaposi's sarcoma may involve the ocular adnexa, including eyelids, conjunctiva, lacrimal glands, and orbit. Ocular lesions usually develop after the appearance of tumors on the extremities, but conjunctival tumors have been reported in the absence of other manifestations. Such involvement has been seen more frequently in patients with the epidemic form of Kaposi's sarcoma. Conjunctival involvement by this tumor is characteristically more evident in the bulbar conjunctiva and may result in focal areas of hemorrhage, with extensive injection and thickening of the conjunctival tissues. The conjunctival tumor may appear as circumscribed subepithelial nodules or diffuse infiltrative lesions, usually involving the palpebral or fornical conjunctiva.

THERAPY

Irradiation. The treatment of choice for the isolated nonaggressive lesions of Kaposi's sarcoma of the ocular adnexa is radiation therapy. Low-dose x-ray treatment ranging from a few hundred to a few thousand rads has been given in divided doses over 4 to 8 weeks and has been shown to be effective.

Surgical. Isolated conjunctival or orbital lesions of Kaposi's sarcoma may also be surgically excised or treated with electrosurgery.

Systemic. Single or combination chemotherapy is generally used for aggressive Kaposi's sarcoma with visceral involvement. Recently recombinant alpha interferon has been approved for the treatment of AIDS-associated Kaposi's sarcoma.

Topical. Immunotherapy with topical agents, such as dinitrochlorobenzene[†] or intralesional purified protein derivative,[†] has been used for localized disease. In the new epidemic of Kaposi's sarcoma, a variety of immune-modulating agents are being tried because the patients are immune deficient. The results of these trials, although promising, are still inconclusive.

PRECAUTIONS

Since most ocular lesions in Kaposi's sarcoma are indolent, conservative management is recommended unless there is clear evidence of aggressive disease.

COMMENTS

In the new epidemic of Kaposi's sarcoma, more than half of the patients have exhibited intraretinal exudates, nerve fiber layer hemorrhages, and cotton-wool spots on ocular examination. Similar findings as well as cytomegalovirus retinitis have also been described. These lesions were usually adjacent to and sometimes obscured the vessels in the peripapillary retina. The cotton-wool spots are seen in a variety of illnesses, such as diabetes mellitus, systemic lupus erythematosus, dermatomyositis, hypertension, anemia, and leukemia. They appear to be the result of focal retinal ischemia. Although the cause of the cotton-wool spots in these patients is unclear, infections with cytomegalovirus or high levels of circulating immune complexes should be considered. The cotton-wool spots do not correlate with the course of the systemic disease.

References

DiGiovanna JJ, Safai B: Kaposi's sarcoma. Retrospective study of 90 cases with particular emphasis on the familial occurrence, ethnic background and prevalence of other diseases. Am J Med 71:779–783, 1981.

Epidemiologic aspects of the current outbreak of Kaposi's sarcoma and opportunistic infections. N Engl J Med 306:248–252, 1982.

Giraldo G, Beth E, Huang ES: Kaposi's sarcoma and its relationship to cytomegalovirus (CMV). III. CMV, DNA and CMV early antigens in Kaposi's sarcoma. Int J Cancer 26:23–29, 1980.

Giraldo G, et al: Antibody patterns to herpes viruses in Kaposi's sarcoma. II. Serological association of American Kaposi's sarcoma with cytomegalovirus. Int J Cancer 22:126–131, 1978.

Harwood AR, et al: Kaposi's sarcoma in recipients of renal transplants. Am J Med 67:759–765, 1979.

Howard GM, Jakobiec FA, DeVoe AG: Kaposi's sarcoma of the conjunctiva. Am J Ophthalmol 79:420–423, 1975.

Jakobiec FA, Jones IS: Vascular tumors, malformations, and degenerations. *In* Duane TD (ed): Clinical Ophthalmology. Hagerstown, MD, Harper & Row, 1982, Vol II, pp 37:27–31.

Lieberman PH, Llovera IN: Kaposi's sarcoma of the bulbar conjunctiva. Arch Ophthalmol 88:44–45, 1972.

Myskowski PL, Niedzwiecki D, Shurgot BA et al: AIDS-associated Kaposi's sarcoma: Variables associated with survival. J Am Acad Dermatol 18:1299–1306, 1988.

Nadji M, et al: Kaposi's sarcoma. Immunohistologic evidence for an endothelial origin. Arch Pathol Lab Med 105:274–275, 1981.

Nicholson DH, Lane L: Epibulbar Kaposi sarcoma. Arch Ophthalmol 96:95–96, 1978.

Safai B: Pathophysiology and epidemiology of epidemic Kaposi's sarcoma. Semin Oncol 6:7–12, 1987.

Safai B, Lynfield R, Lowenthal DA, Koziner B: Cancers associated with HIV infection. Anticancer Res 7:1055–1068, 1987.

Safai B, Good RA: Kaposi's sarcoma: A review and recent developments. Cancer J Clin 31:2–12, 1981.

Safai B, et al: Association of Kaposi's sarcoma with second primary malignancies. Possible etiopathogenic implications. Cancer 45:1472–1479, 1980.

Siegal FP, et al: Severe acquired immunodeficiency in male homosexuals, manifested by chronic perianal ulcerative herpes simplex lesions. N Engl J Med 305:1439–1444, 1981.

Taylor J, et al: Kaposi's sarcoma in Uganda: A clinicopathological study. Int J Cancer 8:122–135, 1971.

Urmacher C, et al: Outbreak of Kaposi's sarcoma with cytomegalovirus infection in young homosexual men. Am J Med 72:569–575, 1982.

LIPOSARCOMA

RICHARD M. CHAVIS, M.D.

Washington, District of Columbia

Liposarcomas are usually aggressive, malignant neoplasms of lipogenic cells. They show a marked predilection for the intermuscular fascial planes of deeper soft tissues, such as the thigh, retroperitoneum, leg, and groin. Metastasis occurs most frequently to lungs, liver, lymph nodes, and periosteum. Liposarcomas of the orbit may occur at any age, which is consistent with the incidence of liposarcoma occurring in other parts of the body. However, this neoplasm is most common in the fifth decade, rarely appears before 30 years of age, and has a slight male predominance. The average age of the patients appears to vary with the histologic type of tumor; patients with the more malignant tumors are much older on the average than those with the less malignant, pure, differentiated, myxoid tumors.

Primary liposarcomas in the orbit are not common, and some metastatic liposarcomas to the orbit have been reported. Prompt diagnosis is especially possible in the orbit, and early appropriate therapy can result in a higher survival rate.

THERAPY

Surgical. Complete surgical excision with wide margins is desirable. For the smaller orbital tumors, this may be possible. A wide excision must be emphasized; reliance on frozen-section diagnosis of clear margins is condemned, since many liposarcomas are irregularly encapsulated. Recurrence in patients undergoing incomplete excision of the liposarcoma at sites other than the orbit is nearly 100 per cent. However, if the liposarcoma is large and in the posterior orbit, complete excision will be compromised by vital orbital structures, and exenteration must be advised.

Irradiation. Prophylactic irradiation following local excision appears to provide the highest 5-year survival rate (87.5 per cent). This combination of treatment modalities should be considered in patients with orbital liposarcoma. Radiation therapy alone should be used only in the case of inoperable tumor.

Ocular or Periocular Manifestations

Extraocular Muscles: Paresis.
Eyelids: Edema.
Globe: Proptosis.
Orbit: Liposarcoma.

PRECAUTIONS

Liposarcomas may be divided into four groups: well-differentiated myxoid tumors, poorly differentiated myxoid tumors, round cell tumors, and pleomorphic tumors. Survival is considerably more favorable with the highly differentiated myxoid types than with the more aggressive and frequently metastatic round cell and pleomorphic types. There is a correspondingly lower incidence of metastasis with the more differentiated myxoid tumors.

COMMENTS

The prognosis for the patient with liposarcoma is dependent upon the histopathology, with variations in malignancy producing various clinical pictures. The prognosis is also dependent upon the location and the modality of therapy used. The growth rate is variable, although most often it is rapid and unrelenting and can reach considerable size within a relatively short period of time.

References

Abdalla MI, Ghaly AF, Hosni F: Liposarcoma with orbital metastases. Case report. Br J Ophthalmol 50:426–428, 1966.

Bartley GB, et al: Spindle cell lipoma of the orbit. Am J Ophthalmol 100:605–609, 1985.

Henderson JW: Orbital Tumors, 2nd ed. New York, Brian C Decker, 1980, pp 253–258.

Miser JS, Pizzo PA: Soft tissue sarcomas in childhood. Pediatr Clin North Am 32:779–800, 1985.

Mortada A: Rare primary orbital sarcomas. Am J Ophthalmol 68:919–925, 1969.

Nasr AM, et al: Standardized echographic-histopathologic correlations in liposarcoma. Am J Ophthalmol 99:193–200, 1985.

Schroeder W, Kastendieck H, von Domarus D: Primäres myxoides Liposarkom der Orbita. Klinischer und histopathologischer Fallbericht. Ophthalmologica 172:337–345, 1976.

LYMPHOID TUMORS
(Inflammatory Pseudotumor, Malignant Lymphoma, Neoplastic Angioendotheliomatosis, Pseudolymphoma, Pseudotumor, Reactive Lymphoid Hyperplasia)

F.T. FRAUNFELDER, M.D.
Portland, Oregon

Lymphoid neoplasms can be divided according to their cell surface membrane characteristics into two broad categories: those that are immunologically heterogeneous (polyclonal) and those that are immunologically homogeneous (monoclonal). The benign (idiopathic) inflammatory pseudotumors and reactive lymphoid hyperplasias (pseudolymphomas), despite diverse histopathologic features, are united by their strikingly similar polyclonal profile. Malignant orbital lymphomas have been described in immunologic cell surface marker studies as monoclonal B-cell proliferations.

Idiopathic orbital inflammation (pseudotumor) is a localized orbital disease frequently referred to as pseudotumor because it causes proptosis due to diffuse multifocal infiltrations of lymphocytes and only rarely forms a discrete localized mass. The clinical disease is typified by the acute onset of pain, conjunctival injection and chemosis, periocular and lid edema and erythema, extraocular motility disturbances, and the rapid development of proptosis. Inflammatory involvement of the perioptic connective tissues can produce visual disturbances. There is a light dispersal of lymphocytes, plasma cells, and occasionally eosinophils (particularly in children) around blood vessels and interstitially within the orbital fat, extraocular muscles, Tenon's space, and lacrimal gland. The involved tissue is variably fibrotic, and the lymphoid component is not hyperplastic or sheet-like. Systemic disease is rarely associated (less than 5 per cent of cases); these associated diseases are either vasculitis or lymphomas.

Patients with reactive lymphoid hyperplasia (pseudolymphoma) present with painless, slowly progressive lesions of the orbit, lacrimal gland, or conjunctiva, and extremely rarely, of the uvea. These tumors are formed by sheet-like hyperplastic, hypercellular accumulations of benign lymphocytes, devoid of a significant stroma or pronounced fibrosis. Histopathologically, these lesions are composed of mature lymphocytes, with intermixed plasma cells, histiocytes, and prominent endothelial cell proliferation. Eosinophils may occasionally be dispersed as well. Approximately 20 per cent of patients with this condition may later develop a systemic lymphoma. A subtype of lymphoid hyperplasia, termed atypical lymphoid hyperplasia, may be associated with systemic disease in up to 50 per cent of cases.

Malignant lymphomas develop insidiously and most often painlessly. They are composed of cytologically malignant and immature lymphocytic cells. Ninety-nine per cent of such lesions involving the ocular adnexa are non-Hodgkin's lymphomas. The non-Hodgkin's lymphomas are classified into well-differentiated lymphocytic, intermediate, and poorly differentiated types. The reticulum cell sarcoma has been shown to be a large cell lymphoma, although it was once believed to be of histiocytic origin. Evidence of follicular or nodular architecture in a lymphoma offers a better prognosis for life and for response to chemotherapy. Otherwise, the lymphoma is termed diffuse.

Most conjunctival lymphoid tumors present as flesh or salmon-colored patches with a predilection for the fornices, although the epibulbar surface may be involved. Lymphoid tumors of the conjunctiva tend to have an onset around 50 years of age and are distinctly rare in childhood. Most lesions are asymptomatic, with patients primarily seeking medical care because of cosmetic appearance or fear of an unknown disease. Over 80 per cent of conjunctival lymphoid tumors are benign; the remainder are malignant lymphomas showing frank cytologic atypia and are associated with systemic lymphoma.

In addition to lymphoid tissue being found in the subconjunctival mucosa, there are also lymphoid tissue masses in the orbital cavity, the lacrimal gland and sac, and the lid. Both the benign and malignant lymphoid tumors produce a slowly developing proptosis that is generally painless. There is a distinct propensity for anterior orbital involvement with a palpable rubbery mass. CT scan reveals a mass lesion that displays a tendency to conform to pre-existing anatomic structures or tissue planes. As a rule, these tumors do not cause the bone destruction apparent on x-rays.

A specific type of orbital lymphoma is Burkitt's lymphoma. This is the only lymphosarcoma that is likely to involve the orbits of children. In the African type, there tends to be involvement of the maxilla, with secondary encroachment on the orbit; hepatosplenomegaly and central nervous system involvement are also typical, with relative sparing of the superficial lymph nodes. This form of lymphoma is curable with chemotherapy, provided that therapy is introduced before evidence of central nervous system disease develops.

Intraocular lymphomas fall into four groups: primary malignant lymphomas, malignant lymphomas of the uvea, reactive lymphoid hyperplasia of the uvea, and neoplastic angioendotheliomatosis. Primary malignant lymphomas (reticulum cell sarcoma or microgliomatosis) of the central nervous system mainly involve the retina and optic nerve, a dispersion of cells into the vitreous is often associated with these tumors. The patient often has cerebral lesions, but only exceptionally are the lymph nodes or other noncentral nervous system tissues affected. Malignant lymphomas of the uvea occur most frequently in patients who have involvement of the lymph nodes, liver, spleen, or other viscera, but rarely is the central nervous system affected. Pseudolymphomas of the uvea are typically isolated lesions, not associated with malignant lymphomas in the central nervous system or other viscera. Neoplastic angioendotheliomatosis is a variant of large cell malignant lymphoma with widespread intravascular proliferation of malignant cells of endothelial origin. Although the most common signs and symptoms relate to skin and central nervous system involvement, ophthalmic manifestations of neoplastic angioendotheliomatosis may include decreased vision, iridocyclitis with keratic precipitates, vitreitis, retinal vascular alterations (retinal hemorrhages, retinal arterial occlusions), papilledema, homonymous hemianiopsia, visual agnosia, and orbital involvement by tumor cells may resemble a malignant lymphoma.

When orbital pseudotumors are bilateral, the chances that a systemic disorder will subsequently be discovered are greatly increased, especially in adults. The ocular signs of hyperthyroidism can not only mimic or produce the clinical picture of an orbital pseudotumor but the histopathologic appearance is also remarkably similar to that of inflammatory pseudotumor. Likewise, pseudotumor of the orbit can occur as the initial manifestation of Wegener's granulomatosis. Orbital cellulitis of bacterial origin can usually be ruled out by obtaining sinus x-rays to demonstrate absence of a primary sinus infection.

THERAPY

There are presently three major modalities of therapy for *idiopathic orbital inflammation:* systemic steroids, surgery, and radiotherapy. Because of the tendency of pseudotumor toward spontaneous remission, it is probably inaccurate to ascribe all of the improvement noted to the efficacy of treatment.

Systemic steroids appear to be most helpful in patients with acute or subacute lesions and least effective in those exhibiting histologic features of a chronic phase. High doses of prednisone, 80 mg daily, should be continued for a total of 3 weeks and tapered slowly to prevent a rebound.

Conflicting data with regard to the efficacy of radiation therapy for this condition have been recorded. Likewise, repeated and extensive surgical intervention appears to be harmful.

Irradiation. If the diagnosis is *benign lymphoid hyperplasia,* radiotherapy is the preferred mode of therapy. Generally, 3000 to 3500 rads are administered. Smaller amounts of radiotherapy can be used, but recurrences may be encountered. Chemotherapy should not be instituted. A noninvasive, systemic workup should include a general physical examination, chest x-ray for hilar adenopathy, a complete blood count, and a serum protein immunoelectrophoresis. Patients should be followed at periodic intervals because even a benign diagnosis does not rule out an associated systemic lymphoma, which have been discovered in up to 20 per cent of cases of benign lymphoid orbital tumors.

If the diagnosis is *malignant lymphoma,* 4000 to 6000 rads of radiotherapy should be administered. Patients who have been diagnosed as having a malignant lymphoma of the orbit have a 75 per cent chance of having an associated systemic malignancy. This malignancy is usually discovered concomitantly or develops a short time after the ocular adnexal presentation, generally within 2 years. In 25 per cent of patients with a diagnosis of malignant orbital lymphoma, there will be no further trouble after radiotherapy to the orbit. These cases probably represent successfully treated primary orbital lymphomas.

For suspected *intraocular reticulum cell sarcoma (microgliomatosis),* a diagnostic vitrectomy with cytologic evaluation can establish the diagnosis. Radiotherapy to the globe and neuraxis is the chief form of therapy for intraocular reticulum cell sarcoma and *neoplastic angioendotheliomatosis.*

Systemic. Patients with the diagnosis of *malignant orbital lymphoma* should have a more thorough systemic workup than those with benign diagnoses. This would include, in addition to the workup outlined earlier for benign lymphoid hyperplasias, a bone marrow biopsy, liver and bone scans, and lymphangiography, possibly coupled with CT scanning for the detection of subclinical retroperitoneal disease. Patients should probably not be subjected to staging laparotomies unless they have abdominal findings or symptoms.

If *systemic lymphoma* is identified, chemotherapy should be entrusted to a general oncologist. Although orbital lesions can be expected to shrink during chemotherapy, radiotherapy should be added because of the need for rapid relief from the vision-threatening orbital deposits. Patients who are found to have an isolated orbital lymphoma without evidence of systemic disease should not receive systemic chemotherapy until widespread disease has been diagnosed.

Combination therapy for nodular lymphomas includes cyclophosphamide, vincristine, and prednisone (COP). Although dosages vary, the preferred regimen is 200 to 300 mg/square meter of oral cyclophosphamide daily for 5 days, a single dose of 1 to 2 mg of intravenous vincristine, and 100 mg of oral prednisone daily for the first 5 days of each cycle. This combination is administered every 3 to 4 weeks, depending on blood counts. Therapy for diffuse lymphomas is more aggressive. Although many drug combinations have been used to treat these lymphomas, an effective combination includes cyclophosphamide, doxorubicin, vincristine, and prednisone (CHOP). Cyclophosphamide is given intravenously in a dosage of 750 mg/square meter in combination with 50 mg/square meter of intravenous doxorubicin and 1 mg/square meter of intravenous vincristine, and 100 mg of oral prednisone is given daily for the first 5 days of each cycle. This is repeated every 3 to 4 weeks, depending on the clinical course.

For cases of suspected *reactive lymphoid hyperplasia of the uvea*, a diagnostic iris biopsy (if heterochromia is present) or a transcleral needle biopsy with cytologic studies may enable diagnosis, which can be extremely elusive. Prolonged doses of 80 to 100 mg of prednisone daily can shrink the choroidal masses; if this form of therapy should fail, 2500 rads of radiotherapy might be tried.

Surgery. Topical ophthalmic corticosteroid eyedrops are relatively ineffectual in melting large conjunctival lymphoid masses; however, intralesional injections of 110 mg of triamcinolone acetonide in an aqueous suspension in four divided doses over a 10-week period may cause some tumors to regress. Surgery alone is less likely to remove all of the tumor and should be conjoined with a wide field or radiotherapy or cryotherapy to the surgical bed. The cryoprobe should be applied "cold" and applied twice to the surgical bed and "normal" surgical margins. If liquid nitrogen is used, contact time is only 1 second. If other cryogens are used, 2 to 3 seconds of contact are necessary. The excision site is usually not closed.

Precautions

Some clinical findings previously regarded with grave suspicion, such as recurrences, bilaterality, and concomitant lymphadenopathy, are common features of benign lymphoid lesions and should not be interpreted as signs of malignancy. Because there is no clinical way of being absolutely certain that one is dealing with a benign or a malignant discrete lymphoid tumor of the lids, orbit, or conjunctiva, and because CT scan results are similar to those of metastatic carcinomas and infiltrating primary neoplasms of the orbit, a biopsy of all of these lesions is required. An incisional biopsy should not be overly aggressive; because of the radiosensitivity of these tumors, one need not attempt to remove all of the lesional tissue. The specimen should be analyzed both histopathologically and immunohistochemically. Special fixation is required for correct evaluation; therefore, a surgical pathologist should be consulted before performing the biopsy. The specimen should be evaluated to see if it is a monoclonal or polyclonal lymphocytic infiltrate. A monoclonal infiltrate is supportive of a diagnosis of malignant lymphoma. In most instances, a polyclonal infiltrate is benign. However, it has recently been reported that, by using molecular genetic techniques, gene rearrangements characteristic of small B-cell clones are found in some tumors that are polyclonal by cell surface markers.

Cryosurgery with liquid nitrogen should be done with a probe if performed in an open wound because a spray will dissect the loose periocular tissue, causing cryoinjury well away from the intended site.

The usual precautions in short- or long-term corticosteroid management are essential. Histologic sections should be read by pathologists well versed with hematologic disorders, and only lesions manifesting frank cytologic atypia should be diagnosed as malignant lesions. These patients must also be periodically examined by a hematologist.

Comments

Neither the lacrimal gland nor the orbital soft tissues contain fully formed lymph nodes or substantial amounts of lymphoid tissue on a normal anatomic basis. The intraocular tissues also lack a standing population of lymphoid cells. The conjunctiva, however, possesses dispersed lymphoid aggregates, particularly in the fornices. Any collection of lymphoid tissue in the orbit is therefore abnormal; fewer than 3 per cent of systemic lymphomas will involve the ocular adnexa at some time during their clinical course. The choroid may rarely become involved by a systemic lymphoma or be the site of localized reactive lymphoid hyperplasia. The latter may mimic a diffuse choroidal melanoma.

References

Baumann MA, et al: Treatment of intraocular lymphoma with high-dose Ara-C. Cancer 57:1273–1275, 1986.

Char DH, et al: Primary intraocular lymphoma (ocular reticulum cell sarcoma) diagnosis and management. Ophthalmology 95:625–630, 1988.

Elner VM, et al: Neoplastic angioendotheliomatosis. A variant of malignant lymphoma. Immunohistochemical and ultrastructural observations of three cases. Ophthalmology 93:1237–1246, 1986.

Freeman LN, et al: Clinical features, laboratory investigations, and survival in ocular reticulum cell sarcoma. Ophthalmology 94:1631–1639, 1987.

Jakobiec FA, et al: Ocular adnexal monoclonal lymphoid tumors with a favorable prognosis. Ophthalmology 93:1547–1557, 1986.

Jakobiec FA, Neri A, Knowles DM II: Genotypic monoclonality in immunophenotypically polyclonal orbital lymphoid tumors. A model of tumor progression in the lymphoid system. Ophthalmology 94:980–994, 1987.

Jereb B, et al: Radiation therapy of conjunctival and orbital lymphoid tumors. Int J Radiat Oncol Biol Phys 10:1013–1019, 1984.

McNalley L, Jakobiec FA, Knowles DM II: Clinical, morphologic, immunophenotypic, and molecular genetic analysis of bilateral ocular adnexal lymphoid neoplasms in 17 patients. Am J Ophthalmol 103:555–568, 1987.

Orcutt JC, et al: Treatment of idiopathic inflammatory orbital pseudotumours by radiotherapy. Br J Ophthalmol 67:570–574, 1983.

Trudeau M et al: Intraocular lymphoma: Report of three cases and review of the literature. Am J Clin Oncol 11:126–130, 1988.

MYCOSIS FUNGOIDES
(Cutaneous T-Cell Lymphoma, Lymphomatoid Papulosis, Sézary Syndrome, T-Cell Lymphoma-Leukemia)

KRISTIAN THOMSEN, M.D.

Copenhagen, Denmark

Mycosis fungoides is a malignant cutaneous lymphoma, and the Sézary syndrome is the rare leukemic form in which the lymphoma originates in the skin. These T-cell disorders also include T-cell lymphoma-leukemia and lymphomatoid papulosis, the latter being a peculiar papular skin eruption with a benign clinical course but with a malignant lymphoma-like histology. The neoplastic T-cell is a hyperconvoluted lymphoid cell that seems to be a helper T-cell. Also Langerhans cells play a role in these T-cell disorders, as they are invariably present in the pleomorphic dermal cell infiltrate that invades the epidermis as the so-called Pautrier abscesses. Mycosis fungoides is rare, with two new cases per million yearly. Usually, the course is long lasting, and durations of 10 to 20 years are frequently seen.

Mycosis fungoides begins in the skin and stays there for long periods of time; eventually, extracutaneous organ involvement appears, and the prognosis becomes grave, as 50 per cent of patients die between 1 and 2.5 years. The initial phases of mycosis fungoides are uncharacteristic, with features of psoriasis, eczema, and seborrheic dermatitis. Often years later, the diagnostic red, scaly, skin plaques appear; a histologic examination is now able to confirm the diagnosis. In advanced stages, lymphomatous tumors develop with spontaneous ulceration of the skin. At this stage, involvement of lymph nodes and viscera occurs. Death is caused by infection or complications to therapy.

In the Sézary syndrome, the skin is erythrodermic and full of the neoplastic lymhpoid cells that swarm into the bloodstream, lymph nodes, and viscera. The cause of the disease is unknown, but recently, a human T-lymphoma virus has been discovered in some of these patients. Ocular manifestations are not rare. The lids may develop plaques and nodules, and tumor involvement may result in destruction of the lid. Lymphomatous involvement of the uvea, cornea, and sclera is rare. Ectropion occurs often in the Sézary syndrome.

THERAPY

Topical. Topical nitrogen mustard is very effective in the plaque stage. Application of 10 to 40 mg of mechlorethamine* dissolved in 40 ml water may be made to the entire skin. Photochemotherapy with psoralens[‡] and ultraviolet light (PUVA) is apparently of an equal efficacy in early stages of the disease. Electron beam is used in plaque and tumor stages with doses of 2.5 to 4.0 MeV for a total dose of 3000 rads. Conventional x-rays can be used on isolated tumors.

Systemic. Extracutaneous stages are treated with chemotherapy, usually in combination with topical therapy. The chemotherapeutic agents are usually given in combination, and the most effective regimen includes cyclophosphamide, methotrexate with leucovorin, bleomycin,[‡] doxorubicin, and prednisone. Maintenance therapy should be given for at least 1 year.

Ocular. Intraocular involvement should be treated with x-rays in dosages dependent on the size of the tumors. Often, these tumors respond to rather low doses of radiation. The least amount of radiation should be applied in order to prevent radiation damage.

Tumors on the lids may be irradiated or removed by plastic surgery with transplantation.

Ocular or Periocular Manifestations

Conjunctiva or Cornea: Chemosis; marginal interstitial keratitis; opacity; tumor.

Eyelids: Ectropion; edema; necrosis; nodules; plaques; tumor.

Optic Nerve: Papilledema.

Orbit: Exophthalmos; necrosis.

Retina: Edema; exudates; hemorrhages; vascular engorgement.

Other: Endophthalmitis; scleritis; uveitis.

PRECAUTIONS

Contact allergy frequently develops following topical use of nitrogen mustard. When the solution is applied to the skin, contact of the eye with the solution should be avoided by the use of protective glasses.

There is a theoretic risk of cataract development in patients receiving PUVA. Therefore, ultraviolet-blocking glasses should be worn during the day of treatment outdoors, as well as indoors.

Side effects of electron beams may include erythema and edema of the skin with chronic radiation damage. The eyes should be shielded during treatment periods.

COMMENTS

In many Western countries, cooperative mycosis fungoides study groups have been established, and these groups should be consulted concerning evaluation of the patient and the appropriate treatment modality. However, it should be emphasized that treatment of extracutaneous stages of mycosis fungoides still is very difficult, although early stages can be controlled by effective topical measures.

References

Brehmer-Andersson E: Mycosis fungoides and its relation to Sézary's syndrome, lymphomatoid papulosis, and primary cutaneous Hodgkin's disease. A clinical, histopathologic and cytologic study of fourteen cases and a critical review of the literature. Acta Derm Venereol 56(Suppl):1–142, 1976.

Brewitt H, Hartung J, Hoffmann K: Lid- und Orbitabe-

teiligung bei Mycosis fungoides. Klin Monatsbl Augenheilkd *164*:345–349, 1974.
Catovsky D, et al: Adult T-cell lymphoma-leukaemia in blacks from the West Indies. Lancet *1*:639–643, 1982.
Deutsch AR, Duckworth JK: Mycosis fungoides of upper lid. Am J Ophthalmol *65*:884–888, 1968.
Edelson RL: Cutaneous T cell lymphoma: Mycosis fungoides, Sézary syndrome, and other variants. J Am Acad Dermatol *2*:89–106, 1980.
Epstein EH Jr, et al: Mycosis fungoides. Survival, prognostic features, response to therapy, and autopsy findings. Medicine *51*:61–72, 1972.
Jimbow K, Takami T: Cutaneous T-cell lymphoma and related disorders. J Int Dermatol *25*:485–497, 1986.
Keltner JL, et al: Mycosis fungoides. Intraocular and central nervous system involvement. Arch Ophthalmol *95*:645–650, 1977.
Lange Wantzin G: Cutaneous T-cell lymphomas and retrovirus infection. Dermatologica *176*:221–223, 1988.
Zachariae H, Thestrup-Pedersen K: Combination chemotherapy with bleomycin, cyclophosphamide, prednisone and etretinate in advanced mycosis fungoides: A six-year experience. Acta Derm Venereol *67*:433–437, 1987.
Zackheim HS: Cutaneous T-cell lymphomas. A review of the recent literature. Arch Dermatol *117*:295–304, 1981.

NEUROBLASTOMA

DEVRON H. CHAR, M.D.
San Francisco, California

Neuroblastoma is a neoplasm derived from immature sympathetic ganglion cells; it can develop anywhere this primitive neural tissue is located. Metastatic orbital disease is the most common ophthalmic manifestation of neuroblastoma; however, there are isolated case reports of primary neuroblastoma involving the ciliary ganglion.

Neuroblastoma has the highest incidence of spontaneous regression of any human malignancy. It is estimated that as many as 1 : 200 neonates may have an in situ tumor that spontaneously regresses. Previous studies may have overestimated this occurrence because immature neuroblasts are present in the fetal adrenal gland. Neuroblastoma is one of the three most common malignancies in young children. There are approximately 500 new cases annually in the United States. There is no sexual predilection. More than 50 per cent of cases develop in children under 2 years of age, with a range from birth to 62 years of age.

The vast majority of metastatic orbital neuroblastomas present after the discovery of the primary neoplasm. In approximately 3 per cent of cases, orbital metastases may be the first manifestation of the disease; often, the characteristic puffy lids with ecchymosis can mimic a battered child syndrome. Orbital metastases in neuroblastoma can be either unilateral or bilateral, but there is a slight predominance of bilateral involvement. The differential diagnosis of orbital proptosis in this age group includes sinusitis with contiguous orbital involvement, leukemia, lymphoma, rhabdomyosarcoma, and orbital spread of retinoblastoma.

Metastatic blastomas have increased our understanding of the prognosis in this tumor oncogene, amplification is observed in poor risk tumors.

THERAPY

Surgical. The diagnosis of orbital neuroblastoma can often be made presumptively if the patient has known metastatic neuroblastoma. All patients require a medical evaluation if there is no history of neuroblastoma. Body CT, bone scan, and bone marrow aspiration are the initial studies necessary in a patient suspected of having neuroblastoma. In patients who present first with an orbital metastasis, an incisional biopsy or fine needle is indicated. Since the vast majority of patients with ophthalmic involvement have widespread disease, the mainstay of palliation is chemotherapy and irradiation. Total resection of an orbital metastasis does not improve survival. In the extremely rare situation in which there is a primary neuroblastoma of the ciliary ganglion, local surgical resection with adjunct chemotherapy may be useful.

Irradiation. Irradiation is a useful palliative adjunct therapy in the management of neuroblastoma. Most patients with orbital metastases respond to 1500 to 3000 rads given over a 2-week period. The effect of radiation on survival is minimal.

Systemic. Combination chemotherapy appears to have greater efficacy than single drug treatment in the management of metastatic neuroblastoma. Current chemotherapeutic agents used in the management of neuroblastoma include cyclophosphamide, vincristine, decarbazine,[‡] doxorubicin, cisplatin,[‡] mechlorethamine,[‡] papaverine,[‡] and trifluridine.[‡] Usually these agents are given in cycles. The two most commonly used drugs are vincristine and cyclophosphamide. Vincristine is used intravenously at a dose of 1.5 mg/square meter for 2 days of every month along with 750 mg/square meter of cyclophosphamide for 1 day of every month. There is also some experimental therapy being performed using monoclonal antibodies[†] and antibodies to ferritin.[†] Other newer therapies include high-dose chemo/radiotherapy followed by bone marrow transplantation and ^{131}I-methiodobenzylguanidine (MIBG); neither of these approaches has yet produced marked improvement in survival.

Ocular. The use of artificial tears following orbital irradiation may be useful in patients who develop dry eye.

Ocular or Periocular Manifestations

Conjunctiva: Chemosis; subconjunctival hemorrhages.

Eyelids: Ecchymosis; edema; ptosis.

Globe: Exophthalmos; proptosis.

Optic Nerve: Atrophy; edema; optic neuritis; papilledema.

Orbit: Metastatic or rarely primary tumor.

Retina: Dilated veins; edema; exudates; hemorrhages; striae.

Other: Absent pupillary reaction to light; convergent strabismus; mydriasis; paralysis of the sixth or seventh nerve.

PRECAUTIONS

The response of patients with metastatic orbital neuroblastoma to either chemotherapy or radiation is transient; there is less than 10 per cent long-term survival in children over 2 years of age. Younger children less than 1 year of age with stage IV-S do quite well. The chemotherapeutic agents used have marked hematologic and, in the case of doxorubicin, cardiac toxicities. In addition, rapid destruction of tumor cells by these agents may produce high blood or renal levels or uric acid, which can lead to subsequent renal shutdown and death. Ocular changes secondary to irradiation of the orbit include erythema, loss of eyelashes or eyebrows, conjunctivitis, conjunctival contraction, keratitis, lens opacities, uveitis, vitreous hemorrhage, retinal pigment epithelial hyperplastic changes, and secondary glaucoma.

COMMENTS

Although it is unusual for neuroblastoma patients to present first to the ophthalmologist because of an orbital mass, unilateral or bilateral orbital swelling and lid ecchymosis in a young child should be evaluated for neuroblastoma. Children with orbital neuroblastoma should have an extensive metastatic evaluation because approximately 70 per cent of these patients have widespread disease at the time of diagnosis. This evaluation should include a general physical examination, complete blood count and SMA-12, bone marrow aspirate and biopsy, brain and body CT scans, urinary catecholamine levels, bone scan, skeletal bone survey, and an intravenous pyelogram.

The prognosis in neuroblastoma is dependent on the age and stage of disease. Patients less than 1 year of age or those older than 6 years of age at the time of diagnosis have a substantially better prognosis than children between the ages of 1 and 5. Although chemotherapy and radiation have had a palliative effect on metastatic disease, they do not appear to have improved the prognosis of widespread neuroblastoma. The mean survival after the diagnosis of orbital neuroblastoma metastases is approximately 3.5 months. Although results with early, localized neuroblastoma (stage I and II) are promising, the prognosis for survival with advanced disease remains dismal.

References

Albert DA, Rubenstein RA, Scheie HG: Tumor metastasis to the eye. Part II. Clinical study in infants and children. Am J Ophthalmol 63:727–732, 1967.

Alfano JE: Ophthalmological aspects of neuroblastomatosis: A study of 53 verified cases. Trans Am Acad Ophthalmol Otolaryngol 72:830–848, 1968.

Breslow N, McCann B: Statistical evaluation of prognosis for children with neuroblastoma. Cancer Res 31:2098–2103, 1971.

Coldman AJ, et al: Neuroblastoma: Influence of age at diagnosis, stage, tumor site, and sex on prognosis. Cancer 46:1896–1901, 1980.

Dousvaros A, Kirks D, Grosseman H: Imaging of neuroblastoma: An overview. Pediatr Radiol 16:89–106, 1986.

Evans AE: Staging and treatment of neuroblastoma. Cancer 45:1799–1802, 1980.

Exelby PR: Retroperitoneal malignant tumors: Wilms' tumor and neuroblastoma. Surg Clin North Am 61:1219–1237, 1981.

Maurer HM: Current concepts in cancer. Solid tumors in children. N Engl J Med 299:1345–1348, 1978.

Nitschke R, et al: Intensive chemotherapy for metastatic neuroblastoma: A Southwest Oncology Group Study. Med Pediatr Oncology 8:281–288, 1980.

Reese AB: Tumors of the Eye, 3rd ed. Hagerstown, MD, Harper & Row, 1976, pp 167–169.

Smith SD: Advances in the pharmacology of cancer chemotherapy. Pediatr Clin North Am 28:145–160, 1981.

OCULAR METASTATIC TUMORS

FREDERICK H. DAVIDORF, M.D.
Columbus, Ohio

Metastatic disease to the eye is a grave prognostic sign, with death commonly occurring within 2 years after the ocular involvement. Breast cancer, being the most common primary malignancy, represents 60 to 70 per cent of all metastatic tumors to the choroid. In females, metastatic carcinoma of the breast accounts for nearly 90 per cent of choroidal metastases. In males, the most common neoplasm is lung cancer, representing nearly 50 per cent of the metastatic tumors to the eye. Genitourinary and gastrointestinal metastases each represent approximately 13 per cent of the metastatic tumors to the choroid in males. The route of metastasis is via the blood. Therefore, the uveal tract is the site of the majority of the ocular metastasis because of its rich blood supply. Usually, uveal metastasis is unilateral, but bilateral tumors occur approximately 25 per cent of the time. Rarely do metastases occur to the optic nerve or retina.

The time between the diagnosis of the primary malignancy and discovery of ocular metastasis varies. Uveal metastasis usually occurs within 2 years, but there are reports in the literature of metastatic uveal disease occurring as long as 22 years after treatment for the primary tumor.

Rarely are metastatic lesions diagnosed without symptoms. Although pain, inflammation, and glaucoma may occur with ocular metastatic disease, the usual presenting symptoms are photopsia and decreased vision.

A typical metastatic tumor to the uvea presents as a pale choroidal elevation with an irregular undulating surface. The overlying pigment epithelium is destroyed, and a retinal detachment is present with shifting subretinal fluid.

Since the most common primary tumor of the choroid is a malignant melanoma, the distinction between these two lesions is important. The clinical appearance of these two tumors differ in many respects. Although most choroidal melanomas are at least partially pigmented, ocular metastases are generally amelanotic. Since metastatic tumors usually grow more rapidly than primary choroidal melanomas, which may lie dormant in the eye for many years, the pigment changes in metastatic lesions are more profound. The pigment epithelium and choriocapillaris overlying the metastatic lesion undergo more complete destruction, and the pigment disruption is profound. A malignant melanoma produces gradual destruction, manifested by islands of pigment atrophy adjacent to areas of completely intact pigment epithelium.

The vasculature of these two lesions also appears different clinically. Virtually all melanomas have an intrinsic blood supply, and these vascular channels frequently can be seen on ophthalmoscopy and with fluorescein angiography. Because metastatic lesions grow more rapidly, their vasculature is usually not as prominent. Finally, the two lesions differ in their growth patterns. Melanomas have two growth phases. During the slow growth phase, the lesion appears dome shaped; the rapid phase is characterized by a collar button lesion produced as the tumor breaks through Bruch's membrane and the pigment epithelium. Metastatic lesions, although dome-shaped when small, are characterized by an irregular surface as the tumor enlarges.

Ophthalmoscopy is the best clinical means to distinguish melanomas from metastatic lesions, but other diagnostic modalities also are beneficial in differentiating these lesions. Quantitative A-scan ultrasonography is one of the most useful tests available. Since melanomas are composed of tightly packed, homogenous cells, there is minimal internal reflectivity to sound as it passes through the tumor. Metastatic lesions are composed of much more heterogeneous cells that are less tightly packed. As sound passes through these tumors, there is much more interference, resulting in significant internal reflectivity.

THERAPY

Systemic. The treatment of choroidal metastasis depends on the type of tumor and whether there is other evidence of metastatic disease. If the patient has recently begun chemotherapy for metastatic disease at other sites, the choroidal mass should be monitored every 3 to 4 weeks. In this situation, the choroidal metastasis frequently responds to systemic treatment.

Irradiation. If the patient has been on chemotherapy for some time (several months) before the diagnosis of the ocular lesion, one should consider focal radiotherapy. In individuals whose ocular lesion is the only site of active metastasis, local radiotherapy is recommended. Administration of 4000 cGy over a 3-week period (20 treatments with 200 cGy) is a sufficient dose to destroy a metastatic breast tumor in the choroid, with usually minimal complications. Generally, metastatic breast carcinoma is quite radiosensitive, whereas metastatic lung lesions are relatively radioresistant.

COMMENTS

When confronted with a choroidal mass, metastatic disease should always be considered, and a metastatic evaluation should be performed. The differentiation between a metastatic mass and a malignant melanoma of the choroid on the basis of ophthalmoscopy and quantitative ultrasound studies is 98 per cent reliable. If the choroidal mass is an isolated metastasis, the treatment of choice is local radiation therapy. If the patient has other evidence of metastasis and is on chemotherapy, the mass should be observed at monthly intervals. Frequently, the uveal metastasis will respond in a similar manner as the other sites. If it fails to regress, radiation therapy is recommended.

References

Char DH, et al: Ocular metastases from systemic melanoma. Am J Ophthalmol 90:702–707, 1980.

Dobrowsky W: Treatment of choroid metastases. Br J Radiol 61:140–142, 1988.

Ferry AP, Font RL: Carcinoma metastatic to the eye and orbit. I. A clinicopathologic study of 227 cases. Arch Ophthalmol 92:276–286, 1974.

Ferry AP, Font RL: Carcinoma metastatic to the eye and orbit. II. A clinicopathological study of 26 patients with carcinoma metastatic to the anterior segment of the eye. Arch Ophthalmol 93:472–482, 1975.

Halpern J, et al: Choroidal metastases arising from carcinoma of the breast. Review and analysis of five cases. J Med 17:1–11, 1986.

Jaeger EA, et al. Effect of radiation therapy on metastatic choroidal tumors. Trans Am Acad Ophthalmol Otolaryngol 75:94–101, 1971.

Letson AD, Davidorf FH, Bruce RA Jr: Chemotherapy for treatment of choroidal metastases from breast carcinoma. Am J Ophthalmol 93:102–106, 1982.

Maor M, Chan RC, Young SE: Radiotherapy of choroidal metastases. Breast cancer as a primary site. Cancer 40:2081–2086, 1977.

Shields JA, Young SE: Malignant tumors of the uveal tract. Curr Probl Cancer 5:1–35, 1980.

ORBITAL METASTASES

DEVRON H. CHAR, M.D.

San Francisco, California

Metastases to the orbit are uncommon and account for only 10 to 15 per cent of ophthalmic metastases. In either adults or children, orbital metastases are often the initial presentation of a systemic malignancy. In children, orbital metastases usually occur before the age of 2 years. In the United States, the most frequent cause of pediatric orbital metastases is neuroblastoma. Acute myelomonocytic leukemia (AMML), although a disseminated disease process and not truly a metastatic tumor, can also present in the orbit of infants or young children as the initial sign of malignancy. Other neoplasms, including Wilm's tumor and Ewing's sarcoma, can secondarily involve the pediatric orbit, but they are much less common. Involvement of orbital bones is common with metastatic pediatric tumors, especially neuroblastoma; the differential diagnosis of orbit bony destruction in this age group includes primary orbital rhabdomyosarcoma and the histiocytosis syndromes.

Approximately 3 to 7 per cent of adult orbital biopsies demonstrate metastatic tumors. The orbit is approximately ten times less frequently involved than the choroid as a site for adult metastatic disease. Metastases to the orbit can involve the extraocular muscles, the intraconal space, the globe and contiguous orbit, the orbital bones, or the orbit and contiguous central nervous system or sinus structures. Overall, approximately 50 per cent of orbital metastases are the initial sign of the systemic neoplasm; however, in females, the primary tumor is usually a previously treated breast carcinoma. In adult males, the most common primary neoplasms include lung carcinoma, renal carcinoma, and gastrointestinal tract tumors. In the former two tumors, as many as 85 per cent of patients present to the ophthalmologist with ocular or orbital symptoms before the diagnosis of the primary neoplasm. Rarer causes of orbital metastases include pancreatic carcinoma, hepatoma, pheochromocytoma, testicular carcinoma, carcinoid, prostate and bladder carcinomas, cardiac myxoma, bile duct carcinoma, and squamous cell carcinoma. Although metastases to the orbit can be the initial sign of systemic disease, there are reports with a latency as long as 30 years between primary tumor treatment and development of orbital disease.

CT or MRI is the diagnostic modality of choice to demonstrate orbital metastases. Metastases in the orbit often produce bone involvement, although they can produce focal enlargement of an extraocular muscle or a more diffuse pattern that can simulate a pseudotumor. In adults, other causes of orbital bony destruction include infection, mucocele, midline lethal granuloma, Wegener's granuloma, histiocytosis syndromes, sarcomas, hematic cysts, epithelial lacrimal gland tumors, lymphoid lesions, and sinus carcinomas. Less commonly, enophthalmos occurs, usually in association with either a scirrhous breast or gastric carcinoma.

In approximately 50 per cent of orbital metastases, an elevation of the plasma CEA (greater than 10 mg/ml) is found, which is consistent with the diagnosis of a metastasis, especially if there is a typical CT/MRI pattern or a history of a known primary tumor. In some cases, orbital inflammatory (pseudotumor) can be differentiated from metastatic tumors on the basis of T_1- and T_2-weighted MR images. Inflammatory (pseudotumor) orbital masses usually are isodense with respect to muscle on a T_1-weighted scan and isodense with respect to fat on the T_2-weighted image. In contrast, metastases are isodense to muscle on T_1-weighted images, but hyperintense to central nervous system on T_2-weighted scans.

Fine needle aspiration biopsy is the most useful ancillary diagnostic modality in uncertain cases. Usually fine needle aspiration biopsy under CT control is diagnostic for a metastatic tumor. Rarely, a false-negative biopsy can occur in a patient with either scirrhous carcinoma or in those with a marked lymphocytic infiltration of a metastatic tumor. The performance of this technique using both CT guidance and documentation is especially important in posterior orbital tumors and in lesions with a presumed false-negative result. If the needle is in the tumor on CT, yet insufficient material is obtained, an open biopsy is indicated.

If a metastatic orbital tumor is diagnosed, consultation with an oncologist is mandatory. If the orbital lesion represents either the first evidence of widespread disease or disease recurrence after a quiescent period, a thorough metastatic evaluation is indicated, including central nervous system imaging and cerebral spinal fluid cytology. A few disastrous cases have been observed where subtle simultaneous frontal lobe metastases were not recognized at the time of diagnosis of an orbital metastasis. In both cases, external beam irradiation was given at other institutions, and failure to image and recognize the CNS disease resulted in two courses of radiation with significantly increased, unnecessary morbidity.

THERAPY

There are three general treatments for orbital metastases.

Systemic. Some of these patients respond to chemotherapy, since there is no blood-brain or blood-ocular barrier present. If an orbital lesion is discovered and there is new or progressive systemic disease, chemotherapy is often a reasonable first option.

Surgical. If a focal symptomatic lesion is found, it can be surgically removed. However, most commonly, patients have either diffuse or nonresectable orbital tumors.

Irradiation. External beam irradiation is useful for many orbital metastases. If there is no other site of metastasis and a nonresectable orbital lesion is symptomatic or if the patient is not responsive to chemotherapy, radiation is indicated. Radiation dose and fraction schedule depend on the tumor type and disease status. Generally, patients receive approximately 40 Gy of photon irradiation over a 5-week period. In some malignancies, especially melanoma and Kaposi's sarcoma, higher daily fractions (more than 400 cGy), are more effective. Similarly, if a patient has a life expectancy of less than 6 months, large daily fractions can decrease the number of times a patient must return for radiation with acceptable morbidity in a shortened life span.

Precautions

The risk of ocular radiation vasculopathy is increased with daily fractions above 200 cGy; however, the mean latency for radiation retinopathy and similar complications is 18 months. Diabetic patients and those on chemotherapy are at greater risk for ocular radiation complications.

Comments

Orbital metastases are associated with poor survival. In our experience, these patients have a mean survival of 8 months after diagnosis of a metastatic orbital tumor.

References

Albert DM, Rubenstein RA, Scheie HG: Tumor metastasis to the eye. II. Clinical study in infants and children. Am J Ophthalmol 63:727–732, 1967.
Bullock JD, Yanes B: Ophthalmic manifestations of metastatic breast cancer. Ophthalmology 87:961–973, 1980.
Char DH: Clinical Ocular Oncology. New York, Churchill Livingstone, 1988.
Char DH, Unsold R: Ocular and orbital pathology. Clinical aspects. In Newton TH, Hasso AN, Dillon WP (eds): Modern Neuroradiology. Computed Tomography of the Head and Neck. New York, Clavadel Press, Vol 3, 1988, pp 910–964.
Font RL, Ferry AP: Carcinoma metastatic to the eye and orbit. III. A clinicopathologic study of 28 cases metastatic to the orbit. Cancer 38:1326–1335, 1976.
Huh SH, et al: Value of radiation therapy in the treatment of orbital metastasis. Am J Roentgenol Radium Ther Nucl Med 120:589–594, 1974.

PERIOCULAR SQUAMOUS CELL CARCINOMA

ROBERT M. DRYDEN, M.D.

Tucson, Arizona

Although squamous cell carcinoma of the eyelids is a relatively rare tumor, it must be diagnosed as early as possible and correctly managed. This tumor accounts for approximately 7 per cent of all eyelid malignancies and 1 to 2 per cent of all eyelid lesions and tends to occur in fair-skinned, elderly patients with a history of sun exposure. It is found in association with actinic keratosis and areas exposed to irradiation. The most common periocular location is the lower lid with a high incidence of canthal involvement.

Periorbital squamous cell carcinoma is an invasive carcinoma of the surface epidermis that usually appears as a discrete, flat, infiltrative, faintly erythematous lesion with overlying telangiectatic vessels and epidermal scaling. Its development is characterized by a fairly rapid and locally destructive growth, with possible extension into surrounding connective tissue and ocular structures. Later, the tumor develops a shallow ulcer surrounded by a wide, elevated, and indurated border. Cilia are frequently lost in the involved area, and bleeding may occur with minor trauma. Although squamous cell carcinoma may metastasize to regional lymph nodes and internal organs, metastasis rarely occurs (0.5 per cent) in carcinomas arising in sun-damaged skin.

The clinical presentation of squamous cell carcinoma, especially early, is very similar to actinic keratosis, basal cell carcinoma, or other benign and malignant skin lesions. Diagnosis, therefore, depends upon careful biopsy and histologic examination, which must be performed before management can be determined.

THERAPY

Surgical. The treatment of choice for periocular squamous cell carcinoma is surgical excision that is monitored by frozen-section control of the tumor margins. Fresh-frozen section technique provides the best chance of complete tumor removal. After excising the entire tumor mass, including a generous margin of normal tissue, a thin layer of tissue approximately 2 mm thick is excised from the entire base and edges of the resected tissue or from the remaining wound. If the lesion is tissue other than a full-thickness eyelid resection, the peripheral borders and base of the tumor should be examined for deep extension. Histologic examination is performed on each specimen utilizing frozen sections. The specimens are sectioned parallel to the outer painted edge so that the entire periphery is microscopically examined. Margins containing tumor are marked on the map, and further specimens are obtained in the involved area until all margins are free of tumor.

The success of this method directly relates to the care devoted by the surgeon and the pathologist. Reconstruction of the wound is not considered until all margins are determined to be free of tumor.

If the tumor is extensive, orbital invasion may have occurred. Preoperative radiologic examination helps determine the extent of tumor involvement. Exenteration is indicated for orbital extension with fresh-frozen tissue technique monitoring of the periocular skin margins.

Cryosurgery of eyelid squamous cell carcinoma is indicated only when the patient is unable to withstand surgical excision. Based on experience with fresh-frozen technique, clinical accuracy in determining the amount of tissue involved with tumor is poor. Frequently, a much larger surgical resection must be performed than anticipated preoperatively. Cryosurgical technique requires freezing the tumor and a 5 to 6 mm margin or surrounding normal tissue to a temperature of −40° to −50° C, allowing it to thaw, and refreezing. The surgeon must rely entirely on clinical impression in determining the extent of the tissue to be frozen. Not only is this an inaccurate method of determining the extent of tumor involvement but cryosurgery also frequently produces a much poorer functional and cosmetic result than surgical excision with frozen-section control followed by plastic reconstruction.

If metastasis to regional lymph nodes has occurred, a radical neck dissection should be considered along with chemotherapy or irradiation.

Irradiation. Success has been reported with radiation therapy for squamous cell carcinomas. This form of therapy should be reserved for extensive squamous cell carcinoma that is surgically inaccessible, usually after tumor debulking.

Ocular or Periocular Manifestations

Conjunctiva: Squamous cell carcinoma.
Cornea: Exposure keratitis; hypopyon ulcer; squamous cell carcinoma.
Eyelids: Chronic inflammation; ectropion; hemorrhages; madarosis; pain; squamous cell carcinoma.
Other: Fixed globe; pain (rare); vision loss.

PRECAUTIONS

As does basal cell carcinoma, squamous cell carcinoma often presents a benign-appearing lesion. Such lesions are often overlooked by the physician unless his or her clinical suspicion for malignancy is high. Any unknown lesion on periocular skin should be biopsied to determine its nature. Only an adequate biopsy of a representative portion of an epidermal tumor can provide the information required to make an accurate diagnosis. A relative quick and easy method to obtain a tissue specimen is to perform a shave biopsy. Shave biopsies are allowed to re-epithelialize; thus, they do not need surgical closure nor do they leave a scar. Shave biopsies usually provide enough tissue for the pathologist to make a diagnosis. If, however, a specimen proves to be inadequate for diagnosis, a larger, deeper biopsy that requires surgical closure can be performed.

Topical fluorouracil[‡] should not be used to treat squamous cell carcinoma. Although it is an effective medication to treat solar keratosis, it is rarely curative in squamous cell carcinoma and may mask deep extension.

Patients who have had one skin malignancy are at greater risk of having a new primary malignancy and are at constant risk of having a recurrence. It should be emphasized that the patients must be encouraged to limit their ultraviolet exposure (sunshine particularly) and must be re-evaluated periodically for the remainder of their lives.

COMMENTS

The goals of periocular cancer surgery in descending order of preference are complete tumor elimination, maintenance of periocular and ocular function, and obtaining satisfactory cosmesis. Although other modalities of therapy have been reported to achieve acceptable cure rates, complete tumor resection with appropriate reconstructive repair provides the highest cure rate and best functional maintenance and cosmetic appearance.

References

Anderson RL, Ceilley RI: A multispecialty approach to the excision and reconstruction of eyelid tumors. Ophthalmology 85:1150–1163, 1978.
Aurora A, Blodi F: Lesions of the eyelids: A clinicopathologic study. Surv Ophthalmol 15:94, 1970.
Beard C: Management of malignancy of the eyelids. Am J Ophthalmol 92:1–6, 1981.
Lederman M: Radiation treatment of cancer of the eyelids. Br J Ophthalmol 60:794–805, 1976.
Lever WF, Schaumburg-Lever G: Histopathology of the Skin, 5th ed., Philadelphia, JB Lippincott, 1975.
Lund HZ: How often does squamous cell carcinoma of the skin metastasize? Arch Dermatol 92:635–637, 1965.
Wilkes TDI, Fraunfelder FT: Principles of cryosurgery. Ophthalmic Surg 10:21–30, 1979.
Zacarian SA (ed): Cryosurgical Advances in Dematology and Tumors of the Head and Neck. Springfield, IL, Charles C Thomas, 1977.

RETINOBLASTOMA
ROBERT M. ELLSWORTH, M.D.
New York, New York

Retinoblastoma is a malignant tumor arising in one or both retinas of young children, usually under the age of 2 years. When the tumor is encountered initially in older individuals, a spontaneous regression is suspected. Overall, spontaneous regressions occur in 1.8 per cent of patients. The tumor arises once in approximately 20,000 new births and occurs bilaterally in about 30 per cent of cases. All bilateral cases and those with a family history represent a germinal mutation. Seventy per cent of all retinoblastomas affect only one eye. Of these unilateral cases, 20 per cent are germinal mutations proved by the transmission of the disease to their progeny; the remaining 80 per cent of unilateral cases may be somatic mutations, since the mode of transmission is much different. Overall, patients with bilateral involvement transmit the disease to 50 per cent of their progeny, while patients with unilateral involvement pass the disease on to 10 per cent of their children. Retinoblastoma usually remains confined to the eye for a relatively long period of time, several months to years, but it may then metastasize rapidly by various routes. The first route is along the optic nerve to gain access to the subarachnoid space, followed by spread over the base of the brain to produce variable pictures of basal meningitis. Hematogenous spread, commonly to bone marrow, is frequently seen. Thirdly, tumor may extend outside the globe to the orbit and then through lymphatics to the regional nodes. Untreated, the tumor is about 99 per cent fatal. The most common presenting sign of retinoblastoma, seen in over 60 per cent of patients, is a white reflex in the pupil (leukokoria), often referred to as a "cat's eye reflex." The second most common sign is strabismus, which is present in 20 per cent of cases and is due to macular involvement by the tumor. In 10 per cent of children afflicted, inflammatory signs of a red painful eye with or without glaucoma are seen. Retinoblastoma within the eye has a poorly developed collagenous and vascular stroma, which tends to break apart with seeding into the vitreous as the tumors become larger. These seeds then multiply on the retinal surface below to establish implantation growths.

THERAPY

Supportive. The most significant factor in the treatment of retinoblastoma is the stage of the disease at the time treatment is undertaken. The approach depends upon whether the tumor is confined to the eye, whether it has extended locally to the orbit, or whether metastasis has already occurred. When a patient with retinoblastoma is seen for the first time, examination should be conducted under anesthesia with full mydriasis and with the indirect ophthalmoscope. It is important to make a detailed drawing of both eyes, charting the precise size and location of all tumors.

Irradiation. When small tumors are discovered at an early age, they may be treated with radiation or other modalities, even though the fellow eye is normal. The following four groups of tumors are treated with radiation alone. Group I includes solitary tumors less than 4 disc diameters in size at or behind the equator and multiple tumors none over 4 disc diameters in size all at or behind the equator. Group II consists of solitary tumors 4 to 10 disc diameters in size at or behind the equator and multiple tumors 4 to 10 disc diameters in size behind the equator. Group III includes any lesion anterior to the equator and solitary tumors larger than 10 disc diameters behind the equator. Group IV includes multiple tumors larger than 10 disc diameters and any lesions extending anteriorly to the ora serrata.

Group V includes massive tumors involving over half of the retina and vitreous seeding. Children with the most advanced tumors in group V should be treated with a combination of radiation plus chemotherapy, using cyclophosphamide and vincristine.[‡]

Radiation treatments are given 3 days a week with a daily dose of 400 rads and a weekly dose restricted to 1200 rads. The total tumor dose is 3500 to 4000 rads in 3 weeks for tumors in groups I through IV and 4000 to 4500 rads in 4 weeks for group V tumors. Tumor regrowth is managed with light coagulation, cryotherapy, or cobalt plaques and, with the greatest reluctance, by a second course of supervoltage radiation.

Photocoagulation and cryotherapy are both valuable adjuncts in the treatment of retinoblastoma. Small tumors can be treated primarily with these modalities to avoid exposure to external-beam radiation. Such clinical situations are, however, rare. Following external-beam radiation, the children are examined at intervals of 6 to 8 weeks, and any tumors anterior to the equator remaining suspicious can be treated with light coagulation or cryotherapy. Tumors up to 6 mm in diameter can be easily treated by either technique. It is generally easier to treat posterior tumors with light coagulation and anterior tumors with cryotherapy. If either of these modalities is used, treatment must be repeated at intervals of 3 to 4 weeks until all vessels to the involved area have been obliterated and the scar is completely flat with no tumor rest.

Supervoltage apparatus with an energy of over 4 MeV is recommended. A linear accelerator or betatron is most satisfactory, but cobalt-60 teletherapy units produce a beam with a penumbra that is difficult to trim, and cataracts usually supervene. A single 3 × 4 temporal portal is combined with a round anterior portal when the tumor is situated anteriorly near the lens. An attempt is always made to keep the dosage to the anterior segment less than 1500 rads.

The use of radioactive cobalt applicators is most satisfactory for the treatment of solitary tumors up to a diameter of 12 mm. If choroidal extension is suspected, cobalt applicators are the best solution to that problem. The tumor is accurately localized, and a cobalt applicator is sutured to the sclera directly over the tumor and allowed to remain in place until the tumor apex receives a dose of 4000 rads, when the plaque is removed at a second operation.

Systemic. Combined radiation and chemotherapy are used in the treatment of tumors in group V and for the treatment of orbital and systemic disease. Because of the complicated chemotherapeutic and radiation management of children with orbital and systemic disease, an oncologist should be consulted to manage these patients. Therapy involves the use of orbital and brain radiation combined with doxorubicin,[‡] cyclophosphamide, vincristine,[‡] and intrathecal methotrexate.[‡]

Surgical. Unilateral retinoblastoma is best treated by prompt enucleation after the fellow eye has been thoroughly studied and the search for metastasis is negative. In bilateral retinoblastoma, the eye in which the disease was detected is usually far advanced and requires enucleation, while treatment is directed to the remaining eye.

Ocular or Periocular Manifestations

Anterior Chamber: Hyphema; hypopyon.

Choroid: Extension of retinoblastoma across the lamina vitrea.

Cornea: Tumor cells on the posterior surface.

Eyelids: Edema (if inflammatory signs are present).

Globe: Endophthalmitis; exophthalmos; intraocular calcification.

Iris: Heterochromia; neovascularization; retinoblastoma cells.

Optic Nerve: Papilledema; retinoblastoma.

Orbit: Panophthalmitis; retinoblastoma extension.

Pupil: Cat's eye reflex; leukokoria; mydriasis.

Vitreous: Hemorrhage; tumor seeding.

Other: Esotropia; exotropia; ocular pain; secondary glaucoma; visual loss.

PRECAUTIONS

Because of the strong hereditary factors in retinoblastoma, all siblings, parents, and children of survivors must have a thorough examination of the retina. In general, these examinations are conducted under general anesthesia at 3-month intervals during the first year of life and at intervals of 4 months during the second year. If no tumor is present by age 3, it is unlikely that one will arise; after this age, examinations are conducted biannually without anesthesia.

One course of external-beam radiation with a tumor dose below 5000 rads is attended by few significant complications. If a second course of radiation is necessary, with a cumulative dose of approximately 8000 rads, there is at least a 90 per cent chance that the eye function will be lost as a result of radiation vascular complications, the most common of which is vascular necrosis leading to intraretinal, preretinal, and vitreous hemorrhage. When the latter is complicated by secondary glaucoma, useful vision in the eye almost never survives. When the retina is detached at the time of radiation, marked salt-and-pepper pigmentary changes supervene, although the retina usually functions well when it spontaneously reattaches. Arrest of bone growth centers is unusual at dosage levels of 3500 to 4500 rads but does occasionally occur. The most serious complication of radiation is the induction of tumors in children with the germinal mutation. It is projected that perhaps 10 per cent of all children with retinoblastoma will eventually develop a radiation-induced tumor, most commonly osteogenic sarcoma, or a second primary neoplasm unrelated to retinoblastoma or the treatment thereof.

The complications of chemotherapy have been markedly reduced in recent years as clinicians have become more familiar with the uses of cyclophosphamide and vincristine. If doxorubicin is employed, its cardiotoxic potential must be recognized; and all chemotherapy must be constantly monitored by a competent oncologist.

The immediate complications of photocoagulation are retinal edema, detachment, and hemorrhage. Occasionally after heavy treatment, fatty yellow exudate may be seen several days following coagulation. Cryotherapy can also produce retinal edema and detachment.

COMMENTS

It should be emphasized that the treatment of retinoblastoma must be tailored to the individual patient, depending on size and location of the tumor. Radiation alone or radiation combined with chemotherapy is the primary approach in the majority of cases, complemented by light coagulation, cryotherapy and radioactive plaques when needed. Small tumors should be treated by these physical agents alone, if possible, to avoid the late effects of external-beam radiation.

Retinoblastoma is the most common intraocular tumor among children and represents about 2 per cent of all childhood malignancies. It is extremely unusual to see a new tumor arise after the age of 3 years in children who have been followed by serial examinations under anesthesia.

References

Abramson DH, Ellsworth RM: The surgical management of retinoblastoma. Ophthalmic Surg *11*:596–598, 1980.

Abramson DH, Ellsworth RM, Rozakis GW: Cryotherapy for retinoblastoma. Arch Ophthalmol *100*:1253–1256, 1982.

Abramson DH, et al: Retreatment of retinoblastoma with external beam irradiation. Arch Ophthalmol *100*:1257–1260, 1982.

Abramson DH, et al: The management of unilateral retinoblastoma without primary enucleation. Arch Ophthalmol *100*:1249–1252, 1982.

Bishop JO, Madson EC: Retinoblastoma. Review of the current status. Surv Ophthalmol *19*:342–366, 1975.

Cowell JK, Thompson E, Rutland P: The need to screen all retinoblastoma patients for esterase D activity: Detection of submicroscopic chromosome deletions. Arch Dis Child *62*:8–11, 1987.

Ellsworth RM: Current concepts in the treatment of retinoblastoma. *In* Peyman GA, et al (eds): Intraocular Tumors. New York, Appleton-Century-Crofts, 1977, pp 335–355.

Ellsworth RM: The practical management of retinoblastoma. Trans Am Ophthalmol Soc *67*:462–533, 1969.

Haik BG, et al: Retinoblastoma with anterior chamber extension. Ophthalmology *94*:367–370, 1987.

Kopelman JE, et al: Multivariate analysis of risk factors

for metastasis in retinoblastoma treated by enucleation. Ophthalmology 94:371–377, 1987.

Reese AB: Tumors of the Eye. 3rd ed, Hagerstown, Md., Harper & Row, 1976, pp 89–132.

RHABDOMYOSARCOMA

HILARY J. RONNER, M.D.,
and IRA SNOW JONES, M.D.
New York, New York

Although rhabdomyosarcoma represents only 4 per cent of all orbital tumors, it is the most common malignant orbital neoplasm of childhood. The tumor characteristically produces rapidly evolving proptosis and is also known for its high fatality rate. It may also present as a palpable nodular subconjunctival or lid mass with injection of the eye and edema of the lids. Most rhabdomyosarcomas occur in children under the age of 10 years. Several cases of congenital and infantile orbital rhabdomyosarcomas have also been reported. The lesion is more commonly seen in males in the ratio of 5:3.

Four major histologic types of rhabdomyosarcoma are recognized: pleomorphic, embryonal, alveolar, and botryoid. Most cases of orbital rhabdomyosarcomas are embryonal tumors, frequently located superonasal to the globe or in the retrobulbar space and resulting in a forward, downward, and outward proptosis of the affected eye. The alveolar variety has a predilection for the inferior orbit; any quadrant, however, may be involved in orbital rhabdomyosarcoma. The majority of orbital rhabdomyosarcomas appear to arise from connective tissue planes within the orbit, rather than from an already differentiated extraocular muscle. Retinal changes produced by the tumor include hyperemia of the optic nerve head with fullness of the retinal veins. Optic atrophy is usually never seen initially, owing to the rapidity with which the neoplasm progresses.

A tissue diagnosis of orbital rhabdomyosarcoma is essential before initiation of therapy and should be obtained as quickly as possible after the patient is examined. It should be stressed that the clinical picture of this disease is so typical that the diagnosis should be suspected at first presentation. In certain cases, growth is truly rapid and grossly obvious over a period of days. Further evaluation of a patient with a suspected lesion should include tomograms of the orbit, as well as a CT or MRI scan. Polytomography is essential, as it may reveal subtle signs of bone erosion and destruction that are highly suggestive of a malignant process. Benign lesions, such as lymphangioma or hemangioma, may rapidly enlarge in the orbit but rarely produce destruction of bone. A chest x-ray should be performed to disclose any possible metastases, and careful inspection and palpation of the cervical and preauricular lymph nodes should be carried out. A bone marrow biopsy is also indicated to rule out involvement of widespread metastases.

As stated earlier, the biopsy should be performed as quickly after presentation as possible. To achieve access to an anterior lesion, a brow incision should be performed. If the mass is retrobulbar in location, the approach should be via a lateral orbitotomy. No attempt should be made to remove all of the suspected tumor, and all maneuvers should be as delicate as possible.

THERAPY

Radiotherapy and chemotherapy are the preferred modes of therapy for the majority of cases of primary orbital rhabdomyosarcoma. Because the function of the eye is at stake and because the tumor is highly radiosensitive, many ocular oncologists believe that prompt biopsy should be followed by immediate radiotherapy, rather than waiting until the first cycle of chemotherapy has been completed.

Irradiation. Most radiotherapists treat patients with 5000 to 6000 rads delivered from combined lateral and anterior portals. The current challenge is to reduce the dose of radiation to a level of 4500 to 5000 rads, which the eye can generally handle without devastating complications. The radiotherapy is delivered in divided doses of 200 rads for 5 days a week over a 6-week period. Two patterns of response to the radiotherapy have been clinically recognized: a rapid resolution of the tumor over a period of days or weeks, and a slower response in which gradual shrinkage of the lesion is detected over several months.

Systemic. In addition to radiotherapy, adjuvant chemotherapy is now given to all patients for 1 year. The current protocol for children with orbital rhabdomyosarcoma consists of only two-drug chemotherapy, utilizing dactinomycin and vincristine. It must be emphasized that these agents should be administered at a major oncology center by a pediatric oncology team in conjunction with an ophthalmologist and a radiotherapist. It is mandatory that patients be carefully monitored with respect to their hemoglobin, leukocyte, and platelet counts. The role of chemotherapy in destroying cryptic micrometastases is encouraging, but its ability to control established metastatic disease is inadequate at the present time.

Surgical. In the past, exenteration of the orbit was the favored treatment of choice for orbital rhabdomyosarcoma. When this mode of treatment was used, survival rates of patients ranged between 30 and 40 per cent. With the introduction of radiotherapy and chemotherapy, local cure has progressed to over 90 per cent of cases, and 5-year survival is up to 80 per cent. Exenteration, obviously, is no longer the preferred mode of therapy and should be reserved for recurrent tumor formation.

SECTION 16

MECHANICAL AND NONMECHANICAL INJURIES

Burns

ACID BURNS

HARVEY H. SLANSKY, M.D.
Boston, Massachusetts

Acid burns of the eye produce a relatively uniform clinical picture of a sharply demarcated area of damage. Since the corneal epithelium is immediately coagulated and opacified by contact with an acid, further penetration of the acid is slowed, unlike alkaline burns. Unless the injury destroys the cornea throughout its whole thickness, the damaged epithelium will gradually slough and be replaced by new transparent cells. The acute phase of an acid burn lasts for about 3 days after the injury, and the eye presents with chemosis and injection, possible limbal blanching, denuded corneal epithelium, and decreased corneal transparency. The patient complains of severe ocular pain, photophobia, and impaired visual acuity. In the intermediate phase from 3 to 7 days after the injury, there may be a prolonged period of active inflammation with an anterior uveitis. If the burn is severe, corneal ulceration and subsequent perforation may occur. In the chronic phase, which occurs in severe burns, vascularization of the cornea and cicatrix formation between the globe and lids may occur.

THERAPY

Ocular. The single most important treatment in the management of the eye injured by acid is copious irrigation immediately after the injury with the closest available water. Irrigation should then be continued with saline or Ringer's solution until litmus paper indicates neutrality when touched to the fornix. Continuous irrigation of the conjunctival sac can be accomplished by an intravenous delivery system. Both the upper and lower fornices should be irrigated, and eversion of the upper lid should be done, whenever possible.

Since bacterial infection, especially staphylococcus and *Pseudomonas*, is often a problem following chemical burns to the eye, topical antibi-

312

otics, such as 0.3 per cent gentamicin solution every 3 hours and 0.5 per cent erythromycin or bacitracin ointment four times daily, should be applied at least until epithelialization is complete. Systemic antibiotics are not usually necessary in mild burns, but may be required in burns with severe ocular infections.

Cycloplegics, such as 1 per cent cyclopentolate or atropine, should be given several times daily to minimize posterior synechiae that may accompany iritis.

Several daily applications of 0.1 per cent dexamethasone will help control anterior uveitis during the first 3 or 4 days after a chemical burn. Initial dosage should depend on the severity of the burn.

Re-epithelialization of the corneal epithelium may be enhanced by using a therapeutic soft contact lens that is large enough to cover the entire cornea. The epithelium grows beneath the lens, free from trauma caused by the burned lids. If corneal perforation threatens, a cyanoacrylate adhesive has proved useful in emergency sealing of the perforation. The bed of the corneal ulcer adjacent to the thin area should be débrided of necrotic material before the adhesive is applied.

The use of collagenase inhibitors is still under investigation, but a 20 per cent solution of acetylcysteine* can be added to the regimen in desperate situations to retard ulceration.

Surgical. If corneal thinning occurs, a lamellar keratoplasty may be performed. The procedure should not be viewed as an attempt to restore vision, but rather as a preparatory step for later surgery. Penetrating keratoplasty can be performed to restore vision. The results have been only fair owing to wound healing problems, but with the use of postoperative soft lenses, collagenase inhibitors, and new suture materials, the results are improving.

If frank corneal perforation has occurred, a blowout patch of preserved or fresh cornea may be applied. The patch is sutured in place and covered by a silicone membrane. This is a temporary procedure to maintain the integrity of the anterior chamber until more definitive surgery can be done. Mucosal grafts can likewise be performed to maintain the integrity of the fornices.

Precautions

Topical corticosteroids should be used with caution in the acid-burned eye, since they retard wound healing and may enhance ulceration. If the corneal epithelium has not managed to spread over existing defects by the end of the fifth to seventh day following injury, corticosteroids should be withheld or used with caution.

Comments

Acid burns of the eyes are generally less severe than alkali burns. Since acids have less ability to penetrate, the overall prognosis in mild to moderate acid burns is good. The most important therapeutic measure is prompt and copious irrigation to dilute the offending agent.

References

Duke-Elder S (ed): System of Ophthalmology. St. Louis, CV Mosby, 1972, Vol XIV, pp 1055–1064.
Paton D, Goldberg MF: Management of Ocular Injuries. Philadelphia, WB Saunders, 1976, pp 163–171.
Ralph RA, Slansky HH: Therapy of chemical burns. Int Ophthalmol Clin 14:171–191, 1974.
Zagora E: Eye Injuries. Springfield, IL, Charles C Thomas, 1970, pp 290–307.

ALKALINE INJURY
ROSWELL R. PFISTER, M.D.
Birmingham, Alabama

Splash of an alkaline solution into the eye causes an immediate rise in the pH, resulting in damage and death of the external ocular tissues (corneal and conjunctival epithelium), the protective envelope (cornea and sclera), and the intraocular tissues (trabecular meshwork, iris, and ciliary body and lens). Alkalis rapidly penetrate cornea and sclera, causing saponification and lysis of cell membranes and denaturation of collagen. The severity of the burn is dependent on the anion concentration, the duration of exposure, and the pH of the solution. The degree of injury may vary from simple epithelial loss to diffuse corneal stromal opacity and perilimbal whitening. Accurate classification of the burn is the key to prognosis.

THERAPY

Ocular. The eyes should immediately be irrigated with copious volumes of an innocuous aqueous solution available at the scene of the injury and on the way to the hospital. Ocular irrigation with lactated Ringer's or other available intravenous solutions should be continued in the emergency facility for at least 2 hours or until the pH of the cul-de-sac is returned to neutrality. The intravenous tubing may be handheld, or alternately, a scleral shell with an inflow tube (Mediflow lens) may provide a more efficient method to deliver fluid to the eye.

The sticky paste of lime (calcium hydroxide) may be removed from the conjunctiva with cotton-tipped applicators soaked in 0.01 M edetate calcium disodium.* Mydriasis and cycloplegia should be induced with 1 per cent atropine instillation twice a day. Antibiosis is effected by topical application of chloramphenicol or gentamicin four times a day as long as an epithelial defect persists. Analgesics and sedatives may be required for patients who sustain a severe burn.

The pressure rise occurring after the burn frequently responds to the oral administration of carbonic anhydrase inhibitors, such as 125 mg of acetazolamide four times a day, or topical ophthalmic 0.5 per cent timolol twice daily. Extensive burns of the palpebral conjunctiva or eyelid skin may cause lagophthalmos, a condition poorly tolerated by the burned cornea. In these cases, coverage of the affected eye with Saran wrap or a bubble provides a moist chamber to protect the cornea. Patching is only occasionally helpful in less severe burns, when the redevelopment of epithelial defects simulates recurrent corneal erosions. The persistence of corneal epithelial defects enhances the incidence of ulcerations and increases the likelihood of infection. Soft contact lenses may facilitate re-epithelialization by acting as a bandage to protect fresh epithelium from exposure to the air and by reducing the shearing stress of blinking. Soft contact lenses with intermediate water content but some inherent rigidity, such as Softcon or Hydrocurve, are preferred. The use of 0.5 N saline drops hourly and lubricants four times daily helps maintain adequate hydration and lens mobility. If the epithelium can be encouraged to recover the cornea, stromal healing is accelerated and the incidence of corneal ulceration is reduced.

In experimental animal studies, inhibitors of collagenase applied topically to the cornea reduced the incidence of corneal ulceration from 80 to 20 per cent. Although cysteine[†] and acetylcysteine* are both effective inhibitors of this enzyme, the latter is more desirable because of its stability, efficacy, availability, and safety. Although it is suspected that 20 per cent acetylcysteine has a favorable effect in the human alkaline-burned cornea, this has not been proved by a clinical trial.

Early insertion of a methylmethacrylate ring designed to fit into the cul-de-sacs may prevent fibrinous adhesions and reduce subsequent fibrotic contracture of the conjunctiva. An alternate approach is to suture Saran wrap over the palpebral and fornix conjunctiva. Such treatments are not clearly advantageous, since it is not unusual for severely burned eyes to undergo total ankyloblepharon. Later, lysis of these adhe-

314 / ALKALINE INJURY

sions with or without mucous membrane grafts, insertion of a symblepharon ring, and placement of intermarginal lid adhesions can restore the cul-de-sacs, improve lid mobility, and reduce or eliminate corneal exposure.

Surgical. Animal studies by Grant have suggested that early paracentesis of the eye did not alter the outcome after an alkaline burn. However, the finding of a severely elevated pH in the aqueous humor of rabbits up to 2 hours after a 2 N sodium hydroxide burn appears to offer a compelling reason for removal of aqueous humor and reformation of the anterior chamber with a buffered solution. This procedure may be performed safely under topical anesthesia by an ophthalmologist. A No. 11 Bard-Parker blade is initially used to facilitate entry of a 27- or 30-gauge needle into the eye.

There is no way known to re-establish cornea clarity after a moderately severe, severe, or very severe alkaline injury. Extensive scarring and vascularization of the cornea, without other complications, are the best possible outcome. Corneal transplantation with fresh tissue may be considered no sooner than 12 to 18 months after injury. Such a transplant cannot survive without the normal blink mechanism and an adequate tear film. For this reason, operative procedures to lyse symblephera, expand cul-de-sacs, and eliminate lagophthalmos are often required to re-establish a more normal external anatomy and physiology before transplantation.

If an epithelial defect persists in a monocular injury, conjunctival transplantation is indicated to stabilize and renew the corneal surface. Removal of the residual epithelium, peritomy and conjunctival recession, and, if necessary, superficial keratectomy prepare the recipient eye. Three conjunctival autographs from the uninjured eye are delineated with a wet field cautery 3 mm on a side and equally based around the limbus. The autographs are oriented the same way they were in the donor eye and evenly spaced and sutured around the recipient limbus.

The success of transplants in alkaline-burned eyes is lower than usual (30 to 50 per cent) because of the high incidence of secondary glaucoma, immunologic rejections, and recurrent epithelial erosions. The necessity for cataract extractions and glaucoma filtering procedures in these eyes after multiple procedures often complicates management.

Ocular or Periocular Manifestations

Conjunctiva: Edema; ischemia; necrosis; scarring; symblepharon.
Cornea: Edema; infiltration; neovascularization; opacity; perforation; ulcer.
Eyelids: Lagophthalmos; scarring.
Iris or Ciliary Body: Chemical mydriasis; hypopyon; iridocyclitis; ischemic necrosis; phthisis bulbi.
Other: Cataract; secondary glaucoma.

PRECAUTIONS

Topical ophthalmic application of steroids after alkaline burns is extremely controversial. In mild or moderate ocular burns, the anti-inflammatory effects may be beneficial throughout the acute phase without enhancing the chance for corneal ulceration. Use of topical steroids in these cases, as well as the more severe burns, for the first 7 days after injury might decrease the inflammatory reaction of the entire anterior segment, possibly reducing some of the late side effects, such as glaucoma. The advantage of such treatment, however, must be weighed against the retardation of wound healing, a consequence of fibroblast inhibition. Topical steroids interfere with the repair process and result in corneal ulcerations and perforations when used for more than 7 days after the injury. It seems most reasonable to avoid topical steroids if possible, but especially later than 7 to 10 days after the burn. The use of systemic steroids soon after the burn has certain theoretic advantages, but its efficacy is unproved.

COMMENTS

It may take 48 to 72 hours after the burn to assess correctly the degree of the ocular damage and to offer an accurate prognosis. The basis of such an evaluation is the degree of corneal opacification and perilimbal whitening. If mild corneal epithelial erosion, faint anterior stromal haziness, and no ischemic necrosis of perilimbal conjunctiva or sclera are present, healing with little or no corneal scarring will result and the visual loss will usually be no greater than 1 to 2 lines. When moderate corneal opacity and little or no significant ischemic necrosis of perilimbal conjunctiva result, the epithelium will slowly heal with moderate scarring and peripheral corneal vascularization, and a visual loss of 2 to 7 lines may occur. Moderate to severe damage following an alkaline burn is noted by corneal opacity blurring iris details and ischemic necrosis of conjunctiva limited to less than one third of perilimbal conjunctiva. Corneal healing will be prolonged with significant corneal vascularization and scarring; the prognosis for visual acuity will usually be limited to 20/200 or less. Blurring of pupillary outline, ischemia of approximately one third to two thirds of perilimbal conjunctiva, and often marbleized cornea indicate severe damage. A very prolonged corneal healing with inflammation and a high incidence of corneal ulceration and perforation are common. In the best cases, severe corneal vascularization and scarring will result in counting-finger vision. When the pupil is not visible, greater than two thirds of perilimbal conjunctiva is ischemic, and the cornea is completely marbleized, a very poor prognosis results. Although corneal healing may be prolonged with frequent conversion of stroma into necrotic sequestrum and very severe corneal vascularization and scarring, corneal ulceration and perforation are frequent. Phthisis bulbi may also occur with or without ulceration or perforation.

Promising new research focuses on orthomolecular approaches, including supplemental sodium ascorbate[‡] to stimulate collagen production from corneal fibroblasts and sodium citrate[‡] to inhibit the respiratory burst, enzyme release, and superoxide radical production from the invading polymorphonuclear leukocytes. A randomized clinical trial of sodium ascorbate and sodium citrate in the treatment of the alkaline burned eyes is currently in progress.

References

Donshik PC, et al: Effect of topical corticosteroids on ulceration in alkali-burned corneas. Arch Ophthalmol 96:2117–2120, 1978.
Kramer S: Late numerical grading of alkali burns to determine Keratoplasty prognosis. Trans Am Ophthalmol Soc 81:97–106, 1983.
Paterson CA, Pfister RR, Levinson RA: Aqueous humor pH changes after experimental alkali burns. Am J Ophthalmol 79:414–419, 1975.
Pfister RR, Paterson CA: Ascorbic acid in the treatment of alkali burns of the eye. Ophthalmology 87:1050–1057, 1980.
Thoft RA: Conjunctival transplantation as an alternative to Keratoplasty. Ophthalmology 86:1084–1092, 1979.

DIRECT AND PHOTOSENSITIZED ULTRAVIOLET RADIATION

SIDNEY LERMAN, M.D.
Atlanta, Georgia

The eye is the only organ or tissue in the body (other than the skin) that is particularly sensitive to the nonionizing wavelengths of radiation (>280 nm) normally present in the environment. The human being is constantly exposed to ultraviolet radiation (solar and man-made) throughout life; it is estimated that approximately 8 per cent (11 mW/cm^2) of solar radiation above the atmosphere falls in the ultraviolet region (280 to 400 nm). At sea level, this is decreased to 2 to 5 mW/cm^2, depending on geographic location and season. Aside from solar radiation, man-made ultraviolet radiation may also play a role in ocular phototoxicity, albeit a relatively small one under normal circumstances. The spectral output of fluorescent lamps is relatively low at these wavelengths and should not pose a problem, except for patients who are being treated with photosensitizing drugs and in aphakes and pseudophakes. However, exposure to floodlights or the blacklight lamps frequently used in various laboratories might present a potential hazard, since their output can approach approximately 5 to 10 per cent of the average level of solar radiation in the atmosphere. Furthermore, a much more significant hazard exists in certain industries that utilize ultraviolet radiation in catalytic polymerization processes.

Ultraviolet-induced changes in human and animal ocular tissues can be attributed to two mechanisms: a direct or intrinsic process in which the radiation is absorbed by specific naturally occurring chromophores within these tissues (nucleic acids or aromatic amino acid residues), or an indirect or photosensitized process in which the radiation is initially absorbed by photosensitizing drugs or other extraneous compounds.

A typical example of corneal photodamage from direct ultraviolet radiation is snow blindness. This type of photokeratitis is due to the relatively high levels of ultraviolet radiation that can be reflected by snow (80 to 90 per cent) compared with less than 5 per cent from earth or grass. In addition to the well-known solar and industrial photokeratitis, ultraviolet radiation has also been implicated in a variety of conjunctival and corneal lesions. These include pingueculae and pterygiums, exposure keratosis (which involves epithelial changes related to actinic radiation and is analogous to actinic keratosis of the skin), nodular band-shaped keratopathy, experimentally induced tumors in animals, and the relatively rare dysplasia and intraepithelial carcinoma. Certain corneal diseases, such as herpes simplex keratitis and recurrent corneal erosions, can also be triggered by exposure to ultraviolet radiation. Experimental ultraviolet photokeratitis is generally associated with an action spectrum showing a major peak at 280 nm and a minor one at approximately 260 nm.

The normal human cornea and aqueous humor transmit almost all of the ultraviolet radiation longer than 300 nm, although there is a small but progressive decrease in the percentage of ultraviolet radiation transmitted as the cornea ages (this may be due to an accumulation of ultraviolet-induced fluorescent chromophores in the cornea as it ages). Thus, the human ocular lens is constantly exposed to ambient ultrviolet radiation (300 to 400 nm) throughout life. One consequence of cumulative photochemical damage is an increasing absorption of ultraviolet radiation and visible light because of the presence of intrinsic and photochemically generated lens chromophores.

Ultraviolet radiation can markedly affect the intact lens by direct absorption both in vivo and in vitro. During the past decade, a considerable amount of evidence has accumulated implicating ultraviolet radiation (between 300 and 400 nm) as a significant factor in the in vitro generation of fluorescent compounds and in protein cross-linking associated with lens aging and cataractogenesis in the animal and human lenses. In vivo studies have demonstrated that ultraviolet radiation of wavelengths longer than 300 nm are capable of generating experimental and human cataracts. The consequences of cumulative photochemical damage are 1) an increasing absorption of ultraviolet radiation and some visible light due to the presence of photochemically generated chromophores that increase in concentration and number as the lens ages; 2) the lens nucleus becomes yellower; and 3) there is a progressive decrease in the transmission of visible light, as well as ultraviolet radiation. The discoloration is mainly confined to the lens nucleus, since the cortex has much higher levels of glutathione and other compounds capable of aborting most of these photochemical reactions. Extreme examples of this age-related photochemical generation of lens pigments are the brown and black cataracts.

Although only a small amount of ultraviolet radiation from the sun enters the eye under normal circumstances, the cumulative effect of many years of exposure is significant, particularly when one considers our ever increasing life span. Epidemiologic surveys provide some support for the thesis that sunlight plays a role in lenticular aging and the development of senile nuclear cataracts. For example, the incidence of cataracts and the rate of cataract extraction are much higher in India, Pakistan, certain areas of Africa and particularly Nepal than in the temperate zones. A recent epidemiologic investigation into the relationship between sunlight and cataract in the United States reported that cataract to control ratios for persons aged 65 years or older were significantly larger in locations with large amounts of sunlight. Obviously, other factors play a role in cataractogenesis, including heredity, nutrition, and metabolism.

Thus, it is now generally accepted that chronic exposure to ultraviolet radiation (300 to 400 nm) over an individual's lifetime leads to the generation and increased accumulation of various pigments in the lens that are, to some extent, responsible for the increased yellow color of the lens nucleus as it ages. In about 10 per cent of the population, this process progresses at a more rapid pace, resulting in the development of the brown (nuclear) cataract. This type of discoloration, in moderation, is actually beneficial because it enables the lens to become a very effective filter for ultraviolet and short wavelength visible radiation (by the second to third decade), thus protecting the retina from cumulative photochemical damage that could occur during one's lifetime. Studies have shown that such radiation can cause irreversible retinal photodamage in the aphakic Rhesus monkey and even in humans. It is interesting that nature has provided humans with the ability to develop a lenticular ultraviolet filter to protect the retina from continuous radiation exposure that could be harmful, particularly in the older individual where the retinal metabolism and repair processes are no longer as effective as in the young. Long wavelength ultraviolet radiation may play a role in certain retinal diseases (cystoid macular edema) that tend to occur in older patients after removal of their cataractous lenses and even in degenerative processes (macular degeneration and retinitis pigmentosa).

In addition to the effects of chronic exposure to ambient ultraviolet radiation, acute exposure to ultraviolet radiation can produce cortical opacities in human and animal lenses. Thus, more intense ultraviolet radiation (300 nm and longer) can induce lens changes involving the cortex, whereas chronic exposure mainly affects the lens nucleus. These effects appear to be dose and time related.

The vitreous is normally protected from ultraviolet radiation by the filtering action of the cornea (up to 295 nm) and by the lens as it ages (>295 nm); however, aphakic and pseudophakic patients lose a significant and protective intraocular filter. The normal vitreous is a gel-like material composed mainly of water, collagenous protein, and long-chain carbohydrates, but these compounds do not have any significant absorption above 250 to 260 nm. Thus, the cornea plays a more significant role as an ultraviolet filter, since it prevents ultraviolet radiation below 295 nm from entering the eye. However, the vitreous does contain some tryptophan residues and several cell types—the hyalocytes and fibrocytes. Thus, the vitreous is also capable of absorbing ultraviolet radiation longer than 295 nm, provided that the filtering action of the ocular lens is removed. There is some experimental evidence that exposure of the vitreous to ultraviolet radiation up to 320 nm results in shrinkage of the vitreous gel and denaturation of the collagen network. There is also a decrease in the viscosity of hyaluronic acid preparations derived from ultraviolet-exposed vitreous, which can be attributed mainly to a decrease in molecular weight and length. It would thus appear that the cornea, which filters all ultraviolet radiation shorter than 295 nm, plays a major role in protecting the vitreous from ultraviolet damage. There is still insufficient experimental evidence to assess the effect of ultraviolet radiation longer than 295 nm, but there are indications that the vitreous is also sensitive to longer wavelength ultraviolet radiation. Thus, the 295- to 400-nm filtering action of the ocular lens may also be of significance in protecting the vitreous.

The fact that visible light is required in the cyclic process of shedding and renewal of the outer membrane discs that contain visual pigments might explain the findings that even moderate but prolonged exposure to visible light, at thresholds of illumination well below those required to cause thermal damage to the retina, is capable of causing retinal pathology in a variety of experimental animals. In the retina, aging is known to be characterized by a loss of rod and cone cells. Recent observations that photic trauma can damage the receptors as well suggest a potential cumulative action of light, resulting in an enhanced loss of visual cells over a period of years. That is, phototoxic effects may be cumulative in the normal aging process of the retina. Photon energies in the electromagnetic spectrum increase as the wavelength decreases, from

1.6 eV at 750 nm to 3.3 eV at 400 nm and higher energies in the ultraviolet wavelengths capable of penetrating to the retina in the young eye and aphakic or pseudophakic eyes. One would anticipate that photic damage would be greatest for ultraviolet radiation (320 to 390 nm) and short wavelength visible light in the blue region and would decrease with increasing wavelengths of light, with the least damage occurring with red light. Recent studies strongly implicate long wavelength ultraviolet and short wavelength visible radiation (320 to 450 nm) as a significant factor in retinal photodamage. These data are of particular concern in young patients as well as aphakes and pseudophakes who are on photosensitizing drugs and all patients exposed to prolonged or above ambient levels of UVA radiation.

The spectral sensitivity of the human retina influences the efficiency of a specific wavelength in producing retinal damage. The ocular lens also protects the retina from visible as well as ultraviolet radiation because it filters more of the short wavelengths of visible light (blue) as compared with the longer wavelengths. Thus, the aging retina, which metabolically should be more susceptible to photic damage caused by visible light (as well as ultraviolet radiation), is in fact protected by the ocular lens that increasingly filters out the ultraviolet and short wavelengths of the visible spectrum as the person ages. This might explain why human retinas are normally capable of withstanding much higher thresholds of radiation intensity as compared with other animals, such as the rat, rabbit, and pigeon. The retinas of these animals can be damaged by levels of environmental light that are not damaging to the normal human eye.

In addition to the demonstrated direct photochemical action of ultraviolet radiation on the ocular lens, there is the possibility of photobiologic damage by means of photosensitized reactions caused by the accumulation of certain drugs within this organ. After the 13 mm stage of development, the ocular lens is completely encapsulated and never sheds its cells throughout life. Thus, photobinding a drug to the lens proteins and nucleic acids ensures its lifelong retention within the lens, with the potential for enhanced photodamage if the photoproducts are capable of acting as photosensitizing agents.

The psoralen compounds are well-known photosensitizing agents and have been used (under controlled conditions) in many dermatology clinics to treat psoriasis and vitiligo. This form of phototherapy, commonly referred to as PUVA therapy, involves the ingestion of methoxsalen or related compounds followed by exposure to UVA radiation (320 to 400 nm) for short periods of time. Methoxsalen can be found in a variety of ocular tissues within 2 hours after an animal (rat, dogfish, or monkey) is given a single dose (equivalent to a human therapeutic level) and can become photobound to lens proteins and DNA if there is concurrent exposure to ambient levels of UVA radiation. Since the mature ocular lens is a very effective filter for UVA radiation in most mammals (including humans), there can be no photobinding of methoxsalen in the retina. However, UVA radiation can penetrate to the retina in aphakic and pseudophakic experimental animals and in young eyes (where the ocular lens still permits significant penetration of UVA radiation), and methoxsalen photobinding can also occur in these retinas.

PUVA therapy has been shown to be associated with cataract formation in humans and experimental animals. There is objective proof that this drug can generate specific PUVA photoproducts in human lenses that have been shown to be associated with the formation of PUVA cataracts in experimental animals. These data are the first objective demonstration of methoxsalen lens protein photoproducts in material derived from human PUVA patients and provide further evidence to substantiate the previous clinical reports of presumptive PUVA cataracts. However, this observation should not deter anyone from prescribing such therapy for psoriasis, since simple and effective preventive measures are available. It should be noted that methoxsalen can be found in the lens *for only 24 hours, provided* that the eye is protected from UVA radiation. Thus, many dermatologists are now providing proper ultraviolet-filtering glasses to all their PUVA patients, with instructions to put them on as soon as they ingest the drug and continue to wear them for at least 24 hours. They must be worn indoors, as well as out of doors, since there is sufficient UVA radiation in ordinary fluorescent lighting to photobind the methoxsalen. A 2-year follow-up study using ultraviolet slitlamp densitography has proven the efficacy of this approach. All the patients were provided with proper ultraviolet-filtering glasses for at least 24 hours after drug ingestion, and none developed enhanced or abnormal lens fluorescence levels. In contrast, patients whose eyes had not been properly protected (those treated prior to 1978) had anomalous and enhanced lens fluorescence, and three of them developed PUVA cataracts. PUVA therapy could pose a potential hazard not only to the ocular lens but also to the retina in young people whose lenses are not effective ultraviolet absorbers or in aphakic or pseudophakic individuals, particularly if they are exposed to repeated PUVA therapy. The clear PMMA intraocular lenses currently in use are excellent transmitters of ultraviolet radiation and thus provide less protection from UVA radiation than the natural lens. Ultraviolet-absorbing intraocular lenses are now being tested by several manufacturers and should provide a simple means to prevent potential UVA photodamage to the pseudophakic retina.

Allopurinol is a commonly used antihyperuricemic agent in treating gout. Scattered reports have appeared regarding the possible relationship between the development of lens opacities in relatively young patients (second to fourth decade) and chronic ingestion of this drug. Photobound allopurinol has been demonstrated in

318 / DIRECT AND PHOTOSENSITIZED ULTRAVIOLET RADIATION

11 cataracts derived from patients who had been on chronic allopurinol therapy for 2 years or more. These data (and other experimental studies) demonstrate that allopurinol can be photobound to lens proteins and thus become permanently retained in the lens. Such material can now act as an additional photosensitizer within the lens, thereby exerting a cataractogenic action. However, this cataractogenic action only occurs when the allopurinol becomes bound to lens proteins. Noncataractous lenses derived from patients on chronic allopurinol therapy do not contain the allopurinol photoproduct, suggesting that only the bound material can be damaging to the lens.

A new slitlamp densitographic apparatus based on the Scheimpflug principle, capable of accurately and reproducibly recording visible changes in lens density as it ages, was recently introduced. This apparatus has been modified to utilize ultraviolet radiation (300 to 400 nm), to excite the ultraviolet-absorbing chromophores in the lens and, to photograph the ensuing fluorescence. This permits utilization of ultraviolet radiation to measure and quantitate the age-related fluorescence levels in the normal lens in vivo and correlate them with in vitro data. This method can also detect abnormal fluorescence levels in patients exposed to above-ambient levels of ultraviolet radiation or photosensitizing agents because lenticular fluorescence directly reflects the cumulative effects of photobiologic changes in this organ. Results of in vivo ultraviolet slitlamp densitography are very encouraging. Such data will permit objective monitoring of at least one aging parameter in this organ (fluorescence) and determination of abnormal levels months to years before lens changes become manifest by conventional slitlamp examinations. This data will enable the clinician to institute protective measures in patients who have abnormal photochemically induced lens changes as monitored by their fluorescence levels. Ultraviolet-absorbing or reflecting lenses are now available to prevent further ultraviolet-induced photochemical damage to the lens.

In order to utilize in vivo lens fluorescence measurements as a monitoring device to determine which patients have enhanced or abnormal lenticular fluorescence (which can predict potential cataract formation months to years before the actual opacity becomes manifest), it is important to develop a "normal lens fluorescence aging index." This index should be correlated with geographic location because ambient solar ultraviolet radiation levels vary significantly in different regions.

These data, although requiring further study to better evaluate the role of ambient solar ultraviolet radiation in the generation of nontryptophan fluorescent chromophores within the ocular lens, demonstrate that such a relationship exists. These data clearly demonstrate that a useful and reproducible lens fluorescence aging index can be obtained with in vivo Scheimpflug measurements, verifying the fact that one objective parameter of lenticular aging is an increase in nontryptophan fluorescence.

A recent study has demonstrated a definite enhancement of total lens fluorescence peaks in patients with early to moderate cortical opacities compared with age-matched individuals who did not have cortical lens changes (as evaluated by the conventional slitlamp). Although their fluorescence enhancement is not as great as is generally seen in patients with brunescent cataracts, these data clearly demonstrate that such lenses do show increased (nontryptophan) fluorescence and suggest that the in vivo lens fluorescence monitoring method can provide a useful and objective parameter in epidemiologic studies. It should, however, be stressed that this approach requires concomitant data on normal age- (and sex-)matched people in the specific location being evaluated in order to be able to delineate those with enhanced lens fluorescence levels.

Although enhanced lens fluorescence in diabetics has been reported years ago, such data provide clear-cut objective measurement that the process of lens aging as monitored by its fluorescence levels is accelerated in the diabetic state, again corroborating the well-known observation regarding a generalized accelerated aging process in such patients.

Similar studies on patients undergoing PUVA therapy further demonstrate that certain photosensitizing drugs cause photochemical changes in the lens. These changes can be easily demonstrated in vivo well before they have advanced to the stage of manifest opacities (capable of being viewed with the conventional slit lamp). Thus, monitoring such patients with this method will enable one to prevent further progression by the simple expedient of prescribing proper ultraviolet absorbing glasses. It is important to stress that most commercial sunglasses are not adequate (irrespective of their color) because they transmit varying amounts of ultraviolet radiation. Even the low-level irradiance from standard household fluorescent lighting can cause photobinding of some photosensitizers within the lens, thereby ensuring their permanent retention.

In addition to detecting abnormal levels or wavelengths of lens fluorescence in the living eye, one can also test the hypothesis that the ultraviolet-filtering capacity of the lens in certain patients with degenerative retinal disease is lower than normal. That is, the ocular lens in such individuals has not developed sufficient chromophores to enable it to absorb all the ultraviolet radiation. In 80 per cent of the population, the lens has become a very effective filter for ultraviolet and short wavelength visible radiation (320 to 450 nm) by the second to third decade, thereby protecting the aging (and metabolically less efficient) retina from potential photodamage. Such wavelengths can cause retinal photodamage as demonstrated by experiments in primate eyes. Clinical retinal pathology has recently been reported in some patients undergoing extracapsular cataract extraction in which an unfiltered operating microscope was employed. Measuring lens fluorescence levels in patients provides values directly related to the ultraviolet-filtering capacity of the patient's own ocular lens. Preliminary results demonstrate a significantly lower level of lens fluorescence in patients with retinal degenerative diseases (compared with the usual values for their age group), indicating that these lenses are less effective in filtering out the 320 to 450 nm wavelengths of radiation. In view of the increasing use of plastic intraocular lenses, which transmit much more ultraviolet radiation than glass (even wavelengths shorter than 320 nm), questions have been raised regarding potential ultraviolet and short wavelength visible (320 to 450 nm) radiation damage to pseudophakic patients. Protecting patients with ultraviolet-absorbing glasses significantly reduces the incidence of postoperative cystoid macular edema.

THERAPY

Supportive. The best and simplest treatment for direct ultraviolet photodamage to ocular tissues is prevention. Because of the confusion and controversial claims regarding the efficacy of commercially available sunglasses in protecting the eye from ultraviolet photodamage, an analysis of a large series of such lenses was made to determine their transmission characteristics. These studies are in general agreement with an earlier report and demonstrate a wide variation in the ultraviolet transmission characteristics of the sunglasses evaluated, ranging from 1.5 to 40 per cent, with similar transmission values noted when tested for more discrete wavelengths (340 to 380 nm). Only the NOIR, Spectra-Shield, Silor, Univis, and UV/400 lenses were more than 99 per cent effective in filtering all the ultraviolet radiation. The Spectra-Shield is a coating for glass lenses, and the Silor, Univis and UV/400 are ultraviolet-absorbing plastic lenses that can be ordered with the patient's correction. For those who do not require corrective lenses, plano spectacles made of any of the foregoing materials can be ordered. For patients on phototherapy, goggles with sidepieces are preferred to prevent reflected radiation. The Blak Ray goggle and those made from the foregoing materials are recommended. These lenses transmit more than 90 per cent of visible light; therefore, patients can wear them with comfort indoors as well as outdoors and thereby protect themselves from all sources of ambient ultraviolet radiation, such as fluorescent lighting and sunlight. They are particularly recommended for patients who, by virtue of their occupations, are exposed to abnormal levels of ultraviolet radiation (in certain industries utilizing ultraviolet polymerization techniques, sailors, roofers, or lifeguards) as well as those undergoing phototherapy (PUVA therapy for psoriasis and vitiligo). In addition, ultraviolet-absorbing glasses in patients with retinal degenerative diseases have been shown to reduce significantly the incidence of postoperative cystoid macular edema. Ordinary commercial sunglasses are not necessarily effective absorbers of ultraviolet radiation longer than 320 nm and are not recommended unless their transmission characteristics are such that they remove 99 per cent or more of all ultraviolet radiation. Although visible radiation is significantly decreased in darkly tinted sunglasses while still permitting some long wavelength ultraviolet transmission, a 50 per cent or more decrease in visible radiation can result in pupillary enlargement of 0.10 to 0.25 mm in patients with blue, gray and hazel eyes, thereby increasing the effective dose of radiation incident on the intraocular tissues.

Despite recent claims by some intraocular lens manufacturers that their lenses absorb ultraviolet radiation, there are as yet no proven products available. Since clear glass absorbs ultraviolet up to 320 nm and some intraocular lenses are made of materials that contain some absorbing chromophores, the manufacturer can claim that their lenses are ultraviolet filters even though they do not remove the longer wavelengths. In order to be truly effective, the intraocular lens must at least filter all radiation up to 400 nm and preferably a significant percentage of the short wavelength visible light (400 to 450 nm). Such lenses will probably become available in the near future. It is hoped that any lenses claiming to be ultraviolet-filtering intraocular lenses will have their true absorption and transmission characteristics clearly noted as a package insert in order to avoid half-truths and questionable claims.

PRECAUTIONS

The recent controversy regarding ocular problems in workers using visual display terminals may turn out to be beneficial and opportune. In contrast with the indifference and ignorance with which the development of the x-ray was embraced in the not too distant past, the community at large, as well as the scientific specialists, are now well aware of possible dangers in misusing electromagnetic radiation. Humans now have the ability to monitor radiation emission levels from technologic marvels and obtain reasonably accurate measurements on most wavelength emissions of interest. A considerable body of ever-expanding scientific knowledge enables one to correlate specific radiation emission levels with threshold doses for possible photobiologic damage. Such measurements have been performed by scientists at the Bureau of Radiological Health, Bell Laboratories, and NIOSH. Scientists at the Bureau of Radiological Health measured ionizing radiation (x-ray) emission levels on 125 video display terminals; of these, 34 video display terminals were also measured for nonionizing radiation emission (ultraviolet, visible, infrared, microwave, and other radiofrequency emissions). A smaller number of video display terminals were similarly evaluated by the Bell Laboratory scientists. These data indicate that the video display terminals emit little or no harmful ionizing or nonionizing radiation under normal operating conditions. The specific emissions that were detectable were all well below the current national and international safety standards.

In addition to "ocular fatigue," questions have been raised regarding a possible relationship between video display terminal radiation emission and "organic" ocular photodamage, particularly to the ocular lens. In the laboratory, the lowest levels of ultraviolet radiation (at specific wavelengths) that have been shown to be capable of producing direct ultraviolet photodamage to the ocular lens, although considerably lower than ambient (solar) ultraviolet radiation, are still significantly larger (at least by a factor of 10) than the ultraviolet radiation emission levels emitted by the video display terminals. Thus, the best available current experimental and epidemiologic evidence does not indicate that the level of ultraviolet radiation emitted by the video display terminals is capable of exerting any deleterious effects on the ocular lenses of personnel using these terminals. However, more attention should be paid to the workplace with respect to the types of lighting (their ultraviolet emission levels) used in these environments and the reflectance level of work surfaces (including ultraviolet reflectance of painted walls, desks, etc.) in order to maintain total ambient ultraviolet radiation exposure at minimum levels. The human ocular lens serves us well as a natural filter for removing the ultraviolet radiation that penetrates into the eye, thereby protecting the underlying retina, which has been shown to be quite sensitive to rather low levels of ultraviolet radiation. Thus, particular care must be taken to protect aphakic and pseudophakic individuals from potential low-level ultraviolet radiation damage. A similar situation pertains to some patients who are receiving photosensitizing drugs. Fortunately, the levels of ultraviolet radiation emitted by the video display terminals are lower by a factor of 100 than the amount shown to cause retinal photodamage in experimental primate studies.

Finally, the ability of protecting the eye from potential ultraviolet photodamage is now possible with special eyeglasses, and similar ultraviolet-absorbing materials could be employed at the manufacturing end to prevent ultraviolet radiation emission from the ever-increasing array of technologic products.

COMMENTS

Ambient ultraviolet radiation is capable of inducing damage to various ocular tissues, particularly the cornea, lens, and retina. The latter two organs are protected from short wavelength ultraviolet radiation by the cornea, which acts as a very effective filter for the 280 to 300 nm wavelengths. However, longer wavelength ultraviolet radiation (>300 nm) has now been shown to play a significant role in the generation of at least one form of aging cataract, the brown (nuclear) cataract, and is one of the risk factors in senile cataractogenesis. In aphakic or pseudophakic individuals (who have lost the filtering protection of their own lenses), the retina can also be susceptible to photochemical damage. Furthermore, photochemical damage to ocular tissues is potentiated by certain photosensitizing drugs and chemical reagents. It should also be noted that visible radiation is significantly decreased in darkly tinted sunglasses, while still permitting some long wavelength ultraviolet transmission. In patients with blue, gray, and hazel eyes, a 50 per cent or more decrease in visible radiation can result in pupillary enlargement of 0.10 to 0.25 mm, thereby significantly increasing the effective dose of radiation incident on the intraocular tissues.

References

Anderson WJ, Gebel RKH: Ultraviolet windows in commercial sunglasses. Appl Optics 16:515–517, 1977.

Hiller R, Giacometti L, Yuen K: Sunlight and cataract: An epidemiologic investigation. Am J Epidemiol 105:450–459, 1977.

Hockwin O, Lerman S: Clinical evaluation of direct and photosensitized ultraviolet radiation damage to the lens. Ann Ophthalmol 14:220–223, 1982.

Lerman S: Photosensitizing drugs and their possible role in enhancing ocular toxicity. Ophthalmology 93:304–318, 1986.

Lerman S: Radiant Energy and the Eye. New York, MacMillan, 1980, pp 29–186.

Lerman S: UV slit lamp densitography of the human lens. An additional tool for prospective studies of changes in lens transparency. In Aging of the Lens Symposium. Munich, Integra, 1982, pp 139–154.

Lerman S, Megaw J: Transmission characteristics of commercially available sunglasses. J Toxicol—Cut Ocular Toxicol 2:47–61, 1983.

Lerman S, Megaw J, Willis I: Potential ocular complications from PUVA therapy and their prevention. J Invest Dermatol 74:197–199, 1980.

Weiss MM, Petersen RC: Electromagnetic radiation emitted from video computer terminals. Am Ind Hyg Assoc J 40:300–309, 1979.

Zigman S, Datiles M, Torczynski E: Sunlight and human cataracts. Invest Ophthalmol Vis Sci 18:462–467, 1979.

ELECTRICAL INJURY

F.T. FRAUNFELDER, M.D.
Portland, Oregon

Electrical injury occurs when an electric current passes through the body. The current may arc between an electrode and the body at voltages ranging from that of lightning, which may be 100 million volts, to as low as 380 volts. Contact with a conductor has also caused electrical burns at potentials less than 6 volts. However, significant ocular injuries have not occurred at potentials of less than 200 volts.

The size of the burn has minimal relationship to the long-term outcome. Small skin burns may cause severe multisystem injury, involving the cardiovascular, central nervous, and musculoskeletal systems as well. Extensive tissue necrosis and vascular injury can also result from small entry wounds.

The most common ocular injury from electricity seems to be opacity of the crystalline lens, which often appears after current flow through the head with the input either at or near the eye.

The cataract formation is usually unilateral on the side proximal to the point of contact, but the contralateral eye may also be involved.

THERAPY

Supportive. Treatment for electrical burns includes relief of pain, strict asepsis and care of the wound, prevention or relief of shock, and control of infection. Analgesia is best provided by meperidine. The usual dose is 25 to 100 mg, which may be repeated every 3 to 4 hours as necessary. Some patients may need psychiatric support with tranquilizers.

Prophylactic treatment of a major burn wound should include an injection of 0.5 ml of absorbed tetanus toxoid to all patients who have not had a booster within the past year. In nonvaccinated subjects, immunization will be completed by two further injections at 4 to 6 weeks and then at 6 months.

Systemic. While dead tissue remains, bacterial activity is heightened, and while the wound remains open, bacterial invasion may occur. *Pseudomonas aeruginosa* and *Staphylococcus aureus* are the predominant organisms present in the majority of significant burn wound infections; streptococci and *Proteus* are less frequent. The administration of gentamicin is recommended for treatment or prevention of burn infections. The usual daily dosage is 3 mg/kg given intravenously or intramuscularly in three divided doses.

Ocular. If the burn wound is around the eye, exposure is the most practical, efficient, and effective means of yielding a cool, dry, and clean wound environment. A topical antibacterial ointment, such as gentamicin, should generally be applied after an initial gentle cleansing with a dilute solution of soap and normal saline, rinsing-irrigation of the burned surface with saline, and gentle drying with sterile cotton-free gauze pads or lint-free sterile towels. Such gentle washing is done two to three times a day. Crust formation may be anticipated in the superficial injury, and crust separation and spontaneous healing may be completed within 2 to 4 weeks after injury. Eschar development, accompanied later by curling, cracking, and separation with thick drainage, occurs in deep wounds. At this point, exposure may need to be abandoned, and daily surgical débridements, washing, and dressing procedures should be instituted. Every 4 hours, the sterile cotton-free gauze dressing with topical antibiotics is changed to maintain free drainage of infected material and promote eschar separation. This process is continued until satisfactory granulation tissue is achieved.

Depending on the severity of the electrical injury, an attack of anterior uveitis may develop. Anterior uveitis may be treated by an application of 1 or 2 per cent atropine one to four times daily. Early and constant pupillary dilation lessens the likelihood of synechiae. One drop of 0.1 per cent dexamethasone may be applied two to four times daily in severe uveitis.

Surgical. If a cataract develops, lens extraction may be necessary. The same operative procedures as for nontrumatic cataracts of particular age groups apply to electrical cataracts.

A split-thickness skin graft may be necessary for achieving burn wound closure of the eyelids. The transplanted skin provides the essential epithelial cover for the granulating surface from which no spontaneous re-epithelialization is possible.

Ocular or Periocular Manifestations

Choroid: Atrophy; rupture.
Cornea: Cicatrization; necrosis; perforation.
Eyelids: Blepharospasm; burns, necrosis.
Lens: Anterior or posterior subcapsular cataract; anterior or posterior subcapsular vacuoles.
Optic Nerve: Atrophy; optic neuritis.
Retina: Attenuated arteries; cysts; dilation of retinal veins; edema; exudates; hemorrhages; holes; pigmentary degeneration.
Other: Anterior uveitis; hyphema; hypotony; increased intraocular pressure; night blindness; nystagmus; paralysis of extraocular muscles; photophobia; visual field defects; visual loss.

Precautions

The best treatment for electrical injury to the eye is prevention; actual treatment is supportive and aimed at preventing infection and tissue loss. Surgical procedures are performed as indicated to restore the eye as nearly as possible to its original state.

Comments

Initial changes in the formation of electrical cataracts are multiple vacuoles beneath the anterior chamber. These vacuoles are replaced by anterior subcapsular streaks in an irregular pattern. Scale-like gray opacities may appear in the subcapsular layers of the extreme anterior cortex. Vesicles and amorphous opacities, as well as crystalline formations, may also appear in the posterior subcapsular area. Although the lens changes may appear to resolve, they are generally progressive. The onset of cataracts may be almost immediate or several years may elapse; average time of onset is 2 to 6 months after injury. If only a few vacuoles are present in the anterior lens cortex within the first few postinjury weeks, there is a high probability that no significant cataract requiring surgery will occur.

Part of the injury may be heat-related as much as true electrical damage. Retinal damage is more likely to be a thermal injury unless the exit point of the electrical injury indicated that the electrical current passed through the posterior segment of the eye.

References

Alexandridis A, et al: Electrophysiological and CT findings in a case of optic neuropathy caused by lightning. Klin Monatsbl Augenheilkd *190*:56–58, 1987.

Al Rabiah SM, et al: Electrical injury of the eye. Int Ophthalmol *11*:31–40, 1987.

Gans M, Glaser JS: Homonymous hemianopia following electrical injury. J Clin Neuro-Ophthalmol *6*:218–221, 1986.

Saffle JR, Crandall A, Warden GD: Cataracts: A long-term complication of electrical injury. J Trauma *25*:17–21, 1985.

Van Johnson E, Kline LB, Skalka HW: Electrical cataracts: A case report and review of the literature. Ophthalmic Surg *18*:283–285, 1987.

HYPOTHERMAL INJURY
(Cryoinjury, Frostbite)

DENNIS L. WINGFIELD, M.D.

North Little Rock, Arkansas

Loss of body heat occurs normally as the body's response to its environment through convection, conduction, radiation, respiratory water loss, and evaporation of perspiration. Local cold injury or frostbite is caused by freezing of tissue and resembles heat injury in pathologic and clinical effects. Initially, one can differentiate only between superficial and deep injury. After several days, the lesions may be categorized into four degrees of severity. First-degree injuries result in hyperemia with edema, mottling, cyanosis, and poor capillary refill. Second-degree frostbite injuries result in hyperemia with superficial vesicles, which form black eschars that eventually separate to reveal soft, easily traumatized, but intact skin. In third-degree frostbite, the entire thickness of the skin is involved, with extension into the subcutaneous tissue. Vesicles, when present, are frequently hemorrhagic and smaller than in second-degree frostbite. Edema is severe but slower to appear. Fourth-degree frostbite destroys the entire thickness of the extremity and usually proceeds to mummification and dry gangrene.

THERAPY

Supportive. The field management of freezing injury varies according to the severity of the injury and the availability of support after institution of treatment. For milder degrees of frostbite, simple rewarming of the affected part is sufficient. This can be accomplished by placing frostbitten hands in the axilla or putting other affected parts of the body on the exposed torso of a partner. For a more serious freezing injury, rewarming should be instituted if the part can be subsequently protected and adequate facilities are available. The affected part should be rapidly rewarmed at temperatures of 38° to 44° C, preferably by immersion in a whirlpool bath. Rewarming should be continued until tissue turgor returns to normal. After rewarming, the part should be dried carefully and rested on sterile sheets. Physiotherapy should always be instituted on a daily basis to facilitate débridement of ruptured blebs and help maintain a sterile wound.

Systemic. After thawing, analgesic drugs may be required for a period of 3 to 5 days, depending on the extent of injury. Antibiotics are not required in uncomplicated cases. The use of low-molecular weight dextran[‡] as an "anti-sludging" agent has shown some promise in clinical trials, although this agent is not presently approved for such use by the Food and Drug Administration. Other drugs directed at the prevention of platelet aggregation and capillary thrombosis, such as heparin and aspirin,[‡] have shown some beneficial effects.

Ocular. When mild frostbite is noted early on the lids or in the periocular area, simple measures, such as the application of warm (not hot) towels, should be sufficient. However, in severe cases in which tissue destruction has taken place, treatment is the same as that for severe frostbite in any area of the body. Areas of partial-thickness skin loss should be protected to prevent contamination and encourage epithelialization. Replacement of areas with total skin loss should be by grafting, when possible.

Ocular or Periocular Manifestations

Choroid or Retina: Atrophy; exudative posterior uveitis; hemorrhages; hyperpigmentation.

Conjunctiva or Cornea: Edema; endothelial damage; epithelial dysplasia; erosion; folds in Descemet's membrane; immune ring; neovascularization; subconjunctival hemorrhages.

Eyelids: Bullae; cicatrization; contracture deformity; depigmentation; discharge; ectropion; edema; hemorrhages; hyperemia; hypesthesia; madarosis; pseudoepitheliomatous hyperplasia.

Other: Anterior uveitis; iris atrophy; paresis of extraocular muscles.

PRECAUTIONS

Since hypothermal injury is usually preventable, counseling individuals on prophylactic measures is of utmost importance. Prophylaxis includes wearing adequate, loose-fitting, dry clothing and protective goggles, limiting exposure to cold to brief periods, and avoiding smoking.

The intent in cryosurgery is, however, to induce a therapeutic "frostbite" for beneficial purposes. Nevertheless care should be taken to prevent excessive freeze. All patients who have cryosurgery to the periorbital area can expect hyperemia, edema, bullae, eschar formation, and a serous or serosanguineous discharge. Counseling patients before cryosurgery on what to expect in the postoperative period and reassuring them that the problem usually lasts for approximately 2 weeks are most important. If proper techniques are followed, little care will be required with injuries secondary to cryosurgery.

Massage, high temperatures, and reactive hyperemia should be avoided in the rewarming of serious frostbite injuries, as these measures enhance tissue damage. Early débridement of vesicles, blebs, or eschar is to be avoided, since it frequently results in contracture and allows for secondary bacterial invasion. However, blebs should be observed closely for signs of secondary infection. Sympathectomy has been used in frostbite with varying success, but with no compelling evidence that the level of demarcation is changed.

Comments

Hypothermal injuries resemble burn injuries both clinically and pathologically, but their management is different. In most cases of hypothermal injury, little or no treatment is necessary, but therapy can prevent loss of viable tissue, especially in the more severe grades of frostbite. Clinical cases of frostbite of the eyes are rare because of the protection afforded by the richly vascular lids and the care usually taken to avoid injury to the eyes. However, severe injury may occur if blinking is diminished or the eyes remain open persistently. The eye may occasionally suffer superficial damages, such as corneal erosion, opacity, or ulceration, as a result of extended exposure.

References

Fraunfelder FT, et al: The role of cryosurgery in external ocular and periocular disease. Trans Am Acad Ophthalmol Otolaryngol 83:713–724, 1977.
Jarrett F: Frostbite: Current concepts of pathogenesis and treatment. Rev Surg 31:71–74, 1974.
Petersdorf RG: Disturbances of heat regulation. In Isselbacher KJ, et al (eds): Harrison's Principles of Internal Medicine, 9th ed. New York, McGraw-Hill, 1980, pp 53–60.
Wingfield DL, Fraunfelder FT: Possible complications secondary to cryotherapy. Ophthalmic Surg 10:47–55, 1979.
Zacarian SA (ed): Cryosurgical Advances in Dermatology and Tumors of the Head and Neck. Springfield, IL, Charles C Thomas, 1977.
Zagora E: Eye Injuries. Springfield, IL, Charles C Thomas, 1970, pp 415–417.

RADIATION
(Gamma Rays, Infrared Rays, Microwaves, Radiowaves, X-rays)

BUDD APPLETON, M.D.

St. Paul, Minnesota

The shortest wavelengths of electromagnetic radiation (gamma rays, x-rays, and short ultraviolet) possess very high photon energy (6 electron volts and greater). This level of energy is sufficient to cause ionization in biologic tissues; consequently, this range is referred to as ionizing radiation. Longer wavelengths containing less than 6 electron volts are referred to as nonionizing radiation; long ultraviolet, visible light, and short infrared energy (with photon energies between 3 and 6 electron volts) are capable of rupturing certain chemical bonds and are therefore described as being photobiologically active. The longest wavelengths (long infrared, microwaves, and radiowaves), having such low photon energies (1 electron volt and less), are capable only of causing molecular agitation (heating) and are therefore considered to have only thermal effects.

Strongly ionizing radiation (gamma rays and x-rays) is well known for its ability to cause human cataract. There is some evidence that the weakly ionizing short ultraviolet rays play at least a contributory role in that condition, but little is known about thresholds and variations in susceptibility to any of those radiation injuries. The same generalization can be made about the role of those energies in causing lid cancers. Ionizing radiation usually has a latent period for biologic effect and may cause a variety of lesions throughout the eye, depending upon the dose. Radiation retinopathy following therapeutic irradiation of paraorbital malignancies has been reported. Decreased or absent lacrimal secretion with consequent drying of the surface of the eye has also been described following irradiation, in addition to atrophy of the Meibomian glands.

Infrared radiation is capable of causing thermal burns. Radiation in this range has also been implicated in a specific type of cataract seen almost exclusively in glassblowers and other workers chronically exposed to these wavelengths. This so-called glassblower's cataract has been reported in individuals with lifelong exposure to extremely intense and prolonged levels of infrared radiation. The opacity starts in the posterior subcapsular region and is often accompanied by a splitting of the layers of the anterior capsule, called true exfoliation (as distinguished from the syndrome of pseudoexfoliation).

The question of "microwave cataract" has received much attention in recent years, especially in connection with allegations that human cataracts have resulted from microwave ovens and from radar. Although it is possible to cause cataracts experimentally in dogs and rabbits using microwave energy, these appear to be purely thermal effects. Thus far, attempts to cause similar cataracts in rhesus monkeys, which have a more effective thermal regulating mechanism, have been unsuccessful. As to human microwave cataract, there is no valid evidence that this condition exists, and all the evidence to date indicates that it does not.

Longer wavelengths, including those in the short and long wavelength radio bands, appear to pass through the human body without depositing any energy and therefore have never been seriously implicated as a cause of ocular injury. The even longer wavelengths associated with 60-cycle and lower frequency emanations seem to be similarly devoid of any human biologic effect. The effects of ultraviolet and visible lights are

324 / RADIATION

covered separately under the sections on ultraviolet radiation and solar retinopathy.

THERAPY

Supportive. The best form of therapy for ocular injuries from energies in the electromagnetic spectrum is prevention. Despite the theoretical value of substances that might protect the lens and skin enzyme systems from radiation damage, there is not yet available "an ionizing radiation protection pill" for this purpose. In the case of occupational exposure to infrared, the use of infrared-absorbing lenses has become an occupational requirement for individuals so exposed. Treatment of thermal burns from infrared radiation exposure is described in the following section on thermal burns.

Surgical. The only known treatment of radiation cataract is surgical removal of the opaque lens.

Ocular or Periocular Manifestations

Conjunctiva: Cicatrization; hyperemia; symblepharon.
Cornea: Epithelial loss; keratoconjunctivitis sicca; necrosis; opacity; punctate keratitis; ulcer; vascularization.
Eyebrows or Eyelids: Blepharitis; carcinoma (?); depigmentation; ectropion; entropion; madarosis; poliosis.
Iris or Ciliary Body: Anterior uveitis; ciliary spasm.
Lacrimal System: Atrophy of lacrimal gland.
Lens: Cataracts; true exfoliation of lens capsule.
Orbit: Necrosis.
Retina: Burns; exudates; hemorrhages; macular degeneration; macular holes; neovascularization; vascular occlusion.
Other: Secondary glaucoma.

PRECAUTIONS

Without any doubt, the lens of the eye is one of the most radiosensitive tissues and therefore can be damaged by relatively low doses of conventional radiation. Other parts of the eye may also become injured as a result of inadequate protection during radiotherapy or by direct exposure after irradiation for intraocular malignancy and for lesions located adjacent to the eye. To avoid such complications, eliminating or at least minimizing radiation exposure of the eyes is of decisive importance.

COMMENTS

Because many of the radiation cataracts are situated near the posterior pole of the lens, the opacity has a very damaging effect upon vision. Fortunately, since the ocular tissues are other-wise healthy, the postoperative results of cataract extraction are usually good.

References

Appleton B, et al: Microwave lens effects in humans. II. Results of five-year survey. Arch Ophthalmol 93:257–258, 1975.

Bagan SM, Hollenhorst RW: Radiation retinopathy after irradiation of intracranial lesions. Am J Ophthalmol 88:694–697, 1979.

Geeraets WJ: Radiation effects on the eye. Ind Med 39:441–450, 1970.

Karp LA, Streeten BW, Cogan DG: Radiation-induced atrophy of the Meibomian glands. Arch Ophthalmol 97:303–305, 1979.

Macfaul PA, Bedford MA: Ocular complications after therapeutic irradiation. Br J Ophthalmol 54:237–247, 1970.

THERMAL BURNS

ARDEN H. WANDER, M.D.
Cincinnati, Ohio

The thermally burned patient may present a difficult and challenging management problem for the ophthalmologist. Although many seriously burned individuals with large, total body burns may initially escape direct damage to the globe, complications from the overall injury can have a devastating effect on the ocular system. Many severely burned patients may well escape direct injury to the cornea and conjunctiva because of the Bell's phenomenon and protection from the eyelids. On the other hand, many do suffer direct corneal and conjunctival injuries that may be thermal in nature from the flame itself or from hot gases. Some corneal injuries may also be toxic in nature from the combustion of toxic chemicals that are released when synthetic materials burn. Finally, severe corneal and ocular injuries may occur if hot liquids or molten metal explode into the eye. These more severe, direct ocular injuries behave much like toxic alkaline burns, with resultant avascular necrosis in some cases and symblepharon formation as well. These more severe, direct ocular injuries are managed similarly to those of toxic chemical injuries.

THERAPY

Supportive. It is imperative to analyze the extent of the ocular injury itself and assess the patient's overall condition and degree of the total body burn. The ophthalmologist must assume that the patient will survive the injury no matter how severe it appears. Initial supportive therapy is directed at resuscitation. This includes the maintenance of the airway, management of shock, and replacement of fluids.

Systemic. Severely burned victims are susceptible to endogenous endophthalmitis from bacterial or fungal septicemia. Hence, the fundi should be checked periodically, especially if blood cultures for fungus or bacteria are positive. *Candida albicans* is a common invader of the bloodstream in such patients because they are often on hyperalimentation, have many open areas, and often are on broad-spectrum antibiotics. Early detection of intraocular infection with *Candida* helps facilitate treatment of the ocular infection, as well as the potential meningitis and encephalitis that may develop. If the funduscopic examination is not possible because of tarsorrhaphies, B-scan ultrasound can be performed periodically if blood cultures become positive. Mucormycosis may also occur in these patients, especially when acidosis is present. One should be alert to this possibility if orbital cellulitis or proptosis occurs. Cultures and biopsy should be performed to make this diagnosis so that systemic therapy with amphotericin B can be initiated.

Ocular. With respect to the ocular injury, the major goal of therapy is to promote the re-epithelialization of the corneal and conjunctival epithelium and then maintain its health and integrity. In order to accomplish this goal, initial examination is important to determine the state of each eye. The eyelids may be swollen shut initially, but may be examined with use of local anesthetics and Desmarres lid retractors, even when severe chemosis is present. The cornea should be evaluated with the application of fluorescein instilled into the conjunctival sac. Foreign bodies need to be removed. Gentle débridement of devitalized lid epithelium may be helpful. Assessment of the lid is very important because both ectropion and spastic entropion may occur. For spastic entropion, a soft bandage contact lens may be used to protect the cornea from the eyelashes until resolution of the edema and reassessment of the lid function are achieved. Thermal corneal and conjunctival burns may be pressure patched daily over antibiotic ointment until re-epithelialization is complete. If facial, brow, or eyelid burns are also present, pressure patching may not be possible. Bandage contact lenses may be used to promote epithelial healing in this situation. When the lids are swollen closed, the eye becomes in essence patched, which is helpful for a corneal burn that should be treated like a corneal abrasion.

First- and second-degree burns to the eyelids and face should be treated with a conservative approach with sterile wet compresses and antibiotic ointment. Third-degree burns to the eyelids will lead to cicatricial contractures of the lids and cicatricial ectropion. These conditions result in exposure keratitis, which by itself can lead to scarring of the cornea, as well as serious corneal infection. Such contractures are best treated with skin grafting after relaxing incisions are made to replace the lost tissue. In large severe burns, split-thickness grafting is recommended for this purpose.

If the total body burn is more than 50 to 60 percent and mostly third degree, there may not be enough normal skin to allow initial eyelid skin grafting, since the burned area must be replaced with skin from the unburned areas. In such cases, a large, almost total tarsorrhaphy should be performed early, allowing healing time before the onset of contractures. It is wise to leave an opening of several millimeters at the medial aspect of each eye for examination and to allow cross-fixation for children who may be in the amblyopic age group. If contractures have already developed before tarsorrhaphy, sufficient relaxing incisions in the contracted tissue will allow the eyelid margins to come together without traction so that tarsorrhaphy may be performed successfully. Split-thickness skin grafts can be put into the tarsal bed thus created. If not enough skin is available from the patient to perform this lid grafting, time may be bought to allow the tarsorrhaphy to heal by placing either donor skin or pigskin into the tarsorrhaphy defect. Later, during the reconstructive phase of therapy, the tarsorrhaphies may be released as the eyelids are rebuilt. It must be emphasized that although the corneas may not be injured initially, serious third-degree burns of the face and eyelids in the presence of a large, total body burn can lead to severe cicatricial contractures and ectropion. Exposure keratitis can ensue if tarsorrhaphy is not performed. *Pseudomonas* or other bacteria, as well as fungus, on many of the burned areas may find their way to the exposed cornea and cause serious corneal infection. This infection may be prevented by the use of aggressive early tarsorrhaphies. Prophylactic antibiotics do not always prevent corneal infections in such a case. This is especially true when the patient is upside down on a rotating bed, when minimal therapy can be given to the eyes. A good tarsorrhaphy will protect the corneas during this phase of the therapy in a severely burned patient.

During the initial assessment of the injury, associated ocular injuries, such as corneal lacerations and intraocular foreign bodies, must also be assessed and treated. This is especially true in explosive-type injuries.

For severe conjunctival burns caused by exploding liquids or molten metal, severe necrosis of the conjunctiva may occur. Local mucosal grafts may be applied in such cases, and the use of symblepharon rings may also help prevent symblepharon. These cases are similar to severe chemical burns, and the articles on acid burns and alkaline burns will provide further information on management of such injuries.

Ocular or Periocular Manifestations

Conjunctiva: Avascular necrosis; chemosis; symblepharon.
Cornea: Avascular necrosis; cicatrization; exposure keratitis (secondary to ectropion); infection; lacerations and foreign bodies; ulcer (secondary to infection).
Eyelids: Avascular necrosis; cicatricial ectro-

pion; contracture deformity; edema; spastic entropion.

Globe: Endophthalmitis; intraocular foreign bodies; proptosis.

Lacrimal System: Chronic epiphora; dacryocystitis; occlusion of the puncta.

Orbit: Cellulitis.

PRECAUTIONS

Scar tissue that may result from the burned cornea will not be prevented by corticosteroids. Furthermore, corticosteroids may delay the re-epithelization and increase the chance of secondary infection.

COMMENTS

In large, total body burns, the acute phase of the injuries requires frequent operations for débridement, as well as skin grafting. Until these patients are totally covered with skin, they are susceptible to infections both systemically and topically. The patients need very frequent follow-up care subsequent to the application of large tarsorrhaphies. Once tarsorrhaphies are healed, examinations may be less frequent, provided the blood cultures remain negative and signs of orbital cellulitis do not occur. When the entire burned area is covered, the reconstructive phase of therapy can begin. When reconstruction of the eyelids with skin grafting is successful, tarsorrhaphies may be released. Significant corneal complications, such as *Pseudomonas* corneal ulcers, may be prevented by tarsorrhaphies; this technique is preferable to treating such an infection, especially in combination with lid retraction and exposure keratitis. For this reason, the need for adequate and early tarsorrhaphies to protect the corneas in the severely burned patient cannot be overemphasized.

References

Asch MJ, et al: Ocular complications associated with burns: Review of a five-year experience including 104 patients. J Trauma 11:857–861, 1971.

Bloom SM, Gittinger JW Jr, Kazarian EL: Management of corneal contact thermal burns. Am J Ophthalmol 102:536, 1986.

Deutsch TA, Feller DB: Paton and Goldberg's Management of Ocular Injuries, 2nd ed. Philadelphia, WB Saunders, 1985, pp. 99–103.

Duke-Elder S (ed): System of Ophthalmology. St. Louis, CV Mosby, 1972, Vol XIV, pp 747–774.

Guy RJ, et al: Three-years' experience in a regional burn center with burns of the eyes and eyelids. Ophthalmic Surg 13:383–386, 1982.

Huang TT, Blackwell SJ, Lewis SR: Burn injuries of the eyelids. Clin Plast Surg 5:571–581, 1978.

Kaufman HE, Thomas EL: Prevention and treatment of symblepharon. Am J Ophthalmol 88:419–423, 1979.

Silver B, et al: Ophthalmic plastic surgery. Am Acad Ophthalmol Otolaryngol Manual, 3rd ed, 1977, pp 116–123.

Zagora E: Eye Injuries. Springfield, IL, Charles C Thomas, 1970.

Foreign Body

INTRAOCULAR FOREIGN BODY—COPPER*
(Chalcosis)

FLEMING D. WERTZ, M.D.,
and THOM S. THOMASSEN, M.D.
Washington, District of Columbia

The incidence of copper-containing intraocular foreign bodies has risen as a result of the increased use of nonmagnetic metal in industries, warfare, and recreation. The presence of an intraocular copper-containing foreign body can lead to suppurative endophthalmitis, recurrent nongranulomatous inflammation, fibrous encapsulation, and dissemination of copper throughout the intraocular structures. The inflammatory response may be acute and suppurative or more chronic and less intense. Either the intensity or the chronicity of the inflammation can cause disorganization and atrophy of the ocular structures, resulting in phthisis. However, not all eyes develop inflammation as a sequela of a copper intraocular foreign body. In those that do not develop inflammation, copper ions may be disseminated throughout the eye, particularly in the limiting membranes of the eye. The deposition of copper produces the clinical picture of chalcosis.

The influence of copper ion in the eye may be extensive. Copper ion participates in two basic processes. The first is a result of copper's tendency to be a reagent for and catalyst of oxidation-reduction reactions. Copper, which has a relatively low Redox potential, has the tendency to remove electrons from appropriate organic donors. An example of this is the oxidation of ascorbic acid by cuprous ion to produce hydrogen peroxide. In addition, copper participates in superoxide and hydrogen peroxide chemistry, resulting in the formation of superoxide and hydroxyl radicals. These attack polyunsaturated fatty acids, resulting in lipid peroxidation and the formation of alkoxy and peroxy radicals. This reaction may simultaneously lead to 1) the initiation of arachidonic acid metabolism that produces prostaglandins and leucotrienes resulting in inflammation, and 2) the incapacitation and

---

* The opinions contained herein are the private views of the authors and are not to be construed as official or as reflecting the views of the Department of the Army or the Department of Defense.

death of cells resulting from the radicals' attack on lipid-containing membranes. The second process involves the complexing of critical enzymes with copper ion, which either displaces key molecules or distorts their stereo configuration, rendering them unable to participate in intracellular metabolism. An example of this process is copper's ability to inactivate carbonic anhydrase, producing a persistent reduction in ocular pressure as long as the copper ion is present.

Patients who retain small copper intraocular foreign bodies and do not have recurrent intraocular inflammation may have a relatively benign course. Several benign functional effects may be noted. These sequelae need not be permanent, as removal of the foreign body will be followed by clearing of copper from the ocular structures.

THERAPY

Ocular. The need to administer ocular therapy depends on the purity of the copper foreign body, its location in the eye, its size and shape, and the associated ocular damage. Alloyed copper foreign bodies in which the copper content is less than 85 per cent do not incite as severe an intraocular inflammatory response as those containing more than 85 per cent copper. The location of the foreign body is critical. If placed in the anterior midvitreous where the oxygen tension is low, it may not incite an inflammatory response. As the location moves progressively toward the ocular coat, the probability of a severe inflammatory response increases. Those foreign bodies adjacent to or in contact with the anterior or posterior segment structures induce an inflammatory or encapsulating fibrotic response in nearly all cases. Finally, the associated ocular damage may well direct the initial therapy. Eyes in which the anterior and posterior segments are disrupted require repair. Lensectomy and vitrectomy, as well as closure of a primary wound, may be required in addition to removal of the foreign body. However, if there is little in the way of ocular damage, the therapy may be directed solely at the presence of inflammation. As in the management of any trauma case, precautions are required to prevent endophthalmitis. These may range from cultures of the ocular fluids to the application of intraocular, periocular, and systemic antibiotics.

After primary repair, therapy should be directed at the copper-induced intraocular inflammation. Small visible shiny foreign bodies in the midvitreous may not induce an inflammatory response; therefore, these cases need not be treated. Systemic steroids, such as prednisone in the range of 60 to 100 mg per day, will suppress the general inflammatory response and inhibit migration of polymorphonuclear leukocytes. Periocular steroids have been shown to be effective in suppressing intraocular inflammation in general. Specifically, periocular injection of dexamethasone* has been shown to retard both inflammation and encapsulation.

Surgical. The therapeutic plan should be flexible. First, the steps necessary to ensure the short-term retention of the eye should be undertaken. Open wounds should be closed, and mixtures of lens, hemorrhage, and vitreous should be removed as the situation dictates. Depending on the location, size, and shape of the foreign body, it may be immediately removed. Further surgical procedures should be directed at repair of ocular damage (cataract, retinal detachment) or removal of the foreign body if serious sequelae follow. Accurate localization of the intraocular foreign body is now possible using the Berman locator, ultrasound devices, computed tomography, and x-ray localization techniques. After the appropriate preoperative maneuvers, bimanual vitrectomy techniques with modern instrumentation can be utilized to remove most intraocular foreign bodies safely.

Subsequent surgical intervention is undertaken if the surgeon judges that the foreign body is inciting a severe inflammatory response that if left unchecked could produce ocular destruction or the foreign body is producing functional impairment (decreased visual acuity, visual field changes, electrophysiologic changes) from the dissemination of copper within the ocular structure. If the foreign body is small and located in the midvitreous with little concomitant ocular damage, serial observation every 3 to 6 months with measurement of the visual acuity, color vision, intraocular pressure, visual field, and ERG may be all that is required. If there is intraocular dissemination of copper or the foreign body is inciting destructive or recurrent inflammation or is adjacent to the ocular coat, the foreign body should be removed by employing modern surgical techniques.

In those patients who are followed, the foreign body should be watched closely for corrosion or tarnishing of the surface and migration of the foreign body. One may be able to predict whether copper is being deposited in the eye from the appearance of the foreign body. Corrosion or tarnishing of its surface has been associated with an increased aqueous copper level and heavy generalized deposition of intraocular copper. In those eyes that harbor an encapsulated foreign body, softening of the capsule and migration or release of the foreign body from the capsule must be watched for and subsequent action taken.

Supportive. Either therapeutic plan—observation or surgery—may be associated with complications, and the patient should be counseled accordingly. The patient who is observed should be made aware that the potential exists for subsequent cataract, hypotony, uveitis, decreased visual function, and migration of the foreign body with subsequent acute inflammation or copper deposition. If the patient undergoes surgery, the procedure and its complications of cataract, aphakia, retinal breaks, retinal detachment, intraocular hemorrhage, and infection should be carefully explained. The patient should be made to feel like an integral part of the managing team, and that ultimately, the decision for enactment of any plan will rest with him or her.

Systemic. Experimental long-term penicillamine‡ has been reported to be of some benefit in reducing the amount of copper deposited intraocularly. If treatment is undertaken, serum and urinary copper levels, renal function tests, and ceruloplasmin levels should be carefully monitored.

Ocular or Periocular Manifestations

Anterior Chamber: Cells and flare/hypopyon; hyphema; multitude of floating metallic particles.

Cornea: Deep stromal deposits; Kayser-Fleischer ring (usually superior and/or inferior but may be circumferential).

Globe: Endophthalmitis; phthisis bulbi.

Iris: Greenish tinge; poor response to mydriatics.

Lens: Brownish-red, small, round deposits on zonules; displacement; sunflower cataract; yellowish opacity (with intraocular lenticular copper foreign body).

Optic Nerve: Papillitis.

Retina: Copper-colored macular sheen; detachment; edema; gliosis; "gold-leaf" granular deposits in macula or adjacent vessels in the posterior pole; hemorrhages.

Sclera: Abscess; softening.

Vitreous: Abscess; fibrillar degeneration; greenish-brown or reddish-brown deposits; opacity; organization.

Other: Decreased visual acuity; encapsulation of foreign body with possible simulation of growing intraocular tumor with or without evidence of chalcosis; nonspecific color vision defect; ocular hypotension (secondary to possible carbonic anhydrase inhibition from metallosis); secondary glaucoma; subconjunctival foreign body from intraocular extrusion (rare); sympathetic ophthalmia (rare); variable disturbance in ERG amplitude; variable elevation in dark adaptometry rod and cone thresholds; variable isopter constriction in visual field testing.

Precautions

Those foreign bodies containing a high percentage of copper (usually greater than 85 per cent) often cause a severe suppurative response leading to phthisis bulbi, unless surgical intervention is performed swiftly. Less pure copper-containing foreign bodies can cause severe retinal toxicity if located near the wall of the eye, or they may become encapsulated and cease to be toxic. Encapsulated foreign bodies may migrate and produce a suppurative reaction long after the original injury. A pure or alloy copper foreign body may remain free of inflammation for an indefinite period if located anteriorly in the midvitreous. In such cases, a conservative policy of observation for macular changes and vitreous opacification is probably justified before attempting the difficult surgical removal of a nonmagnetic foreign body, with the possibility of eventual loss of vision as a direct result of the surgical maneuver. Even after the foreign body has been extracted, an intensification of the chalcosis may occur due to dissemination from microfragmentation of the particle. Use of penicillamine‡ has yielded equivocal results, and if used, the patient must be observed for possible serious hematologic and renal adverse reactions. In diagnostic dilemmas, the presence of abnormal amounts of intraocular copper can be determined by diagnostic x-ray spectrometry, which may also prove advantageous over conventional electrophysiologic tests in the early detection of chalcosis.

Comments

The clinical course of chalcosis can be highly variable, being dependent on the copper content, as well as the location of the foreign body. Increased use of alloys as opposed to the pure form may make the chronic form of chalcosis more common in the future. In chronic chalcosis, inevitable blindness, as is the rule in siderosis, tends not to occur, owing to the fact that deposition of copper in the eye is primarily extracellular. However, the tendency is for gradual diminution of vision and for the clinical picture of chalcosis to occur over a period of months or years. Recent advances in surgical technique have made the removal of such foreign bodies less hazardous than in the past. Nonetheless, surgical removal of these nonmagnetic foreign bodies is difficult and potentially fraught with serious complications and is best left to surgeons experienced in the latest technique of their removal.

References

Gorodetsky R, et al: Noninvasive copper measurement in chalcosis. Comparison with electroretinography and ophthalmoscopy. Arch Ophthalmol 95:1059–1064, 1977.

McGahan MC, Bito LZ, Myers BM: The pathophysiology of the ocular microenvironment. II. Copper-induced ocular inflammation and hypotony. Exp Eye Res *42*:595–605, 1986.

Mittag T: Role of oxygen radicals in ocular inflammation and cellular damage. Exp Eye Res *39*:759–769, 1984.

Neubauer H: The Montgomery Lecture, 1979. Ocular metallosis. Trans Ophthal Soc UK *99*:502–510, 1979.

Paton D, Goldberg MF: Management of Ocular Injuries. Philadelphia, WB Saunders, 1976, pp 134–137.

Peyman GA, Schulman JA: Intravitreal Surgery Principles and Practice. New York, Appleton-Century-Crofts, 1986, pp 239–278.

Rosenthal AR, Eckhert C: Copper and zinc in ophthalmology. *In* Karcioglu ZA, Sarper RM (eds): Zinc and Copper in Medicine. Springfield, IL, Charles C Thomas, 1980, pp 595–609.

Rosenthal AR, et al: Chalcosis: A study of natural history. Ophthalmology *86*:1956–1969, 1979.

Soyeux, A.: Traitement de corps étrangers intraoculaires cuivriques par la D.-pénicillamine (dans deux cas avec 1 et 2 ans ½de recul). Bull Soc Ophthalmol Fr *80*:727–729, 1980.

Zeimer R, et al: Experimental chalcosis. A comparison between in vivo and in vitro findings. Arch Ophthalmol 96:115–119, 1978.

INTRAOCULAR FOREIGN BODY—NONMAGNETIC CHEMICALLY INERT

WILLIAM H. HAVENER, M.D.
Columbus, Ohio

A variable degree of uncertainty accompanies all intraocular foreign bodies. Inferences as to their nature are usually made from the circumstances of the accident. Such substances as stone, coal, lead, glass, silicone, and polymethyl methacrylate are generally nonreactive and nontoxic. Chemical nonreactivity is the common denominator of such substances. For practical purposes, most items that would be relatively undamaged by lying exposed to the weather for 5 years will not be toxic or reactive within the eye. Such materials include porcelain, silver, platinum, aluminum, stainless steel, tantalum, pottery fragments, and the like.

Inasmuch as the title of chemically inert foreign body excludes toxic manifestations, the manifestations of such injury will be purely mechanical, such as hemorrhage or cataract, or due to secondary infection. Significant, persistent, or newly developing signs or symptoms other than would be expected from the mechanical injury itself must be suspected as evidence of possible intolerance of the foreign body or development of infection. Exceptions to this are the well recognized late manifestations of injury itself. Late corneal decompensation, progressive corneal opacification, or even band keratopathy may follow injury. Traumatic iritis is common after a contusion, even if there has been no perforating wound. Delay in cataract formation is the typical course of a small injury to the lens. Contraction of vitreous bands may cause vitreous hemorrhage, retinal tears, and retinal detachment many years after a penetrating injury.

THERAPY

Supportive. Careful use of the usual clinical methods of biomicroscopy, ophthalmoscopy, gonioscopy, a metal detector, x-rays, or computed tomography will provide the information necessary for identification of the location of a foreign body and the damage resulting from its trajectory. If the foreign body can be visualized, simple inspection is one of the best methods of evaluation. The careful approach of a magnet to an eye as the foreign body is observed helps determine its magnetic properties. The density and configuration of the x-ray picture of a foreign body are helpful. Metallic density is unique, differentiating such materials from stone, glass, or plastic.

Continuing observation of the tolerance of the eye for a presumably inert foreign body is an essential part of the evaluation of such a case. For example, a small piece of brass from a dynamite cap may be perfectly tolerated for many years. On the other hand, a supposedly inert glass splinter may be toxic.

Without question, many perforated eyes will not develop infection even if no antibiotic therapy is instituted. Unfortunately, once a frank intraocular infection has developed, substantial scarring or even complete loss of the eye is the rule. Therefore, immediate and vigorous systemic antibiotic therapy as soon as possible is recommended for every case of penetrating ocular injury. Careful and close observation may be a reasonable alternative, but this observation must be as frequent as every 8 hours or less if the earliest stages of infection are to be recognized in time for effective treatment.

The selection and dosage of antibiotic must be arbitrarily chosen, unless a positive culture from the laceration is obtained at the time of surgery. Chloramphenicol should be considered because of its differential solubility characteristics and wide-spectrum effectiveness.

The status of tetanus immunization should be ascertained and appropriate booster or primary immunization given, as with any penetrating wound.

Surgical. In most cases, the surgical procedure required to remove a small, nonmagnetic, chemically inert foreign body from within the eye is considerably more hazardous and destructive than the continuing presence of the inert particle. By definition, if the intraocular foreign body is chemically inert, it does not in itself justify any surgery, except closure of the penetrating wound (if it is not spontaneously self-closing). This is not to deny the incidental removal of a foreign body if it is reasonably accessible to grasping with a forceps during repair of the laceration.

Optical consideration may require removal of a large foreign body suspended in the axial vitreous. Nonmagnetic particles imbedded in the retina or choroid or very near these layers can easily be removed through an incision made precisely at the location of the foreign body. In the instance of a foreign body at or anterior to the equator, such an approach may be less damaging than a transvitreal approach. Similarly, an intralenticular foreign body should be removed at the time of a cataract extraction.

Secondary problems may require surgery. Corneal edema resulting from endothelial irritation may indicate the removal of a glass splinter from the inferior chamber angle, or retinal detachment surgery may be required if the particle has sufficiently damaged the vitreous and retina.

Ocular. Cycloplegic therapy is advised, as indicated by the presence and severity of accompanying traumatic iridocyclitis.

There is an unfortunate tendency to equate a red eye (from almost any cause) to a need for corticosteroid therapy. This is to be deplored. Very little, if any, evidence indicates that any eye with a small penetrating wound will heal significantly better with corticosteroid therapy than without. One of the most certain of all clinical facts is that immunologic incompetence is a consequence of corticosteroid therapy. Corticosteroid treatment of an injured eye enhances the probability that it will succumb to whatever fungus, virus, bacterium, or coccus has been introduced by the injury.

PRECAUTIONS

The tentative diagnosis of inert foreign body should be recognized as being subject to revision. A false sense of security may be induced by such a diagnosis, and one may neglect a proper follow-up. Until the test of time has shown that an unexplained loss of visual acuity or other problem has not occurred, the diagnosis of inertness is an unproved assumption and must be treated as such. Such cases should be followed at regular intervals for a considerable time, at least several years or more if significant intraocular structural injury has been sustained.

Dangerous materials may be misclassified as inert. Many varieties of thorns contain toxins that elicit a severe intraocular response. Wood splinters and other hard plant fragments are not generally well tolerated. Chemical additives may cause some types of plastic material to be toxic.

One should be persistently suspicious of the presence of an intraocular foreign body in any type of injury. Small and radiolucent particles are especially difficult to detect. Re-evaluation of the status of an injured eye may be necessary if its course of recovery is not as prompt and uneventful as expected. The most distressing cases are those in which an apparently minor injury of no real significance finally results in an eye blinded by siderosis bulbi or endophthalmitis.

COMMENTS

In theory, the management of an intraocular nonmagnetic chemically inert foreign body can be described in two words: do nothing. In practice, a considerable amount of judgment is required. The most difficult decision is whether the foreign body under consideration is inert or toxic. A well-tolerated small inert intraocular foreign body does not require surgery and should be left alone. The strong temptation to cut just because it is there should be resisted.

References

Duke-Elder S (ed): System of Ophthalmology. St. Louis, CV Mosby, 1972, Vol XIV, pp 459–460, 500–508.

Havener WH: Ocular Pharmacology, 5th ed. St. Louis, CV Mosby, 1983.

Havener WH, Gloeckner SL: Atlas of Diagnostic Techniques and Treatment of Intraocular Foreign Bodies. St. Louis, CV Mosby, 1969, pp 168–175.

Neubauer H: Intraocular foreign bodies. Trans Ophthalmol Soc UK 95:496–501, 1975.

INTRAOCULAR FOREIGN BODY—STEEL OR IRON
(Siderosis)

PHILIP P. ELLIS, M.D.
Denver, Colorado

An intraocular iron or steel foreign body usually does not produce an immediate violent reaction, apart from mechanical trauma. As with all other deep perforating injuries, intraocular hemorrhage and inflammation may occur, leading to fibrous proliferation. The after effects of retained iron foreign bodies are usually serious and consist of a delayed chronic degenerative process, which may result in blindness. Siderosis is produced by oxidation and absorption of iron or steel with distribution of ferric ions throughout the eye, including the cornea, trabeculum, suprachoroidal space, iris epithelium, ciliary body, lens epithelium, and retina. The severity of ocular siderosis varies with the size and chemical composition of the particle, as well as its position in the eye. The locations in which the most severe reactions develop are the ciliary body and the posterior segment when encapsulation has not developed. A better prognosis follows lodgement in the anterior chamber, and the best prognosis occurs when the particle is deposited within the substance of the lens. Intracellular deposits can develop in the cornea, causing brown or rust-colored rings; brownish-yellow spots may develop in the lens, usually resulting in a total cataract. Retinal degeneration is the most serious consequence and may initially include a pigmentary degeneration. Retinal detachment is a common sequela. A marked concentric contraction of the visual fields and night blindness are prominent symptoms. In the later stages, complete amaurosis may gradually develop. Secondary glaucoma is common in the absence of irritative or inflammatory episodes.

THERAPY

Surgical. Removal of an iron or steel foreign body as soon as possible is the best treatment if the foreign body is accessible. With modern surgical techniques, most foreign bodies can be removed satisfactorily. However, if removal is going to compromise vision seriously, the foreign body may be left. Deterioration of the eye is not inevitable, as encapsulation may prevent the diffusion of toxic substances. Steel and iron are magnetic, and removal of the intraocular foreign body can be accomplished with magnetic extraction or the use of vitrectomy instruments. The method of removal depends on the location, the duration of foreign body retention, and the degree of inflammatory reaction.

If the foreign body is in the anterior chamber or lens, extraction should be through a limbal incision. Siderosis is unlikely with a steel or iron foreign body in the lens; cataract formation may not occur, especially if the lenticular perforation is less than 2 mm. Small or medium-sized foreign bodies may be removed along the site of entry.

If the foreign body is lodged in the vitreous, pars plana vitrectomy and removal of the foreign body under direct visualization with the use of currently available fine intravitreal instruments increasingly are becoming the surgical procedures of choice. A fine probe, containing a rare earth magnet, may be inserted intraocularly to remove the foreign body, or the foreign body may be grasped with fine forceps. Intravitreal foreign body extraction with an electromagnet applied on the surface of a pars plana incision, with or without a preceding vitrectomy, is an approach preferred by many surgeons. If not performed initially, a secondary vitrectomy may be required later to treat vitreous hemorrhage, which can serve as a scaffold for fibrous proliferation. With either surgical approach, extraction of the foreign body and repair of the wound should be performed immediately. Magnetic extraction through the anterior route may be performed if the lens is damaged, or alternatively, the lens can be removed through a pars plana vitrectomy approach, followed by foreign body extraction. However, unless damage to the lens is severe, it is usually best not to remove a traumatized lens at the time of foreign body extraction. In some patients with large posterior foreign bodies that cannot be removed through the pars plana wound, extraction through a limbal wound may be advantageous after lens removal and vitrectomy have been performed.

If the foreign body is in one of the coats of the eye, it is extracted across sclera through an incision directly over the foreign body. Prophylactic cryotherapy or diathermy to prevent retinal detachment may be desirable.

Double perforation is rare, and a second site of impact may be present on the retina with the foreign body in a pool of blood inferiorly. All eyes should be examined carefully for retinal breaks, which should be treated either primarily or during secondary surgical procedures.

When steel is in the orbit, it usually elicits no symptoms. Treatment is conservative, unless there are severe inflammatory signs, compression effects with pseudotumor, or a communication with a paranasal sinus or intracranial space.

If there is no hope for sight and the globe has been severely traumatized, enucleation should be considered to prevent sympathetic ophthalmia.

Systemic. Deferoxamine is used in the treatment of many iron storage diseases. It combines with iron to form a stable chelate that prevents the iron from entering into further chemical reactions. The chelate is readily soluble in water and excreted in the urine. It can help prevent siderosis, but does not reverse the existing process. The usual dose is 1 gm given intramuscularly, followed by 500 mg every 4 hours for two doses.

Ocular. Topical ophthalmic deferoxamine may be used in the treatment of siderosis involving the cornea. For the treatment of superficial iron deposits in the cornea, a 10 per cent solution of deferoxamine* in 1 per cent methylcellulose is applied topically four times a day for several weeks. Alternatively, the drug may be applied in a 5 per cent concentration in any ointment base. For iron deposits in the deeper layers of the cornea or the iris and lens, 0.5 ml of a 10 per cent solution is injected subconjunctivally* twice a week for 8 to 10 weeks.

Although it is uncommon for these intraocular foreign bodies to cause infections, antibiotic chemoprophylaxis is recommended. Atropine is also recommended to minimize iritis.

Ocular or Periocular Manifestations

Anterior Chamber: Cells and flare; hypopyon.
Conjunctiva: Rusty discoloration; subconjunctival hemorrhages.
Cornea: Edema; Fleischer's ring; Hudson-Stähli line; interstitial keratitis; neovascularization; opacity.
Iris: Iridoplegia; rusty discoloration; synechiae; uveitis.
Lens: Brown discoloration; cataract; luxation or subluxation.
Retina: Detachment; macular edema; pigmentary degeneration; rusty discoloration; sclerosis.
Other: Dyschromatopsia; night blindness; phthisis bulbi; secondary glaucoma; syneresis; visual loss.

PRECAUTIONS

It is imperative that therapy be instituted as soon as possible. Although siderotic deposits may clear after the intraocular foreign body is removed or has become encapsulated, surgery seldom helps once siderosis has become fully established. Late surgery may even accelerate the onset of phthisis bulbi. Small particles absorbed into the ocular structures may oxidize to nonmagnetic particles of rust, which cannot be localized or extracted.

Objects penetrating the eye may passively carry along not only bacteria and fungi but also additional foreign bodies, such as particles of bone or eyelashes. Organic foreign bodies are most likely to produce a considerable inflammatory reaction. In every case, infection must be considered a potential occurrence. Prophylactic and therapeutic measures should be administered preoperatively and postoperatively for the control of severe inflammation.

Deferoxamine is contraindicated in patients with severe renal disease and should probably not be administered to women in early pregnancy because of possible teratogenic effects. Long-term use of deteroxamine for treatment of iron storage diseases has been linked with the development of retrobulbar neuritis. The visual loss is usually reversible after the medication is discontinued.

ORBITAL IMPLANT EXTRUSION

MARK R. LEVINE, M.D.
Cleveland, Ohio

Loss of an eye from enucleation is emotionally traumatic. Subsequent extrusion of the orbital implant complicates the problem even more. Extrusions may occur early or many years after the initial implant. The causes of early extrusions are edema, infection, hemorrhage, too large an implant, and faulty surgical technique. Late extrusion occurs because of erosion of tissue covering the anterior surface of the implant from friction by a rough prosthesis. This erosion causes either a secondary infection and extrusion, or epithelialization of the cavity around the implant and contraction of the orbital tissues that lead to extrusion. A secondary implant is always desirable to maintain orbital volume, minimize supratarsal sulcus deformity, promote motility, and maximize cosmetic acceptability.

THERAPY

Surgical. For implant replacement after complete extrusion, the method of choice is immediate replacement with patching, unless the socket is infected. If the socket is infected, it is packed with antibiotic-impregnated gauze, which is replaced until the socket infection has been resolved, which may take 7 to 10 days. The conjunctiva is dissected from the rest of the orbital contents, taking care not to injure the superior or inferior rectus muscles. A cavity may be present within the muscle cone if the extrusion occurred within 2 to 3 weeks of the implant; however, the extraocular muscles and Tenon's capsule will usually have retracted into a small fibrotic mass. A cavity is created in this mass by sharp dissection only in the oblique meridian to avoid severing the rectus muscle, which may or may not be visualized. Excision of scar tissue posteriorly or posterior dissection is carried out until Tenon's capsule and the muscles can stretch easily over the implant. For the patch itself, autogenous fascia lata femoris taken from the lateral thigh is wrapped around a 14- to 16-mm spherical implant and sutured together with 4-0 Vicryl. This adds 2 mm more to the 14- or 16-mm implant. Sutures of 4-0 double-armed Vicryl are placed in each of four quadrants of the fascia-enveloped sphere. The implant is placed in the socket, and the sutures are brought out from each socket quadrant between the rectus muscle and fixed externally. Doing so helps position the implant. Tenon's capsule posterior to the recti is sutured over the fascial ball with interrupted 5-0 Vicryl, taking bites of the fascia lata, creating a barrier, and centrally fixing the implant. The recti are gently approximated with 5-0 Vicryl suture, and the anterior Tenon's capsule is closed with 6-0 Vicryl suture. The conjunctiva is closed with a continuous 6-0 chromic catgut suture. A con-

COMMENTS

Topical ophthalmic administration of deferoxamine does not penetrate the eye in sufficient concentrations to do much good. Subconjunctival administration of the drug has been used in experimental animals and has prevented the development of siderosis when iron was implanted into the vitreous. Systemic deferoxamine has been reported to improve discoloration and glaucoma associated with siderosis. There is some doubt whether it can prevent electroretinogram changes, although there was one clinical report that it did. Iron usually enters the eye in the metallic nonoxidized form. It is then oxidized through the ferrous state and is usually present in the eye in the ferric state. Ferrous iron is the most toxic to the eye. Deferoxamine has a strong affinity for the ferric form and removes the ferrous form at a slower rate.

In industry, most of the foreign bodies that enter the eye are particles from highly tempered steel tools. These particles strike the eye with great force, accounting for the fact that 85 percent of iron-containing ocular foreign bodies are found in the posterior segment of the globe. Siderosis is not inevitable if the steel is retained. Different types of steel are not equally destructive, owing to lower ferrous contents. However, the difficulty of extraction is greater with particles containing less iron, owing to a diminution of magnetic properties.

Occasionally, steel fragments remain in the posterior segment of the eye for months without the patients being aware of their presence until impaired vision forces them to seek medical advice. In other cases, encapsulated intraocular metallic foreign bodies that have long remained dormant may shift location and cause inflammatory reaction, resulting in hypopyon, plastic endophthalmitis, and atrophy of the globe.

References

Appel I, Barishak YR: Histopathological changes in siderosis bulbi. Ophthalmologica 176:205-210, 1978.

Benson WE: Intraocular foreign bodies. *In* Duane TD (ed): Clinical Ophthalmology. Hagerstown, MD, Harper & Row, 1984, Vol V, pp 15:1-15.

Deutsch TA, Feller DB: Paton and Goldberg's Management of Ocular Injuries, 2nd ed. Philadelphia, WB Saunders, 1985, pp 75-84.

Ellis PP: Ocular Therapeutics and Pharmacology, 7th ed. St. Louis, CV Mosby, 1985, p 247.

Gardner HB: Deferoxamine: Effects on intravitreal iron. Exp Eye Res 23:333-339, 1976.

Michels RG: Vitrectomy methods in penetrating ocular trauma. Ophthalmology 87:629-645, 1980.

Spoor TC, Nesi FA (eds): Management of Ocular Orbital and Adnexal Trauma. New York, Raven, 1988, pp 113-127.

former is then inserted. Two 4-0 silk suture tarsorrhaphies are performed. A pressure patch is then applied, which is not removed for 5 days.

An alternate method is the use of dermis fat graft that is obtained from the lateral thigh near the buttock. A dermatome is used to remove the epidermis, and the dermis fat graft is then fashioned to the appropriate size (25 mm by 25 mm) and placed into the orbital socket with the dermis facing anteriorly. The dermis is then sewn to the rectus muscles and Tenon's capsule. If there is sufficient conjunctiva, it may be closed over the dermis, but if conjunctiva is in short supply, the dermis may be left bare. The conjunctiva will migrate over the dermis in 4 to 6 weeks. The donor site is closed by using 5-0 Vicryl sutures to close the dermis and 5-0 nylon to close the skin.

PRECAUTIONS

Any implant not covered by conjunctiva will ultimately extrude if not repaired. Also, any oversized or irregularly placed implant is bound to extrude eventually. The exposure of an orbital implant should be repaired immediately. Freshening the edges of conjunctiva and Tenon's capsule and resuturing them generally are only temporary measures in early extrusion.

COMMENTS

Implant extrusion is prevented by using basic surgical principles and good surgical technique. Meticulous hemostasis is essential to prevent hematoma formation and tension on the suture line. A well-positioned, centrally placed implant with layered closure (fascia lata, posterior Tenon, rectus muscle, anterior Tenon, and conjunctiva) will act as a barrier to early and late extrusion and will enhance motility and cosmesis.

References

Levine MR: Extruding orbital implant: Prevention and treatment. Ann Ophthalmology 12:1384–1386, 1980.
Levine MR, Older JJ: Enucleation surgery and treatment of the extruding orbital implant. In Stewart WB, et al: Ophthalmic Plastic Surgery. A Manual Prepared for the Use of Graduates in Medicine, 4th ed. San Francisco, American Academy of Ophthalmology, 1983.

Fractures

EXTERNAL ORBITAL FRACTURES

BYRON SMITH, M.D.,
and RICHARD D. LISMAN, M.D.
New York, New York

External fractures of the orbit involve direct disjunction of any portion of the orbital rim and may also involve the walls of the orbit. Naso-orbital fractures are one of the most common external orbital fractures; these fractures of the medial aspect of the orbit commonly involve the lacrimal system. Trauma in this region usually includes the severance of the medial canthal tendon, which displaces and widens the medial canthus and severs the lacrimal excretory apparatus by direct laceration or bony fragments. As a consequence of damage to the medial canthal tendon, the lid margins may relax and evert the lacrimal punctum away from the globe. This results in epiphora caused by the abnormal evacuation of tears. A direct injury to the lacrimal sac or nasolacrimal duct caused by displaced bony fragments results in a more serious disturbance of the lacrimal outflow system. Repeated bouts of acute dacryocystitis often follow such injuries.

Orbital rim fractures commonly occur through bony sutural lines. The zygomaticofrontal suture superolaterally and the zygomaticomaxillary suture infranasally are the weakest portions of the orbital rim. Fractures through these sites produce a displaced zygoma, often referred to as a tripod fracture.

Fractures to the supraorbital rim are usually seen in addition to severe head trauma and accompanying cerebral injury. The orbital roof is quite thin and can be penetrated by any long sharp foreign bodies that pass through the upper eyelid avoiding the globe. Finally, infraorbital rim fractures often involve an associated zygomatic fracture.

THERAPY

Supportive. After the extent of the injury has been evaluated by clinical and radiographic examination, triage is in order. Isolated rim fractures with minimal edema and hemorrhage and without cutaneous anesthesia represent the mildest end of the spectrum of fractures that are simply observed. At the other end of the spectrum, neurosurgical emergencies include those fractures involving the orbital roof that can produce orbital emphysema, epistaxis due to involvement of the frontal or ethmoidal sinuses, and cerebrospinal rhinorrhea due to fracture of the frontal sinus or cribriform plate. In any fracture that apparently has intracranial complications, immediate action is the rule.

More commonly, though, external orbital fractures result in cosmetic deformities. The only midfacial fractures that involve the orbit are LeFort II and LeFort III fractures. "Pure" LeFort fractures are rare in ophthalmologic practice. More commonly, they involve naso-orbital fractures, classically obtained during automobile accidents when the victim's face hits the dash-

334 / EXTERNAL ORBITAL FRACTURES

board of the car. Medial canthal deformities, lacrimal obstruction, and a widened interpalpebral distance are all repaired late. Immediate supportive therapy includes antibiotics, radiographic examination, and clinical evaluation of the fracture.

Fractures of the lateral wall of the orbit, most commonly zygomatic fractures, present clinically as a flattening of the malar prominence. Often, gaps or fracture deformities of the rim can easily be palpated. Concomitant hemorrhage and edema vary according to the extent of the trauma. Emphysema of the soft tissues is not found with lateral fractures. If the lateral wall of the oribit is displaced at the zygomaticofrontal process, the lateral orbital tubercle is displaced downward and the lateral canthal tendon follows with it. Further, a depressed zygomatic arch may rarely press on the coronoid process of the mandible, creating pain and dysfunction upon opening the mouth. These fractures are more easily repaired after resolution of the edema that occurs during the acute phase of the injury.

Surgical. Only those fractures that produce cosmetic deformities or functional defects are explored and repaired. The more serious of the external orbital fractures are those involving the medial and lateral canthal regions. Fractures through these extremities of the orbit require a significant restoration of orbital contour, as well as functional components of the orbit. Repair of both medial canthal and lacrimal defects are performed through vertical or curvilinear skin incisions made over the frontal process of maxilla. The dissection is carried down through subcutaneous tissue and periosteum. The periosteum should be raised from the bone with a small elevator along the medial orbital wall over the lacrimal groove and across the lamina papyracea. Bony fragments that protrude are resected; the lacrimal sac or its remnants are elevated and retracted laterally. If the medial orbital wall is excessively thickened by overlapping or malunion of bony fragments, it is thinned with a Hall drill to allow repositioning of the medial canthal structures. Next, the medial canthal tendon should be isolated and the lacrimal system reconstituted. Severed canaliculi may be repaired with silicone intubation and a nasolacrimal duct obstruction restored with a dacryocystorhinostomy. The medial canthal tendon should be reinserted at or immediately behind the anterior lacrimal crest. The medial canthal tendon may be wired, or a transnasal wiring may be necessary to reform the medial canthal angle.

Zygomatic fractures may be approached most easily through a horizontal lateral canthal incision. This approach offers favorable visualization of the fracture site but not a cosmetically pleasing scar. The more favorable cosmetic approach to zygomatic fractures is through a Gillies incision posterior to the hair line in the temporal region. The incision is made parallel and posterior to the hair line and is carried down to the temporal fascia. The temporal muscle is exposed, and a surgical plane is dissected bluntly between the temporal fascia and the temporal muscle, usually with a Bristoe elevator. This elevator is pushed through this surgical space down to the overhanging bone of the zygoma, and minimal pressure is exerted on the temporal bone, lifting the fractured zygoma into place. This is usually performed as a bimanual procedure. The surgeon's hand is used over the zygoma to push the fractured bone up into position while the Bristoe elevator is used from beneath and above.

If there is significant displacement of the fracture or the fragments are comminuted, direct visualization is preferable. Tripod fractures most often have to be reduced and wired only at the zygomaticofrontal fracture site. Only if a great deal of displacement is evident at the zygomaticomaxillary fracture site would reduction and wiring be necessary at both positions. A third alternative for the incision for repair of a zygomaticofrontal fracture is in the lateral one third of the brow. Reduction of fractures of the inferior orbital rim are performed through a blepharoplasty-type of incision.

Standard procedure for wiring an orbital rim is to create two opposing drill holes on either side of the fracture. It is usually most difficult to carry a drill hole from the external side of the orbital rim through to the internal portion; it is far easier to create two drill holes 90° to one another that will meet within the bony confines of the orbital rim. Twenty-eight or 30-gauge stainless steel wire is threaded through the holes and twisted externally until good apposition of the bony fragments is obtained. The free ends of the wire are twisted away from the incisional area and buried deep in the subcutaneous tissue. When the Gillies approach is used laterally, the fragments are not directly aligned, and no wiring is performed. However, if significant displacement of the fracture is evident and a fair amount of instability is obvious, a direct approach with wiring is preferable.

Ocular or Periocular Manifestations

Extraocular Muscles or Eyelids: Displacement; downward displacement of the lateral canthus; ecchymosis; edema; laceration; ptosis; telecanthus.

Lacrimal System: Avulsion; dacryocystitis; epiphora; laceration; mucocele; obstruction.

Orbit: Cicatrization; damage of soft tissue; edema; enophthalmos; emphysema; exophthalmos; fracture; hemorrhages; step deformity of the inferior orbital rim.

Precautions

Contusion and orbital hemorrhage may mimic orbital fracture. In these patients, careful observation frequently reveals marked improvement within a week. Failure to diagnose fractures that require early treatment may result in complications caused by fibrosis, contracture, and malunion. The mere presence of an orbital fracture without a functional or cosmetic defect is not necessarily an indication for surgery. In many cases, a surgeon can be of greatest assistance to the patient by conservatively following the clinical findings to determine whether surgery may later become necessary.

COMMENTS

Orbital fractures are of particular interest to the ophthalmologist because of the frequency with which the eye and ocular adnexa are damaged. Fractures in the orbital region are unique; the bones are closely associated with many fragile anatomic structures. These areas of bone are subject to severe comminution. Orbital fractures are usually in close approximation to the paranasal sinuses, which compounds the clinical problems for the surgeon.

Solitary rim fractures may be wired in place if the cosmetic defect is significant. Exploration of an orbital roof with a communication superiorly should be performed by a neurosurgeon.

References

Bedrossian EH, Della Rocca RC: Management of zygomaticomaxillary (tripod) fractures. *In* Smith BC (ed): Ophthalmic Plastic and Reconstructive Surgery. St. Louis, CV Mosby, 1987, pp 506–522.

Converse JM, Smith B: Naso-orbital fractures and traumatic deformities of the medial canthus. Plast Reconstr Surg 38:147–162, 1966.

Converse JM, Smith B, Lisman RD: Differential diagnosis and its influence on the treatment of orbital blow-out fractures. *In* Aston SJ, et al (eds): Third International Symposium of Plastic and Reconstructive Surgery of the Eye and Adnexa. Baltimore, Williams & Wilkins, 1982, pp 96–104.

Dortzbach RK, Soll DB, McCord CD: Orbital fractures. *In* Silver B (ed): Ophthalmic Plastic Surgery. Rochester, NY, American Academy of Ophthalmology and Otolaryngology, 1977.

Smith B: Reduction of nasal orbital fracture and simultaneous dacryocystorhinostomy. American Academy of Ophthalmology 1976 Instruction Section.

Smith B, Lisman RD: Blow-out fractures of the orbit. *In* Harley RD: Pediatric Ophthalmology, 2nd ed. Philadelphia, WB Saunders, 1983, pp 388–395.

Smith B, Nightingale JD: Fractures of the orbit: Blowout and nasoorbital fractures. Int Ophthalmol Clin 18:137–147, 1978.

INTERNAL ORBITAL FRACTURES
(Blowout Fractures)

BYRON SMITH, M.D.,
and RICHARD D. LISMAN, M.D.
New York, New York

An internal orbital fracture, commonly called a blowout fracture, involves the roof, floor, or walls of the orbit, but does not include an orbital rim fracture. Blowout fractures frequently occur as an isolated event, but they can be seen in conjunction with naso-orbital, zygomatic, or rim fractures. These fractures can be divided into "pure" blowout fractures, which involve only the internal orbital bony structure, and "impure" blowout fractures, which have associated rim fractures. As with any bony injury, fractures may be displaced, compounded, or telescoped. A keen understanding of the mechanism and theory underlying this unique type of fracture is important in predicting the outcome of the injury; further, a good understanding of the anatomy of this region is essential.

A "pure" blowout fracture can be produced when the orbit is struck by an object of greater diameter than the anterior orbital bony dimension. Circular objects, such as a fist or a ball, of a dimension larger than the horizontal diameter of the anterior opening of the orbit are typical of the type of objects that can increase intraorbital pressure and produce fractures at the weakest point of the bony orbit.

The orbital rims are quite strong, but the walls of the orbit are mostly comprised of thin bones. The most common site of a blowout fracture is the ethmoidal plate or that part of the floor weakened by the infraorbital groove, which is directly in front of the inferior orbital fissure. These areas are in close approximation to the extraocular muscles and connective tissue. If the fracture is located lateral to this groove, the muscles may not be affected. The medial wall is by far the thinnest of the orbital walls; fractures through the medial walls produce variable amounts of inflammation and hemorrhage. After such fractures, the possible sequelae are enophthalmos, cranial nerve dysfunction, ptosis, disruption of ocular motility, and superior sulcus deformities.

THERAPY

Supportive. Although the radiographic analysis is most important, it is secondary to clinical impressions. The Caldwell frontal view is most helpful in evaluation of the margin walls, superior orbital fissure, sphenoid ridges, and temporal, ethmoid, frontal and nasal fossae. The Waters' view shows the orbital floor and roof, the zygomatic bone, and temporal arch. The lateral view is used to interpret anteroposterior relationships. Finally, tomography is extremely useful in equivocal cases. When in doubt, high-resolution computed tomography in axial and coronal planes is most helpful.

Patients are managed by x-ray studies, repeated exophthalmometry, repeated diplopia fields, and repeated muscle measurements. Obviously, forced ductions play a significant role in the establishment of the diagnosis, and measurement of the interpalpebral distances can be a useful adjunct to exophthalmometry. All patients present with a variable amount of edema and ecchymosis, depending on soft tissue damage.

The management of blowout fractures is somewhat controversial. No two fractures are alike; the first 7 to 14 days after the fracture are usually spent in conservative management. All patients

336 / INTERNAL ORBITAL FRACTURES

are symptomatic to some degree upon initial presentation. Patients with persistent diplopia in primary position, which has not improved by direct diplopia field examinations, are also explored at that time. Patients with an increasing amount of enophthalmos over a period of 10 to 14 days fall into the same category. The most difficult patients to manage are those who have no diplopia but have noticeable enophthalmos that has not improved during the initial 7- to 14-day period. The surgical possibilities should be presented to these patients so they understand that the enophthalmos will remain and possibly worsen without surgical intervention. It is further noted that surgery may produce the complication of diplopia, which is not present at initial presentation. Finally, "old" blowout fractures without diplopia but with significant enophthalmos are a most vexing problem. Bone is grafted to the orbital floor of these patients only after a guarded prognosis is given. Obviously, patients without diplopia or enophthalmos or those with improving diplopia or stable enophthalmos are not surgically explored. Patients with diplopia in upward gaze only are not subjected to surgery.

Surgical. Fracture reduction and plating of the inferior floor defects are done only within the above general guidelines. A subciliary or a lateral canthal approach is cosmetically superior to incisions directly over the inferior orbital rim. A skin or skin-orbicularis flap is created in the fashion of a blepharoplasty. The inferior orbital rim is identified and the periosteum is incised and elevated to explore the orbital floor. A hand-over-hand method is used to free the orbital contents from the defect and elevate the contents from the maxillary antrum. If necessary, the rim is mobilized and wired. The orbital floor can be restored with cartilage, bone graft, or inorganic implants. Gel film has been used for small defects; Teflon, Silastic, or supramid are preferred as implants.

The inferior rectus muscle is identified, and forced ductions document the inferior rectus muscle to be free from entrapment. After the implant is placed, periosteum is closed; care is taken not to include the orbital septum in the skin closure. A modified Frost lid suture is used to prevent eyelid retraction; it is taped to the skin above the brow and removed after a few days.

Ocular or Periocular Manifestations

Extraocular Muscles: Pain; positive forced duction test; restriction of elevation and depression.

Eyelids: Hypesthesia; ptosis.

Globe: Enophthalmos; exophthalmos.

Orbit: Ecchymosis; edema; emphysema; pain; retro-orbital hemorrhage.

Pupil: Mydriasis.

Other: Decreased vision; diplopia.

PRECAUTIONS

Visual acuity should be checked frequently in the postoperative period. Significant decreases in vision should be explored for evidence of postoperative hemorrhage into the orbit. Late permanent muscle imbalances are observed until measurements are consistent and stabilized for a period of at least 3 months. Surgery is advocated for muscles controlled motility in the field of action of greatest deviation. Most often, the operation is performed on the sound eye.

Contraction of the inferior rectus is almost invariably responsible for limitation in the fields of monocular fixation. Retraction of the globe may occur when the patient looks upward. Resection of the antagonistic superior rectus in the presence of a fibrotic inferior rectus may create or augment the extent of the enophthalmos. Horizontal and vertical deviations are less troublesome than torsional deviations. Fortunately, most patients with persistent diplopia learn to cope by the acquisition of monocular suppression. Contracture of the extraocular muscles other than the inferior rectus or inferior oblique occurs less frequently. The anatomic relationship of the muscles near the floor of the orbit renders them more vulnerable to ischemic involvement.

If pseudoptosis is present, it is not treated until maximal muscle recovery has been obtained. Levator resection or tarsal shortening usually rectifies the residual lid problems. Severe enophthalmos requires orbital floor implantation; excellent results with bone grafting are obtained, even in seeing eyes. Mild enophthalmos can be cosmetically corrected with implants into the upper lids, such as scleral strips or collagen injections, to augment and create the appearance of a lid fold in an enophthalmic socket.

Although orbital hemorrhage is dreaded, a defect in the inferior floor remains with most floor implant procedures. This defect allows drainage through to the maxillary antrum, leaving the orbit decompressed. Infection and allergy to the implant are rare. More common, though is displacement or migration of the implant. Ectropion, entropion, or vertical shortening of the lower lid is possible. Muscle deviation may be improved or exacerbated by the surgery; visual disturbances are caused by the pressure of the plate upon the optic nerve or tissue in the apex of the orbit. Late complications include enophthalmos, pupillary abnormalities, blepharoptosis, ptosis of the globe, abnormalities of the interpalpebral fissure, sinus disease, lacrimal obstruction, and chronic lid edema.

COMMENTS

It has long been recognized that the inferior rectus muscle is quite fibrotic in some patients with "old" blowout fractures. An ischemic type of contraction has been postulated as responsible for this finding. This is similar to a Volkmann's ischemic contracture, which orthopedic surgeons have long recognized. With some defects of the inferior orbital floor, not only is the inferior rectus muscle entrapped in the bony fragments and maxillary antrum but hemorrhage and edema within the compartment of the inferior rectus muscle are also responsible for the eventual infarction and fibrosis. Blowout fractures with large floor defects may produce a ptotic globe, but if the globe is well supported by the periorbita, diplopia may not be present.

Without entrapment of the inferior rectus, hemorrhage and edema apparently expand into the maxillary antrum. However, in small defects of the orbital floor, the osseofascial planes around the inferior rectus form a compartment. Edema and hemorrhage reside in this compartment, and pressure increases; this is similar to a Volkmann's contracture in the small muscles of the hands or limbs. The vascular supply to the extraocular muscles is both from distal and proximal; these fine vessels can be occluded when the pressure in the inferior rectus "compartment" rises from 20 to 40 mm Hg. Normal and fibrotic inferior recti muscles have low compartment pressures, 0 to 2 mm Hg. In acute blowout fractures, pressure rises from 2 to 60 mm Hg. This is a useful adjunct to management of blowout fractures. There is a definite group of patients with minimal diplopia or enophthalmos and high inferior rectus pressures who should be explored within 7 days. This group with small floor defects is the one that may go on to inferior rectus fibrosis. Systemic steroids normally are indicated in this small group. Patients with small floor defects and high inferior rectus pressure are given 100 mg of systemic steroids daily for short duration.

Not every practitioner has the equipment to measure the pressure within the inferior rectus muscle sheath. However, systemic steroids are helpful in patients with small floor fractures and an excessive amount of edema and ecchymosis; the ophthalmologist should be wary of the possibility of compartment syndrome and resultant inferior rectus fibrosis.

References

Converse JM, Smith B: Enophthalmos and diplopia in fractures of the orbital floor. Br J Plast Surg 9:265–274, 1957.
Converse JM, Smith B: Blowout fracture of the floor of the orbit. Trans Am Acad Ophthalmol Otolaryngol 64:676, 1960.
Converse JM, smith B, Lisman RD: Differential diagnosis and its influence on the treatment of orbital blow-out fractures. In Aston SJ, et al (eds): Third International Symposium of Plastic and Reconstructive Surgery of the Eye and Adnexa. Baltimore, Williams & Wilkins, 1982, pp 96–104.
Lisman RD, Smith BC, Rudgers R: Volkmann's ischemic contractures and blowout fractures. Adv Ophthalmol Plastic Reconstruct Surg 7:117–131, 1988.
Nathog RH: Traumatic enophthalmos. In Smith BC (ed): Ophthalmic Plastic and Reconstructive Surgery. St. Louis, CV Mosby, 1987, pp 491–505.
Putterman AM, Smith BC, Lisman RD: Blowout fractures. In Smith BC (ed): Ophthalmic Plastic and Reconstructive Surgery. St. Louis, CV Mosby, 1987, pp 477–490.
Putterman AM, Stevens T, Urist MJ: Nonsurgical management of blow-out fractures of the orbital floor. Am J Ophthalmol 77:233–239, 1974.
Smith B, Lisman RD: Blow-out fractures of the orbit. In Harley RD: Pediatric Ophthalmology, 2nd ed. Philadelphia, WB Saunders, 1983, pp 388–395.

OPTIC FORAMEN FRACTURES

A.J.M. VAN DER WERF, M.D.
Amsterdam, The Netherlands

Fracture of the optic foramen is a rare traumatic condition that is usually caused by a closed head injury. It may occur with no evidence of laceration or abrasion; an amaurotic or Marcus Gunn pupil may be the only immediate clinical sign. Profound primary optic atrophy is usually noted within 3 weeks if the optic nerve has been severed. Optic atrophy may be caused by injury to the eyeball itself, injury to the optic nerve inside the orbital cavity, damage to the optic nerve between the chiasm and the optic foramen, or lesions near or inside the optic canal. The following mechanisms may also be involved in optic nerve injury caused by fractures of the optic foramen: tearing of the nerve at the entrance of the cranial cavity, mechanical trauma from bony fragments, tearing of the nerve inside the canal, bleeding inside the optic nerve, and hyperostosis at the site of a fracture.

THERAPY

Surgical. The indications for decompression must depend upon the mechanism involved. When there is immediate and complete loss of function, decompression is useless and any future improvement that may occur is due to the incompleteness of the optic nerve injury. On the other hand, if the functional impairment is only partial with or without progression of the visual loss and there is evidence or a strong suspicion of partial bony compression or intraneuronal hemorrhage based on tonofilm EMI scans, decompression may be indicated. Decompression of the optic canal can be done either by the subfrontal or transethmoidal approach. The latter may be carried out under local anesthesia, which permits control of vision during the operation. The greater part of the wall of the optic canal, notably the medial wall, can be removed. This procedure comprises a pansinusectomy, but is undoubtedly less traumatizing to the brain than the subfrontal route. The better the initial vision, the more improvement may be expected.

Ocular or Periocular Manifestations

Extraocular Muscles: Paralysis of sixth nerve.
Optic Nerve: Atrophy; compression; hemorrhages; pallor.
Pupil: Marcus Gunn pupil.
Retina: Retinal artery occlusion.
Other: Exophthalmos; hemianopsia; scotoma; visual loss.

PRECAUTIONS

One should be careful in reducing orbital fractures in the presence of fractures of the paranasal sinuses, especially when the frontal sinus is involved. Such a reduction may enlarge a dural tear already present, and rhinorrhea may become apparent. Before any attempt is made to reduce an orbital fracture, careful x-ray examination of the paranasal sinuses is necessary. In the case of a fractured frontal sinus, neurologic advice should be sought. It has been postulated that optic nerve lesions might result secondarily from reduction of orbital fractures associated with a fracture of the optic canal.

COMMENTS

Optic nerve lesions occur less frequently with a fracture of the optic canal than they do without such a fracture. Complete and immediate loss of vision is usually permanent, and a decompression operation is useless. Partial impairment of vision and progressive loss of vision may be indications for surgery if there is strong suspicion of nerve compression. Restoration of vision by natural healing is possible even in the amaurotic patient, but chances are better when the initial loss is not very severe.

References

Smith JL: Some neuro-ophthalmological aspects of head trauma. *In* Proceedings of the Congress of Neurological Surgeons. Baltimore, Williams & Wilkins, 1966, pp 181–192.
van der Werf AJM: Fractures of the optic foramen. *In* Bleeker GM, Lyle TK (eds): Fractures of the Orbit. Baltimore, Williams & Wilkins, 1970, pp 153–156.

Laceration, Tear, or Contusion

CHORIORETINAL CONCUSSIONS AND LACERATIONS

DAVID J. WILSON, M.D.
Portland, Oregon

A concussion is a condition that results from a violent shake or jar of a tissue; in the case of the eye, it usually results from the contact of some type of missile with the globe. A concussion may result in a contusion, an injury without rupture of the tissue, or it may result in a laceration, which is defined as a tear.

When a missile strikes the globe, the amount of damage that is done is dependent on the kinetic energy transferred to the globe. The kinetic energy is a function of the mass of the missile and the square of the velocity of the missile. The perturbations of the globe following missile impact have been described in four stages: compression, decompression, overshooting, and oscillation. During compression, the cornea indents and pushes the lens posteriorly. The anterior sclera expands to compensate for the decrease in volume caused by the corneal indentation. Decompression follows as the cornea or sclera pushes the missile outward. The equatorial diameters continue to expand, and the vitreous moves posteriorly. During compression and decompression, the combined effects of the expanding anterior and equatorial sclera and posterior movement of the lens and vitreous result in traction on the retina at the vitreous base. During overshooting, the antero-posterior diameter exceeds its original dimension, and the equatorial diameter decreases. A series of oscillations follow, during which the antero-posterior and equatorial diameters expand and contract periodically.

THERAPY

Surgical. Retinal tears are a well-known complication of concussive injuries. The most common type of tear is a retinal dialysis, which may occur anterior or posterior to the vitreous base. Also, large ragged retinal holes with pieces of necrotic retina in the adjacent vitreous may result from retinal necrosis at the site of severe retinal contusion. In addition, horseshoe tears may occur at sites of vitreous attachment, and macular holes may develop secondary to contrecoup forces. The treatment of retinal tears without detachment is cryopexy or laser photocoagulation. When an associated retinal detachment is also present, a retinal reattachment operation is indicated.

Choroidal damage following concussive injuries usually takes the form of subretinal hemorrhage or choroidal rupture. Choroidal ruptures appear as white curvilinear streaks concentric to the optic nerve head. They occur more commonly on the temporal side of the optic nerve head. If the choroidal rupture occurs directly beneath the fovea, the visual prognosis is poor.

However, if the fovea is spared, central vision may be unaffected. There is no treatment for choroidal ruptures, but choroidal neovascular membranes can develop as a late complication of choroidal rupture. If recognized early, these membranes may be amenable to treatment with laser photocoagulation.

Ocular or Periocular Manifestations

Anterior Chamber: Hyphema.
Ciliary Body: Cyclodialysis.
Choroid: Hemorrhage; rupture.
Lens: Cataract.
Retina: Commotio retinae; dialysis; hemorrhage; tears.
Sclera: Laceration.
Vitreous: Detached vitreous base; hemorrhage.
Other: Decreased vision; pain.

PRECAUTIONS

At the time of the initial examination, care should be taken to document the full extent of the injury. If no initial treatment is required, the patient should be warned about the symptoms of possible late complications, such as retinal detachment and choroidal neovascular membranes.

COMMENTS

A thorough examination of both the injured and fellow eye should be accomplished to ascertain the extent of the injury. The initial visual acuity should be recorded, and appropriate x-rays, CT, or MRI scanning should be obtained to evaluate for associated orbital or head injuries and for intraocular foreign bodies. In the presence of vitreous hemorrhage, ultrasonography may be helpful in delineating the extent of the ocular damage. It is essential to determine if a scleral rupture is present; if this is suspected, an exploration of the globe and repair of the laceration should be performed.

The most common retinal injury following nonpenetrating blunt trauma is commotio retinae (Berlin's edema). The milky-white appearance of the retina in this condition has been shown experimentally to be caused by disruption of the photoreceptor outer segments. There is no treatment. RPE hyperplasia occurs in response to the disruption of the photoreceptor outer segments, which may result in a corpuscular intraretinal pigmentary pattern similar to that seen in retinitis pigmentosa. The visual prognosis following commotio retinae depends on the location and the extent of the photoreceptor outer segment regeneration.

References

Bloome MA, et al: Acute retinal necrosis. Ann Ophthalmol 11:723–728, 1979.
Cox MS, Stephens CI, Freeman HM: Retinal detachment due to ocular contusion. Arch Ophthalmol 76:678–685, 1966.
Delori F, Pomerantzeff O, Cox MS: Deformation of the globe under high speed impact: Its relation to contusion injuries. Invest Ophthalmol 8:290–301, 1969.
Kelley JS, Hoover RF, George T: Whiplash maculopathy. Arch Ophthalmol 96:834–835, 1978.
Russell SR, Olsen KR, Folk JC: Predictors of scleral rupture and the role of vitrectomy in severe blunt ocular trauma. Am J Ophthalmol 105:253–257, 1988.
Sipperley JO, Quigley HA, Gass JDM: Traumatic retinopathy in primates, the explanation of commotio retinae. Arch Ophthalmol 96:2267–2273, 1978.

CILIARY BODY CONCUSSIONS AND LACERATIONS
JOHN E. READ, M.D.
Chesterton, Indiana

Injury resulting from blunt trauma to the globe may present a constellation of findings in various areas of the globe, including involvement of uveal tissue. Mild injuries may produce an iridocyclitis, with the usual findings of anterior chamber flare and cells, relative hypotony, and occasionally anterior vitreous cells. As the force of the injury to the globe is increased, rupture of the pupillary sphincter, iridodialysis, angle recession, or traumatic cyclodialysis may occur separately or in combinations and in various degrees of severity. Traumatic cleavage of the tissues of the ciliary body and iris, especially involving the angle, may create an anterior chamber hyphema with or without hemorrhagic or exudative detachment of the ciliary body. The latter rarely may extend posteriorly, producing a choroidal detachment. Abnormal location of uveal pigment may produce evidence of recent or previous blunt trauma in the form of a Vossius ring, a complete or partial ring of pigmentary debris on the anterior surface of the lens capsule representing an imprint of the iris border as it was compressed against the lens during trauma. The anterior vitreous may have pigmentary debris seen on slitlamp examination as small flecks of brownish pigment. In the early postinjury period, hypotony is the usual finding. However, as the amount of exudation and cellular content of the anterior chamber increases and as the direct effect of the trauma on the trabecular meshwork reduces its rate of outflow, ocular hypertension may alternatively be encountered.

Nonpenetrating trauma caused by forces of higher velocity may produce contrecoup injuries. These may include Berlin's edema of the retina, peripheral retinal dialysis, posterior pole retinal hemorrhages, choroidal ruptures, and a retinitis sclopetaria. During the early period after injury, these complications may be difficult to differentiate from the papilledema or cystoid macular edema resulting from profound hypotony.

Late manifestations of blunt trauma include secondary glaucoma associated with major circumferential areas of angle recession. Extensive ciliary body injuries may involve necrosis of major portions of the pars plicata. This may result in extensive fibrosis or atrophy. Massive fibrosis and organization of the vitreous may follow with subsequent retinal detachment. Decreased function of the ciliary body may also lead to significant amounts of hypotony, decreased accommodation, and, subsequently, phthisis bulbi.

Lacerations of the ciliary body most often have associated corneoscleral laceration, hyphema, injury of the lens capsule, or vitreal hemorrhage. Lacerations involving the uveal tissue more often are secondary to perforating or penetrating objects from an obvious anterior source that produce a laceration of the cornea or anterior sclera. However, some penetrating objects that have their initial injury site through the skin of the lid at or even outside the orbital rim may bypass the conjunctival sac and produce scleral and uveal penetration more posteriorly in an occult choroidal injury. Major lacerations of the ciliary body ordinarily have a poor prognosis for a visual recovery.

Penetrating injuries caused by small projectiles may create anterior as well as posterior lacerations. Orbital x-rays and especially computed tomography may be used to locate precisely the retained foreign body in the orbit or surrounding tissues.

THERAPY

Supportive. The ciliary body injured by blunt trauma should be protected from further injury by using a Fox shield. A patch may be added under the shield for increased comfort from photophobia and to absorb ocular secretions. Topical ophthalmic cycloplegics, such as 1 per cent atropine or 5 per cent homatropine solution (for minor trauma), may be administered four times daily. Topical ophthalmic corticosteroids in 0.125 to 1.0 per cent solutions may be applied two to six times a day to help decrease the inflammatory reaction. Administration of 100 mg/kg of aminocaproic acid every 4 hours (maximum, 30 gm) has been shown statistically to prevent recurrent hemorrhage in the presence of anterior chamber hyphema. A topical antibiotic may be added for prophylaxis of epithelial injuries, such as abrasions, if they are present. Sedation and medication for pain may be added as required for patient comfort.

Prolonged hypotony from choroidal effusions rarely requires a posterior sclerotomy for drainage of the suprachoroidal space.

Repair of a large iridodialysis may be undertaken at a later time for correction of visual symptoms, such as diplopia or photophobia. These and other blunt separations of the iris and angle structures do not ordinarily require early surgical repair.

Injury that presents as a laceration of the conjunctiva should be considered a perforating injury until proved otherwise. Protection of the injured globe should be considered of paramount importance during the evaluation period before repair. Tetanus immunization and parenteral administration of broad-spectrum antibiotics should be instituted early in the course of contaminated wounds.

Surgical. When surgical repair of a ciliary body laceration is performed, cultures should be taken of the wound. Because the traumatized eye does not tolerate a cyclectomy well, ciliary body tissue is excised only if it is necrotic, severely traumatized, or grossly contaminated. If a cyclectomy is necessary, encircling trans-scleral diathermy may be indicated to decrease bleeding and subsequent ciliary body detachment. Penetrating injuries that extend into the choroid from the ciliary body should receive encircling cryotherapy to minimize postoperative retinal detachment. Meticulous reconstruction of corneal and scleral lacerations, preferably by microsurgical techniques, should be undertaken as soon as practical after careful evaluation. Every effort to maintain the contour of the eye and to obtain a liquid-tight seal should be made. Loss of corneal or scleral tissue may require replacement with patch grafting in order to restore the contour of the globe. Fine nylon sutures may be used for corneal closure; 7-0 or 8-0 white virgin silk may be preferred for scleral repair. Suturing of the ciliary body laceration rarely is indicated. In all areas, nonabsorbable sutures should be used for contaminated or potentially contaminated wounds.

In the past, ciliary body injuries were repaired with as much cleansing of the anterior chamber and wound lips as possible through the injury site, followed by local reconstruction. A period of recovery was planned, followed by a subsequent discission of secondary membranes or enucleation, as indicated. Because of the large amounts of blood and lens material mixed with vitreous, these eyes often have prolonged and violent episodes of uveitis, complicated by ciliary body detachment, hypotony or glaucoma, and vitreous traction. However, with the availability of automated vitreous suction, cutting, and infusion devices, the extensive removal of vitreous, lens debris, and anterior chamber blood may improve the chances for survival of the globe. Viscoelastic material may be used to protect the corneal endothelium and reconstruct the anatomic contours of the intraocular structures. After the initial wound repair, a second entry is made into the globe through a pars plana incision for introduction of the automated vitreous apparatus. If the lens capsule has been interrupted, lens remnants and debris are removed and any remaining hyphema is irrigated out. Vitreous-containing blood and lens cortex are then removed, taking care that a previously undiagnosed detached retina is not included. Closure of the pars plana incision completes the combined procedure.

It is believed that eyes repaired in this manner early in the posttraumatic period have less chronic irritation and an earlier recovery. Postoperative care includes a patch and shield, as well as topical antibiotics, corticosteroids, and cycloplegics. Glaucoma may be controlled by carbonic anhydrase inhibitors and topical timolol.

Secondary surgical procedures may be required later in the postinjury period to correct retinal detachment, further reconstruct iris or corneal injuries, add encircling Argon laser photocoagulation to areas of threatened retinal detachment, or to use the Neodymium Yag laser to sever fibrotic bands or remove obstructions from the visual axis.

Major ocular injuries that include large areas of choroidal involvement may present what appears initially to be a hopelessly disrupted globe. Primary enucleation should be avoided and considered only as a rare event. Every effort should be made to salvage the injured globe, with maximal effort to reconstruct the injury in nearly every case. The rare exception may be where there is obviously irreparable loss of uveal tissue in major amounts, preventing adequate reconstruction. The postponement of enucleation and the maximal effort to salvage the eye will be appreciated by the patient, and the surgeon may occasionally be rewarded by some return of visual potential. With present-day methods of microsurgical reconstruction, sympathetic ophthalmia is now a rare event and should be of minimal concern in planning the repair of a major ocular injury, at least for an initial 9-day period.

Ocular or Periocular Manifestations

Anterior Chamber: Angle recession; hyphema; shallow; Tyndall effect and cellular debris.
Choroid: Detachment; rupture.
Ciliary Body: Cyclodialysis cleft; hemorrhagic or exudative detachment.
Iris: Atrophy; iridodialysis; sphincter rupture; uveitis.
Retina: Berlin's edema; dialysis; hemorrhages.
Other: Decreased accommodation; hypotony; macular edema; papilledema; secondary glaucoma; vitreal hemorrhages.

Precautions

The presence of swollen periorbital tissues and eyelids must not deter the examiner from a meticulous evaluation of the globe and orbital contents at the earliest opportunity. In addition to recognizing major ocular injuries that would otherwise go undetected until the edema subsides, it is important to take advantage of the clarity of the ocular structures that may opacify later. The initial inclination is to make only a cursory assessment, intending a more extensive evaluation later. However, the subsequent occurrence of secondary hemorrhage from an initially small hyphema, further edema and clouding of a severely contused cornea, and rapid development of a cataract or vitreal hemorrhage may totally obscure all posterior structures that would have been visualized initially.

The surgeon must exert more than the usual amount of care in examining the patient with a possible ciliary body laceration. The exact location of the injury must be identified without placing undue pressure on the globe and risking the further extrusion of intraocular contents.

Comments

During the acute phase, patients with known blunt trauma to the eye should be examined for angle recession with maximal care using the gonioscopy mirror, or the examination should be deferred until after healing has progressed so that this procedure will not induce additional injury. If angle recession is found, periodic examinations to detect latent glaucoma will be necessary for the rest of the patient's life. Angle recession of any amount may aggravate any ocular hypertension already present in an eye with open-angle glaucoma. A recent study indicates that angle recessions may close up or disappear during the healing phase of blunt trauma. This imposes an additional requirement for the gonioscopist to examine carefully the injured eye by comparison to the normal, fellow eye for subtle residual evidence of angle damage. Similarly, all patients with known ocular blunt trauma deserve a complete, dilated, indirect ophthalmic examination in the early postinjury period in order to rule out a retinal dialysis before its extension into a subsequent retinal detachment.

References

Agapitos PJ, Noel LP, Clarke WN: Traumatic hyphema in children. Ophthalmology 94:1238–1241, 1987.
Britten MJA: Follow-up of 54 cases of ocular contusion with hyphaema. With special reference to the appearance and function of the filtration angle. Br J Ophthalmol 49:120–127, 1965.
Herschler J: Trabecular damage due to blunt anterior segment injury and its relationship to traumatic glaucoma. Trans Am Acad Ophthalmol Otolaryngol 83:239–248, 1977.
Kutner R, et al: Aminocaproic acid reduces the risk of secondary hemorrhage in patients with traumatic hyphema. Arch Ophthalmol 105:206-B, 1987.
Mooney D: Anterior chamber angle tears after nonperforating injury. Br J Ophthalmol 56:418–424, 1972.
Paton D, Goldberg MF: Management of Ocular Injuries. Philadelphia, WB Saunders, 1976, pp 235–239.
Read JE: Trauma Ruptures and bleeding. In Duane TD (ed): Clinical Ophthalmology. Hagerstown, MD, Harper & Row, 1982, Vol IV, pp 61:3–12.
Read J, Goldberg MF: Comparison of medical treatment for traumatic hyphema. Trans Am Acad Ophthalmol Otolaryngol 78:799–815, 1974.
Runyan TE: Concussive and Penetrating Injuries of the Globe and Optic Nerve. St. Louis, CV Mosby, 1975, pp 66–72.
Russell SR, Olsen KR, Folk JC: Predictors of scleral rupture and the role of vitrectomy in severe blunt ocular trauma. Am J Ophthalmol 105:253–257, 1988.
Thomas MA, Parrish RK II, Feuer WJ: Rebleeding after traumatic hyphema. Arch Ophthalmol 104:206–210, 1986.

CONJUNCTIVAL LACERATIONS AND CONTUSIONS

L.F. RICH, M.S., M.D.
Portland, Oregon

Traumatic injuries to the conjunctiva are usually not serious in themselves. However, they may mask an underlying ocular injury or retained foreign body. Every conjunctival laceration potentially overlies a scleral laceration or rupture. Associated conjunctival hemorrhage and edema may obscure the presence of transparent gelatinous vitreous, black uveal tissue, or gray, slime-like retina, any of which may have herniated through a scleral laceration. Complications may occur if a conjunctival laceration contains an embedded foreign body that goes unnoticed. Such an occurrence may result in corneal erosion, tissue reactions, conjunctival cysts or granuloma, and membrane formation. Likewise, contusion injuries of the conjunctiva are seldom of major clinical importance. However, late sequelae from extensive necrosis may occur, including loss of fornices or changes in the tear film.

THERAPY

Supportive. Because conjunctival hemorrhage and chemosis following contusions are usually not serious, treatment requires only supportive therapy, such as ice packs to minimize swelling in the acute phase. Subconjunctival hemorrhage following contusive injuries may at times result in a chemosis so severe that the conjunctiva balloons out between the lids. In this situation, treatment does not relieve the edema, but may be directed at relief of discomfort. This distended conjunctiva should be covered with ointment or a plastic sheet until swelling subsides. At some point, the use of a muscle hook may allow an infolding of the conjunctiva into the fornices to a degree that will allow a pressure patch. Rarely is it necessary to attempt to find the source of hemorrhage.

In the case of conjunctival laceration, the wound should be carefully examined, usually under topical anesthesia, to determine the extent of injury and to search for retained foreign bodies. Any foreign bodies that are found and removed should be cultured for bacterial and fungal growth. Dental film is most useful for detecting nonmetallic foreign bodies. A Berman metal locator is also of value in selected instances. Prophylactic use of topical antibiotic solutions is advisable for all conjunctival lacerations.

Surgical. Surgical repair is rarely necessary if the laceration is less than 1 cm in length. If surgical reapproximation of a gaping wound is deemed necessary, interrupted or continuous 6-0 or 7-0 gut sutures are sufficient for this purpose. Careful attention should be given to reapproximation of lacerated conjunctival edges in order to exclude Tenon's capsule from the wound. If Tenon's fascia is included in a sutured conjunctival laceration, a chalky-white herniation will result. On rare occasions, extensive loss of conjunctiva may require a conjunctival graft from the fellow eye or a mucous membrane graft from the mouth. However, even injuries that have resulted in loss of a considerable amount of tissue can usually be closed satisfactorily because of the elasticity of the conjunctiva.

If tissue necrosis has resulted from a severe contusive injury, excision of the necrotic tissue will facilitate more rapid wound healing and will also decrease the possibility of infection.

Ocular or Periocular Manifestations

Conjunctiva: Chemosis; cicatrization; cysts; granulation; hemorrhages; hyperemia; keratinization; necrosis; nodules; pseudo-membrane. Conjunctivitis.

PRECAUTIONS

In the exploration of conjunctival lacerations, care must be taken to eliminate any pressure on the globe, as this may lead to prolapse of intraocular contents through an unsuspected scleral penetration. If laceration of the globe is detected at the time of this exploration, it is desirable to proceed immediately with all necessary surgical repairs. A fracture of one of the paranasal sinuses allows air to be trapped within the conjunctival tissues, which can be diagnosed by crepitus as well as a roentgenographic study. Fractures involving the ethmoidal sinuses are probably the most common cause of traumatic conjunctival emphysema. Care must be taken to ensure that any prolonged course of conjunctival edema is not associated with an infectious process, a retained subconjunctival or orbital foreign body, or even a scleral rupture.

Knowledge of the normal anatomy of the plica semilunaris and the caruncle is required to prevent an unsightly surgical repair. Traction on the plica by tight closure to inadequately mobilized bulbar conjunctiva may produce a disfiguring appearance of the eye caused by persistent redness of the conjunctiva. The implantation of conjunctival epithelium in the subconjunctival space may produce inclusion cyst formation.

COMMENTS

Most conjunctival wounds involve the bulbar conjunctiva in the interpalpebral zone. Less frequently, the superior and inferior palpebral areas are lacerated, and in these instances, painstaking inspection must be performed. These tears are commonly seen in association with lid lacerations or perforations, and meticulous examination of the underlying sclera and a thorough fundus examination are essential. The possibility of scleral perforation always exists in these cases, and proper management depends on an immediate and accurate diagnosis.

retrobulbar injections, particularly if the laceration is large or possible expulsion of the internal contents is anticipated. After careful scrupulous cleaning of the skin and lids and copious irrigation of the fornices, any prolapsed uveal or lenticular tissue should be excised to free the wound margins. The wound should then be sutured with interrupted 10-0 silk or nylon sutures, avoiding placement of sutures across the visual axis and burial of knots in the central cornea, if possible. Jagged irregular lacerations may occasionally be closed with 10-0 nylon sutures. An initial suture well placed in the center of the laceration stabilizes the wound so that less prolapse of eye contents will occur as the wound is sutured. After the wound has been sutured, the anterior chamber should be reformed by introducing saline between the sutures with a 30-gauge irrigating needle or through a paracentesis tract. If iris or lens material is adherent to the back of the wound, the injection of a large air bubble and a sweep of the anterior chamber with a very fine cyclodialysis spatula may be required. The spatula should be introduced through a paracentesis site usually placed across from the wound at right angles to the line of the laceration. The sutures should be left in place until wound healing is certain. In general, fine corneal sutures should be left for at least 2 to 3 months before being removed, particularly if the eye is quiet and uninflamed. The sutures should be removed only if they become loose, if the vessels bridge the wound, or if the wound develops the characteristic scar of healing.

Extensive perforating injuries with avulsion or melting of tissue may require lamellar or penetrating keratoplasty. A blowout patch or modified keratoplasty may be required when other methods are contraindicated or the peripheral cornea or limbus is involved. The decision to remove traumatized iris at the same time must be made on an individual basis. Vitreous cutting instruments, such as the ocutome, should be available in such cases for use in the anterior segment. Systemic broad-spectrum antibiotics should be considered in all such wounds. Viscous material, such as sodium hyaluronate, should also be available to maintain the anterior chamber during repair.

Precautions

Topical corticosteroids should not be used in the eye with a corneal abrasion, since these medications allow for delayed wound healing and overgrowth of fungal and bacterial infections. Topical anesthetics should not be given to the patient suffering from corneal abrasion or a foreign body, since they can retard healing, aggravate the keratitis, and cause the patient to become dependent upon the drug.

No matter how severe or penetrating a corneal laceration, primary repair should be attempted. Enucleation should not be done until it is obvious that the eye will not have any function. A traumatic blind eye may have better appearance than the best prosthesis that can be fitted. However, primary enucleation is justified when the globe is totally disorganized or the retina has prolapsed.

Comments

The sooner surgery is performed in patients with corneal lacerations, the better the chance of good recovery. Corneal wounds rapidly become edematous, making strict anatomic repair more difficult. Iris prolapse and lens damage lead to an increasingly fibrinous reaction and inflammation, and scleral and uveal wounds may ooze blood into the vitreous.

References

Boruchoff SA: Corneal surgery. In Duane TD (ed): Clinical Ophthalmology. Hagerstown, MD, Harper & Row, 1982, Vol V, pp 6:1–10.

Duke-Elder S (ed): System of Ophthalmology. St. Louis, CV Mosby, 1972, Vol XIV, pp 313–321.

Paton D, Goldberg MF: Management of Ocular Injuries. Philadelphia, WB Saunders, 1976, pp 193–225.

Read JE: Trauma: Ruptures and bleeding. In Duane TD (ed): Clinical Ophthalmology. Hagerstown, MD, Harper & Row, 1982, Vol IV, pp 61:1–16.

Runyan TE: Concussive and Penetrating Injuries of the Globe and Optic Nerve. St. Louis, CV Mosby, 1975, pp 8–23.

Schlaegel TF Jr, Giles CL: Trauma: Inflammations. In Duane TD (ed): Clinical Ophthalmology. Hagerstown, MD, Harper & Row, 1982, Vol IV, pp 62:1–4.

Stamper RL, et al: Glaucoma, Lens and Anterior Segment Trauma. Basic and Clinical Science Course, Section 8. San Francisco, American Academy of Ophthalmology, 1987–1988.

Wilson FM II, et al: External Disease and Cornea. Basic and Clinical Science Course, Section 7. San Francisco, American Academy of Ophthalmology, 1987–1988.

EXTRAOCULAR MUSCLE LACERATIONS

EUGENE M. HELVESTON, M.D.

Indianapolis, Indiana

Laceration of an extraocular muscle without globe or eyelid involvement is rare; most injuries of this nature also involve adjacent structures. The inferior rectus muscle is the most frequently injured extraocular muscle. The rectus muscles are injured more frequently than the oblique muscles, probably because there is less protective anatomy separating the rectus muscles from the environment. In addition, when the eye is threatened, forced eyelid closure is accompanied by upward and usually outward movement of the eyes. This places the inferior and medial rectus muscles more anteriorly, causing them to be more prone to injury. The superior oblique may be lacerated along with the upper lid if it is avulsed by an object, such as a store display hook.

References

Norton AL, Green WR: Foreign bodies as a cause of conjunctival pseudomembrane formation. Br J Ophthalmol 55:312–316, 1971.

Paton D, Goldberg MF: Management of Ocular Injuries. Philadelphia, WB Saunders, 1976, pp 181–190.

Runyan TE: Concussive and Penetrating Injuries of the Globe and Optic Nerve. St. Louis, CV Mosby, 1975, pp 1–7.

CORNEAL ABRASIONS, CONTUSIONS, LACERATIONS, AND PERFORATIONS

ROGER L. HIATT, M.D.

Memphis, Tennessee

The most important corneal injury is an epithelial abrasion following a contusive force or a direct contact injury to the epithelium. It is associated with pain, lacrimation, blepharospasm, and photophobia. Concussive injuries involving the cornea may result in either localized or generalized edema. Folds may be present at the level of Bowman's or Descemet's membrane or both. A contusive injury of the cornea may result in multiple focal areas of corneal erosion associated with epithelial and endothelial edema but without observable stromal changes. Late recurrent corneal erosion may result and should be anticipated. If the blow is severe enough, hyphema may result from associated uveal tract injury.

Compression injuries are the most common corneal injuries associated with birth. Usually, the localized edema or corneal clouding disappears within a few hours. More severe trauma causes a residual astigmatism or even tears in Descemet's membrane running in a parallel fashion across the posterior corneal surface. These tears may result in marked visual loss because of the irregular refraction produced.

Superficially embedded bodies generally produce no lasting symptoms other than transient irritation. Corneal scarring results only when a foreign body has penetrated Bowman's membrane. A partial-thickness corneal laceration involving the stroma is frequently the result of a tangentially directed cutting force, such as a fingernail. If infection does not supervene and the laceration does not involve the visual axis, the only sequela is usually minimal linear corneal scar. However, many severe complications may be associated with penetrating corneal lacerations, including loss of the anterior chamber, penetration of the lens capsule, cataract, vitreous hemorrhage, iris incarceration, uveal prolapse, epithelial or stromal ingrowth, corneal astigmatism, corneal opacities, and endophthalmitis.

THERAPY

Ocular. In any corneal abrasion or lac meticulous inspection of the eye for th ence of a foreign body is necessary. A anesthetic, such as 0.5 per cent propa may be needed for the examination but therapy. The cornea should be examined biomicroscope using oblique illumination should be attempted even in a child, but focal illumination with magnification ob from a head loop may have to be substitu some patients. All damage to intraocular tures should be documented and t promptly. Pressure should never be appli the globe. Desmarres retractors, sterile bei per clips, or a small wire speculum may be to retract the lids. In a cooperative patient severe blepharospasm, a modified lid block as that performed by the Atkinson's techn may be necessary to facilitate examination treatment. Foreign bodies should be remc with a moistened cotton-tipped applicator fine sterile hypodermic needle attached to a ringe. Foreign bodies embedded in the cor should be removed with care so as not to disr the deeper layers of the cornea, thereby prod ing unnecessary scarring. If no foreign body c be found, fluorescein staining may locate abrasion.

Treatment of a corneal abrasion consists of topical broad-spectrum antibiotic ointment fo lowed by firm patching for 24 to 48 hours, de pending upon the size of the epithelial defect. I ocular discomfort or inflammation is significant, a drop of a cycloplegic, such as 2 per cent homatropine, will relieve ciliary spasm until the patient can be seen again the following day. Significant abrasions should always be re-examined within 24 to 48 hours to ensure that epithelial healing is complete and that no infection, iritis, or other complication develops. If a rust ring is present upon re-examination, it may be removed with a fine needle or peeled from the cornea with fine forceps. Again, topical antibiotics and patching are applied. A central deep rust ring may be allowed to work its way to the surface, until it extrudes spontaneously. Another alternative is to try to remove it with an electrically powered burr applied to the site of the rust ring with the aid of the slitlamp. This should be treated with antibiotic drops or ointments several times a day and followed at frequent intervals until the epithelium is completely healed. Antibiotic drops or ointments should be continued for several days after surface healing, as much for their lubricating properties as for their antibacterial properties.

Surgical. Partial-thickness corneal lacerations with well-apposed margins and no tendency toward gaping may be managed by placement of an ultra-thin bandage soft contact lens. Antibiotic coverage and careful follow-up are essential. Full-thickness lacerations larger than 2 or 3 mm or irregular lacerations usually require direct suturing under a microscope. General anesthesia is employed to obviate the necessity for

THERAPY

Surgical. Surgical treatment consists of reattachment of the lacerated ends of the muscles or tendon as soon as possible after exploration of the injury site. When a muscle is lacerated either at or near the insertion, the muscle capsule and attachment to the posterior Tenon's capsule prevent the muscle from retracting deeply into the orbit. If no muscle tissue can be found for reattachment to the insertion or cut end of the muscle, a muscle transfer may be indicated.

Full tendon transfer of the two adjacent rectus muscles may be done with retention of the anterior ciliary artery in the remaining rectus muscles. If any reason exists for concern about postoperative anterior segment ischemia, a muscle tendon splitting technique with the muscle bellies joined by a slip of proline-reinforced bank sclera might be indicated. If the passive duction test is restricted, disinsertion of the antagonist of the transected muscle, followed by a scleral augmented muscle transfer, should be done, even in a young patient. This allows retention of at least one anterior ciliary artery. Injection of 2.5 to 10 units of botulinum A toxin may be made at the myoneural junction of the antagonist muscle instead of carrying out a recession. Laceration of the superior oblique tendon may be treated as a superior oblique paralysis.

Ocular or Periocular Manifestations

Anterior Chamber: Abnormal angle; hyphema.
Conjunctiva: Chemosis; laceration; subconjunctival hemorrhages.
Cornea: Edema; opacity.
Extraocular Muscles: Paralysis of third or sixth nerve.
Eyelids: Blepharospasm; ecchymosis; edema.
Other: Blowout orbital fracture; cataract; diplopia; ocular pain; optic nerve or retinal hemorrhages; photophobia; strabismus.

PRECAUTIONS

Dilation of the pupil and meticulous examination of the globe are necessary to rule out associated injury to the globe. Determination of visual acuity and retinal examination should always be done. If foreign bodies or fractures are suspected, x-ray studies should be considered.

COMMENTS

One of the major problems facing an ophthalmologist in the diagnosis of extraocular muscle laceration is whether a muscle is lacerated or trauma to the nerve has occurred. A lacerated muscle requires immediate attention. On the other hand, trauma to the nerves may spontaneously recover with time. Patients who have normal binocular cooperation before extraocular muscle injury can withstand significant insult to motility and retain good fusion if alignment is reestablished in a portion of the field.

References

Helveston EM: Atlas of Strabismus Surgery, 2nd ed. St. Louis, CV Mosby, 1977, p. 96.
Helveston EM, Grossman RD: Extraocular muscle lacerations. Am J Ophthalmol 81:754–760, 1976.
Helveston EM, Merriam W, Ellis FD: Extraocular muscle-tendon transfer with scleral augmentation. Am J Ophthalmol 89:819–823, 1980.
Mailer CM: Avulsion of the inferior rectus. Can J Ophthalmol 9:262–266, 1974.

EYELID CONTUSIONS, LACERATIONS, AND AVULSIONS

ROBERT C. DELLA ROCCA, M.D., F.A.C.S.,
and John Nassif, M.D.
New York, New York

Eyelid contusions, lacerations, and avulsions associated with blunt or sharp trauma to the adnexa and orbital region may lead to permanent and severe functional or structural abnormalities. Prompt evaluation, recognition, and treatment will allow for appropriate repair, satisfactory healing, renewed lid function, and ocular protection.

Lacerations or avulsion of the lids and canthi can lead to sequelae, such as lid malposition, severe scarring, lacrimal dysfunction, ptosis, and chronic ocular problems. Effective treatment may minimize these secondary problems. Definitive repair of traumatic ptosis, lacrimal obstruction, and motility problems can be delayed up to 6 to 12 months after injury because partial or complete resolution may occur during this period. If motility abnormalities or globe malposition is seen, an orbital floor fracture should be suspected and appropriately managed.

THERAPY

Supportive. A careful history determining the time, circumstances, and type of injury is obtained. Ocular evaluation is essential. Evaluation of visual acuity, pupillary reaction, motility status, slitlamp microscopy, and ophthalmoscopy should be completed. Initial evaluation of the patient 8 to 12 hours after injury requires delayed primary repair of the laceration or avulsion. If there is the suspicion that an ocular or orbital foreign body exists, ultrasonography, radiography, and CT scanning are indicated. Orbital x-rays including Waters' and intermediate views, are done when periorbital and adnexal trauma is severe to rule out orbital fractures.

Although each wound is somewhat different, the application of a few basic principles of wound management is useful. Initially, attempts to alleviate pain, reduce swelling, and prevent drying of the wound should be made. Plain gauze moistened with saline is useful in preventing dryness of the wound; detergent solutions should be avoided.

With a relatively clean wound, débridement can be accomplished with irrigation, using copious amounts of saline. The heavily contaminated wound (with debris) may be cleaned with saline and perhaps a small brush. Foreign material should be removed from the wound. Irregularities at the wound margin should be smoothed. Doing so may require excision of a small amount of tissue and should be judiciously done when the laceration is near important structures, such as the lacrimal gland or canaliculi.

It is necessary to ask the patient or family when tetanus immunization was last received. Tetanus may occur even in patients with minor lesions, but is more common after contamination of deep wounds that contain devitalized tissue. The need for active immunization with tetanus toxoid or passive immunization with tetanus immune globulin is determined both by the patient's immunization history and nature of the wound. Except in individuals with three or more doses of recent tetanus immunization, tetanus toxoid is administered when the wound is cleaned and relatively minor. It is combined with tetanus immune globulin when the wound is severe. If it has been 5 years since the last immunization, tetanus toxoid should be given again after injury, even though the patient has received three or more doses of tetanus immunization in the past.

Human and animal bites that cause lacerations of the adnexa present special problems. With animal bites, primary repair of the laceration or avulsion can be done after prompt irrigation and débridement. Repair of human bites, which are more dangerous, is delayed for several days. The use of deep sutures should be avoided when possible with human bites. Tetanus prophylaxis and broad-spectrum antibiotics are used when treating these problems.

Surgical. Surgical technique should include adequate subcutaneous closure, careful eversion of the skin edges, and good approximation of the wound margins. Tension at the wound surface should be avoided.

Whenever possible, primary repair is recommended. If significant bacterial contamination as in crushing injuries, neglected wounds (wounds evaluated 12 or more hours after injury), and human bites is suspected, delayed primary repair is advised. In this instance, the wound is cleaned with forced saline irrigation, left open, and dressed. Three to four days later, surgical débridement and delayed primary repair are completed. If marked lid edema or facial swelling obscures the extent and details of the injury, delayed repair is considered. Secondary repair allowing for the formation of granulation tissue may be necessary when there is extensive tissue loss. Secondary reconstruction can be delayed if the globe is appropriately protected.

Partial-thickness lid lacerations are repaired with 6-0 silk or 6-0 nylon interrupted sutures. Rarely is it necessary to suture lacerated orbicularis muscle or orbital septum. Vertical traction near the lid margin should especially be avoided to limit the possibility of late ectropion.

Full-thickness lid lacerations require a three-layered closure. First, the lid margin is repaired with 5-0 or 6-0 silk sutures. The first deep suture is placed near the mucocutaneous junction to approximate the posterior aspect of the lid margin. The second suture is placed through the anterior aspect of the lid margin. One or two more sutures complete repair of the margin. The anterior tarsal margins are approximated with 5-0 plain sutures. They are passed partial thickness through the tarsal wound edge margins and tied. With this technique, sutures are not placed through the conjunctiva. The skin is closed with 6-0 silk sutures.

Full-thickness tissue loss involving more than one third of the lid requires the use of lateral cantholysis. The inferior crux of the tendon in the lower lid is lysed to facilitate mobilization of the lid. A skin flap is made to help relax the posterior aspect of the lid (muscle, tarsus, and conjunctiva). Tissue loss involving more than one third of the lid may require a temporal sliding myocutaneous flap after cantholysis. Pedicle lid grafts (modified Hughes or Beard procedures) may be necessary if there has been more extensive loss of lid substance, including the lid margins. The modified Hughes and Beard procedures are used for reconstruction of the lower and upper lids, respectively.

Late contracture and secondary lid malposition of the lids following repair of complicated lacerations can be avoided. With extensive lid lacerations, a temporary tarsorrhaphy or modified Frost suture passed through the involved lid margin for traction may be helpful in maintaining fornix depth while limiting lid retraction. The tarsorrhaphy or sutures may be left in place for 14 to 21 days as indicated.

If there is minimal postoperative wound elevation or irregularity, massaging the wound can be helpful. This can be done with moist cotton or gauze, perhaps over a drop of mineral oil. If scar hypertrophy or perhaps early keloid formation is detected, the use of intradermal steroids can be effective. When intralesional injection with steroids is indicated, triamcinolone is used (40 mg/ml for lesions involving the lids). For 5 mm of scar, 0.1 ml of steroid is injected with a tuberculin syringe. It may be necessary to repeat the injection up to five times, once every 3 to 4 weeks. Treatment of the scar should be uniform. Depigmentation is a complication of this treatment, and darkly pigmented individuals should be alerted to this possibility. The results of steroid injection, sometimes combined with surgical scar removal, can be rewarding.

Lacerations in the medial canthal region are repaired primarily with 5-0 nylon or silk sutures. Inferior traction on the medial aspect of the lid on commissure should be avoided. If this should develop, the use of full skin grafts from the upper lids or postauricular region is necessary. Subcutaneous cicatrical tissue must be excised before the graft can be sutured into position. A succession of Z-plasties is useful in treating scars that are away from the lid margin.

If the lid is avulsed medially, the avulsed portion should be attached to the medial canthal tendon with 4-0 or 5-0 prolene suture. Wire wedged on a spatula needle can be effective in stabilizing the lid position medially.

Lacrimal sac or common canalicular injury is suspected with severe eyelid contusions, lacerations, or avulsions that occur medially. After assessing the degree of injury and anatomic disruption, the lacrimal system is evaluated. Canalicular lacerations are repaired with the aid of surgical microscope by monocanalicular or bicanalicular intubation. With monocanalicular intubation, the tubing is passed through the identified margins of the lacerated canaliculus and into the lacrimal sac. It is then fixed in position. Repair of the lid laceration is completed after the intubation has been completed.

Definitive repair of lacrimal sac obstruction secondary to trauma is delayed until at least 4 to 6 months after injury. Of course, the onset of recurrent acute dacryocystitis may require earlier repair. A dacryocystorhinostomy or perhaps conjunctival dacryocystorhinostomy may be necessary at that time.

If a laceration through the upper lid has involved the levator aponeurosis, immediate repair of the aponeurosis should be attempted. Careful separation of the anatomic layers and identification of the medical and lateral horns of the superior transverse (Whitnall's) ligament are helpful in completing this repair. If the patient with ptosis is evaluated several weeks after injury, delayed repair of ptosis is advised. It should be done at least 6 months after injury.

If there is extensive or deep tissue loss in the medial canthal region, advancement glabella flaps or combined advancement and rotation myocutaneous flaps are useful. If tissue loss extends down to bone, median frontal flaps are reasonably effective.

Laceration or avulsion of the lateral aspect of the lower lid may lead to severe ectropion and displacement of the lids. Restoration of lid position is contingent upon re-establishing lateral support. When the injury is extensive, it is very difficult to identify the torn lateral canthal tendon. A substitute tendon can be made by reflecting a tongue of periosteum from the zygoma at a level above the lateral commissure and attaching the lateral lid margin to the periosteum with 4-0 prolene suture or fine gauge wire. The repaired lateral canthal angle may initially be higher than normal, allowing for some sagging within a few months.

The establishment of satisfactory medial and lateral canthal position is very important. This is a necessary step in the reconstruction process and will avoid such problems as ectropion, lid retraction, and possibly epiphora.

Ocular or Periocular Manifestations

Eyelids: Edema; lid malposition and globe exposure; scarring; traumatic ptosis.

Other: Keratoconjunctivitis sicca; lacrimal obstruction; orbital hemorrhage; restricted motility.

PRECAUTIONS

Careful suturing techniques with good wound approximation are of paramount importance in limiting unsatisfactory scarring and perhaps secondary lid deformities. Initially, sacrificing tissue should be avoided, although its vitality may be questionable.

Orbital compression secondary to hemorrhage must be promptly treated. A lateral canthotomy, allowing for some relaxation of the lids, may not be completely successful. If there is marked or resistant compression, a 1.5-cm incision extending laterally from the lateral commissure is made down to the periosteum.

The periosteum over the anterior aspect of the zygoma is incised vertically. An incision is made through the periorbita, and the retrobulbar hemorrhage and clot are evacuated.

COMMENTS

When significant injury to the lids has occurred, the extent of tissue loss should be determined first. Although avulsed lid tissue may be discolored and appear devitalized, it can usually be grafted back into the lid. Fortunately, adnexal circulation is excellent, thereby enhancing lid reconstruction even when the tissues have been severely traumatized. If avulsions or lacerations are extensive, the use of 4-0 silk sutures to fix tissue in proper position is helpful in an emergency room setting. The wound should be covered with a slightly moistened dressing (sterile saline) before definitive surgery is scheduled.

Protection of the globe, maintenance of tissue vitality, and re-establishment of lid function are important priorities. Further reconstructive and cosmetic procedures, such as skin grafting, scar revision, and ptosis repair, can be scheduled at a later date as indicated.

References

Chang WHJ: Wound management. *In* Chang WHJ (ed): Fundamentals of Plastic and Reconstructive Surgery. Baltimore, Williams & Wilkins, 1980, pp 9–63.

Smith BC, et al (eds): Ophthalmic Plastic and Reconstructive Surgery. St. Louis, CV Mosby, 1987, pp 417–472.

Tessier P, et al: Symposium on Plastic Surgery in the Orbital Region. St. Louis, CV Mosby, 1976, pp 8–17, 39–78, 129–140.

Tessier P, et al: Plastic Surgery of the Orbit and Eyelids. New York, Masson, 1981, pp 328–362.

INDIRECT GLOBAL RUPTURES AND SHARP SCLERAL INJURIES

WILLIAM H. COLES, M.D., M.S.
Buffalo, New York

Indirect scleral rupture results from concussive injuries to the globe with subsequent tears in the ocular coats, usually the sclera. The presence of hyphema (especially if the blood has clotted), increased depth of the anterior chamber, and low intraocular pressure are important signs in the diagnosis of indirect scleral ruptures. Low intraocular pressure may be variable, and the presence of normal or high intraocular pressure does not rule out the possibility of a scleral rupture if other signs are present. Other important signs include limitation of gaze in the field of rupture near the rectus muscle insertion, which is a common site for rupture, and chemosis of the conjunctiva, which may be localized or generalized. This chemosis is fairly distinctive and is usually not associated with direct trauma to the conjunctival area. Ultrasound and CT scanning can help locate the site of rupture and degree of associated damage. With CT scans, a flattening of the normal curved posterior globe, a thickened sclera, intraocular air, vitreous hemorrhage and opacification, or disruption of the scleral coat should be sought.

Direct scleral injuries are the result of penetrating injuries from a sharp or pointed object. Penetrating scleral wounds are usually accompanied by a history of trauma that the patient readily provides. Penetration of the globe by objects most commonly occurs anteriorly because the orbital bones protect posteriorly. Posterior penetrating injuries can occur from bones fractured in the surrounding orbit. Penetrating objects through the brow or lids or from gunshot wounds to the temple region may be responsible for posterior wounds.

THERAPY

Supportive. Immediate management of scleral injuries includes the following: protection of the eye by a firm shield until repair is possible; tetanus protection if indicated; and systemic antibiotics, although the need for them is not proved.

Surgical. After the initial suturing, surgical therapy for blunt injuries with rupture usually requires a secondary procedure. The extent of retinal and choroidal damage is determined, and repair is undertaken if the prognosis indicates its need. If vitreous hemorrhage is present, aggravation of the fibrotic process may make surgery more urgent. These operations require vitrectomy instrumentation inserted through a pars plana approach. Scleral buckles are almost routine after this type of surgery.

Sharp penetrating injuries anterior to the equator are always repaired. In double perforating injuries with small posterior exit wounds after suturing the anterior wounds, repair is frequently not necessary if the posterior wound is smaller than 2 to 3 mm. Scleral wounds are usually sutured with nonabsorbable sutures.

Systemic. Systemic steroids to delay reaction are used in injuries with high risks of fibrotic contraction.

PRECAUTIONS

The most important precaution in both penetrating and blunt injury is recognition of the presence of hemorrhage as a poor prognostic factor. Hemorrhage is both a source of fibrosis and an aggravating influence on fibrosis in the posterior part of the eye. If this dense contracting fibrosis is not treated, it can cause total disruption of the structural integrity of the eye and eventual visual loss.

COMMENTS

Penetrating and blunt trauma with rupture of the globe can be a devastating process. In both types of injury, the initial insult is followed by a healing process. It is this healing process that gets out of control and eventually causes loss of the eye. Tracks through the vitreous provide sources of fibroblast growth and a framework for subsequent organization. This process can be significantly established within a few week. If the vitreous is not removed sooner than 14 days postinjury, the technical aspects of removal become more difficult.

Whether immediate or delayed vitrectomy is correct for penetrating injuries is controversial. In penetrating injuries where there is little associated contusive injury, immediate surgery can be done with few risks of complications. However, when a significant contusive injury has occurred as in a blunt rupture or penetrating injury with a blunt foreign object, early surgery can be complicated by bleeding during the surgery. The vitreous detachment that will occur in these injuries after a few days can make removal of the vitreous technically easier, especially in younger patients. In these cases, waiting up to 10 days is advised before initiating surgery.

Injury in children can be more devastating than in adults for a number of reasons. The fibrosis can be far more massive and rapid. Even more important is the need to establish the best visual stimulus early to prevent amblyopia. In children, aggressive therapy without delay is often indicated.

References

Abrams GW, Topping TM, Machemer R: Vitrectomy for injury. The effect on intraocular proliferation following perforation of the posterior segment of the rabbit eye. Arch Ophthalmol 97:743–748, 1979.

Cherry PMH: Indirect traumatic rupture of the globe. Arch Ophthalmol 96:252–256, 1978.

Cleary PE, Ryan SJ: Experimental posterior penetrating eye injury in the rabbit. II. Histology of wound, vitreous, and retina. Br J Ophthalmol 63:312–321, 1979.

Cleary PE, Ryan SJ: Vitrectomy in penetrating eye injury. Results of a controlled trial of vitrectomy in an experimental posterior penetrating eye injury in the rhesus monkey. Arch Ophthalmol 99:287–292, 1981.

Coles WH, Haik GM: Vitrectomy in intraocular trauma. Its rationale and its indications and limitations. Arch Ophthalmol 87:621–628, 1972.

Conway BP, Michels RG: Vitrectomy techniques in the management of selected penetrating ocular injuries. Ophthalmology 85:560–583, 1978.

Hanscom T, Kreiger AE: Late vitrectomy in double perforating ocular injuries. Ophthalmic Surg 10:78–80, 1979.

Meredith TA, Gordon PA: Pars plana vitrectomy for severe penetrating injury with posterior segment involvement. Am J Ophthalmol 103:549–554, 1987.

Michels RG, Conway BP: Vitreous surgery techniques in penetrating ocular trauma. Trans Ophthalmol Soc UK 98:472–480, 1978.

Pilkerton AR, et al: Experimental vitreous fibroplasia following perforating ocular injuries. Arch Ophthalmol 97:1707–1709, 1979.

Russell SR, Olsen KR, Folk JC: Predictors of scleral rupture and the role of bitrectomy in severe blunt ocular trauma. Am J Ophthalmol 105:253–257, 1988.

Tolentino FO, et al: Vitrectomy in penetrating ocular trauma: An experimental study using rabbits. Ann Ophthalmol 11:1763–1771, 1979.

IRIS LACERATIONS, HOLES, AND IRIDODIALYSIS

HELLMUT F. NEUBAUER, M.D.
Cologne, West Germany

Iris lacerations, holes, and iridodialysis usually occur secondary to concussive or penetrating injuries. Although tears or holes in the stromal or interstitial tissues of the iris are frequent, they are often difficult to locate unless they are at lest 1 mm in size and the defect includes the pigment epithelium. These tears or holes are usually of little clinical significance unless they are of considerable size. If bleeding should occur in conjunction with the tear, it is often minimal and self-limited. Wounds in the iris form fibrous tissue slowly following trauma; therefore, healing is minimal and occurs primarily when the wound margins are in apposition. Tears or lacerations in the pupillary zone most commonly involve the sphincter, stromal, and pigmented epithelial layers. If only the stromal layer is torn, no permanent pupillary dysfunction will result, and only a few residual iris frills or tags will be detected. However, if the sphincter is involved, a characteristic triangular defect will be seen, with the apex toward the periphery. The pupil is typically irregular, is dilated or semidilated, and has abnormal sphincter reactions to stimulation. The portion of the sphincter not involved in the laceration functions normally. Hyphema may be associated with a tear of the sphincter, but if this is the sole origin of bleeding, it usually causes no major problems. A flattened or misshapen pupil results from iridodialysis. Severe hemorrhages may be associated with iridodialysis, resulting from tears in the iris feeder vessels, which cross this zone in a radial fashion or from extension of the laceration into the ciliary body. Iridodialysis may be small and slitlike or large, and single or multiple. Areas of iris atrophy may accompany these tears.

THERAPY

Supportive. Rest and observation are preliminary measures in patients with iridodialysis. The iridodialysis itself seldom requires treatment, unless the dialysis is of sufficient size to cause visual confusion owing to the irregular diffusion of light or unless the dialysis, acting as a second pupil, allows the formation of a second image, with the development of uniocular diplopia. In these patients, operative measures may be indicated, but such corrective measures should be deferred until the vision is stable. Since McCannel's technique for refixation of the iris has only minor risks, this operation may also be done for cosmetic reasons in special cases. However, an opaque contact lens with clear optic may be tried before surgical measures are undertaken.

Surgical. Treatment depends on the individual situation and the extent of tissue damage. However, in all cases one needs to restore optimal optic conditions. Reposition of the iris is certain in the smaller fresh incarceration without basic tissue damage. If the iris continues to incarcerate in the limbal area after an otherwise favorable reposition, a small basal iridectomy should be done in that area.

A primary iris suture without tissue excision should be considered when a smooth radial laceration is present. If the iris injury is irregular and a large portion of the iris tissue is damaged with loss of the pigment layer, the iris suture should be performed after excision of the damaged tissue. The purposes of these measures are to restore a reasonably useful pupil and avoid constant blurring.

The sector iridectomy should be considered only when a large iris incarceration persists for longer than 24 hours. Considerable loss of pigment and the impossibility of restoration of a useful pupil should also be evident. The decision is easier when a sector iridectomy occurs under the upper lid. Iris bleeding can be controlled either by wet-field cautery, by grasping the small vessel with Barraquer iris forceps and touching the forceps with diathermy, or by a 10-0 nylon suture.

For iridodialysis occurring in a blunt injury without cataract, McCannel's operation should be performed secondarily, when the eye has recovered from the injury. A repair can be made by passing a 10-0 monofilament suture on its needle into the iris angle under a small conjunctival flap opposite the dialysis tear. The needle is continued from the angle root, into the posterior chamber, and under the edge of the torn iris and proceeds vertically across the anterior chamber and through the cornea. A small, narrow limbal keratome incision is made beside the suture, just at the corneoscleral junction. A small blunt iris hook is slipped through this incision and moved across the anterior chamber to engage the previously placed vertical suture, which is drawn out in a loop. The corneal suture is then cut flush at its exit, and its loop is pulled out in a single strand. The two ends are then tied, and as the knot is drawn down firmly, it pulls the torn edge of the iris securely into the iris root cleft. A second suture can be placed in a similar manner, and even a third and fourth if the iridodialysis is large. If the distance between the iris root and the natural place of its fixation is large, the filling of the anterior chamber by transient sodium hyalonurate will stretch the iris and facilitate the maneuver. This technique may also help in primary wound surgery (e.g., in closing a subconjunctival scleral rupture) to bring the incarcerated iris into its normal position by a spatula.

If a contusion cataract is present, iridopexy is performed together with the cataract extraction. Only in corneoscleral lacerations with or without cataract should one consider performing the iridopexy at the same time as the wound is treated.

Ocular or Periocular Manifestations

Anterior Chamber: Cells and flare; hyphema.
Iris or Ciliary Body: Anterior uveitis; atrophy; hemorrhages; iridoplegia; pigmentary deposits; sphincter stromal tear.
Lens: Pigmentary deposits; Vossius' ring.
Pupil: Constriction; cycloplegia; deformed margins; dilation; notching.
Other: Corneal pigmentary deposits; decreased accommodation; diplopia; photophobia.

PRECAUTIONS

Often, injuries resulting in a torn or lacerated iris also involve other areas of the eye. These areas must be identified. In the case of serious damage to the anterior segment, injuries involving the cornea, sclera, iris, lens, vitreous, and even the retina must be handled in the correct order. The surgeon must be able to devise a plan for each individual case.

The presence and exact location of an iridodialysis should be noted in the record, since recurrence of bleeding or hyphema may arise from the ciliary body at the site of the iridodialysis. One should be certain to perform McCannel's operation for iridodialysis only after the eye has recovered from the injury, because functional success is endangered by the traumatic iritis. In treating iridodialysis, there is a risk of producing a recurrent hyphema, since the incision may have to pass through a proliferative scar from the original injury. A period of observation is usually necessary following iridodialysis to determine if associated ocular injuries are present. The iridodialysis itself rarely causes problems; however, recessed-angle glaucoma may occur months or years after the initial injury.

COMMENTS

The mechanism of the production of iris lacerations following contusions involves several factors. The most important of these are dilation of the corneoscleral ring occurring in compensation for the anteroposterior compression of the globe; the prompt and marked contraction of the sphincter of the iris, which occurs immediately on the application of blunt trauma to the cornea whether or not a posttraumatic mydriasis develops; the impact of the compression wave of aqueous that forces the iris into the lens and the lateral displacement of the aqueous; and possibly a rebound of the lens from the vitreous against which it is thrust, an action that may distend the iris. It is possible that some or all of these forces acting simultaneously and momentarily may produce different end results, depending on the relative strength of each in a particular case.

One should not forget that even cyclodialysis may be observed following concussive injury. In cases of marked hypotony, refixation of the ciliary body could become necessary.

References

Foster CS, Mark DB: Uveal prolapse. *In* Heilmann K, Paton D (ed): Atlas of Ophthalmic Surgery, Vol II, New York, Thieme Medical Publishers, 1987, pp 5.23–5.25.

Hanna C, Roy FH: Iris wound healing. Arch Ophthalmol 88:296–304, 1972.

Mackensen G: Korrektur einer postkontusionellen Iridodialyse. *In* Mackensen G, Neubauer H (ed) Augenaerztliche Operationen, Vol I, Berlin, Springer, 1988, pp. 623–626.

McCannel MA: A retrievable suture idea for anterior uveal problems. Ophthalmic Surg 7:98–103, 1976.

Neubauer H: Treatment of major trauma of the anterior segment: With a discussion of more radical primary surgery. Trans Ophthalmol Soc UK 95:322–325, 1975.

Paton D, Craig J: Management of iridodialysis. Ophthalmic Surg 4:38–39, 1973.

Runyan TE: Concussive and Penetrating Injuries of the Globe and Optic Nerve. St. Louis, CV Mosby, 1975, pp 61–63.

Waubke Th N, Mellin KB: Behandlung von Irisverletzungen. *In* Mackensen G, Neubauer H (ed) Augenaerztliche Operationen, Vol II. Berlin, Springer, pp. 570–573.

LACRIMAL SYSTEM CONTUSIONS AND LACERATIONS

BENJAMIN MILDER, M.D.
St. Louis, Missouri

Because of the superficial location of the lacrimal canaliculi, any traumatic insult to the medial canthus may interrupt the lacrimal drainage system. Any laceration of the nasal one third of the eyelids may likewise impair tear drainage as a result of direct injury to the puncta, the canaliculi, or the lacrimal sac. Eyelid injuries may also disrupt lacrimal excretion indirectly by interfering with the "pumping action" of the orbicularis muscle or by altering the position of the punctum in relation to the globe. Cicatrization following injuries to the lids may produce ectropion or stenosis of the punctum. Fractures of the orbit may produce deformity or obliteration of the lacrimal sac or nasolacrimal duct, with subsequent obstructive dacryocystitis. Nasomaxillary fractures resulting from frontal injury and involving the lacrimal bone may result in a purulent dacryocystitis and fistulization to the skin surface. Discontinuity of the membranous nasolacrimal duct may result in the formation of fistulas emptying into the antrum or the nasal cavity. Although occasional cysts or fistulas occur in the lacrimal gland, such injury is rare, since the gland is protected by the bony orbital rim and the secretion occurs from multiple sources.

THERAPY

Systemic. Although the principal concern of the surgeon is the repair of damaged tissues and restoration of function, the first considerations in severe trauma should be medical. In grossly contaminated injuries, prophylactic broad-spectrum antibiotics should be administered at the outset. A suitable broad-spectrum program would include daily intravenous administration of 5 mg/kg of gentamicin. This should be combined with 250 mg of oral cephalexin four times daily. The surgeon must judge whether 0.5 ml of tetanus toxoid is indicated.

Surgical. All severed canaliculi must be repaired over a stent. Silicone tubing is currently favored for this purpose. It is not essential that a lacerated canaliculus be repaired immediately. In fact, waiting for 6 to 24 hours may allow for reduction of edema and some retraction of tissue so that the medial cut end of the canaliculus is better exposed to view. If this proximal cut end of the canaliculus cannot be readily identified, the intact canaliculus may be irrigated with a colored solution, such as fluorescein solution. This is instilled through the intact canaliculus under increased pressure. Although the Worst pigtail probe has disappeared, for the most part, from the surgical armamentarium, it may be helpful in identifying the cut end of the canaliculus when it is severed at or near the common canaliculus.

When silicone tubing is used, one end of the tube is threaded through the punctum and distal end of the canaliculus, continued on across the severed gap through the proximal end of the divided canaliculus and brought through the nasolacrimal duct, emerging in the inferior meatus of the nose. The free end of the silicone tube is then threaded through the intact canaliculus and brought through the nasolacrimal duct in the same fashion, so that at the conclusion of the procedure both free ends emerge from the nares and the tube is looped between the two puncta at the nasal angle of the lids. After this silicone stent is in position, the severed ends of the canaliculus are then approximated under microscopic control, using three interrupted 8-0 absorbable sutures. The lid margin is then approximated, and the posterior and skin surfaces of the lid laceration are closed. Finally, a mattress suture is threaded into the nasal end of the tarsus and drawn across the laceration, to be anchored at the periosteum in the region of the insertion of the medial canthal tendon. This mattress suture and the stent should remain in place for 3 weeks.

After the lacerated canaliculus has been intubated, if the free end of the silicone stent cannot be drawn through the intact canaliculus, it may be fastened to the end emerging from the naris at the nasolabial fold.

If the punctum is involved in a canalicular laceration, careful repair around the stent should be undertaken. If the punctum remains patent, but is open and in contact with the tear lake, adequate function may be restored. Compression of the canaliculus in the act of blinking is a more significant physiologic element in tear excretion than is the capillary action at the punctum.

Stenosis of the canaliculus may result from injury. If the axial extent of the stenosis is minimal, it may be possible to penetrate this occlusion with a punctum dilator, insert a stent, and leave it in place for 3 to 8 weeks in order to ensure continued patency. If the stenosis is more extensive or if a large section of the canaliculus is missing, reconstructive surgery is rarely successful. Careful evaluation of lacrimal outflow function is required because the patient may have adequate outflow through the intact punctum and canaliculus of the opposite lid. If this is not possible, an alternate route for tear elimination must be established. The preferred method is conjunctivodacryocystorhinostomy, after the method of Jones, with insertion of a Pyrex glass tube as a permanent stent.

In patients with stenosis of the punctum and a relatively intact canaliculus, every effort should be made to re-establish patency of the punctum. Once again, the silicone stent is indicated. If it is unsuccessful in keeping the punctum open, a punctumplasty should be performed using the three-snip method or the punch technique. In the three-snip operation, the punctum is dilated and a snip 2 mm long is made with scissors in the canaliculus, parallel to and near the inner margin of the lid. Two more snips are made, beginning at opposite ends of the initial cut and continued downward so as to meet inferiorly. These snips produce a gaping opening on the posterior surface of the eyelid, involving the punctum and the vertical limb of the canaliculus and placing this opening in contact with the tear lake. The same result can be achieved using a Holth scleral punch, by inserting the male blade of the punch into the vertical limb of the canaliculus and the female blade on the conjunctival aspect of the eyelid.

If the common canaliculus is stenosed by trauma, the silicone tubing technique should be employed after first penetrating the stenotic area with a slender punctum dilator or a stainless steel lacrimal probe. Here, too, the silicone tube should be left in place for an extended period of time, usually 3 to 8 weeks. If the canaliculus closes after removal of the stent, it can be reinserted for an additional period.

If the lower punctum is everted, with or without stenosis, the three-snip or Holth punch punctumplasty may be effective in restoring the drainage of tears. The ectropion of the lower punctum may require excision of a diamond-shaped or spindle-shaped segment of conjunctiva and tarsal plate. The excised segment should be 8 mm long and 5 mm wide and the defect closed with 6-0 silk sutures.

If the medial canthal tendon is avulsed and displaced in a fracture, it should be reattached either by direct or transnasal wiring. If there was no accompanying dacryocystitis after restoration of the position of the medial canthus, lacrimal excretory function should be tested, dacryocystograms performed, and a decision made on the basis of these findings as to whether or not dacryocystorhinostomy is necessary. If dacryocystitis is present, these procedures may be performed at the same operative session.

If the nasolacrimal duct is deformed or obliterated with subsequent dacryocystitis, a probe should be passed through the upper canaliculus, tear sac, and nasolacrimal duct and identified in the inferior meatus of the nose at the time of fracture reduction. This method aids in determining whether the bones are adequately positioned. The dacryocystitis is managed by dacryocystorhinostomy.

The surgical treatment of traumatic lacrimal fistula is dacryocystorhinostomy with excision of the fistulous track. It is important to stress that traumatic lacrimal fistulas, or diverticulae, require careful dacryocystography to establish the site of obstruction and the course of the fistula.

Ocular or Periocular Manifestations

Lacrimal System: Avulsion of medial canthal tendon; cicatrization; cyst of lacrimal gland; dacryocystitis; disruption of nasolacrimal duct; ectropion of puncta; epiphora; fistula of lacrimal gland or sac; stenosis of canaliculi or puncta.

Precautions

Interruption of the nasolacrimal duct should be suspected in any injury involving the middle third of the face, especially the ocular adnexa. Early recognition and prompt treatment are the keys to successful results. In particular, any injury in the medial canthal area should be carefully inspected. The disturbance caused by complete stenosis of the lacrimal canaliculus may be minimal in elderly persons, and if this is confirmed by low Schirmer readings, surgery may not be required.

Comments

Because injury to the lacrimal apparatus usually produces gross abnormality of the tissue or obvious functional disturbances, the sensitive tests of drainage function are not often required for immediate diagnosis. Repair of a canaliculus is not always successful, but is worth attempting. However, the closer the laceration is to the punctum, the higher the probability is for a successful surgical repair. If only the upper canaliculus is injured, there is little likelihood of epiphora resulting. Occasionally, a patient whose lower canaliculus has been irreversibly damaged manages well with the upper canaliculus alone.

References

Bennett JE: The lacrimal drainage system. *In* Duane TD (ed): Clinical Ophthalmology. Hagerstown, MD, Harper & Row, 1982, Vol V, pp 11:1–8.
Bohigian GM: Handbook of External Diseases of the Eye. Fort Worth, Alcon, 1980, p 163.
Haik BG: Teflon sleeve cannalicular. AJO *106*:367, 1988.
Harris GJ, et al: Lacrimal intubation in the primary repair of midfacial fractures. Ophthalmology 94:242–247, 1987.
Nagashima K, et al: Relative roles of upper and lower lacrimal canaliculi in normal tear drainage: Jpn J Ophthalmol 28:259–262, 1984.
Paton D, Goldberg MF: Management of Ocular Injuries. Philadelphia, WB Saunders, 1976, pp 52–58.
Romano PE: Single silicone intubation for repair of single canaliculus laceration. Ann Ophthal *18*:112, 1986.
Zagora E: Eye Injuries. Springfield, IL, Charles C Thomas, 1970, pp 164–168.

STRIPPING OR DETACHMENT OF DESCEMET'S MEMBRANE
RICHARD P. KRATZ, M.D.
Newport Beach, California

Detachment of Descemet's membrane is usually one of the unreported complications of ocular surgery because it seldom results in a visual complication. Small detachments are frequently not noticed, and since the endothelial cells enlarge and cover the defect, it is spontaneously repaired before a final refraction is completed. The incidence has been listed by Hessburg as 1.4 per cent with anterior chamber implants. A 0.5 per cent incidence was reported by Emery in phacoemulsification, and Dowlut and Brunet reported a 0.5 per cent incidence in intracapsular surgery without any intraocular lens implantation.

Descemet's membrane is the basement membrane of the cornea and increases in thickness with age. It inserts at Schwalbe's line, which is approximately at the location of the limbal blood vessel arcade. It is loosely attached to the overlying stroma and is covered by a single layer of endothelial cells that probably do not undergo mitosis and have the important function of maintaining corneal clarity. Usually, there are about 2000 cells/square millimeter, but corneal decompensation occurs when the number drops to about 500 cells/square millimeter. Therefore, it is important not to detach Descemet's membrane because of the resultant loss of endothelial cells.

By far, the most common time for occurrence of Descemet's membrane *detachment* is *during cataract surgery*. A mechanical stripping of Descemet's membrane may occur as instruments enter the anterior chamber, and the frequency is increased when blunt instruments are used. Descemet's membrane is very tough; however, if blunt pressure is applied, it can be separated readily from the overlying stroma. Scissors used during enlargement of the section or irrigating cannulas injecting viscoelastic substances, balance salt solution, or acetylcholine may strip Descemet's membrane. One of the most common causes is stripping by the sleeve of the phacoemulsification tip or the irrigating aspirating tip. Therefore, the silicone sleeve should be tapered. Repeated entries through the incision to remove cortex increase the chance of detachment. The bevel of an irrigating cystitome may engage and strip the membrane. Therefore, whenever any instrument is inserted, one should ensure that the incision is large enough to accommodate the instrument, and the instrument should be gently pressed against the posterior lip of the incision to avoid contact with Descemet's membrane. Intraocular lenses may also engage Descemet's membrane during insertion, and detachment of Descemet's membrane can also occur during cyclodialysis, trabeculectomy, penetrating keratoplasty, or anterior chamber taps. In addition, *nonsurgical detachments* have been reported in birth injury, blunt or sharp trauma, congenital glaucoma, and keratoconus.

THERAPY

Surgical. Very small detachments often go unnoticed and are seldom seen unless there is a good red reflex. The location of the detachment is usually at the anterior edge of the surgical incision and often is not noted until a small fragment has been torn off. This usually heals without visual impairment. A slightly larger fragment may be triangular or rectangular in shape and will still be attached on one side. It is important not to mistake it for a fragment of anterior capsule and remove it by aspiration. The detached Descemet's membrane can be returned to its normal position by gentle irrigation with viscoelastic substances, balanced salt solution, or an air bubble. Viscoelastic material and an air bubble in the anterior chamber at the conclusion of the surgery also assist in the reduction of the tear. Larger detachments can be more challenging. For example, one eye with a Binkhorst intraocular lens had folded the Descemet membrane on itself so that the superior margin of the membrane was adherent to the inferior part of the iris. After 8 months and decompensation of the superior half of the cornea had occurred, the patient was referred for a corneal transplant. A puncture wound at the 6:00 o'clock limbus with gentle teasing of a cannula and instillation of air into the anterior chamber restored the membrane to its normal position; in 3 weeks, the cornea had cleared, and vision had returned to 20/30. Sometimes, it is necessary to use a blunt hook to reposition the membrane; this is best done with the aid of viscoelastic material. To hold Descemet's membrane in place, it is occasionally necessary to use a double-armed 10-0 nylon suture through and through the cornea with a knot tied on the corneal surface. In graft failure, the old graft may be removed by blunt dissection only to find the iris firmly adherent to the Descemet's membrane. It is possible to strip the Descemet's membrane free from the overlying stroma. This will create an artificial angle and restore an anterior chamber to the eye after the new graft has been sutured in place.

COMMENTS

Sometimes, a scroll of Descemet's membrane may be seen in the anterior chamber in the postoperative period. Occasionally, this scroll is attached to the iris, and sometimes a small fragment is flatly attached to the endothelium. These fragments seldom create a problem. Sometimes, a scroll of Descemet's membrane may be seen at 6:00 o'clock, touching both the iris and the endothelium. Fragments in this location should be carefully observed because they sometimes result in corneal decompensation. This can be recognized by seeing microcystic edema overlying the site of the Descemet scroll. If the microcystic edema appears to be increasing, it is necessary to remove the small fragment (which is not an easy procedure) or else complete corneal decompensation may occur.

References

Dowlut SM, Brunet M: Detachment of Descemet's membrane in cataract surgery. Can J Ophthalmol 15:122–124, 1980.

Emery JM, Wilhelmus KA, Rosenberg S: Complications of phacoemulsification. Ophthalmology 85:141–150, 1978.

Hessburg PC: Implantation of flexible anterior chamber intraocular lenses. *In* Stark W, Terry AC,

Maumenee AE (eds): Anterior Segment Surgery. IOLs, Lasers, and Refractive Keratoplasty. Baltimore, Williams & Wilkins, 1987, p 110.
Mackool RJ, Holtz SJ: Descemet membrane detachment. Arch Ophthalmol 95:459–463, 1977.
Makley TA Jr, Keates RH: Detachment of Descemet's membrane. (An early complication of cataract surgery). Ophthalmic Surg 11:189–191, 1980.
Makley TA Jr, Keates RH: Detachment of Descemet's membrane with insertion of an intraocular lens. Ophthalmic Surg 11:492–494, 1980.
O'Donnell FE Jr: Surgical techniques for extracapsular cataract extraction with expression of the nucleus. In Steele AD McG, Drews RC (eds): Cataract Surgery. London, Butterworths, 1984, pp 90, 107.
Polack FM, Binder PS: Detachment of Descemet's membrane from grafts following wound separation: Light and scanning electron microscopic study. Ann Ophthalmol 7:47–54, 1975.
Raber IM, Yanoff M: Effect of intraocular lens surgery on the cornea. In Rosen ES, Haining WM, Arnott ED (eds): Intraocular Lens Implantation. St Louis, CV Mosby, 1984, p 577.
Sugar HS: Prognosis in stripping of Descemet's membrane. Am J Ophthalmol 63:140–143, 1967.
Waring GO, Laibson PR, Rodrigues M: Clinical and pathologic alterations of Descemet's membrane: With emphasis on endothelial metaplasia. Surv Ophthalmol 18:325–368, 1974.

TRAUMATIC CATARACT
GEORGE M. GOMBOS, M.D.
Brooklyn, New York

Cataract is by far the most common complication causing loss of vision after any type of ocular injury. Traumatic cataract may result from nonperforating and perforating injury to the globe. Nonperforating trauma to the eye includes contusive or concussive injuries. Cataract development after such injuries is not unusual and may occur without any detectable damage to the lens capsule. The exact mechanism of this type of cataract is not known. Contusive or concussive forces produce waves of pressure changes that may injure the epithelial cells, lens capsule, lens fibers, or zonules. Lenticular opacifications present in a variety of forms, such as discrete punctate, scattered subepithelial changes, or rosette-shaped opacities. Most commonly, the location of these changes is anterior, frequently segmental or localized. Occasionally, late rosette opacities deep in the cortex may occur many years after the acute trauma. Contusive injury may cause a full or partial circle of iris pigment on the anterior surface of the lens capsule, which is called the Vossius ring. Opacities caused by concussive or contusive injury may be transient, static, or progressive. Such cataracts may mature suddenly any time.

In addition to the lens opacities, blunt trauma to the globe can cause subluxation or complete luxation of the lens. The striking force tears the zonules holding the lens in place behind the iris. Any contusive or concussive injury may cause instant rupture of the lens capsule, which will result in a rapid development of cataractous changes.

Perforating injury of the lens always involves other tissue injury, such as corneal or scleral perforation. Injury to any other intraocular tissue is always a possibility, although perforating injury of the globe may rupture the anterior lens capsule only. Needles, wires, darts, and other sharp objects can cause puncture wounds of the eyeball with minimal evidence of entry and anterior lens capsule damage. Occasionally, such injury causes partial opacity of the lens material but it is not progressive in nature, and the eye may retain very good visual acuity. If both the anterior and the posterior capsules are damaged, full-blown cataract formation is a strong likelihood. The progress is usually rapid. Sudden deterioration of vision to hand movement or light perception can be expected.

Traumatic cataract may present as the only significant pathology (simple traumatic cataract) or as part of an overall perforating ocular injury (complicated traumatic cataract). In the latter case, lens material is mixed with vitreous or blood or both. A secondary inflammatory process develops in almost every case. Swelling of the lens material may induce pupillary-block glaucoma. Also, lens material causes a characteristic macrophage reaction in the anterior segment of the globe. Proteinaceous material and cellular debris clog the outflow channels of the aqueous humor and raise the intraocular pressure. This condition, the combination of severe uveitis and extremely high intraocular pressure, is called phacolytic glaucoma.

THERAPY

Supportive. If the visual acuity is 20/40 or better, the cataract is nonprogressive, and the eye is quiet, no specific treatment is required. Periodic re-evaluations are suggested.

Surgical. Traumatic cataract should be operated on if visual acuity deteriorates or ocular complications exist. In cases where the traumatic cataract is part of an extensive perforating injury, immediate surgical intervention is essential. Extracapsular cataract extraction or manual or automated irrigation-aspiration techniques, are the procedures of choice. However, these simple surgical techniques are not always feasible. If the lens capsule is badly ruptured and the lens material is mixed with vitreous and blood, complete lensectomy and anterior vitrectomy are indicated. The "open sky" approach or pars plana techniques are equally acceptable; however, the open sky approach in experienced hands results in less postoperative morbidity and better visual acuity. Limbal lens extraction may be employed when the cataractous lens is subluxated or dislocated. If vitreous is present in the anterior chamber, anterior vitrectomy in conjunction with cataract extraction is the preferred surgical approach.

The use of an intraocular lens after traumatic cataract surgery is controversial. As most traumatic cataracts occur in younger ages, lens implantation might be hazardous because biodegradation of the plastic material may cause UGH (uveitis, glaucoma, hemorrhage) syndrome in later stages of life. Such advances as epikeratophakia and keratomileusis in surgical techniques and new generations of contact lenses have led to excellent visual results in unilateral aphakia, and the newer contact lenses could be excellent substitutes for an intraocular lens. However, in some selected cases, an intraocular lens is the only alternative enabling both rapid visual rehabilitation and treatment of amblyopia. In conclusion, one should remember that each traumatic injury is different, and, therefore, no dogmatic techniques or rules could apply to cataract surgery in cases of trauma.

Ocular or Periocular Manifestations

Anterior Chamber: Flare and cells; lens particles; shallow anterior chamber.
Conjunctiva: Chemosis; hemorrhage, hyperemia.
Cornea: Corneal edema; possible perforation site.
Pupil: Leukokoria.
Sclera: Possible perforation site.

PRECAUTIONS

A complete history and circumstances of the trauma must be obtained. Documentation of the place, date, and time of the injury, as well as the visual acuity, is important for medical and medicolegal purposes. The possibility of an intraocular foreign body should always be considered. Therefore, appropriate x-ray films and CT scans have to be performed when the clarity of the media does not allow complete evaluation or the history suggests an intraocular foreign body.

COMMENTS

In severe or extensive injury to the eye, almost all structures of the eye (cornea, sclera, lens, uvea, vitreous, and retina) can be involved. A recent concept, the so-called primary overall repair, is considered an important development in the management of ocular trauma. It seems to be an obsolete idea that trauma of the eyeball or traumatic cataract must be handled first by a so-called cataract specialist and that later the case is referred to a retinal or a "foreign body" specialist. The ophthalmologist who handles the anterior segment should take care of the entire eye as soon as possible. All necessary repairs should be treated in one surgical session, if feasible.

References

Bellows JG, Bellows RT: Cataract due to trauma, cataracta complicata, and displacement of the lens. A. Traumatic cataract. In Bellows JG (ed): Cataract and Abnormalities of the Lens. New York, Grune & Stratton, 1975, pp 265–272.
Bhatia IM, Panda A, Sood NN: Management of traumatic cataract. Ind J Ophthalmol 31:290–293, 1983.
Billore OP, Shroff AP, Dubey AK: Evaluation of lensectomy in traumatic cataract with perforated and non perforated eye injuries. Ind J Ophthalmol 31:585–587, 1983.
Charles S: Vitreous Microsurgery. Baltimore, Williams & Wilkins, 1981, pp 33–42.
Gombos GM: Handbook of Ophthalmologic Emergencies. New Hyde Park, NY, Medical Examination Publishing, 1977, pp 112–113, 168–169.
Jain IS, et al: Prognosis in traumatic cataract surgery. J Pediatr Ophthalmol Strabismus 16:301–305, 1979.
Morgan KS, et al: Epikeratophakia in children with traumatic cataracts. J Pediatr Ophthalmol Strabismus 23:108–114, 1986.
Paton D, Goldberg MF: Management of Ocular Injuries. Philadelphia, WB Saunders, 1976, pp 239–254.

Venom

BEE STING OF THE CORNEA
IRA G. WONG, M.D.,
and GILBERT SMOLIN, M.D.
San Francisco, California

Bee sting of the cornea occurs when the toothed lancet of the stinging apparatus penetrates the cornea. Attached to the stinger are poison sacs containing as much as 0.3 mg venom, which can produce both a toxic and immunologic reaction in the cornea. The venom contains toxin, such as melittin, apamin, and formic acid, and a potent allergen, phospholipase A.

The corneal response depends upon the amount of venom and the patient's immunologic reaction to the venom. When free of venom, the stinger is inert and can be tolerated for a long period of time. If a small amount of venom penetrates the cornea, the reaction may be minimal corneal edema and conjunctival chemosis, and hyperemia. If a large amount of venom is introduced or the patient has a hypersensitivity to the venom, a dense cellular infiltration may occur at the sting site, as well as an iritis and iridoplegia.

THERAPY

Systemic. A systemic reaction to a bee sting of the cornea has not been reported. However, a patient may have additional stings elsewhere and develop a systemic reaction. If anaphylaxis or laryngeal edema develops in a hypersensitive patient, 0.5 ml of 1:1000 epinephrine should be given intramuscularly and repeated in 5 minutes for as often as necessary. In severe reactions, the same dosage of epinephrine may be given intravenously in 10 ml of saline. Intravenous administration of 5 to 20 mg of diphenhydramine may be given after the epinephrine. Patients with severe laryngeal edema should be given 500 mg of hydrocortisone intravenously every 6 hours, and tracheostomy should be strongly considered. The patient is placed in shock position and kept warm.

Ocular. Topical instillation of one drop of 0.1 per cent epinephrine and one drop of 1 per cent prednisolone solution in the conjunctival sac should be made immediately. The prednisolone drops are continued every 2 to 3 hours, and cold compresses are applied to the eye. The stinger should be removed from the wound, with care not to express more venom into the wound by squeezing the poison sac. A prophylactic topical antibiotic may also be prescribed.

Ocular or Periocular Manifestations

Conjunctiva: Chemosis; hemorrhage; hyperemia.
Cornea: Abscess; epithelial and stromal keratitis.
Eyelids: Edema; induration.
Iris: Depigmentation; iridoplegia; iritis.
Other: Irritation; lacrimation; ocular pain.

PRECAUTIONS

If the stinger cannot be removed from the cornea or is in the anterior chamber, surgical intervention may not necessarily be needed, as the stinger is inert when free of venom. Intensive anti-inflammatory therapy should be given to treat the effects of the venom.

COMMENTS

The order Hymenoptera contains over 60,000 species that are found throughout the world. All insects of this order have a stinging apparatus located at the rear of the abdomen, through which venom is ejected. In some species, such as the honey bee, the venom apparatus may be torn away from the insect's body and remain in the prey. Stings from other Hymenoptera, such as wasps, hornets, and ants, may be treated in the same manner.

References

Duke-Elder S (ed): System of Ophthalmology, St. Louis, CV Mosby, Vol XIV, 1972, pp 1204–1207, 1346–1348.
Smolin G, Wong I: Bee sting of the cornea: Case reports. Ann Ophthalmol 14:342–343, 1982.

SPIDER BITES
F. HAMPTON ROY, M.D.
Little Rock, Arkansas

The bite of several different spiders can cause severe, even fatal systemic poisoning in humans. The most numerous of the venomous spiders are members of the genus *Latrodectus*. The venom of this genus (which includes the American black-widow spider) and of the genus *Phoneutria* is a nonhemolytic, noncytotoxic neurotoxin that produces diffuse central and peripheral nervous excitement, autonomic activity, muscle spasm, hypertension, and vasoconstriction in humans. Other symptoms may include marked abdominal rigidity, intense pain, paresthesia, headache, sweating, nausea, and facial congestion.

The venom of spiders of the *Loxosceles* genus (which includes the brown recluse spider) is a mixture of hemolysin and cytotoxin that causes ischemic necrosis at the site of the bite. The bite is often relatively painless, and the lesion is initially surrounded by a bluish-white halo of vasoconstriction that may later develop extensive gangrene. Systemic symptoms may include chills, malaise, or a scarlatiniform rash. In cases of severe envenomation, massive intravascular hemolysis, convulsions, hemoglobinuria, and acute renal failure may occur. Bites from spiders of the genus *Chiracanthium* cause similar, though milder symptoms. Tarantulas or wolf spiders of various genera, including *Lycosa* and *Phidippus*, may also cause local necrosis and ulceration in humans.

Severe systemic envenomation by the black-widow spider occasionally results in edema of the eyelids, ptosis, conjunctivitis, and constriction of the pupils. The venom of spiders of the *Phoneutria* genus may cause visual disturbances, including blindness. The bite of Australian funnel-web spiders (*Atrax robustus* and *A. formidabilis*) also results in pupillary constriction. A unique type of ocular injury is the ejection of venom into the eye by the green lynx spider (*Peucetia viridans*).

THERAPY

Supportive. For *Latrodectus* poisoning, measures should include a hot tub bath, which provides prompt, thorough temporary relief. Intravenous injection of 10 ml of 10 per cent calcium gluconate may relieve muscle cramps. However, the action of this drug is often brief, and subsequent doses have less effect than the first dose. Alternative intravenous treatment with 10 to 20 ml of methocarbamol, followed by oral administration, has been indicated. In some cases, if pain is severe, opiates may be necessary.

Persons bitten by *Loxosceles* spiders should be observed carefully and should be hospitalized if severe sequelae develop. Administration of 100 mg of hydroxyzine four times a day may alter the necrotic local lesions. Renal functions, white count, and abnormalities in coagulation should be followed. If severe hemolysis develops, renal dialysis should be begun within the initial 48 to 72 hours. Maintenance of an alkaline urine and transfusion may also be beneficial in patients with hemolysis. Broad-spectrum antibiotics given early may help localize inflammation and control secondary infection.

Nonspecific treatment consists of broad-spectrum antibiotics (systemic and local) after the wound is cleaned. Tetanus prophylaxis is indicated.

Surgical. Surgery should be considered only for large (greater than 1 cm) and deep necrotic bites of the *Loxosceles* genus, especially those extending into fat. The affected area should be excised and saucerized. Excision at the fascial level is usually sufficient. Resurfacing with split-thickness grafts, skin flaps, or pedicles are seldom indicated in orbital or lid lesions. Plastic surgery may be performed if the bite results in a cosmetically disfigured area.

Systemic. Systemic treatment of *Latrodectus* or *Loxosceles* envenomation consists of the administration of 2.5 ml of reconstituted antiserum. This is usually quite effective within a few hours.

For *Loxosceles* bites for which antivenin is unavailable, 100 mg of prednisone or 16 mg of dexamethasone should be given orally for large bites and always at the first indication of systemic envenomation. This dosage may be used daily for the first 3 days, with gradual tapering. In severe cases, an intralesional injection of 2.5 mg/ml of triamcinolone may be administered; no more than 5 mg should be infiltrated into the lesion. Antihistamines may be useful for milder lesions. The administration of heparin appears to give some protection against disseminated intravascular coagulation.

Ocular or Periocular Manifestations

Conjunctiva: Chemosis; conjunctivitis; cyanosis; edema; subconjunctival hemorrhages.
Eyelids: Edema; gangrene; necrosis; paralysis; ptosis; purpura.
Pupil: Constriction.
Retina: Cyanosis.
Other: Visual disturbances; visual loss.

PRECAUTIONS

Early excision of spider bites should only be undertaken when the spider has been identified as a brown recluse. However, only few cases require surgical care. For early surgery to be acceptable, it must be proven that the bite is destined to become one of the very rare, large, deep bites.

Potential problem cases should be recognized early. Patients at risk, such as older hypertensive patients and young children, should be hospitalized and expectantly treated with antivenin. Close supervision during the first 12 hours after the bite is important in this high-risk group; deaths due to cardiac or respiratory failure have occurred.

Because of the excellent blood supply to the eyelids, the lid margin may be spared in gangrenous eyelid processes. There is sparing of the marginal lid strip and a propensity for self-repair for lid bites.

COMMENTS

Most spiders bite humans defensively. Only a few types, including the black widow, the wandering spider, and the funnel-web spider, appear to be aggressive to any degree.

The brown recluse spider is the most dangerous of North American arachnoids and appears to be most abundant in the mid-Southern states of the United States. Bites cause only local itching without systemic signs, or there may be a local vesicle with an area of necrosis. If the area of necrosis is greater than 1 cm, there usually are mild to moderate systemic signs; if the area of necrosis is greater than 4 cm, there is definite systemic envenomation and sometimes secondary infection.

References

Edwards JJ, Anderson RL, Wood JR: Loxoscelism of the eyelids. Arch Ophthalmol 98:1997–2000, 1980.
Grant WM: Toxicology of the Eye, 2nd ed. Springfield, IL, Charles C Thomas, 1974, pp 938–939.
Minton SA Jr: Venom Diseases. Springfield, IL, Charles C Thomas, 1974, pp 37–57.
Wallace JF: Disorders caused by venoms, bites, and stings. *In* Isselbacher KJ, et al (eds): Harrison's Principles of Internal Medicine, 9th ed. New York, McGraw-Hill, 1980, pp 923–924.
Zeligowski AA, Peled IJ, Wexler MR: Eyelid necrosis after spider bite. Am J Ophthalmol 15:101:254–255, 1986.

SECTION 17

UNCLASSIFIED DISEASES OR CONDITIONS

AMYLOIDOSIS
JAY H. KRACHMER, M.D.,
Iowa City, Iowa
and STEVEN P. DUNN, M.D.
Southfield, Michigan

Amyloidosis is a disease complex resulting in the accumulation of an extracellular, amorphous, eosinophilic substance that is readily identified by its staining with Congo red and its distinctive ultrastructure. In recent years, two major protein components have been identified, enabling classification of various forms of the disease on biochemical grounds.

Immunocytic amyloidosis (including primary systemic amyloidosis and amyloidosis associated with multiple myeloma) is characterized by amyloid deposits of immunoglobulin (AL) protein origin. It frequently presents in the seventh decade with symptoms of weakness, fatigue, weight loss, dyspnea, paresthesias, ankle edema, and dysphonia. Multisystem involvement of characteristic, with renal, cardiac, and hepatic disease in a high proportion of affected patients. Ocular involvement has been estimated to occur in 8.4 per cent of patients with primary systemic amyloidosis. The eyelids are the most commonly involved site. Discrete of confluent, bilateral, yellow-white, xanthoma-like nodules, occasionally with petechiae and hemorrhage, may be the initial features. Proptosis has been reported. Involvement of the lacrimal and parotid glands may produce dryness of the eyes and mouth. Ptosis and external ophthalmoplegia have been attributed to amyloid deposits in the extraocular muscles. Pupillary abnormalities are thought to be due to amyloid neuropathy or possibly secondary to deposits in the iris sphincter and dilator muscles. Linear and veil-like vitreous opacities associated with slowly progressive visual loss are virtually diagnostic of amyloid disease.

Nonimmunologic, reactive, or localized amyloidosis is characterized by amyloid deposits of unknown origin (AA protein). The most common forms of amyloidosis affecting the eye and adnexa fall into this group. Its onset is more variable than immunocytic amyloidosis, with some forms presenting as early as the third decade. Localized orbital amyloidosis is extremely rare. Most lesions are unilateral, firm, and associated with slowly progressive proptosis and impairment of motility. Conjunctival amyloidosis occurs as an asymptomatic, yellow, waxy mass involving the superior palpebral or fornical conjunctiva. Bulbar and limbal involvement has been reported. Enlargement or swelling of the eyelid with ptosis, epiphora, or subconjunctival hemorrhage may be accompanying manifestations. Corneal amyloid has been demonstrated in lattice dystrophy, polymorphic amyloid degeneration, gelatinous drop-like dystrophy, and occasional cases of corneal trauma, keratoconus, and chronic inflammation.

Rarely, patients in families with systemic amyloidosis can present with lattice accumulation of amyloid. A familial form of amyloidosis characterized by flat or protuberant subepithelial deposits has been described as well.

THERAPY

Supportive. Therapy of systemic amyloidosis is presently unsatisfactory. The disease is almost invariably fatal. Because some amyloid fibrils have an immunologic origin, therapeutic trials using a combination of melphalan[‡] and prednisone[‡] have been tried. Preliminary reports have been unimpressive.

Colchicine[‡] has proved to be a major advancement in the therapy of patients with familial Mediterranean fever, preventing the development of amyloidosis in this disease. Its use in other disorders has been disappointing. Similarly, studies with dimethyl sulfoxide (DMSO),[‡] an amyloid fibril denaturing agent have been discouraging.

Thus, supportive medical care becomes very important. All patients in this group deserve a thorough evaluation and search for an underlying cause of their amyloidosis. Partial or complete resorption of amyloid deposits with improvement of symptoms has been reported with treatment of the underlying inflammatory or neoplastic process.

Surgical. The surgical management of amyloidosis is usually directed at localized disease. There is a strong tendency, however, for recurrence, which should be explained to the patient. Local discomfort, marked proptosis, diplopia, and poor vision are the usual reasons for surgical therapy. Excision of orbital amyloid is useful in cases where it is well circumscribed. In most cases, though, the infiltration is diffuse and impossible to remove completely. Surgical therapy often proves more diagnostic than therapeutic. Mucous membrane grafting is frequently necessary after the excision of conjunctival amyloid deposits. Reduced vision often leads to penetrating keratoplasty by the fourth or fifth decade in patients with lattice dystrophy. Though the success rate exceeds 90 per cent in this group, there may be recurrences. Keratoplasty may be helpful in patients with gelatinous drop-like dystrophy and diffuse familial amyloidosis as well. Polymorphic amyloid degeneration does not require therapy. Total vitrectomy appears to be the treatment of choice for amyloid patients with these dense vitreous opacities interfering with vision.

Ocular or Periocular Manifestations

Conjunctiva: Amyloid deposits; hemorrhages.
Cornea: Familial amyloidosis; gelatinous drop-like dystrophy; lattice dystrophy; polymorphic amyloid degeneration; secondary amyloid deposits.
Extraocular Muscles: Convergence insufficiency; paresis or paralysis.
Eyelids: Amyloid deposits; edema; petechial hemorrhages; ptosis; thickening.
Iris or Ciliary Body: Amyloid deposits; choriocapillaris occlusion; Fuchs' epithelioma; perivascular sheathing.
Orbit: Amyloid deposits; proptosis.
Pupil: Anisocoria; irregularity.
Retina: Arterial occlusion; hemorrhages; perivascular sheathing.
Sclera: Amyloid deposits.
Vitreous: Glass-wool or sheet-like opacity; pseudopodia lentis.

PRECAUTIONS

A high incidence of recurrent amyloid deposits after surgery should be borne in mind by the ophthalmologist and the patient. This is particularly important when cosmetic surgery is planned. Regrafting and repeat vitrectomy are options available to the patient with visual deterioration or recurrent corneal and vitreal amyloidosis.

COMMENTS

Localized amyloid deposits are by far the most common form of ocular amyloidosis. In some cases, amyloid deposits involving the eye may actually be an early localized manifestation of a generalized amyloidosis. This is particularly true with eyelid and vitreal amyloid deposits. The possibility that these deposits may be associated with an underlying disease process or immunologic abnormality must always be considered.

References

Doughman DJ: Ocular amyloidosis. Surv Ophthalmol 13:133–142, 1969.
Glenner GG: Amyloid deposits and amyloidosis. The B-fibrilloses. (First of two parts). N Engl J Med 302:1283–1292, 1980.
Glenner GG: Amyloid deposits and amyloidosis. The B-fibrilloses. (Second of two parts). N Engl J Med 302:1333–1343, 1980.
Henderson JW: Orbital Tumors, 2nd ed. New York, Brian C Decker, 1980, pp 547–552.
Hitchings RA, Tripathi RC: Vitreous opacities in primary amyloid disease. A clinical, histochemical, and ultrastructural report. Br J Ophthalmol 60:41–54, 1976.
Knowles DM II, et al: Amyloidosis of the orbit and adnexae. Surv Ophthalmol 19:367–384, 1975.
Kyle RA: Amyloidosis: Part 1. Int J Dermatol 19:537–539, 1980.
Kyle RA: Amyloidosis: Part 2. Int J Dermatol 20:20–25, 1981.
Kyle RA: Amyloidosis: Part 3. Int J Dermatol 20:75–80, 1981.
Mannis MJ, et al: Polymorphic amyloid degeneration of the cornea. A clinical and histopathologic study. Arch Ophthalmol 99:1217–1223, 1981.
Zemer D, et al: Colchicine in the prevention and treatment of the amyloidosis of familial Mediterranean fever. N Engl J Med 314:1001, 1986.

BEHÇET'S DISEASE
(Silk Road Disease)
KANJIRO MASUDA, M.D.
Tokyo, Japan

Behçet's disease is a systemic disease of unknown etiology, and its diagnosis is based on a combination of major and minor symptoms. The major symptoms are recurrent aphthae in the mouth; skin lesions, such as erythema nodosum, acne, and subcutaneous thromboangiitis; ocular lesions, such as hypopyon iritis and retinal vasculitis with hemorrhages and exudates; and genital ulcer. During the chronic course of the disease, these major symptoms recur as attacks, but not necessarily in concurrence. The minor symptoms include arthritis, epididymitis, intestinal lesions, and vascular, neuropsychologic, lung, or kidney involvement.

The disease has been seen all over the world, but it is especially frequent in Japan, the eastern Mediterranean, and Middle East, where it is known as the Silk Road disease. Immunogenetically, HLA-BW51 is closely related to this disease.

The onset of the disease usually occurs in the third and fourth decades. The course of the disease shows exacerbations and remissions, and symptoms may subside within several years or linger for more than 20 years.

The visual prognosis is usually poor. From the ophthalmologic point of view, Behçet's disease may be classified into two groups: the anterior type, which chiefly involves the anterior segment of the eye (iridocyclitic type), and the posterior type involving the posterior segment of the eye (fundus type).

THERAPY

Ocular. A good visual acuity can be maintained in the anterior type of Behçet's disease for a much longer time than in the posterior type. At the time of attack, 1 per cent atropine once or twice a day and topical corticosteroids two to four times daily should be used. After severe attacks showing distinct hypopyon iritis, subconjunctival injection* of corticosteroids is indicated.

Systemic. Long-term systemic administration of corticosteroids results in an unfavorable visual prognosis. Consequently, immunosuppressive agents are the main drugs currently used in the posterior type of Behçet's disease. Systemic steroids should be used only in cases with macular involvement and only for a short period of time (7 days). As soon as the attacks subside, corticosteroids must be tapered. The immunosuppressive agents are used both to treat the attacks and to reduce the number of attacks. A daily dosage of 0.5 to 1.5 mg of colchicine‡ or 50 to 150 mg of cyclophosphamide‡ or both is recommended. Oral administration of chlorambucil‡ has also been reported to be beneficial. Since these agents reduce the motility and number of leukocytes, especially neutrophils, blood cell counts are recommended every 2 weeks. When leukocytes in the peripheral blood are maintained between 3000 to 5000 cells per cubic millimeter, the number of the attacks is reduced. In severe cases, cyclosporine is used with an initial dose of 5 mg/kg daily. The dose may be increased or decreased according to the clinical manifestations and side effects, such as kidney or liver dysfunction.

Ocular or Periocular Manifestations

Anterior Chamber: Angle hypopyon; cells and flare; hypopyon.
Choroid: Cell infiltration; choroiditis.
Cornea: Keratic infiltration; keratic precipitates.
Globe: Phthisis.
Iris or Ciliary Body: Iridocyclitis; posterior synechia.
Lens: Cataracts.
Optic Nerve: Atrophy.
Retina: Cystoid macular edema; exudates; hemorrhages; macular hole; thromboangiitis.
Sclera: Episcleritis; scleritis.
Vitreous: Cells; hemorrhages; opacity.
Other: Glaucoma.

PRECAUTIONS

Side effects of the immunosuppressive agents must be carefully checked. Cyclophosphamide induces azoospermia, which may continue for a long time even after cessation of its use. Colchicine and chlorambucil also have toxic effects on reproductive cells and bone marrow. Regular blood cell counts must be carried out, and the dosage of these drugs should be controlled, depending on the results. Cyclosporine causes liver and kidney dysfunction. Therefore, kidney and liver function and blood pressure must be checked regularly.

COMMENTS

Before the introduction of immunosuppressive agents, the visual prognosis of Behçet's disease had been very poor. In more than 80 per cent of the cases with ocular involvement, particularly those involving the posterior segment, severe decrease in vision occurred by 5 years after the onset. However, use of the immunosuppressive agents has greatly improved the visual prognosis; only 5 per cent of cases now show severe visual acuity loss 5 years after the onset. In males, 84 per cent of cases are of the posterior type, whereas 36 per cent of cases in females are of the anterior type. Consequently, visual prognosis is usually better in females than in males. The cause of death is often neuropsychologic, intestinal, or cardiovascular involvement.

References

Graham E et al: Cyclosporin A in the treatment of severe Behçet's uveitis. *In* Lehner T, Barnes CG (eds): Recent Advances in Behçet's Disease, New York, Royal Society of Medicine Services, 1986, p 351.
Hayashi K, et al: Long-term treatment of severe Behçet's disease with cyclosporin A. *In* Lehner T, Barnes, CG (eds): Recent Advances in Behçet's Disease, New York, Royal Society of Medicine Services, 1986, p 347.
Masuda K, et al: A nation-wide survey of Behçet's disease in Japan. 2. Clinical survey. Jpn J Ophthalmol 19:278–285, 1975.
Masuda K, et al: Cyclosporin A treatment of Behçet's disease—A multicentre double-masked trial. *In* Lehner T, Barnes CG (eds): Recent Advances in Behçet's Disease. New York, Royal Society of Medicine Services, 1986, pp 327–331.
Mishima S, et al: Behçet's disease in Japan: Ophthalmologic aspects. Trans Am Ophthalmol Soc 77:225–279, 1979.
Pisanti S, et al: Oral health parameters in Behçet's disease. A comparison between conventional therapy and cyclosporin A treatment. *In* Lehner T, Barnes CG (eds): Recent Advances in Behçet's Disease. New York, Royal Society of Medicine Services, 1986, pp 337–341.

COGAN'S SYNDROME
BARTON F. HAYNES, M.D.
Durham, North Carolina

Typical Cogan's syndrome is a rare clinical entity of unknown etiology that is characterized by nonsyphilitic interstitial keratitis and is associated with vestibuloauditory dysfunction. It occurs primarily in young adults. The vestibuloauditory symptoms are simultaneous onset of hearing loss, nystagmus, tinnitus, and vertigo, which usually progress rapidly to complete nerve deafness and persistent labyrinth dysfunction when untreated. Ten per cent of patients with Cogan's syndrome may present with scleritis or episcleritis instead of interstitial keratitis and vestibuloauditory dysfunction. This manifestation of the disease has been termed "atypical Cogan's syndrome."

The primary systemic complication of typical Cogan's syndrome (manifested by interstitial keratitis and vestibuloauditory dysfunction) is life-threatening aortic valvular disease with acute aortitis in up to 10 per cent of patients. Systemic vasculitis, once thought to be a complication of typical Cogan's syndrome, is rarely seen in typical Cogan's syndrome, but has been observed in up to 25 per cent of cases with atypical Cogan's syndrome (manifested by scleritis, episcleritis, or types of inflammatory eye disease other than interstitial keratitis associated with vestibuloauditory dysfunction).

The primary ocular manifestation of typical Cogan's syndrome is chronic bilateral interstitial keratitis, which may vary in intensity from day to day and from eye to eye. The keratitis is manifested by patchy infiltrates of the deep corneal stroma, followed by a variable degree of corneal vascularization; in the acute stage, it is often associated with pain, photophobia, hyperemia, and mild uveitis.

THERAPY

Ocular. Topical 1 per cent atropine solution or ointment is often necessary in the management of acute uveitis and keratitis and may be applied three times daily. Topical steroids may be indicated to control ocular inflammation. A solution of 1 per cent prednisolone may be applied every 2 hours during acute stages of the disease and then tapered after symptoms resolve. Between flares of interstitial keratitis, no topical ophthalmic therapy is usually necessary. Systemic corticosteroid therapy is only rarely indicated to control the symptoms of acute interstitial keratitis.

Systemic. Corticosteroids are indicated in the early treatment of acute deafness associated with Cogan's syndrome. When treated early in the course of vestibuloauditory dysfunction, some patients with Cogan's syndrome do respond to corticosteroid therapy with improved hearing. Therefore, a course of daily oral corticosteroids, such as 1 to 2 mg/kg of prednisone[‡] for 2 to 4 weeks, is warranted for patients with Cogan's syndrome with recent onset of severe hearing impairment. If hearing is improved by this treatment, corticosteroids should be continued on an alternate-day regimen, followed by gradual tapering. If hearing does not improve after 2 to 4 weeks of daily prednisone, the corticosteroid should be rapidly tapered and discontinued.

Corticosteroids may also be of use in treatment of systemic manifestations of Cogan's syndrome. Daily doses of 1 to 2 mg/kg of prednisone[‡] may be beneficial. If clinical response ensues, this dose should be gradually changed to an alternate-day regimen.

If aortitis with aortic insufficiency or a Takayasu-like large vessel vasculitis is present, treatment should be instituted with 2 mg/kg of prednisone[‡] and 2 mg/kg of cyclophosphamide.[‡] Such therapy should be continued until manifestations of aortitis or large vessel vasculitis are stable or quiescent, and then treatment should be continued for an additional year. In cases of hemodynamically significant aortic insufficiency, aortic valve replacement should be considered. In Takayasu's arteritis-like syndromes, vascular bypass surgery may be indicated to prevent ischemic tissue damage. If cyclophosphamide cannot be tolerated because of side effects or the large vessel vasculitis syndromes do not completely respond to the drug, consideration should be given to discontinuing cyclophosphamide and instituting therapy with 5 mg/kg of oral cyclosporine[‡] daily. In the setting of Cogan's syndrome and large vessel vasculitis, treatment with either cyclophosphamide or cyclosporine should be accompanied by prednisone therapy, initially every day and subsequently in alternate-day doses.

In patients with atypical Cogan's syndrome with documented systemic necrotizing vasculitis, both prednisone[‡] and 1 to 2 mg/kg of cyclophosphamide[‡] daily may be necessary. Data are now available that show that both remissions and long-term cures of systemic necrotizing vasculitis can be effected by the judicious use of short courses of prednisone and prolonged courses of low oral dosages of cyclophosphamide.

Ocular or Periocular Manifestations

Conjunctiva: Catarrhal conjunctivitis; chemosis; hyperemia.
Cornea: Infiltration; interstitial keratitis; opacity; vascularization.
Iris: Anterior uveitis.
Other: Nystagmus; ocular pain; photophobia.

PRECAUTIONS

Corticosteroids can be dangerous if improperly used; thus, patients must be closely supervised and the dosage individualized in accordance with the severity of the disorder, the response of the patient, and the anticipated duration of therapy. Corticosteroids should be given in the smallest dosage that will control a specific symptom and should be used for the shortest time possible. Frequently, use of an alternate-day regimen of corticosteroids will give therapeutic results while minimizing severe side effects. The tapering of corticosteroid therapy should be effected gradually and cautiously.

The side effects of systemic corticosteroid administration are numerous and serious and include osteoporosis, immunosuppression and susceptibility to infection, weight gain, cataracts, myopathy, and psychosis. Strict criteria, therefore, should be used for systemic steroid administration in Cogan's syndrome. Steroids should be used in a therapeutic trial to alleviate hearing loss as early as possible in the course of the disease. Months to years later in the course of Cogan's syndrome, corticosteroids may exacerbate hearing fluctuation if cochlear hydrops is present. Thus, steroids should be administered late in Cogan's syndrome only if the hearing loss is suddenly severe or if manifestations of the original inflammatory process return, such as an elevated erythrocyte sedimentation rate, anemia, or leukocytosis. If hearing loss is complete or hearing fluctuations do not respond to steroids, there is no evidence to warrant the continuation of steroids. Two diuretics that are commonly used to treat cochlear hydrops in Cogan's syndrome are chlorthalidone and hydrochlorothiazide. The common side effects of both drugs are potassium depletion and volume depletion, as well as a variety of manifestations of drug allergy.

Cyclophosphamide is indicated for the rare patients with systemic necrotizing vasculitis and atypical Cogan's syndrome or typical Cogan's syndrome associated with large vessel vasculitis. Cyclophosphamide, an alkylating drug, is associated with severe bone marrow suppression and infection, hemorrhagic cystitis, gonadal dysfunction, gastrointestinal disturbances, and myeloid and other malignant diseases. Therefore, this drug should be used only for immune-mediated hearing loss and eye disease associated with biopsy-proven systemic necrotizing vasculitis or with the large vessel vasculitis syndrome associated with typical Cogan's syndrome. When used, the dosage should be titered to keep the white blood cell count greater than 3000 cells per cubic millimeter and the polymorphonuclear leukocyte count greater than 1000 to 2000 cells per cubic millimeter.

Cyclosporine is a potent immunosuppressive drug that profoundly inhibits normal T-cell activation and function. The primary toxic effects of cyclosporine include opportunistic infections and renal toxicity. The renal toxicity involves primarily drug-induced interstitial nephritis and subsequent irreversible renal fibrosis. Therefore, careful monitoring of serum cyclosporine levels should be undertaken, keeping the trough serum levels below 200 ng/ml. The serum creatinine level should be followed monthly and the dosage of cyclosporine reduced or stopped, according to the magnitude of creatinine rise. Renal biopsy should be performed after 18 months of therapy to monitor renal damage during long-term cyclosporine therapy. Other potential side effects of cyclosporine are an increased risk of lymphoid malignant disease, hypertension, tremor, paresthesia, seizures, hypomagnesemia, anorexia, and nausea.

Comments

Cogan's syndrome consists of nonsyphilitic interstitial keratitis associated with vestibuloauditory dysfunction. The etiology of the syndrome is unknown, and the clinical course is extremely variable. Rare patients with atypical Cogan's syndrome have died within months of onset, usually in relationship to the systemic vasculitis. However, most often, the syndrome appears to be characterized by an acute phase lasting months to years and a low-grade, chronic phase lasting indefinitely. Most patients with Cogan's syndrome regain and retain good vision, but varying degrees of deafness is the rule. Topical ophthalmic corticosteroid therapy usually controls the symptoms of keratitis associated with Cogan's syndrome. Systemic corticosteroids may be of benefit in preventing deafness, and all patients with Cogan's syndrome should be given a trial of oral corticosteroids at the first sign of vestibuloauditory dysfunction. Careful periodic evaluation for signs and symptoms of systemic vasculitis should be made.

Since typical Cogan's syndrome has an excellent prognosis, corticosteroid therapy in most cases poses the greatest threat to long-term patient survival. Thus, it is imperative to continue to attempt to taper corticosteroid dosages in Cogan's syndrome, preferably with the use of intermittent rather than continuous long-term administration. Most patients require steroids only for the first 2 to 6 months after the onset of the disease, with chronic hearing fluctuations caused by cochlear hydrops, rather than by active cochlear inflammation. Intermittent topical ocular administration of corticosteroids nearly always controls interstitial keratitis. Because of the risk of herpetic keratitis, intermittent rather than long-term continuous ocular steroid administration is preferred.

References

Cogan DG, Dickersin GR: Nonsyphilitic interstitial keratitis with vestibuloauditory symptoms. A case with fatal aortitis. Arch Ophthalmol 71:172–175, 1964.
Haynes BF, et al: Cogan syndrome: Studies in thirteen patients, long-term follow-up, and a review of the literature. Medicine 59:426–441, 1980.
Haynes BF, et al: Successful treatment of sudden hearing loss in Cogan's syndrome with corticosteroids. Arthritis Rheum 24:501–503, 1981.
Haynes BF, et al: Pathogenesis and immunotherapy of Cogan's syndrome. In Eisenbarth GS (ed): Immunotherapy of Diabetes and Selected Autoimune Diseases. Boca Raton, FL, CRC Press, 1989.

FAMILIAL DYSAUTONOMIA
(Riley Day Syndrome)
FELICIA B. AXELROD, M.D.,
and ROBERT D'AMICO, M.D.
New York, New York

Familial dysautonomia is a congenital condition of autonomic dysfunction and decreased sensory appreciation. It is inherited as an autosomal recessive trait and occurs almost exclusively among Jews of Eastern European ancestry (Ashkenazi).

Consistent neuropathologic findings include low populations of sympathetic neurons and terminals, severe depletion of parasympathetic neurons in sphenopalatine ganglia but minimal depletion in ciliary ganglia, and paucity of unmyelinated sensory neurons in sural nerves and dorsal root ganglia. Biochemical data indicate diminished norepinephrine and epinephrine excretion but normal amounts of dopamine products.

Clinical manifestations of familial dysautonomia are caused by deficits in autonomic homeostatic function and sensory appreciation of peripheral pain and temperature. Prominent early manifestations include feeding difficulties, hypotonia, delayed developmental milestones, labile body temperature and blood pressure, absence of overflowing tears and corneal hypesthesia, marked diaphoresis with excitement, and breath-holding episodes. Recurrent pneumonias are frequent and caused by repeated aspiration. Intractable vomiting crises occur in 40 per cent of patients on a cyclical basis and are associated with hypertension, tachycardia, diffuse sweating, personality changes, and occasionally, hyperpyrexia. Spinal curvature occurs in 95 per cent of patients by adolescence. Ocular complications occur primarily as a result of decreased lacrimation and corneal hypesthesia and often worsen during acute illnesses as a result of hypertension, fever, and dehydration. Convergence insufficiencies and exodeviations are frequently associated with familial dysautonomia, and there is a higher than normal incidence of myopia. Optic pallor and abnormal visual evoked potentials have also been noted and indicate further involvement of cranial sensory nerves. The optic neuropathy worsens with age and is compatible with a progressive neurologic disorder.

Diagnosis is confirmed by lack of an axon flare following intradermal injection of histamine phosphate (1 : 10,000), miosis with dilute parasympathomimetic agents, decreased or absent deep tendon reflexes, and absence of fungiform papillae on the tongue.

THERAPY

Systemic. Treatment is directed to specific symptoms and complications. For infants with feeding problems, dietary therapy and thickened foods are used. In some cases, "gavage" feeding or gastrostomy is indicated to maintain nutrition, avoid dehydration, and prevent aspiration. Pulmonary hygiene, consisting of postural drainage, is helpful for children who have had recurrent pneumonias. Suctioning of tracheal secretions may be needed because of ineffective cough. Prophylactic antibiotics are not indicated.

Vomiting crises are managed in the hospital with intravenous fluids and parenteral diazepam. Diazepam‡ at 0.2 mg/kg is given intravenously every 3 hours until the crisis is resolved. If the patient is hypertensive 15 minutes after diazepam, chlorpromazine at 1.0 mg/kg can be given as a rectal suppository. Induction of a deep sleep is necessary for resolution of the crisis. Chloral hydrate (30 mg/kg) can be given as a rectal suppository with diazepam to induce sleep and can be repeated every 6 hours as needed.

Ocular. Fundamental to the therapy of all dry eye syndromes is the regular use of tear substitutes. Frequency of instillation depends on the child's own baseline eye moisture, environmental conditions, and whether the child is febrile or dehydrated. The wetting effect of saline solutions may be prolonged by the addition of viscosity-increasing, large molecular weight polymers, such as methylcellulose or polyvinyl alcohol. Increasing corneal surface wettability by the addition of mucomimetic polymers also may be beneficial. Ointments are preferred for nighttime applications.

Corneal hypesthesia compounds the problem, as it results in decreased blink frequency and indifference to corneal trauma. Epithelial erosions of the exposed cornea and conjunctiva are the hallmarks of dry eye states. These lesions may become confluent, leading to patchy areas of de-epithelialization. Early treatment of corneal epithelial erosions includes increased frequency of tear substitutes, prophylactic topical antibiotics, patching the eye, attention to the general state of hydration, and search for a precipitating systemic factor that may have disturbed the patient's fragile catecholamine homeostasis. Persistent erosions or ulcerations may require more vigorous and innovative approaches, such as moisture chamber spectacle attachments, swim goggles or taped-on "bubbles" for sleep, bandage lenses, occlusion of the lacrimal puncta, stimulation of tear flow by systemically administered cholinergic agents (bethanechol), or small lateral tarsorrhaphies that limit the area exposed to surface evaporation. Bipedicled tarsorrhaphies and conjunctival flaps are disfiguring and visually limiting. These procedures should be reserved for unresponsive cases in which the integrity of the globe is threatened.

All epithelial defects are at risk for secondary infection, and corneal and conjunctival cultures should be obtained when clinical signs suggest contamination. In addition, lack of the irrigating function of tear flow and its bacteriostatic elements predisposes the eye to chronic blepharitis.

Calcium deposition in the region of the palpebral fissure may be seen in persistent corneal ulcerations. Dense, white, anterior stromal infiltrates accompanied by interstitial vascularization are occasionally noted. These are sterile and appear to be caused by tissue anoxia and usually respond to a short course of topical steroids. A dry eye is often a congested eye, and topical steroids may give a false picture of improvement by their anti-inflammatory action. The risks of long-term steroid therapy, such as lens opacification, secondary glaucoma, and susceptibility to infection, far outweigh any symptomatic benefits derived.

The dry anesthetic cornea is an unfavorable environment for a corneal graft. Delayed re-epithelialization, recurrent erosions, and late opacification frequently complicate and limit the final visual result.

Ocular or Periocular Manifestations

Cornea: Hypesthesia; ulcer.
Eyelids: Blepharitis.
Lacrimal System: Decreased tear secretion.
Other: Hyperreactivity to sympathetic and parasympathetic agents; myopia; optic pallor; strabismus.

PRECAUTIONS

Systemic dehydration compounds the problem of the dry eye. Vomiting crises, febrile episodes, and severe diarrhea should be considered situations that pose potentially increased risk to the cornea.

If surgical procedures are performed, special precautions are required in administration of anesthesia. Dysautonomic patients have labile blood pressures and diminished responsiveness to variations in blood gases. Local anesthesia is preferred. However, if general anesthesia is indicated, the patient should be hydrated preoperatively, as well as intraoperatively. Inhalation anesthetics are tolerated best, and there should be constant intraoperative monitoring of blood pressure and heart rate.

COMMENTS

Corneal pathology is complicated. The relatively dry eye and corneal hypesthesia predispose to de-epithelialization, but systemic autonomic dysfunction and disturbed catecholamine homeostasis may precipitate acute problems, complicate management, and inhibit normal healing processes.

Vigorous attention to systemic problems, avoiding chronic and acute dehydration, and early attention to corneal problems through education of parents and patients have helped preserve corneal integrity and resulted in a decreased need for tarsorrhaphies.

References

Axelrod FB: Familial dysautonomia. In Gellis SS, Kagan BM: Current Pediatric Therapy 10. Philadelphia, WB Saunders, 1982, pp 80–82.
Axelrod FB, Nachtigal R, Dancis J: Familial dysautonomia: Diagnosis, pathogenesis and management. Adv Pediatr 21:75–96, 1974.
Brunt PW, McKusick VA: Familial dysautonomia. A report of genetic and clinical studies, with a review of the literature. Medicine 49:343–374, 1970.
Diamond GA, D'Amico RA, Axelrod FB: Optic nerve dysfunction in familial dysautonomia. Am J Ophthalmol 104:645–648, 1987.
Ginsberg SP, et al: Autonomic dysfunction syndrome. Am J Ophthalmol 74:1121–1125, 1972.
Goldberg MF, Payne JW, Brunt PW: Ophthalmologic studies of familial dysautonomia. The Riley-Day syndrome. Arch Ophthalmol 80:732–743, 1968.
Howard RO: Familial dysautonomia (Riley-Day syndrome). Am J Ophthalmol 64:392–398, 1967.
Pearson J, Axelrod F, Dancis J: Current concepts of dysautonomia: Neuropathological defects. Ann NY Acad Sci 228:288–300, 1974.
Rizzo JF III, Lessell S, Liebman SD: Optic atrophy in familial dysautonomia. Am J Ophthalmol 102:463, 1986.
Smith AA, Dancis J, Breinin G: Ocular responses to autonomic drugs in familial dysautonomia. Invest Ophthalmol 4:358–361, 1965.

HISTIOCYTOSIS X
(Eosinophilic Granuloma,
Hand-Schüller-Christian Disease,
Letterer-Siwe Disease)

DAVID J. APPLE, M.D.,
HUGH L. HENNIS, M.D., Ph.D.,
Charleston, South Carolina

and KEVIN MILLER, M.D.
Las Vegas, Nevada

The term "histiocytosis X" refers to a spectrum of diseases of unclear etiology, that are characterized by an abnormal proliferation of histiocytes. These histiocytic syndromes have been recently reorganized into three groups based primarily on their pathologic features. The first of these three groups includes the Langerhans' cell histiocytes. Included under this category are Letterer-Siwe, Hand-Schüller-Christian syndrome, and eosinophilic granuloma of bone. Until recently, these three diseases were referred to as histiocytosis X, a term first proposed by Lichtenstein in 1952. The second category includes histiocytes that are not Langerhans' cells. Included in this group is juvenile xanthogranuloma. The final group encompasses malignant disorders of histiocytes, including histiocytic lymphoma and acute monocytic leukemia.

Langerhans' cells are characterized by a dendritic pattern, clear cytoplasm, and ultrastructurally by Birbeck granules. These cells are derived from the bone marrow. By studying cell surface markers, these cells have been identified as belonging to the monocyte/macrophage group. They may be detected in tissue sections by monoclonal antibodies directed against cell surface antigens, including T_4 and T_6 markers, class II histocompatibility antigens, and an intracytoplasmic marker, the S100 protein.

The widespread location of the histiocytic system in the human body explains the numerous clinical manifestations of this disease. Letterer-Siwe disease, sometimes termed "acute differentiated histiocytosis" when the hallmark of the disease is a *moderate degree of cellular differentiation,* is typically much more "malignant" than the former two entities, both in the cytologic and clinical sense. Some authors consider eosinophilic granuloma and Hand-Schüller-Christian disease as variants of the same disease process, i.e., proliferative histiocytic diseases with *well-differentiated cells*. However, highly disseminated forms of Hand-Schüller-Christian disease may occur that may more closely resemble the findings of Letterer-Siwe disease. Therefore, since histiocytosis X may exhibit such a wide variety of clinical manifestations, it does not always fit precisely into one of the above three categories.

Eosinophilic granuloma of bone, the most "benign" disease in this group, may occur over a wide age range, from the preschool years to adulthood. Most cases are diagnosed before the age of 10 years, but onset well into adult life is not unusual; therefore, these patients are on the average slightly older than those in the other two categories. The hallmark of the disease is bone infiltrates, which may be unifocal or multifocal. They most commonly affect the skull, ribs, vertebrae, pelvis, scapula, and proximal long bones. These lesions may be visible or palpable and may be associated with pain or tenderness. So-called extraosseous forms of eosinophilic granuloma, most commonly affecting the gastrointestinal tract and lung, have also been described.

Unifocal eosinophilic granuloma behaves almost invariably as a benign lesion and responds readily to excision or radiation therapy. With multifocal disease, there is clear overlap in symptoms with Hand-Schüller-Christian disease, and the two entities may be difficult to separate by either clinical or histologic criteria.

Hand-Schüller-Christian disease is an intermediate form between eosinophilic granuloma and Letterer-Siwe disease. It includes a combination of the bony lesions that are more typically associated with eosinophilic granuloma and some of the visceral and soft tissue lesions that are the hallmark of Letterer-Siwe disease. The classic clinical triad of Hand-Schüller-Christian disease is bony lesions in the skull, exophthalmos, and diabetes insipidus. Actually, the full triad occurs in only a small percentage of patients. This disease occurs during childhood, usually presenting before the age of 4 years. This is a slightly older age group than that seen in Letterer-Siwe disease, which typically occurs in infancy. As one might expect, it often has a clinical course intermediate in character between that of Letterer-Siwe disease and eosinophilic granuloma.

The most severe form of histiocytosis X, Letterer-Siwe disease (acute differentiated histiocytosis), is usually seen in children under 2 years of age. In addition, congenital forms have been described. The disease is rapidly progressive, often fatal, and characterized by widespread tissue involvement with cellular infiltration. Most commonly involved are the skin, lungs, lymph nodes, liver, spleen, bone marrow, and gingival mucosa. The disease is not uniformly fatal, however. In one series, a mortality rate of 70 per cent in children under the age of 6 months was reported. In general, the younger the child at the onset of the disease, the worse the prognosis. The bony involvement, typically seen in eosinophilic granuloma, is less prominent. These patients may develop liver, lung, or bone marrow dysfunction, all of which are poor prognostic signs. Most deaths are secondary to hepatic or lung failure or complications, such as bleeding or infection.

The widespread effects of histiocytosis X sometimes lead to infiltration of ocular and periocular structures. Several studies have shown that the incidence of orbital involvement is about 20 per cent. In addition, only about half of these patients developed proptosis. The most commonly seen signs of eye involvement are unilateral and bilateral proptosis, and less frequently papilledema with optic atrophy.

Exophthalmos is usually caused by involvement by lytic lesions of the orbital bones but, rarely, may be due to involvement of the orbital soft tissues. On rare occasions, the globe may be directly involved by infiltrates as with the choroidal infiltrates seen in Letterer-Siwe disease. In addition, secondary open-angle glaucoma, bilateral perforating corneal ulcers, nystagmus, secondary intracranial palsies, posterior scleritis, eyelid infiltration, and secondary infection all have been reported.

When confronted with a questionable case of histiocytosis X, appropriate studies include a chest x-ray, bone scan, bone marrow biopsy, and liver function tests. In addition, appropriate consultation should be sought. Orbital x-rays may reveal evidence of a lytic lesion that frequently shows a narrow zone of sclerosis. The gold standard of diagnosis is still a detailed histopathologic examination of appropriate biopsy specimens.

THERAPY

Irradiation. Single bony lesions and even cases with multifocal lesions affecting bone carry an excellent prognosis. Spontaneous clearing may actually occur in some cases. When therapy is required, lesions are often best treated with curettage or local low-dose irradiation or both. If a lesion is easily accessible and asymptomatic, a diagnostic biopsy followed by a simple curettage or excision is often all that is needed. If the lesion recurs or does not improve clinically or radiographically after curettage, local irradiation is indicated.

If curettage is difficult or is required in a location that may lead to dysfunction or disfigurement, a diagnostic biopsy followed by irradiation is the preferred initial treatment. Biopsy with irradiation is also preferred over curettage for large lesions in weight-bearing bones because it lessens the likelihood of pathologic fractures.

Vertebral lesions present a special situation and may require radiation therapy if there is partial collapse of lytic involvement. Only low-dose irradiation is needed for bony lesions. A dose of 400 to 600 rads given in 150- to 200-rad fractions daily is usually effective.

The most common ophthalmic complications of histiocytosis X is localized orbital and periorbital lesions with or without exophthalmos. These complications can be treated much like other localized lesions. Low-dose radiation therapy with 300 to 600 rads or curettage or both are often effective.

Systemic. The optimal treatment regimen for disseminated histiocytosis X (usually connoting severe forms of the Hand-Schüller-Christian disease variant, as well as Letterer-Siwe disease) has not been established. The variable clinical presentation or course and the fact that this disease sometimes undergoes spontaneous remission have made evaluation of therapy difficult. Evaluation has been further complicated by the disease's response to a wide variety of therapeutic modalities. These include steroids, vinca alkaloids (vincristine or vinblastine), alkylating agents, antimetabolites, antibiotics, radiation, and thymic extract.[†]

It remains to be determined what drug or drug combination will be most effective for a given patient with disseminated histiocytosis X. Some authors have shown that vinblastine used as a single agent can be effective in treating severe forms of this disease. It may be given intravenously once a week at an initial dose of 0.15 mg/kg. This dose is increased by 0.05 mg/kg weekly until the white blood cell count drops below 3000/cubic millimeter. Thereafter, the maximum dose that does not cause leukopenia is given weekly. If the disease clears in 12 weeks, the medication is discontinued and the patient observed. If there is improvement in the majority of the initial organs involved but not complete remission, the patient continues with the maximum tolerated dose given every 2 weeks for 3 to 6 months. If the patient is started on vinblastine and there is no improvement or improvement in less than 50 per cent of the initial organs involved after 12 weeks of therapy, the patient should be started on another regimen.

Prednisone may be administered in conjunction with the above regimen for vinblastine. Prednisone has often been helpful in reducing exophthalmos. It is administered orally in a daily dosage of 2 mg/kg in three divided doses for 6 weeks. This is followed by 1 mg/kg daily for 4 weeks, and it is then gradually reduced over a 2-week period and discontinued.

More aggressive therapy is justified in patients with the most severe forms of disseminated histiocytosis X, particularly infants with Letterer-Siwe disease and severe organ dysfunction. A few of these patients have been treated with a combination of vinblastine, prednisolone, methotrexate,[‡] and cyclophosphamide.[‡] Vinblastine is given in an intravenous dose of 6.5 mg/square meter once a week for 8 weeks. The daily dose of prednisolone is 40 mg/square meter, given orally once a day for 6 weeks. The weekly dose for methotrexate is 20 mg/square meter, administered intravenously once a week 1 day after vinblastine for 8 weeks. Administration of 200 mg/square meter of intravenous cyclophosphamide once a week for 8 weeks may be given 2 days after methotrexate. After this 8-week induction phase is completed, weekly cyclophosphamide and methotrexate are continued in the above doses. The patient is also given consolidation courses of vinblastine; this is defined as daily doses of 6.5 mg/square meter for 1 week and is repeated every 4 weeks. The therapy is discontinued if all measurable lesions disappear. If there is resolution of 50 per cent or more of the initial lesions, the treatment is continued for 6 more months.

Irradiation can be combined with chemotherapy in treating disseminated histiocytosis X. The severity of gingival and cutaneous lesions may be reduced by giving 450 to 600 rads in 2 or 3 fractions during the time period while the response to chemotherapy is being evaluated.

Ocular. Intraocular infiltrates, usually manifested as an anterior or posterior uveitis or less commonly as a scleritis, must be treated according to the standard regimens that are well known to ophthalmologists. In addition, the cornea must be protected from exposure by frequent instillation of lubricants and ointments, cellophane patching, or lateral tarsorrhaphy.

Supportive. Supportive care is also very important in treating disseminated histiocytosis X. Appropriate antibiotics, blood products, nutrition, skin care, physical therapy, and orthopedic care are often required.

Ocular or Periocular Manifestations

Anterior Chamber: Cells and flare due to anterior uveitis; hypopyon; spontaneous hemorrhage.

Choroid: Extramedullary hematopoiesis (rare); infiltration by histiocytic cells leading to a rather diffuse, flat thickening.

Conjunctiva: Chemosis; dilated vessels.

Cornea: Bullous keratopathy; endothelial atrophy; infiltration; pannus; perforation; scarring; ulcer; vascularization.

Eyelids: Edema; infiltration; rash; xanthoma, especially in patients with icterus.

Globe: Exophthalmos, luxation.

Iris or Ciliary Body: Cellular infiltration with possible secondary increased intraocular pressure; infiltration; iridocyclitis or cyclitis with possible formation of a cyclitic membrane; nodular lesions mimicking tumors or juvenile Xanthogranuloma; pigmentary changes, including heterochromia; secondary atrophy; uveitis or iridocyclitis with potential for synechiae formation.

Lens: Cataract.

Optic Nerve: Atrophy and gliosis; infiltration of surrounding meninges; papilledema.

Orbit: Infiltrates; periorbital bone lesions.

Retina: Degeneration; detachment and retinal folds; edema; histiocytic infiltration.

Sclera: Episcleritis; scleritis.

Vitreous: Histiocytic infiltration, often leading to liquefaction.

Other: Glaucoma; nystagmus; phthisis bulbi; poor pupillary dilation with mydriatics; visual loss.

Precautions

Although many of the chosen therapeutic agents have significant associated morbidity, the severe forms of histiocytosis X may show such severe extremes of morbidity and mortality that radical treatment may be required. Therapy should be undertaken only by physicians experienced in the use of such chemotherapeutic agents (usually pediatric oncologists) and closely monitored with frequent blood counts and periodic evaluations of liver and renal function.

Systemic steroids are also useful in reducing exophthalmos. Nevertheless, depending on the severity of the disease, the side effects associated with their use must be carefully considered.

Low-dose irradiation of the eye carries the risk of producing radiation cataracts.

Comments

Diabetes insipidus is a classic complication of histiocytosis X, and local radiation therapy may be beneficial in preventing its progression. This treatment is most effective in patients with at least partial urinary concentrating ability. Low doses of 800 to 1200 rads delivered to the hypothalamic-pituitary region are probably sufficient for this treatment. Vasopressin is important in the management of patients who retain some degree of pituitary dysfunction. Intrathecal methotrexate‡ has also been used to treat diabetes insipidus, but the results have been disappointing.

Some patients have been shown to have decreased levels of human growth hormone associated with impaired linear growth. Therapy with human growth hormone is therefore indicated in selected patients.

Infections are common in patients with histiocytosis X, both because of the nature of the disease and its treatment. Otitis media is a frequent complication that may result in loss of hearing. The physician should watch for and be prepared to treat these infections. However, prophylactic antibiotics are not useful because they predispose the patient to opportunistic infections.

References

Basset F, Nezelof C, Ferrans VJ: The histiocytosis. Pathol Ann: 17:27–78, 1982.
Crocker AC: The histiocytosis syndromes. In Gellis SS, Kagan BM: Current Pediatric Therapy 10. Philadelphia, WB Saunders, 1982, pp 661–662.
Giller RH, et al: Xanthoma dissemination. Am J Pediatr Hematol Oncol 10:252–257, 1988.
Greenberger JS, et al: Results of treatment of 127 patients with systemic histiocytosis (Letterer-Siwe syndrome, Hand-Schüller-Christian syndrome and multifocal eosinophilic granuloma). Medicine 60:311–338, 1981.
Harrist TJ, Bhan AK, Murphy GF: Histiocytosis X: In situ characterization of cutaneous infiltrates with monoclonal antibodies. Am J Clin Pathol 79:294–300, 1983.
Jakobiec FA, Jones IS: Lymphomatous, plasmacytic, histiocytic, and hematopoietic tumors. In Duane TD (ed): Clinical Ophthalmology. Hagerstown, MD, Harper & Row, 1982, Vol II, pp 39:28–37.
Lahey, M.E.: Histiocytosis X. In Spittell JA Jr: Clinical Medicine. Hagerstown, MD, Harper & Row, 1980, Vol V, pp 1–6.
Lahey ME: Prognostic factors in histiocytosis X. Am J Pediatr Hematol Oncol 3:57–60, 1981.
McMillan EM, Humphrey GB, Stoneking C: Analysis of histiocytosis X infiltrates with monoclonal antibodies directed against cells of histiocytic, lymphoid and myoloid lineage. Clin Immunol Immunopathol 38:295–301, 1986.
Moore AT, Pritchard J, Taylor DSI: Histiocytosis X: An ophthalmological review. Br J Ophthalmol 69:7–14, 1985.
Richter MP, D'Angio GJ: The role of radiation therapy in the management of children with histiocytosis X. Am J Pediatr Hematol Oncol 3:161–163, 1981.
Starling KA: Chemotherapy of histiocytosis. Am J Pediatr Hematol Oncol 3:157–160, 1981.
Wood CM, et al: Globe luxation in histiocytosis X. Br J Ophthalmol 72:631–633, 1988.

REITER'S DISEASE
K. MATTI SAARI, M.D.
Turku, Finland

Reiter's disease is a symptom complex with varying degrees of expression. Patients have a high incidence of HLA-B27 antigen. The disease has been reported more frequently in males than in females during the years of maximum sexual activity. It may occur as a complication of nonspecific urethritis, postgonococcal urethritis, or dysentery and following *Yersinia, Salmonella,* or *Campylobacter* infection. Commonly, a first attack in the male consists of nonspecific urethritis (with or without complications of hemorrhagic cystitis or epididymitis), conjunctivitis, anterior uveitis, latex negative erosion polyarthritis with marked periarthritis, and fasciitis. Characteristic keratodermic involvement of skin and mucous membrane occurs in about 25 per cent of patients. Circinate balanitis may develop first after the nonspecific urethritis and is a sign that arthritis is about to develop. There may also be cardiac or neurologic involvement. Sequelae may include painful deformed feet, ankylosing spondylitis, and, rarely, aortic incompetence or amyloid disease. In recurrent attacks of the venereal form, genital infection may sometimes be absent following systemic treatment. *Chlamydia* has been isolated from urethral material in about 50 per cent of the cases, but *Ureaplasm urealyticum* (T. strain) may also be found.

Ocular manifestations in Reiter's disease are common and nonspecific; over 50 per cent of patients develop eye lesions. The conjunctivitis, which is usually bilateral and mucopurulent, occurs in 30 to 50 per cent of patients and is occasionally the presenting complaint, but usually causes little discomfort. Anterior uveitis occurs in severe attacks, which may last 6 weeks or more; although the disease usually follows a self-limiting course, recurrences are common. There is a strong association of anterior uveitis with sacroiliitis; 50 per cent of patients with sacroiliitis develop iritis, and only about 10 per cent of patients without sacroiliitis develop iritis.

THERAPY

Systemic. The urethritis associated with Reiter's disease warrants administration of a 3- to 4-week course of oral tetracyclines. The usual adult dosage of tetracycline or oxytetracycline is 250 to 500 mg, given four times daily after meals. Alternatively, 100 mg of doxycycline can be given one to two times daily after meals; this drug is well absorbed and causes little gastrointestinal upset. While urethritis persists, other manifestations remain or may recur. Tests of overnight urethral secretion will show when the urethritis has cleared. It is epidemiologically vital that all sexual partners be examined for genital infection. If treatment is necessary, it should be given concurrently to prevent "ping-pong" reinfection. When *Chlamydia* infection is affecting the whole family, oral erythromycin is the drug of choice for children (daily dosage 40 mg/kg) and for pregnant women (500 mg administered every 8 hours).

Septic cases of *Salmonella*, *Shigella*, and *Yersinia* infections triggering Reiter's disease can be treated with a mixture of trimethoprim and sulfamethoxazole; the suggested adult oral dosage is 160 mg of trimethoprim and 800 mg of sulfamethoxazole twice daily. The recommended daily dose for children is 6 mg/kg of trimethoprim and 30 mg/kg of sulfamethoxazole. *Yersinia* infection in adults is usually treated with 250 mg of oral tetracycline every 6 hours for 10 days. *Campylobacter* infection is treated, when needed, with erythromycin; the oral dosage for adults is 250 to 500 mg every 6 hours and 40 mg/kg daily for children.

Ocular. The anterior uveitis usually responds gradually to standard therapy with cycloplegics and corticosteroids. This regimen usually includes topically administered corticosteroids, such as 0.1 per cent dexamethasone or 0.5 to 1.0 per cent prednisolone, every hour daily and corticosteroid ointment for the night, and 1 per cent atropine or 0.25 per cent scopolamine three times daily. In severe cases with fulminant onset of intraocular inflammation, 60 mg of oral prednisolone daily with subsequent lowering of dosage or anterior subconjunctival depot corticosteroid injection* (into the lower fornix or beneath Tenon's capsule) may be used. Another alternative in severe cases is the anterior subconjunctival injection of a soluble corticosteroid, such as 1 ml of dexamethasone* solution containing 4 mg/ml, which is repeated every 1 to 2 days. Conjunctivitis does not usually require treatment, but the lubricating action of 1 per cent chlortetracycline ophthalmic ointment is comforting.

Supportive. The patient with arthritis and a high erythrocyte sedimentation rate should be admitted to the hospital for rest. Symptomatic therapy for arthritis associated with Reiter's disease includes nonsteroidal anti-inflammatory drugs and modalities of physical therapy. Indomethacin is the agent of choice, administered in a dosage of 25 to 50 mg three times daily. If indomethacin is not tolerated, other nonsteroidal anti-inflammatory drugs can be used. These agents relieve pain, reduce swelling and tenderness of the joints, and increase grip strength.

Ocular or Periocular Manifestations

Anterior Chamber: Cells and flare; fibrinous exudate.
Conjunctiva: Chemosis; follicles; hyperemia; mucopurulent conjunctivitis; subpalpebral papillary conjunctivitis.
Cornea: Edema; epithelial erosion; fine keratic precipitates; punctate keratitis.
Iris: Acute anterior uveitis; posterior synechiae; vasodilation of iris vessels.
Optic Nerve: Disc edema; optic neuritis.
Other: Cells in vitreous; macular edema.

PRECAUTIONS

Photosensitivity may follow the intake of tetracyclines, particularly doxycycline; therefore, patients taking such drugs should limit their exposure to the sun. Any product containing aluminum, magnesium, or calcium ions (antacids, milk, and milk products) should not be taken 1 hour before or 2 hours after an oral dose of a tetracycline, since it can decrease the absorption by as much as 25 to 50 per cent. An exception to this is doxycycline, which is well absorbed in the presence of milk and milk products and is best taken with milk after meals. Tetracyclines should be avoided during pregnancy and in children younger than 8 years of age because of irreversible deposition of the substance in growing teeth and bones.

Local side effects of topical corticosteroids may include a rise in intraocular pressure. This rise can usually be handled by the addition of topically administered 1 per cent epinephrine or 0.5 per cent timolol eyedrops twice daily or by oral carbonic anhydrase inhibitors. Fluorometholone is of value in such patients, since it rarely causes an increase in intraocular pressure.

In Reiter's disease, the urethritis, balanitis, conjunctivitis, and mouth ulcers are often clinically silent, and these components of the disease are frequently missed. "Formes frustes" of the syndrome are becoming more clearly recognized, and the condition will be diagnosed more often also in females. In children, the diagnosis may be made during an epidemic of dysentery or enteritis, with Reiter's syndrome affecting many members of the family.

COMMENTS

Recurrences without urethritis should probably still be treated with tetracycline. The conjunctivitis is usually painless, clears by itself within days, and is not affected by treatment.

The keratitis, although self-limited, may be temporarily incapacitating.

Many individuals develop an exacerbation or relapse without obvious reason, and the disease is frequently disturbing for the patient with feelings of guilt and anxiety about sexual misconduct. Therefore, one of the major considerations in treatment is explanation of the recurrent nature of the condition: the patients have a genetically determined susceptibility to develop Reiter's disease after contact with an unrecognized (or recognized) precipitating event.

References

Calin A: Reiter's syndrome. Med Clin North Am 61:365–376, 1977.
Harris JRW (ed): Recent Advances in Sexually Transmitted Diseases. New York, Churchill Livingstone, 1981.
Kousa M: Clinical observations on Reiter's disease with special reference to the venereal and non-venereal aetiology. Acta Derm Venereol 58 (Suppl.):1–36, 1978.
Ostler HB, et al: Reiter's syndrome. Am J Ophthalmol 71:986–991, 1971.
Rosenberg AM, Petty RE: Reiter's disease in children. Am J Dis Child 133:394–398, 1979.
Saari KM, Kauranen O: Ocular inflammation in Reiter's syndrome associated with *Campylobacter jejuni* enteritis. Am J Ophthalmol 90:572–573, 1980.
Saari KM, et al: Ocular inflammation in Reiter's disease after *Salmonella* enteritis. Am J Ophthalmol 90:63–68, 1980.

SARCOIDOSIS

DANIEL H. GOLD, M.D.
Galveston, Texas

Sarcoidosis is a systemic inflammatory disease characterized by the development of noncaseating epitheliod cell granulomas in tissues and organs throughout the body. It may take an acute or chronic course and is often a benign self-limited disorder. Its clinical manifestations are protean and depend upon the specific site(s) of inflammation in any given patient. Intrathoracic involvement occurs in close to 90 per cent of cases, with granulomas in the lungs or intrathoracic lymphoid tissue. Ocular involvement occurs in about 25 per cent of cases and produces some of the most serious complications of this disorder.

Although its etiology is unknown, sarcoidosis is associated with a number of immunologic abnormalities. Immunohistopathologic studies have demonstrated a high ratio of T-helper to T-supressor lymphocytes in the lungs, lymph nodes, and eyes of patients with active sarcoidosis. Lymphokines produced by these activated T-helper cells may attract other inflammatory cells, resulting in the subsequent development of a typical granuloma. They may also affect the humoral immune system by stimulating B-lymphocytes to produce a polyclonal increase in circulating immunoglobulins, as well as a variety of autoantibodies.

THERAPY

Ocular. Most of the ophthalmologic complications of sarcoidosis are secondary to inflammatory involvement of ocular or periocular structures and respond quite well to steroid therapy. Topical steroids may suffice in the treatment of anterior uveitis. During waking hours, 1 per cent prednisolone eyedrops are used every 1 to 2 hours, with gradual tapering of the dose as the inflammation subsides. This treatment must be combined with mydriatic/cycloplegic drops to avoid development of posterior synechiae with a small bound-down pupil. Long-acting drugs, such as 1 per cent atropine twice daily or 2 to 5 per cent homatropine four times daily, are preferred in acute or severe uveitis, whereas shorter-acting mydriatics (1 per cent tropicamide) can be used once daily to keep the pupil moving in patients with low-grade, chronic inflammatory disease. A combination of mydriatic agents, including 2.5 or 10 per cent phenylephrine, may be used in an attempt to break pre-existent posterior synechiae.

When anterior segment inflammation is very severe or does not respond quickly to topical medication, this treatment should be supplemented by anterior subtenon steroid injection; 40 mg of triamcinolone,* 40 mg of methylprednisolone,* or 24 mg of dexamethasone* may be used. Triamcinolone has the greatest anti-inflammatory activity, is well absorbed, produces little discomfort when injected, and lasts 2 to 3 weeks. The periocular injection may be repeated in 3 to 4 weeks, if needed.

Glaucoma may develop as a result of the underlying disease or may occur as a response to the topical steroid therapy. If the patient is a steroid responder, fluorometholone drops may produce a sufficient anti-inflammatory response without as much pressure-elevating effect as topical prednisolone. Regardless of its etiology, the glaucoma may be treated with topical 0.25 or 0.5 per cent timolol every 12 hours or carbonic anhydrase inhibitors, such as 250 mg of acetazolamide four times daily or long-acting 500 mg sequels two times a day.

Systemic. Systemic steroid therapy is indicated for control of posterior segment inflammation, orbital disease, the neuro-ophthalmologic complications of sarcoidosis, or anterior segment inflammatory disease that is not responsive to topical or periocular steroids. Treatment should begin with 60 to 80 mg of prednisone daily (or equivalent doses of prednisolone or dexamethasone). The drugs may be given as a single daily dose before breakfast or in divided doses four times daily. The dosage should be slowly tapered as the inflammation subsides. Alternate-day therapy with twice the usual daily dose may avoid some of the complications of prolonged systemic steroid therapy. It may be useful in patients requiring long-term treatment for chronic inflammatory disease, but should not be employed in the initial stages of treatment when rapid control of significant inflammation is desired.

No other drugs can approach the effectiveness of systemic steroids in the treatment of sarcoidosis. In patients requiring treatment and in whom strong contraindications to the use of systemic steroids are present, such drugs as chlorambucil,[‡] azathioprine,[‡] methotrexate,[‡] or cyclosporine[‡] may be of value, either alone or in combination with systemic steroids. The drugs are given orally in daily doses. They should be considered only under unusual circumstances and given in consultation with physicians thoroughly familiar with their use. Nonsteroidal anti-inflammatory agents, such as oxyphenbutazone[‡] or indomethacin,[‡] may be of value in selected patients with ocular or systemic inflammation but are not widely used.

Surgical. Since the initial ocular complications of sarcoidosis are inflammatory in nature, surgery plays little role in their management. However, surgery may be required in the management of late complications, such as cataract formation that occurs secondary to the chronic uveitis or steroid therapy. Surgical or laser iridectomy may be needed to relieve pupillary block with iris bombé if the synechiae cannot be broken with mydriatic therapy. Filtering surgery is a last resort in uncontrolled glaucoma secondary to chronic angle closure with peripheral anterior synechiae, though the inflammatory nature of the underlying disease decreases the chance of a successful outcome.

Argon laser photocoagulation is of value in treating the retinal neovascularization seen in sarcoid patients. Scatter (modified panretinal) photocoagulation to areas of retinal nonperfusion can produce regression of the neovascularization. Focal treatment directly to the neovascular fronds has also been effective, although more widespread photocoagulation is preferred in the presence of significant zones of nonperfused retina. Disc neovascularization, without extensive areas of peripheral retinal vascular nonperfusion, may regress promptly with systemic steroid therapy. A 4- to 6-week trial of systemic steroids is appropriate before attempting laser photocoagulation.

Vitrectomy may be required for nonclearing vitreous opacities, hemorrhage, or traction retinal detachment.

Ocular or Periocular Manifestations

Choroid: Chorioretinal scarring; granuloma; subretinal neovascular membranes (juxtapapillary and macular).
Conjunctiva: Granuloma; nonspecific conjunctivitis; phlyctenules.
Cornea: Band keratopathy; hypesthesia (secondary to fifth nerve paralysis); interstitial keratitis; keratoconjunctivitis sicca.
Extraocular Muscles: Granulomatous infiltration of muscles; paralysis of third, fourth, or sixth cranial nerve with diplopia.
Eyelids: Cutaneous granuloma (lupus pernio); paralysis (secondary to seventh nerve palsy); ptosis (secondary to paralysis of third nerve).
Iris: Anterior and/or posterior synechiae; anterior uveitis (usually chronic granulomatous, but may be acute nongranulomatous); nodules (intrastromal lesions or surface keratic precipitate-like deposits).
Lacrimal System: Dacryoadenitis; dacryocystitis (may produce obstructive disease of lacrimal drainage system); lacrimal gland enlargement.
Lens: Cataracts.
Optic Nerve: Atrophy; neovascularization over disc; papilledema (secondary to elevated intracranial pressure); retrobulbar or optic neuritis (usually associated with granuloma formation within the optic nerve).
Orbit: Granuloma; proptosis.
Pupil: Amaurotic pupillary signs; internal ophthalmoplegia.
Retina: Detachment; edema; granuloma; hemorrhages; neovascularization; perivasculitis; pigmentary loss, clumping, or mottling (gross or subtle change); retinal vein occlusions (usually peripheral); superficial exudative "candle-wax" lesions.
Sclera: Episcleritis; scleritis.
Vitreous: Granulomas (snowball or string of pearls configuration, usually inferior); hemorrhages; vitreitis (associated with inflammation of adjacent structures).
Other: Phthisis; secondary glaucoma (may be due to peripheral anterior synechiae, iris bombé, or nodular infiltration of trabecular meshwork); visual field defects (secondary to granulomatous involvement of optic nerves, chiasm, or tracts).

Precautions

The major complications of the treatment of sarcoidosis are related to the adverse effects of steroid therapy. Systemic steroids produce a host of potentially serious side effects and should be used in consultation with the patient's internist. Salt and water retention may cause problems in patients with cardiac disease or hypertension. Potential aggravation or unmasking of diabetes mellitus, peptic ulcer, gastritis, esophagitis, or chronic infections (especially tuberculosis) requires particular attention. Other serious side effects include steroid-induced myopathy, osteoporosis with vertebral collapse, psychiatric problems, and adrenal insufficiency secondary to rapid withdrawal of the drugs after prolonged treatment. Ocular complications of both systemic and topical therapy include the development of posterior subcapsular cataracts and elevated intraocular pressure.

Chloroquine, sometimes used as adjunctive therapy to control the hypercalcemia and hypercalcinuria associated with sarcoidosis, can produce macular pigmentary changes progressing to bull's-eye maculopathy with loss of central vision. Serial visual acuity testing, funduscopic examinations, and central visual field studies with an Amsler grid should be performed on patients receiving chloroquine. Fluorescein angiography, color vision testing, and electro-oculography may also be useful in following these patients.

Sarcoid inflammatory disease tends to be recurrent, especially as therapy is decreased or withdrawn. Both the patient and the treating physician must be aware of this pattern, and careful follow-up evaluations are essential. Synechiae and their complications may develop fairly rapidly; if significant inflammation is present, weak mydriatics, such as tropicamide, are not strong enough to prevent their development or to break them once they occur. Patients should be encouraged to seek attention at the first sign of a change in their ocular status. At the same time, the physician must not "overtreat" the disease. Many uveitis patients develop a chronic "breakdown" in their blood-ocular barrier, with mild flare and an occasional cell in the anterior chamber. Distinguishing this situation from a chronic, active, ongoing inflammatory process may be difficult. The absence of new synechiae, keratic precipitates, and increasing anterior chamber reaction allows the ophthalmologist to observe the patient without reinstituting or increasing the therapy.

Every patient with anterior segment sarcoidosis should be carefully evaluated for posterior segment disease. Care must be taken to avoid a situation in which topical therapy is producing a satisfactory regression of anterior uveitis while leaving a serious, progressive, posterior inflammatory process untouched. Although most patients have bilateral ocular disease, the extent of involvement and degree of inflammation may be quite asymmetric. Both eyes must be carefully evaluated.

Comments

The ocular complications of sarcoidosis are part of a *systemic* disorder, and a coordination of effort between the ophthalmologist and other physicians caring for the patient is essential. Almost all patients with ocular sarcoidosis have evidence of active disease elsewhere in the body. Although there has been widespread debate in the medical literature as to when sarcoidosis should be treated, the presence of ocular inflammatory disease is almost universally accepted as an absolute indication for initiating therapy.

The diagnosis of sarcoidosis is made with greatest confidence by histopathologic demonstration of noncaseating epithelioid granulomas in affected tissues. Conjunctival biopsy may reveal typical granulomas, but the incidence of positive biopsies varies greatly among the series reported in the literature. Other important diagnostic aids include typical findings on chest x-rays, elevated levels of serum angiotensin-converting enzyme, and positive gallium uptake scans. Although not absolutely diagnostic, a positive scan in the presence of elevated angiotensin-converting enzyme levels is very strongly suggestive of the presence of sarcoidosis. Although anterior uveitis is the most common clinically observed manifestation of ocular sarcoidosis, conjunctival biopsy studies and lacrimal gland gallium uptake studies suggest that asymptomatic lacrimal gland and conjunctival granulomas are actually the most common forms of ocular involvement. Ocular changes are more likely to occur in patients with sarcoidosis of the skin, peripheral lymphadenopathy, hypercalcemia, neurologic involvement, parotid enlargement, and joint disease. Band keratopathy is strongly associated with an underlying hypercalcemia. Other reported associations include posterior segment inflammation (especially optic nerve involvement) with central nervous system sarcoidosis, and upper respiratory involvement with sarcoidosis of the lacrimal sac.

There are, within the broader clinical spectrum of sarcoid disease, several widely recognized syndromes with ocular components. These include Heerfordt's syndrome (uveitis, parotid enlargement, a chronic febrile course, and cranial nerve palsies, especially seventh) and Löfgren's syndrome (erythema nodosum, bilateral hilar adenopathy, acute iritis, and parotitis). Löfgren's syndrome is generally considered to have a relatively benign, self-limiting course. Another sarcoid "syndrome" includes chronic uveitis, cutaneous sarcoidosis, bone cysts, and pulmonary fibrosis and is considered a more persistent and troublesome clinical complex.

Treatment of ocular sarcoidosis requires both diligence and patience. Therapy in this condition is seldom a quick "one-shot" proposition. The patient's clinical response is the ultimate determinant in making decisions as to the type, route, and duration of therapy. Recurrences may develop after long periods of quiescence, and these patients must be followed indefinitely.

References

Aaberg TM: The role of the ophthalmologist in the management of sarcoidosis. Am J Ophthalmol 103:99–101, 1987.

Beardsley TL, et al: Eleven cases of sarcoidosis of the optic nerve. Am J Ophthalmol 97:62–77, 1984.

Chan CC, et al: Immunohistopathology of ocular sarcoidosis. Report of a case and discussion of immunopathogenesis. Arch Ophthalmol 105:1398–1402, 1987.

Hoover DL, Khan JA, Giangiacomo J: Pediatric ocular sarcoidosis. Surv Ophthalmol 30:215–228, 1986.

Jabs DA, Johns CJ: Ocular involvement in chronic sarcoidosis. Am J Ophthalmol 102:297–301, 1986.

James DG: Ocular sarcoidosis. Ann NY Acad Sci 465:551–563, 1986.

Johns CJ (ed): Tenth International Conference on Sarcoidosis and Other Granulomatous Disorders. Ann NY Acad Sci 465:1–746, 1986.

Karma A, Huhti E, Poukkula A: Course and outcome of ocular sarcoidosis. Am J Ophthalmol 106:467–472, 1988.

Karma A, Poukkula AA, Ruokonen AO: Assessment of activity of ocular sarcoidosis by gallium scanning. Br J Ophthalmol 71:361–367, 1987.

Palestine AG, Nussenblatt RB, Chan CC: Treatment of intraocular complications of sarcoidosis. Ann NY Acad Sci 465:564–574, 1986.

Stone LS, Ehrenberg M: Bilateral nodular sarcoid choroiditis with vitreous hemorrhage. Br J Ophthalmol 68:660–666, 1984.

VOGT-KOYANAGI-HARADA SYNDROME
(Harada's Syndrome, Uveitis-Vitiligo-Alopecia-Poliosis Syndrome, Vogt-Koyanagi Syndrome)

ALAN H. FRIEDMAN, M.D.,
New York, New York

The Vogt-Koyanagi-Harada (VKH) syndrome is a multisystem disorder characterized by headache, fever, bilateral uveitis (granulomatous or nongranulomatous), vitiligo, poliosis, alopecia, tinnitus, neck stiffness, loss of hearing, and pleocytosis of the cerebrospinal fluid. The etiology of the VKH syndrome is unknown, despite reports implicating viruses, bacteria, and fungi. A genetic predisposition has been suggested by the finding of the syndrome in three siblings. The syndrome has a definite predilection for darkly pigmented races or those with Oriental ancestry and affects adults, usually between 20 and 50 years of age. The first symptoms of the disease may be headache, nausea, vomiting, stiffness, and pain in the back of the neck that is sometimes associated with a meningeal syndrome or encephalitic signs. In the later stage, there is a hearing decrease or tinnitus, which is often caused by involvement of the eighth cranial nerve. Skin involvement manifested by poliosis, alopecia, or vitiligo may occur after the central nervous system and ocular signs of the disorder have subsided. This is usually within 2 to 3 months after onset, but the earliest signs of depigmentation can be found in the perilimbal area about 1 month after onset.

Initially, ocular involvement is characterized by posterior uveitis, which is manifested by bilateral serous retinal detachment with congestive papillary edema that rapidly becomes severe. As the inflammation progresses, the retinal detachment tends to predominate in the inferior segment of the eye. Fluorescein angiography reveals characteristic leakage of the dye from the choroid into the subretinal space. Subsequently, inflammatory reaction spreads toward the anterior uvea and produces various signs of anterior uveitis, such as flare and cells in the anterior chamber, mutton-fat keratic precipitates, and iris nodules. The severity of the anterior segment reaction varies from almost no reaction (Harada type) to severe reaction (Vogt-Koyanagi type). Marked decrease in visual acuity is noted early in the course of the disease. Impairment of visual fields is variable and corresponds to the extent of the retinal detachment. Rarely, cataracts or secondary glaucoma may develop. The usual course of events with prompt and adequate therapy is for the vision to return eventually to normal. However, many patients have some permanent impairment of vision. Following resolution of the retinal detachments, a diffuse depigmentation of the entire fundus is seen that has been characterized in the choroid as "the sunset glow" sign with associated changes at the level of the retinal pigment epithelium, namely depigmentation and hyperpigmentation.

THERAPY

Systemic. In the VKH syndrome, systemic corticosteroid therapy is the most effective agent. One regimen is to prescribe 100 mg of prednisone orally at breakfast each day for the first week, then decrease the dosage to 100 mg at breakfast every other day during the second week. The dosage should be tapered according to the therapeutic response. Particular attention should be directed toward detection of acute ocular inflammatory recurrence, which is liable to occur as early as 3 to 6 weeks or up to 9 months after systemic corticosteroid therapy has been discontinued. The clinical signs during the flare-up are almost identical to those during the initial attack. In the case of such a flare-up, the same therapeutic regimen should be reinstituted.

Ocular. The cornerstone of ocular therapy is systemic and local corticosteroids. One per cent prednisolone drops are instilled hourly during the first several days (while awake), with tapering to four to six times daily. Concomitant periocular injection of dexamethasone* or methylprednisolone* should be given.

Ocular or Periocular Manifestations

Choroid: Edema: exudative choroiditis; depigmentation (sunset glow fundus); multiple areas of leakage on fluorescein angiography.

Conjunctiva: Perilimbal vitiligo (Sugiura's sign).

Eyelids: Poliosis; vitiligo.

Iris: Anterior uveitis; nodules.

Optic Nerve: Edema; hemorrhages; optic disc hyperemia.

Retina: Exudative retinal detachment; macular edema; macular scarring; retinal pigment epithelial depigmentation and hyperpigmentation; retinal vascular sheathing; subretinal neovascularization.

Vitreous: Exudates; haze.

Other: Cataracts; mutton-fat keratic precipitates; phthisis bulbi; secondary glaucoma.

Precautions

The ocular inflammatory reactions in this disease are severe and can be chronic. Unless adequately treated, they often result in severe visual impairment or blindness.

Corticosteroids should be used cautiously to avoid the side effects of these drugs. The lowest possible dosage should be utilized to control the inflammation; when reduction in dosage is possible, the reduction should be gradual.

Comments

In the VKH syndrome, the retinal detachments usually start in the macular area, extend inferiorly, and finally extend to involve the entire retina. Without treatment, the neuroretinitis and posterior uveitis regress slowly, taking from 6 to 12 months. Visual prognosis is poor without treatment. Less than 30 per cent of patients who have not been treated regain useful vision because of secondary glaucoma, cataract, or phthisis bulbi. Although varying in intensity, the clinical signs and symptoms closely simulate those occurring in the sympathized eye in sympathetic ophthalmia.

References

Friedman AH, Deutsch-Sokol RH: Sugiura's sign: Perilimbal vitiligo in the Vogt-Koyanagi-Harada syndrome. Ophthalmology 88:1159–1165, 1981.

Ohno S, et al: Vogt-Koyanagi-Harada syndrome. Am J Ophthalmol 83:735–740, 1977.

Shimizu K: Harada's Behcet's, Vogt-Koyanagi syndromes—Are they clinical entities? Trans Am Acad Ophthalmol Otolaryngol 77:281–290, 1973.

Snyder DA, Tessler HH: Vogt-Koyanagi-Harada syndrome. Am J Ophthalmol 90:69–75, 1980.

Sugiura S: Vogt-Koyanagi-Harada disease. Jpn J Ophthalmol 22:9–35, 1978.

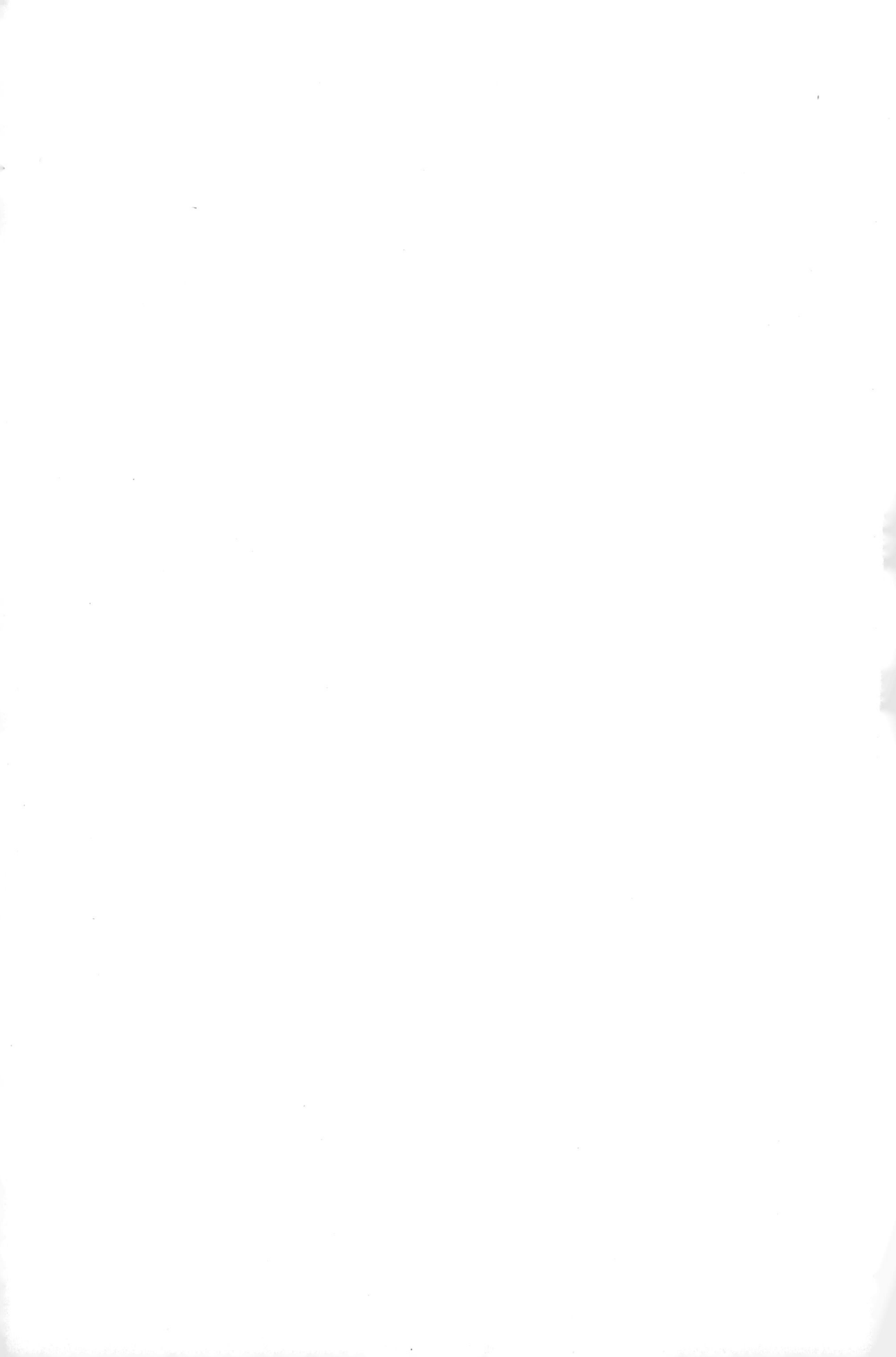

Part II

EYE AND ADNEXA

SECTION 18

ANTERIOR CHAMBER

EPITHELIAL INGROWTH
(Epithelial Downgrowth)

PATRICIA W. SMITH, M.D.,
Charlottesville, Virginia

and WALTER J. STARK, M.D.,
RONALD G. MICHELS, M.D.
Baltimore, Maryland

Sheet-like epithelial invasion of the anterior chamber is a rare, dreaded complication of ocular trauma or anterior segment surgery. Its diagnosis, often delayed, is based on a constellation of signs and symptoms together with an awareness of the disease. Its presence should be suspected after surgery or trauma complicated by wound leak, hypotony, persistent inflammation, and, later, intractable glaucoma.

Fortunately, the incidence of epithelial ingrowth after cataract surgery appears to have decreased, from an incidence of 1.1 per cent reported 40 years ago to less than 0.2 per cent in recent reports. The onset of symptoms of epithelial ingrowth—usually within 3 years after surgery—may be insidious, with the patient complaining of tearing, dull aching pain, photophobia, and blurred vision. On examination, wound gap, a bleb, or a fistula may be seen with judicious pressure on the globe. These conditions are sometimes seen more clearly after instillation of 2 per cent fluorescein. On retroillumination, the ingrowth itself appears as a translucent posterior corneal membrane demarcated by a gray line. This leading gray line is often scalloped, with focal pearl-like areas of thickening. No keratic precipitates are present. Diminished corneal sensation, corneal edema overlying the ingrowth, stromal vascularization, and striae are variably present. Glaucoma is present in half of the cases. Gonioscopy may show wound-incarcerated tissue, a fistula or suture tract, and obliteration of the angle by the epithelial sheet or by peripheral anterior synechia. Anterior chamber cell and flare are frequently present. Involvement of the iris is more extensive than that of the cornea and is seen clinically as an immobile, distorted area with obscured details. Precise delineation of iris involvement using the argon laser (500-μm spot, 100 mW, 0.1 second) can be done preoperatively; the normal iris sustains a well-demarcated slight burn, whereas epithelium overlying iris shows a characteristic fluffy white appearance. Iris biopsy or corneal endothelial curettage provides histologic confirmation of the diagnosis. Membranes over the pupil, over the vitreous face, and enveloping the intraocular lens may be seen in advanced cases.

THERAPY

Supportive. There is no effective medical treatment for epithelial ingrowth. Topical corticosteroids may suppress inflammation and its symptoms indefinitely, but do not prevent progression of the ingrowth.

Surgical. Surgical intervention for epithelial ingrowth has been reported to result in 25 per cent of eyes retaining good vision (greater than 20/40). Before operation, the site of invasion, any fistula or bleb, and the extent of iris involvement are determined. At surgery, a peritomy is performed, and any leaking fistula is closed using a partial-thickness, limbus-based scleral flap dissected just posterior to the site, reflected anteriorly, and secured with 10-0 nylon suture. Vitrectomy instruments are introduced using a pars plana approach, and involved iris and vitreous tissues are excised. The anterior vitreous is then removed as well to provide space for the subsequent fluid-gas exchange. With a sterile air bubble in the anterior segment, any retinal breaks are localized and treated. Cryotherapy is then applied in a transcorneal and transscleral fashion to devitalize any epithelium remaining on the posterior cornea, in the angle, and on the ciliary body. On the cornea, a single freeze-thaw is applied sufficient to form ice crystals on the posterior surface of the cornea. The air bubble is replaced, if it is not needed to tamponade any retinal breaks.

Ocular or Periocular Manifestations

Conjunctiva: Bleb; ciliary flush; fistula.
Cornea: Edema; hypesthesia; neovascularization; posterior corneal membrane.
Iris: Corectopia; decreased mobility; iritis; loss of details; peripheral anterior synechiae.
Lens: Ciliary body, vitreous: epithelial sheet covering; inflammation; intraocular lens cocoon.
Other: Blur; glaucoma; pain; photophobia.

PRECAUTIONS

Closure of a leaking fistula in an eye thought otherwise inoperable may lead to intractable glaucoma.

On preoperative evaluation, photocoagulation of the iris to delineate its involvement is done within 24 hours of surgery, since it produces moderate anterior chamber inflammation.

Cryotherapy will destroy corneal endothelium so the freeze should be limited to the involved area of cornea. The presence of air in the anterior chamber enables such precise treatment. Penetrating keratoplasty may be needed later for visual rehabilitation if extensive corneal cryotherapy is required.

Comments

The differential diagnosis of epithelial ingrowth includes 1) an anteriorly shelved cataract incision, seen as a diagonal, posterior-to-anterior intrastromal line on careful slitlamp examination; 2) fibrous ingrowth, distinguished by its slow growth and vascularity; 3) vitreocorneal adhesions, which may cause corneal edema and have a grayish appearance; 4) detachment of Descemet's membrane; 5) peripheral corneal edema caused by surgical or traumatic endothelial damage; 6) reduplication of Descemet's membrane over the cornea, angle, and iris ("glass membrane"), in which the photocoagulation test is negative.

Once epithelial ingrowth is proven by biopsy or photocoagulation, early treatment is recommended because the necessary surgery is often less extensive and its results may be better at that stage. Observation of the corneal area of involvement is not advocated, since it may remain stationary while angle, iris, and ciliary body involvement progresses.

Portions of this text were excerpted from Smith PW, Stark WJ, Maumenee AE, Green WR: Epithelial, fibrous, and endothelial proliferation. *In* Ritch R, Krupin T, Shields MB (eds): The Glaucomas. St. Louis, CV Mosby, 1989. Used with permission.

References

Bernardino VB, Kim JC, Smith TR: Epithelialization of the anterior chamber after cataract extraction. Arch Ophthalmol 82:742–750, 1969.

Calhoun FP Jr: An aid to the clinical diagnosis of epithelial ingrowth into the anterior chamber following cataract extraction. Am J Ophthalmol 61:1055–1059, 1966.

Maumenee AE, et al: Review of 40 histologically proven cases of epithelial downgrowth following cataract extraction and suggested surgical management. Am J Ophthalmol 69:598–603, 1970.

Smith PW, et al: Epithelial, fibrous, and endothelial proliferation. *In* Ritch R, Krupin T, Shields MB (eds): The Glaucomas. St. Louis, CV Mosby, 1989, pp 1299–1335.

Stark WJ, et al: Surgical management of epithelial ingrowth. Am J Ophthalmol 85:772–780, 1978.

FIBROUS INGROWTH
(Fibroblastic Ingrowth, Fibrocytic Ingrowth, Fibrous Metaplasia, Stromal Ingrowth, Stromal Overgrowth)

KENNETH C. SWAN, M.D.
Portland, Oregon

Fibrous ingrowth is a condition in which connective tissue grows into the anterior chamber during abnormal wound healing following penetrating wounds in the cornea or limbus. The connective tissue invasion may clothe the back of the cornea, the chamber angle, the surface of the iris, and the anterior face of the vitreous. It may infiltrate the vitreous and even adhere to the retina. Factors predisposing the eye to this complication include poor wound apposition, recurrent hemorrhage, uveitis, tissue incarceration, and bulky, poorly placed, or tight sutures. Retrocorneal membranes are not uncommon after penetrating keratoplasty. Clinically, fibrous membranes appear to be frayed, gray or white, mesh-like structures, with irregular tongue-like strands on the advancing edge. Associated findings may include detachment of Descemet's membrane, bullous keratopathy, corneal edema, glaucoma, or phthisis bulbi, and retinal detachment may result in severe impairment of vision. Frequently, the patient experiences little discomfort, although chronic irritative changes may eventually ensue. Contraction of this newly formed tissue may pull upon the corneal scar and deform the globe until the eye becomes atrophic or until recalcitrant secondary glaucoma appears.

THERAPY

Ocular. There is no specific treatment for fibrous ingrowth into the anterior chamber. Although topical ocular corticosteroids are frequently prescribed, they seldom are of significant value. Currently available antimetabolites[‡] exert toxic effects on the endothelium, but new agents hold promise. Some manifestations of fibrous ingrowth may be treated. For example, the thin fibrous membrane covering the pupillary aperture may be surgically excised or penetrated by YAG laser; however, this manipulation should be undertaken only if there is little evidence of continuing fibrous ingrowth. Otherwise, it may aggravate the process and cause increased proliferation. If the fibrous ingrowth extends posteriorly into the vitreous and causes retinal detachment by direct traction, the prognosis generally is unfavorable, but an effort should be made to save these globes by removing the traction employing vitreous surgery techniques.

Ocular or Periocular Manifestations

Cornea: Bullous keratopathy; detachment of Descemet's membrane; edema; retrocorneal membrane.

Globe: Atrophy; deformity; phthisis bulbi.
Other: Pupillary distortion; retinal detachment; secondary glaucoma.

PRECAUTIONS

Proper operative and postoperative techniques are important in minimizing fibrous ingrowth. Endothelial bridging of the inner wound after cataract surgery seems to block migration of fibroblasts in the eye; therefore, care must be taken not to injure this layer, especially in those patients with an endothelial dystrophy. During the critical period when the limbal wound is fragile, a precisely closed flap that contains both conjunctiva and Tenon's capsule provides considerable support. These layers seal down rapidly. Secondly, the limbal incision should be directed to enter the anterior chamber in the region of the Schwalbe line. Incisions that enter posteriorly are more likely to result in serious bleeding and to heal with more proliferative reactions than are anterior incisions. Limbal wound closure should be precise; multiple bulky knots incite undue fibroplasia. Improperly placed sutures actually may hold the wound edges apart. Too tightly tied sutures exaggerate errors made in placement, as well as incite reaction caused by pressure necrosis.

COMMENTS

The pathogenesis of fibrous ingrowth is not fully understood. The most likely sources are subepithelial connective tissue, corneal or limbal stroma, and metaplastic endothelium. Fibrous ingrowth is often confused with epithelial downgrowth, although the appearance of the membrane is different. Fibrous ingrowth tends to be self-limiting in many cases. Estimating the incidence of fibrous ingrowth is difficult, since many of these cases remain unrecognized until the globe is enucleated.

References

Friedman AH, Henkind P: Corneal stromal overgrowth after cataract extraction. Br J Ophthalmol 54:528–534, 1970.
Jaffe NS: Fibrous ingrowth. *In* Cataract Surgery and Complications, 3rd ed. St. Louis, CV Mosby, 1981, pp 537–550.
Jaffe NS: Cataract Surgery and Its Complications, 2nd ed. St. Louis, CV Mosby, 1976, pp 428–441.
Swan KC: Fibroblastic ingrowth following cataract extraction. Arch Ophthalmol 89:445–449, 1973.
Yanoff M, Fine BS: Stromal ingrowth. Ocular Pathology, 2nd ed. Philadelphia, Harper & Row, 1983, pp 157–159.

INTRAOCULAR EPITHELIAL CYSTS

PATRICIA W. SMITH, M.D.,
Charlottesville, Virginia
and WALTER J. STARK, M.D.
Baltimore, Maryland

Cystic invasion of the anterior chamber may occur after trauma, cataract surgery, penetrating keratoplasty, or perforating corneal ulcer. Delayed or inadequate wound closure, perhaps complicated by incarceration of the iris, lens capsule, or vitreous, predisposes to cyst formation.

Clinically, it is important to differentiate epithelial cysts from sheet-like epithelial ingrowth, since their courses and prognoses differ greatly. The translucent or gray epithelial cyst appears to connect at one end with the wound. Transillumination and tremulousness, as well as lack of vascularity, which is demonstrable on fluorescein angiography, attest to its cystic nature. The cyst appears on the iris surface, in contrast to the stromal or iris pigment epithelial origin of primary iris cysts; however, a cyst that has grown through a peripheral iridectomy and presents in the posterior chamber may appear to arise from the iris stroma. Pupillary distortion, iridocyclitis, glaucoma, and encroachment on the visual axis may accompany growth of the cyst and indicate treatment. The course of these lesions varies tremendously; some lie dormant for years before enlarging, and others grow to considerable size before stabilizing.

THERAPY

Supportive. If periodic observation of the epithelial cyst shows sight-threatening complications, antiglaucoma and anti-inflammatory medications are used as temporizing measures before definitive treatment.

Surgical. Intervention is warranted only when growth, glaucoma, or iritis affect vision because the cyst can recur as sheet-like epithelial ingrowth.

The current surgical technique is wide excision of the intact cyst, if possible. If the cyst is adherent to the cornea, iris, or vitreous face, it is first collapsed by aspiration, using a 25-gauge needle through the limbus at the cyst attachment. A vitreous sweep through a separate limbal wound may be used to peel the cyst away from the cornea. If small, the collapsed cyst is frozen through the cornea and limbus after an insulating air bubble is introduced into the anterior chamber. Larger cysts may require the use of

---

Portions of this text were excerpted from Smith PW, Stark WJ, Maumenee AE, Green WR: Epithelial, fibrous, and endothelial proliferation. *In* Ritch R, Krupin T, Shields MB (eds): The Glaucomas. St. Louis, CV Mosby, 1989, pp 1299–1335. Used with permission.

vitrectomy instruments, introduced through the limbus or the pars plana, to excise iris and vitreous that are firmly adherent to the cyst. Freezing over air is then performed that is sufficient to cause the brief formation of an ice ball involving the adherent epithelial cells. Corneal edema may ensue after cyst excision and freezing; penetrating keratoplasty has been done to restore good vision in some of these cases.

Photocoagulation has been used to puncture and shrink epithelial cysts, although multiple applications are necessary. In one report, three cases of epithelial cysts were treated with sessions of photocoagulation to the pigmented base; four to six sessions were required before rapid movement of fine particles within the cyst or iris constriction was noted. The three cysts resolved without sequelae, except for updrawn pupils, at less than 1-year follow-up. Other authors have reported cyst resolution in small series with up to 5-year follow-up. Photocoagulation has the advantage of being relatively less invasive than some surgical procedures. However, when the cyst is not pigmented, is firmly adherent to cornea or vitreous, or presents in the posterior chamber, photocoagulation may not be useful.

Ocular or Periocular Manifestations

Anterior Chamber: Cell and flare; cyst; obliteration of angle.
Conjunctiva: Bleb; ciliary flush; fistula.
Cornea: Edema.
Iris: Corectopia; immobility; mass (if presenting from posterior chamber.)
Other: Blur; glaucoma; photophobia.

PRECAUTIONS

Cryotherapy should be limited to the cornea involved with adherent cyst, since it will destroy endothelium, as well as epithelium. Air tamponade enables precise treatment of the intended area and insulates other anterior segment structures. A single freeze-thaw, sufficient to form ice crystals on the posterior surface of the cornea, is recommended.

In treating a cyst with laser, care should be taken not to perforate the cyst, since externalizing it may convert it into sheet-like epithelial ingrowth.

COMMENTS

Cystic and sheet-like epithelial invasion of the anterior chamber differs only in mechanical factors, with epithelial cysts entering the anterior chamber as a loop and expanding in a balloon fashion in the anterior chamber. Clinically, evidence for this theory is found in the conversion of cyst to sheet-like ingrowth after surgical intervention. Occasionally, the cyst may be free floating within the anterior chamber, which is thought to result from implantation of viable epithelial cells by anterior segment instrumentation.

References

Harbin TS, Jr, Maumenee AE: Epithelial downgrowth after surgery for epithelial cyst. Am J Ophthalmol 78:1–4, 1974.
Okun E, Mandell A: Photocoagulation treatment of epithelial implantation cysts following cataract surgery. Trans Am Ophthalmol Soc 72:170–183, 1974.
Scholz RT, Kelley JS: Argon laser photocoagulation treatment of iris cysts following penetrating keratoplasty. Arch Ophthalmol *100*:926–927, 1982.
Smith PW, et al: Epithelial, fibrous, and endothelial proliferation. *In* Ritch R, Krupin T, Shields MB (eds): The Glaucomas. St. Louis, CV Mosby, 1989, pp 1299–1335.

POSTOPERATIVE FLAT ANTERIOR CHAMBER
E. MICHAEL VAN BUSKIRK, M.D.
Portland, Oregon

Collapse of the anterior chamber after anterior segment surgery is a serious complication that may lead to corneal decompensation, cataract, or intractable glaucoma due to peripheral anterior synechiae. It may immediately follow glaucoma or cataract surgery or may be delayed for days, weeks, or even months into the postoperative period. Shallowing of the anterior chamber is relatively more common after filtering surgery for glaucoma, particularly when the full-thickness procedures are chosen over the partial-thickness "trabeculectomy" procedures. The latter technique reduces the incidence, but does not eliminate flat chamber as a complication.

The flat anterior chamber almost invariably results from one or a combination of the following events: wound leak, serous or hemorrhagic choroidal detachment, pupillary block, or posterior entrapment of aqueous humor (malignant glaucoma or ciliary-block glaucoma). Identification of pathogenesis is essential to plan the safest and most effective therapy. Occasionally, the appropriate etiologic diagnosis only becomes clear during operative intervention so that the surgeon must be prepared to follow a logical series of surgical steps to do the least necessary to correct the problem and prevent its recurrence.

The wound should be carefully examined to identify any possible leak. In an eye that does not appear to be extremely soft, the intraocular pressure can be carefully measured using a sterilized applanation tonometer. A very soft eye suggests a wound leak or choroidal detachment, whereas a normotensive or firm eye is more suggestive of pupillary block or posterior aqueous entrapment. However, pupillary block can also occur with a soft eye, if wound leak or choroidal detachment coexists.

Excess aqueous runoff through the filtration site commonly occurs during the first few days after filtering procedures, resulting in shallowing of the anterior chamber and choroidal detachment, which, in turn, leads to further flattening of the anterior chamber. Pupillary block rarely occurs after filtration surgery if an adequate iridectomy has been performed. This condition occurs more commonly after cataract surgery, especially with anterior chamber intraocular lenses when vitreous or lens material can block one or more iridectomies. In some cases, particularly when pupillary block has been allowed to persist, the aqueous humor may be diverted into the vitreous cavity, driving the vitreous forward and blocking access to both the anterior and posterior chambers, leading to so-called malignant glaucoma.

Hemorrhagic choroidal detachment also occasionally follows any intraocular procedure, but is more common in eyes that have had multiple intraocular procedures. It may occur intraoperatively and be heralded by rapid shallowing of the anterior chamber and prolapse of ocular contents into the wound site. Patients under local anesthesia will complain of pain. After filtration surgery, hemorrhagic choroidal detachment more commonly occurs during the early postoperative period and again is heralded by severe pain and loss of vision with flattening of the anterior chamber. These postoperative suprachoroidal hemorrhages are now seen more frequently than in previous decades, because more difficult eyes are being subjected to filtration surgery with the availability of adjunctive chemotherapy or tube implants. Aphakic eyes that have undergone vitrectomy are especially prone to suprachoroidal hemorrhage after filtration surgery. Although many suprachoroidal hemorrhages will absorb spontaneously, prompt diagnosis will permit the institution of appropriate therapy that can save vision.

THERAPY

Ocular. Therapy is entirely dependent upon correct determination of pathogenesis. Wound leaks usually require surgical repair, but very tiny wound leaks sometimes heal spontaneously with a pressure dressing and administration of systemic carbonic anhydrase inhibitors used to reduce aqueous flow.

When a flat anterior chamber results from excess filtration, the Simmons scleral shell tamponade applied with a pressure dressing often proves useful if applied before extensive choroidal detachment is well established. The anterior chamber usually deepens within 2 to 3 hours, but the Simmons shell should then be left in place for at least 48 hours, "weaning away" the pressure dressing and then the shell tamponade. Maximum mydriasis and cycloplegia are also helpful to retrodisplace the lens-iris diaphragm and prevent complicating pupillary block.

Pupillary block rarely follows filtration surgery if an adequate iridectomy has been performed, but more commonly occurs after cataract surgery or after filtration in aphakic or pseudophakic eyes. These eyes invariably require a laser or surgical iridectomy, but the attack should initially be broken medically to reduce the intraocular pressure and to allow clearing of the cornea. Maximum mydriasis should be achieved using 1 per cent atropine in combination with 2.5 per cent phenylephrine. In some cases, a combination of 4 per cent cocaine and 1 per cent epinephrine may augment mydriasis. Vitreous dehydration with osmotic agents, such as oral glycerin, oral isosorbide, or intravenous mannitol, is useful in combination with ocular mydriatic/cycloplegics to reverse some cases of pupillary block and posterior entrapment of aqueous humor.

A flat anterior chamber, associated with visible patent iridectomy, a high intraocular pressure, and a visible red fundus reflex, should raise the specter of posteriorly entrapped aqueous humor or malignant glaucoma. In previous years, these cases required surgical intervention, and the diagnosis was often made on the operating table. With the current availability of the neodymium YAG laser, malignant glaucoma in the aphakic or pseudophakic eye can be readily treated without returning to the operating room. In the aphakic or pseudophakic eye with malignant glaucoma, the vitreous face appears to be tightly adherent to the entire posterior surface of the posterior capsule, the intraocular lens, and the iris. The iris appears to be bulging forward into the anterior chamber under posterior tension. Vitreous is seen bulging through a patent iridectomy. Careful slitlamp examination of the vitreous cavity reveals vitreous fibrils densely compacted against the posterior capsule or anterior hyaloid face with clear fluid-containing space entrapped posteriorly. This can also be documented with ultrasonic examination in some cases. Disruption of the anterior and posterior vitreous surface with the YAG laser allows a pathway for posteriorly entrapped aqueous humor to enter the anterior chamber and exit the eye. This YAG "vitrotomy" results in a dramatic deepening of the anterior chamber and lowering of intraocular pressure. Malignant glaucoma in the phakic eye is more difficult to treat with YAG vitrotomy because of poor visibility; it usually requires surgical intervention as described later.

Vitreous dehydration with osmotic agents, such as oral glycerin, oral isosorbide, or intravenous mannitol, is useful in combination with ocular mydriatic/cycloplegics to reverse some cases of pupillary block and posterior aqueous entrapment.

Surgical. Surgical wound leaks should usually be repaired under general anesthesia. If the wound leak is present under a conjunctival flap but draining sufficiently to cause flattening of the anterior chamber, it may sometimes be sealed with cryosurgery or various chemical agents, such as trichloroacetic acid (100 per cent solution applied with an orange stick barely moistened with the acid).

Leaking filtration blebs with a flat anterior chamber usually need to be surgically repaired.

Tapered noncutting needles with 10-0 suture permit surgical closure with minimal further disruption of delicate conjunctiva. Leaking cystic blebs at the limbus may be locally excised, sliding adjacent conjunctiva over to cover the resultant defect. To provide a smooth limbal area and to anchor the new conjunctiva firmly, a very small corneoscleral groove can be prepared to recess the conjunctival flap edge for suturing.

In the absence of a wound leak, surgical anterior chamber reformation following filtration surgery almost always includes drainage of suprachoroidal fluid from a choroidal detachment. Most moderately shallow anterior chambers after filtering surgery will reform spontaneously without any intervention. Deepening the chamber at the slitlamp is rarely necessary and subjects the patient to the risk of infection and lens injury. If surgical intervention must be undertaken, it is best performed with good anesthetic control and visibility in the operating room. After surgically reforming the anterior chamber through a corneal paracentesis wound, suprachoroidal fluid should be drained completely from two inferior posterior sclerotomies. If no suprachoroidal fluid is present and the anterior chamber remains flat, especially with increased intraocular pressure, pupillary block or posterior entrapment of aqueous humor is likely to be present. In this case, an additional peripheral iridectomy should be performed. If the anterior chamber remains shallow even after peripheral iridectomy, malignant glaucoma from posterior diversion of aqueous humor is the most likely diagnosis. In this case, liquid vitreous may be aspirated through the pars plana as described by Simmons and Chandler. Alternatively, a vitrectomy may be performed via the pars plana in phakic eyes, if visibility permits, or through the limbus in the aphakic eye.

If pupillary block is strongly suspected, probably the safest procedure is laser iridotomy. An incomplete iridectomy is readily opened with argon laser applied to the underlying intact iris pigment epithelium. An occluded iridectomy requires additional laser iridotomies to be placed using 50-μM spot size, varying the duration and power for the color and thickness of the iris. Two iridotomies, one on each side of the intraocular lens, should be performed in patients with pupillary block associated with anterior chamber intraocular lenses.

Ocular or Periocular Manifestations

Iris or Ciliary Body: Anterior displacement of iris; ciliary body detachment.
Vitreous: Anterior displacement; hemorrhages.
Other: Choroidal detachment; nonrhegmatogenous retinal detachment; orbital hemorrhages; scleral invagination.

Precautions

The flat anterior chamber should not be allowed to persist longer than 10 to 14 days, depending on its etiology and the degree of intraocular inflammation. Increased intraocular pressure, collapse of the filtration bleb, lens-corneal trough "kissing," choroidal detachments, or excess inflammation all mandate earlier surgical intervention. Their absence permits watchful waiting. Eyes with wound leaks usually require surgical repair if other measures do not correct the problem promptly. Pupillary block requires prompt iridectomy to prevent the development of permanent angle-closure glaucoma from peripheral anterior synechia. Laser iridotomy should be performed away from the visual axis to reduce the possibility of macular laser burns.

After filtration surgery, the surgeon should shun the temptation to operate simply because the anterior chamber is shallow. Nearly all shallow anterior chambers related to excess aqueous runoff, even with choroidal detachment, resolve spontaneously over 7 to 10 days. Management during this critical period is designed to prevent compromise of the other intraocular structures. *Usually, watchful waiting is the safest course.* Deepening of the anterior chamber at the slitlamp is almost never necessary. If the chamber is shallow enough to threaten the lens or cornea, such deepening under poorly controlled conditions runs a significant risk of lens injury and, with lesser degrees of shallowing, is unnecessary.

Comments

During draining of either serous or hemorrhagic choroidal detachment, one must ensure that as much of the suprachoroidal fluid is removed as possible to prevent rapid recurrence of large choroidal detachment and flattening of the anterior chamber. After initial drainage of suprachoroidal fluid from both sclerotomy sites, the anterior chamber should be reformed to greater than normal depth through a corneal paracentesis wound. The sclerotomy sites should then be reinspected with further drainage of any additional fluid. At the conclusion of the procedure, the anterior chamber should again be deepened to slightly greater than normal depth and the eye left tacitly normotensive.

If the hemorrhage is more than a few hours old, it may be expected to have layered out within the suprachoroidal space, with the red cells most dependent. Hence, only xanthochromic fluid may at first appear, with thick wine-colored material following later. In many of these cases, a large portion of the blood dissects interstitially within the choroid, making its complete removal technically impossible. Hence, a large, choroidal, hemorrhagic mass with obscuration of the red fundal reflex may be present, even after all suprachoroidal blood has been removed. The blood-engorged choroid will be visible at the sclerotomy site. At that stage, no further attempts should be made for fluid drainage, and the overlying Tenon's and conjunctival incisions should be closed. The interstitial blood will gradually absorb with time.

References

Bellows AR, Chylack LT Jr, Hutchinson TT: Choroidal detachment. Clinical manifestation, therapy and mechanism of formation. Ophthalmology 88:1107–1115, 1981.

Brubaker RF: Intraocular surgery and choroidal hemorrhage. Arch Ophthalmol 102:1753–1754, 1984.

Brubaker RF, Pederson JE: Ciliochoroidal detachment. Surv Ophthalmol 7:281–289, 1983.

Chandler PA: V. Complications of surgery. Causes of failures and methods of prevention and correction. Trans Am Acad Ophthalmol Otolaryngol 53:224–231, 1949.

Chandler PA, Maumenee AE: A major cause of hypotony. Am J Ophthalmol 52:609–618, 1961.

Gressel MG, Parrish RK II, Heuer DK: Delayed nonexpulsive suprachoroidal hemorrhage. Arch Ophthalmol 102:1757–1760, 1984.

Shields MB: Trabeculectomy vs. full-thickness filtering operation for control of glaucoma. Ophthalmic Surg 11:498–505, 1980.

Simmons RJ: Malignant glaucoma. Br J Ophthalmol 56:263–272, 1972.

Simmons RJ, Kimbrough RL: Shell tamponade in filtering surgery for glaucoma. Ophthalmic Surg 10:17–34, 1979.

Watkins PH Jr, Brubaker RF: Comparison of partial-thickness and full-thickness filtration procedures in open-angle glaucoma. Am J Ophthalmol 86:756–761, 1978.

RECURRENT LATE HYPHEMA FROM FOCAL WOUND VASCULARIZATION

KENNETH C. SWAN, M.D.
Portland, Oregon

Focal vascularization of the stromal wound may result in recurrent hyphema months to as long as 15 years (mean, 4 to 5 years) after cataract or glaucoma surgery. It results from the ingrowth of episcleral vessels that terminate in capillaries at the inner edge of the incision site. In one series, this ingrowth was observed in 12 per cent of 58 eyes examined 5 to 10 years after cataract extraction. Bleeding from these capillaries may occur spontaneously or result from physical strain or minimal trauma, such as gonioscopy or insertion of contact lenses. Bleeding usually is minimal and therefore is easily overlooked or mistaken for iridocyclitis. Blurred vision is the major symptom, but occurs only during the bleeding episode, unless the blood extends into the anterior vitreous. Pain is minimal or absent. During bleeding episodes, blood cells can be observed streaming down through the anterior chamber or on the iris. Enough blood may accumulate to produce a visible hyphema, but the diagnosis usually requires gonioscopy. Collections of old or new blood cells or their pigmented remnants in the lower chamber angle confirm that bleeding has occurred. A tuft of capillaries visible in the lips of the wound identifies the bleeding site. The entity may be innocuous, but recurring hyphemas may lead to angle-closure glaucoma or serious visual disturbance, if there is recurrent bleeding into the anterior vitreous. Patients who have had bleeding only after physical strain or trauma have the best prognosis.

THERAPY

Supportive. Initially, treatment should be by conservative measures, including protecting the eye from trauma, avoiding the prone position in sleep, wearing a protective shield at night, and discontinuation of contact lenses if insertion or removal precipitates bleeding.

Surgical. Recurrent bleeding, especially into the vitreous, requires intervention, but no form of treatment has been universally successful. Argon laser applications applied through a gonioscope and surface applications with the cryoprobe have been most useful, but recurrences have been reported with both techniques. Identification and surgical excision or direct coagulation of the indipping vessel should be reserved for recalcitrant bleeding.

Ocular or Periocular Manifestations

Anterior Chamber: Angle-closure glaucoma; floating cells (red blood cells); hyphema; pigment and synechia in lower angle.

Cornea: Focal tufts of capillaries in inner edges of old wound.

Vitreous: Old and new collections of blood cells on surface or in anterior vitreous.

Other: Transient blurring of vision.

PRECAUTIONS

To avoid alarm, patients suspected of having this condition should be warned that gonioscopy may precipitate bleeding and transitory blurring of vision. If cryotherapy is used, the probe should be applied and withdrawn gently; otherwise, significant bleeding may be precipitated.

COMMENTS

The pathogenesis of wound vascularization has not been fully established, but poor wound apposition, especially gaping of the interior edges of the wound at the bleeding site, has been observed in many patients. Posterior placement of the incision in the sclera may also predispose to wound vascularization, but this has not been well documented. Although most cases have been observed after intracapsular extraction, wound vascularization with late hyphema is now appearing in patients who have had extracapsular extractions through relatively small incisions, as well as after iridectomy, filtrations, and trabeculectomies. The entity should be suspected in patients who have recurrent transitory blurring of vision after operative procedures requiring incisions in the limbal area.

References

Jarstad JS, Hardwig PW: Intraocular hemorrhage from wound vascularization years after anterior segment surgery. (Swan Syndrome) Can J Ophthalmol 22:271–275, 1987.

Swan KC: Hyphema due to wound vascularization after cataract extraction. Arch Ophthalmol 89:87–90, 1973.

Swan KC: Late hyphema due to wound vascularization. Trans Am Acad Ophthalmol Otolaryngol 81:138–144, 1976.

Watzke RC: Intraocular hemorrhage from wound vascularization following cataract surgery. Trans Am Ophthalmol Soc 72:242–252, 1974.

Watzke RC: Intraocular hemorrhage from vascularization of the cataract incision. Ophthalmology 87:19–23, 1980.

TRAUMATIC HYPHEMA

PAUL E. ROMANO, M.D., M.S.O.,
and JERRY N. SHUSTER, M.D.
Gainesville, Florida

Hyphema, an accumulation of blood within the anterior chamber, is most commonly the result of trauma. The typical injury is a direct blow to the cornea from a fist or low-velocity missile. The force is transmitted to the aqueous humor, pushing the iris-lens diaphragm posteriorly, which results in a tear in the root of the iris or the face of the ciliary body. Bleeding that follows from torn blood vessels is usually self-limited because of the tamponade of such bleeding into the closed space of the anterior chamber. The intraocular pressure may be elevated acutely due to the mechanical block of the trabecular meshwork by blood.

Approximately 2 days after the onset of the hyphema, the clot begins to retract, and the risk of rebleeding begins. With recurrent hemorrhage, the risks of such complications as elevation of intraocular pressure, corneal endothelial decompensation, and progressive blood staining of the corneal stroma increase. Additionally, the indications for surgical intervention are more likely to be encountered with a secondary hemorrhage.

THERAPY

Before undertaking therapy, sickle cell anemia (including trait) must be ruled out because the patient who also has that blood dyscrasia, must be treated much more carefully, and at times more aggressively. (See below under Surgical therapy and under Precautions.)

Supportive. The patient with *initial bleed* should be hospitalized at bedrest for 6 days, which covers the period of greatest risk of rebleeding, days 2 through 5; the patient should be allowed progressive ambulation on the sixth day in preparation for discharge. This hospitalization protects the young patient from further or repeat trauma, facilitates the frequent observations that are appropriate, ensures the administration of systemic treatment, and seems to produce better overall results. The head of the bed may be elevated to facilitate settling of the hyphema, clearing of the superior filtering angle, and earlier visualization of the fundus. Allowing bathroom privileges seems not to affect the situation deleteriously.

The size of the hyphema does not alter these recommendations; most studies suggest that the rebleeding rate is the same regardless of the size of the initial hyphema. Although small hyphemas (less than one third) show no greater rebleed rate with modest ambulation than bedrest, larger ones do. In addition, bedrest seems to accelerate clearing of the hyphema.

Ocular occlusion seems unnecessary. Certainly, it has been demonstrated that binocular occlusion has no advantage over monocular, and the former is hazardous psychologically. Likewise as seen in more recent studies, patching does not seem to have any effect at all on the outcome.

A perforated aluminum shield should be prescribed to prevent accidental reinjury of the eye. Otherwise limiting the use of the eyes seems a futile exercise and has not been demonstrated as having any effect upon the outcome.

Although some studies have suggested that the rebleed rate is higher for some age and ethnic groups, and the inference has been made that different age and ethnic groups might therefore be treated differently, that evidence is weak and far from providing any definitive medical indication for treating these different groups differently. For the present, then, all traumatic hyphemas should be treated identically, as above and as follows.

Sedatives or tranquilizers may be useful in some patients. However, aspirin is contraindicated, as its antiplatelet action may facilitate a rebleeding episode.

Systemic. Recent studies strongly support the use of systemic antifibrinolytic agents, such as corticosteroids and aminocaproic acid, and one of these should be given for 5 days in all cases. The recommended daily dose of prednisone is the equivalent of 40 mg for an adult or 0.6 mg/kg for children, given in divided doses. Aminocaproic acid should be given in dosages of 100 mg/kg every 4 hours for 5 days. Both drugs may be discontinued at that time without tapering dosages, if there has been satisfactory resolution of the initial bleed. Both drugs have been demonstrated to reduce the rebleeding rate to virtually zero in this condition. Corticosteroids are favored over aminocaproic acid because most physicians are intimately familiar with prescribing steroids, undesirable side effects from aminocaproic acid have been reported occasionally, and aminocaproic acid has also been demonstrated to retard clot reabsorption slightly. Steroids also have an anti-inflammatory effect not found in aminocaproic acid.

If there is a *rebleed*, the foregoing treatment is simply continued for an additional 5 days, with closer observation for complications (glaucoma and corneal blood staining) that occur much more frequently following rebleeds than after primary bleeds.

Significant pressure evaluation of greater than 50 mm Hg for more than 5 days or 35 mm Hg for more than 7 days may increase the possibility of optic nerve damage. A healthy, normal, young eye can withstand the following pressures without damage to the optic nerve: 50 mm Hg for 5 days, 45 mm Hg for 7 days, or 35 mm Hg for 14 days. Since the pressure will go down when the angle clears, it is not necessary therefore to treat elevated pressure per se. However, if treatment is needed, 250 mg of oral acetazolamide may be given four times daily (30 mg/kg daily in divided doses in children, total dose not to exceed 1000 mg/day). In addition, topical ophthalmic 0.25 or 0.5 per cent timolol or 1 to 2 per cent epinephrine may be applied twice daily. Osmotic agents may be added, if necessary. A 50 per cent solution of glycerin may be administered orally in a dosage of 2 to 3 ml/kg, or a 20 per cent solution of mannitol may be given intravenously in a dosage of 1 to 2 gm/kg.

Surgical. There is rarely an indication for surgical intervention before the fourth day after the initial bleed, except for patients with sickle cell anemia. Increased intraocular pressure in these patients may be a result of increased sickling of red blood cells in the anterior chamber, which blocks the trabecular meshwork and renders medical therapy ineffective. Therefore, the optic nerve can be damaged at lower pressures because of sickling, and earlier surgical intervention is needed. The rule for patients with sickle cell anemia is "24 × 24": any pressure elevation greater than 24 mm Hg for 24 hours is cause for aggressive treatment because of danger to the optic nerve.

Otherwise, the indications for surgical intervention in patients with hyphema include 1) sustained pressure elevation that is unacceptable given the baseline health of the optic nerve or is unresponsive to medical management, 2) early corneal blood staining demonstrated by an orange granular appearance to the posterior corneal stroma, or 3) a greater than 50 per cent hyphema that shows no evidence of clearing after 4 days because the risk of peripheral anterior synechiae and secondary glaucoma increases.

Many techniques have been advocated, and all are hazardous because blood clots and uveal tissue are easily confused and the hyphema limits visibility. An irrigating and aspirating technique may be used to wash out free blood. This may be combined with the use of fibrinolysins. An ocutome may be used to aspirate and cut the clot from the anterior chamber. Sears described a technique to express the clot in toto on the fourth day, at which time the clot begins to retract. A cryoprobe or forceps have also been recommended to extract the clot; these procedures have the disadvantage of necessitating a large incision and involving the risk of loss of lens, uvea, and vitreous. Removing the blood from the anterior chamber usually halts corneal blood staining and alleviates the glaucoma. If persistent bleeding occurs during the procedure, the involved area of the ciliary body can be treated transclerally with diathermy.

Ocular or Periocular Manifestations

Conjunctiva: Injected secondary to initial trauma, or iritis and uveitis from hyphema.

Cornea: On presentation, clear; or with manifestations of blunt or abrading trauma such as an epithelial abrasion. After one or more days, corneal blood staining, manifest initially by a translucent diffuse reddish granular apperance to the posterior stroma; changing with time to an opaque green (bile-colored) stain which may last for a year or two.

Anterior Chamber: On presentation may be clear or contain various quantities and forms and colors of either or both clotted and unclotted blood; from and including a small dark horizontally layered, almost invisible clot at the bottom of the chamber, to larger layered amounts of dark blood; to a chamber completely filled with almost black clot, the so called "eight ball hyphema". The blood may also be unclotted bright red and diffusely fill the chamber. Combinations of the above maybe seen.

Later, residuae of clots may be seen including whitish fibrin membranes.

Iris: May be obscured by anterior chamber blood. Traumatic lesions may be apparent such as dialysis or recesion of the angle. Pupil may be occluded or secluded by fibrin. Iritis, peripheral anterior and posterior synechiae.

Vitreous and Retina: Usually uninvolved but may have suffered any of a variety of traumatic lesions from the initial trauma. Even when directly untraumatized, in severe hyphemas, blood often enters and fills the vitreous body as well as the anterior chamber (viz. "eight ball hyphema").

Other: Ocular pain, secondary glaucoma (until hyphema clears, or permanently secondary to angle recession and scarring); visual loss.

Precautions

There is no specific indication for any topical ocular medication in the management of the initial bleed. Contraindications include rapidly acting cycloplegics and mydriatics that may occasionally precipitate rebleeding episodes and the use of miotics that may cause vascular dilation and congestion in the iris and ciliary body, thereby increasing the risk of rebleeding.

It is usually neither necessary nor possible to examine the posterior pole ophthalmoscopically in most hyphemas. Although postponement of pupillary dilation for this is recommended, there may be reasons, such as scleral rupture, intraocular foreign body, or retinal detachment, when atropine only should be used. Atropine appears to have no deleterious effect on the course of traumatic hyphema. The less manipulation of the eye, the better. Daily tonometry and slitlamp examination are not required unless one has reason to suspect a significant elevation of pressure or blood staining. This is especially true for the young patient in whom sedation may be required or a struggle may be anticipated. Some pressure elevation on the first day should be expected, but it is usually transient and not very high and does not specifically require treatment. Acetazolamide should not be routinely given because it slows clot reabsorption and may facilitate rebleeding by lowering intraocular pressure too far.

If the clot reabsorbs without complication, no further therapy is necessary. Eye examination is completed 2 weeks after discharge. Gonioscopy, which can be traumatic, must be performed at some point to identify angle recession. The timing of gonioscopy depends on the instrument to be used, the skill of the examiner, the cooperation of the patient, and the fact that early gonioscopy most reliably identifies angle recession. Regular long-term follow-up of all hyphema patients is indicated for the detection of late-onset secondary glaucoma.

All persons who might have sickle cell anemia should have the appropriate studies performed on admission because the management of these patients with traumatic hyphema has much narrower limits with regard to elevated pressure. Use of acetazolamide in patients with sickle cell disease is contraindicated because of its concomitant acidosis, which may trigger sickling.

Comments

Significant pressure elevation or blood staining of the cornea occasionally occurs with a severe initial bleed, but usually follows a rebleed. Additional treatment may be required; however, both pressure elevation and corneal blood staining tend to be self-limiting or transient.

Corneal blood staining is more significant in the child under 6 years of age, as a functional amblyopia is likely to result. In addition, the probability of developing secondary strabismus is greater in the child under 8 or 10 years of age who will have more difficulty regaining fusion when the blood has cleared months or years later. The blood staining itself is a significant cosmetic defect as well.

Since the pressure will go down when the angle clears, it is not necessary therefore to treat elevated pressure per se. This is an especially important principle when almost every agent used to lower pressure may have a deleterious effect on the primary problem, delaying clot reabsorption, removing the tamponade effect of elevated pressure, or promoting rebleeding episodes through iris vascular congestion and engorgement.

References

Crouch ER Jr, Frenkel M: Aminocaproic acid in the treatment of traumatic hyphema. Am J Ophthalmol 81:355–360, 1976.

Edwards WC, Layden WE: Monocular versus binocular patching in traumatic hyphema. Am J Ophthalmol 76:359–362, 1973.

Goldberg MF: The diagnosis and treatment of sickled erythrocytes in human hyphemas. Trans Am Ophthalmol Soc 76:481–501, 1978.

Rakusin W: Traumatic hyphema. Am J Ophthalmol 74:284–292, 1972.

Read J, Goldberg MF: Comparison of medical treatment for traumatic hyphema. Trans Am Acad Ophthalmol Otolaryngol 78:799–815, 1974.

Romano PE: Pro steroids for systemic antifibrinolytic treatment for traumatic hyphema. *In* Rosenbaum AL (ed): Controversies in Pediatric Ophthalmology, Vol 23, No 2, pp 92–95.

Rynne MV, Romano PE: Systemic corticosteroids in the treatment of traumatic hyphema. J Pediatr Ophthalmol Strabismus 17:141–143, 1980.

Sears ML: Surgical management of black ball hyphema. Trans Am Acad Ophthalmol Otolaryngol 74:820–826, 1970.

Wilson FM II: Traumatic hyphema: Pathogenesis and management. Ophthalmology 87:910–919, 1980.

Yasuna E: Management of traumatic hyphema. Arch Ophthalmol 91:190–191, 1974.

SECTION 19

CHOROID

ANGIOID STREAKS
FUMIO KAYAZAWA, M.D.
Osaka, Japan

Angioid streaks are the fundal appearance produced by pathologic alterations of the pigment epithelium, Bruch's membrane, and the choriocapillaris. The primary focus lies in the elastic lamina that occupies the midsegment of the Bruch's membrane. The streaks are observed only in the peripapillary area or radiate from the peripapillary chorioretinal atrophy in the asteroid-like fashion throughout the fundus bilaterally. In particular, they have a distinct tendency to involve the macula. The color of the streaks is variable and may be reddish-brown, gray, or combinations of these. Several fundal appearances are frequently observed along with the streaks: mottled fundus (peau d'orange), focal chorioretinal atrophy (salmon spot), and pigment proliferation. Disciform macular degeneration induced by subretinal neovascularization, leading to permanent visual loss, is the complication of greatest concern.

A number of systemic diseases are associated with angioid streaks: pseudoxanthoma elasticum, Paget's disease, sickle cell anemia, senile elastosis, Marfan's syndrome, and Ehlers-Danlos syndrome. In pseudoxanthoma elasticum, autosomal recessive inheritance may be demonstrated. Aging is another important etiologic factor.

The fundal appearance of angioid streaks resembles involutional macular degeneration, choroidal sclerosis, myopic chorioretinal degeneration (lacquer cracks), and presumed ocular histoplasmosis. Although differential diagnosis is not difficult to make in typical cases, diagnosis may be more difficult when streaks are subtle. Genetic traits, systemic abnormalities, other fundal appearances, and fluorescein angiography are aids in arriving at an early diagnosis.

THERAPY

Supportive. Angioid streaks are benign fundal lesions, unless subretinal neovascular ingrowth occurs. Spontaneous resolution of neovascular tufts does not naturally take place. Hemostatic or eutrophic agents are not effective in improving disciform exudative response.

Surgical. When fluorescein angiography discloses neovascular membranes located outside the fovea, positive photocoagulation is effective in closing it. Heavily overlapped photocoagulation with energy settings of 200 to 300 mW, spot size of 100 to 200 μm, and time exposure of 0.1 to 0.2 second is required. Retrobulbar anesthesia is preferable in some cases. A careful follow-up study with fluorescein angiography should be made at 1- to 2-week intervals after photocoagulation. If neovascularization recurs, immediate treatment should be readministrated in the newly developed sites.

Ocular or Periocular Manifestations

Choroid: Atrophy; neovascularization; vascular sclerosis.
Retina: Focal chorioretinal lesions (salmon spot); hemorrhages; macular degeneration (exudative or nonexudative); pigmentary mottling (peau d'orange).
Other: Visual loss.

PRECAUTIONS

Subretinal neovascularization associated with angioid streaks frequently appears in the papillomacular area and tends to involve the fovea. In such cases, photocoagulation is counteractive because inadequate therapy accelerates the exudative response. When fluorescein angiography discloses the neovascular tuft located about 500 μm away from the center of the fovea, thorough, heavily overlapped photocoagulation should be administered. Most of the regrowth may develop 6 to 8 weeks after apparently successful photocoagulation and progress rapidly.

A serious complication is arcuate scotoma, which is caused when heavily overlapped photocoagulation with a longer exposure time is administered in the papillomacular area. Other complications that may occur include macular puckers and retinal hemorrhages. The prophylactic treatment of angioid streaks before the development of choroidal neovascularization is not recommended.

COMMENTS

The condition of angioid streaks is relatively benign and requires no active therapy, unless exudative macular degeneration or serious systemic diseases accompany it.

In a few cases, seemingly beneficial results have been achieved using laser photocoagulation. However, the tendency for widespread macular involvement and foveal proximity of the subretinal neovascular membrane has led to discouraging results in many cases. Thus, careful consideration is essential when such tendencies are identified. Once determined to be present, prompt photocoagulation and adequate follow-up may increase chances for effective treatment.

Krypton or dye laser appears to be more promising than argon laser because energy loss into the blood is smaller due to a longer wavelength. However, its use must be studied in further detail.

References

Clarkson JG, Altman RD: Angioid streaks. Surv Ophthalmol 26:235, 1982.
Deutman AF, and Kovács B: Argon laser treatment in complications of angioid streaks. Am J Ophthalmol 88:12–17, 1979.
Fine SL: Angioid streaks. Int Ophthalmol Clin 17:173–182, 1977.
Hamilton AM, Pope FM, Condon PI, et al: Angioid streaks in Jamaican patients with homozygous sickle cell disease. Br J Ophthalmol 65:341, 1981.
Kayazawa F: A successful argon laser treatment in macular complications of angioid streaks. Ann Ophthalmol 13:581–584, 1981.
Meislik J, et al: Laser treatment in maculopathy of pseudoxanthoma elasticum. Can J Ophthalmol 13:210–212, 1978.
Peabody RR, Warren H: Angioid streaks in macular disease. In L'Esperance FA Jr (ed): Current Diagnosis and Management of Chorioretinal Diseases. St. Louis, CV Mosby, 1977, pp 527–539.
Singerman LJ, Hatem G: Laser treatment of choroidal neovascular membranes in angioid streaks. Retina 1:75, 1981.
Wessing A, Meyer-Schwickerath G: Lichtchirurgische Behandlung und sonstige chirurgische Massnahmen bei Maculaaffektionen. Ber Dtsch Ophthalmol Ges 73:585–594, 1975.
Wilkinson CP: Stimulation of subretinal neovascularization. Am J Ophthalmol 81:104–106, 1976.

CHOROIDAL DETACHMENT
(Ciliochoroidal Detachment)

A. ROBERT BELLOWS, M.D.
Boston, Massachusetts

Choroidal detachment is the clinical term used to describe the accumulation of fluid in the potential space between the choroid and sclera. The entity has been referred to as a ciliochoroidal detachment, implicating the ciliary body as well as the choroid, and the terms are often used interchangeably. The suprachoroidal space is anteriorly limited by the scleral spur and posteriorly in the region of the four vortex veins. When fluid accumulates in this space, it produces a characteristic internal ballooning of the choroid that appears as large, brown, quadrantic mounds that are delimited posteriorly by the ampullae of the vortex veins. Often as fluid accumulates in the suprachoroidal space, there is an anterior displacement of the ciliary body and the lens-iris diaphragm, resulting in shallowing of the anterior chamber. The major significance of a choroidal detachment occurs when shallowing of the anterior chamber causes architectural disruption that can result in irreversible pathology.

The entity of choroidal detachment has been recognized since Waldrop recalled the histopathology in 1818 initially described by Zinn in 1755. Although Von Graefe in 1858 described the clinical characteristics using his ophthalmoscope, it was 10 years before Knapp enucleated an eye following cataract surgery for the suspicion of a malignant melanoma and discovered a benign choroidal detachment. The mechanism of this disorder has remained controversial, but Fuchs in 1900 believed that aqueous contributed to a choroidal detachment through an unsuspected cyclodialysis cleft. A few years later, Meller and Verhoeff each suggested that, after surgery or trauma, intraocular pressure decreased and remained low to encourage a transudation of fluid from the choroidal vasculature into the suprachoroidal space and that this was responsible for the development of a choroidal detachment.

It has been shown that the accumulation of fluid in the suprachoroidal space that produces a characteristic choroidal detachment can occur during or immediately after an operation and as late as 6 years after an uneventful surgery. Ocular and periorbital trauma can be responsible for choroidal detachment, as are the more unusual causes of nanophthalmos and the uveal effusion syndrome. Other etiologies include local inflammation (scleritis), systemic inflammation (Vogt-Koyanagi-Harada syndrome) and systemic vascular disorders (carotid cavernous fistula and eclampsia).

Although the mechanism of fluid formation is still not completely understood, it is clear that hypotony and transudation from the vascular network are the main contributors. When the ciliary body is detached, aqueous secretion can be decreased and may prolong ocular hypotony. Capper and Leopold have demonstrated that both surgical trauma and hypotony are necessary to produce suprachoroidal fluid accumulation in experimental rabbits, whereas in monkeys, aqueous may actually contribute to an experimental choroidal effusion through the mechanism of uveal scleral flow. In humans, it is apparent that in the presence of a wound leak or intentional fistulization following glaucoma surgery the intraocular pressure drops near zero and osmotic pressure alone cannot prevent the transudation of fluid from the choroidal capillaries. A dynamic example of the physiology involved is noted during glaucoma surgery in patients with high episcleral venous pressure. In these patients when the intraocular pressure has been lowered to zero during surgery, high venous pressure creates a large transcapillary pressure differential, rapidly forcing fluid out of the vascular network into the suprachoroidal space. This form of effusion has been noted to occur acutely during the course of an operation and mimics the dreaded surgical complication of expulsive hemorrhage. When this fluid has been analyzed, it contains very little serum protein of small molecular-weight particles, indicating that the mechanism of molecular sieving contributed to the rapid formation of fluid in the suprachoroidal space. It is postulated that the differential created by elevated episcleral venous pressure across an intact isoporous membrane produces this rapid accumulation of fluid.

Ocular Manifestations

Three distinct forms of suprachoroidal detachment have been characterized: serous choroidal detachment, hemorrhagic choroidal detachment, and intraoperative choroidal effusion. *Serous choroidal detachment*, the most common form of choroidal effusion, occurs approximately 5 to 7 days after glaucoma surgery, 10 days after combined glaucoma and cataract surgery, and 2 to 4 weeks after cataract surgery. Serum protein makes up about two-thirds of the suprachoroidal fluid, with normal electrolyte and ascorbic acid concentrations, and exclusion of all very high molecular-weight proteins. During the postoperative phase, intraocular pressure remains very low, and the pressure differential across the capillary bed permits fluid to escape with small- and medium-sized protein molecules through an isoporous membrane and to collect in the interstitium and the suprachoroidal space.

Hemorrhagic choroidal detachment occurs most frequently after combined cataract and glaucoma surgery and in eyes with multiple surgical procedures. This dramatic form of effusion frequently occurs after an inadvertent increase in orbital venous pressure, such as Valsalva maneuver, cough, or straining at stool. The patient often reports a sudden onset of excruciating pain that is accompanied by elevated intraocular pressure, flat anterior chamber, large ciliochoroidal effusion, and prominent ocular hyperemia. Surgical drainage of the suprachoroidal space reveals a large quantity of dark unclotted blood, and reformation of the anterior chamber can potentially save the eye.

A subacute form of hemorrhagic choroidal effusion can also occur and is heralded by transient ocular pain and marked ocular hyperemia with inflammation. Blood in the suprachoroidal space is often accompanied by increased ocular inflammation that can induce peripheral anterior synechia and contribute to failure of a glaucoma filtering bleb. When a choroidal tap is indicated, usually large amounts of maroon unclotted fluid are evacuated, and occasional pockets of clear xanthochromic fluid can be released. This form of choroidal effusion is very similar to the serous choroidal detachment, and the clinical course is identical.

Intraoperative choroidal effusion can occur at the time of cataract extraction, penetrating keratoplasty, or glaucoma surgery in patients with elevated episcleral venous pressure. The rapid onset of fluid accumulation can mimic an expulsive hemorrhage, but only clear xanthochromic fluid is recovered in the suprachoroidal space. Anticipation of this potential complication or recognition when it occurs can prompt a posterior sclerotomy and immediate evacuation of fluid, which have been shown to reduce the operative and postoperative complications.

THERAPY

Ocular. When a clinically significant choroidal detachment is present, medical management should be started immediately with topical cycloplegic-mydriatic drops and frequently applied ophthalmic steroids. The use of systemic steroids is controversial. Although there may be no evidence of inflammatory cells in the suprachoroidal fluid, it has been observed that an inflammatory component is usually present and may prolong the hypotony. Systemic steroids can decrease capillary permeability, which may diminish the accumulation of fluid in the suprachoroidal space. In the presence of excessive filtration after glaucoma surgery or in an active wound leak, a firmly applied pressure patch may be effective in decreasing an aqueous leak and producing a transient elevation in intraocular pressure. Both of these mechanisms may reverse the accumulation of fluid in the suprachoroidal space and enhance the reattachment of the ciliary body. The role of nonsteroidal anti-inflammatory medications, such as indomethacin[‡] or salicylates,[‡] has not been clinically tested, but they may prove to be valuable.

Surgical. When invasive surgery is indicated, a conjunctival incision 4 mm from the limbus in the inferotemporal and inferonasal quadrants can be made after achieving adequate anesthesia by local injection along the orbital floor or into the retrobular space. A radial incision through sclera will release a copious amount of clear xanthochromic fluid. Release of fluid alternated with repeated reformation of the anterior chamber with drain the suprachoroidal space. At the completion of the drainage, the ciliary body should be in apposition with the sclera and the anterior chamber reformed with fluid. The conjunctival incisions are closed with 10-0 nylon sutures.

PRECAUTIONS

Inflammation and risk of infection remain the major complications following choroidal tap and reformation of the anterior chamber. The incidence of cataract formation in phakic patients after glaucoma surgery and choroidal tap is approximately 33 per cent. This incidence is similar to a series of patients after filtering surgery in which 30 per cent required cataract surgery after successful filtration.

A number of surgical advances have decreased the incidence of choroidal detachment and have therefore made it a less frequent complication. The use of the operating microscope, microsurgical techniques, and multiple fine nylon or silk sutures has decreased the incidence of wound leak and shallow anterior chambers. Also, glaucoma surgery has been improved by microsurgical techniques, and guarded filtering procedures (trabeculectomy) minimize the transient hypotony caused by overfiltration and therefore reduce the incidence of choroidal detachment.

The fundamental question of how a ciliary body detachment is associated with aqueous hyposecretion has not yet been answered. If this mechanism could be established, a controlled, therapeutic detachment of the ciliary body should produce aqueous hyposecretion and result in hypotony, which might be an effective form of therapy for glaucoma. Additional work on the passage of fluid across ocular tissues, particularly the sclera, could result in noninvasive methods to treat significant choroidal detachments.

Comments

The clinical course of the choroidal detachment is usually self-limited. Frequently, it follows an uncomplicated surgical procedure, and spontaneous absorption is the rule. When a choroidal detachment is associated with a shallow or flat anterior chamber, it may cause persistent peripheral anterior synechiae, which could result in severe secondary angle-closure glaucoma. The additional possibility of corneal-lenticular touch with development of cataract or corneal edema is a serious sequela of choroidal detachment and must be remedied. Additional indications for surgical intervention with drainage of fluid from the suprachoroidal space and reformation of the anterior chamber include the following: lens-cornea touching with progressive corneal edema, flat anterior chamber with inflammation and failing bleb, hemorrhagic choroidal detachment with flat anterior chamber, and increased ocular inflammation, flat anterior chamber and aphakia with no improvement in 3 to 5 days, appositional kissing choroidals for greater than 48 hours, would leak with flat anterior chamber and choroidal detachment, and choroidal detachment in apposition to lens with flat anterior chamber and pupillary block. The latter may require a possible iridectomy.

References

Bellows AR, et al: Choroidal effusion during glaucoma surgery in patients with prominent episcleral vessels. Arch Ophthalmol 97:493–497, 1979.
Bellows AR, Chylack LT Jr, Hutchinson BT: Choroidal detachment. Clinical manifestation, therapy, and mechanism of formation. Ophthalmology 88:1107–1115, 1981.
Berke SJ, et al: Chronic and recurrent choroidal detachment after glaucoma filtering surgery. Ophthalmology 94:154–162, 1987.
Brubaker RF, Pederson JE: Choroidal Detachment Survey. Ophthalmology 27:281–289, 1983.
Burton TC, Stevens TS, Harrison TJ: The influence of subconjunctival depot corticosteroid or choroidal detachment following retinal detachment surgery. Trans Am Acad Ophthalmol Otolaryngol 79:845–850, 1975.
Capper SA, Leopold IH: Mechanism of serous choroidal detachment. A review and experimental study. Arch Ophthalmol 55:101–113, 1956.
Chandler PA, Maumenee AE: A major cause of hypotony. Am J Ophthalmol 52:609–618, 1961.
Chylack LT Jr, Bellows AR: Molecular sieving in suprachoroidal fluid formation in man. Invest Ophthalmol Vis Sci 17:420–427, 1978.
Peyman GA, et al: Computed tomography in choroidal detachment. Ophthalmology 91:156–162, 1984.
Pederson JE, Gaasterland DE, MacLellan HM: Experimental ciliochoroidal detachment. Effect on intraocular pressure and aqueous humor flow. Arch Ophthalmol 97:536–541, 1979.
Ruiz RS, Salmonsen PC: Expulsive choroidal effusion. A complication of intraocular surgery. Arch Ophthalmol 94:69–70, 1976.
Sugar HS: Postoperative cataract in successfully filtering glaucomatous eyes. Am J Ophthalmol 69:740–746, 1970.

CHOROIDAL NEOVASCULAR MEMBRANES
(Disciform Macular Degeneration, Hemorrhagic Disciform Detachment, Subretinal Neovascularization)

ROBERT E. KALINA, M.D.
Seattle, Washington

Choroidal neovascularization is a sheet of new capillaries, with or without a fine connective tissue network, that extends from the choroid either through a break in Bruch's membrane or around the peripapillary end of Bruch's membrane into the subretinal pigment epithelial or subretinal space. Although neovascular membranes may occur anywhere in the fundus, they are most common in the posterior pole and often cause permanent loss of central vision secondary to serous and hemorrhagic detachment of the macula. Clinical examination reveals a dirty gray or yellow subretinal membrane or a pigmented mound beneath the retina. Subretinal blood may be present along the outer edge of the neovascular membrane.

If a pigmented ring can be seen, the neovascular membrane often is confined to the ring. Fluorescein angiography permits accurate localization of the extent of the neovascular membrane, except when it is obscured by blood or other opacity. The membrane often assumes the configuration of a wheel, including radial vessels and larger peripheral arcades.

Choroidal neovascularization is associated with a wide variety of clinical syndromes affecting Bruch's membrane and adjacent tissues. Most important among these associations are macular drusen and presumed ocular histoplasmosis. Less common, but still important, predisposing causes are angioid streaks, choroidal ruptures, myopia, drusen of the optic disc, choroidal tumors, and many other inflammatory or degenerative disorders of the posterior pole of the eye. Idiopathic cases are not rare.

THERAPY

Systemic. A wide variety of vitamin[‡] and mineral preparations[‡] have been advocated for macular diseases, but there is no scientific or clinical evidence to suggest that these are beneficial. Anticoagulants[‡] have been advocated by some authorities based on the mistaken belief that the observed process was related to circulatory deficiency, but these agents actually may be harmful by predisposing to intraocular hemorrhage. Oral corticosteroids[‡] often have been prescribed and still are advocated by some, but there is no evidence that the final visual result is altered by such therapy.

Surgical. Choroidal neovascular membranes can be destroyed by laser photocoagulation. Moderately intense burns must be applied to cover the entire neovascular network. The side of the neovascular membrane closest to the fovea should be treated first. Small (50- or 100-μm) spots may be used to outline the margin of the area to be treated, but the entire membrane should be treated with larger (200- to 500-μm) spots at up to 0.5-second exposures. Treatment should extend beyond the edge of the membrane by at least 100 μm in all directions. The surgeon must make reference to a recent fluorescein angiogram, and retrobulbar anesthesia and akinesia often are required. The patient should be reexamined at intervals to detect incomplete treatment or recurrence. Fluorescein angiography should be repeated at about 3 weeks or with any change in symptoms.

Although photocoagulation of choroidal neovascular membranes is thought to be beneficial, treatment is not without risk, and some cases may undergo spontaneous involution. In general, the prognosis for vision in eyes with choroidal neovascular membranes improves with increasing distance of the membranes from the center of the macula with or without treatment. A collaborative clinical trial has established the effectiveness of argon (blue-green) laser photocoagulation for idiopathic choroidal neovascular membranes and for those associated with drusen in older patients (aging macular degeneration) or the presumed ocular histoplasmosis syndrome. Laser therapy for other causes of subretinal neovascularization remains under study, as does the use of other wavelengths.

Supportive. Choroidal neovascular membranes are a leading cause of visual loss. Fortunately, peripheral vision is retained in most patients and total blindness does not ensue, a prognostic fact that can be comforting to the patient and that should be stressed by the ophthalmologist. The responsibility of the physician does not end with such reassurance for bilaterally affected patients, but should include assessment of the potential usefulness of low-vision aids and services for the partially sighted.

Ocular or Periocular Manifestations

Retina: Chorioretinal scars; detachment of retinal pigment epithelium or retina; drusen; subretinal hemorrhage or lipid.

Other: Central scotoma; metamorphopsia; micropsia.

PRECAUTIONS

Since photocoagulation of choroidal neovascular membranes can contribute to visual loss, patients should be selected carefully for treatments. Choroidal neovascular membranes farther than 2500 μ from the center of the fovea probably do not require treatment. Treatment of neovascularization closer than 200 μm to the center of the foveal avascular zone usually presents unacceptable risks of visual loss because of damage to the fovea or its vascular supply. Absorption of light by xanthophyll in the foveal area increases damage to the sensory retina. Photocoagulation in the papillomacular bundle may produce nerve fiber layer damage, particularly if the retina is not elevated by serous fluid. Partial treatment of a choroidal neovascular membrane generally is unsuccessful and is not recommended.

Neither treatment nor study by fluorescein angiography is indicated for advanced stages of macular scarring caused by choroidal neovascularization. Treatment should be considered only for symptomatic eyes in which there is reasonable hope of preserving useful central vision. Since recurrence in the treated eye or involvement of the fellow eye is common, patients should report promptly if new symptoms are observed. Home use of an Amsler grid may be helpful for early detection. Ophthalmoscopic or fluorescein angiographic detection of a pigment epithelial defect in the foveal area of the fellow eye in the presumed ocular histoplasmosis syndrome is a risk indicator for that eye.

COMMENTS

Choroidal neovascular membranes always should be suspected when detachment of the macula occurs. Their presence is particularly likely when the subretinal fluid contains blood or lipid.

Photocoagulation of choroidal neovascular membranes became possible after the introduction of fluorescein angiography permitted their precise localization. The xenon arc photocoagulator was used initially, but soon was supplanted by the widely available argon (blue-green) laser. More recently, lasers emitting other wavelengths have been introduced and are being studied in the treatment of choroidal neovascular membranes and other retinal diseases. Theoretical advantages of these wavelengths include reduced damage to retinal blood vessels and reduced absorption by yellow pigment in the lens and fovea. The effectiveness of these new modalities for treatment of choroidal neovascular membranes, particularly those very close to the center of the fovea, remains to be proven in clinical trials.

Since this chapter was originally written, krypton red laser photocoagulation has been shown to be effective for the treatment of choroidal neovascularization 1 to 199 μm from the center of the foveal avascular zone in patients with the presumed ocular histoplasmosis syndrome.

References

Gass JDM: Stereoscopic Atlas of Macular Diseases: diagnosis and Treatment, 3rd ed. St. Louis, CV Mosby, 1987.
Macular Photocoagulation Study Group: Krypton laser photocoagulation for neovascular lesions of ocular histoplasmosis. Results of a randomized clinical trial. Arch Ophthalmol 105:1499–1507, 1987.
Macular Photocoagulation Study Group: Argon laser photocoagulation for neovascular maculopathy. Three-year results from randomized clinical trials. Arch Ophthalmol 104:694–701, 1986.
Young RW: Pathophysiology of age-related macular degeneration. Surv Ophthalmol 31:291–306, 1987.

CHOROIDAL RUPTURES

RONALD E. SMITH, M.D.
Los Angeles, California

Direct choroidal ruptures are relatively rare and are probably caused by direct concussive necrosis of the choroid. They are usually found anterior to the equator. They appear as large, broad, and usually irregular lesions lying near the periphery exposing the sclera, bordered initially by hemorrhage and eventually by heavy pigment changes. Indirect choroidal ruptures, however, are a common complication of contusive injuries to the eye and appear as a yellowish-brown streak. The edges of direct choroidal ruptures may be associated with an edematous hemorrhagic retina. Rents in the choroid and Bruch's membrane usually occur temporal to the disc in a concentric fashion and are often associated with intrachoroidal, subretinal, and intraretinal hemorrhages. Multiple tears of various sizes may be encountered. If the macula has not been directly involved, good visual acuity is to be expected; central vision usually improves within the first 10 days. Late subretinal neovascularization may occasionally occur with hemorrhagic or serous detachment of the retina in the macular area.

THERAPY

Supportive. The common sequence of events after choroidal rupture is gradual clearing of localized hemorrhage and retinal or choroidal edema, followed by formation of a gliotic scar and pigment epithelial alterations in the area of the choroidal tear. This scar may develop into a sharply defined white streak, which is usually a third or less of the diameter of the disc in width and is bordered by heavily pigmented edges. No treatment is recommended, except possibly rest, topical mydriatics, and a pad and bandage.

Surgical. When complicating subretinal neovascularization occurs, photocoagulation may be indicated. Treatment should consist of heavy confluent laser burns of the entire neovascular membrane. Argon laser photocoagulation is preferred for convenience and accuracy of energy delivery.

Ocular or Periocular Manifestations

Choroid: Atrophy; edema; hemorrhages; necrosis.
Retina: Detachment; edema; elevation; hemorrhages; macular detachment; subretinal neovascularization.
Other: Central scotoma; decreased visual acuity; visual loss.

PRECAUTIONS

Small circumscribed areas of subretinal new vessels in an area of long-standing choroidal rupture may not require any therapy at all. Until the natural course of these lesions is defined, photocoagulation should only be considered for patients with progressive serous or hemorrhagic detachments associated with subretinal neovascularization.

A marked loss of central vision persisting longer than 2 months usually indicates a permanent condition. Patients with choroidal rupture should be followed with potential complications in mind.

COMMENTS

Fluorescein angiography is an important modality in the management of choroidal rupture, since the late development of subretinal neovascularization may cause secondary serous or hemorrhagic macular detachments. Photocoagulation may be indicated in these instances. However, there is disagreement whether all such patients should be treated, and adequate clinical trials have not been performed.

References

Duke-Elder S (ed): System of Ophthalmology. St. Louis, CV Mosby, 1972, Vol XIV, pp 151–158.
Smith RE, Kelley JS, Harbin TS: Late macular complications of choroidal ruptures. Am J Ophthalmol 77:650–658, 1974.
Zagora E: Eye Injuries. Springfield, IL, Charles C Thomas, 1970, pp 21–23.

EXPULSIVE HEMORRHAGE
(Subchoroidal Expulsive Hemorrhage)

DANIEL M. TAYLOR, M.D.
New Britain, Connecticut

Expulsive hemorrhage may take the form of a localized subchoroidal hemorrhage, a massive subchoroidal hemorrhage with a break into the vitreous, or a hemorrhage that proceeds to extrusion of the contents of the globe. It is the most serious and devastating complication of intraocular surgery, but fortunately is uncommon with an incidence of approximately 0.25 per cent. The author has experienced 20 expulsive hemorrhages in over 8000 intraocular procedures performed from 1951 through 1988. It is most often encountered during cataract extraction in elderly patients with arteriosclerosis and/or hypertensions and glaucoma, but may also occur in young patients, particularly when glaucoma is present. The author has experienced a high incidence of expulsive hemorrhage during extensive keratoplasty procedures, with a total of 9 occurrences in about 1500 keratoplasties. The eye is most vulnerable and treatment least effective when the hemorrhage occurs during penetrating keratoplasty. The author has also experienced extensive subchoroidal bleeding during the first 24 hours after filtering surgery for uncontrollable glaucoma.

The immediate cause of expulsive hemorrhage during intraocular surgery is a sudden change in the intraocular pressure gradient when the eye is opened. These changes are greater if the arterial pressure is chronically elevated because of hypertensive cardiovascular disease or is acutely elevated at the time of surgery because of anoxia, CO_2 build-up, pressor drugs, or venous obstruction (Valsalva maneuver—vomiting, bucking, coughing). The underlying cause is the presence of arterial necrosis of the short and long posterior ciliary arteries. The arterial necrosis may be caused by degenerative vascular disease, such as hypertensive arteriosclerotic cardiovascular disease and diabetes. It may also occur on a nutritional basis in an otherwise normal eye, since the vessel walls of the small arterials are nourished by filtration only. The average filtration pressure of 30 mm Hg is the difference between the average intraocular arterial pressure of approximately 50 mm Hg minus the intraocular pressure of 20 mm Hg. Chronic glaucoma, by reducing the differential between the intraocular arterial pressure and the intraocular pressure, may result in inadequate nutrition of the vascular wall and subsequent arterial necrosis. It is estimated that expulsive hemorrhage occurs ten times more frequently in glaucomatous eyes than in nonglaucomatous eyes. The most common site is just after the vessel emerges from the scleral wall to enter the subchoroidal space.

The first sign of this complication is the sudden unexplained presentation of vitreous from the wound. Later, the choroid and retina may bulge through the incision, and blood breaks into the vitreous cavity. If the subchoroidal bleeding spontaneously stops or is exteriorized by sclerotomy, the choroid and the retina may not rupture. If bleeding, continues, the entire contents of the eye may extrude. The choroid and retina are dissected from the sclera by the arterial hemorrhage, and other short ciliary arteries and vortex veins are torn in rapid sequence, thus compounding the problem. With severe bleeding from multiple sites, the condition rapidly becomes irreversible. In the author's experience, 75 per cent of expulsive hemorrhages occurred at the time of surgery and 25 per cent during the first 24 hours postoperative. Some of the latter may represent hemorrhages of small magnitude that require additional time to manifest changes.

THERAPY

Surgical. Immediate and rapid closure of the corneal scleral wound with temporary 7-0 or 8-0 interrupted black silk sutures is mandatory to permit a rapid build-up of the intraocular pressure, which, in turn, tends to tamponade bleeding from the ruptured arterial vessel. A posterior sclerotomy should be done approximately 8 to 10 mm behind the limbus over the site of the suspected subchoroidal hemorrhage, and this incision should be kept open until bleeding stops. A T- or V-shaped sclerotomy is preferred, as it results in more adequate drainage. The lips of the wound may be cauterized to cause shrinkage, thereby keeping the wound open, possibly for days, to allow continuous drainage. If the first sclerotomy does not find the bleeding site, a second or third sclerotomy should be done in the opposite quadrants. These procedures usually provide sufficient drainage of the subchoroidal space to prevent massive prolapse and rupture of the choroid and retina. When the bleeding is extremely brisk, it may be necessary to aspirate the subchoroidal blood with a syringe and a cannula for as long as 1 hour. On occasion, the blood loss may exceed 100 ml.

When the bleeding stops, the initial operative incision can be reopened, and a vitrectomy can be performed to remove carefully all formed vitreous from in front of the iris and from the wound. These steps should be performed meticulously to prevent shallowing of the anterior chamber with peripheral anterior synechiae formation and severe secondary angle-closure glaucoma. The cataract incision can then be carefully reclosed with nonabsorbable sutures of nylon and interrupted silk. The globe should be reformed with an intravitreal balanced salt solution to increase the intraocular pressure with the effect of expressing the residual blood through the sclerotomy site. Before closure, it may even be possible to insert an intraocular lens if the bleeding appears to be completely under control. If the hemorrhage occurs during keratoplasty shortly after removal of the button, it will be impossible to close the eye quickly enough. Under these circumstances, the assistant can place a thumb over the keratoplasty opening to tamponade the eye while the surgeon performs the posterior sclerotomy. When all bleeding has ceased, it will then be possible to suture in the donor button. With these techniques, the author has salvaged 62 per cent of all eyes experiencing expulsive hemorrhage during surgery. Evisceration or enucleation may be necessary in rare instances, if the contents of the eye have been extruded and the bleeding cannot be stopped.

Systemic. After the surgical treatment of an expulsive hemorrhage, systemic and topical ophthalmic corticosteroids may be given to control inflammation and suppress secondary uveitis and vitreitis. Oral administration of 40 mg of prednisone and 1 per cent topical ophthalmic prednisolone solution four times daily is helpful. Cycloplegics, consisting of 1 per cent atropine or 5 per cent homatropine, may be given twice daily.

PRECAUTIONS

Any procedure that abruptly reduces intraocular pressure may precipitate expulsive hemorrhage. Patients with hypertension should be well controlled with their blood pressure lowered before surgery. Patients with chronic glaucoma should also have their intraocular pressures brought under control by the usual glaucoma medications. Patients on anticoagulants or aspirin should refrain from using these medications for at least 5 days before surgery. Epinephrine and other pressor agents should be avoided. Immediately before surgery the intraocular pressure should be reduced to a minimum by the use of intravenous hypotensive agents, such as 150 to 250 ml of 20 per cent mannitol given one half-hour before surgery. The globe and orbit should also be decompressed by a mercury bag or thorough massage before surgery. The head of the operating table can be slightly elevated to avoid elevation of venous pressure. General anesthesia should be avoided whenever possible to eliminate the possibility of the Valsalva effect, produced by bucking on the tube, coughing, or vomiting. Postoperatively, if the chamber remains shallow and peripheral anterior synechiae develop, intractable glaucoma may occur with ultimate loss of the eye. Trabeculectomy or cyclocryotherapy may prove effective in controlling postoperative angle-closure glaucoma.

COMMENTS

Unfortunately, there is no way to avoid completely an expulsive hemorrhage. They will occur despite the best efforts. However, a heightened index of suspicion does permit one to operate more efficiently and effectively should an expulsive hemorrhage occur. One must be particularly wary of any patient who has had a previous expulsive hemorrhage, as it has been amply documented that expulsive hemorrhages can recur in both eyes on successive occasions. One must be willing to accept the risk of a higher incidence of expulsive hemorrhage in extensive reconstructive procedures, including total penetrating keratoplasties, on seriously diseased eyes. In the surgical management, speed is more important than accuracy. A few moments of delay may be the difference between success and failure. Unfortunately, the neophyte surgeon is usually ill prepared to cope with a sudden massive expulsive hemorrhage. Late recognition and inability to perform efficiently and effectively the proper surgical maneuvers will usually result in total loss of the eye. With experience, it is possible to salvage the eye in approximately two thirds of the cases and even to obtain useful or excellent vision. Early recognition and immediate steps to close the eye and to externalize the bleeding are mandatory.

References

Freiwald MJ: Recovery from severe traumatic ocular hemorrhage. J Albert Einstein Med Ctr 20:87–90, 1972.
Gerard LJ, et al: Expulsive hemorrhage during intraocular surgery. Trans Am Acad Ophthalmol 77:119–125, 1973.
Payne JW, et al: Expulsive hemorrhage: Its incidence in cataract surgery and the report of four bilateral cases. Trans Am Ophthalmol Soc 83:181–196, 1985.
Shaffer RN: Posterior sclerotomy with scleral cautery in the treatment of expulsive hemorrhage. Am J Ophthalmol 61:1307–1311, 1966.
Taylor DM: Expulsive hemorrhage. Am J Ophthalmol 78:961–966, 1974.
Taylor DM: Expulsive hemorrhage: Some observations and comments. Trans Am Ophthalmol Soc 72:157–169, 1974.
Taylor DM: Discussion of Payne, et al: Expulsive hemorrhage: Its incidence in cataract surgery and the report of four bilateral cases. Trans Am Ophthalmol Soc 83:198–201, 1985.

MALIGNANT MELANOMA OF THE POSTERIOR UVEA
(Choroidal Melanoma, Ciliary Body Melanoma)
JERRY A. SHIELDS, M.D.,
and CAROL L. SHIELDS, M.D.
Philadelphia, Pennsylvania

Malignant melanoma of the uvea is the most common primary intraocular malignancy. This tumor arises from the uveal melanocytes, which are derived embryologically from the neural crest. Melanomas that occur in the ciliary body and peripheral choroid frequently attain a large size before they are diagnosed clinically. Choroidal melanomas that arise in the macular region are usually smaller at the time of diagnosis because they produce earlier visual symptoms.

The goal of the ophthalmologist in the management of a patient with a posterior uveal melanoma is to control the tumor and to salvage the patient's vision when this can be achieved without endangering the patient's overall health. The method of treatment should be carefully selected so as to meet these goals. Important considerations that should be taken into account when recommending specific management for a patient with a malignant melanoma of the posterior uvea include the size, extent, location, and activity of the tumor; the condition of the opposite eye; and the patient's age, general health, and psychologic status. Once all of the factors that influence the therapeutic choice have been assessed thoroughly, the patient with a posterior uveal melanoma can be managed by any of several methods, depending upon the overall clinical situation.

THERAPY

Supportive. In recent years, many authorities have begun to recommend only *periodic observation* to manage initially selected melanomas of the posterior uvea. This approach seems to be particularly justifiable in the case of many small or medium-sized melanocytic tumors that are presumably malignant melanomas, but that have dormant characteristics on ophthalmoscopic examination. The relative indications for managing a posterior uveal melanoma by periodic observation include the following: 1) any small melanoma that appears dormant on the initial examination and that has been documented with fundus photography or ultrasonography not to have grown; 2) some medium-sized melanomas that appear dormant on the initial examination, 3) small or medium-sized melanomas in elderly or seriously ill patients, even though the tumor shows signs of slow growth; and 4) most small or medium-sized melanomas if the tumor is located in the patient's only useful eye, even though the tumor shows signs of slow growth. The definitions of dormant characteristics and size categories are cited in the literature.

The diagnostic tests used and the frequency of follow-up examinations depend upon the size category and the apparent activity of the tumor. If a patient has a tumor that is classified as a suspicious nevus, he or she should have fundus photographs and be re-examined in 3 months. If no growth is detected, examination should be repeated every 6 months thereafter. If a lesion is classified as a small melanoma that has dormant characteristics, the patient should have baseline fundus photographs, fluorescein angiography, and A-scan and B-scan ultrasonography. The photographs should be repeated in 3 to 4 months. If the lesion shows no apparent change at that time, fundus photography should then be repeated every 6 months. If growth is suspected on the basis of clinical examination, then fundus photography, fluorescein angiography, and ultrasonography should be repeated to confirm any change, and the patient should be considered for one of the therapeutic methods to be described later.

Medium-sized melanomas that have dormant characteristics, especially if they are found in elderly patients, can usually be safely managed by periodic observation. Because of their greater tendency to show subsequent growth, they should have initial fundus photography, fluorescein angiography, and ultrasonography. The photographs and ultrasonography should be repeated every 3 to 6 months, and therapy should be considered if the growth is documented.

Surgical. *Photocoagulation* is another method of treating selected small choroidal melanomas. However, it cannot be used in the treatment of ciliary body melanomas. The relative indications for treatment of a choroidal melanoma by photocoagulation are as follows: 1) a small melanoma that shows unequivocal evidence of growth by both serial photography or ultrasonography; 2) some small melanomas that have not necessarily been documented to grow but that show features of activity on the initial examination, particularly if the tumor margin is more than 2 mm from the foveola or optic disc margin, and 3) selected medium-sized melanomas that are more than 2 mm from the optic disc or fovea. To utilize photocoagulation, the ocular media should be clear. Either argon laser or xenon photocoagulation can be employed. If the xenon arc is used, retrobulbar anesthesia is preferable. When one uses the argon laser, topical anesthesia is usually sufficient.

Any of several available contact lenses can be used. During the first treatment session, burns are applied in two confluent rows around the margins of the tumor. The settings necessary to obtain adequate burns around the tumor vary with the degree of fundus pigmentation. Using the argon laser, however, a spot size of 200 to 500 μm, an intensity of 500 to 1000 mW, and duration of 0.5 second, usually suffice.

About 3 weeks later, the tumor is surrounded again using similar settings. After two or three surrounding treatments, most of the choroidal vessels around the tumor become obliterated or incorporated into scar tissue. In subsequent sessions about 3 to 5 weeks apart, the surrounding area is retreated, and the surface of the tumor is treated heavily. Using the argon laser, it may require up to 1500 mW with a duration of 1.0 to 1.5 seconds to obtain sufficient destruction of the tumor. After a total of four to ten treatments, the area of the tumor is usually replaced by a depressed scar, consisting of a thin layer of fibroglial tissue overlying the bare sclera. In many cases treated by this method, a central area of flat pigmentation is often left in the center of the scar. It is not necessary to continue treatment once the central pigment is flat, less than 1.5 mm in diameter, and hypofluorescent with fluorescein angiography.

With the advent of low-energy radioactive plaques, photocoagulation is rarely used today in the management of choroidal melanomas. Although *radiotherapy* was once believed to be ineffective in the treatment of uveal melanomas, it has recently become the most widely employed method in the management of melanomas of the choroid and ciliary body. In view of the recent controversy regarding enucleation for posterior uveal melanomas, the indications for radiotherapy are increasing. The relative indications will probably continue to change as more follow-up data on treated patients become available. The most widely employed method of radiotherapy has been the application of an episcleral radioactive plaque. The isotopes employed include Cobalt-60, Iridium-192, Iodine-125, and Ruthenium-106, depending on the size and extent of the tumor. Heavy ion radiotherapy, using proton beam or helium ions, also has its advocates. However, the authors believe that the overall complications are fewer when radioactive plaques are employed.

The current indications for treating a posterior uveal melanoma with an episcleral plaque are as follows: 1) selected small melanomas that are documented to be growing; 2) most medium-sized and large choroidal and ciliary body melanomas that are less than 10 mm in thickness and that show evidence of growth in an eye that has useful or salvagable vision; and 3) most medium-sized and large melanomas that occur in the patient's only useful eye, regardless of the visual acuity. Initially, use of episcleral plaque radiotherapy was preferred on medium-sized melanomas that were located in the nasal portion of the fundus and that were at lest 3 mm from the optic disc. As further information regarding more favorable mortality rates became available, larger melanomas and those located closer to the disc and fovea have been treated successfully by episcleral plaque radiotherapy. Today, specially designed episcleral plaques can be used for juxtapapillary melanomas and subfoveal melanomas. For patients who have a large melanoma located in their only eye, episcleral plaque radiotherapy is generally used, despite the large size of the tumor.

The surgical application of an episcleral plaque should be performed as gently as possible to minimize the theoretic possibility of systemic dissemination of tumor cells during the surgical manipulations. The current policy is to expose gently and inspect the sclera to detect any extrascleral extension of the tumor and then to localize the lesion with transcleral transillumination. The shadow of the tumor is outlined on the sclera with a sterile marking pencil, and a dummy plaque is used to align the scleral sutures. The dummy plaque is then removed, and the radioactive plaque is inserted and tied securely in position. The plaque is left in position long enough to deliver about 8000 to 10,000 cGy to the tumor apex, after which it is removed under local anesthesia and the patient discharged.

Theoretically, an ideal approach to the management of a melanoma of the ciliary body or choroid is to perform *local resection* to remove the tumor and salvage the eye, particularly, if this can be achieved without worsening the patient's prognosis for life expectancy. Several years ago, a penetrating sclerochorioretinectomy (full-thickness eyewall resection) was performed, but in recent years, a partial lamellar sclerouvectomy has been preferred. This technique removes the tumor and inner sclera while leaving intact the retina and the outer sclera. This procedure is described in the recent literature.

The relative indications for local resection of a posterior uveal melanoma are as follows: 1) a growing ciliary body melanoma or a ciliochoroidal melanoma that does not cover more than one third of the pars plicata; and 2) a choroidal melanoma that is not greater than 12 mm in diameter, which is centered near the equator and which is documented to be growing. It should be stressed that melanomas that meet these criteria can also be managed by episcleral plaque radiotherapy in most instances. The preferred method of therapy in these instances is unresolved, and each case must be evaluated individually.

As mentioned earlier, the role of *enucleation* in the management of patients with posterior uveal melanomas remains controversial. There are definite indications for enucleation, although the indications for this procedure are fewer than they were in the past. Current indications for enucleation to treat posterior uveal melanomas are as follows: 1) most ciliary body or choroidal melanomas that have produced visual loss, but that are too large to manage with either radiotherapy or local resection; 2) most posterior uveal melanomas that have produced total retinal detachment or severe secondary glaucoma; and 3) most small and medium-sized choroidal melanomas that are documented to be growing and that are invading the tissues of the optic nerve.

In enucleation, the so-called no-touch technique is used less frequently today. The value of this technique in reducing the mortality rate from uveal melanomas remains unproven, although some authorities believe that adherence to this technique does reduce the mortality rate. A gentle enucleation with minimal manipulation of the globe should be adequate.

In the last few years, pre-enucleation radiotherapy (PERT) has been employed by some authorities in hopes of decreasing the chances of metastases. Recent studies have suggested that PERT is of little or no value, and the technique has been largely abandoned.

Exenteration of the orbital contents is considered by some authorities to be an acceptable method of treating uveal melanomas with extraocular extension into the orbit. Others believe that orbital exenteration does not improve the patient's life expectancy in such cases. The current indications for orbital exenteration for a uveal melanoma are extensive extraocular involvement by the melanoma at the time of initial presentation (provided there is no evidence of systemic metastasis) or orbital recurrence of a uveal melanoma some time after enucleation (provided there is no evidence of systemic metastasis). With improved diagnostic techniques and earlier recognition of uveal melanomas, it has become uncommon for patients to present initially with extensive extraocular involvement.

Ocular or Periocular Manifestations

Ciliary Body: Tumor.
Choroid: Tumor.
Conjunctiva: Injection.

Episclera: Extrascleral extension; sentinel vessels (ciliary body tumor).
Iris: Neovascular glaucoma; tumor-induced dialysis (from ciliary body tumor).
Optic Nerve: Atrophy.
Retina: Hemorrhage; nonrhegmatogenous retinal detachment.

Precautions

There appears to be little or no danger in periodical observation of small to medium-sized melanomas that show dormant features. Most of these tumors have little, if any, tendency to grow and a low potential to metastasize. Although no long-term data are yet available concerning periodic observation of choroidal melanomas, up to 50 per cent of small to medium-sized melanomas that show dormant features can be documented to grow during a 5-year follow-up. Lesions located within 2 mm of the optic disc or foveola should be followed more frequently. If growth toward either of these structures is documented, either plaque radiotherapy or photocoagulation should be considered.

The complications of photocoagulation for choroidal melanomas include branch retinal vein obstruction, cystoid macular edema, preretinal membrane formation with retinal traction, choroidovitreal neovascularization, vitreous hemorrhage, and retinal detachment. All of these complications are more frequent after xenon arc photocoagulation and are relatively uncommon or less severe when argon laser is used. Treatment of choroidal melanomas by photocoagulation is most often successful if the tumor is in the small size category, being less than 3 mm in thickness as measured by A-scan ultrasonography.

There are very early complications of episcleral plaque radiotherapy, including ocular irritation and diplopia. Diplopia can occur if a rectus muscle is disinserted to properly position the plaque. It is rarely necessary, however, to disinsert a rectus muscle to position the plaque. Later complications of episcleral plaque radiotherapy include radiation retinopathy, radiation papillopathy, neovascular glaucoma, vitreous hemorrhage, radiation cataract, punctal occlusion with epiphora, keratoconjunctivitis sicca, radiation anterior uveitis, sclera necrosis, and persistent diplopia.

Tumors treated by episcleral plaque radiotherapy can sometimes show a rather dramatic response to treatment. Most posterior uveal melanomas show either stabilization or a decrease in tumor size during a follow-up period of 2 to 6 years. The visual results have been satisfactory, and the complications have been relatively few. The mortality rate during this relatively short follow-up period appears to be the same for patients treated with episcleral plaques and those with comparable-sized tumors treated with enucleation.

Episcleral plaque radiotherapy usually is not associated with immediate visual morbidity. The early complications of sclerochorioretinal resection, however, are greater than those of plaque radiotherapy. The most important early surgical complications of sclerochorioretinal resection are hypotony, wound leak, vitreous bleeding, and retinal detachment. Postoperative or late complications of local resections include vitreous fibrosis, cataract, and ischemic inflammation in the anterior segment. The vitreosis fibrosis can lead to chronic traction on the retina and a delayed retinal detachment. In many cases, removal of a ciliochoroidal tumor necessitates removal of a large portion of the zonular support to the lens. This can lead to postoperative shifting of the lens, with inflammation, corneal edema, or glaucoma. To avoid this complication, the lens should generally be removed at the time of surgery when the tumor covers more than 4 clock hours of the pars plicata.

Unfortunately, the mortality rate for patients with posterior uveal melanomas remains rather high following enucleation. Approximately 30 to 45 per cent of patients who undergo enucleation for choroidal melanoma will eventually die of metastasis, despite the fact that no evidence of metastasis is detected on the systemic evaluation before enucleation. The mortality rate for patients treated with the so-called no-touch technique or for those who have PERT appears to be no different from those who have had a standard gentle enucleation.

Comments

The management of malignant melanoma of the posterior uvea has recently become a topic of great controversy. The traditional treatment of enucleation of the tumor-containing eye has recently been challenged by a number of authorities, and clinicians are more frequently using alternative methods of management when possible. Current management ranges from periodic observation and fundus photography of selected small lesions that appear dormant to photocoagulation, radiotherapy, or local resection of growing tumors in eyes with useful or salvageable vision. In cases in which the tumor is far advanced and there is no hope of useful vision, enucleation is generally advisable.

The choice of therapy is a complex one, and each case must be individualized. In selecting a therapeutic approach, certain factors must be carefully weighed. These include the size of the melanoma, its extent and location, its apparent activity, the status of the opposite eye, and the age, general health, and psychologic status of the patient.

Periodic observation is believed to be the treatment of choice for most small and many medium-sized melanomas of the posterior uvea that have not been documented to grow. If such lesions are documented to grow or if they show ophthalmoscopic evidence of progressive growth on the initial examination, then photocoagulation or episcleral plaque radiotherapy may be employed. Laser photocoagulation may be done if the tumor is not greater than 10 mm in diameter or 3 mm in thickness. In the case of medium-sized or large tumors that are growing, the patient can be managed with either scleral plaque radiotherapy or local resection of the tumor. Because radiotherapy has less immediate visual morbidity than local resection, more patients are being managed today by radiotherapy, most commonly in the form of a radioactive plaque using Cobalt-60, Iodine-125, Iridium-192, or Ruthenium-106.

Patients with large tumors that have produced severe visual loss are currently managed by enucleation. It appears that the so-called no-touch technique of enucleation and pre-enucleation radiotherapy do not favorably alter the prognosis. If there is extrascleral extension on initial examination or orbital recurrence after enucleation, exenteration of the orbit or one of its modifications seems advisable.

Patients who have known systemic metastases, either before or after enucleation or other treatment, have a poor prognosis. In such case, palliative irradiation, chemotherapy, or immunotherapy may be employed.

The management of posterior uveal melanomas will probably remain controversial for several years. It is hoped that with the accumulation of further knowledge of the various therapeutic alternatives, the physician will be able to recommend a specific form of therapy in an individual case with more certainty and confidence. Randomized clinical trials are difficult to accomplish for cases of uveal melanomas because there are so many factors involved in making the therapeutic choice. Unless such studies provide definitive information, each case should be evaluated independently, and the physician should choose the form of therapy that seems most appropriate in view of the overall clinical situation.

References

Brady LW, et al: Malignant intraocular tumors. Cancer 49:578–585, 1982.
Fraunfelder FT, et al: No-touch technique for intraocular malignant melanomas. Arch Ophthalmol 95:1616–1620, 1977.
Shields JA: Accuracy and limitations of the P-32 test in the diagnosis of ocular tumors: An analysis of 500 cases. Ophthalmology 85:950–966, 1978.
Shields JA: Diagnosis and Management of Intraocular Tumors. St. Louis, CV Mosby, 1982.
Shields JA: Counseling the patient with posterior uveal melanoma. Editorial. Am J Ophthalmol 106:88–91, 1988.
Shields JA, Shields CL: Massive extraocular extension of posterior uveal melanoma. Am J Ophthalmol (Submitted for publication).
Shields JA, et al: Cobalt plaque therapy for posterior uveal melanomas. Ophthalmology 89:1201–1207, 1982.
Zimmerman LE, McLean IW, Foster WD: Does enucleation of the eye containing a malignant melanoma prevent or accelerate the dissemination of tumor cells? Br J Ophthalmol 62:420–425, 1978.

SYMPATHETIC OPHTHALMIA
(Sympathetic Uveitis)

GEORGE E. MARAK, JR., M.D.
Alexandria, Virginia

Sympathetic ophthalmia is a bilateral nonnecrotizing uveitis that is believed to represent an autoimmune response to an unidentified ocular antigen suspected to be of retinal or retinal pigment epithelial origin. A perforating wound is important in the pathogenesis of the disease, since it allows antigens to escape from the "immunologic privilege" of the intraocular compartment. The contamination introduced with a perforating wound may have an adjuvant effect that helps account for the 30 to 50 times more frequent incidence of sympathetic ophthalmia after accidental compared to surgical penetrating wounds.

Sympathetic ophthalmia, as with any inflammatory disease, may present with varying degrees of severity. This creates problems in the differential diagnosis. The textbook description of sympathetic ophthalmia is well recognized and need not be repeated; however, it may also present as a mild anterior uveitis, pars planitis, peripapillitis, or focal choroiditis, which is not easily confused with multifocal placoid pigment epitheliopathy (in the author's experience).

Fluorescein angiography presents a characteristic picture in sympathetic ophthalmia. Ultrasonography can demonstrate choroidal thickening. A peau d'orange appearance seen on slitlamp examination indicates variations in the choroidal infiltrate that may be helpful in distinguishing sympathetic ophthalmia from bilateral phacoanaphylactic endophthalmitis.

THERAPY

Systemic. The objective of therapy in sympathetic ophthalmia is to control the inflammation as soon as possible. A combination of systemic, subtenon,* and topical corticosteroids in doses proportionate to the severity of the inflammation is the treatment of choice. Severe disease may require initial daily doses of 200 mg of oral prednisone. This is given as a single morning dose for 3 to 10 days. Depending upon the patient's response, alternate-day therapy may be initiated. The steroids may be gradually tapered with clinical monitoring of the inflammation. In the absence of systemic complications, treatment should be maintained 3 to 6 months after all signs of inflammation have cleared. Exacerbations are unpredictable and may occur several years after a preceding episode of inflammation. Regular lifetime observation of the patient is necessary.

Patients unresponsive or intolerant of steroids require highly individualized management. A variety of anti-inflammatory agents have been employed with irregular success. Combinations of steroids and immunosuppressive drugs are the most promising alternative approach in difficult cases. Various immunosuppressive drugs have been employed alone in systemic treatment of sympathetic ophthalmia with anecdotal success in problem patients. Most recently, cyclosporine‡ has been fashionable, but it may cause permanent renal damage, and it is a potential neoplastic agent. Appropriate precautions and patient consent are essential in problem cases when individualized management includes treatment with immunosuppressive drugs.

Ocular. Subtenon injections of soluble steroids, such as 4 mg of dexamethasone,* may be employed several times a week in the initial treatment of severe disease. Topical corticosteroids can be used hourly in severe disease and reduced as the inflammation resolves.

Careful attention should be given to mydriasis. In severe uveitis, long-acting agents, such as atropine and scopolamine, often do not provide adequate dilation to prevent posterior synechia formation. Moving the pupil with pilocarpine and obtaining maximum dilation with phenylephrine and cyclopentolate should be appropriately employed at office visits to ensure against synechia formation.

Surgical. Cataract surgery has been performed successfully in a number of patients with sympathetic ophthalmia. There appear to be no unusual risks if it is done during a remission. Additional steroid coverage has conventionally been employed when cataract surgery is performed on patients with sympathetic opthalmia.

The success of glaucoma surgery in uveitis is not widely discussed. Many enucleated eyes have had previous glaucoma surgery, but there are no reliable data on the complications of glaucoma surgery in either sympathetic ophthalmia or other forms of severe uveitis.

Ocular or Periocular Manifestations

Choroid: Chorioretinal scarring and adhesions; focal obliteration of choriocapillaris.

Iris: Focal to diffuse nonnecrotizing granulomatous uveitis.

Optic Nerve: Edema; infiltration around pia septa; meningeal inflammation; perivasculitis.

Retina: Dalen-Fuchs' spots; exudative detachment; inflammation; perivasculitis.

Other: Cataracts; focal scleritis; phthisis bulbi; poliosis; secondary glaucoma; vitiligo.

Precautions

Continued lifelong observation of patients with sympathetic ophthalmia is necessary. Relapses occur in most patients, and the interval between relapses has been as long as 13 years.

It is important not to produce an exacerbation of the inflammation by tapering medication too rapidly. Patients should be re-examined within a few days after any medication reduction. Continuing systemic or topical medication for 3 to 6 months after all inflammation has cleared is important in avoiding exacerbations.

The usual complications and ocular side effects of systemic steroids are to be anticipated, and therapy should be modulated accordingly. Immunosuppressive agents are reserved for those patients who cannot tolerate or do not respond to steroid treatment.

Comments

Although two recent reports resurrect the idea that early enucleation of the injured eye is helpful to the sympathizing eye, this conclusion is not supported by the authors own data. As in all other reports, no statistically significant difference in the visual outcome of the sympathizing eye is related to the time of enucleation of the inducing eye once sympathetic ophthalmia has developed.

One would not treat glomerulonephritis or multiple sclerosis by removing one kidney or half of the brain. The idea of removing a noxious influence by enucleating the sympathizing eye is of historic interest but inconsistent with current concepts of autoimmunity. It is not justifiable to remove a potentially functional eye in established cases of sympathetic ophthalmia for the purpose of improving the prognosis of the sympathizing eye. The injured eye may eventually achieve better vision.

Every attempt should be made to save potentially useful eyes. However, with the development of sympathetic ophthalmia in eyes after vitrectomy, those eyes that have no hope for useful vision in the opinion of the surgeon should be enucleated after discussion with the patient.

The only known prevention for sympathetic ophthalmia is enucleation within 2 weeks of injury (before the development of the autoimmune response). Prophylactic steroids do not prevent sympathetic ophthalmia. The potential increased incidence of infection outweighs any potential benefit of prophylactic steroids.

References

Andrasch RH, Pirofsky B, Burns RP: Immunosuppressive therapy for severe chronic uveitis. Arch Ophthalmol 96:247–251, 1978.

Ben Ezra D, Nussenblatt RB, Timonen P: Optimal Use of Sandimmune in Endogenous Uveitis. Berlin, Springer-Verlag, 1988.

Croxatto JO, et al: Atypical histopathologic features in sympathetic ophthalmia. A study of a hundred cases. Int Ophthalmol 4:129–135, 1982.

Makley TA, Azar A: Sympathetic ophthalmia. A long-term follow-up. Arch Ophthalmol 96:257–262, 1978.

Marak GE Jr: Recent advances in sympathetic ophthalmia. Surv Ophthalmol 24:141–156, 1979.

Rao NA, et al: The role of the penetrating wound in the development of sympathetic ophthalmia. Arch Ophthalmol 101:102–104, 1983.

SECTION 20

CONJUNCTIVA

ALLERGIC CONJUNCTIVITIS
(Atopic Conjunctivitis, Hay Fever Conjunctivitis)

MATHEA R. ALLANSMITH, M.D., and ROBERT N. ROSS, Ph.D.

Boston, Massachusetts

Several ocular diseases bear a clinical resemblance to allergic diseases of other organs; they are characterized by inflammation, recurrence, and chronicity. Inflammation (redness, pain, swelling, and warmth) is a hallmark of ocular allergy as it is of anaphylactic reactions of the nasal mucosa, bronchi, or skin. Signs and symptoms of ocular allergy recur, often waxing and waning seasonally, as they do in such allergic diseases as hay fever or asthma. Finally, allergic disease is chronic. Clinical severity of allergic disease may change over the course of years, but once established, the allergic diathesis is usually detectable throughout life. This chronicity is as true of ocular allergy as it is of other allergic diseases.

Of those diseases that might have an allergic component, only hay fever conjunctivitis has been proven to be an IgE-mediated ocular allergy. This most common ocular atopy is characterized by itching, redness, and swelling of the lids and conjunctiva. Hay fever conjunctivitis is a recurrent seasonal (occasionally perennial) disease associated with air-borne allergens, such as pollen, mold, house dust, and animal dander.

Itchy, irritated eyes can result from a cascade of events triggered by activation and degranulation of conjunctival mast cells. There are an estimated 50 million mast cells in the ocular and adnexal tissues of one human eye. Each mast cell contains at least several hundred granules. On the surface of the mast cell membrane are 100,000 to 500,000 receptors for IgE, of which approximately 10 per cent are occupied at any time.

Animal studies of ocular anaphylaxis and human studies of inflammatory cells present in tears suggest that an immediate anaphylactic reaction of conjunctiva may be followed by a more prolonged and more damaging late-phase reaction. Leukotrienes almost certainly play a role in producing the conjunctival late-phase reaction. Direct application of leukotriene B_4 (LTB_4) was found to increase the number of eosinophils and neutrophils in rat conjunctiva. Interpretation of this research is complicated, however, by the failure to observe *clinical* signs of a late-phase reaction in human conjunctiva.

Ocular allergic diseases are characterized by several features:

1. The presence of large *papillae*: Hay fever conjunctivitis does not produce papillae; giant papillary conjunctivitis (GPC), vernal keratoconjunctivitis (VKC), and atopic keratoconjunctivitis (AKC) do produce abnormally large conjunctival papillae.
2. *Seasonal* nature of the disease: Hay fever (allergic rhinitis or, more properly, allergic rhinoconjunctivitis) may be caused by seasonal blooms of pollen-producing plants. If so, the signs and symptoms of hay fever conjunctivitis will be seasonal. Vernal keratoconjunctivitis is worse in the spring and summer than during other times of the year. Signs and symptoms of atopic keratoconjunctivitis are usually perennial.
3. *Natural history* of the disease: Hay fever conjunctivitis usually begins early in life and continues as long as the hay fever continues. Vernal keratoconjunctivitis is primarily a disease of childhood and young adulthood. Atopic keratoconjunctivitis persists through life.
4. *Threat to the visual axis*: Atopic keratoconjunctivitis poses a serious threat to vision. Vernal keratoconjunctivitis usually does not, but is so intensely uncomfortable that patients have considerable trouble seeing. Hay fever conjunctivitis usually poses no threat to vision.

Hay fever conjunctivitis (seasonal allergic conjunctivitis) is a mild inflammation of the conjunctiva that is usually associated with allergic rhinitis (hay fever). Air-borne allergens—for instance, pollen, molds, dust, and animal danders—can trigger an immediate allergic response in the nose (rhinitis) and conjunctiva (conjunctivitis). The mechanism of hay fever conjunctivitis is still not completely understood. Most likely, allergens dissolve in the tear film and react with specific IgE receptors bound to conjunctival mast cells and basophils. As with hay fever itself, hay fever conjunctivitis is usually seasonal. Yet, when the offending allergen is perennial—for instance, house dust or molds—signs and symptoms are also likely to be perennial.

Hay fever conjunctivitis is a type I hypersensitivity response to air-borne allergens. The ocular itching, conjunctival edema, and tearing are the result of mast cell degranulation and the release of histamine and other inflammatory mediators into tissue and the tear film. Local tissue eosinophilia may be a feature of hay fever conjunctivitis, but few, if any, eosinophils reach the surface of the conjunctiva and are not detected in laboratory studies of conjunctival tissue.

THERAPY

Supportive. Avoiding offending allergens remains an essential approach to minimizing the discomforts of allergic disease. Patients with seasonal hay fever can take precautions during the hay fever season to avoid pollens in the air by staying indoors; using air conditioners, air filters, or electrostatic precipitators; avoiding areas where plants producing offending pollens grow; and reducing the total allergenic load. Reducing the total allergenic load is important because the physiologic effects of allergens are additive. People with perennial hay fever conjunctivitis can take precautions to minimize their exposure to such year-long allergens as house dust, molds, and animal danders.

One of the most effective treatments of vernal keratoconjunctivitis is to reduce exposure to allergens. VKC patients are often advised to move to cooler climates where the cooler temperatures and the relatively lower concentrations of airborne allergens give relief. Avoidance is not as effective in controlling AKC.

Other hygienic treatments are available for treating the general symptoms and signs of ocular allergy. Cold compresses on the eyes, topical astringents, avoidance of light, and wearing cotton gloves to prevent rubbing and scratching are all possible approaches.

Medical. *Pharmacologic* treatments are now available to give relief from many of the symptoms of ocular allergy. Cromolyn sodium stabilizes the mast cell, thereby inhibiting degranulation and the release of histamine and other mediators of the allergic response. It has been prescribed to treat VKC, AKC, and hay fever conjunctivitis. Good results have been obtained with a schedule of one drop of 4% cromolyn sodium ophthalmic solution administered to each eye four times daily. Clinical signs and symptoms of VKC, AKC, and hay fever conjunctivitis are significantly reduced. Pretreatment with cromolyn sodium is also an effective prophylactic measure for hay fever conjunctivitis when administered several hours before anticipated exposure to known allergens.

Topical steroids (and even systemic steroids for some conditions) have a significant place in the treatment of allergic disease by reducing the effects of inflammatory processes. One drop of 1 per cent prednisolone or 0.1 per cent dexamethasone may be applied every 2 hours during the day for 4 days. In the most troublesome cases of AKC and occasionally in VKC, patients may be placed on a 2-week course of systemic corticosteroids. However, this is a last-resort effort to protect the patient's sight.

Yet, although topical corticosteroids give considerable relief from inflammatory disease, serious adverse reactions can occur. Physicians are generally reluctant to prescribe corticosteroids unless the visual axis is in jeopardy. Ophthalmologists may be more willing to take the risk in treating VKC and AKC where the cornea may be involved than in treating hay fever conjunctivitis. Used as a topical preparation on the eye, corticosteroids may produce such unwanted complications as cataracts, glaucoma, and increased susceptibility to infections.

Systemic *histamine antagonists* (antihistamines) are prescribed in ocular allergy to reduce the immediate effects of circulating histamine released by degranulating mast cells. In hay fever conjunctivitis, oral antihistamines help reduce the nasal and ocular symptoms. Although oral antihistamines may be prescribed in VKC and AKC, they are not completely effective because the signs and symptoms of these diseases are caused by more factors than simply release of histamine. H_1 antihistamines frequently cause drowsiness, dizziness, and difficulty concentrating. They may also dry mucous membranes. The newer antihistamine preparations (for instance, terfenadine) are reported to have fewer unwanted side effects.

Immunotherapy and hyposensitization are often successful in reducing the severity of nasal symptoms of allergic rhinitis. They have not been as successful in reducing the ocular signs and symptoms. Therefore, hyposensitization and immunotherapy are not recommended for patients suffering from hay fever conjunctivitis primarily without associated nasal disease. In hay fever conjunctivitis, immunotherapy reduces about 80 per cent of the symptoms about 80 per cent of the time. Likewise, if testing for allergens discloses the role of specific allergens in VKC, immunotherapy may help. The success rate is not high, however, and immunotherapy for VKC is usually considered as a last resort.

Ocular or Periocular Manifestations

The following tissues of the ocular adnexa are affected by atopic conjunctivitis (A) and hay fever conjunctivitis (H).

Conjunctiva: Chemosis; ciliary flush; vasodilation (A,H).
Cornea: Superficial punctate keratitis (A).
Eyelids: Edema; maceration of medial and lateral canthi; pruritis (A,H); thickening (A).
Lacrimal System: Excessive lacrimation (A,H).
Other: Anterior uveitis (A,H); cataracts (A).

PRECAUTIONS

When used chronically, topical vasoconstrictors may produce rebound hyperemia. These agents are also capable of producing pupillary dilation in the face of corneal epithelial defects, which allow a pharmacologic concentration to penetrate the cornea. Thus, they should be used with caution in patients with both corneal lesions and narrow angles. Patients with cardiac irregularities and hypertension who use local vasoconstrictors should also be monitored carefully.

Because of the damaging effects on the corneal epithelium, therapeutic use of local anesthetics is contraindicated.

During the allergy season, contact lenses are often poorly tolerated in patients with allergic conjunctivitis. In symptomatic patients, lens wear may be resumed when the pollen season has passed.

Comments

Hay fever conjunctivitis is caused by type I immediate hypersensitivity to air-borne antigens. In this reaction, the antigen is captured by an IgE molecule that is bound to a mast cell membrane. The result is the release from mast cells of a cascade of preformed mediators (e.g., histamine) and newly formed mediators, such as, prostaglandins, leukotrienes, and chemotactic factors, that increase conjunctival vessel permeability and trigger immediate and (perhaps) late-phase inflammatory reactions.

Other ocular reactions, seen in GPC and vernal conjunctivitis, have features of both type I and type IV hypersensitivity reactions. Therefore, mast cell-mediated reactions are not the sole contributors to ocular allergic disease. Much remains to be learned about these conditions.

References

Abelson MB, Baird RS, Allansmith MR: Tear histamine levels in vernal conjunctivitis and other ocular inflammations. Ophthalmology 87:812–814, 1980.
Allansmith MR: Introduction: Ocular allergy. In Suran A, Grey I, Nussenblatt RB (eds): Immunology of the Eye; Workshop III. Immunologic Aspects of Ocular Diseases: Infection, Inflammation, and Allergy. Washington, DC, Information Retrieval, 1981, pp 347–352.
Beetham WP: Atopic cataracts. Arch Ophthalmol 24:21–37, 1940.
Patterson R: Investigations of spontaneous hypersensitivity of the dog. J Allergy 31:351–363, 1960.
Prausnitz C, Kustner H: Studien uber die Ueberempfindlichkeit, Zentralbl. Bakteriol. 86:160–169, 1921.
Rachelefsky GS, et al: Defective T cell function in atopic dermatitis. J Allergy Clin Immunol 57:569–576, 1976.
Smolin G, O'Connor GR: Ocular Immunology. Philadelphia, Lea & Febiger, 1981, p. 112.

BACTERIAL CONJUNCTIVITIS
(Mucopurulent Conjunctivitis, Purulent Conjunctivitis)

DOUGLAS J. COSTER, F.R.C.S.
Adelaide, Australia

Bacterial infection of the conjunctiva usually produces a purulent or mucopurulent conjunctivitis. Most but not all cases of purulent conjunctivitis are caused by bacteria. The infective process is usually of an acute nature, but occasionally bacteria produce a low-grade chronic reaction. For the most part, the condition is a mild affliction.

A wide range of bacteria can infect the conjunctiva, and there is considerable variation with the age of the patient, locality, and season. Staphylococci; *Hemophilus; Pseudomonas;* enteric gram-negative rods, such as *Proteus* and *Escherichia coli;* and streptococci, in particular the pneumococcus, are the principal bacteria responsible for purulent conjunctivitis. In developed countries, *Neisseria gonorrhoeae* is an unusual cause of ophthalmia neonatorum; *Chlamydia trachomatis* is the usual agent. Between the ages of 3 months and 8 years, pneumococcal infection is frequent. *Hemophilus* conjunctivitis also occurs most often in this age group. In the elderly or infirm, *Moraxella* conjunctivitis is common.

The only certain way to implicate an etiologic agent is to isolate it in the laboratory. Management of bacterial conjunctivitis involves recognition of the disease at a clinical level, identification of the etiologic agent, appreciation of the importance of the case from a public health point of view, and the administration of antimicrobial chemotherapy.

THERAPY

Ocular. Antibiotics are often begun before specimen collection or before laboratory results become available. Commonly used topical ophthalmic agents are sulfacetamide, erythromycin, bacitracin, chloramphenicol, neomycin, polymyxin B, gentamicin, and tobramycin. A satisfactory agent would be active against expected pathogens, have low local and systemic toxicity, and have low allergenicity. Polymyxin B and bacitracin are toxic at the site of delivery, neomycin is allergenic, and the topical use of chloramphenicol has been implicated in several cases of aplastic anemia. The indiscriminate use of aminoglycosides has resulted in the emergence of resistant strains of bacteria. Fortunately, most cases of bacterial conjunctivitis will respond to a low dose of any broad-spectrum antibiotic applied topically. Severe fulminating cases and those not responding to initial therapy deserve bacteriologic investigation. All conjunctivitis in children should be investigated.

If a case of purulent conjunctivitis fails to respond to initial antimicrobial measures, medication should be withdrawn for 24 hours after which material is collected for cytologic and microbiologic examination. On the basis of culture and susceptibility tests, appropriate chemotherapy should be instigated.

Patients infected with *N. gonorrhoeae, Moraxella,* or streptococci should be treated with fortified sodium penicillin G* eyedrops at a concentration of 100,000 units/ml. Those with *Hemophilus* infection should receive topical 0.5 per cent chloramphenicol or 0.5 per cent neomycin. Prolonged treatment with chloramphenicol should be avoided. Infections with gram-negative bacilli are best treated with 0.3 per cent gentamicin eyedrops unless sensitivity tests suggest otherwise. Topical therapy for conjunctivitis should be given every 2 hours for 2 or 3 days until the process is controlled and then four times a day for another week.

Systemic. The only indication for systemic therapy is severe conjunctivitis caused by *N. gonorrhoeae* or *H. influenzae* in children or when there is a suspicion of involvement of underlying tissues. Patients with *Neisseria* infections should receive 4.8 million units of procaine penicillin G intramuscularly divided into two doses at one visit plus 1 gm of oral probenecid. Patients allergic to penicillin and those over 8 years of age can be treated with 1.5 gm of intramuscular tetracycline initially, followed by 0.5 gm orally four times a day for 4 to 7 days. Children younger than 8 years of age who are allergic to penicillin can be treated with 40 mg/kg of oral erythromycin daily. A parenteral alternative to penicillin for adults is 2 to 4 gm of intramuscular streptomycin. Children from whom *H. influenzae* is isolated should be treated with systemic ampicillin, unless the strain is ampicillin-resistant and thus requires systemic chloramphenicol.

Ocular or Periocular Manifestations

Conjunctiva: Purulent or mucopurulent conjunctivitis.

PRECAUTIONS

A patient with purulent conjunctivitis may fail to respond to topical medication for a number of reasons. The condition may not be caused by free-living bacteria, but by an intracellular agent, such as *C.trachomatis,* or by a noninfective process, such as occurs with erythema multiforme or Reiter's syndrome. If the condition is caused by bacterial infection, the agent may not be sensitive to the drug used. Alternatively, the conjunctival sac may be loaded with organisms from the lacrimal sac or from other nonocular sites under various circumstances. A persistent, uniocular purulent discharge should alert the ophthalmologist to the possibility of a foreign body. Another reason for treatment failure is poor patient compliance. Occasionally in mucopurulent disease, mucus may protect organisms from chemotherapeutic agents. This protection can be overcome by the combined use of topical antibiotics and mucolytic agents. Ten per cent acetylcysteine* eyedrops used twice a day are very effective in this common situation.

COMMENTS

The need for bacteriologic investigation is debatable. Two approaches to bacterial conjunctivitis can be followed. A broad-spectrum antibiotic may be administered on suspicion of bacterial infection, with laboratory investigation reserved for refractive cases. Alternatively, more specific chemotherapy can be prescribed based on the bacteria isolated if cultures are initiated as a first step. In favor of broad-spectrum therapy is the excellent response achieved in most cases. Against this approach is the fact that not all purulent conjunctivitis is caused by bacteria, and not all bacteria will respond to simple broad-spectrum therapy. When a case has not responded to a trial of chemotherapy, the chances of achieving a microbiologic diagnosis may have been lost. In most situations, broad-spectrum antibiotics are used based on a clinical diagnosis of bacterial conjunctivitis. Severe purulent conjunctivitis, however, requires initial laboratory investigation.

References

Bradley J: Immune responses to bacteria. *In* Watts J McK, et al (eds): Infection in Surgery: Basic and Clinical Aspects. New York, Churchill Livingstone, 1981, pp 68–78.

Fraunfelder FT, Bagby GC, Kelly DJ: Fatal aplastic anemia following topical administration of ophthalmic chloramphenicol. Am J Ophthalmol 93:356–360, 1982.

CICATRICIAL PEMPHIGOID
(Benign Mucous Membrane Pemphigoid, Ocular Cicatricial Pemphigoid)

LYNNE H. MORRISON, M.D.,
and KENNETH C. SWAN, M.D.
Portland, Oregon

Cicatricial pemphigoid is a relatively rare, chronic inflammatory disease affecting primarily the mucous membranes. Patients are usually 60 years of age or older, and females are more frequently affected than males. The conjunctiva and oral mucosa are the most frequently affected areas, but the oropharynx, nasopharynx, esophagus, genitalia, and rectal mucosa may also be involved. Cutaneous lesions are present in approximately 25 per cent of cases. Although the primary lesions are subepithelial bullae that heal with scarring, erosions rather than blisters are most often observed in the mucous membranes. Ocular involvement of cicatricial pemphigoid often begins with a conjunctivitis accompanied by subepithelial fibrosis. Progressive fibrosis results in foreshortening of the fornices and eventually leads to the development of symblepharon. The fibrotic process can cause trichiasis and entropion. Reduced numbers of conjunctival goblet cells produce altered tear composition, which combined with tear insufficiency caused by lacrimal duct compromise, contributes further to corneal exposure, resulting in corneal ulceration, keratinization, and neovascularization. Blindness has occurred in approximately 25 to 33 per cent of patients with ocular involvement.

Cicatricial pemphigoid is thought to be mediated by autoantibodies directed against an antigen in the basement zone. These antibodies are detectable in the vast majority of cases in conjunctival biopsies made for immunofluorescent studies. Direct immunofluorescent studies on conjunctival biopsies are the most reliable means of establishing a diagnosis.

THERAPY

Systemic. The disease is best controlled with systemic therapy. Topical treatment alone provides little benefit. Most experience has been gained with systemic corticosteroids, usually in the form of prednisone. Starting doses are usually in the range of 40 to 60 mg of prednisone daily. After initial control, the dose is tapered to the lowest level possible, with the goal of achieving alternate-day therapy. Steroids act as a suppressive agent and do not produce long-term remission of the disease. When they are discontinued or tapered, the process is likely to be reactivated. Unfortunately, high doses of prednisone are often required on a long-term basis to maintain control, although some patients can be tapered to low doses. Maintenances doses range from 2.5 to 60 mg of prednisone daily. Another problem with the use of prednisone as sole therapy is its possible failure to halt the progression of disease. In one series, 25 per cent of patients on systemic corticosteroids progressed to blindness. Despite these problems, prednisone can be considered for patients with mild, nonprogressive, early ocular disease. If they show evidence of continued scarring, require high doses of prednisone for control, or manifest unacceptable steroid side effects, alternate therapy should be considered.

The sulfone derivative dapsone[‡] has been shown to be effective in controlling cicatricial pemphigoid. It is a reasonable therapeutic choice for mild to moderately active cicatricial pemphigoid that is not rapidly progressive. It is strikingly effective in oral lesions, but also has been found to stop progression of ocular disease. In one series, 88 per cent of patients with mild to moderately active ocular cicatricial pemphigoid responded to dapsone with evidence of improvement in 4 weeks. A usual and expected side effect of dapsone is hemolytic anemia, which is dose dependent and is accompanied by a compensatory reticulocytosis. To allow time for this compensation to occur and to allow for assessment of drug tolerance, dapsone is started at a low dose and increased to the therapeutic range. The usual starting dose is 50 mg daily for 1 to 2 weeks; the dose is then increased to 50 mg twice a day and is adjusted thereafter based on the therapeutic response and level of anemia. Successful maintenance doses range from 50 to 150 mg of dapsone daily. Patients should have glucose-6-phosphate dehydrogenase levels checked before starting therapy. If these levels are deficient, marked degrees of hemolysis can occur with the use of dapsone.

Patients with rapidly progressive or extremely active disease require more aggressive therapy. A very successful form of treatment appears to be the use of immunosuppressive drugs either alone or in combination with prednisone. Cyclophosphamide[‡] in combination with prednisone has been shown to be highly effective for controlling disease activity. Rather than simply suppressing disease activity, this regimen has the potential to induce a sustained remission. Azathioprine[‡] can be used as an alternative immunosuppressive agent, but may be less effective than cyclophosphamide and is less likely to induce a long-term remission. Cyclophosphamide is started at a dose of 1 to 2 mg/kg daily together with prednisone 1 mg/kg daily. Prednisone may be deleted if there are contraindications to its use, but control of the disease activity will be slower. The patients are treated with this combination of drugs for 1 month and then re-evaluated clinically. If significant disease activity is still present, the dose of cyclophosphamide can be increased in 25-mg amounts monthly as tolerated. The prednisone dose is tapered rapidly to 40 mg daily and then over the course of a month is tapered to 40 mg every other day. The alternate-day dose is then tapered and finally discontinued over the course of about 2 months. Once the disease is well controlled, the cyclophosphamide is continued for another 12 months. Usually a total of 18 months is required to complete the course of therapy.

Ocular. Ocular surface lubrication is an important part of therapy in patients with sicca syndrome secondary to advanced ocular cicatricial pemphigoid. Ointment lubricants without preservatives are preferred and should be used frequently enough to provide surface protection (every 2 to 4 hours and at bedtime). Artificial tears without preservatives can be used between ointment applications as needed.

Routine lid hygiene is useful adjunctive therapy, especially in patients with chronic blepharitis.

Surgical. Corneal clarity and integrity are best preserved by control of entropion and trichiasis, adequate lubrication, and prevention of infection. Destruction of aberrant lashes is an important part of patient management not only because it reduces the damage to the ocular surface epithelium but it also removes a source of ocular inflammation, which may be confused with inflammation caused by the underlying immunologic disease. The aberrant lashes are best removed by cryotherapy. This should be performed precisely and freezing limited to the lid margin, since freezing of the conjunctival surface may incite a marked inflammatory reaction. Punctal occlusion is essential in cases where tear flow is deficient.

Oculoplastic procedures may be useful to correct conjunctival shrinkage and thereby minimize corneal exposure and blinding sequelae. These procedures can exacerbate the existing inflammation and therefore should generally be deferred until the disease activity has been adequately controlled. Incisions made directly through the contractured conjunctiva into the fornices have been disappointing, even with stents and grafts. Cicatricial entropion generally can be corrected by sliding the conjunctiva off the tarsal plates into the fornices. Although this procedure can be performed under topical anesthesia, subconjunctival injections* of anesthetic solution serve the dual purpose of deep anesthesia and establishment of a line of dissection. The addition of epinephrine minimizes the bleeding. Under the operating microscope, an incision is made through the conjunctiva at the lid margin. Thickened conjunctiva is dissected off the tarsus and allowed to retract into the fornices. This allows the lids to return to their normal positions and leaves the bulbar conjunctiva undisturbed. The tarsus re-epithelializes rapidly. During healing, patients are instructed to stretch the skin of the lids over the orbital margins while rotating their eyes. This maneuver helps preserve the fornices.

Both lamellar and penetrating keratoplasties have been used to restore clarity and substance to the cornea, but the outcome may be disappointing. Cataracts are also common in these patients and may progress to maturity. Cataract extractions have been performed through limbal incisions under limbal base flaps on patients with ocular pemphigoid. Such surgical procedures can exacerbate disease activity and, in general, are best performed once the disease activity has been brought under control.

Ocular or Periocular Manifestations

Conjunctiva: Chronic inflammation with cicatrization and symblepharon; keratinization.
Cornea: Mechanical irritation and infection; pannus; recurrent keratitis secondary to exposure, stromal thinning; ulcers.
Eyelids: Ankyloblepharon; entropion; trichiasis.
Lacrimal System: Cicatricial closure of the ducts.

PRECAUTIONS

A number of diseases may mimic cicatricial pemphigoid. Severe conjunctival inflammation caused by erythema multiforme, toxic epidermal necrolysis, or alkali burns may result in a scarring conjunctivitis similar to what is seen with cicatricial pemphigoid. Additionally, topical application of ocular medication, such as echothiophate, pilocarpine, epinephrine-containing compounds, and idoxuridine, can produce toxic effects of the conjunctival epithelium that are difficult to distinguish from cicatricial pemphigoid. These cases of pseudopemphigoid are best distinguished from idiopathic cicatricial pemphigoid by direct immunofluorescent studies. A biopsy taken from uninvolved tissue immediately adjacent to a lesion shows linear deposition IgG and C3 along the basement membrane zone in cases of cicatricial pemphigoid but not in pseudopemphigoid. A conjunctival biopsy is preferred when ocular involvement is present, but a biopsy from other perilesional sites may also be equally useful.

Patients in whom long-term use of systemic steroids is contemplated should be questioned regarding the presence of diabetes mellitus, hypertension, history of peptic or duodenal ulcers, and history of tuberculosis, since high doses of corticosteroids can exacerbate these conditions. A chest x-ray, skin test for tuberculosis, and fasting blood sugar should be obtained before placing patients on long-term high-dose corticosteroids. They should be managed in association with an internist or endocrinologist who can provide preventive measures for and evaluate osteoporosis.

The side effects of cyclophosphamide include hemorrhagic cystitis, alopecia, leukopenia, anemia, thrombocytopenia, and possibly an increased risk of developing a malignancy. The most common side effect is that of leukopenia. Patients should be managed in conjunction with an internist, oncologist, or rheumatologist familiar with the use and side effects of this drug. They should have a weekly complete blood cell count with differential, platelet count, and urinalysis. If the dose of cyclophosphamide is unchanged after several months, these parameters may then be monitored every 2 weeks and then subsequently every month if parameters remain stable. The white blood cell count should not fall below 3000 cells/cubic millimeter, with at least 1500 granulocytes/cubic millimeter while on immunosuppressive agents. Azathioprine has the same adverse effects as cyclophosphamide, except that it has not been associated with hemorrhagic cystitis; however, it has been associated with hepatic damage. Initially patients on azathioprine should have a complete blood cell count with differential, platelet count, and liver functions monitored weekly.

The most common adverse effects of dapsone are hemolytic anemia and methemoglobinemia. The anemia is dose related, generally occurring in patients taking 50 mg or more daily, and is compensated by a reticulocytosis. Although the anemia is usually well tolerated by most patients, it may cause problems for those with cardiopulmonary disease. Patients should have G-6-PD levels checked before starting dapsone; if they are deficient in this enzyme, a marked hemolytic anemia may occur. Less common side effects include periperal neuropathy and toxic hepatitis. Complete blood cell counts should be done routinely in patients on dapsone.

COMMENTS

The natural history of untreated cicatricial pemphigoid is that of a progressive disease, which generally does not have a spontaneous remission. It most frequently affects ocular and oral mucous membranes, but may involve the skin, esophagus, rectal, vaginal, or pharyngeal mucous membranes. Because of the chronic nature of the disease and the potential for various organ system involvement, these patients require long-term care that may involve a variety of specialists, including dermatologists, gastroenterologists, and otorhinolaryngologists. The disease activity may be suppressed by corticosteroids or dapsone, but cytotoxic agents offer the possibility of disease remission. Because of the potentially serious adverse effects associated with these medications, patient management is best done in conjunction with an internist, dermatologist, or rheumatologist familiar with their use.

References

Fiore PM, Jacobs IH, Goldberg DB: Drug-induced pemphigoid. A spectrum of diseases. Arch Ophthalmol 105:1660–1663, 1987.

Foster CS: Cicatricial pemphigoid. Trans Am Ophthalmol Soc 84:527–663, 1986.

Mondino BJ, Brown SI: Immunosuppressive therapy in ocular cicatricial pemphigoid. Am J Ophthalmol 96:453–459, 1983.

Rogers RS, Seehafer JR, Perry HO: Treatment of cicatricial pemphigoid with dapsone. J Am Acad Dermatol 6:215–223, 1982.

CONJUNCTIVAL MELANOTIC LESIONS
(Benign Congenital Melanosis, Benign Nevi, Melanoma, PAM, Precancerous and Cancerous Melanosis, Primary Acquired Melanosis)

F.T. FRAUNFELDER, M.D.

Portland, Oregon

Melanotic conjunctival lesions can be divided into benign congenital melanosis, benign nevus, primary acquired melanosis (PAM) with or without atypia, melanoma in situ, and melanoma. Melanomas may be also differentiated into those occurring with and those occurring without primary acquired melanosis. Primary acquired melanosis was formerly known as Reese's precancerous melanosis, benign acquired melanosis, idiopathic acquired melanosis, and intraepithelial atypical melanocytic hyperplasia. Recent major contributions in this confusing and controversial area have been made by Jakobiec, Zimmerman, and their co-workers.

Benign congenital melanosis simply denotes increased production of melanin granules, which are distributed by normal numbers of melanocytes to the surrounding epithelial cells of the conjunctiva. Clinically, they are brown flat macules or patches without thickening or vascularity. These lesions occur most frequently in black patients near the limbus in the interpalpebral space, because their melanocytes can readily produce extra melanin granules when irritated by external stimulation. In Caucasians, similar lesions can develop idiopathically. In skin pathology, such lesions are called ephelides (freckles) or lentigines, the latter implying a mild increase in the number of benign melanocytes, in addition to increased pigment production.

Benign nevus is the most common melanocytic tumor of the conjunctiva. Nevi are characteristically located in the interpalpebral space from the limbus to the caruncle, but they may arise anywhere in the palpebral conjunctiva or the lid margins. Nevi are proliferative disorders of benign melanocytes and commence generally within the first two decades of life; they almost always make their appearance by the end of the third decade. These lesions begin as intraepithelial nests of benign melanocytes (junctional nevi). During the second and third decades, the intraepithelial cells drop off into the connective tissue of the substantia propria (compound nevi). Finally, the intraepithelial portion burns out, and one is left with nests of subepithelial melanocytes (dermal or subepithelial nevi). Epithelial inclusion cysts, which become more prominent with expansion of the subepithelial component, are a helpful diagnostic finding. Nevi are not necessarily pigmented, and up to 30 per cent of them are poorly pigmented or nonpigmented so that identification of the typical inclusion cysts is very important. It is worth emphasizing that any melanocytic lesion that first appears after the third or fourth decade and that was assuredly not present during the first two should be regarded with suspicion.

Primary acquired melanosis (PAM) is a condition that is most common in the middle-aged Caucasian population. It usually appears as a unilateral, multifocal, flat pigmentation in various patterns and colors. In contrast to junctional nevi, which are almost always found only in childhood, PAM is acquired after childhood. Primary acquired melanosis can be histologically differentiated into presence (high risk) or absence (low risk) of atypia; however, these two entities cannot be differentiated clinically. The recognition and management of acquired pigmentation in middle age are critical. Primary acquired melanosis may result in malignant melanoma if not accurately and promptly treated, as seen with some series reporting a 25 per cent mortality rate with this disease.

Malignant melanoma of the conjunctiva is a rare disease. Conjunctival melanomas may arise in one of three ways: as a de novo lesion, probably springing up from the malignant transformation of an individual intraepithelial melanocyte, as a malignant degeneration within a pre-existent benign nevus, or as a nodule arising from a primary acquired melanosis.

When a melanoma arises de novo, there is presumably a period of intraepithelial horizontal proliferation of atypical melanocytes, followed by an invasive vertical growth phase into the underlying connective tissue of the substantia propria. This type of melanoma often develops on the epibulbar surface, frequently next to the limbus, and generally can be excised with wide margins and the performance of a superficial keratectomy or sclerectomy if necessary due to fixation.

The second type of melanoma, that arising in a nevus, also tends to be a localized lesion, but one will often obtain the history of a pre-existent pigmented lesion developing in childhood that was stationary for many years. In this case, it is presumed that persistent junctional intraepithelial nests, which are a site of ongoing mitotic activity, spawned a malignant clone. In excised specimens of such cases, one can see a mixture of the benign pre-existent nevus cells in the substantia propria and the new clone of cells proliferating both within the epithelium and as an invasive melanoma component. These lesions also should be treated by adequate local excision.

The third type of conjunctival melanoma develops in primary acquired melanosis that may wax and wane; it usually appears in middle-aged or elderly individuals. In this disease, there is widespread radial intraepithelial proliferation of melanocytes that progresses slowly over large geographic regions of the conjunctiva for many years and sometimes for decades. The lesion is granular brown in coloration, and at its outset is flat. There may be skip areas with foci of involvement of the lid margins and superior and inferior bulbar tarsal conjunctiva; at times, the entire conjunctiva may be involved. The flat, golden-brown pigmentation can be differentiated from the benign melanosis described earlier by its progressive character and its appearance in later life. Furthermore, it tends to involve Caucasians more than blacks, whereas benign melanosis more commonly affects blacks.

Although malignant melanomas arising without primary acquired melanosis seem to grow more rapidly than those with primary acquired melanoma, the mortality rates are the same. Approximately 75 per cent of malignant melanomas occur with primary acquired melanosis, and 20 to 30 per cent occur in prior nevi with or without primary acquired melanosis. The average age of patients with this condition is 52 to 53 years. Conjunctival melanomas are extremely rare in blacks and those younger than 20 years of age.

THERAPY

Supportive. Benign congenital melanoses do not need therapy, unless the patient desires their removal for cosmetic reasons.

Surgical. Because of the persistence of junctional activity and the drop off of melanocytes into the connective tissue in the formation of compound and subepithelial nevi, it is part of the natural history of nevi to enlarge and acquire thickness. However, nevi should be excised only if they become so large as to produce foreign body sensations or corneal wetting problems, are cosmetically undesirable, or their enlargement leads one to suspect a possible malignant degeneration into a melanoma. A malignant degeneration will be signalled by increased vascularity around the lesion, homogeneous nodule formation within it, fixation to underlying sclera, or hemorrhage and bleeding. A biopsy should be performed on any suspicious conjunctival nevus for histopathologic evaluation because it has been shown that nevi are a potential precursor lesion; 20 to 30 per cent of conjunctival melanomas arise from nevi. The development of a conjunctival melanoma in the first or second decade is fortunately rare; suspicious lesions in this age group generally turn out to be epithelioid or spindle cell nevi, which can grow rapidly and provide some diagnostic difficulty for pathologists.

The management of primary acquired melanosis requires close cooperation with a pathologist familiar with ophthalmology. Excisional biopsy is preferred for small lesions. If a quadrant of conjunctiva is involved, a biopsy should be done of the central area, especially the thickest area. Biopsies may have to be done on multiple areas because microinvasive melanomas may be clinically flat. Primary acquired melanosis with atypia requires complete eradication of the entire lesion. Predominantly epithelioid lesions or growth patterns other than basilar hyperplasia carry the worst prognosis. The author's preferred method of treatment is essentially the same as described for conjunctival or corneal intraepithelial neoplasia and squamous cell carcinoma. Small areas are surgically excised and treated with cryotherapy to the surgical bed, causing a highly successful superficial freeze. Larger lesions require multiple treatments so the most atypical areas are treated first. A quadrant of primary acquired melanosis can be treated with cryotherapy by ballooning up the conjunctiva with a local anesthetic and lightly freezing the involved area with cryogen spray; freezing should not be deep enough to touch the sclera. Treatment of more than one quadrant at a time is seldom helpful because sicca and significant symblepharon may occur. The carbon dioxide laser can also be used to eradicate superficial juxtalimbal disease without causing untoward damage. If there is evidence postoperatively of intraocular inflammation, administration of 80 mg of oral prednisone daily for 1 to 2 weeks helps suppress the potentially damaging inflammation and cataractogenic effects. Since new lesions of primary acquired melanosis without atypia may appear, close observation with drawings to map the areas of pigmentation and examination with a Wood's light two to three times a year are essential.

The management of malignant melanoma of the conjunctiva requires total eradication followed by close observation (three to four times a year). Enucleations are rarely indicated because the bulk of the conjunctiva still remains. Exenteration is usually reserved for bulky tumors of the anterior segment and often is only palliative. Metastatic spread is usually to the preauricular or submandibular lymph nodes. The treatment of choice is wide surgical excision with cryotherapy of the surgical bed. Multifocal disease carries a worse prognosis than unifocal disease.

PRECAUTIONS

Pigment surrounding the lacrimal duct or punctum suggests the spread of tumor cells along these ducts and indicates that cancer is more extensive than clinically apparent. In the management of conjunctival melanotic lesions with corneal involvement, care is required not to damage Bowman's layer, unless the lesion is a malignant melanoma, since this layer may act as a barrier to primary acquired melanosis invasion. In this situation, superficial abrading with secondary cryotherapy or chemical cautery may suffice. Although palpebral lesions may be flat in appearance, they may in reality have undergone significant vertical growth because the conjunctiva is adherent to the tarsal plate, thereby fooling the unwary clinician. Since nevi are rare in the fornix and palpebral conjunctiva, pigmented lesions in these areas are more prone to be malignant.

COMMENTS

Primary acquired melanosis with atypia and malignant melanoma of the conjunctiva may be best managed by the collaborative efforts of an ophthalmic oncologist and an experienced ophthalmic pathologist; however, ophthalmologists with cryotherapy experience may have the best cure rates. Clearly, there is no place for observation of conjunctival melanomas as is possible in the management of choroidal melanomas.

References

Cochran AJ, et al: Assessment of immunological techniques in the diagnosis and prognosis of ocular malignant melanoma. Br J Ophthalmol 69:171–176, 1985.

Codere F, et al: Carbon dioxide laser treatment of the conjunctiva and the cornea. Ophthalmology 95:37–45, 1988.

Dutton JJ, Anderson RL, Tse DT: Combined surgery and cryotherapy for scleral invasion of epithelial malignancies. Ophthalmic Surg 15:289–294, 1984.

Folberg R, McLean IW, Zimmerman LE: Conjunctival melanosis and melanoma. Ophthalmology 91:673–678, 1984.

Folberg R, McLean IW, Zimmerman LE: Malignant melanoma of the conjunctiva. Hum Pathol 16:136–143, 1985.

Jakobiec FA, et al: Unusual melanocytic nevi of the conjunctiva. Am J Ophthalmol 100:100–113, 1985.

Jakobiec FA, et al: Secondary and metastatic tumors of the orbit. In Duane TD (ed): Clinical Ophthalmology. Philadelphia, WB Saunders, 1987, Vol 2, pp 46:23–65.

Jakobiec FA, et al: Cryotherapy for conjunctival primary acquired melanosis and malignant melanoma. Experience with 62 cases. Ophthalmology 95:1058–1070, 1988.

Jakobiec FA, Folberg R, Iwamoto T: Clinicopathologic characteristics of premalignant and malignant melanocytic lesions of the conjunctiva. Ophthalmology 96:147–166, 1989.

Jeffrey IJ, et al: Malignant melanoma of the conjunctiva. Histopathology 10:363–378, 1986.

Lederman M, Wybar K, Busby E: Malignant epibulbar melanoma: Natural history and treatment by radiotherapy. Br J Ophthalmol 68:605–617, 1984.

Spencer WH, Zimmerman LE: Conjunctiva: Neoplasm and related conditions. In Spencer W (ed): Ophthalmic Pathology: An Atlas and Textbook, 3rd ed. Philadelphia, WB Saunders, 1985, Vol 2, pp 192–228.

CORNEAL AND CONJUNCTIVAL CALCIFICATIONS
(Band Keratopathy)

MARK S. DRESNER, M.D.,
DAVID J. SPENCE, M.D.,
and DAVID J. SCHANZLIN, M.D.
St. Louis, Missouri

Corneal and conjunctival calcification may occur as an isolated condition or in association with a variety of disease entities, although the source and mechanism of the calcium deposition are not clear. The corneal involvement is most commonly described as calcific band keratopathy because of the band-like configuration of the deposits in the interpalpebral area. Band keratopathy is seen in association with local ocular and systemic disease. Chronic uveitis of any etiology and ocular trauma, along with its accompanying chronic inflammation, are the most common ocular causes of band keratopathy. Systemic disease with altered calcium metabolism, such as hyperparathyroidism, vitamin D toxicity, and uremia, are also commonly associated with calcific band keratopathy. Calcific band keratopathy has also been described in individuals treated with or exposed to organomercurials, such as phenylmercuric nitrate or thimerosal. Band keratopathy has recently been reported following the use of Viscoat (chondroitin sulfate, sodium hyaluronate, and phosphate buffer) during routine cataract extraction. Inborn errors of metabolism, such as hypophosphatasia, may predispose patients to develop corneal and conjunctival calcification.

Clinically, calcific band keratopathy appears as a superficial corneal opacity resembling frosted or ground glass, with white flecks and holes in the band that give a Swiss cheese appearance. It is covered by a clear epithelium and is usually localized to the area of exposed cornea in the interpalpebral fissure. The band is concentric with the limbus, but separated from it by a clear interval. Histologically, calcium salts are deposited in the extracellular space, when the disorder is secondary to local ocular disease, and in the intracellular space, when the condition is secondary to systemic alterations of calcium metabolism. The epithelial basement membrane,

Bowman's layer, and superficial stroma are all involved. As calcification progresses, fragmentation and even destruction of Bowman's membrane may ensue. Early in its course, as the calcific band approaches the pupillary area, there is no immediate effect on visual acuity. With progression, however, plaques composed and coalesced calcium replace the epithelial and subepithelial layers of the cornea, resulting in marked irritation and pain. Eventual involvement of the central cornea and pupillary axis results in decreased visual acuity. A fibrous pannus may also be occasionally associated. In calcific band keratopathy, calcium salts precipitate in Bowman's membrane, the basement membrane of corneal epithelium, and anterior stroma. Calcareous degeneration, in contrast, usually spares the basement and Bowman's membranes and is characterized by clumps of calcium salts in the superficial and deep stroma. Calcareous degeneration can occur rapidly, especially with anterior segment ischemia.

Conjunctival calcification appears as small, hard, white or yellow elevated concretions in the palpebral conjunctiva. These conditions are usually products of cellular degeneration, but may also be associated with any chronic conjunctival inflammation. They may be accompanied by hyperemia and symptoms of irritation.

THERAPY

Surgical. Treatment of band keratopathy is indicated in patients with symptomatic irritation or decreased vision. The surgical goal is to remove the opaque calcium deposits while avoiding stromal scarring. The initial approach is to attempt chelation of the calcium salt deposits with edetate disodium (EDTA).* Topical anesthetic is first instilled into the conjunctival culde-sac, and the epithelium is mechanically removed. The distal end of a Weck-Cel sponge is saturated with 0.5 per cent EDTA* and held against the area of calcium deposition. A to-and-fro abrasive action is used to help remove the calcium deposits; this is best accomplished at the slitlamp. If significant clearing has not occurred after 10 minutes of treatment, one should move to higher concentrations of EDTA (1.0 or 1.5 per cent). Sometimes, the treatment must be continued for 20 to 30 minutes. In refractory cases, gentle curettage with a scalpel may be necessary. An antibiotic solution and weak cycloplegic are then placed in the eye; a patch or bandage lens may be used for comfort and to facilitate epithelial healing. If the opacification cannot be removed by chelation or curettage, lamellar keratoplasty should be considered. A technique using EDTA and a diamond burr on a Fisch drill has been shown to be effective in removing deposits without significant scarring.

Conjunctival concretions causing irritation and a foreign body sensation can often be shelled out with a sharp pointed knife or broad needle. Occasionally, this procedure may be difficult.

The success of medical and surgical therapy may be limited if the underlying disease process itself causes decreased vision. Also, unless the underlying disease is controlled, the calcium deposition may recur and the treatment may need to be repeated.

Ocular or Periocular Manifestations

Conjunctiva: Palpebral conjunctival calcific deposits or concretions.
Cornea: Calcific band-shaped keratopathy; opacity.
Other: Decreased visual acuity; irritation.

PRECAUTIONS

Patients should be questioned concerning excessive vitamin D ingestion. Although corneal and conjunctival calcification may be reversible with discontinuation of the vitamin, nephrocalcinosis may still develop. A general medical workup is advisable.

COMMENTS

Although the exact cause of calcific band keratopathy is not clear, a combination of factors is felt to be responsible. One theory suggests that the combination of a metabolically altered tissue from mechanical or chemical trauma in the presence of local alkalosis and chronic exposure facilitates deposition of calcium salts in the interpalpebral fissure. A correlation also exists between metastatic calcification and an elevated concentration of a product of serum calcium and phosphorus.

References

Bokosky JE, Meyer RF, Sugar A: Surgical treatment of calcific band keratopathy. Ophthalmic Surg 16:645–647, 1985.
Duffey RJ, LoCascio JA: Calcium deposition in a corneal graft. Cornea 6:212–215, 1987.
Galin MA, Obstbaum SA: Band keratopathy in mercury exposure. Ann Ophthalmol 6:1257–1261, 1974.
Kennedy RE, Roca PD, Landers PH: Atypical band keratopathy in glaucomatous patients. Am J Ophthalmol 72:917–922, 1971.
Kennedy RE, Roca PD, Platt DS: Further observations on atypical band keratopathy in glaucoma patients. Trans Am Ophthalmol Soc 72:107–122, 1974.
Lembach RG, Keates RH: Band keratopathy: Its significance and treatment. Perspect Ophthalmol 1:13–16, 1977.
Lemp MA, Ralph RA: Rapid development of band keratopathy in dry eyes. Am J Ophthalmol 83:657–659, 1977.
Lessell S, Norton EWD: Band keratopathy and conjunctival calcification in hypophosphatasia. Arch Ophthalmol 71:497–499, 1964.
O'Connor GR: Calcific band keratopathy. Trans Am Ophthalmol Soc 70:58–81, 1972.
Schechter EL, Keates RH: Treatment of band keratopathy. Ophthalmic Surg 2:75, 1971.

FILTERING BLEBS
(Leaking and Inadvertent Nonleaking)

GISSUR J. PETURSSON, M.D.

Little Rock, Arkansas

A filtering bleb is a blister-like postoperative scar through which aqueous drains from the anterior chamber to the subconjunctival space. Often such a scar is created following glaucoma surgery to allow a permanently open channel for drainage. However, a filtering conjunctival bleb can be an unplanned complication following cataract surgery, especially when a limbus-based conjunctival flap is used. A leaking filtering bleb can be immediate, such as in incomplete repair of conjunctival flap buttonholing or closure, or delayed, wherein a thin-walled bleb or flap incision ruptures at a later time. Except when secondary to immediate and obvious wound dehiscence, the exact etiology of postcataract blebs has not yet been established.

Although spontaneous resolution of this type of bleb is most common, the continued presence of an unplanned filtering bleb can have grave consequences. Delayed intraocular infection may occur; use of a corneal contact lens may become problematic both from a mechanical viewpoint and from an increased risk of infection; and rarely, maculopathy may follow bleb-induced hypotony. Normally, postcataract and almost all filter surgery blebs are asymptomatic and without noteworthy manifestations. Symptoms with leaking blebs are usually those associated with extreme hypotony. Additionally, excessive precorneal "tear" pooling is frequently seen. Hypotony with the absence or near absence of the anterior chamber with no visible filtering bleb following glaucoma surgery is highly suggestive of a leak.

THERAPY

Surgical. During filtering glaucoma procedures, buttonholing typically takes place more easily close to the limbus where conjunctiva and Tenon form a single layer; peritomy and suturing of the conjunctiva onto the cornea are advisable under such circumstances. Another way to deal with such a hole at or near the limbus is to close it with a suture and then to suture the folded-over conjunctiva in the hole area down off to the side in a wing suture-like manner.

Conjunctival closure by use of coaptation wet-field cautery has been suggested, but healthy tissue margins are essential for this procedure. Direct suturing of a leaking bleb away from the limbus can be tricky. If the conjunctiva is very thin in the hole area, this procedure may fail unless suture material and needle are selected carefully. The tapered point needles BV100-4 or BV75-4 make a very tight tract that will hold a leak in the most delicate tissue. This needle is intended for microsurgery and labeled as such, but is not listed with ophthalmic sutures. The needle comes with black monofilament 9-0 or 10-0 nylon suture. Owing to the delicate nature of the needle, a delicate needle holder is necessary. The suture can be left in place indefinitely or removed in 1 to 3 months if it causes irritation. Similar absorbable sutures are now available.

For the nonleaking bleb with extreme hypotony or high risk of infection, trichloroacetic acid and cautery of various kinds have been used successfully in the past. However, cryosurgery for these blebs is more practical. Three freeze-thaw applications with the retina or preferably the glaucoma probe at temperature of $-65°$ to $-80°$ C for 3 seconds each time seem to be effective. Tenon's and episcleral tissue of the entire bleb area must be involved in the freezing. Up to 8 weeks must be allowed for full results.

For stubborn persistent blebs, the following suturing method seems to work. One 7-0 chromic catgut suture is passed from the cornea, deep across the corneoscleral wound and either beyond or through the bleb, depending on its size. The suture is tied snugly, compressing the bleb beneath the knot. In the same manner, 8-0 or 7-0 black silk can be used and left in place for 2 to 4 weeks until the bleb has disappeared. This suture method is felt to work largely by virtue of its inflammatory response. The patient is placed on topical cycloplegics and antibiotics. This procedure is performed under microscopic control after either local subconjunctival injection[*] or 2 per cent lidocaine with epinephrine in the adjacent area or, alternatively, retrobulbar block.[*]

For the immediate large bleb with obvious wound dehiscence, direct surgical revision is required.

Supportive. For a delayed leak discovered postoperatively, conservative treatment consisting of topical antibiotics, pressure dressings, and oral acetazolamide may be indicated initially. This treatment will sometimes allow spontaneous closure of the fistula in 1 to 2 days. Tissue adhesives have also been used successfully, but results are unpredictable.

Ocular or Periocular Manifestations (Leaking blebs)

Conjunctiva or Sclera: Marked uniformly diffuse hyperemia.

Cornea: Edema; folds in Descemet's membrane.

Lacrimal System: Increased lacrimation; precorneal accumulation of "tears."

Other: Irritation; markedly decreased intraocular pressure or frank hypotony; photophobia; shallow or flat anterior chamber.

PRECAUTIONS

Acid and heat cautery of postcataract blebs may cause tissue necrosis. In some instances, heat or acid cautery of a bleb has resulted in endophthalmitis, originating at the site of the bleb in a bed of tissue necrosis.

Surgical revision of leaking blebs sometimes involves major mobilization and pull down of conjunctiva, especially if the leaky area is very thin walled and ischemic. Leaks, sometimes intermittent, are also caused by inadequately closed conjunctival incisions of limbal-based or poorly fixed fornix-based flaps.

COMMENTS

True postcataract filtering blebs should be distinguished from the occasional cystic, sterile, inflammatory reactions surrounding sutures, especially 8-0 virgin silk and chromic catgut. The true postcataract filtering bleb always resembles the bleb created intentionally in glaucoma surgery.

When compared to other methods of bleb elimination, such as heat cautery or chemical cauterization, cryotherapy appears to be preferable. With cryosurgery, tissue destruction is minimal. Thus, one avoids the problem of aqueous leakage and necrosis, which may predispose the eye to more dreaded complications, such as loss of the anterior chamber, epithelial downgrowth, and intraocular infection. However, there may be mild anterior chamber cellular reaction after cryotherapy.

References

Bruner WE, Maumenee AE: A simple method of repairing inadvertent filtering blebs after cataract surgery. Am J Ophthalmol 91:794–796, 1981.

Clesby GW, Fung WE, Webster RG Jr: Cryosurgical closure of filtering blebs. Arch Ophthalmol 87:319–323, 1972.

Coyle JT: Outpatient repair of unintentional filtering blebs. Ocul Ther Surg 1:35, 1982.

Kirk HW: Cauterization of filtering blebs following cataract extraction. Trans Am Acad Ophthalmol Otolaryngol 77:573–580, 1973.

Hoskins H Jr, Kass M: Becker-Shaffer's Diagnosis and Therapy of Glaucomas, 6th ed. St Louis, CV Mosby, 1989, pp 583–586.

Petursson GJ, Fraunfelder FT: Repair of an inadvertent buttonhole or leaking filtering bleb. Arch Ophthalmol 97:926–927, 1979.

Yannuzzi LA, Theodore FH: Cryotherapy of postcataract blebs. Am J Ophthalmol 76:217–222, 1973.

GIANT PAPILLARY CONJUNCTIVITIS

MATHEA R. ALLANSMITH, M.D., and ROBERT N. ROSS, Ph.D.

Boston, Massachusetts

The long-term presence of ocular prostheses, the relatively short-term presence of monofilament suture barbs in contact with the conjunctiva, and contact lens wear have been associated with a cluster of signs and symptoms now known as giant papillary conjunctivitis. With an estimated 20 million people in the United States wearing contact lenses, this popular alternative to wearing eyeglasses is the most common factor in the etiology of giant papillary conjunctivitis. In addition to the large number of elective wearers of contact lenses, a smaller number of people must wear contact lenses for adequate correction of their visual deficits.

Giant papillary conjunctivitis (GPC) is a reversible ocular inflammatory syndrome that is often contact lens related. It is characterized by such symptoms as itchy eyes, discomfort, and reduced tolerance of the worn contact lens and by such signs as abnormally large conjunctival papillae, excess mucus production, and hyperemia.

Evidence suggests that GPC may be the result of mechanical trauma, repeated with each excursion of the upper eyelid over the worn contact lens, plus a hypersensitivity reaction to antigens trapped on the surface of the worn contact lens, or some combination of these factors and others still to be discovered. Because GPC occurs in wearers of soft, hard, and rigid gas-permeable contact lenses, it is unlikely that the lesions of GPC associated with contact lens wear are caused by a reaction to the contact lens material itself.

Signs and symptoms of GPC range along a continuum from minimal to severe. They may be reversed when the contact lens (or other insult to the conjunctiva) is removed or altered. The chances of successful treatment therefore depend upon the earliest possible recognition of the disease process and initiation of the appropriate treatment.

The presence of the contact lens in repeated contact with the conjunctiva alters conjunctival surfaces. This is a normal response to the presence of a foreign body on the eye. In some patients, however, enlarged papillae erupt on the upper tarsal conjunctiva, displacing the normal (less than 0.3 mm diameter) conjunctival papillae. Furthermore, in GPC mucous vesicles in nongoblet epithelial cells of the conjunctiva contribute to dramatically increased production of mucus.

In clinical appearance, giant papillary conjunctivitis closely resembles vernal conjunctivitis. Both conditions are characterized by ocular irritation, itching of the eye, and increased production of mucus, which decreases visual acuity. The appearance of enlarged papillae (greater than 0.3 mm in diameter) on the upper tarsal conjunctiva and thick coatings of mucus on worn contact lenses are characteristic features of contact-lens-associated GPC. Limbal and corneal lesions have been observed, but always in association with lesions on the upper tarsal conjunctiva.

Symptoms of GPC usually antedate signs. Itchy eyes when lenses are removed, accumulations of mucus in the nasal corner of the eye, and slight blurring of vision caused by coatings on the lens are common early symptoms of GPC. These symptoms are so common and may be so minor that many patients may neglect to bring them to the attention of the lens fitter. The later stages of GPC are usually severe enough, however, to demand attention. Patients with advanced GPC complain of a foreign body sensation when wearing the contact lens, and sheets of mucus (occasionally strings of mucus) may glue the eyes during sleep. Lenses become visibly coated soon after being inserted.

The earliest sign of GPC is mild hyperemia of the upper tarsal conjunctiva. Small strands of mucus may be observed across the otherwise smooth conjunctiva. The conjunctiva is usually still translucent in appearance early in the progress of GPC, but careful observation reveals that the conjunctiva is somewhat thickened. As GPC progresses, infiltration by inflammatory cells may render the conjunctiva opaque.

Later in the development of GPC, wearing contact lenses produces significant pain and other discomfort, and production of mucus increases. In the absence of appropriate corrective action, the patient develops intolerance to wearing the contact lenses, production of mucus is copious, and hyperemia is marked. Pseudoptosis may be seen in some patients. Patients with advanced GPC ordinarily find it impossible to wear their contact lenses.

Concurrent with opacification of the upper tarsal conjunctiva, enlarged collagen structures begin to emerge from the tarsal plate. Papillae greater than 0.3 mm in diameter are abnormal; as they grow, they push aside the normal smaller papillae. As enlarged papillae grow, their apexes flatten. Because ulceration of the conjunctiva may accompany the other inflammatory processes of GPC, fluorescein staining is a critical diagnostic sign.

Although the description of the clinical signs generally holds true for all instances of GPC, the appearance of papillae and their location in various zones of the upper tarsal conjunctiva differ somewhat depending on the type of contact lens being worn by the patient. Papillae associated with wearing soft contact lenses tend to appear first in the upper zone of the tarsal area and progress toward the lid margin. In advanced GPC associated with wearing soft contact lenses, enlarged papillae are more numerous throughout the upper tarsal conjunctiva. Papillae associated with wearing hard contact lenses are fewer in number, smaller in size, may have crater-like or flattened (rather than rounded) tops, and usually appear first along the lid margins.

Although the etiology and pathogenesis of GPC are not yet fully understood, it is recognized that increased coatings on worn contact lenses exacerbate the signs and symptoms of existing cases of GPC and may contribute to the onset of the disease. These factors that increase the patient's exposure to lens coatings may increase the signs and symptoms of the disease: 1) wearing lenses for long periods during the day, 2) wearing the same lenses for months or years without changing them, 3) wearing larger lenses that present a greater area to the conjunctival epithelium, and 4) inadequate cleaning of the lenses.

THERAPY

Treatment and prevention of GPC depend on three therapeutic strategies: 1) establishing adequate lens hygiene, 2) finding appropriate lens design and material, and 3) treating the inflamed conjunctiva with effective pharmacotherapy.

Supportive. Signs and symptoms of GPC can be resolved in many cases by improving the patient's lens hygiene. Cleaning agents should be free of preservatives, e.g., thimerosol. Saline solution for rinsing and storing lenses should likewise be nonpreserved. Sterilization by hydrogen peroxide has been found to be the method best tolerated by the compromised conjunctiva. Cold overnight disinfection presents the compromised conjunctiva with too great an insult when the lenses are returned to the eye. Heat disinfection may bake coatings onto the lens surface and further traumatize the compromised conjunctiva when the contact lenses are reinserted. Enzymatic cleaning of the lens is essential to minimize the accumulation of lens coatings and to remove accumulated environmental antigens. Papain preparations seem to be more effective and better tolerated by the compromised conjunctiva than other enzymatic preparations for lens cleaning.

Even with improved lens hygiene, some patients with GPC may be unable to tolerate their present lenses, but can tolerate lenses of another design or material. In some cases, however, patients must stop wearing their contact lenses entirely until signs and symptoms of GPC resolve. Fluorescein staining of the apexes of enlarged papillae, the appearance of heavy mucus on the conjunctiva, significant tarsal hyperemia, and decentering of the contact lens on blinking are all indications that the lenses must be removed. Lenses may be reintroduced 3 to 5 days after the hyperemia, excessive mucus production, and itching have resolved even though the enlarged papillae are still observable. Enlarged papillae may not regress for several months or even years.

Ocular. Topical corticosteroids have not proved particularly effective in the management of GPC. In cases of florid GPC, however, a short course of topical corticosteroids may be appropriate to quiet the eye before beginning the long-term management of the disease.

Because of the involvement of conjunctival mast cells in GPC, the mast cell stabilizer—cromolyn sodium—has had a beneficial effect on the course of GPC. Along with rigorous lens hygiene, 4 per cent cromolyn sodium ophthalmic solution applied four times daily (even while the lens is in place) may help resolve early GPC before it progresses. Advanced GPC is not amenable to treatment with cromolyn sodium alone. However, once the signs and symptoms of advanced GPC are brought under control by means of better lens hygiene, refitting with a better tolerated lens, and resting the inflamed conjunctiva, cromolyn sodium may be introduced as part of regular maintenance therapy.

Comments

In order to follow the progression or regression of the clinical signs of GPC with contact lens wear and therapy, it is necessary to describe accurately the appearance of the upper tarsal conjunctiva on each visit. A record should be made indicating the zones of involvement, the size and elevation of the papillae, fluorescein staining pattern of the tops of papillae, and the presence of mucus. The progression of these signs and symptoms in the initial disease state has some prognostic value. The earlier GPC is treated, the more likely treatment will arrest progress of the disease while maintaining long-term tolerance of the contact lens.

References

Allansmith MR, Ross RN: Ocular allergy and mast cell stabilizers. Surv Ophthalmol 30:229–244, 1986.

Allansmith MR, Ross RN: Giant papillary conjunctivitis. In Duane T (ed): Clinical Ophthalmology. Philadelphia, Harper & Row, 1987, pp 1–10.

Allansmith MR, Ross RN: Giant papillary conjunctivitis. "Ocular Allergy" issue of International Ophthalmol Clin 28:309–316, 1988.

Allansmith MR, et al: Giant papillary conjunctivitis in contact lens wearers. AM J Ophthalmol 83:697–708, 1977.

Allansmith MR, Baird RS, Greiner JV: Contact lens-associated giant papillary conjunctivitis as a model for vernal conjunctivitis. In Silverstein AM, O'Connor GR (eds): International Symposium on Immunology and Immunopathology of the Eye. New York, Masson, 1979, pp 346–349.

Allansmith MR, Baird RS, Greiner JV: Number and type of inflammatory cells in conjunctiva of asymptomatic contact lens wearers. Am J Ophthalmol 87:171–174, 1979.

Allansmith MR, Baird RS, Greiner JV: Vernal conjunctivitis and contact lens-associated giant papillary conjunctivitis compared and contrasted. Am J Ophthalmol 87:544–555, 1979.

Allansmith MR, Korb DR, Greiner JV: Giant papillary conjunctivitis induced by hard or soft contact lens wear: Quantitative histology. Ophthalmology 85:766–778, 1978.

Fowler SA, Greiner JV, Allansmith MR: Soft contact lenses from patients with giant papillary conjunctivitis. Am J Ophthalmol 88:1056–1061, 1979.

Greiner JV, et al: Conjunctiva in asymptomatic contact lens wearers. Am J Ophthalmol 86:403–413, 1978.

Greiner JV, et al: Mucus secretory vesicles in conjunctival epithelial cells of wearers of contact lenses. Arch Ophthalmol 98:1843–1846, 1980.

Greiner JV, Covington HI, Allansmith MR: Surface morphology of giant papillary conjunctivitis in contact lens wearers. Am J Ophthalmol 85:242–252, 1978.

Korb DR, et al: Prevalence of conjunctival changes in wearers of hard contact lenses. Am J Ophthalmol 90:336–341, 1980.

Mackie IA, Wright P: Giant papillary conjunctivitis (secondary vernal) in association with contact lens wear. Trans Ophthalmol Soc UK 98:3–9, 1978.

Price MJ, et al: Tarsal conjunctival appearance in contact lens wearers. Contact Lens 8:16–22, 1982.

Richmond PP: Giant papillary conjunctivitis: An overview. J Am Optom Assoc 50:343–347, 1979.

Srinivasan BD, et al: Giant papillary conjunctivitis with ocular prostheses. Arch Ophthalmol 97:892–895, 1979.

IRRITATIVE CONJUNCTIVITIS
(Toxic Conjunctivitis)
RONALD E. SMITH, M.D.
Los Angeles, California

Direct contact of the eye with many agents in the environment can result in irritative or toxic conjunctivitis. A wide variety of drugs, chemicals, foreign bodies, pollutants, and such organic matter as pollens can cause significant symptoms if prolonged direct contact with the eye occurs. Ocular symptoms are often very acute, with onset soon after contact. The initial reaction in ocular tissues involves the conjunctiva, lid margins, and cornea and varies from a very mild burning or foreign body sensation to severe photophobia and pain. Objective findings may range from mild hyperemia to frank necrosis and ulceration of the conjunctiva, depending upon the potency and degree of toxicity of the offending irritant. Long-term exposure to an environmental irritant may cause the same symptoms over a prolonged period and can lead to chronic cicatrization in the conjunctiva or cornea.

THERAPY

Supportive. Removal of the environmental irritant, if detected, is the primary treatment for toxic conjunctivitis. In the case of air-borne toxic agents, use of air conditioning, special ventilation techniques, or safety goggles may prevent irritation if removal is impractical. If an ophthalmic drug is the offending toxic agent, then tapering or discontinuing the medication would be appropriate. Different manufacturers use various preservatives in similar eye medications, and use of an alternative brand may alleviate the problem. Many household and industrial chemical products are extremely toxic to the eye and require prompt and copious irrigation of the conjunctival sac. If available, sterile normal saline or balanced salt solution is the treatment of choice for any type of acute chemical injury to the cornea or conjunctiva; however, tap water, which is almost always readily accessible, is also an ideal irrigating solution.

Ocular. In general, the toxic effect will gradually disappear with removal of the irritating agent from the environment. However, if moderate to severe external ocular inflammation is present, a low concentration of topical corticosteroid preparation, such as 0.12 per cent prednisolone or 1 per cent medrysone, may be used to reduce more quickly the conjunctival inflammation. Concomitant use of a topical ophthalmic broad-spectrum antibiotic is also indicated to prevent superinfection. The usual administration of both drugs is one to two drops applied three to four times daily, depending on severity of the inflammation. The patient should be seen every few days, especially if corticosteroids are used. It is unusual for toxic conjunctivitis to require the use of systemic medications.

If the environmental agents have resulted in a chronic irritative conjunctivitis, such as that associated with air pollutants, then topical astringents, vasoconstrictors, or artificial tears containing methylcellulose may offer symptomatic relief. These agents may be instilled two to three times daily, but can themselves occasionally result in toxic conjunctivitis if used over a long period of time.

Ocular or Periocular Manifestations

Conjunctiva: Edema; follicles and papillae; hyperemia; necrosis (rare); watery discharge.
Cornea: Epithelial erosion and punctate staining; late scarring and vascularization with severe irritants (rare); mild epithelial and rarely stromal edema; stromal infiltration and ulceration in severe cases (rare).
Other: Foreign body sensation; irritation; photophobia.

Precautions

If the offending agent cannot be removed from the environment, action must be taken to reduce direct corneal and conjunctival exposure. Such preventive measures as goggles or improved ventilation may be helpful.

As in all instances of corticosteroid use, patients must be followed for complications that may ensue from the steroids themselves, including cataract and glaucoma. As corticosteroids simply suppress the inflammatory signs but do not alter the basic etiologic mechanism of this ocular problem, removal of the offending environmental agent is the long-term treatment of choice.

Comments

Toxic or irritative conjunctivitis resulting from exposure to environmental irritants is a nonspecific inflammatory reaction. Careful history taking is an important aspect in the management of such cases, as occupational or home-related exposure may be important considerations in patients in whom the causal agent cannot be identified. An additional diagnostic consideration is the patient who uses long-term instillation of topical ocular medications, including nonprescription drugs, such as artificial tears, astringent drops, or vasoconstrictors.

References

Allansmith MR: The Eye and Immunology. St Louis, CV Mosby, 1982.
Boerner CF, et al: Electron Microscopy for the diagnosis of ocular viral infections. Ophthalmology, 88:1377, 1981.
Kowalski RP, Harwick JC: Incidence of Moraxella conjunctival infection. Am J Ophthalmol, *101*:437–440, 1986.
Leibowitz HM, et al: Human conjunctivitis: II. Treatment. Arch Ophthalmol *94*:1752–1756, 1976.
Roy FH: Ocular Syndromes and Systemic Diseases, 2nd ed. New York, Grune & Stratton, 1989.

LIGNEOUS CONJUNCTIVITIS

JULES FRANCOIS, M.D., F.A.C.S., F.R.S.M.,
Ghent, Belgium
and JEROME KAZDAN, M.D., F.R.C.S.(C)
Toronto, Ontario

Ligneous conjunctivitis is a rare form of chronic conjunctivitis that is characterized by ligneous induration of the lids, membrane formation on the tarsal conjunctiva, and occasional corneal complications. Induration of the palpebral conjunctiva tends to be localized to the upper lid in the tarsal region, although both upper and lower lids can be involved. The lid gradually loses its flexibility and gives the impression of wood or cartilage. The lesion can also present as a tumor-like thickening in the lid. A thick whitish membrane of 1 to 2.5 mm inserting into the tarsal conjunctiva with a free periphery is almost always present. Corneal complications are rarely bilateral and may include opacification, vascularization, and keratomalacia with possible perforation.

Typically, the disease begins in early infancy and is usually bilateral and more prevalent in females. It has been reported as persisting in mild form without impairing vision for 38 years, and relapse has been recorded up to 25 years after spontaneous clearing. Systemic disturbances are rare, although occasionally other mucous membranes may be affected.

Histologically, the primary changes are localized in the conjunctival stroma where amorphous hyaline plaques with a marked vascularization are found. Histochemically, these plaques, which are of connective tissue origin, contain a hyaluronidase-sensitive mucopolysaccharide, either hyaluronic acid or chondroitin sulphate A or C.

The pathogenesis of ligneous conjunctivitis, as well as the nature and origin of the hyaline-like material, remains unknown. Many causes have been postulated, including bacterial infection, trauma, disturbance of the immune system, abnormal vascular permeability, deposition of tonofibrils from degenerating epithelial cells, and abnormal collagen synthesis. The fact that it is sometimes found within families underlies the assumption of an hereditary disturbance of the metabolism of the connective tissue of the mucosa. Numerous mast cells and eosinophils have been noted; in this respect, ligneous conjunctivitis resembles vernal conjunctivitis, a known hypersensitivity disease process. The increased vascular permeability and inflammatory cells, particularly eosinophils, may result from the release of mediator from mast cell granules. It is also conceivable that the deposition of hyaline material is related to mast cell degranulation. Increased fibrogenesis is a feature of mast cell tumors, as hyalinization of bronchial basement membrane is of asthma; both conditions are related to mast cell abnormalities.

THERAPY

Ocular. Topical enzyme treatment with either hyaluronidase‡ or chymotrypsin‡ has been reported to be successful in some but not all cases. Two drops of 1.5 mg of hyaluronidase* (750 IU) dissolved in 1 ml physiologic saline may be instilled every hour. If improvement is obvious, instillation every 3 hours may be sufficient. However, the enzyme should be continued two or three times a day indefinitely, since the condition may recur as hyaluronidase is only substitutive and not curative.

Marked improvement has been reported after surgical excision combined with topical application of 4 per cent cromolyn.‡ A dosage of one or two drops of cromolyn four times daily is recommended. More experience with this form of therapy is needed to confirm its efficacy.

Recently favorable responses have been obtained after surgical excision combined with topical application of cyclosporine drops 20 mg/ml initially given every 1 to 2 hours while awake for a few weeks, and then every 4 hours while awake for up to 1 year. Serum cyclosporine levels during treatment were not significant.

It is also advisable to apply an appropriate topical broad-spectrum antibiotic into the conjunctival sac three or four times daily, as associated bacterial infection is common.

Topical corticosteroids have not usually been of benefit.

Surgical. During the enzyme treatment, it is advisable to destroy the granulomatous tissue by diathermy coagulation to hasten recovery. This coagulation should be done only after institution of the enzyme treatment in order to prevent postoperative recurrences. Cryosurgery has been tried on this entity without consistent success.

Ocular or Periocular Manifestations

Conjunctiva: Fibrosis; membrane and pseudomembrane.

Cornea: Clouding; keratomalacia; opacity; perforation; vascularization.

Eyelids: Induration; ligneous membrane.

PRECAUTIONS

Even with the use of overlying grafts, surgical stripping of the membrane in ligneous conjunctivitis uniformly leads to severe bleeding and prompt recurrence, even as early as 48 hours. Removal may not be of benefit.

COMMENTS

Enzymatic therapy of ligneous conjunctivitis is usually effective. As cromolyn is a known inhibitor of mediator release from mast cell granules, the success of this therapy supports the suggestion that mast cells are involved in the pathogenesis of ligneous conjunctivitis.

Results of the immunohistochemical studies before and after topical cyclosporine treatment support the hypothesis of local immune response in the pathogenesis of this disorder.

The prognosis is graver when the condition is bilateral, accompanied by a pseudomembrane, or associated with systemic manifestations. An upper respiratory tract infection often accompanies ligneous conjunctivitis, and such symptoms as stomatitis, nasopharyngitis, otitis, bronchitis, vulvovaginitis, fever, nephritis, and inflammation of the joints may also be present.

References

Bateman JB, Pettit TH, Isenberg SJ, Simons KB: Ligneous conjunctivitis. An autosomal recessive disorder. J Pediatr Ophthalmol Strabismus 23:137, 1986.

Chambers JD, et al: Ligneous conjunctivitis. Trans Am Acad Ophthalmol Otolaryngol 73:996–1004, 1969.

Cooper TJ, Kazdan JJ, Cutz E: Ligneous conjunctivitis with tracheal obstruction. A case report, with light and electron microscopy findings. Can J Ophthalmol 14:57–62, 1979.

Eagle RC Jr, Brooks JSJ, Katowitz JA, et al: Fibrin as a major constituent of ligneous conjunctivitis. Am J Ophthalmol 101:493, 1986.

Firat T: Ligneous conjunctivitis. Am J Ophthalmol 78:679–688, 1974.

Francois J, Victoria-Troncoso V: Treatment of ligneous conjunctivitis. Am J Ophthalmol 65:674–678, 1968.

Friedlaender M, Ostler HB: Treatment of ligneous conjunctivitis with cromolyn: A case report. Proctor Bull 1:3, 1978.

Hidayat AA, Riddle PJ: Ligneous conjunctivitis: A clinicopathologic study of 17 cases. Ophthalmology 94:949, 1987.

Holland EJ, et al: Immunohistologic findings and results of treatment with cyclosporine in ligneous conjunctivitis. Am J Ophthalmol 107:160–166, 1989.

Kanai A, Polack FM: Histologic and electron microscope studies of ligneous conjunctivitis. Am J Ophthalmol 72:909–916, 1971.

Melikian HE: Treatment of ligneous conjunctivitis. Ann Ophthalmol 17:763, 1985.

McGrand JC, Rees DM, Harry J: Ligneous conjunctivitis. Br J Ophthalmol 53:373–381, 1969.

Spaeth GL: Chronic membranous conjunctivitis. A persisting problem. Am J Ophthalmol 64:300–305, 1967.

OPHTHALMIA NEONATORUM
(Conjunctivitis of Newborns, Neonatal Ophthalmia)

EARL A. PALMER, M.D.
Portland, Oregon

Although the term "ophthalmia neonatorum" connotes gonorrheal infection, it designates a syndrome including any conjunctivitis, affecting one or both eyes, that occurs during the first month of life. Thus, it is not a single disease. Frequently, purulent exudate occurs out of proportion to erythema and edema; hence comes the pediatric colloquialism, "sticky eye." This syndrome varies in severity from the mild chemical conjunctivitis caused by instillation of prophylactic 1 per cent silver nitrate to the fulminating corneal perforation and panophthalmitis that can complicate infection with *Neisseria gonorrhoeae* or *Pseudomonas aeruginosa*. Even mild or moderate eye infection in the newborn may be rarely associated with grave systemic complications.

Inclusion conjunctivitis (inclusion blennorrhea) caused by *Chlamydia trachomatis* is the most common infectious ophthalmia neonatorum seen in the United States. The majority of bacterial cases, in contrast, result from infection with *Staphylococcus aureus, Pneumococcus,* or species of *Neisseria* or *Hemophilus*. One of an assortment of generally saprophytic organisms may be occasionally isolated from milder cases. Anaerobic organisms may be more commonly at fault than is generally appreciated. Even herpes simplex virus can infect the newborn eye.

Infectious keratitis may produce visual damage through corneal scarring. Bacterial keratitis (especially *Pseudomonas* or gonococcal) may perforate to cause endophthalmitis. Herpes simplex keratoconjunctivitis may accompany an encephalitis that can produce brain damage. Chlamydial (inclusion) conjunctivitis is associated with a neonatal pneumonia syndrome, with prominent tachypnea, absent febrile response, and diffuse infiltrates on x-ray. This association must be appreciated by the ophthalmologist and pediatrician, even though the conjunctivitis itself generally responds well to topical erythromycin. Neonatal infection may be derived in utero, during passage through the birth canal, or postpartum from external fomites and personal contact. A number of pyogenic organisms are dangerous to the newborn because they may be associated with septicemia. These include gram-positive diplococci (pneumococcus), and gram-negative diplococci (*N. gonorrhoeae* and *N. meningitidis*). Newborn infants may not show a febrile response to sepsis and have an immature microbial defense system.

THERAPY

Ocular. Specific treatment depends upon knowledge of the infecting agent. For this reason, a culture for sensitivity should be obtained, in case the chosen treatment proves ineffective. A gram-stained smear should be examined microscopically to guide initial therapy. If no organisms are found, a Giemsa preparation may show the intracytoplasmic inclusions of chlamydial infection.

The following pertinent subjects are discussed elsewhere in this volume: Bacterial conjunctivitis; Candidiasis; *Escherichia coli;* Gonorrhea; *Hemophilus influenzae;* Herpes simplex; Inclusion conjunctivitis; Irritative conjunctivitis; Koch-Weeks bacillus; Pneumococcus; Proteus; *Pseudomonas aeruginosa;* Staphylococcus; Streptococcus.

Chemical conjunctivitis caused by 1 per cent silver nitrate prophylaxis is typically mild and begins clearing spontaneously within 24 hours. If concentrations of silver nitrate over 2 per cent are erroneously given, necrotic keratoconjunctivitis may result. In such cases, the accumulated exudate should be removed from the fornices by frequent irrigations, and any synechiae should be broken with a glass rod as they form.

Candida conjunctivitis of the newborn may be suggested by associated thrush of the oral cavity and a thrush-like pseudomembrane on the conjunctiva. It may be substantiated by microscopic examination of a scraping. The condition is usually self-limited.

In acute purulent conjunctivitis caused by coliform organisms, topical 0.5 per cent neomycin or 0.3 per cent gentamicin is usually suitable. The drops or ointment should be instilled every hour on the first day and then every 4 hours for the next 10 to 14 days. Since corneal invasion and perforation can result from *Pseudomonas* conjunctivitis, treatment must be initiated rapidly and aggressively, especially in the premature infant. Topical 0.3 per cent gentamicin or 0.25 per cent polymyxin B instilled every half-hour is recommended. Frequency of drops is gradually reduced to every 4 hours as inflammation subsides. The eyelids may be cleansed or gently irrigated with saline as often as necessary. Coliform organisms can invade the bloodstream of newborns, particularly premature infants, and result in death, with or without meningitis.

Hemophilus species may be treated with either topical 10 or 15 per cent sulfacetamide or 0.3 per cent gentamicin drops instilled each hour until clinical resolution begins and then tapered to every 4 hours for about another 5 days.

Conjunctivitis caused by gram-positive cocci and diplococci is treated with 0.5 per cent erythromycin ointment every 2 hours the first day and four times a day for the next 7 days.

Herpes keratoconjunctivitis in newborn infants is sometimes associated with a severe systemic illness that has a high mortality rate. Effective treatment for the disseminated infection is still being sought. When conjunctivitis occurs in an infant born to a mother with genital herpes, topical prophylactic idoxuridine instilled five times daily should be strongly considered. Treatment of herpetic keratitis is discussed elsewhere.

Inclusion conjunctivitis is treated systemically as noted in the following section.

Systemic. Where systemic complications occur, care should be directed by a pediatrician. The systemic drug dosages in newborn infants may vary depending upon renal or hepatic function, level of maturity, concomitant medications, state of hydration, and other systemic variables that are best evaluated by the pediatrician.

Inclusion conjunctivitis is treated with oral erythromycin 50 mg/kg daily in four divided doses for 14 days. Topical erythromycin does not improve the response rate. Recurrent or persistent disease should be treated with an additional 1 to 2 weeks of oral erythromycin. Prophylaxis of the newborn with topical erythromycin is effective in preventing chlamydial conjunctivitis, but does not prevent nasopharyngeal infection or chlamydial pneumonia.

Gonorrheal ophthalmia neonatorum signifies probable venereal disease in the mother. Possible complications include disastrous invasion of the globe, septicemia, arthritis, and meningitis. It typically appears as an acute purulent conjunctivitis after the first 24 hours and before 72 hours after birth. It may, however, be acquired prenatally by ascending invasion. A culture with sensitivities is initiated. After treatment is begun, hospital care under isolation for 24 hours is indicated. Aqueous crystalline penicillin G is given intravenously for 7 days at a dose of 100/mg/kg daily in four divided doses. The World Health Organization has recommended a single intramuscular dose of kanamycin 7.5 mg (followed by topical tetracycline ointment) for areas of the world with a prevalence of penicillin-resistant gonococci of 1 per cent or more. In the United States, it may be preferable to use a single dose of 125 mg of ceftriaxone intramuscularly, without a topical anti-infective. Topical antibiotics may be superfluous in the absence of corneal ulceration. Exudates should be gently removed with saline periodically.

Supportive. All newborn infants should receive the benefit of prophylactic treatment. Good prepartum care of the mother is the first step. For the infant, treatment is logically directed against gonorrhea, but ideally, as many other microbes as possible should also be covered. The following alternatives have been found highly effective. A 1 per cent silver nitrate solution (from a single-use ampule and not rinsed out), 1 per cent tetracycline, or 0.5 per cent erythromycin ophthalmic ointment should be instilled as soon as practical after delivery, ideally in the first 15 minutes and whenever possible within the first hour postnatally. Even infants born by cesarean section should receive prophylaxis. An infant born to a mother known to be infected with gonorrhea should be given a single dose of parenteral aqueous crystalline penicillin G: 50,000 units for full-term infants and 20,000 units if birth weight is under 2000 gm.

Ocular or Periocular Manifestations

Conjunctiva: Bloody discharge; catarrhal, membranous, or pseudomembranous conjunctivitis; chemosis; cicatrization; follicles; hyperemia; mucopurulent or purulent exudates; necrosis.

Cornea: Infiltration; keratitis; micropannus; necrosis; perforations; staphyloma; ulcer.

Eyelids: Blepharitis; edema; hyperemia; vesicles.

Globe: Endophthalmitis; panophthalmitis.

Other: Iris atrophy; peripheral posterior uveitis; photophobia; visual loss; vitreitis.

PRECAUTIONS

The appearance of localized or generalized corneal haze in this condition should be taken as a serious sign of potential corneal ulceration.

Silver nitrate prophylaxis is safe unless untrained personnel erroneously administer a solution not intended for the eye. No silver nitrate solution more concentrated than 2 per cent should be placed in the eye; 1 per cent concentration is sufficient.

Systemic infection with herpes simplex can be thoroughly devastating and is often fatal to the newborn. Fortunately, this is rare as there is no proven effective treatment. Herpetic keratoconjunctivitis can rarely be present at birth, although more typically it is acquired during passage through an infected birth canal. Thus, even infants born by cesarean operation can exhibit this entity.

The "venereal" causes of ophthalmia neonatorum also require treatment of the parents. These causes include gonorrhea, herpes simplex type 2, and *Chlamydia trachomatis*.

COMMENTS

The exact time of onset may be helpful in clinically distinguishing among the causes of ophthalmia neonatorum. Silver nitrate irritation is evident within hours after the drops are instilled, but abates dramatically within 24 hours and disappears within 72 hours.

Gonorrheal conjunctivitis is most likely to appear in newborns at 2 to 6 days of age. A severe purulent conjunctivitis appearing at this time should suggest gonorrhea. Inclusion conjunctivitis develops from 5 to 14 days postnatally; herpetic keratoconjunctivitis follows about the same pattern, but can appear even earlier. *Pseudomonas* conjunctivitis or corneal ulcer may appear acutely at any time in debilitated infants, particularly premature infants on mechanical ventilation.

References

Beem MO, Saxon EM: Respiratory-tract colonization and a distinctive pneumonia syndrome in infants infected with *Chlamydia trachomatis*. N Engl J Med 296:306–310, 1977.

Burns RP, Rhodes DH: Pseudomonas eye infection as a cause of death in premature infants. Arch Ophthalmol 65:517–525, 1961.
Hammerschlag MR, et al: Erythromycin ointment for ocular prophylaxis of neonatal chlamydial infection. JAMA 244:2291–2293, 1980.
Laga M, et al: Single-dose therapy of gonococcal ophthalmia neonatorum with ceftriaxone. N Engl J Med 315:1382–1385, 1986.
Miller ME, Stiehm ER: Introduction. Host defenses in the fetus and neonate. Pediatrics 64(Suppl):708, 1979.
Nahmias AJ, et al: Eye infections with herpes simplex viruses in neonates. Surv Ophthalmol 21:100–105, 1976.
Nishida H, Risemberg HM: Silver nitrate ophthalmic solution and chemical conjunctivitis. Pediatrics 56:368–373, 1975.
Oriel JD: Ophthalmia neonatorum: Relative efficacy of current prophylactic practices and treatment. J Antimicrob Chemother 14:209–219, 1984.
Sexually transmitted disease treatment guidelines. MMWR 34(Suppl):75S–108S, 1985.
Whitley RJ, Ch'ien LT, Alford CA Jr: Neonatal herpes simplex virus infection. Int Ophthalmol Clin 15:141–149, 1975.

PTERYGIUM AND PSEUDOPTERYGIUM

L.F. RICH, M.S., M.D.
Portland, Oregon

A pterygium is a triangular elevated mass of thickened bulbar conjunctiva that extends onto the cornea in the interpalbebral zone. Its name is derived from the Greek word meaning wing, which describes its characteristic shape. Within the interpalpebral fissure, a pterygium is most commonly found on the nasal aspect of the globe and less often on the temporal aspect. If present outside the interpalpebral fissure area, it is considered an atypical pterygium, and other diagnoses, such as phlyctenular keratoconjunctivitis or malignancies, must be considered.

Environment and heredity are thought to play important roles in the pathogenesis of pterygium. Its incidence is higher in tropical or subtropical areas of the world and in individuals frequently exposed to sunlight, air-borne allergens, wind, dust, fumes or other noxious stimuli. Frequently, a pingueculum precedes the pterygium. The elevated conjunctival tissue may lead to tear film defects and may form a dellen or an area of dryness in the adjacent tissue. Inflammation and vascularization are thereby initiated, and the patient may have symptoms of irritation or itching. Recurrent episodes of exposure may irritate the mass of tissue, enlarge it, and produce another dellen, which continues the advancement. Eventually, the lesion grows beyond the limbus, invades cornea, may progress into or beyond the visual axis, and may result in blindness.

Pseudopterygium is similar in appearance to a true pterygium, but bridges the limbus so that a probe may be passed beneath the lesion at the limbus. It is often the result of damage to the cornea with a chemical, thermal or physical insult. Pseudopterygium is more likely to occur in atypical locations (i.e., outside the interpalpebral fissure area) than a true pterygium. As with a true pterygium, recurrences are more aggressive than the primary lesion.

THERAPY

Supportive. Unless the patient specifically requests surgery, it is best to avoid intervention and limit treatment to medical modalities. Advice can be given to help minimize the progression of the pterygium. Specifically, protection against sunlight and dryness is important. Episodes of irritation should be treated with topical lubricants, such as artificial tears or ointments; if inflammation and edema occur, a mild vasoconstrictor drop may prevent elevation and dellen formation. Mild corticosteroids, such as medrysone, can be prescribed for short-term usage. More potent steroids, particularly those with good ocular penetration, should be avoided if possible to minimize complications associated with corticosteroid use.

When outdoors, the patient should be encouraged to wear sunglasses or protective goggles. Occlusive goggles are of value in dusty windy environments. If a patient has a known sensitivity to an air-borne allergen and anticipates exposure to that allergen, systemic antihistamines before exposure may prevent an allergic response. Once the response has occurred, however, antihistamines are of little value.

Surgical. Surgical intervention is indicated when the patient requests removal of the pterygium for cosmetic reasons, the progression of the lesion threatens vision, or symblepharon limits ocular motility. If none of these indications exists, it is best to treat the pterygium medically, because if the pterygium recurs following surgery, it is often worse than the primary lesion.

There are multiple surgical techniques for removal of pterygium. Avulsion of the head of the pterygium from the cornea may be possible if the lesion is loosely attached. This technique has the advantage of being relatively noninvasive to corneal tissue. Leaving a smooth area with little or no removal of corneal and limbal tissue may lessen the chances of recurrence. Many surgeons smooth the base of the cornea where the pterygium had been removed, using a diamond burr or scalpel blade. If the pterygium is firmly attached and cannot be avulsed from the cornea, a delineating keratotomy with partial lamellar keratectomy will aid removal. This procedure is best done under the microscope to minimize removal of corneal tissue and to avoid perforation into the anterior chamber. Once the head of the pterygium has been removed from the cornea and is beyond limbus, its body and tail should be excised to avoid the insertion of the rectus muscle. Some surgeons prefer to remove as little of the body of the pterygium as possible and attach the cut ends of conjunctiva to the sclera or to one another. Others prefer to leave the sclera bare. Control of bleeding is essential, and all feeder vessels should be cauterized.

Local anesthesia is preferred over general anesthesia unless the patient is unable to cooperate or is extremely anxious about ocular surgery. Subconjunctival injection* of lidocaine without hyaluronidase is preferred. Epinephrine may be added to the anesthetic to inhibit bleeding. A topical anesthetic, such as cocaine, may also be used to prevent pain when the eye is grasped in an area other than where the lidocaine had been injected. Occasionally, retrobulbar anesthesia is necessary if the patient is unable to control ocular movements. In such patients, akinesia of the eyelids may be necessary as well.

After the lesion has been excised, it is wise to submit it to the pathologist for evaluation. Occasionally, malignancies may mimic a typical pterygium; in these cases, surgery may spread or stimulate its growth.

Several postoperative adjunctive measures lower the recurrence rate after excision of a pterygium or pseudopterygium. Many ophthalmic surgeons advocate the use of strontium[90] beta irradiation immediately after excision of the pterygium. Between 1000 and 1500 reps, preferably in divided doses, may be applied at and near the limbus in three adjacent points. Another treatment modality that has become less popular in recent decades is the topical application of thiotepa. This antineoplastic agent is applied four to six times daily for 6 to 8 weeks in the postoperative period. Once the epithelium has been regenerated, topical corticosteroids may be useful in managing the fibrovascular healing response and minimizing cicatrization.

Primary excision of pterygium is followed by recurrence in 40 to 50 per cent of cases. Recurrent pterygium is more difficult to treat and is more likely to recur after a second excision than a primary pterygium. Simple excision may be used, but adjunctive irradiation or antimetabolite therapy is highly advised. If symblepharon is present or the remaining conjunctiva is insufficient to permit adequate ocular motility, a mucous membrane or conjunctival graft may be needed to cover the bare area. A conjunctival graft may be used from the same or the fellow eye and is preferably taken from a vicinity outside the interpalpebral fissure area.

Corneoscleral grafts with or without mucous membrane or conjunctival grafts have been advocated in cases of recurrent pterygium. Their use is advised in cases where the limbal architecture has been disturbed from one or more surgical interventions. They are best accomplished with partial-thickness grafts incorporating corneal and scleral donor tissue in the same configuration as the tissue resected from the recipient eye. The grafted area can be trephined or cut freehand and the donor tissue similarly dissected to fit the outline. If cornea and scleral tissue is used, it can be incorporated as a single graft to maintain the architecture of the limbal sulcus. A clear corneal graft that bridges the limbus has also been advocated, but it has the disadvantage of producing a single contour without providing a limbal sulcus. A corneal graft alone is likely to allow vascularization at the graft-host interface, so it is probably best to avoid leaving the edge of the graft at the limbus. Grafting is necessary if multiple excisions have left the corneal tissue thin, and perforation or ocular weakness is imminent.

Ocular or Periocular Manifestations

Conjunctiva: Temporal displacement of semilunar fold; symblepharon; wing-shaped fleshy, vascularized growth.
Cornea: Conjunctival (encroachment); gray infiltrates; elevated mass; keratitis, iron pigment line.
Other: Astigmatism; decreased visual acuity; diplopia; restriction of ocular motility.

PRECAUTIONS

Surgical excision of a pterygium is the most common form of therapy employed today. The surgical process and the pterygium itself destroy limbal tissue and predispose the eye to recurrence of the lesion. In addition, the elevation of conjunctiva and the irregular corneal and limbal tissue resulting from surgery may reinitiate the pathologic process of localized dryness, vascularization, and regrowth. Furthermore, an acute inflammatory process after surgery may produce granulation tissue that can contract and stimulate conjunctivalization of the limbus and cornea. Excessive postoperative inflammation and irritation from exposure during the early postoperative period encourage regrowth. Recurrences may be seen as early as 2 weeks or several years after excision. The size of the original lesion may play a role in the probability of recurrence. A large, fleshy, vascularized, primary pterygium with inflammation indicates activity and should not be approached surgically until the inflammation has been minimized. In addition, large pterygia require more extensive surgery, which produces greater injury to underlying and surrounding tissue than occurs when smaller lesions are removed.

COMMENTS

Each surgical intervention may produce a greater cosmetic blemish and a more difficult management situation than the previous lesion. A pterygium is more likely to return following a recurrence than after removal of a primary lesion. Symblepharon is often a sequela of pterygium surgery; restriction of ocular motility and pain with extraocular movements, particularly abduction of the globe, may result.

References

Bahrassa F, Datta R: Postoperative Beta radiation treatment of pterygium. Int J Rad Oncology Biol Phys 9:679–684, 1983.

Ehrlich D: The management of pterygium. Ophthalmic Surg 8:23–30, 1977.

Kleis W, Picó G: Thio-tepa therapy to prevent postoperative pterygium occurrence and neovascularization. Am J Ophthalmol 76:371–373, 1973.

Talbot AN: Complications of beta ray treatment of pterygia. Trans Ophthalmol Soc NZ 31:62–63, 1979.

Tarr KH, Constable IJ: Late complications of pterygium treatment. Br J Ophthalmol 64:496–505, 1980.

Vastine DW, et al: Reconstruction of the periocular mucous membrane by autologous conjunctival transplantation. Ophthalmology 89:1072–1081, 1982.

Vorkas AP: Pterygium. Choice of operation. Trans Ophthalmol Soc UK 101:192–194, 1981.

VERNAL KERATOCONJUNCTIVITIS

M.M. EL HENNAWI, M.Ch.

Alexandria, Egypt

Vernal keratoconjunctivitis is a severe perennial form of allergic conjunctivitis involving the cornea and conjunctiva. The condition is found predominantly in children or young adults and commonly in atopic individuals, who may also suffer from eczema, asthma, or hay fever. It is characterized by intermittent exacerbations, which are often seasonal.

The disease generally affects the upper tarsal conjunctiva, which shows a papillary hypertrophy and has a cobblestone appearance in severe cases. The limbal conjunctiva may also be affected, either as localized edema and hyperemia or as fleshy isolated vegetations. The main symptoms are intense photophobia, severe itching, and the production of tenacious stringy mucous discharge. It is considered to be an atopic disease and has been classified as a type I allergic disease of the outer eye.

THERAPY

Supportive. Desensitization to inhalant allergens has been used in the treatment of this disease, but has not generally been found to be helpful. Iced compresses and dark glasses may produce marked amelioration of ocular symptoms in most cases.

Systemic. Corticosteroid therapy is of great help in severe perennial cases. In addition, long-acting antihistamines may be required. Sustained-release preparations of pheniramine may be used for administration once daily at bedtime.

Ocular. Cromolyn sodium is a valuable drug both in the prophylaxis and treatment of vernal keratoconjunctivitis. As a prophylactic agent, a 2 per cent solution of cromolyn sodium may be used three times daily for 1 month before the expected season of exacerbation. As a therapeutic agent, marked improvement is attained with administration four times daily in mild and moderate cases. In severe cases or acute exacerbation, additional therapy is recommended. Topical ophthalmic corticosteroids are very effective in the treatment of vernal keratoconjunctivitis. Prednisolone or dexamethasone may be required three or four times daily. Dosages are applied according to severity; in acute exacerbation, steroid eyedrops may be required very frequently, every 2 or 3 hours during the day. Vasoconstrictors may also be helpful in decreasing hyperemia.

Surgical. Shaving of papillae, combined excision of tarsus and conjunctiva, and cryotherapy have been used, but none appears to give long-lasting relief. Plano-T contact lenses may be helpful in persistent epithelial keratitis. In epithelial plaques, superficial keratectomy and iodine cautery usually result in healing of the epithelium.

Ocular or Periocular Manifestations

Conjunctiva: Cobble-stone appearance; palpebral hyperemia; perilimbal hyperemia; stringy mucous discharge; "Tranta's spots"; vegetations that encroach to the cornea.

Cornea: Erosion; keratitis epithelialis vernalis; plaques; vernal ulcer.

Other: Decreased visual acuity; persistent lacrimation; photophobia.

PRECAUTIONS

Although stinging may occur as an adverse reaction to cromolyn sodium, the eyedrops do not cause significant adverse effects, such as the rise in ocular tension found with steroid eyedrops. In addition to reducing the risk of steroid-induced glaucoma, cromolyn sodium also reduces the possibility of herpetic keratitis or cataract.

If increased intraocular pressure persists in chronic topical corticosteroid users, the optic nerve may become damaged, and severe or total loss of sight may result from steroid-induced glaucoma. Periodic measurement of the intraocular pressure is obligatory in those patients using corticosteroids.

COMMENTS

Chronic vernal keratoconjunctivitis in children is usually one of the very difficult problems of management. Continuous and persistent observation is very essential, especially in children receiving chronic steroid therapy.

This risk of steroid-induced glaucoma should always be considered. Although the various forms of therapy available may give rise to marked amelioration of symptoms in most cases, they are not curative. Further research is needed to clarify the etiology of vernal keratoconjunctivitis and to establish a more effective, safer, and curative therapy.

References

Dart JKG, Buckley RJ, Monnickenda M, Prasad J: Perennial allergic conjunctivitis: definition, clinical characteristics and prevalence. A comparison with seasonal allergic conjunctivitis. Trans Ophthalmol Soc UK 105:513–520, 1986.

El Hennawi M: Thesis. Study of the effect of disodium cromoglycate in spring cattarh as compared with other certain anti-allergic drugs. The effect of disodium cromoglycate on locally administered radioactive histamine concentration. Alexandria, University of Alexandria, 1974.

El Hennawi M: Clinical trial with 2% sodium cromoglycate (Opticrom) in vernal keratoconjunctivitis. Br J Ophthalmol 64:483–486, 1980.

Jones BR: Allergic disease of the outer eye. Trans Ophthalmol Soc UK 91:441–447, 1971.

Rice NSC, et al: Vernal kerato-conjunctivitis and its management. Trans Ophthalmol Soc UK 91:483–489, 1971.

SECTION 21

CORNEA

Degenerative Changes

CORNEAL MUCOUS PLAQUES
(Keratitis Mucosa)

RAMESH C. TRIPATHI, M.D., Ph.D.
Chicago, Illinois

Corneal mucous plaques are abnormal collections of a mixture of mucus, epithelial cells, and proteinaceous and lipoidal material that adhere firmly to the corneal surface. The plaques may also enmesh calcareous granules and bacteria, as well as dust particles and other foreign bodies. The mucous plaques are translucent to opaque and may vary in size and shape from multiple small islands to bizarre patterns involving more than half the corneal surface. The presence of an abnormality of the exposed surface of the superficial corneal epithelial cells, excessive mucus formation, and the presence of epithelial receptor sites predispose to this condition. The normal desquamation of epithelial cells beneath the plaque is thus retarded. The plaque is formed when high viscosity mucus and proteinaceous material become adherent to the deeper squamous cells of the cornea or to Bowman's layer through the intercellular spaces and even through abnormally formed transcellular apertures; this material enmeshes the desquamated epithelial cells. The viscosity of the mucus may increase because of dehydration, an increase in its sialomucin component, or secondarily because of infection by staphylococci, the enzymes of which destroy the mucoprotein and mucopolysaccharide components of normal mucus. Corneal mucous plaques occur primarily in patients with keratoconjunctivitis sicca, but may also be seen with herpes zoster keratitis. Ciliary or conjunctival injection, mild iritis, profuse keratic precipitates, and epithelial and stromal edema are associated findings.

Symptoms associated with the plaques vary from blurring of vision to foreign body sensation with marked pain and, except when severe, are often indistinguishable from the symptoms of keratoconjunctivis sicca with or with Sjögren's syndrome. These symptoms may also be seen with herpes zoster keratitis and in patients using extended-wear soft contact lenses. There appears to be an association of the entity with systemic disease, primarily rheumatoid arthritis or other collagen diseases.

THERAPY

Ocular. Topically applied 10 to 20 per cent acetylcysteine drops,* one to four times daily usually prevents corneal mucous plaques. Existing plaques can also often be rapidly loosened and dissolved with this treatment. Mucous plaques causing severe symptoms may be removed surgically by scrapping, followed by a bandage soft contact lens. In some patients, a soft contact lens is also of therapeutic or preventive value.

Staphylococcal blepharitis may occur in association with corneal mucous plaques and may predispose patients to this condition. Therefore, treatment should also include the control of associated local microbial infections.

Artificial tear preparations may be indicated for the treatment of dry eye. In the presence of filamentary keratitis and excessive mucus formation, hypotonic artificial tear substitutes (rather than the mucoid type of tear substitutes) may be combined with acetylcysteine.

Ocular or Periocular Manifestations

Cornea: Filamentary keratitis; keratoconjunctivitis sicca; mucous plaques.
Conjunctiva: Conjunctivitis; fornix filaments; hyperemia; mucoid discharge.
Eyelids: Blepharospasm; chronic blepharitis.

PRECAUTIONS

Because of variation in the frequency and severity of corneal mucous plaques, the use and concentration of topical acetylcysteine should be individualized.

The bandage soft lens may often be subject to deposit formation and spoilage secondary to alterations in tear function (including rapid tear break-up time), associated necrosis of keratoconjunctival tissue, and the plaque exposure. Periodic cleaning or change of the soft contact lens may be required.

COMMENTS

In some cases, the corneal mucous plaques recur when acetylcysteine is discontinued. Plaques may occur even in those patients receiving acetylcysteine, but usually the mucous adherences are smaller or remain on the cornea for shorter periods of time than if the patient did not receive therapy. In some patients, plaques may recur if the soft contact lens is discontinued.

Multiple plaques, which are frequently bilateral, are common. When a plaque has adhered to the cornea, it remains for a few days or weeks; recurrences may appear but seldom in the same location. Thickened plaques with a dry surface may appear elevated well above the tear film.

References

Fraunfelder FT, Wright P, Tripathi RC: Corneal mucus plaques. Am J Ophthalmol 83:191–197, 1977.
Marsh RJ, Fraunfelder FT, McGill JI: Herpetic corneal epithelial disease. Arch Ophthalmol 94:1899–1902, 1976.
Shaw EL, Gasset AR: Management of an unusual case of keratitis mucosa with hydrophilic contact lenses and N-acetyl-cysteine. Ann Ophthalmol 6:1054–1056, 1974.

FUCH'S DELLEN
(Facets, Fuchs' Dimples)
F. LAGOUTTE, M.D.
Bordeaux, France

Dellen are paralimbal corneal ulcerations occurring at the base of abnormal conjunctiva or corneal elevations. These ellipsoid depressions or dells in the cornea are a quite common but not well-known phenomenon. Dellen are usually elliptical and saucer-shaped with clearly defined edges. Although transient dellen are superficial and purely epithelial, they may last several weeks and sometimes become deep. Cicatrization normally follows, often with reduction of corneal thickness (facets). Abnormal paralimbic conjunctival elevation most commonly is associated with filtering bleb, hematoma, chemosis, conjunctival tumor, rectus muscle surgery, conjunctival autograft, or pterygium. Abnormal corneal elevations can be seen secondary to localized graft displacement or edema, too tight corneal sutures, or corneal tumor. Poor palpebral congruence prevents the lids from normally spreading the tears, which causes a break in the oily film. This break and the resulting dessication can be aggravated by a trapped air bubble that sometimes bursts when the lids open.

THERAPY

Ocular. Treatment consists of elimination of the cause. In most cases, a pressure dressing is sufficient to control any abnormal conjunctival or corneal elevation. Rarely, an elevated growth may require conjunctival surgery. If there is an inflammatory elevation (such as a granuloma), topical corticosteroids may be of value, but should be used with caution because of the corneal ulcer.

Further treatment should be directed toward the secondary complications that may result. The area of dellen formation should be treated three times daily with ocular lubricants, preferably in ointment form; drops are less effective because they do not maintain prolonged protective coating over the dellen. Antibiotics may be necessary to avoid secondary infections.

Recently, the depression of the cornea has been "filled" with a fibrin sealant, i.e., TISSUCOL®. The sealant is covered with a bandage lens, and the cicatrization forms in a few days.

Ocular or Periocular Manifestations

Conjunctiva: Ectasia.
Cornea: Cicatrization; keratoconjunctivitis sicca; marginal keratitis; paralimbal elevation; thinning; ulcer.

PRECAUTIONS

Elimination of the cause of the elevation should be the primary focus of therapy. Use of corticosteroids should be limited and closely supervised because of the possibility of corneal ulcer.

COMMENTS

Dellen are more frequent than is commonly thought. They are usually benign, but occasionally present difficulties. In almost all cases, they heal well with the use of the simple techniques described earlier.

References

Baum JL, Mishima S, Boruchoff SA: On the nature of dellen. Arch Ophthalmol 79:657–662, 1968.
Fuchs A: Pathological dimples ("dellen") of the cornea. Am J Ophthalmol 12:877–883, 1929.
Insler MS, Tauber S, Packer A: Descemetocele formation in a patient with a postoperative corneal Dellen. Cornea 8:129–130, 1989
Lagoutte F, Gauthier L, Comte P: A fibrin sealant for perforated and preperforated corneal ulcers. Br J Ophthalmol (In press).
Lagoutte F, Lebur J: Un phénomène méconnu: Les ulcérations cornéennes à l'aplomb des reliefs conjonctivaux exagérés ("dellen de Fuchs"). A propos de 7 cas. Bull Soc Ophthalmol Fr 80:1033–1035, 1980.
Mackie IA: Localized corneal drying in association with dellen, pterygia and related lesions. Trans Ophthalmol Soc UK 91:129–145, 1971.
Nauheim JS: Marginal keratitis and corneal ulceration after surgery on the extraocular muscles. Arch Ophthalmol 67:708–711, 1962.
Tragakis MP, Brown SI: The tear film alteration associated with dellen. Ann Ophthalmol 6:757–761, 1974.

MOOREN'S ULCER
THOMAS O. WOOD, M.D.,
and AUDREY W. TUBERVILLE, M.D.
Memphis, Tennessee

Mooren's ulcer is a chronic painful ulceration of the cornea that begins in the periphery with an elevated, de-epithelialized leading edge and progresses centrally and circumferentially. If untreated, it is usually relentlessly progressive and may invade the entire cornea. As the ulcer progresses, a vascularized pannus forms in its wake. Between wakes and iritis, perforation may occur. Iritis can be severe enough to result in posterior synechiae, cataracts, and glaucoma.

Two types of Mooren's ulcers are recognized: 1) unilateral ulcers that tend to be mild and responsive to therapy and 2) bilateral ulcers that may occur simultaneously or nonsimultaneously. Bilateral simultaneous ulcers are the most refractory to therapy.

Associated trauma or corneal inflammation, such as caused by corneal foreign body, abrasion, or cataract surgery, is antecedent in about one third of cases. Herpes simplex keratitis, herpes zoster ophthalmicus, chemical burns, and connective tissue/vasculitis diseases, such as rheumatoid arthritis and polyarteritis nodosa, may also lead to Mooren's or Mooren's-like ulcers.

The basic etiology of Mooren's ulcer is unknown. Recent evidence indicates, however, that autoimmune processes, both humoral and cell mediated, may play a role. Accidental or surgical trauma, which is often the precipitating event, may alter a portion of the cornea (probably the epithelium) and cause it to become recognized as foreign tissue. The finding of many plasma cells and lymphocytes in the adjacent conjunctiva is supportive of an autoimmune etiology.

THERAPY

Ocular. The use of frequent topical steroids (initially every 30 to 60 minutes), and tapering over 2 months as the ulcer heals, is of benefit. If there is no response to topical steroids, conjunctival resection should be considered.

Mooren's ulcers that develop after cataract surgery may respond to soft contact lens therapy. Some cases require topical steroids and soft contact lenses.

Topical antibiotics may be used to protect the eye from secondary infection while the ulcer is healing.

Surgical. Conjunctival excision is the therapeutic procedure of choice if topical steroids and soft lens therapy have failed. A 3-mm conjunctival resection adjacent to the ulcer with débridement of the ulcer bed and leading epithelial edge is usually adequate. Tarsorrhaphy may be combined with conjunctival resection to assist epithelial healing. Surgery performed at an early stage of the disease may preserve vision.

Glue or lamellar grafting may be necessary if the ulcer perforates. In end-stage ulcers, removal of the remaining central island of stroma can facilitate healing.

Systemic. Cyclosporine[‡] or immunosuppression[‡] should be considered when local therapy fails.

PRECAUTIONS

Although a few cases of successful penetrating keratoplasty have been reported, Mooren's ulcer is often reactivated after keratoplasty or cataract surgery.

COMMENTS

The visual acuity in patients with Mooren's ulcer that has progressed across the central cornea may improve when the disease becomes inactive. The eyes develop a vascularized flap of conjunctival origin covering a markedly thin stroma. Because of the risk of reactivating the ulcer in the graft after surgery, these patients are usually best served with the vision provided by their thinned vascularized cornea.

References

Berkowitz PJ, et al: Presence of circulating immune complexes in patients with peripheral corneal disease. Arch Ophthalmol 101:242–245, 1983.

Brown SI, Mondino BJ: Penetrating keratoplasty in Mooren's ulcer. Am J Ophthalmol 89:255–258, 1980.

Brown SI, Mondino BJ: Therapy of Mooren's ulcer. Am J Ophthalmol 98:1–6, 1984.

Foster CS: Systemic immunosuppressive therapy for progressive bilateral Mooren's ulcer. Ophthalmology 92:1436–1439, 1985.

Hill JC, Potter P: Treatment of Mooren's ulcer with cyclosporin A: report of three cases. Br J Ophthalmol 71:11–15, 1987.

Martin NF, Stark WJ, Maumenee AE: Treatment of Mooren's and Mooren's-like ulcer by lamellar keratectomy: Report of six eyes and literature review. Ophthalmic Surg 18:564–569, 1987.

Murray PI, Rahi AHS: Pathogenesis of Mooren's ulcer: Some new concepts. Br J Ophthalmol 68:182–187, 1984.

Smolin G, O'Connor GR: Ocular Immunology. Philadelphia, Lea & Febiger, 1981, pp 171–178.

Wakefield D, Robinson LP: Cyclosporin therapy in Mooren's ulcer. Br J Ophthalmol 71:415–417, 1987.

Wood TO, Tuberville AW, Murrah W: Corneal problems following cataract surgery. *In* Emery JM, Jacobsen AC (eds): Current Concepts in Cataract Surgery. New York, Appleton-Century-Crofts, 1981, pp 193–199.

Supported by the Baptist Memorial Hospital Clinical Innovations Research Fund.

PELLUCID MARGINAL CORNEAL DEGENERATION
(Corneal Piriformis)

MARK S. DRESNER, M.D.,
and DAVID J. SCHANZLIN, M.D.

St. Louis, Missouri

Pellucid marginal corneal degeneration or corneal piriformis affects the inferior peripheral cornea bilaterally and results in marked thinning of the cornea. There is usually no evidence of scarring, infiltration, vascularization, iron ring, or lipid deposition. This condition is most commonly diagnosed between the ages of 20 and 40 years and occurs equally in males and females. Patients usually present with high degrees of irregular astigmatism. The 1- to 2-mm wide band of corneal thinning is characteristically located near the inferior limbus, causing an area of cylindrical protrusion of the cornea. Concentric Descemet's folds can develop near the inferior limbus, and acute hydrops is an infrequent complication.

The etiology of pellucid marginal corneal degeneration is unknown; however, heredity does appear to be a factor. Recently, similar changes in the epithelium and basement membrane have been reported in pellucid marginal corneal degeneration and keratoconus; similarly, collagen, such as the fibrous long-spacing (FLS) type with a periodicity of 100 to 110 nm versus 60 to 64 nm in normals, is seen in this entity, as well as advanced keratoconus. Some authors suggest that the pellucid marginal corneal degeneration most likely represents a peripheral form of keratoconus. Bowman's layer may be normal, focally disrupted, or completely absent in the area of the thin band. Descemet's membrane and endothelium are usually normal.

THERAPY

Ocular. Spectacle correction is usually unsatisfactory because of the irregular and high astigmatism. Contact lenses are difficult to fit because of the degree of astigmatism; however, when they can be worn, their use results in good vision. When the disease has progressed to such an extent that hard contact lenses cannot be worn, fitting with a piggyback contact lens system (therapeutic bandage lens with overlying hard lens) is frequently successful.

Surgical. Penetrating keratoplasty has provided good results for the treatment of the cylindrical corneal protrusion and, for this reason, is considered a viable treatment in advanced cases of pellucid marginal degeneration of the cornea. Alternative modes of therapy include corneal wedge resection and thermokeratoplasty. Additionally, inferior lamellar patch grafts have been successful in reducing the inferior ectasia of the cornea, which results from the marked corneal thinning, and have not only allowed patients to resume contact lens wear but have also reduced the degree of high astigmatism.

PRECAUTIONS

Penetrating keratoplasty frequently tends to be accompanied by more complications when performed for pellucid marginal corneal degeneration than when used for keratoconus, primarily because of the larger graft that must be positioned to reach the limbus inferiorly. Surgery with such large penetrating grafts has a greater tendency to vascularize and results in erosion of the sutures. Thermokeratoplasty remains an unproven procedure for this disorder; this technique should be approached with caution, since it has been shown to cause endothelial damage, as well as persistent epithelial healing problems. In cases where there has been contact lens failure, an inferior lamellar patch graft to stabilize the structurally weakened inferior cornea and to steepen the flat vertical meridian should be considered.

COMMENTS

Pellucid marginal corneal degeneration is an infrequently diagnosed disorder. The condition is rare, and most of the literature on this condition is from Europe. Pellucid degeneration of the cornea affects the inferior portion of the cornea and does not extend into the limbus; it is without vascularization or lipid infiltration, and the cornea retains normal sensitivity, thus differentiating it from other peripheral corneal thinning diseases, such as Terrien's marginal degeneration, Mooren's ulceration, or senile marginal degeneration. The central cornea retains normal thickness, and the high astigmatism results from the inferior weakening and bowing forward of the inferior cornea, also serving to differentiate this condition from other corneal disorders that result in high irregular astigmatism and corneal thinning, such as central keratoconus, posterior keratoconus, keratoglobus, and keratotorus.

References

Kolker AE, Hetherington, J Jr: Becker-Shaffer's Diagnosis and Therapy of the Glaucomas. 4th ed, St. Louis, CV Mosby, 1976, p 397.

Krachmer JH: Pellucid marginal corneal degeneration. Arch Ophthalmol 96:1217–1221, 1978.

Krachmer JH, Feder RS, Belin MW: Keratoconus and related non-inflammatory corneal thinning disorders. Surv Ophthalmol 28:293–322, 1984.

Petursson GJ, Fraunfelder FT: Repair of an inadvertent buttonhole or leaking filtering bleb. Arch Ophthalmol 97:926–927, 1979.

Rodrigues MM, et al: Pellucid marginal corneal degeneration: A clinicopathologic study of two cases. Exp Eye Res 33:277–288, 1981.

Yannuzzi LA, Theodore FH: Cryotherapy of post-cataract blebs. Am J Ophthalmol 76:217–222, 1973.

TERRIEN'S MARGINAL DEGENERATION
(Furrow Dystrophy, Marginal Ectasia, Peripheral Furrow Keratitis)

MARK J. MANNIS, M.D.

Sacramento, California

Terrien's marginal degeneration is an uncommon condition of unknown etiology that is characterized by slowly progressive, marginal corneal thinning and ectasia. It is most often bilateral but may be asymmetric, and it occurs most commonly in the 20- to 30-year-old age group with predominance in males. Progression of the disease is slow and occurs over a period of years. The furrowing and ectasia of the cornea are commonly seen at the superior limbus and are preceded by fine peripheral vascularization and marginal opacification. These changes are followed by progression to marginal furrowing or gutter formation which steadily deepens. Irregular deposits of lipid appear at the leading edge of the furrow. The paralimbal thinning may also involve the inferior limbus or progress circumferentially, although the interpalpebral cornea is most commonly spared. This slow process is nonulcerative, and patients are not commonly symptomatic with pain. Clinical symptoms develop when the continued thinning produces blurred vision from high degrees of against-the-rule astigmatism. As the limbal thinning progresses, the cornea flattens in the vertical meridian, producing high degrees of corneal astigmatism. Severely thinned and ectatic areas may perforate spontaneously or with minor trauma.

THERAPY

Supportive. No medical therapy is effective in preventing progression of the disease. Supportive therapy in the initial stages consists of spectacle correction of the astigmatic refractive error. Rigid toric contact lenses or piggyback soft/rigid lens systems may be necessary as the astigmatism progresses.

Surgical. In advanced cases of Terrien's marginal degeneration, contact lens fitting may no longer be possible. In addition, ectatic areas may become dangerously thin. In such cases, surgery may be indicated both to correct the astigmatism and to prevent rupture of the globe through structural reinforcement. A variety of surgical approaches have been suggested, including excision of the ectatic tissue followed by suturing of the walls of the furrow, annular full-thickness keratoplasty, crescentic lamellar keratoplasty, and large eccentric penetrating grafts.

Ocular or Periocular Manifestations

Cornea: Flattening of the corneal curvature in the vertical meridian; perforation; peripheral thinning and ectasia; peripheral vascularization and lipid deposition.

Other: Episodic irritation; high astigmatism with blurred vision.

PRECAUTIONS

In the majority of cases, conservative management is indicated. Because of the thinning and ectasia in more advanced cases, mild trauma can result in rupture of the thinned area. Such patients should therefore be instructed to avoid situations in which the eye might be traumatized. The dispensing of protective eyewear may be warranted. Patients should be cautioned to seek attention for any abrupt change in their visual status or for the development of pain in the eye.

COMMENTS

Although a rare disorder, Terrien's degeneration typically comes to the attention of the ophthalmologist either when the patient becomes visually symptomatic because of progressive astigmatism or after recurrent episodes of ocular irritation. This slowly progressive, generally noninflammatory disease can most often be managed conservatively, but must be followed periodically for progression to thinning, which might threaten the integrity of the globe.

References

Brown AC, Rao NG, Aquavella JV: Peripheral corneal grafts in Terrien's marginal degeneration. Ophthalmic Surg 14:931–934, 1983.

Caldwell DR, et al: Primary surgical repair of severe marginal ectasia in Terrien's marginal degeneration. Am J Ophthalmol 97:332–336, 1984.

Goldman KN, Kaufman HE: Atypical pterygium: A clinical feature of Terrien's marginal degeneration. Arch Ophthalmol 96:1027–1029, 1978.

Robin JB, et al: Peripheral corneal disorders. Surv Ophthalmol 31:1–36, 1986.

Suveges I, Levai G, Alberth B: Pathology of Terrien's disease: Histochemical and electron microscopic study. Am J Ophthalmol 74:1191–1200, 1972.

Dystrophies Affecting Primarily the Corneal Epithelium

EPITHELIAL BASEMENT MEMBRANE DYSTROPHY
(Cogan's Microcystic Corneal Dystrophy, Map, Dot, Fingerprint Dystrophy)

and RECURRENT EROSION
(Recurrent Epithelial Erosion)

PETER R. LAIBSON, M.D.
Philadelphia, Pennsylvania

Corneal erosion and recurrent corneal erosion are common ocular disorders that are sometimes preceded by trauma but at other times occur spontaneously. In the spontaneous cases of corneal erosion, the underlying disease process may be an epithelial basement membrane corneal dystrophy.

Epithelial basement membrane dystrophy is usually a bilateral epithelial disorder characterized by various patterns of intraepithelial dots, linear changes that mimic the appearance of maps, and other corneal irregularities, such as parallel lines, which may bring to mind fingerprints. The intraepithelial dots consist of opaque putty-gray intraepithelial cysts that are located usually in the central two thirds of the cornea. These cysts are made up of cytoplasmic and nuclear debris and range in size from a pinpoint lesion to a cyst measuring up to 2 mm across. They may be oval, oblong, or comma shaped and are associated with the map and the fingerprint patterns in most cases. Microcysts are rarely found alone, but map and fingerprint changes are commonly seen without the presence of microcysts (dots).

This disorder occurs in adults of both sexes, although somewhat more commonly in females and usually after the fourth decade. It is probably hereditary, with variable penetrance, although in 6 per cent of a large study population, these changes were present in some form.

Map and fingerprint alterations are not rare and can be found in asymptomatic individuals without prior history of trauma or ocular disease. They are frequently seen in conditions where there is corneal edema, such as near the healing incision of a cataract wound or in the central cornea in Fuchs' corneal dystrophy.

Fingerprint lines histologically are similar to map-like changes, since both have an aberrant or multilaminar basement membrane produced by the basal epithelial cells of the corneal epithelium. At least 80 to 90 per cent of patients who have epithelial basement membrane dystrophy are asymptomatic. Symptoms, when they are present, consist of slightly blurred vision when the epithelial and basement membrane changes are in the visual axis or foreign body sensation with recurrent erosion when the epithelium is loose.

Recurrent corneal erosions may follow corneal trauma that involves the epithelium and basement membrane. Recurrent epithelial erosions probably occur as a result of inadequate basement membrane healing, either because the basal epithelial cells fail to produce a proper basement membrane that attaches to Bowman's membrane and stroma or because of faulty basement membrane adherence.

Recurrent epithelial erosions tend to recur in the early morning during sleep and often awaken the patient with a sharp pain. In rare cases, patients so fea. the pain on awakening that they are unable to sleep well at night. The very common sharp pain on opening the eyelids either during sleep or on awakening in the morning may be fleeting, lasting only seconds, or it may last for minutes to an hour or two. In most cases, this sharp pain is only fleeting and is a warning that the epithelium is not completely healed. Continued use of precautionary measures, such as not rubbing the eyes through the lids on awakening, and medications to prevent recurrent erosion, are necessary as long as the fleeting, sharp pain occurs in the morning.

THERAPY

Ocular. The greatest problem facing patients with epithelial basement membrane dystrophy is pain from recurrent corneal erosion. If the erosion is small, it will usually heal spontaneously or with the aid of a pressure patch placed on the eye for a day or two. Usually, a lubricating or an antibiotic ointment, such as bacitracin or erythromycin, is used beneath the pressure patch. Resistant cases may well require mechanical débridement, depending on the size of the defect or the amount of ocular irritation. Local cycloplegics may be necessary. The minor corneal erosion may be treated with lubricating ointments alone for several weeks to several months to control symptoms.

Soft contact lenses have been helpful in cases with multiple recurrent corneal erosions. However, concern about extended soft contact lens use persists because of the fear of corneal infectious disease.

In some cases, very mild corneal erosion may be prevented by using 2 or 5 per cent sodium chloride drops during the day and 5 per cent sodium chloride ointment at bedtime. Many patients believe that sodium chloride ointment is no more effective than a lubricant ointment or an ointment without preservatives. Each person must establish a regimen of drug use that seems, to control symptoms most effectively. It might involve the use of medication only when symptoms recur or, in some instances, daily application for many months after the termination of a recurrent episode to prevent further recurrences.

With the more severe cases of recurrent corneal erosion that do not seem to heal with any of the above regimens, the use of anterior stromal puncture has been advocated. Anterior stromal puncture may be used for patients with severe multiple erosions that fail to heal with all previous therapeutic regimens. Forty to fifty puncture marks through the epithelium and Bowman's membrane are created into the anterior stroma, using a sharp 27-gauge needle. The needle is inserted through loosened epithelium and indents the cornea in order to enter the stroma. Patients who have had multiple recurrences and were not helped by débridement alone or débridement with cautery showed significant improvement with anterior corneal puncture.

Anterior corneal puncture is usually the final treatment for the most severe patients; in almost every case where this procedure is done, patients do respond to this treatment. Most patients respond after the first episode of anterior corneal puncture, but a few may require repeated anterior corneal puncture. This is a relatively innocuous but very helpful way to treat the most severe cases of recurrent corneal erosion.

The use of fibronectin[†] epidermal growth factor[†] or other locally active macromolecules are still experimental.

Ocular or Periocular Manifestations

Cornea: Epithelial blebs; opacity (punctate, striate, map, dot, geographic, fingerprint).
Other: Astigmatism; irritation; visual loss.

PRECAUTIONS

Treatment should be as simple as possible with as few drugs as necessary. Some drugs, such as local anesthetics, have been shown to delay epithelial wound healing. For this reason, it is imperative never to prescribe a topical anesthetic for the patient's own use, even when symptoms are severe.

Indications for chemical cautery or lamellar keratectomy for resistant erosions have become almost nonexistent with the advent of therapeutic soft contact lenses and now anterior stromal puncture. Owing to the cost of the lens and frequent follow-up visits, the use of long-term therapeutic soft contact lenses should be delayed, and anterior corneal puncture should be relied on for treatment of the most severe cases.

COMMENTS

Systemic disease does not appear to play a role in epithelial basement membrane dystrophy or recurrent corneal erosion.

References

Cogan DG, et al: Microcystic dystrophy of the corneal epithelium. Trans Am Ophthalmol Soc 62:213–225, 1964.
Laibson PR: Microcystic corneal dystrophy. Trans Am Ophthalmol Soc 74:488–531, 1976.
McLean EN, MacRae SM, Rich LF: Recurrent erosion. Treatment by anterior stromal puncture. Ophthalmology 93: 784–788, 1986.
Trobe JD, Laibson PR: Dystrophic changes in the anterior cornea. Arch Ophthalmol 87:378–382, 1972.

JUVENILE CORNEAL EPITHELIAL DYSTROPHY
(Meesmann's Corneal Dystrophy)

ROBERT P. BURNS, M.D.
Columbia, Missouri

Juvenile corneal epithelial dystrophy is a rare, autosomal dominant dystrophy of the corneal epithelium with minimal severity. The dystrophy is present in the first few months of life, but may go unnoticed, since discomfort and visual loss are minimal. In later life, some irritation and diminishing visual acuity may appear. Slitlamp observation reveals bilateral epithelial cysts, which appear as tiny gray-white punctate opacities distributed profusely in the interpalpebral zone of the cornea. Examination of the cysts by focal illumination demonstrates mainly debris, which is small in proportion to the volume of the cysts themselves. Retroillumination shows regular and spherical cysts, occasionally fused and varying in diameter from 10 to 50 μ. The corneal epithelium as a whole does not appear edematous, although a slight haze may be seen between cysts. In time, the whole epithelium may be diffusely affected by the dystrophy. Sometimes, a whorl-shaped pattern is seen, and opacities at the level of Bowman's membrane may occur. The toxic changes in corneal epithelium induced by tetracaine anesthesia resemble Meesmann's dystrophy.

THERAPY

Surgical. Treatment of juvenile corneal epithelial dystrophy is usually unnecessary, since the visual acuity of many patients remains unimpaired. If visual acuity is significantly impaired, lamellar keratoplasty may be indicated. It should include removal of the diseased epithelium and basement membrane, as well as Bowman's layer and the superficial corneal stroma, which contain an "inducing factor" for the epithelial dystrophy.

Ocular or Periocular Manifestations

Cornea: Cicatrization; epithelial cysts; haze; opacity in Bowman's membrane.
Other: Decreased visual acuity; irritation; lacrimation; photophobia.

PRECAUTIONS

Medical therapy does not seem to be of any help, since the abnormality responsible for the degeneration of the epithelial cells has not been identified. Eugenic control seems unnecessary for such a nondisabling hereditary disorder.

Epithelial scraping is an ineffective procedure in the treatment of this disorder, since it does not remove the "inducing factor" in Bowman's membrane. In time, juvenile corneal epithelial dystrophy may return in an area of prior superficial keratectomy.

Recently, the symptoms and epithelial microcysts in Meesmann's dystrophy were reported to be greatly reduced by prolonged wear of soft contact lenses.

Comments

The exact pathogenic mechanism in this disorder is not yet known. Current evidence seems to implicate a chemically unknown substance deposited in the corneal epithelial cells, possibly under the influence of an "inducing factor" in the superficial corneal stroma. This substance leads to cell death and cyst formation in the epithelium, with rapid regrowth of epithelium. Clinical diagnosis is not difficult, but laboratory confirmation can be obtained only by transmission electron microscopy.

References

Bourne WM: Soft contact lens wear decreases epithelial microcysts in Meesmann's corneal dystrophy. Trans Am Ophthalmol Soc 84:170–178, 1986.

Bron AJ, Tripathi RC: Cystic disorders of the corneal epithelium. I. Clinical aspects. Br J Ophthalmol 57:361–375, 1973.

Burns RP: Meesmann's corneal dystrophy. Trans Am Ophthalmol Soc 66:530–635, 1968.

Fine BS, et al: Meesmann's epithelial dystrophy of the cornea. Am J Ophthalmol 83:633–642, 1977.

Grayson M: Degenerations, dystrophies, and edema of the cornea. In Duane TD (ed): Clinical Ophthalmology. Hagerstown, MD, Harper & Row, 1982, Vol IV, pp 16:7–8.

Malbran ES: Corneal dystrophies: A clinical, pathological, and surgical approach. Am J Ophthalmol 74:771–809, 1972.

Pülhorn G, Thiel H-J: Licht- und elektronenmikroskopische Untersuchungen über die Zystenbildung bei hereditärer Hornhautepitheldystrophie Meesmann-Wilke. Ophthalmologica 168:348–359, 1974.

REIS-BÜCKLERS' SUPERFICIAL CORNEAL DYSTROPHY
(Bücklers' Annular Corneal Dystrophy)

FRANK M. POLACK, M.D., F.A.C.S.

Gainesville, Florida

Reis-Bücklers' dystrophy is a corneal disease characterized by recurrent epithelial erosions that start early in life and by irregular opacities and thickening of Bowman's membrane. The dystrophy has a dominant mode of transmission, is usually bilateral, symmetric, and becomes evident in the first or second decade of life. The first symptoms are usually those of foreign body sensation. Visual acuity is not affected until the late twenties. Slit lamp examination shows epithelial alterations over areas of Bowman's thickening and interwoven ring-like opacities. Opacities have also been observed in the superficial stromal layers; however, the middle and deeper layers of the stroma and the endothelium are not involved. Corneal sensitivity may be decreased. Histologic studies show destruction of Bowman's layer and replacement by fibrous tissue. Fibroblasts have been seen compromising the superficial corneal stroma, intermixed with layers of regular collagen interspersed with collagen fibrils that acquire a curly configuration. These findings have been considered characteristic of this disease. The recurrent epithelial erosion is caused by the abnormal basement membrane and lack of hemidesmosomes, which are missing where Bowman's membrane has been destroyed.

THERAPY

Ocular. The treatment of Reis-Bücklers' dystrophy in early stages consists of the use of ocular lubricants and patching during the episodes of recurrent erosion. The use of soft (bandage) contact lenses is helpful in some patients with frequent episodes of erosion.

Surgical. When the vision is compromised, a superficial keratectomy is preferable to a lamellar corneal transplant. If necessary, this keratectomy can be performed at least twice in a given patient. Recurrence of the disease may develop in the corneal surface after keratectomy and keratoplasty, but may not appear for 2 to 6 or more years. Abnormal substances in conjunctival or limbal epithelial cells may be responsible for the recurrences following surgery.

Precautions

Penetrating keratoplasty is not indicated in this type of dystrophy.

Comments

There are two hypotheses for the causes of Reis-Bücklers' dystrophy. The first is that the primary changes occur in Bowman's membrane with secondary epithelial changes. The other theory is that an abnormal epithelium leads to degeneration of keratocytes and Bowman's membrane.

References

Hogan MJ, Wood I: Reis-Bücklers' corneal dystrophy. Trans Ophthalmol Soc UK 91:41–57, 1971.

Malbran ES: Corneal dystrophies: A clinical, pathological, and surgical approach. Am J Ophthalmol 74:771–809, 1972.

Dystrophies Affecting Primarily the Corneal Stroma

CRYSTALLINE CORNEAL DYSTROPHY
(Schnyder's Crystalline Corneal Dystrophy)

MALCOLM N. LUXENBERG, M.D.

Augusta, Georgia

Schnyder's crystalline dystrophy is a bilateral corneal disease with little or no progression. It is inherited as an autosomal dominant trait, and onset occurs in early life, possibly being congenital. The lesions are oval or round with irregular borders, and the margins tend to be denser than the center of the lesion. The opacities are usually located in the central cornea and grossly appear yellowish-white. On slitlamp examination, many fine, needle-shaped, colored crystals are seen in the anterior stroma with some involvement of Bowman's membrane, and occasional crystals can be noted in the deeper stroma. The surrounding cornea is usually clear, although there have been cases reported with stromal haze or small, white, scattered punctate opacities. The epithelium, endothelium, and Descemet's membrane are normal. A corneal arcus and Vogt's limbal girdle are frequently present, and corneal sensation is occasionally decreased. There are usually no edema, abnormal vascularization, or signs of previous inflammation. Xanthelasma has been noted in some patients; rarely, there may be associated skeletal abnormalities. Visual acuity is usually good, but in a few cases, vision has been decreased enough to warrant keratoplasty. Except for decreased vision, the lesions are usually asymptomatic. Hyperlipidemia and hyperlipoproteinemia have been noted in some patients, but this is not a universal finding. There is no firm evidence of a direct relationship between abnormal elevation of serum lipids and development of the lesions. Histologic studies have shown that the crystalline material is cholesterol, especially the esterified form; in addition, there is a deposition of neutral fats in the corneal stroma. The pathogenesis of the corneal changes is unknown.

THERAPY

Systemic. Dietary measures and drug therapy to lower serum lipids have not been shown to have any beneficial effects on the lesions.

Surgical. In most patients, surgical treatment is not necessary as the visual acuity is not affected. However, if vision is significantly decreased by the corneal lesion, keratoplasty may be performed.

Ocular or Periocular Manifestations

Cornea: Arcus; hypesthesia; stromal opacities; Vogt's limbal girdle.
Eyelids: Xanthelasma.

PRECAUTIONS

Crystalline corneal dystrophy must be differentiated from other crystalline deposits in the cornea that may be seen in association with cystinosis or the dysproteinemias. Crystals may recur in the cornea after keratoplasty, but it is not known whether these represent the same abnormal materials as those present before transplantation.

COMMENTS

The etiology of the crystalline corneal lesions is unknown. They may be the result of a defect in corneal lipid metabolism that may be modified by abnormally elevated serum lipids.

References

Bron AJ, Williams HP, Carruthers ME: Hereditary crystalline stromal dystrophy of Schnyder. I. Clinical features of a family with hyperlipoproteinaemia. Br J Ophthalmol 56:383–399, 1972.
Delleman JW, Winkelman JE: Degeneratio corneae cristallinea hereditaria. A clinical, genetical and histological study. Ophthalmologica 155:409–426, 1968.
Ehlers N, Matthiessen ME: Hereditary crystalline corneal dystrophy of Schnyder. Acta Ophthalmol 51:316–324, 1973.
Garner A, Tripathi RC: Hereditary crystalline stromal dystrophy of Schnyder. II. Histopathology and ultrastructure. Br J Ophthalmol 56:400–408, 1972.
Luxenberg M: Hereditary crystalline dystrophy of the cornea. Am J Ophthalmol 63:507–511, 1967.
Rodrigues MM, et al: Unesterified cholesterol in Schnyder's corneal crystalline dystrophy. Am J Ophthalmol 104:157–163, 1987.
Weller RO, Rodger FC: Crystalline stromal dystrophy: Histochemistry and ultrastructure of the cornea. Br J Ophthalmol 64:46–52, 1980.

Williams HP, et al: Hereditary crystalline corneal dystrophy with an associated blood lipid disorder. Trans Ophthalmol Soc UK 91:531–541, 1971.

GRANULAR CORNEAL DYSTROPHY
(Bücklers' Type I; Groenouw's Type I)
KAMAL F. NASSIF, M.D.,
and ROBERT A. HYNDIUK, M.D.
Milwaukee, Wisconsin

Granular dystrophy is an autosomal dominant inherited dystrophy that tends to affect both eyes symmetrically. It becomes apparent in the first decade of life as superficial stromal and central irregular white opacities. These opacities, most of which are located under Bowman's membrane, assume different shapes and sizes that do not usually exceed 0.5 mm in diameter. They are nontransparent in direct and retroillumination. At this stage, the intervening stroma is clear, and the epithelium is regular and uninvolved; these patients are therefore asymptomatic. Early in the first and second decade, the visual acuity is normal.

As the affected individual gets older, the opacities enlarge and increase in number and may even coalesce, with loss of the characteristically clear intervening stroma. A diffuse, superficial stromal, ground glass haze develops during the fourth and fifth decades, and visual acuity starts to decline. The opacities progressively involve the deeper stroma and the midperiphery, whereas the far periphery is characteristically clear even late in the disease. A less common confluent superficial form may be confused with the geographic type of Reis-Bücklers' dystrophy, with opacification extending beyond the central area leaving only a peripheral clear vein of uninvolved clear cornea.

The epithelium and basement membrane are usually not clinically affected. When such involvement occurs, it is usually late in the disease and produces an irregularity of the surface with a resultant irregular astigmatism and decreased visual acuity. Depending on the extent of involvement of the epithelium, recurrent erosions may result, causing pain, foreign body sensation, and photophobia.

The lesions of granular dystrophy are eosinophilic accumulations of noncollagenous proteins that histologically stain intensely red with Masson's trichome stain and fail to do so with periodic acid-Schiff. They are sharply demarcated and interdigitate with the collagen fibrils, which retain their normal structure and organization. The lesions appear to concentrate around keratocytes, which often show nonspecific changes consisting of either degenerative or active intracellular changes. This has prompted some investigators to assume that the pathology lies within the keratocytes.

Ultrastructurally, electron-dense, rod-shaped crystals have been found that are 100 to 500 μm in diameter and of variable morphologic organization. Recent reports have shown these rod-shaped granules to be surrounded by microfibrils. The granules stain with protein stains and with Luxol fast blue, suggesting a phospholipid composition possibly from abnormal degradation of corneal epithelial cell membranes containing specific phospholipid-protein complexes. The stromal deposits could result from a genetic defect in processing or assembly of membrane-derived corneal epithelial proteins and phospholipids. Also immunohistologic stains show that the deposits react at the edges with antibodies to form microfibrillar protein. These granules have not only been noted in the superficial stroma but also in the epithelial and subepithelial layers. An epithelial etiology has been suggested by the detection of these granules intraepithelially as well both in primary and recurrent dystrophy.

Granular corneal dystrophy is localized in the cornea without associated ocular or systemic disease. It has, however, been noted to occur coincidentally in a family with retinal degeneration and albinism and in another family with ectodermal dysplasia.

THERAPY

Supportive. Granular dystrophy has variable expressivity and therefore may remain asymptomatic in some patients. Even when it progresses, it does so late in life, starting during the fifth or sixth decade. Recurrent erosions are rare, but when they do occur, they do so late in the disease and are treated symptomatically with lubrication, patching, or even soft contact lenses. The latter may control the recurrence of the erosions and may help improve the visual acuity, as they mask the epithelial irregularity.

Surgical. When the opacities progress and coalesce and the visual acuity decreases sufficiently to interfere with the patient's life-style, surgical treatment is recommended. Since the opacities usually lie in the superficial stroma, Descemet's membrane and endothelium remain unaffected even when the opacities extend deep into the stroma. Therefore, a lamellar keratoplasty should be adequate to achieve a clear cornea devoid of opacities. However, since the visual results obtained with penetrating keratoplasty are superior to those following lamellar keratoplasty, penetrating keratoplasty has become the procedure of choice. The success rate of clear grafts maintained for over 10 years after penetrating keratoplasty for granular dystrophy is over 90 per cent.

Supported in part by an unrestricted grant from Research to Prevent Blindness, Inc. and supported in part by Ophthalmic Research Core Grant EY-01931.

PRECAUTIONS

Recurrence of granular dystrophy, although uncommon, may develop in either a lamellar or penetrating graft between 1 and 19 years after the surgical procedure. This recurrence may be related to repopulation of the donor cornea with "diseased" host epithelium or keratocytes. Recurrence most commonly occurs as a deposition of the hyaline opacities between the epithelium and Bowman's membrane. These subepithelial deposits often can be shaved off with a Bard-Parker blade in the office, with prompt healing following pressure patching in 2 to 3 days.

COMMENTS

The hyaline deposits may represent a metabolic product of corneal epithelial cells, rather than a product of collagen breakdown, since the hyaline material is a noncollagenous protein with an amino acid composition that is similar to keratohyaline. However, these deposits fail to react with antibodies to keratin. They have recently been shown to contain phospholipids and microfibrillar proteins. The location of the deposits, the chemical composition, and the recent demonstration of intracellular changes in the overlying epithelium in primary and recurrent granular dystrophy support the concept that the epithelium, rather than the keratocytes, may be the source of this abnormal material.

The best criterion at present for a definite diagnosis of granular dystrophy is transmission electron microscopy, which reveals the characteristic electron-dense, crystalline, rod-shaped bodies.

References

Akiya S, Brown SI: Granular dystrophy of the cornea, characteristic electron microscopic lesion. Arch Ophthalmol 84:179–192, 1970.

Brownstein S, et al: Granular dystrophy of the cornea. Light and electron microscopic confirmation of recurrence in a graft. Am J Ophthalmol 77:701–710, 1974.

Rodrigues MM, Krachmer JH: Recent advances in corneal stromal dystrophies. Cornea 7:19–29, 1988.

Rodrigues MM, Gaster RN, Pratt MV: Unusual superficial confluent form of granular corneal dystrophy. Ophthalmology 90:1507–1511, 1983.

Rodrigues MM, et al: Microfibrillar protein and phospholipid in granular corneal dystrophy. Arch Ophthalmol 101:802–810, 1983.

Spencer WH: Ophthalmic Pathology. Philadelphia, WB Saunders, 1985, Vol I, pp 320–325.

Waring GO III, Rodrigues MM, Laibson PR: Corneal dystrophies. I. Dystrophies of the epithelium, Bowman's layer and stroma. Surv Ophthalmol 23:71–122, 1978.

LATTICE CORNEAL DYSTROPHY
(Lattice Dystrophy Type I, Lattice Dystrophy Type II, LCD-I, LCD-II, Meretoja's Syndrome)

ROBERT A. HYNDIUK, M.D.
Milwaukee, Wisconsin

Lattice corneal dystrophy type I (LCD-I) is an autosomal dominantly inherited dystrophy that usually affects both eyes symmetrically. It is characterized by a localized corneal deposition of amyloid that is unrelated to systemic disease. It appears in the first or second decade of life as characteristic refractile anterior stromal branching filamentous lines, focal white dots or dashes, or faint central stromal opacities. The deposits are prominent centrally and spare the peripheral 2 to 3 mm of cornea. The dystrophy is slowly progressive, with the lesions involving deeper cornea and the opacity becoming denser and visually disabling usually by the third or fourth decade. Occasionally, the first symptoms of the disease may be noted in childhood or in the sixth or seventh decade; there is a considerable variation among different families in the age at which symptoms appear. Symptoms of photophobia, foreign body sensation, and pain from recurrent corneal epithelial erosions may be prominent in some patients. As corneal sensation decreases, the recurrent epithelial erosions become less painful. Irregular surface corneal astigmatism further decreases functional vision. Clinically, some forms of LCD-I have been misdiagnosed as herpes simplex keratitis during erosion episodes.

The characteristic microscopic finding in the stroma is a fusiform deposit of amyloid that pushes aside the collagen lamellae, probably corresponding to the lattice lines and dots seen clinically. Portions of Bowman's membrane are replaced by the deposits and irregular connective tissue. These changes are associated with recurrent erosions clinically. The stromal deposits appear pink histologically with Congo red and exhibit dichroism and increased birefringence. Electron microscopy of the lesions shows a felt-like mass of fine (8- to 10-nm diameter), nonbranching short fibrils without periodicity that are approximately half the size of adjacent collagen, and are sometimes associated with amorphous, electron-dense elastoid material. The keratocytes often have prominent endoplasmic reticulum, and they show degeneration. Immunohistochemical studies have detected lectin receptors suggesting a variety of amyloid glycoconjugates. The source of amyloid accumulation is unknown, but could be related to keratocytes or activated mononuclear cells.

Lattice corneal dystrophy type II (LCD-II, Meretoja's syndrome) is an autosomal dominant

---

Supported in part by an unrestricted grant from Research to Prevent Blindness, Inc. and supported in part by Ophthalmic Research Core Grant EY-01931.

form of LCD with an onset of clinical signs in the second decade. It is associated with systemic amyloidosis, including signs of progressive cranial and peripheral nerve palsies, dry skin, blepharochalasis, protruding lips, a "mask-like" facies, and bundle branch block. It is more common in Scandinavian countries, and only a few cases have been reported in the United States. Histologically, the corneal deposits are similar to those of LCD-I, with amyloid often surrounding nerve axons in peripheral stroma. Amyloid deposits are also found in conjunctiva below epithelium and in skin often around adnexal appendages and in subepidermal areas.

THERAPY

Ocular. Epithelial irregularities may result in recurrent erosions and cause additional visual loss from the irregular surface. Artificial tears, lubricating ointments, intermittent pressure patching, and soft contact lenses help control the recurrent erosions. Therapeutic soft contact lenses may also be helpful in improving vision, sometimes dramatically, by correcting the irregular surface.

Surgical. Penetrating keratoplasty has become the procedure of choice with a high success rate (approximately 90 per cent). However, the dystrophy may recur in up to 48 per cent of grafts after periods ranging from 3 to 26 years postoperatively, usually taking the form of subepithelial opacities or anterior stromal haze, and rarely lattice figures. In one large series, regrafting was necessary to restore vision in 15 per cent of penetrating keratoplasties for LCD-I.

Ocular or Periocular Manifestations

Cornea: Central stromal opacity; decreased corneal sensitivity; pseudodendritic staining; recurrent epithelial erosion; refractile anterior stromal lines; white stromal dots.

Other: Epiphora; irritation; ocular pain; photophobia; visual loss from opacity and irregular surface.

PRECAUTIONS

Diagnosis may occasionally be a problem, especially in some children. Examination of the child's parents may be helpful. Pseudodendritic corneal lesion during erosion episodes may be misdiagnosed as herpes simplex keratitis.

The patient should be advised about the risk of postoperative recurrence of dystrophy in the graft. Lattice corneal dystrophy recurs more commonly than macular or granular corneal dystrophy.

COMMENTS

Some investigators consider the lattice lines to represent degenerated corneal nerves, but in typical lattice dystrophy type I, there is no clear relationship between the corneal nerves and the amyloid deposits. The electron microscopic findings of a felt-like mass of short, fine, nonbranching fibrils is diagnostic for amyloid. Lattice dystrophy is unrelated to primary or secondary amyloidosis of the cornea. Keratocytes and possibly also corneal epithelial cells may have the ability to elaborate the amyloid material.

References

Klintworth GK: The cornea—structure and macromolecules. Am J Pathol 89:719–808, 1977.
Meisler DM, Fine M: Recurrence of the clinical signs of lattice corneal dystrophy (Type I) in corneal transplants. Am J Ophthalmol 97:210–214, 1984.
Meretoja J: Lattice corneal dystrophy—two different types. Ophthalmologica 165:15–37, 1972.
Panjwani N, et al: Lectin receptors of amyloid in corneas with lattice dystrophy. Arch Ophthalmol 105:688–691, 1987.
Purcell JJ, et al: Lattice corneal dystrophy associated with familial systemic amyloidosis (Meretoja's syndrome). Ophthalmology 90:1512–1517, 1983.
Rodrigues MM, Krachmer JH: Recent advances in corneal stromal dystrophies. Cornea 7:19–29, 1988.
Spencer WH: Ophthalmic Pathology. Philadelphia, WB Saunders, 1985, Vol I, pp 320–325.
Sturrock GD: Lattice corneal dystrophy: A source of confusion. Br J Ophthalmol 67:629–634, 1983.
Waring GO III, Rodrigues MM, Laibson PR: Corneal dystrophies. I. Dystrophies of the epithelium, Bowman's layer and stroma. Surv Ophthalmol 23:71–122, 1978.

MACULAR CORNEAL DYSTROPHY
(Fehr's Macular Dystrophy, Groenouw's Type II)

CLEMENT McCULLOCH, M.D., F.R.C.S.(C)

Toronto, Ontario

Macular dystrophy of the cornea is an autosomal recessive disorder characterized by bilateral multiple grayish-white opacities lying at all levels of the stroma. The corneal changes range in size from minute to 0.5 mm in diameter; they have hazy edges, and there may be stromal scarring between them. The opacities may protrude through Bowman's membrane, break through the epithelium, and result in erosion, with accompanying irritation and photophobia. As a result of the lifting up of epithelium by the lesions, irregular astigmatism may be produced. The changes end at the limbus and do not extend onto conjunctiva or to other ocular structures. The symptoms are those of progressive blurring and visual loss. They usually become noticeable in the early teens, and by middle age they may be severe. By the age of 40 or 50 years, the corneal scarring has usually become diffuse, and there is a loss of acuity below 20/200. There are no apparent systemic manifestations.

THERAPY

Supportive. If the disease is in its early stages and there are irregularities in the corneal surface resulting in irregular astigmatism, improvement in vision may be obtained with contact lenses. A contact lens can be helpful because it covers the irregular corneal surface, but it may not be tolerated.

Surgical. Penetrating keratoplasty is the procedure of choice, and chances of a clear graft are excellent. A 7.5- or 8.0-mm graft is preferable. Over the course of several years, a few opacities may develop in the graft, but the patient will have a number of years of clear vision.

Ocular or Periocular Manifestations

Cornea: Stromal nebulae, corneal leucoma, thickening of Descemet's membrane, stromal thinning.
Other: Visual loss, photophobia.

PRECAUTIONS

Although deep lamellar keratoplasty may improve vision somewhat, the density of the deep stromal opacities in the more advanced cases and the frequent coincidence of the thickening of Descemet's membrane often associated with guttate swelling constitute obstacles to perfect transparency that is difficult to overcome with this technique. Lamellar transplantation is not indicated because of the stromal changes that occur behind the base of a lamellar graft and the rapid extension of the opacities into the graft.

COMMENTS

The diagnosis of macular corneal dystrophy is made because of the appearance of the corneal disease, although the hereditary pattern is of help. The fuzzy edges of the opacities distinguish macular corneal dystrophy from granular corneal dystrophy in which the edges of the stromal granules are sharp and the neighboring stroma is clear without scarring. As time passes, the deep opacities become more marked. Descemet's membrane appears irregular, and it is not possible to assess the endothelium because of the opacities in front of it. If the corneal changes are advanced, the stromal scar will be diffuse. Clinical differentiation from other dystrophies will be difficult, and a firm diagnosis may depend on the pathologic finding of an accumulation of a mucopolysaccharide-like material in the stromal keratocytes. Some of this material appears to be extruded out of the cells and among the corneal fibrils. The material also can raise Bowman's membrane, break through it, and be present under the epithelial cells. It can be found penetrating Descemet's membrane and in the corneal endothelial cells. Involvement of Descemet's membrane may include the presence of guttate excrescences. There is a defect of keratan sulfate in cornea and in serum.

References

Bruner WE, Dejak TR, Grossniklaus HE, et al: Corneal alpha-galactosidase deficiency in macular corneal dystrophy. Ophthal Paediatr Genet 5:179–183, 1985.

Donnenfeld ED, Cohen EJ, Ingraham MJ, et al: Corneal thinning in macular dystrophy. Am J Ophthalmol 101:112–113, 1986.

Ghosh M, McCulloch C: Macular corneal dystrophy. Can J Ophthalmol 8:515–526, 1973.

Klintworth GK, Smith CF: Macular corneal dystrophy. Studies of sulfated glycosaminoglycans in corneal explant and confluent stromal cell cultures. Am J Pathol 89:167–182, 1977.

Klintworth GK, Meyer R, Dennis R, et al: Macular corneal dystrophy: lack of keratan sulfate in cornea and serum. Ophthal Paediatr Genet 7:139–143, 1986.

Lorenzetti DWC, Kaufman HE: Macular and lattice dystrophies and their recurrences after keratoplasty. Trans Am Acad Ophthalmol Otolaryngol 71:112–118, 1967.

Malbran ES: Corneal dystrophies: A clinical, pathological, and surgical approach. Trans Am Acad Ophthalmol Otolaryngol 76:573–624, 1972.

Pouliquen Y, et al: Combined macular dystrophy and cornea guttata: An electron microscopic study. Albrecht Von Graefes. Arch Klin Exp Ophthalmol 212:149–158, 1980.

Snip RC, Kenyon KR, Green WR: Macular corneal dystrophy: Ultrastructural pathology of corneal endothelium and Descemet's membrane. Invest Ophthalmol 12:88–97, 1973.

Dystrophies Affecting Primarily the Corneal Endothelium

CONGENITAL HEREDITARY ENDOTHELIAL DYSTROPHY
(CHED)

IRENE H. MAUMENEE, M.D.
Baltimore, Maryland

Two types of congenital hereditary endothelial dystrophy are recognized. The hereditary disorder can either occur as an autosomal recessive disorder at birth or as an autosomal dominant disorder during early to late childhood or even early adolescence. The clinical symptoms are similar and consist of diffuse corneal haze with significant thickening of the cornea secondary to dysfunction of the endothelium. In this disorder, the corneal endothelium is severely attenuated and may be totally absent. The disorder may be slowly progressive and lead to bullous epithelial changes in adulthood. The visual acuity varies between 20/40 and finger-counting vision. Otherwise, the eyes are normal, and the corneal diameter and the intraocular pressure are normal. There is no excess tearing. These features should help in the differential diagnosis from congenital glaucoma, which is commonly confused with CHED.

THERAPY

Surgical. In patients with severely reduced vision caused by corneal opacification or in those with a painful eye with bullous epithelial changes, corneal grafting is indicated. In milder cases, this procedure should be delayed.

Ocular or Periocular Manifestations

Cornea: Clouding; diffuse thickening or extreme thinness of Descemet's membrane; endothelial dysgenesis; stromal edema; stromal thickening.
Other: Amblyopia; nystagmus; visual loss.

PRECAUTIONS

Differential diagnosis of congenital corneal clouding includes congenital glaucoma, corneal dysgeneses (Peters' anomaly, sclerocornea, anterior staphyloma), posterior polymorphous dystrophy birth trauma with rupture of Descemet's membrane, metabolic diseases (mucopolysaccharidoses, mucolipidoses), and interstitial keratitis (luetic, herpetic).

COMMENTS

Congenital hereditary endothelial dystrophy is a disorder that commonly is misdiagnosed as congenital glaucoma, resulting in unnecessary surgical intervention in these patients. Given that there are two genetic types, the existence of two different pathogenetic mechanisms has to be assumed. However, the basic mechanisms are not known to date.

References

Antine B: Histology of congenital hereditary corneal dystrophy. Am J Ophthalmol 69:964–969, 1970.
Judisch GF, Maumenee IH: Clinical differentiation of recessive congenital hereditary endothelial dystrophy and dominant hereditary endothelial dystrophy. Am J Ophthalmol 85:606–612, 1978.
Kenyon KR, Antine B: The pathogenesis of congenital hereditary endothelial dystrophy of the cornea. Am J Ophthalmol 72:787–795, 1971.
Maumenee AE: Congenital hereditary corneal dystrophy. Am J Ophthalmol 50:1114–1124, 1960.
Pearce WG, Tripathi RC, Morgan G: Congenital endothelial corneal dystrophy. Clinical, pathological, and genetic study. Br J Ophthalmol 53:577–591, 1969.

FUCHS' CORNEAL DYSTROPHY
(Combined Dystrophy of Fuchs, Endothelial Dystrophy of the Cornea, Epithelial Dystrophy of Fuchs, Fuchs' Epithelial-Endothelial Dystrophy)

WILLIAM M. BOURNE, M.D.
Rochester, Minnesota

Fuchs' combined corneal dystrophy is a bilateral, slowly progressive corneal disease. It is characterized by endothelial degeneration that allows accumulation of water in the cornea and is followed by the development of dystrophic changes in the epithelium and eventually in the substantia propria. The condition is usually transmitted dominantly and occurs in elderly females two times as often as in males. All elements of the disease are ultimately caused by endothelial dysfunction that starts very early in life, but this dysfunction may not be manifest itself until the third to sixth decade of life. The first stage is an uncomplicated central endothelial dystrophy (cornea guttata), which progresses in disciform fashion toward the periphery and may extend from limbus to limbus. Fine pigment granules may be found centrally on the posterior surface of the cornea and within the endothelial cells. Symptoms are often absent. The second stage is characterized by edema of the stroma and the epithelium wherein bullae may be formed. Vision becomes affected, and haloes that are usually more serious in the morning, may occur. The third stage of subepithelial connective tissue formation with vascularization and scarring may result in a completely opaque cornea and loss of large superficial areas of epithelium. The final stage is one of complications, particularly glaucoma or infection.

THERAPY

Ocular. In early instances of epithelial edema, 5 per cent sodium chloride drops administered six to eight times a day and at bedtime may be used to decrease corneal edema and allow the patient to see better for a short period of time. This hyperosmotic agent acts primarily on the epithelial edema and has little or no influence on the stromal edema. It is especially useful in the morning when epithelial edema has accumulated during the night as the closed eyes have prevented evaporation. A hair dryer held at arm's length from the corneal surface may help decrease stromal edema. If discomfort is present as a result of bulla formation or rupture, a bandage soft contact lens may be beneficial.

The degree of edema that may appear in a cornea with Fuchs' dystrophy is in direct relation to the level of intraocular pressure. Incipient Fuchs' dystrophy in which the failure of endothelial function is just beginning to produce stromal and endothelial edema may sometimes be controlled temporarily by a reduction in the intraocular pressure, even though it is within normal limits. This reduction may be achieved by the use of miotics, such as 1 per cent pilocarpine three to four times daily or 0.25 per cent timolol twice daily.

These topical ophthalmic measures do not affect the progression of the endothelial dysfunction, however. They are useful as temporary therapy during the early stages of epithelial edema. Eventually, these measures offer no improvement, and keratoplasty offers the only hope for good vision.

Surgical. Over 90 per cent of penetrating corneal transplants for Fuchs' dystrophy are successful, resulting in clear grafts. Even corneas in the most advanced stages of the disease can be successfully operated on. Keratoplasty employing a 7.5- to 8.5-mm graft is the treatment of choice when the visual function is irreversibly compromised and no longer fulfills the patient's needs. Each case must be considered separately. A healthy active individual may merit keratoplasty when the visual acuity has decreased to 20/70 in the worse eye or to 20/40 (the visual acuity needed to drive an automobile) in the better eye when both eyes are affected. On the other hand, an old, infirm, or inactive individual may not benefit from keratoplasty until the visual acuity is less than 20/200 in both eyes. In some patients, a Gundersen-type, thin, conjunctival flap or even cauterization of superficial cornea may be helpful.

Ocular or Periocular Manifestations

Cornea: Bullous keratopathy; cicatrization; endothelial degeneration; epithelial and stromal edema; folds in Descemet's membrane; pigment on posterior surface; striae; vascularization; vesicles.

Other: Irritation; ocular pain; secondary glaucoma.

PRECAUTIONS

Anything that damages corneal endothelial cells, such as iridocyclitis or cataract extraction, can lead to more rapid progression of Fuchs' dystrophy and corneal decompensation.

Any corneal transplant is susceptible to immune rejection episodes, which, if not controlled, lead to graft failure and a permanently cloudy cornea. Transplant failures, however, may be regrafted with success. Rejection episodes should be treated with hourly administration of prednisolone eyedrops for several days, tapering the dosage over the next few weeks. If treated early, most transplants will clear.

COMMENTS

Penetrating keratoplasty is an effective treatment for Fuchs' dystrophy because it replaces the diseased corneal endothelial cells with normal cells. Lamellar corneal transplants are not indicated in this disease because they do not replace the dystrophic endothelial cells that are its cause.

Fuchs' dystrophy progresses slowly over many years, rather than in days or months. Therefore, the conservative topical ocular therapies mentioned earlier may suffice in the early stages of the disease for a year or more, and it may be several more years before keratoplasty is indicated.

References

Bourne WM, Johnson DH, Campbell RJ: The ultrastructure of Descemet's membrane. III. Fuchs' dystrophy. Arch Ophthalmol 100:1952–1955, 1982.

Davison JA, Bourne WM: Results of penetrating keratoplasty using a double running suture technique. Arch Ophthalmol 99:1591–1595, 1981.

Fine M, West CE: Late results of keratoplasty for Fuchs' dystrophy. Am J Ophthalmol 72:109–114, 1971.

Kenyon KR, Fogle JA, Grayson M: Dysgeneses, dystrophies, and degenerations of the cornea. In Duane TD (ed): Clinical Ophthalmology. Hagerstown, MD, Harper & Row, 1982, Vol IV, pp 16:33–35.

Krachmer JH, et al: Corneal endothelial dystrophy. A study of 64 families. Arch Ophthalmol 96:2036–2039, 1978.

Olson RJ, et al: Visual results after penetrating keratoplasty for aphakic bullous keratopathy and Fuchs' dystrophy. Am J Ophthalmol 88:1000–1004, 1979.

Waring GO III, Rodrigues MM, Laibson PR: Corneal dystrophies. II. Endothelial dystrophies. Surv Ophthalmol 23:147–168, 1978.

Wilson SE, Bourne WM: Fuchs' Dystrophy. Cornea 7:2–18, 1988.

Ectatic Conditions

KERATOCONUS
Mark J. Mannis, M.D.
Sacramento, California

Keratoconus is a noninflammatory corneal disorder characterized by bilateral axial thinning and protrusion of the cornea. The etiology of keratoconus has not been determined nor is there a consistent pattern of heredity. Keratoconus occurs in both sexes and is frequently an isolated phenomenon. It is more commonly associated with a history of generalized atopy, contact lens wear, Down's syndrome, ocular fragility syndromes, such as Ehlers-Danlos or Marfan's syndrome, or Leber's familial amaurosis. Onset of the disease is usually around puberty and is asymmetrically progressive.

The process of ectasia and corneal scarring that occurs usually involves the central two thirds of the cornea and is often centered just below the visual axis. Diagnostic findings include central corneal thinning, inferior corneal steepening, vertical striae in the pre-Descemet's stroma, deposition of iron in the basal corneal epithelium (Fleischer ring), and reticular scarring at the level of Bowman's membrane. These corneal changes are accompanied by the development of progressive myopia, irregular corneal astigmatism, and decreased best-corrected vision as scarring develops. Occasionally, Descemet's membrane may rupture, resulting in the sudden influx of aqueous into the corneal stroma (acute hydrops), which produces edema and loss of transparency. This usually resolves with varying degrees of corneal scarring. With advanced disease, marked corneal distortion and scarring occur. Progression of the disease may be erratic and usually spans a 10- to 20-year period before it stops.

THERAPY

Ocular. In its early stages, keratoconus is managed with spectacle correction. When spectacles are no longer practical because of the development of irregular astigmatism, contact lenses are indicated for visual correction. Gas-permeable rigid lenses are optimal for the correction of irregular astigmatism, although other lens systems, such as hybrid lenses or piggyback lens combinations, may be useful in patients who tolerate hard lenses poorly. Advanced disease with steep, irregular cones often requires special keratoconus designs with steep, vaulted posterior curves. Contact lens fit in keratoconus is often a compromise between the ideal lens fit and the patient's requirements for vision and comfort, and the fit is most commonly reached by trial fitting.

Surgical. *Penetrating keratoplasty* has been the mainstay of surgical therapy for keratoconus and is indicated when the patient can no longer tolerate contact lens wear or when the vision, even with a contact lens, is unsatisfactory for visual function. Penetrating grafts in keratoconus remain clear in 90 per cent of cases, but are subject to the complications associated with keratoplasty in general, including graft rejection, high corneal astigmatism, secondary cataract, and glaucoma. A rare but significant complication of penetrating keratoplasty for keratoconus is permanent mydriasis.

Other surgical procedures currently employed for the treatment of keratoconus include *thermokeratoplasty, lamellar keratoplasty,* and *epikeratoplasty.* Thermokeratoplasty achieves flattening of the conical cornea by thermal shrinkage of the corneal collagen at the apex of the cone. Such an approach has been suggested for patients who are poor candidates for penetrating keratoplasty. A probe at 100 to 110° C is applied to the apex of the cone in order to obtain corneal flattening. The degree of flattening is not entirely predictable, and recurrent epithelial breakdown may be a problem after thermokeratoplasty. Lamellar keratoplasty avoids intraocular surgery, but can be technically difficult, especially if there are large areas of thinning. A partial-thickness lamellar graft is sutured into a dissection bed in the host cornea. The level of vision achieved after lamellar keratoplasty is generally not as good as that achieved after penetrating keratoplasty. Epikeratoplasty, a form of onlay grafting, has more recently been advocated as a surgical alternative and may be indicated in patients with corneas too steep for contact lens wear but without central corneal scarring. Using this technique, a lathed corneal button without refractive power is tightly sutured over the apex of the cone to produce central flattening. The advantage of this procedure is that it avoids intraocular surgery and the attendant complications, making it theoretically suitable for patients, such as retarded individuals or active young athletes, in whom penetrating grafts might be a liability. Successful epikeratoplasty provides structural support to the central cornea and flattens the cone to allow successful contact lens wear. Complications of epikeratoplasty include poor epithelialization, infection, dehiscence, and persistent graft haze.

Ocular or Periocular Manifestations

Cornea: Acute hydrops; central corneal thinning; Fleischer ring; inferior corneal steepening; reticular anterior stromal scarring, vertical striae in the pre-Descemet's stroma.

Other: High or irregular astigmatism; photophobia; progressive myopia; visual loss.

PRECAUTIONS

The accurate diagnosis of keratoconus requires careful attention to the retinoscopic reflex, an appreciation of corneal topography using the keratometer or photokeratoscope, and recognition of the corneal diagnostic signs. Patients with keratoconus who are managed with contact

POSTERIOR POLYMORPHOUS CORNEAL DYSTROPHY
(Hereditary Deep Dystrophy, Hereditary Mesodermal Dystrophy, Keratitis Bullosa Interna, Koeppe's Posterior Polymorphous Degeneration, Schlichting's Dystrophy)

S. ARTHUR BORUCHOFF, M.D., and ROGER F. STEINERT, M.D.

Boston, Massachusetts

Posterior polymorphous dystrophy is an uncommon congenital corneal condition that is bilateral but not symmetric. It is characterized by vesicles at the level of Descemet's membrane, which often occur in groups or in a linear-oriented distribution and are surrounded by gray haze. Intervening areas of cornea appear normal. Descemet's membrane is thickened, and localized excrescences project into the anterior chamber or form bands or lines. White patches may be localized, or the entire posterior cornea may appear opacified. Most cases have clear stroma and epithelium, with little or no effect on vision.

Autosomal dominant inheritance with high penetrance and variable expression is suggested by most pedigrees; however, sporadic cases do occur, and pedigrees consistent with autosomal recessive inheritance have also been reported. The condition is generally stable or slowly progressive. Rarely, epithelial and stromal edema may occur and may lead to loss of vision.

Many cases are associated with anomalies of the iris and angle. Glaucoma may occur in association with angles that may appear either normal or abnormal. Posterior polymorphous dystrophy may thus be classified as a mesodermal dysgenesis (anterior cleavage disorder).

THERAPY

Ocular. Patients should be followed for glaucoma and treated appropriately. If corneal edema occurs, topical hypertonic sodium chloride is of little benefit for the edema, but no other medical measures are indicated.

Surgical. Epithelial and stromal edema and opacification of Descemet's membrane sufficient to cause marked impairment of vision are indications for penetrating keratoplasty.

Supportive. The patient and family should be reassured that most cases are mild and nonprogressive, with little or no effect on vision.

Ocular or Periocular Manifestations

Cornea: Band keratopathy; epithelial and stromal edema; focal or diffuse gray-white opacity in Descemet's membrane; linear bands in Descemet's membrane; sclerocorneal posterior embryotoxon; vesicles and excrescences with areolar haze protruding into the anterior chamber.
Eyebrows or Eyelashes: Heterochromia (rare).
Eyelids: Vitiligo.
Iris: Atrophy; corectopia; "glassy" iris membrane; heterochromia; iridocorneal adhesions to Schwalbe's ring or peripheral cornea; prominent iris processes; prominent Schwalbe's ring.

PRECAUTIONS

Because of the frequent association with glaucoma, periodic examinations of the patient are indicated. Elevated intraocular pressure may precipitate edema, which may be reversible with control of pressure. Family members should likewise undergo ophthalmologic evaluation.

COMMENTS

Significant visual impairment in the absence of edema is rare. Periodic examination with pachymetry reveal whether the condition is progressive. Severe edema can obscure the posterior changes, and examination of family members may suggest the diagnosis in such cases.

References

Boruchoff SA, Kuwabara T: Electron microscopy of posterior polymorphous degeneration. Am J Ophthalmol 72:879–887, 1971.
Cibis GW, et al: The clinical spectrum of posterior polymorphous dystrophy. Arch Ophthalmol 95:1529–1537, 1977.
Grayson M: The nature of hereditary deep polymorphous dystrophy of the cornea: Its association with iris and anterior chamber dysgenesis. Trans Am Ophthalmol Soc 72:516–559, 1974.
Johnson BL, Brown SI: Posterior polymorphous dystrophy: A light and electron microscopic study. Br J Ophthalmol 62:89–96, 1978.

tion by intestinal parasites (Metazoa), *Candida albicans, Chlamydia,* coccidioidomycosis, herpes simplex virus, and gonococci. Rarely, phlyctenular keratoconjunctivitis can occur idiopathically.

The symptoms of conjunctival phlyctenulosis are usually mild to moderate itching, tearing, and irritation. A mucopurulent discharge may be seen if secondary bacterial infection has occurred. A rope-like tenacious mucus may be seen when the underlying cause is staphylococcal blepharoconjunctivitis. Although conjunctival phlyctenules may be found anywhere on the bulbar conjunctiva, they typically occur near the interpalpebral limbus as a small pinkish-white nodule in the center of a hyperemic area. In a few days, the superficial part of the nodule becomes gray and soft, the necrotic center sloughs, and the lesion clears rapidly. No scar remains.

The symptoms of corneal phlyctenulosis are usually much more severe. There is extreme photophobia, blepharospasm, foreign body sensation, and tearing. Corneal phlyctenulosis usually begins at the limbus; it rarely develops in the cornea itself. The corneal lesions can be classified into two main groups: corneal (nonvascularized) and limbal (vascularized). The corneal lesions tend to be bilateral. They occur as either a solitary opacity or a generalized nebular opacity. The limbal lesions are usually triangular in shape, with the base at the limbus. In the majority of cases, they occur inferiorly. The old, inactive lesions or scars may be wedge shaped, fascicular, or trapeziform. The typical active limbal phlyctenule lies astride the limbus as a pinkish-white mound bordered on the conjunctival side by a fan of dilated vessels. It may remain at this position and evolve through stages of necrosis, shelling out, and healing. It may also wander toward the center of the cornea as a progressively developing gray, necrotic, superficial ulcer surrounded by a white infiltrated area. The end stage of multiple attacks of phlyctenulosis is a confluent pattern of more or less vascularized superficial corneal scars. Scars on the visual axis may severely limit vision and occasionally produce blindness. Corneal perforation is rare.

Histologic examination of the phlyctenule shows lymphocytes, histiocytes, and plasma cells. Polymorphonucleocytes are found in necrotic lesions. Bacteria are not found in the lesion itself.

The diagnosis of phlyctenulosis is based upon identification of the typical morphologic features. Phlyctenular keratoconjunctivitis can be a potentially serious condition that can, in some cases, result in severe visual impairment or blindness. Therefore, it is the responsibility of the physician to provide adequate, quick diagnosis and, if possible, etiologic identification at the time of presentation. Mucopurulent material should be cultured so the appropriate antibiotic may be selected for treatment of the suprainfection. In endemic areas, a thorough tuberculosis workup is mandatory. Because of the relative infrequency of tuberculosis, evaluation for systemic tuberculosis is not necessary for patients in nonendemic areas if the underlying etiology is obvious.

The diagnosis of *Chlamydia* is suggested by the history of persistent, usually unilateral chronic conjunctivitis in a young, sexually active adult. The diagnosis of herpes simplex virus is usually established by the previous history. The hyperacute onset of gonococcal conjunctivitis usually makes this diagnosis obvious and requires immediate smears, cultures, and treatment. Coccidioidomycosis is usually found only in endemic areas and has distinctive systemic symptomatology.

The diagnosis of acne-rosacea associated keratitis or staphylococcal blepharoconjunctivitis is usually obvious. If all of the preceding diagnoses can be excluded, the stools of the patient should be examined for intestinal parasites or their ova by direct or flotation method. In some cases, serologic tests for parasites may be helpful.

THERAPY

Ocular. For *phlyctenulosis associated with tuberculosis*, systemic antituberculous therapy should be given if tuberculosis is diagnosed as the primary cause (family history, physical examination, skin tests, and chest x-ray). The treatment for the ocular lesion is the application of topical corticosteroids. Until the lesions subside, 1 per cent prednisolone or 0.1 per cent dexamethasone may be administered every 2 hours for the first 2 to 4 days, followed by rapid tapering once improvement begins to occur. A prophylactic broad-spectrum antibiotic, such as bacitracin-polymyxin B ointment, is used topically two or three times daily while steroids are being used.

For *phlyctenulosis associated with acne rosacea* keratitis, the mainstay of therapy in adults and children over the age of 10 is orally administered tetracyclines. The use of 250 mg of oral tetracycline three or four times daily or 100 mg of oral doxycycline two times daily for approximately 2 to 4 weeks is recommended until the patient is less symptomatic. Then maintenance on 250 mg of tetracycline or 100 mg of doxycycline every day is given as long as the patient tolerates the medication. The lesions tend to be quite sensitive to topical corticosteroids; patients usually respond to 1 per cent prednisolone or 0.1 per cent dexamethasone drops four to six times a day for several days, with rapid tapering as the response to therapy permits. An antistaphylococcal antibiotic, such as bacitracin ointment, is applied topically two to four times daily. Although it is quite unusual to see children with phlyctenular keratoconjunctivitis on the basis of acne rosacea alone, it is recommended that children under 8 years of age be treated with erythromycin systemically, rather than tetracycline, to avoid staining of the enamel of the developing permanent teeth that may occur with tetracycline drugs.

In *staphylococcal-induced phlyctenulosis*, the corneal lesions usually respond to topical steroid treatment as outlined for acne rosacea. It is helpful to use a topical antistaphylococcal antibiotic ointment, such as bacitracin, administered initially two to four times daily followed by tapering to bedtime use only. If the lid changes are sufficiently severe, systemic tetracycline or doxycycline should be used. The mainstay of therapy and future prevention is a vigorous program of warm compresses to the lids combined with generous lid hygiene. The lid margins may be cleaned up to four times daily initially with a cotton-tipped applicator moistened either with water or preferentially baby shampoo diluted with water 1:5. With the eyes closed, the lids should be scrubbed with a cotton ball and rinsed with water. Hot compresses should be applied for a period of at least 5 minutes after the cleaning. This should be done initially four times a day, but rapidly tapered to one or two times daily to encourage continued patient compliance.

If the patient is infested with *intestinal parasites*, the specific anthelminthic treatment should be given. Once again, the topical steroid regimen is dictated by the severity of the pathology and the rapidity of response. The appropriate treatment for *chlamydial keratoconjunctivitis with phlyctenulosis* is a 3-week course of oral tetracyclines (250 mg of tetracycline four times daily or 100 mg of doxycycline two times daily) combined with topical steroids that are tapered as soon as the phlyctenular component improves. Treatment for *gonococcal-related phlyctenulosis* consists of proper and rapid diagnosis from conjunctival smears and scrapings combined with the appropriate systemic antigonococcal therapy, as well as intensive topical tetracycline ointment or aqueous pencillin G§ drops (100,000 units/ml). Steroids should be withheld until the ocular surface has been adequately sterilized. *Herpes simplex virus* is treated by judicious concomitant use of topical steroids and topical antivirals. Topical steroids alone are usually sufficient to eradicate and control *idiopathic phlyctenulosis*.

One of the most serious complications of phlyctenular keratoconjunctivitis is frequent recurrent disease with significant corneal scarring and visual disability. Usually, the eradication of the offending organism, such as tuberculosis, Metazoa, *Chlamydia*, or gonococci, is sufficient to prevent subsequent recurrences. More troublesome is the recurrent disease that is often seen in patients with acne rosacea keratitis or staphylococcal blepharoconjunctivitis in which eradication of the sensitizing antigen is impossible. Patients with acne rosacea keratitis require maintenance on systemic tetracycline to prevent progressive corneal vascularization and scarring, as well as recurrent phlyctenulosis. If blepharitis is a significant component, meticulous attention to lid hygiene is necessary. Patients with staphylococcal blepharoconjunctivitis should be maintained on lid hygiene and warm compresses at least once a day indefinitely, supplemented with a topical antistaphylococcal antibiotic during exacerbations. Short-term or long-term tetracycline use may be necessary in some recalcitrant cases.

The use of topical steroids should not be advocated for the long-term suppression of blepharitis-related disease, inasmuch as the possibility of cataract formation and increased intraocular pressure may result in more morbidity than the disease itself.

If significant corneal scarring and visual impairment occur, penetrating keratoplasty may be required for visual rehabilitation. Persistence of the underlying disease complicates the postoperative course and limits the prognosis. The goal of therapy for phlyctenular keratoconjunctivitis is to prevent the disease from progressing to this point.

Ocular or Periocular Manifestations

Conjunctiva: Hyperemia; infiltration; necrosis; nodules; ulcer.
Cornea: Cicatrization; infiltration; perforation; ulcer; vascularization.
Eyelids: Blepharospasm; chronic staphylococcal blepharitis; meibomianitis.
Other: Irritation; lacrimation; ocular pain; photophobia; pruritus; visual loss.

Precautions

All patients receiving tetracycline should be warned of potential gastrointestinal disturbances, phototoxicity, and the risk or oral or genital candidiasis. The risks of topical steroid use should be discussed in advance. Penetrating keratoplasty for visual rehabilitation should be performed only when the ocular surface condition has stabilized and the eye has been noninflamed for several months.

Comments

Acne rosacea keratitis and staphylococcal blepharoconjunctivitis are chronic conditions that are difficult or impossible to eradicate. Both diligent attention by the physician and compliance by the patient are required to maximize comfort, prevent recurrence of phlyctenular keratoconjunctivitis, and minimize long-term disability.

References

Allansmith MR, Ross RN: Phlyctenular keratoconjunctivitis. *In* Duane TD (ed): Clinical Ophthalmology. Philadelphia, Harper & Row, 1986, Vol IV, 8:1–6.

Beauchamp GR, Gillette TE, Friendly DS: Phlyctenular keratoconjunctivitis. J Pediatr Ophthalmol Strabismus 18:220–228, 1981.

Duke-Elder S: System of Ophthalmology. St. Louis, CV Mosby, 1965, Vol VIII, pp 461–475.

Jakobiec FA, Lefkowitch J, Knowles DM: B- and T-lymphocytes in ocular disease. Ophthalmology 91:635–654, 1984.

Mandino BJ, et al: Rabbit model of phlyctenulosis and catarrhal infiltrates. Arch Ophthalmol 99:891–895, 1981.

Zaidman GW, Brown SI: Orally administered tetracycline for phlyctenular keratoconjunctivitis. Am J Ophthalmol 92:173–182, 1981.

SUPERIOR LIMBIC KERATOCONJUNCTIVITIS

(SLK, Theodore's Superior Limbic Keratoconjunctivitis)

ARDEN H. WANDER, M.D.
Cincinnati, Ohio

Superior limbic keratoconjunctivitis (SLK) is a puzzling entity first described by Theodore in 1963. The disease is characterized by inflammation of the upper palpebral conjunctiva that is manifested clinically by a papillary reaction. The upper bulbar conjunctiva becomes thickened and inflamed. Fine punctate fluorescein or rose bengal staining occurs on the upper cornea, limbus, and adjacent conjunctiva. Filaments occur at the superior limbus and cornea in about one third of the cases. The condition is usually bilateral, but may be unilateral and occurs in all age groups. It lasts anywhere from weeks to many years with a characteristic course of remissions and exacerbations; at times it is worse in one eye and at times worse in the other eye. This characteristic history makes evaluation of therapy quite difficult.

The symptoms include burning, foreign body sensation, pain, epiphora, photophobia, blepharospasm, mild decrease in vision, and a pseudoptosis. Some patients also complain of a dry feeling in the eyes. Mucous discharge may also occur. The symptoms are significantly worse when filaments are present. Although superior limbic keratoconjunctivitis is not reported to be associated with dry eyes, 5 of Theodore's original 11 patients with SLK did in fact have diminished tearing. Later, he reported in another study that perhaps 25 per cent or more of his cases had decreased tear secretion. He further reported one case of a patient with keratitis sicca who had filaments of the superior cornea from the SLK and of the inferior cornea from the keratitis sicca. Punctal occlusion cured the lower corneal staining, and the filaments disappeared from the lower portion but not the upper portion of the cornea. In the author's series, this association has been found in about 30 per cent of the cases.

The cause, and thus the definitive treatment, is unknown. There is an associated increased incidence of dysthyroid disease. Diagnosis may be confusing and at times difficult, but is important so that ineffective and often dangerous therapy may be avoided. The diagnosis is made by the characteristic history and clinical findings. In addition, scrapings of the involved bulbar conjunctiva help make the diagnosis. Theodore and Ferry verified Thygeson's observation that Giemsa-stained scrapings demonstrate keratinized epithelial cells. Scrapings of the upper palpebral conjunctiva show polymorphonuclear leukocytes. The author has observed a unique nuclear serpiginous change in Papanicolaou-stained cells scraped from the superior bulbar conjunctiva of patients with typical superior limbic keratoconjunctivitis. Within the preserved nuclear membrane, there is an unusual arrangement of chromatin condensation in the form of a coil or in the shape of the letters *S* or *M*. Biopsy of the involved bulbar conjunctiva reveals keratinization, dyskeratosis, acanthosis, balloon degeneration of the nuclei, and some cells with swollen pale-staining cytoplasm. Serpiginous changes in the nuclei are also seen in histologic sections.

THERAPY

Ocular. Treatment remains a significant problem. Silver nitrate in concentrations from 0.25 to 0.50 per cent applied by cotton-tipped applicators to the upper tarsal conjunctiva and at times the upper bulbar conjunctiva has remained the treatment of choice. This has been the time-honored therapy and may dramatically improve the patient symptomatically. Unfortunately, the signs and symptoms may recur anywhere from a few days to several months later. This therapy can be repeated. Scraping the superior bulbar conjunctiva and tarsal conjunctiva with a platinum spatula seems to accomplish the same purpose. Scraping may relieve symptoms for up to several weeks to a few months.

Pressure patching the worse eye daily for a full week at a time may relieve the symptoms in some patients. The following week, the non-patched eye may be patched for a week at a time, changing the patch each day. This alternate patching technique has also been used successfully in conjunction with the use of a bandage contact lens in the nonpatched eye.

One drop of 10 or 20 per cent acetylcysteine* three to five times a day can be used for the excess mucus that is related to the filament formation. It may help decrease the symptoms when mucus and filaments are prominent. Bandage contact lenses may also be used when the filaments predominate.

Topical application of one drop of 4 per cent cromolyn‡ to the involved eye or eyes every 3 hours has been reported to be beneficial for some patients with SLK. When successful, treatment must be continued on a long-term basis because recurrences may occur upon discontinuing the medication.

Because associated problems, such as chronic blepharitis, may increase the symptoms, these problems should also be treated. Those patients who also have decreased tear secretion and inferior corneal staining should certainly be treated with artificial tears and advised to avoid contributing environmental factors, such as wind, smoke, and polluted environments. Patients with associated significant decreased tearing with inferior corneal staining and filaments may be helped from a symptomatic point of view by hydroxylpropyl cellulose ophthalmic insert used once or twice a day. However, these inserts do not help the superior punctate staining or the superior filaments. Punctal occlusion may also help these patients.

Surgical. A recession or resection of the involved superior bulbar conjunctiva has been recommended for more severe cases. An arcuate segment of conjunctiva and Tenon's is removed from the 10 to 2 o'clock meridian superiorly for 2 to 5 mm after a peritomy incision. The remaining superior edge of the conjunctiva may be sutured to the episclera with interrupted sutures or left alone. Unfortunately, the symptoms may recur as the conjunctival epithelium grows over the resected area. Cryotherapy to the involved superior bulbar conjunctiva has also been advocated for relief of symptoms. As with the use of the silver nitrate and surgical resection, however, the symptoms may recur in days to months after this treatment.

Ocular or Periocular Manifestations

Conjunctiva: Filaments; mucous discharge; punctate staining; thickened; upper bulbar hyperemia.
Cornea: Filaments; pannus; punctate staining.
Eyelids: Blepharospasm; pseudoptosis; upper palpebral conjunctival papillary reaction.
Other: Burning; decreased visual acuity; foreign body sensation; irritation; lacrimation; photophobia.

PRECAUTIONS

Because this condition is chronic, corticosteroids, which have little effect, should be avoided. The condition does not respond to antibiotics or antivirals, and these should also be avoided because of their potential toxic nature. Ptosis surgery performed on SLK patients with pseudoptosis may cause a significant increase in the patient's symptoms. Hence, care should be taken before surgery in evaluation of all ptosis cases to be sure that the ptosis is not a pseudoptosis secondary to SLK.

Extra precautions must be maintained when treating patients who have associated decreased tear production. Close follow-up is necessary when bandage contact lenses are used because the complications from bandage contact lenses are significantly higher in patients with dry eyes. It has also been found that conjunctival recession or resection may not be as successful in patients who also have significantly reduced tearing. A scleral melt may occur in the exposed portion of the sclera after a conjunctival resection in patients with severe dry eyes. Hence, one should be more conservative in managing patients with SLK who also have dry eyes.

COMMENTS

Because the definitive cause of the condition is unknown, definitive therapy is lacking. Therapy is difficult. Also, because of the characteristic natural history of the disease, which includes periods of exacerbation and remission, care and caution must be taken in the evaluation of the therapy for this condition. This is especially true because the condition can in fact disappear untreated. Because these patients often live in pain and discomfort for many years, the ophthalmologist must treat them with strong supportive effort both medically as well as sociologically. These patients often become incapacitated from their condition and need back-up and support from their physician.

References

Cher I: Clinical features of superior limbic keratoconjunctivitis in Australia. A probable association with thyrotoxicosis. Arch Ophthalmol 82:580–586, 1969.

Confino J, Brown SI: Treatment of superior limbic keratoconjunctivitis with topical cromolyn sodium. Ann Ophthalmol 19:129–131, 1987.

Donshik PC, et al: Conjunctival resection treatment and ultrastructural histopathology of superior limbic keratoconjunctivitis. Am J Ophthalmol 85:101–110, 1978.

Grayson M: Diseases of the Cornea. St. Louis, CV Mosby, 1979, pp 86–92.

Mondino BJ, Zaidman GW, Salamon SW: Use of pressure patching and soft contact lenses in superior limbic keratoconjunctivitis. Arch Ophthalmol 100:1932–1934, 1982.

Passons GA, Wood TO: Conjunctival resection for superior limbic keratoconjunctivitis. Ophthalmology 91:966–968, 1984.

Tenzel RR: Comments on superior limbic filamentous keratitis: Part 2. Arch Ophthalmol 79:508, 1968.

Tenzel RR: Resistant superior limbic keratoconjunctivitis. Arch Ophthalmol 89:439, 1973.

Theodore FH: Superior limbic keratoconjunctivitis. Eye Ear Nose Throat Monthly 42:25–28, 1963.

Theodore FH: Further observations on superior limbic keratoconjunctivitis. Trans Am Acad Ophthalmol Otolaryngol 71:341–351, 1967.

Theodore FH: Superior limbic keratoconjunctivitis. A summary. Mod Probl Ophthalmol 9:23–26, 1971.

Theodore FH, Ferry AP: Superior limbic keratoconjunctivitis. Clinical and pathological correlations. Arch Ophthalmol 84:481–484, 1970.

Wander AH, Masukawa T: Unusual appearance of condensed chromatin in conjunctival cells in superior limbic keratoconjunctivitis. Lance 2:42–43, 1981.

Wright P: Superior limbic keratoconjunctivitis. Trans Ophthalmol Soc UK 92:555–560, 1972.

THYGESON'S SUPERFICIAL PUNCTATE KERATOPATHY

HUGH P. WILLIAMS, F.R.C.S., D.O.
London, England

Thygeson's superficial punctate keratopathy is a bilateral, coarse, punctate epithelial keratopathy occurring without conjunctival involvement. The disease runs a chronic course with exacerbations and remissions. Typically, the patient is young, usually under 40 years of age, and complains of foreign body sensation, photophobia, and tearing. The coarse punctate epithelial lesions are faint gray in color, are oval and irregular in shape, and may be seen with magnification. They appear anywhere on the cornea, but commonly in the central area. The lesions are slightly elevated and composed of a multitude of tiny gray dots. There is never any stromal or anterior chamber involvement. Each lesion is transient, undergoing a cyclic enlargement and diminution. Attacks usually undergo spontaneous remission in days to weeks only to recur again within weeks or months. Recurrences may develop over any period of time, and this prolonged morbidity has been observed for up to even 30 years. There are no residual abnormalities between attacks. The etiology of the disorder is not known; no pathogens have been proved to be causative.

THERAPY

Ocular. There is no specific treatment for this disorder, but symptomatic relief from the use of topical ocular corticosteroids is dramatic. The lesions and symptoms begin to clear after 2 to 3 days of treatment. An effective regimen is administration of 0.1 per cent betamethasone* or 0.5 per cent prednisolone five times daily for 5 days, thereafter reducing the treatment in potency and frequency of daily applications until ocular comfort is achieved. Nonsteroidal anti-inflammatory eyedrops, such as fluorometholone or clobetasone,† are helpful. Soft therapeutic contact lenses worn on daily demand can relieve symptoms and avoid complications associated with continuous wear lenses.

Ocular or Periocular Manifestations

Cornea: Punctate epithelial opacities.
Other: Decreased visual acuity; irritation; lacrimation; photophobia.

PRECAUTIONS

Corneal scraping with or without chemical cauterization is ineffective in this disorder; the lesions recur quickly. The keratopathy does not respond to antimicrobials or antiviral therapy. The potential hazards of topical ophthalmic corticosteroid therapy as used in this disorder must always be remembered.

COMMENTS

Thygeson's superficial punctate keratopathy is not common nor communicable, but is frequently misdiagnosed. Characteristically, there is no residual scarring, but it has been observed in coincidental association with vernal keratoconjunctivitis and may occur with other external eye diseases that are capable of causing corneal scarring. The rapid response to corticosteroid therapy suggests a hyperimmune or dyskeratotic mechanism, although this has not been proved.

Decrease in visual acuity is usually minimal; however, exacerbations may reduce it to 20/60. Between attacks, it returns to normal.

References

Abbott RL, Forster RK: Superficial punctate keratitis of Thygeson associated with scarring and Salzmann's nodular degeneration. Am J Ophthalmol 87:296–298, 1979.

Goldberg DB, Schanzlin DJ, Brown SI: Management of Thygeson's superficial punctate keratitis. Am J Ophthalmol 89:22–24, 1980.

Jones BR: Thygeson's superficial punctate keratitis. Trans Ophthalmol Soc UK 83:245–253, 1963.

Williams HP, Mackie IA: Current management of Thygeson's superficial punctate keratopathy. *In* The Cornea in Health and Disease (VIth Congress of the European Society of Ophthalmology). London, Academic Press, 1981, pp 693–698.

SECTION 22

EXTRAOCULAR MUSCLES

ABDUCENS (SIXTH NERVE) PARALYSIS

EUGENE M. HELVESTON, M.D.
Indianapolis, Indiana

Abducens nerve abnormalities produce weakness or paralysis of the lateral rectus muscle, depending upon the extent of involvement of the nerve. The condition may be unilateral or bilateral, causing absence or reduction of lateral rectus function, esotropia, and homonymous or uncrossed diplopia. With total paralysis of the sixth nerve, esotropia is usually present in the primary position. Single binocular vision may be present in such a unilateral involvement if the eyes are directed maximally away from the field of action of the paretic muscle. In some cases, "single" vision occurs because the nose blocks the adducted eye. Bilateral sixth nerve palsy produces diplopia in all fields of gaze. Congenital sixth nerve palsy is rare, but acquired transient sixth nerve palsy in childhood may be more common than has been suspected. Because the long intracranial course of the abducens nerve makes it vulnerable, acquired sixth nerve palsy is not uncommon. It may result from generalized intracranial hypertension, direct pressure caused by space-occupying lesions, localized edema, inflammation, toxic substances, demyelinating diseases, and viruses. Acute sixth nerve palsy can be transient, with recovery occurring in weeks to months. Usually, a period of 6 months is required to ensure maximum recovery. Any deviation from an acquired sixth nerve palsy that is present 6 months after the incident can be considered permanent. Acquired sixth nerve palsy can be aggravated by contraction of the antagonist medial rectus. Hypoplasia of the abducens nucleus has been described at autopsy in cases who had a clinical diagnosis of type I Duane's retraction syndrome.

THERAPY

Ocular. Unilateral sixth nerve palsy may be compensated for by assuming a head posture with the face turned toward the involved side and the eyes directed toward the side opposite the lesion. With bilateral sixth nerve palsy, diplopia can be relieved only by suppressing or closing one eye. The use of base-out prisms can be effective in helping the patient maintain fusion in unilateral sixth nerve palsy. Base-out prism over the sound eye has been suggested as a temporizing technique, which can be effective in reducing the degree of contracture of the antagonist medial rectus on the involved side. Occlusion can also be applied to eliminate the diplopia.

The use of attenuated botulinum A toxin[†] has been suggested for treatment of acute sixth nerve palsy. In this pharmacologic approach, between 2.5 and 10 units is injected into the antagonist medial rectus muscle after a localization of the myoneural junction with an EMG electrode. This treatment weakens the injected muscle for several weeks to months and prevents contraction. When lateral rectus function returns, the recovered muscle works against a normal antagonist.

Surgical. The surgical treatment of sixth nerve palsy should be undertaken only after an adequate workup has been completed. In cases of acquired sixth nerve palsy, a sufficient time, usually 6 months, should elapse before the condition can be considered stable. The deviation is usually incomitant, but does tend to become comitant with time.

The deviation should be measured carefully in the primary position, right gaze, and left gaze. Also up- and downgaze should be measured to determine the presence or absence of vertical incomitance. Saccadic velocity testing of the action of the paretic muscle and the antagonist, done either by observation or with an EOG recording device, can be compared to assess the degree of lateral rectus palsy. In cases where significantly limited abduction is present and sixth nerve palsy is suspected, differential intraocular pressure testing can be carried out. When intraocular pressure increases in the field of *limited* action, intact agonist function can be inferred. If no increase in intraocular pressure is found in the presence of limited ductions, absence of agonist contraction can be diagnosed. Passive ductions, carried out either in the office after the use of topical anesthetic or in the operating room, can determine the presence or absence of mechanical restriction of the antagonist.

With knowledge of the angle of deviation, the degree of weakness of the paretic lateral rectus, and the presence or absence of restriction of the antagonist, surgery may be carried out. In cases where the medial rectus is contracted, it may be recessed. In most instances, this means that the medial rectus should be recessed maximally (to a point approximately 11.0 mm from the limbus), and the overlying conjunctiva and anterior Tenon's capsule should be recessed to the muscle's original insertion. If some lateral rectus function is present, an 8- to 10-mm resection of the lateral rectus muscle in addition to the medial rectus recession may suffice. If no lateral rectus function is present, a muscle transfer procedure may be used to shift action of the superior rectus and the inferior rectus to the lateral rectus. This full tendon transfer should be accompanied by oculinum injection to the medial rectus. This procedure can produce straight eyes in the primary position and improved but never normal abduction in the involved eye. With surgically treated unilateral sixth nerve palsy, some range of fusion with single binocular vision can be obtained. In cases of bilateral sixth nerve palsy, even with successful surgical treatment and straight eyes in the primary position, troublesome diplopia invariably persists. This diplopia is caused by unresolvable and constant recurrent secondary deviations or a poorly understood condition called central disruption of fusion. This latter condition can accompany severe head trauma, which in turn is often a precursor of bilateral sixth nerve palsy.

Precautions

The differential diagnosis of sixth nerve palsy includes several relatively uncommon conditions. Extraocular muscle fibrous syndrome is characterized by esotropia that increases on upgaze, bilateral ptosis, a chin-up position, and autosomal dominant inheritance. In this condition, passive elevation and abduction are restricted. Möbius syndrome is characterized by an esotropia, flat lower face, and atrophy of the distal third of the tongue. It occurs as a result of bilateral sixth and seventh nerve palsy. Class I Duane's syndrome is characterized by unilateral or bilateral esotropia, decreased abduction, and enophthalmos on abduction. It has been shown in certain cases to be associated with hypoplasia of the abducens nerve nucleus. Thyroid ophthalmopathy may involve the medial rectus muscles and produce a unilateral or bilateral mechanical esotropia. Myasthenia gravis may be associated with unilateral or bilateral esotropia. Blowout fracture of the medial wall of the orbit with entrapment of the medial rectus produces limited abduction with or without esotropia in the primary position. Certain cases that have been diagnosed in the past as congenital esotropia may be acquired sixth nerve palsy that has stabilized as an esotropia. Viral illness in childhood or prolonged anesthesia in infancy and childhood has been noted to cause transient sixth nerve palsy.

Comments

Sixth nerve palsy in general does not constitute a diagnostic mystery. Careful evaluation of the patient in the office can usually provide enough information for an accurate diagnosis. Occasionally, an endrophonium test may be employed to rule out myasthenia gravis. However, in most cases of myasthenia, other extraocular muscles are involved. Also, the extraocular muscle response to myasthenia is usually less dramatic than the response of the levator palpebrae or facial muscles. In relatively rare cases for which no satisfactory explanation can be found, further neurologic workup, including CAT scan, may be employed.

References

Ellis FD, Helveston EM: Special considerations and techniques in strabismus surgery. Int Ophthalmol Clin 16:247–254, 1976.
Helveston EM: Atlas of Strabismus Surgery, 2nd ed. St. Louis, CV Mosby, 1977.
Hotchkiss MG, et al: Bilateral Duane's retraction syndrome. A clinical-pathologic case report. Arch Ophthalmol 98:870–874, 1980.
Metz HS, Mazow M: Botulinum toxin treatment of acute sixth and third nerve palsy. Graefes Arch Clin Exp Ophthalmol 226:141–144, 1988.
Scott AB: Botulinum toxin injection of eye muscles to correct strabismus. Trans Am Ophthalmol Soc 79:734–770, 1981.

ACCOMMODATIVE ESOTROPIA

EDWARD L. RAAB, M.D.
New York, New York

Accommodative esotropia is among the most common forms of acquired strabismus. Intermittency and a variable angle of deviation at onset in a child with no generalized neurologic abnormality are characteristics of this condition. The most common age of appearance is between 24 and 30 months, although cases of onset before 1 year of age have been documented. Because presumably there has been an interval of normal binocular visual experience early in life before onset, some degree of fusion capacity usually can be demonstrated by the appropriate clinical office tests. Amblyopia may develop once the deviation becomes constant, but usually it is not severe unless there is accompanying anisometropia. Several series have shown that excessive hypermetropia and a high AC/A ratio are equally prevalent as etiologic factors. Cases showing both characteristics tend to pose more troublesome management problems.

Accommodative esotropia traditionally has been considered an essentially self-limited condition that subsides in the great majority of cases by about age 10 years. Recent reports have indicated, however, that there is a high rate of persistence well beyond that age and that neither this outcome nor the deterioration to a partial or complete nonaccommodative component can be predicted from the presence or absence of any of several associated clinical features, such as family history of strabismus, inferior oblique overaction, or progressive increases in hypermetropia.

THERAPY

Ocular. The basic objectives of treatment of accommodative esotropia are to maintain straight eyes by discouraging excessive accommodative convergence, to prevent or eliminate amblyopia, and to remove or compensate for coexisting misalignments (e.g., oblique muscle dysfunctions) that can act as obstacles to fusion despite adequate control of the esotropia.

A decrease in accommodative convergence, either because of a normal response to an excessive demand or to an exaggerated response to average hypermetropia, can be achieved by optical or pharmacologic means. Generally, spectacles that compensate for the full hyperopic refractive error are well accepted for full-time wear immediately or after a brief period of adjustment. Although for ongoing management, the goal is to provide the *least* assistance that will keep the eyes straight in binocular viewing in order to encourage and expand fusional divergence, usually it is best to gain the fullest control possible at the initial treatment, with subsequent tapering as seems opportune.

Bifocals are given for residual esotropia at near that is greater by 10 or more prism diopters than the distance deviation with hypermetropia compensated, provided that the eyes are realigned at distance to less than 10 prism diopters of residual deviation. Here too, although the minimally necessary addition is to be desired, rapid control of the case involving a high distance/near comparison calls initially for the full add of +2.50 or +3.00 diopters. Since in a one-visit initial examination/treatment scheme, the cycloplegic determination usually is performed after alignment measurements have been completed, obviously it is desirable to estimate in advance the possible need for a bifocal even before it can be known that the esodeviation is entirely accommodative in nature. Generally, it is safe to assume that a bifocal is needed if the esotropia angle at near is greater than at distance by at least 20 prism diopters with no compensation for hypermetropia and before any cycloplegic is administered. The need in patients with differences between 10 and 20 prism diopters is more difficult to predict, but in the author's experience a bifocal is required in at least half of such cases (although when later adjusted, usually in less than full strength). When in doubt, it is probably best for this group to receive the bifocal initially and to remove or reduce it rapidly based on the examiner's subsequent familiarity with the case. The less desirable alternative of omitting the bifocal until the case is re-evaluated results in a large proportion of automatic prescription changes.

Well-controlled patients are seen at intervals of 4 to 6 months, unless their visits must be more frequent because of amblyopia treatment. Once accommodative convergence is controlled, the distance and near (if any) powers can be reduced at intervals of several months by an amount determined by office trial to maintain at least peripheral fusion. The cover/uncover test may show no refixation shift for either eye, or there may be a small refixation (less than 10 prism diopters with the simultaneous prism/cover test). The alternate cover test may, of course, show a larger deviation, e.g., an eso*phoria* response. Unless there has been surgery for a nonaccommodative portion of the deviation, such reductions in spectacle power before age 5 years usually are not possible. Generally, it is best not to prescribe a reduction in power greater than 0.75 diopters at one time, regardless of what may appear to be possible. It is not necessary to verify such a change by an otherwise unneeded cycloplegic refraction, since the least assistance possible is intended, regardless of the total hypermetropia or whether it shows a commensurate change.

Anticholinesterase drugs applied topically act by facilitating accommodative effort for a given level of innervational output. The usually employed agents are 0.06 or 0.125 per cent echothiophate (Phospholine) iodine solution or 0.025 per cent isoflurophate ointment, one drop in each eye once daily. In actual practice, these drugs are considered less reliable than optical correction for both diagnosis and treatment. The "indeterminate" case usually is not better detected by these agents.

Amblyopia is managed by conventional occlusion programs. If on initial evaluation, it appears as though the eyes will be straightened successfully by glasses or miotics, it is permissible to defer occlusion temporarily in children old enough that their visual acuity can be monitored accurately. Restoring proper alignment has been observed to result in some degree of spontaneous visual improvement in several cases. A short delay of 2 or 3 months could lessen considerably the duration of a subsequently employed occlusion regimen and avoid the interruption of the opportunity for fusion that patching would cause.

Surgical. There is a general agreement that during childhood an operation is an inappropriate substitute for optical or pharmacologic control of accommodative convergence. However, some patients with fully compensated accommodative esotropia gradually develop a constant nonaccommodative component as well. There are no reliable predictors of this sequel; various series indicate its occurrence rate to be between 17 and 48 per cent. Surgery is necessary once this complication is present and should be planned for only the residual deviation that is no longer influenced by accommodation.

Comitant vertical deviations of less than 10 prism diopters can be managed by incorporating vertical prism power in the spectacle prescription. Larger deviations, prominent inferior oblique overaction, and dissociated vertical deviation require surgery, occasionally even when the horizontal alignment has been controlled successfully.

Supportive. Formal orthoptic exercises to reduce dependency on glasses or miotics do not play a prominent role in the treatment of accommodative esotropia. Progressively reduced hypermetropia correction or a schedule of decreasing miotic administration is in effect a training of fusional divergence under more natural circumstances. However, the assistance of the orthoptist in several other aspects of management of these patients, such as amblyopia monitoring and treatment reduction, is both appropriate and valuable.

Precautions

In determining the refractive error, there is controversy as to which of several available cycloplegic agents is best. Many ophthalmologists insist that atropine, the most powerful of the group, is the only suitable drug for this purpose. However, the extra visit required to accomplish the refraction, the multiple-dose regimen, the duration of side effects in predisposed individuals, and the prolonged wear-off time with its residual (although temporary) visual handicap suggest the need for an effective compromise. The unreliability attributed to cyclopentolate for refraction in esotropia cases may be due to the common practice of refracting after only 25 to 30 minutes, as is generally done in routine situations. A 45- to 60-minute interval is more suitable and is in keeping with the described properties of this drug. The power of cyclopentolate to "uncover" additional hypermetropia on serial determinations, when used in this manner, is similar to that of atropine. The ability to arrive at a definitive treatment plan, which with either agent often requires a subsequent adjustment of the prescription, in one visit is the overriding advantage of this suggested regimen. It is not necessary to discontinue miotics in order to obtain reliable refraction data with this regimen.

An important limitation to miotic treatment is that these drugs do not substitute for glasses when the refractive errors are anisometropic and therefore do not remove a prominent predisposing factor in amblyopia development. In particular, the author has not found them to be a useful substitute for glasses in noncompliant children; the parent unable or unwilling to enforce firmly the wearing of spectacles is not likely to prevail in the comparably difficult conflict resulting from frequent drop instillation. Anticholinesterase agents also cannot replace glasses if prisms are to be part of the treatment program. If these agents are employed, it is likely that patients unresponsive to three or four doses weekly will not be better with more frequent use. The patient (if old enough) and the responsible adult must be cautioned that succinylcholine employed as a muscle relaxant during general anesthesia can result in apnea if anticholinesterase agents have been taken within the previous several weeks.

Comments

Despite its conceded shortcomings, the distance/near fusion-free alignment comparison remains the most practical method of estimating the AC/A ratio. The ratio as an absolute figure, however, is of little clinical value. Apparent changes in this determination are often noted over several examinations and usually are due to unappreciated variations in accommodative effort. This artifact can be minimized in measuring alignment by employing fixation targets that require accurate and clear observation of fine detail by the patient.

The natural history of accommodative esotropia is marked by two events that are of particular concern to ophthalmologists and to the parents of these patients. One relates to whether surgery will be required. Operation should be reserved for those who, either through delayed or inadequate treatment or in many cases even despite timely and conscientious measures, deteriorate to a partial or complete nonaccommodative component to the deviation. Surgery can restore straight eyes, but usually not without the need for continuing accommodation control.

The other familiar dilemma concerns the likelihood of spontaneous improvement of the condition so that treatment is no longer required. Conventional belief has been that most cases of accommodative esotropia subside uneventfully by about age 10 years. Recent scrutiny of this question has indicated that the age of disappearance is quite variable, that some cases persist into adulthood or indefinitely, and that, as with deterioration, there are no reliable predictive clues.

Accommodative esotropia has been noted as an accompanying feature to many other forms of strabismus. The most important of these combinations occurs in the infant with congenital esotropia. Although accommodative esotropia as a pure deviation occurs infrequently in the early months of life, many authors have described what appears to be a predisposition of the congenitally esotropic infant toward developing a simultaneous or subsequent accommodative strabismus somewhat rapidly after even successful surgery for the former condition. It is particularly important that parents of these infants be forewarned of this possibility.

Many parents are under the misconception that accommodation-controlling measures cure this condition. It is important that they be educated to understand that these treatments compensate rather than cure, that they are effective only when used, and that they are meant to tide the child over until the condition (it is hoped) subsides naturally.

References

Hiles DA, Watson BA, Biglan AW: Characteristics of infantile esotropia following early bimedial rectus recession. Arch Ophthalmol 98:697–703, 1980.

Parks MM: Abnormal accommodation in squint. Arch Ophthalmol 19:364–380, 1958.

Raab EL: Etiologic factors in accommodative esodeviation. Trans Am Ophthalmol Soc 80:657–694, 1982.

Raab EL: Persisting accommodative esotropia. Arch Ophthalmol 104:1777–1779, 1986.

ACCOMMODATIVE INSUFFICIENCY
(Accommodative Effort Syndrome, Ill-Sustained Accommodation)

K. NOLEN TANNER, M.D., Ph.D.
Portland, Oregon

Asthenopia is a very frequent complaint heard by all general ophthalmologists, and all ophthalmologists know that there are a myriad of causes. One common cause, which is so easily treated with great patient satisfaction and has such characteristic features that it deserves a name as a special entity, is accommodative insufficiency. Unfortunately, this cause of asthenopia has not received the attention it deserves in the literature and in ophthalmic training programs. As a result, it is far more often missed than detected, and most patients with this condition either receive no treatment or inadequate treatment.

Stated simply, accommodative insufficiency is the inability to accommodate without the help of convergence. In other words, these patients have almost no accommodative reserve. On the classical accommodative-convergence graph plotted in diopters of accommodation versus meter angles of convergence, the comfortable function zone is narrow and lies almost entirely below the 1:1 accommodative-convergence line.

The patient may be a male or female from about 10 to 35 years of age. In general, the symptomatology and the physical findings change little, if any, over this age range. Over 35 years of age, the condition of accommodative insufficiency begins to blend into presbyopia. The patients are not dyslexic; they can and do read well. Generally, however, prolonged and intensive reading is disliked, and these individuals tend to gravitate to outdoor activities and occupations that require little prolonged close work. Patients often seek help when their job situation changes, and they are suddenly required to spend much of their working day at intensive close work, such as examining computer printouts, or when beginning a course of study in college or graduate school. They typically complain of asthenopic symptoms—headaches, eyestrain, and intermittent blurring after 20 to 40 minutes of reading. If the asthenopic symptoms begin in less than 15 minutes or after an hour or so, they generally do not fit into this classical picture. On examination they generally have 20/20 visual acuity without correction, and their refractive error is negligible, ranging from about −0.50 diopters to about +0.75 diopters with no more than 0.50 diopters of cylinder. Over the years, this refractive error changes very little, if at all. Children who are found to be myopic at 8 to 10 years of age and who become increasingly myopic as they go through adolescence rarely, if ever, are found to have accommodative insufficiency. The typical accommodative-insufficient patient is able to read Jaeger 2 print easily, but may be noticed to squint or frown when reading. In making this diagnosis, the first specific test is applied while the patient is reading Jaeger 2. When +1.00 or +1.25 diopter spheres are placed in front of each eye in the form of loose lenses, an immediate positive response will be elicited from the accommodative insufficient patient. Sometimes, the patient is seen to relax the facial muscles. If the patient says that +1.00 diopter spheres make the print "a little better," this test is considered negative.

After determining that the patient has little, if any, refractive error, the patient is placed behind the refractor with a reading card placed at 35 cm for the second test. With Risley prisms present over both eyes while reading Jaeger 2 print, base-in prisms are slowly wound in over both eyes. The typical accommodative-insufficient patient finds that the print blurs with approximately 2 to 4 diopters of base-in prism over each eye. The blur is relieved by adding bilateral +0.25 to +0.50 diopter spheres in the refractor. As the reading continues, additional prism is turned in. As the print blurs out, it is brought back with plus spheres, +0.25 diopters at a time, until 8 diopters of base-in prism are before each eye for a total of 16 diopters. A patient who has a pupillary distance of exactly 60 mm naturally viewing an object at 33 cm is converging 18 prism diopters. Thus, a patient with approximately 60 mm pupillary distance viewing an object at 35 cm and with 16 diopters of base-in prism has the eyes almost completely straight and with very little remaining convergence. Almost invariably under these conditions, the accommodative-insufficient patient requires +1.00 to +1.50 diopter (usually +1.25 diopter) spheres over each eye to be able to read Jaeger 2 print.

The third test is to place the patient in the refractor without prisms but with −3.00 diopters before each eye gazing at a Snellen chart 20 feet away. The typical accommodative-insufficient patient is unable to resolve any better than 20/100, in spite of all his or her efforts.

THERAPY

Ocular. A patient who is found to have markedly improved vision with +1.00 or +1.25 diopter spheres over both eyes when reading Jaeger 2 print, requires +1.25 diopter sphere to read Jaeger 2 at 35 cm with 16 diopters of base-in prism, and is unable to read better than 20/100 at 20 feet with −3.00 diopter spheres before each eye can certainly be said to have accommodative insufficiency. This patient will benefit greatly with reading glasses. They are usually given as simple half-eye reading glasses, with +1.00 to +1.25 diopter spheres and occasionally +1.50 diopters. The patient should be instructed that the benefit of these glasses will be apparent only after approximately 20 minutes or so of reading. Shorter periods of reading can usually be done comfortably without the reading glasses.

COMMENTS

When all of the features are present as described, there is little doubt as to the diagnosis cells to inhibit burst cells normally. "Voluntary nystagmus" in normal subjects is characterized by small-amplitude saccadic oscillations that cannot be sustained for a long period of time.

Although the types of pathologic nystagmus and saccadic oscillations are numerous, relatively few are frequently encountered by ophthalmologists among outpatients. Most fixation instabilities can be adequately detected and classified by the examiner's unaided eye. Their clinical significance, the need for additional diagnostic tests, and the plan for drug, ocular, or surgical therapy can then be determined.

The important observations necessary to classify nystagmus include examinations for 1) waveform, 2) direction, 3) effect of visual fixation, 4) effect of gaze position, and 5) binocular symmetry. The examiner should ask the following questions: 1) Are there slow movements in one direction and fast movements in the opposite direction (jerk waveform), or do movements in both directions have equal velocity (pendular)? 2) Is the direction horizontal, vertical, oblique (combination of horizontal and vertical), or rotatory (torsional)? 3) Does the amplitude or direction of the nystagmus change in different positions of gaze? 4) If fixation is blocked by high plus lenses (Frenzel goggles), does the amplitude and frequency increase or decrease? 5) Are the amplitude and direction of the nystagmus the same in both eyes?

Vestibular nystagmus results from damage of the vestibular end organs or their central connections in the lower brainstem and vestibulocerebellum (flocculonodular lobes). It is suppressed by fixation, has a jerk waveform, and is horizontal, oblique, and torsional in direction. In addition, vestibular nystagmus caused by acute lesions of the end organs or vestibular nerves diminishes rapidly over several days with fixation and is associated with vertigo, tinnitus, or hearing loss. Blurring vision with high plus lenses enhances the nystagmus. Observation of the fundus of one eye with a direct ophthalmoscope while covering the other eye blocks fixation and magnifies the motion of the fundus caused by the nystagmus. Motion of the fundus is in the opposite direction to movement of the eye. Instructing the patient to rapidly oscillate the head horizontally with the eyelids closed for several seconds, stop the head movements, and open the eyelids can enhance vestibular nystagmus.

Positional vestibular nystagmus is found only when the patient's body is moved from the upright sitting or standing positions to a supine position. The paroxysmal form requires a rapid positioning into a backward, head-hanging position (Barany-Nylen or Hallpike maneuvers). The nystagmus is initially intense, but quickly fatigues over several seconds. *Benign paroxysmal positional nystagmus* is probably caused by degenerative changes in the utricules in which otoconia from the utricular macule fall on the cupula of the posterior semicircular canal, making that cupula sensitive to linear acceleration. These changes can follow viral labyrinthitis, trauma, and vascular occlusion to the end organs or can be idiopathic. The jerk nystagmus is not inhibited by fixation and is disconjugate. It is usually induced by turning the head to the side of the damaged ear in the head-hanging position. The nystagmus in the eye on that side ("lower" eye) is oblique and torsional; the nystagmus in the other eye ("upper" eye) is upbeating. Rapid positioning can also induce other types of pathologic nystagmus, e.g., downbeat nystagmus. However, these types of nystagmus usually are not disconjugate. *Sustained positional nystagmus* can be caused by damage to the end organs, vestibular nerves, or central vestibular pathways. The jerk nystagmus is less intense than benign paroxysmal positional nystagmus, is inhibited by fixation, and persists as long as the supine position is maintained.

Congenital nystagmus, in contrast to vestibular nystagmus, is decreased by blocking fixation and is intensified by the effort to fixate and see clearly. It is not usually associated with other neurologic defects, and its etiology is essentially unknown. The nystagmus has pendular and complex (combinations of pendular and jerk) waveforms, is almost always horizontal (even in vertical gaze), and has a high frequency. A null position of gaze is often present in which the intensity of nystagmus is least and visual acuity is greatest. An associated habitual face turn places the eyes in the null position. In addition, nystagmus is decreased by convergence. *Physiologic end-point nystagmus* is a horizontal jerk nystagmus in the extremes of eccentric gaze (45°) and is found in most normal subjects. There is a fast component in the direction of gaze. The nystagmus is decreased by moving the eyes a few degrees toward center. The nystagmus amplitude can be slightly larger in the abducting eye than in the adducting eye. This slight disconjugacy should be separated from that found in the nystagmus of internuclear ophthalmoplegia. Other signs associated with internuclear ophthalmoplegia (slowing of the velocities of saccades by the adducting eye, overshooting or hypermetria of saccades by the abducting eye, limitation of the range of adduction and skew deviation) are not found.

Gaze-evoked nystagmus results from an inability to maintain eccentric gaze. It is larger in amplitude and is present in less extreme positions of gaze (30°) than physiologic end-point nystagmus. If horizontal, gaze-evoked nystagmus is equal in both directions; it is not localizing diagnostically. Drugs, fatigue, or diffuse central nervous system (CNS) disorders are the usual causes. If the nystagmus is asymmetric, it usually indicates a structural lesion of the cerebrum, brainstem, or cerebellum to the side of greater amplitude. *Rebound nystagmus* is a form of gaze-evoked nystagmus. A gaze-evoked nystagmus gradually decreases as eccentric gaze is maintained for several seconds. On return to center gaze, several beats of jerk nystagmus with fast components in the opposite direction to the previous eccentric gaze are present. Lesions of the cerebellum are usually present.

Upbeat nystagmus is a vertical jerk nystagmus with fast components beating upward. If it is present only in upgaze, drugs, fatigue, or diffuse CNS disorders are often the cause. However, if present in primary gaze, it is usually caused by damage to the lower brainstem or cerebellum. *Downbeat nystagmus* is a vertical jerk nystagmus with fast components beating downward. It is one of the most localizing of all ocular motor signs. The amplitude is usually greatest in lateral gaze. Convergence often increases the nystagmus. The nystagmus might not be seen until rapid positioning of the head is performed. A lesion at the level of the craniocervical junction, involving the cerebellum or lower brainstem, is usually present (Arnold-Chiari malformation, basilar impression, platybasia, multiple sclerosis, cerebellar degenerations, or vascular accidents). Toxicity due to carbamazepine, phenytoin, lithium and amiodarone and deficiencies of thiamine or magnesium can cause downbeat nystagmus.

Periodic alternating nystagmus is a horizontal jerk nystagmus in the primary position with fast components alternately beating in opposite directions. The amplitude of right-beating nystagmus increases and decreases gradually (about 90 seconds). The phase of right-beating nystagmus is followed by a null phase (about 10 seconds) in which no nystagmus is present. A phase of left-beating nystagmus with increasing and decreasing amplitude (about 90 seconds) follows. The cycling of phases is repetitive and regular. This type of nystagmus usually results from lesions of the lower brainstem or cerebellum. Alternating nystagmus can be a form of congenital nystagmus or can be caused by acquired bilateral blindness. However, the phases are usually asymmetric and variable in these types of alternating nystagmus.

Dissociated nystagmus, in which oscillations are greater in amplitude or are present in only one eye, usually results from structural lesions. Monocular forms are often pendular and present in primary gaze. The most common causes are spasmus nutans, uniocular visual loss in childhood, optic nerve glioma, and lesions of the brainstem. Binocular forms are often jerk oscillations and are present in eccentric gaze. The most common form is the abducting nystagmus of internuclear ophthalmoplegia, in which the abducting eye has a larger gaze-evoked nystagmus than the adducting eye. Myasthenia gravis can produce a dissociated gaze-evoked nystagmus, as well as conjugate gaze-evoked, horizontal, or vertical nystagmus, when eccentric gaze is maintained and fatigue of the extraocular muscles occurs.

There are other less common but highly localizing forms of nystagmus. *Convergence-retraction nystagmus* appears as fast phases of convergence (rarely divergence) and retraction of both eyes on attempted upward vertical refixations and is part of Parinaud's syndrome. It is best demonstrated with optokinetic stripes moving downward that induce upward saccadic fast phases and is caused by structural lesions in the pretectal-tectal region of the midbrain, e.g., pinealoma. *See-saw nystagmus* consists of pendular vertical oscillations in which the rising eye intorts as the falling eye extorts. It is usually associated with bitemporal hemianopsia and results from lesions near the optic chiasm. *Superior oblique myokymia* represents pendular and jerk, torsional, and oblique oscillations of one eye, producing monocular oscillopsia. Its amplitude is very small and its frequency high. Observation of conjunctival blood vessels or of the fundus with the direct ophthalmoscope helps detect oscillations. It occurs in otherwise healthy patients and can resolve spontaneously. Successful treatment with carbamazepine has been reported, and surgical procedures to weaken the superior oblique muscle have also been attempted.

The most common and significant ocular effects of nystagmus are reduction of visual acuity, as in congenital nystagmus, and oscillopsia, as in acquired forms of nystagmus. Motion of images across the fovea at velocities of 4°/second or higher due to instability of fixation can decrease visual acuity. Therefore, therapy that reduces the slow-phase velocity of nystagmus can improve visual acuity. The velocities of slow components in congenital nystagmus are very high. However, visual acuity can be normal or nearly normal. The amount of time in the nystagmus cycle during which the image is stationary at the fovea (foveation time) is correlated with visual acuity. Fixation instability and oscillopsia make orientation in space and executing saccades effectively during reading difficult.

Visual acuity is usually not impaired by square wave jerks. Small amplitude saccades carry the eyes away from and back to the target, but the short pauses between saccades (intersaccidic intervals) allows sufficient foveation time for normal levels of acuity. Visual acuity is decreased by ocular flutter and opsoclonus. Large-amplitude to-and-fro saccades do not have intersaccidic intervals. Square wave jerks and ocular flutter are usually horizontal. Saccades in opsoclonus are horizontal, vertical, and oblique and have straight and curved trajectories.

THERAPY

Systemic. The most effective therapy for nystagmus and saccadic oscillations is treatment of the underlying disorder before irreversible damage to the CNS occurs. Detection and identification of the oscillations by the ophthalmologist, referral for neurologic examination when indicated, and obtaining appropriate laboratory tests are required. Improved techniques of computed tomography and magnetic resonance imaging (MRI) enhance detection of CNS lesions. MRI is particularly useful in detecting abnormalities of the brainstem and cerebellum because the bones around the posterior fossa are not imaged. Arnold-Chiari malformations can be detected easily by MRI. Downbeat nystagmus caused by these and other malformations can resolve after surgical decompression of the foramen magnum.

Treatment for patients with vestibular nystagmus is usually aimed at alleviating vertigo. Antivertiginous medications include several classes of drugs, e.g., anticholinergics (scopolamine and atropine), monoaminergics (amphetamine and ephedrine), antihistamines (meclizine, cyclizine, dimenhydrinate, and promethazine), phenothiazines (prochlorperazine and chlorpromazine), benzodiazepines (diazepam), and butyrophenones (haloperidol and droperidol). The dosage and route of administration (oral, parenteral, and transdermal) varying according to the severity and chronicity of vertigo. Compensation exercises have also been recommended in therapy of vertigo. Benign paroxysmal positional vertigo (nystagmus) has been successfully treated with positional exercises that induced the vertigo.

Gamma-aminobutyric acid (GABA) is an inhibitory neurotransmitter in the central nervous system. Baclofen, an analog of GABA, is absorbed after oral administration and has been used to treat spasticity caused by disorders of the spinal cord. Its therapeutic effects might result from inhibiting the release of glutamate, an excitatory CNS neurotransmitter, rather than from augmentation of GABA-ergic pathways. Baclofen‡ has been used to treat several types of nystagmus and has been found to decrease the nystagmus amplitude and oscillopsia. It has been reported to be effective in treating some patients with acquired periodic alternating nystagmus (PAN), congenital PAN, and acquired, nonperiodic alternating nystagmus. The dosage is usually 5 to 20 mg three times daily. Improvement in vision and decreased oscillopsia are noticed several minutes after taking the medication and regress after a few to several hours. Medication should not be administered at bedtime or at other times when use of the eyes is not anticipated. Common side effects include drowsiness fatigue, nausea, headache, and confusion. It has not been recommended for children under age 12.

Adult patients with congenital nystagmus have also been treated with baclofen. In one study, nystagmus intensity (frequency × amplitude) decreased at the null position of gaze, and vision improved subjectively in half of the patients. Only one patient chose to continue the medication for more than 6 months. Baclofen has been reported to be effective in some patients with congenital or see-saw nystagmus, although it was not found to be helpful in patients with downbeat nystagmus. Baclofen alone or in combination with clonazepam was not effective in patients with oculopalatal myoclonus.

Clonazepam is an anticonvulsant that augments GABA-ergic activity in the central nervous system. It has been reported to decrease the amplitude and oscillopsia of downbeat nystagmus. A test dose of 1 to 2 mg of clonazepam‡ given orally can reduce downbeat nystagmus in 45 to 60 minutes. Sustained therapy with 0.25 to 0.50 mg several times a day has been used successfully by several patients. Drowsiness was the most common adverse effect. Cessation of drugs causing downbeat nystagmus and supplementation with thiamine or magnesium when deficiencies exist should be considered. The combination of baclofen and clonazepam has reduced see-saw nystagmus and oscillopsia. Clonazepam has also been reported to be effective in treating opsoclonus. Corticosteroids‡ and corticotropin‡ can decrease opsoclonus in children with myoclonus of the limbs and ataxia, and corticotropin can also reduce opsoclonus in children with neuroblastoma. Clonazepam has been successful in treating myoclonic ocular jerks, but was not useful in treating a few patients with oculopalatal myoclonus.

Ocular. Prisms in spectacle lenses can be useful in improving vision in congenital nystagmus. Base-out prisms induce convergence and can decrease nystagmus (increase foveation time). Prisms with bases oriented in the same direction can move the eyes toward a null position and reduce nystagmus. However, the weight and blurring of prisms that are strong enough to affect nystagmus sufficiently often discourage their use. Contact lenses can be successfully used by patients with congenital nystagmus and can help patients achieve better visual acuity than spectacles. One mechanism by which contact lenses improve vision could be the decrease in nystagmus amplitude by tactile feedback from the inner eyelids. Auditory biofeedback has been reported to be effective in decreasing congenital nystagmus in the laboratory. However, it is not certain if the reduction in nystagmus can persist outside the laboratory setting.

An optical method of stabilizing images on the retina or patients with nystagmus and decreasing oscillopsia has been described. A high plus spectacle lens focuses light rays from images at the center of rotation of the eye. A high minus contact lens moves the focal point to the retina. This method has improved vision in some patients with acquired forms of nystagmus. Patients with congenital nystagmus do not complain of oscillopsia, and this optical method has induced oscillopsia in some patients with congenital nystagmus.

Surgical. Extraocular muscle surgery can be effective in improving visual function in patients with congenital nystagmus and eccentric null positions. A patient assumes a habitual face turn to place the eyes in an eccentric gaze position in which the nystagmus is decreased and vision is improved. Large-amplitude face turns and eccentric gaze positions (30° or greater) can interfere with a patient's effective use of his or her best visual function. Improvement in visual acuity should be demonstrable in the null position. Patients with congenital nystagmus can have associated ocular disorders, such as oculocutaneous albinism and optic atrophy, that are primarily responsible for impairment of vision. In such patients, reduction of nystagmus might not significantly improve visual function. The null positions at distance and at near are often different and can be in opposite directions of gaze. The author has not found that surgery based on the null position at distance has interfered with visual function at near. Recession and resection procedures on the four horizontal recti muscles are performed to rotate the eyes in the direction opposite to that of the horizontal component of the null position. The amount of surgery should be greater than that usually used for a similar strabismic deviation. The null position is moved toward primary gaze, but it can gradually return toward its preoperative position. Simultaneous correction of a horizontal strabismus can also be attempted. Correction of a vertical component to the eccentric null position can be attained by vertical displacement of the horizontal rectus insertions in the direction opposite to that of the vertical component. Successful surgery can enlarge the area of gaze about the null position (null zone) in which nystagmus amplitude remains low and visual acuity is maximized.

Precautions

To date, no serious adverse effects of drug treatment of nystagmus have been reported. However, such drugs as baclofen and clonazepam have been used in relatively few patients. Too, numerous side effects have been reported when these drugs have been used for other medical conditions, some of which can be life threatening, e.g., bone marrow suppression secondary to carbamazepine. Ophthalmologists should be familiar with these side effects. Developmental anomalies in fetuses of rats given more than the maximum human dose of baclofen have been described. Reports have suggested that use of clonazepam for epilepsy might be associated with increased incidence of birth defects. The author does not use baclofen or clonazepam to treat nystagmus in women of childbearing age or in children.

Comments

The ophthalmologist's contribution to the management of nystagmus usually is to identify the type of nystagmus and its diagnostic localizing value. In addition, valuable information can be provided by identifying nonpathologic types of nystagmus, such as physiologic end-point nystagmus and nystagmus that is usually not associated with other neurologic defects, such as congenital nystagmus. Costly diagnostic workups can thereby be avoided. In addition, the ophthalmologist's knowledge of the localizing value of certain types of nystagmus, such as downbeat nystagmus, can result in more effective use of neuroradiologic tests and neurosurgical correction of CNS abnormalities. In selected cases of congenital nystagmus, the ophthalmologist can significantly improve visual function with surgical procedures.

This work was supported by a Development Grant from Research to Prevent Blindness, Inc., to the Department of Ophthalmology, Indiana University of Medicine.

References

Allen ED, Davies PD: Role of contact lenses in the management of congenital nystagmus. Br J Ophthalmol 67:834–836, 1983.

Bagolini B, Penne A, Zanasi MR: Ocular nystagmus: Some interpretational aspects and methods of treatment. Int Ophthalmol 6:37–48, 1983.

Carlow TJ: Medical treatment of nystagmus and ocular motor disorders. Int Ophthalmol Clin 26:251–263, 1986.

Chambers BE, Ell JJ, Gresty MA: Case of downbeat nystagmus influenced by otolith stimulation. Arch Neurol 13:204–207, 1983.

Currie J, Matsuo V: The use of clonazepam in the treatment of nystagmus-induced oscillopsia. Ophthalmology 93:924–932, 1986.

Dell'Osso LF, Daroff RB, Troost BT: Nystagmus and saccadic intrusions and oscillations. In Duane TD (ed): Clinical Ophthalmology. Philadelphia, Harper and Row, 1985, Vol II, pp 11:1–27.

Dell'Osso, LF, et al: Contact lenses and congenital nystagmus. Clin Vis Sci (in press).

Kirschen DG: Auditory feedback in the control of congenital nystagmus. Am J Optom Physiol Opt 60:364–368, 1983.

Leigh JL, et al: Oscillopsia, retinal image stabilization and congenital nystagmus. Invest Ophthalmol Vis Sci 29:279–282, 1988.

Pinel JF, et al: Down-beat nystagmus: Case report with magnetic resonance imaging and surgical treatment. Neurosurgery 21:736–739, 1987.

Rushton D, Cox N: A new optical treatment for oscillopsia. J Neurol Neurosurg Psychiatr 50:411–415, 1987.

Scott WE, Kraft SP: Surgical treatment of compensatory head position in congenital nystagmus. J Pediatr Ophthalmol Strabismus 21:85–95, 1984.

Yee RD, Baloh RW, Honrubia V: Effect of baclofen on congenital nystagmus. In Lennerstrand G, Zee DS, Keller EL (eds): Functional Basis of Ocular Motility Disorders. Oxford, Pergamon Press, 1982, pp 151–157.

OCULOMOTOR (THIRD NERVE) PARALYSIS

HOWARD EGGERS, M.D.,
and PHILIP KNAPP, M.D.
New York, New York

Paralysis of the oculomotor nerve may be congenital or acquired. It typically presents with symptoms of heteronymous diplopia and blurred vision. The findings are ipsilateral to the lesion and include paralysis of four of the six oculorotary muscles (the superior rectus, medial rectus, inferior rectus, and inferior oblique), which produces an exotropia, hypotropia, and incyclotropia of the involved eye; paralysis of the ciliary muscle and iris sphincter, resulting in absent accommodation and a dilated pupil; and paralysis of the levator, resulting in blepharoptosis. A partial form, or paresis, produces any intermediate degree of weakness of these muscles. The upper division can be involved, producing a double elevator paresis with true or pseudoptosis. The lower division may be selectively involved, sparing the superior rectus and levator. A diabetic oculomotor paresis frequently partially involves pupillary function. A sufficiently discrete nuclear lesion may involve the contralateral instead of the ipsilateral superior rectus and may produce bilateral partial ptosis, although these findings are exceedingly rare.

THERAPY

Supportive. Accurate diagnosis and appropriate medical treatment are necessary. Prism therapy is generally of no benefit because fusion is obtained in only one direction. The involved eye is occluded, if necessary, for relief of diplopia. Because spontaneous recovery may occur up to 6 or 9 months after the onset of the paralysis, surgery should be deferred this long. If any recovery occurs, it must be followed to its end; surgery should only be considered for the remaining deviation.

Ocular. Bifocal correction for near vision may be needed. If amblyopia is present at a treatable age, patching is required. Because of the importance of adequate amblyopia therapy, surgical realignment is best deferred until after amblyopia therapy is completed.

Surgical. The goal of surgery is to realign the eye close to primary position. The choice of procedure depends on which muscles are involved and the completeness of the paralysis.

In partial paralysis there may be sufficient medial rectus function to respond well to a resection of the medial and recession of the antagonist lateral rectus.

In complete paralysis of the third nerve, the transposition of a sound superior oblique should be considered. Although this is a difficult procedure, it is worth trying so that a viable muscle will oppose the action of the recessed lateral rectus to keep the eyes aligned. If the tendon can be released from the trochlea by cutting the trochlea with scissors or popping it with a hemostat without creating much trauma, it is worthwhile. If the tendon is severed, then one goes ahead as though the superior oblique muscle also was paralyzed. If the tendon is freed, it is resected until it is snug and sutured to the insertion of the medial rectus, which then does not require any surgery. There is no value to resecting the medial rectus unless there is a small amount of residual function in it or the superior oblique tendon is lost. The lateral conjunctiva and Tenon's capsule are recessed from the vertical corneal meridian all the way to the orbital margin, and the lateral rectus recessed as far as practically possible. The eye is then anchored in a slightly adducted position for 1 month.

Surgical elevation of the lid may be required if ptosis is severe enough; however, ptosis repair should be deferred until after the eye is aligned. A maximal levator resection utilizing the cutaneous approach can suspend the upper lid. However, a frontalis sling is preferred, as it is easier to set the correct lid level. The ptosis should only be corrected to cover half of the cornea with the brow relaxed because the eye cannot rotate upward with a protective Bell's reflex. Frequent blinking and moisturizing drops must be relied on to prevent corneal drying. Children adapt better than adults to this corneal exposure.

In double elevator paresis with a negative traction test for elevation, a transposition of the full tendons of the medial and lateral recti to the corners of the superior rectus is the operation of choice. The ptosis should not be corrected, for it may be pseudoptosis caused by the hypotropia. If it is real ptosis, elevation of the eye will aggravate the ptosis; therefore, the patient or family should be warned preoperatively.

A paralysis of the lower division of the third nerve (affecting the medial rectus, inferior rectus, and inferior oblique) is treated by transferring the functioning superior rectus to the medial rectus, the lateral rectus to the inferior rectus, and tenectomizing the superior oblique.

Ocular or Periocular Manifestations

Extraocular Muscles: Paralysis of superior rectus, medial rectus, inferior rectus, and inferior oblique muscles.

Eyelids: Ptosis.

Other: Decreased visual acuity; diplopia; internal ophthalmoplegia (paralysis of pupillary sphincter and ciliary muscle); mydriasis; paralysis of accommodation.

PRECAUTIONS

Because of the severe loss of function of the oculorotary muscles in third nerve paralysis, the only attainable goal is realignment of the eye in primary position. Cases with incomplete paralysis may obtain a small horizontal and vertical range of fusion. Care must be taken that the lid is not elevated too far and corneal function compromised. Children learn to suppress the double image; however, adults frequently require an opaque contact lens because of the absence of fusion anywhere, except in one direction of gaze.

COMMENTS

Total third nerve paralysis is devastating to oculomotor function, and even the limited goal of repositioning the eye near primary position is no small achievement. Useful function of the eye in a binocular context can only be obtained in some cases of partial paralysis. Accurate diagnosis and ruling out of other neurologic involvement are essential before any consideration is given to surgical repair.

References

Glaser JS: Infranuclear disorders of eye movements. *In* Duane TD (ed): Clinical Ophthalmology. Hagerstown, MD, Harper & Row, 1982, Vol II, pp 12:1–38.

Helveston EM: Atlas of Strabismus Surgery, 2nd ed, St. Louis, CV Mosby, 1977, pp 176–179.

SUPERIOR OBLIQUE MYOKYMIA

WILLIAM T. SHULTS, M.D.
Portland, Oregon

First described by Duane as unilateral rotary nystagmus, superior oblique myokymia is a benign disorder of ocular stabilization. It is characterized by recurrent episodes of monocular vertical and rotary microtremor and is accompanied by torsional shimmering oscillopsia. The affected eye phasically intorts for seconds during each episode. Although episodes may occur without a provoking change in ocular position, they may be precipitated by downward gaze or lateral head tilts in susceptible patients. There are no known associations with other neurologic disease. Disordered activation or inhibition at the level of the trochlear nucleus or both have been proposed as the mechanisms of production of this unique ocular dyskinesia.

THERAPY

Systemic. Carbamazepine[‡] in a dosage from 100 mg twice daily to 200 mg three times daily has provided dramatic relief of symptoms in most patients. The duration of therapy for superior oblique myokymia is rarely longer than 2 or 3 years.

Surgical. Those cases unresponsive to medical therapy have responded to intrasheath tenotomy of the superior oblique muscle and recession of the inferior oblique muscle of the involved eye.

Ocular or Periocular Manifestations

Extraocular Muscles: Vertical and rotary microtremor.
Other: Oscillopsia; sensation of eye movement; torsional diplopia.

PRECAUTIONS

Use of carbamazepine requires periodic laboratory evaluation of various hematologic parameters, as aplastic anemia, agranulocytosis, thrombocytopenia, and leukopenia are rare associated side effects. Before initiating therapy a pretreatment hematologic battery with the following tests should be obtained: complete blood count, platelet count, reticulocyte count, and serum iron. These tests should be repeated monthly for as long as therapy is continued.

COMMENTS

The symptom of episodic monocular torsional oscillopsia is so distinctive for this disorder that the diagnosis can literally be made over the phone. A slitlamp examination is sometimes needed to see the fine tremorous ocular movements of this benign condition. Referral is unnecessary and, in fact, contraindicated lest the patient be subjected to a major battery of unnecessary neurodiagnostic tests by a consultant unfamiliar with this condition.

References

Duane A: Unilateral rotary nystagmus. Ophthalmol Rec 15:465–468, 1906.
Hoyt WF, Keane JR: Superior oblique myokymia. Report and discussion on five cases of benign intermittent uniocular microtremor. Arch Ophthalmol 84:461–467, 1970.
Palmer E, Shults WT: Superior oblique myokymia: preliminary results of surgical treatment. J Ped Ophthalmol Strab 21:96–101, 1984.
Susac JO, Smith JL, Schatz NJ: Superior oblique myokymia. Arch Neurol 29:432–434, 1973.

SUPERIOR OBLIQUE PALSY

EUGENE M. HELVESTON, M.D.
Indianapolis, Indiana

Superior oblique palsy is the most commonly occurring cranial nerve palsy. It occurs so often because the trochlear nerve rootlets exit the tentorium as fragile threads that may be ruptured by the edge of the dura (tentorium) as the brain shifts and resettles after closed head trauma. Superior oblique palsy may be unilateral or bilateral, congenital or acquired. The superior oblique tendon is also the most frequently noted to be congenitally anomalous or absent.

The symptoms of unilateral superior oblique palsy are abnormal head posture in childhood and both intermittent diplopia (both vertical and horizontal) and abnormal head posture in the adult. In bilateral superior oblique palsy, the chin is depressed to avoid diplopia. The head is tilted to the side opposite the involvement in unilateral superior oblique palsy. Spontaneous torsional diplopia is reported with horizontal displacement of the tilted images in many cases of bilateral superior oblique palsy. As with other cranial nerve palsies, acquired superior oblique palsy (bilateral or unilateral) may resolve in weeks to months after the onset. However, any deviation that persists after 6 months may be considered permanent.

Evaluation of the patient suspected of superior oblique palsy should begin with a careful history. Frequently, a history of trauma is elicited, but often it is not. Questions should be directed toward presence or absence of abnormal head posture, vertical diplopia, and torsional diplopia. An initial qualitative evaluation is carried out following a simple two-step test.

Step 1. The patient is asked to look far to the right and then far to the left. In the lateral version of greater vertical tropia, the adducted eye points to the oblique on the same side or the rectus muscle on the opposite side as the two vertically acting muscles that could be paretic.

Step 2. The head is tilted 45° to one side and then 45° to the other side (Bielschowsky head tilt test). If the vertical deviation increases when the head is tilted toward the higher eye, the oblique arrived at in step 1 is considered paretic. If the vertical deviation increases when the head is tilted to the side of the lower eye, the rectus muscle arrived at in step 1 is considered paretic.

This simple test combining lateral versions and the Bielschowsky head tilt test is a satisfactory method for diagnosing a paresis of any of the vertically acting muscles.

Prism and cover testing should then be carried out in the nine diagnostic positions to provide a quantified evaluation. An essential part of evaluation of the patient with suspected superior oblique palsy is the Maddox double rod test. A red Maddox rod, with the cylinders vertically oriented, is placed in front of the right eye, and a white Maddox rod, similarly oriented, is placed in front of the left eye. The patient is asked to view a point source of light in a darkened room. The Maddox rods are then adjusted if necessary so that red and white lines are parallel. The ocular torsion expressed in degrees is read directly from the trial frame holding the Maddox rods.

Superior oblique palsy without measurable torsion and without spontaneous complaint of torsional diplopia is considered congenital or early acquired; superior oblique palsy with measurable torsion less than 15° and without complaint of spontaneous torsional diplopia is acquired unilateral superior oblique palsy; and spontaneous complaint of torsional diplopia indicates bilateral superior oblique palsy. Also, any measured cyclotropia greater than 15° indicates bilateral superior oblique palsy.

THERAPY

Surgical. The prism and cover measurements obtained in the nine diagnostic positions in a patient with superior oblique palsy can be recorded and interpreted according to a scheme devised by Knapp. *Class I* superior oblique palsy has the greatest vertical deviation in the field of action of the antagonist inferior oblique muscle. It is treated with inferior oblique weakening. *Class II* superior oblique palsy has the greatest vertical deviation in the field of action of the underacting paretic superior oblique. It is treated with superior oblique strengthening. *Class III* is an equal vertical deviation in the field of action of the inferior oblique antagonist and the paretic superior oblique. Deviations of less than 20 prism diopters are treated with inferior oblique weakening, and deviations over 20 prism diopters are treated with inferior oblique weakening combined with superior oblique strengthening. As an alternate to superior oblique strengthening, recession of the contralateral inferior rectus or the ipsilateral superior rectus may be carried out. The pattern in *Class IV* superior oblique palsy is characterized by an "L" shape with a vertical deviation in the field of action of the paretic superior oblique, the antagonist inferior oblique, and also the ipsilateral inferior rectus. It is treated with superior oblique strengthening, inferior oblique weakening, and, if needed, at a second procedure, strengthening of the ipsilateral inferior rectus. As an alternative to superior oblique strengthening, the contralateral superior rectus may be recessed. *Class V* superior oblique palsy is characterized by a greater vertical deviation in all fields of downgaze according to Knapp's classification. It may be treated by strengthening the paretic superior oblique and weakening the contralateral superior oblique. Appropriate vertical rectus surgery or superior oblique strengthening and appropriate vertical rectus surgery may represent a prudent alternative. *Class VI* superior oblique palsy is bilateral superior oblique palsy. It is characterized by a "V" pattern, chin depression, bilaterally positive Bielschowsky test, right hyper in left gaze, left hyper in right gaze, and complaints of torsional diplopia with the tilted images separated horizontally. Also, measured cyclotropia is often greater than 15°. It is treated with bilateral superior oblique strengthening. *Class VII* superior oblique palsy, canine tooth syndrome, is characterized by underaction of the superior oblique and underaction of the inferior oblique on the same side. It can be caused by one or three conditions: trauma to the trochlear area, producing a "double Brown's syndrome"; iatrogenic causes, such as an acquired Brown's syndrome secondary to strengthening the superior oblique along with a residual superior oblique palsy; or a combination of local trauma to the trochlea causing restriction to upgaze along with closed head trauma producing a fourth nerve palsy. *Class VII* superior oblique palsy is extremely difficult to treat. If the patient is able to fuse in the primary position and has some range of fusion above and below, probably no treatment is indicated. If the Brown's syndrome is the most severe problem, an attempt may be made to relieve surgically the trochlear restriction with or without recession of the yoke and contralateral inferior rectus to treat the superior oblique palsy. Iatrogenic Brown's syndrome may require reduction of the tuck or recession of the resected superior oblique tendon along with recession of the contralateral inferior rectus.

Certain types of superior oblique palsy are characterized by fairly severe torsional defects with very little vertical tropia. They may occur unilaterally or bilaterally. In such a case, the patient may benefit from anterior transposition of the superior oblique tendon. It may be done by shifting the whole tendon or just the anterior fibers; an adjustable suture may be used in this procedure.

In cases where the superior oblique reflected tendon is absent, recession of the antagonist inferior oblique, recession of the ipsilateral superior rectus, and, if necessary, appropriate treatment of any coexisting horizontal deviation are done. Congenital absence of the superior oblique should be suspected if congenital superior oblique palsy is associated with a significant horizontal deviation, amblyopia, ptosis, or bony asymmetry of the orbits or face.

PRECAUTIONS

Strengthening procedures of the superior oblique frequently produce an iatrogenic mechanical limitation of elevation in adduction or Brown's syndrome. For this reason, shortening of the superior oblique tendon by tuck or resection and advancement should be done in fairly small amounts and should be graded according to the redundance or laxity of the tendon noted at surgery.

In cases of superior oblique palsy after closed head trauma, a high index of suspicion regarding bilateral superior oblique palsy should be maintained. If unsuspected bilateral superior oblique palsy is treated as unilateral superior oblique palsy, a second procedure for superior oblique palsy will invariably be required on the second eye. Because of the complicated nature of the vertical or torsional diplopia associated with superior oblique palsy, prism therapy is often ineffective. Generally, nearly every case of superior oblique palsy can be classified as either congenital, congenital absence, or traumatic acquired. Other causes for superior oblique palsy, such as tumor, vascular abnormalities, toxins, or inflammation, are rarely implicated. A reliable guideline is to suspect a redundant or anomalous tendon in cases of congenital superior oblique palsy on the other hand, acquired superior oblique palsy is more likely to have a more normal-appearing tendon. In the former, superior oblique tendon tuck, resection, or redirection is frequently indicated. In acquired superior oblique palsy, alternatives to superior oblique strengthening should be considered.

Occasionally, patients may present with intermittent symptomatic oscillopsia. Careful evaluation may reveal rhythmic intorsion of one eye accompanied by cyclodiplopia. This condition has been called superior oblique myokymia. It may be transient, or it may be persistent and extremely troublesome. Superior oblique tenectomy has been suggested as a suitable treatment, but such treatment may in turn result in troublesome superior oblique underaction. In this case, inferior oblique weakening may be done at the time of superior oblique myectomy or during a second procedure.

COMMENTS

Superior oblique palsy is not uncommon and is usually a result of trauma or congenital unknown causes. Significant systemic disease is rarely associated with this condition, and therefore, extensive workup is not indicated unless other neurologic complaints warrant it. Surgical treatment can be very successful, and the scheme devised by Knapp has been very useful.

References

Ellis FD, Helveston EM: Superior oblique palsy: Diagnosis and classification. Int Ophthalmol Clin 16:127–135, 1976.
Helveston EM: Atlas of Strabismus Surgery, 3rd ed. St. Louis, CV Mosby, 1985.
Helveston EM, Birchler CCO: Class VII superior oblique palsy: Subclassification and treatment suggestions. Am. Orthopt J. In press.
Helveston EM, Giangiacomo JG, Ellis FD: Congenital absence of the superior oblique tendon. Trans Am Ophthalmol Soc 79:123–135, 1981.
Knapp P: Classification and treatment of superior oblique palsy. Am Orthopt J 24:18–22, 1974.
Metz HS, Lerner H: The adjustable Harada-Ito procedure. Arch Ophthalmol 99:624–626, 1981.
von Noorden GK: Binocular Vision and Ocular Motility. Theory and Management of Strabismus, 2nd ed. St. Louis, CV Mosby, 1980, p 371.
von Noorden GK, Murray E, and Wong SY: Superior oblique paralysis: A review of 270 cases. Arch Ophthalmol 109:1171–1176, 1986.

V-PATTERN ESOTROPIA
HENRY S. METZ, M.D.
Rochester, New York

V-pattern esotropia is an incomitant esotropia in which the deviation is greater in downgaze than in upgaze. By convention, there should be a 15 prism diopter difference between up- and downgaze measurements to classify the patient as having a V-pattern. Many cases are associated with overaction of the inferior oblique muscles and underaction of the superior oblique muscles. Increased abduction in upgaze secondary to inferior oblique overaction may be the cause of the V-pattern. In some patients, oblique muscle function appears normal. A downward slant of the lid fissures has also been noted in some cases. The V-pattern may be associated with any type of esotropia, including accommodative or paralytic varieties. Patients with superior oblique palsy often demonstrate a V-pattern, most likely secondary to superior oblique weakness and thus diminished abduction effect in downgaze. Brown syndrome patients also frequently have a V-pattern.

THERAPY

Ocular. Neither prisms nor orthoptics can be expected to eliminate the V-pattern.
Surgical. When the inferior oblique muscles overact, inferior oblique weakening surgery (recession, myectomy, disinsertion) can collapse the V-pattern. Appropriate surgery on the horizontal recti to correct the esotropia in primary gaze should be planned at the same time.

In cases in which the inferior oblique muscles do not overact, vertical transposition of the horizontal recti, along with recession or resection for the esotropia, can be successful. When planning bilateral surgery, both medial recti should be depressed or both lateral recti elevated. If monocular surgery is performed, the medial rectus insertion should be depressed and lateral rectus insertion elevated. Less than one-half tendon width transposition is usually ineffective, whereas more than one tendon width transposition is rarely indicated. Horizontal transposition of the vertical recti for V-pattern (superior recti moved nasally, inferior recti moved temporally) has been described, but is not commonly utilized because of variability and lack of good predictability of the results.

Ocular or Periocular Manifestations

Extraocular Muscles: Inferior oblique muscle overaction and superior oblique muscle underaction; V-pattern esotropia following superior oblique palsy with antagonist muscle (inferior oblique) overaction.
Other: Chin-down position for upgaze; visual acuity decrease is unusual unless untreated amblyopia is present.

PRECAUTIONS

In the presence of superior oblique overaction (even mild overaction), it may be unwise to perform inferior oblique myectomies or large recessions as an A-pattern may result.

Small degrees of torsion may result from monocular transposition of the horizontal rectus insertions (1 to 1.5°). These are not symptomatic. However, in patients with superior oblique palsy and excyclotorsion, this added cyclotorsion may add to the problem. Therefore, monocular horizontal rectus transpositions are best avoided.

Occasionally, accommodative esotropes with fusion at distance fixation and esotropia at near fixation are mistaken for a V-pattern esotropia. This occurs because the near deviation is measured in downgaze instead of in primary gaze. Attention to proper measurement technique can help avoid this confusion.

COMMENTS

V-pattern esotropia is not only cosmetically unsatisfactory but also a barrier to fusion (both central and peripheral) because of the incomitance of the deviation. Surgery for the esotropia alone usually does not collapse the "V," so that oblique muscle surgery or vertical transposition of the horizontal rectus insertions is useful. Less than 10 prism diopters of V-pattern rarely require attention in surgical planning.

References

Goldstein JH: Monocular vertical displacement of the horizontal rectus muscles in the A and V patterns. Am J Ophthalmol 64:265, 1967.
Jampolsky A: Oblique muscle surgery of the A and V patterns. J Pediatr Ophthalmol 2:31, 1965.
Knapp P: A and V patterns. *In* Symposium on Strabismus. Transactions of the New Orleans Academy of Ophthalmology. St. Louis, CV Mosby, 1971, p 242.
Metz HS, Schwartz L: The treatment of A and V patterns by monocular surgery. Arch Ophthalmol 95:251, 1977.
Parks MM: The weakening surgical procedures for eliminating overaction of the inferior oblique muscle. Am J Ophthalmol 73:107, 1972.
Scott AB, Stella SL: Measurement of A and V patterns. J Pediatr Ophthalmol 5:181, 1968.
Taylor J: The management of A and V patterns in strabismus. Aust J Ophthalmol 4:165, 1976.

V-PATTERN EXOTROPIA
HENRY S. METZ, M.D.
Rochester, New York

V-pattern exotropia is an incomitant exotropia in which the deviation is greater in upgaze than in downgaze. By convention, 15 prism diopters of difference between up- and downgaze should be present to classify the patient as having a V-pattern. Many patients with V-pattern exotropia demonstrate inferior oblique overaction or superior oblique underaction or both. Oblique muscle function may appear normal. An outward and downward slant of the palpebral fissures has been noted in some cases. The V-pattern may be seen with intermittent or constant exotropia. It has also been noted with large-angle long-standing exotropia in which the lateral rectus muscle has become contractured with time, although an X-pattern with all obliques overacting may also be seen.

THERAPY

Ocular. The V-pattern is not affected by orthoptics or prisms.
Surgical. With inferior oblique muscle overaction, a weakening procedure (recession, myectomy, disinsertion) is usually the technique of choice to collapse the V-pattern. Horizontal rectus surgery for correction of the exodeviation should be performed at the same time. If both inferior obliques are overacting, bilateral surgery is indicated even if the overaction is unequal. However, if only one inferior oblique muscle is overacting, unilateral surgery is appropriate, although a second operation may have to be done in the future if the previously normal inferior oblique becomes overactive.

When inferior oblique muscle action is normal or minimally overactive, vertical transposition of the horizontal recti combined with appropriate amounts of recession or resection or both for the exotropia can be helpful. If both lateral recti are recessed, the insertions should be elevated (about one-half tendon width for a small V-pattern to a full tendon width for a large V-pattern) to provide comitance in up- and downgaze. If the medial recti are resected, their insertions should be depressed a similar amount. In cases where monocular recession-resection is planned, the lateral rectus should be elevated and the medial rectus depressed.

Attempts at horizontal displacement of the vertical rectus insertions (inferior recti temporally, superior recti nasally) have generally proven less effective and less predictable, and this approach is rarely indicated.

Ocular or Periocular Manifestations

Extraocular Muscles: Brown syndrome where there is restriction to elevation of the globe in adduction; Duane syndrome, probably due to lateral rectus co-contraction; inferior oblique overaction and superior oblique underaction; superior oblique palsy with antagonist (inferior oblique) overaction.
Other: Chin-up position.

PRECAUTIONS

When superior oblique overaction is present, inferior oblique weakening surgery may be contraindicated as an A-pattern may result.

Monocular vertical transposition of the horizontal rectus insertions may produce small degrees of cyclotorsion (1 to 1.5°). This has not produced symptoms. Patients with superior oblique palsy may have excyclotorsion so any procedure that could accentuate the torsion should be avoided. With bilateral superior oblique palsy, V-pattern, and symptomatic cyclotorsion, a bilateral superior oblique tuck may be the surgery of choice.

COMMENTS

V-pattern exotropia not only causes a cosmetically unsatisfactory eye position but is also an impediment to fusion (many exodeviations have some fusion potential). Surgery for correction of the exotropia alone usually does not collapse the "V," so oblique muscle surgery or vertical transposition of the horizontal rectus insertions may be considered. Tilting the chin 30° upward and downward for measurement has been found to be equally as accurate as moving the target above and below primary gaze.

References

Costenbader F: Symposium: The A and V patterns in strabismus. Trans Am Acad Ophthalmol Otolaryngol 76:354, 1964.
Goldstein JH: Monocular vertical displacement of the horizontal rectus muscles in the A and V patterns. Am J Ophthalmol 64:265, 1967.
Jampolsky A: Oblique muscle surgery of the A and V pattern. J Pediatr Ophthalmol 2:31, 1965.
Knapp P: A and V patterns. *In* Symposium on Strabismus. Transactions of the New Orleans Academy of Ophthalmology. St. Louis, CV Mosby, 1971, p 242.
Metz HS, Schwartz L: The treatment of A and V patterns by monocular surgery. Arch Ophthalmol 95:251, 1977.
Scott AB: V-pattern exotropia. Elecromyographic study of an unusual case. Invest Ophthalmol 12:232, 1973.
Scott AB, Stella SL: Measurement of A-V Patterns. J Pediatr Ophthalmol 5:181, 1968.

SECTION 23

Eyelids

ANKYLOBLEPHARON
DAVID W. VASTINE, M.D.,
and ROBERT L. STAMPER, M.D.
San Francisco, California

Ankyloblepharon is an adhesion between the upper and lower lids along the palpebral margin. It may range in size from a single filamentous band to a rather extensive adhesion. This condition can be either congenital or secondary to severe inflammatory conditions of the lid margins. The usual site of fusion is the outer canthus, in which case the condition is called *external* ankyloblepharon. An *internal* form, with fusion at the inner canthus, is less common. Either form gives the appearance of a pseudostrabismus. Ankyloblepharon is frequently found in conjunction with symblepharon.

THERAPY

Surgical. Surgical therapy is aimed at separating the disturbed epithelial surfaces until re-epithelialization and healing can occur. Usually, the eyelids may be separated easily with scissors. However, if the involvement is extensive, the separation is more effectively done with a scalpel while the underside of the eyelid is supported and separated from the globe with a ribbon retractor or similar instrument to protect the cornea and to facilitate the dissection. The marginal surfaces may be separated by a thin, soft plastic or silicone sheet sutured in place until the lid margins have re-epithelialized. A marginal graft may be necessary in severe cases. In those cases, the margins are lined with conjunctiva, the skin and conjunctival edges are sutured, and the lids are held apart to prevent new adhesions. If the canthi are involved, a canthoplasty may also be required. Associated symblepharon is also repaired by surgical lysis, Z plasty, and autologous conjunctival transplantation.

Ocular or Periocular Manifestations

Eyelids: Adhesions; fusion; symblepharon.
Globe: Anophthalmos; microphthalmos; phthisis bulbi; xerosis.
Lacrimal System: Epiphora; punctal occlusion.

PRECAUTIONS

Bands of scar tissue form most commonly at the outer canthus, but they may also form at the inner canthus. They may also bridge the palpebral aperture. In the severe form, scar tissue may significantly hinder eye opening and may even interfere with vision. Corneal and conjunctival xerosis may develop with severe dryness. In most severe cases, symblepharon must take operative priority. Medial lid adhesion and scarring may incorporate the puncta and the canalicular apparatus. Reconstructive procedures may be required to re-establish the integrity of the lacrimal drainage system, including punctoplasty and the insertion of Quickert-style Silastic tubes.

COMMENTS

The inheritance pattern of congenital ankyloblepharon has been described as dominant in some patients and sporadic in others. Intrauterine injury or inflammation, as well as a primary aberration of growth at either canthus, has been postulated as potential causes of the congenital variety.

Acquired forms of ankyloblepharon may occur during healing of destructive processes involving the palpebral margins. Apposition of upper and lower marginal surfaces that have been denuded of epithelium plays a key role in the pathogenesis of secondary ankyloblepharon. Some of the more common causes of acquired ankyloblepharon are caustic and thermal burns, trauma, ulcerative blepharitis, impetigo, cicatricial pemphigoid, and epidermolysis bullosa. Lupus vulgaris of the skin and eyelids, diphtheritic conjunctivitis, trachoma, vaccinia, smallpox, and other skin and mucous membrane disorders may also result in ankyloblepharon.

References

Beard C: Diseases of the lids. *In* Dunlap EA (ed): Gordon's Medical Management of Ocular Disease, 2nd ed. Hagerstown, MD, Harper & Row, 1976, pp 110–135.

Duke-Elder S (ed): System of Ophthalmology. St. Louis, CV Mosby, 1963, Vol III, pp 867–871; 1974 Vol XIII, pp 590–591.

BENIGN ESSENTIAL BLEPHAROSPASM

JOHN R. SAMPLES, M.D.
Portland, Oregon

Benign essential blepharospasm is a potentially disabling disorder that affects primarily older individuals and is often associated with other evidence of orofacial dyskinesia. It is an involuntary tonic, often forceful closure of the eyelids that may be either intermittent or continuous. Symptoms are typically made worse by stress, fatigue, bright lights, and driving, although this varies among affected individuals. It may be relieved by sleep and relaxation. In some instances, patients may be distracted from their blepharospasm by being given tasks to perform that require a fair amount of concentration. The disease is usually slowly progressive, but a variety of courses may be seen. It is almost always bilateral, although one side may be worse than the other. Involvement of the lower face and the oropharynx, termed Meig's syndrome, is surprisingly common and often overlooked.

It is helpful to differentiate the syndrome of benign essential blepharospasm from other causes of blepharospasm. A thorough neurologic and ophthalmologic examination is required before making the diagnosis. Some individuals have a psychogenic etiology for their blepharospasm. Such individuals are typically young and do not present with a true tonic closure of the eyelids, but rather a flutter or a voluntary squeezing. The chronic closing of the protractor muscles (orbicularis oculi, corrugator, and procerus), in patients with benign essential blepharospasm, can lead to dermatochalasis, brow ptosis, and blepharoptosis. These patients are prone to developing entropion and ectropion. The differential diagnosis also includes dry eye conditions, other types of keratitis, apraxia of lid opening in which the patient is unable to initiate the opening of the eyes, hemifacial spasm, tardive dyskinesia, postencephalic parkinsonism, and other movement disorders. Since some patients with blepharospasm may have Parkinson's disease, referral to a neurologist to rule out that disease may be an important part of the initial evaluation. The pathophysiology of blepharospasm remains uncertain.

THERAPY

Systemic. A large variety of drugs have been recommended or tried for benign essential blepharospasm. Pharmacologic trials need to be limited because many patients will become frustrated after trying several drugs. However, if the patient is found to have diseases or disorders that mimic Parkinson's disease, treatment with a dopamine agonist, such as a carbidopa/levodopa combination, bromocriptine, or amantadine, may be effective.

It is usually best to start with an anticholinergic/antispasmodic, such as trihexyphenidyl, and increase the doses slowly. Many patients will obtain control of their blepharospasm but will not tolerate the associated systemic side effects, including dry mouth, that are seen with the use of trihexyphenidyl. Following anticholinergic therapy, a trial with a benzodiazapine, such as clonazepam, may be worthwhile. Antidepressants have been useful in a very limited number of patients. No medication has been identified as specifically curative for this condition.

Ocular. Some patients who present with blepharospasm have keratitis or evidence of dry eyes. It is important therefore to rule out the presence of a dry eye or blepharitis. These patients may be particularly prone to both of these conditions. In particular, patients are prone to keratitis after surgery or botulinum A toxin injections for this condition.

Botulinum A toxin[†] injections provide effective relief for most patients with benign essential blepharospasm. The toxin works by interfering with acetylcholine release from nerve terminals. It may provide relief from spasm for 3 months or longer. It is generally well tolerated, although some patients will develop ptosis or diplopia. A typical pattern of injection is to place 5 units subcutaneously at each of the two sites over the brow, the upper lid and the lower lid on one side, for a total of six injections per side. Many patterns are used, and these should be tailored to the patient's spasm.

Surgical. Surgery should be reserved for individuals who have failed trials with medication and botulinum A toxin. Older procedures involved sectioning the seventh cranial nerve either at its main trunk or along the peripheral branches. Reinnervation was a frequent problem, and as a result resection of the orbicularis oculi muscles has become more popular using the technique described by Gillum and Anderson. This technique involves the meticulous extirpation of all of the accessible orbicularis oculi, procerus, corrugator, superciliaris and fascial nerves in postorbicular fascia.

Supportive. A foundation exists to deal with the problem of benign essential blepharospasm (Benign Essential Blepharospasm Research Foundation, Inc., 755 Howell Street, Beaumont, TX 77706). These patients are often helped by support groups, although a few patients have been adversely affected by participation, when they have been exposed to patients with disease which is far more advanced than their own. Because there is substantial variability in the severity of blepharospasm, some patients may develop increased anxiety as the result of participating in support groups that include patients with severe truncal ataxia. Therefore, referral of patients needs to be individualized.

Ocular or Periocular Manifestations

Cornea: Keratitis.
Lids: Blepharospasm; dermatochalasis; ectropion; entropion.
Other: Dystonias of the head, neck, and whole body.

PRECAUTIONS

Knowledge and familiarity with the drugs used to treat this condition are essential. The effective use of botulinum A toxin requires experience tailoring the injections to each individual in order to obtain a desirable effect with minimal complications. Every patient receiving the toxin should have a complete eye examination before treatment, since baseline parameters are essential before ptosis or diplopia develops. Patients undergoing botulinum A toxin therapy should be closely monitored for ophthalmic complications, including ptosis and keratitis. Obtaining a careful and appropriate consent before using botulinum A toxin injections is mandatory.

COMMENTS

A therapeutic approach to the patient with benign essential blepharospasm should include a trial of medications before consideration of botulinum A toxin injections or surgery. Rarely, patients respond to medication and require no further therapy. Several patients have been observed to do extremely well with an anticholinergic alone. If systemic medications are ineffective in controlling the medicine, then a trial with botulinum A toxin injections is indicated. The efficacy of such injections has been demonstrated. Repeated injections and the patient's lack of acceptance of them are indications for proceeding with surgery. A variety of surgical approaches have been described. The most effective may be the removal of orbicularis oculi, procerus, and corrugator muscles to limit the effect and extent of the disease.

References

Freuh BR, et al: Treatment of blepharospasm with botulinum toxin. A preliminary report. Arch Ophthalmol 102:1464–1468, 1984.
Gillum WN, Anderson RL: Blepharospasm surgery. An anatomical approach. Arch Ophthalmol 99:1056–1062, 1981.
Jankovic J: Clinical features, differential diagnosis and pathogenesis of blepharospasm and cranial cervical dystonia. *In* Bosniak SL, Smith BC (eds): Advances in Ophthalmic Plastic and Reconstructive Surgery—Blepharospasm. New York, Pergamon Press, Vol 4. 1985.
Jones FTW, Samples JR, Waller RR: The treatment of essential blepharospasm. Mayo Clin Proc 60:663–666, 1985.
Lingua RW: Sequelae of botulinum toxin injection. Am J Ophthalmol 100:305–307, 1985.

BLEPHAROCHALASIS
CROWELL BEARD, M.D.,
and JOHN H. SULLIVAN, M.D.
San Francisco, California

Blepharochalasis is characterized by bilateral episodic swelling of the eyelids and periorbital areas, lasting up to several days and resulting in progressive damage to the eyelid structures. It is sometimes familial, affecting both sexes, with the onset of symptoms usually between the ages of 7 and 20.

As a result of repeated attacks, the skin loses its elasticity, becomes thin, and resembles parchment. Stretching and thinning of the orbital septum cause the preaponeurotic fat and occasionally the orbital lobe of the lacrimal gland to prolapse into the eyelid. The upper nasal fat pad often atrophies, and the overlying skin retracts, causing a typical depression and pseudoepicanthal fold. Moderate to severe ptosis can result from progressive damage to the levator aponeurosis. The lateral canthal tendons may also deteriorate, resulting in horizontal phimosis of the lid slits and rounded lateral canthi.

THERAPY

Supportive. In the acute phase, treatment is symptomatic. If a specific factor that triggers an acute attack can be identified, the only treatment necessary is avoidance. Unfortunately, this is seldom possible. Cold compresses during the acute phase may reduce swelling and tissue damage. Local and systemic corticosteroids are of limited value. Fortunately, the frequency and severity of attacks lessen with age.

Surgical. Surgery is usually necessary to repair damaged eyelid tissue. Removal of redundant skin by blepharoplasty is beneficial. Prolapsed preaponeurotic fat may be excised, and the lacrimal gland may be sutured to the periorbita of the lacrimal fossa if it has been displaced. Horizontal phimosis is treated by reattaching the lateral canthal tissues to the periosteum anterior to the orbital tubercle with a nonabsorbable suture material.

Ptosis repair is frequently necessary and often difficult. The Fasanella-Servat procedure is sufficient to correct minimal ptosis. Disinsertion or dehiscence of the levator aponeurosis is best managed by reattachment or levator tuck. Surgery is often unsatisfactory because recurrent attacks of edema destroy the result. For this reason, ptosis surgery should be delayed until the frequency and severity of attacks have diminished. This is not always possible, particularly if the ptosis is disabling. Delayed repair, although preferable, may be complicated by the presence of severely damaged tissues. Reapproximation or repair of a markedly thinned levator complex can be very challenging and unfortunately is apt to be followed by recurrence.

Precautions

The term "blepharochalasis" is frequently misused by ophthalmologists and plastic surgeons to indicate any of the conditions characterized by "baggy eyelids." Aging redundant eyelid skin is more accurately termed "dermatochalasis." True blepharochalasis is a very rare cause of baggy eyelids.

Comments

The etiology of this rare condition remains unknown. In the acute phase, it resembles angioneurotic edema, which is more common and believed to be allergic in origin. Blepharochalasis has not been shown to be an allergic reaction, although factors that seem to precipitate an acute attack, such as fever or exposure to sunlight, have been observed in some patients. Eosinophilia, urticaria, visceral involvement, laryngeal edema, and respiratory distress are rarely observed. Therefore, blepharochalasis appears to represent a specific localized disease entity that is not the same as angioneurotic edema.

References

Alvis BY: Blepharochalasis. Report of a case. Am J Ophthalmol 18:238–245, 1935.
Collin JRO, et al: Blepharochalasis. Br J Ophthalmol 63:542–546, 1979.
Custer PL, Tenzel RR, Kowalczyk AP: Blepharochalasis syndrome. Am J Ophthalmol 99:424–428, 1985.
Stieglitz LN, Crawford JS: Blepharochalasis. Am J Ophthalmol 77:100–102, 1974.
Sunder TR, Balsam MJ, Vengrow MI: Neurological manifestations of angioedema. Report of two cases and review of the literature. JAMA 247:2005–2007, 1982.

BLEPHAROPHIMOSIS
JAY JUSTIN OLDER, M.D.
Tampa, Florida

Blepharophimosis is the condition in which the palpebral aperture is decreased in height and width. The dominantly inherited tetrad of ptosis, epicanthus inversus, telecanthus, and blepharophimosis is referred to as the blepharophimosis syndrome. Patients with the blepharophimosis syndrome have small palpebral apertures associated with an increased width between the inner canthi (telecanthus) and a fold of skin from the lower lid extending toward the bridge of the nose (epicanthus inversus). The narrow palpebral aperture is a result of the ptosis, which is usually severe. Dominant inheritance with essentially 100 per cent penetrance has been well documented. There appear to be no other associated systemic findings, and intelligence is normal. Ectropion, punctal displacement, low-set ears, strabismus, and optic nerve colobomata have been reported in a few patients with this syndrome. The individual features of short palpebral apertures, telecanthus, and ptosis are sometimes seen as part of the following syndromes: fetal alcohol, Dubowitz, trisomy 18, Williams, cerebro-oculo-facial-skeletal, Carpenter, oral-facial-digital, and Waardenburg. These possibilities should be considered in the absence of a definite dominant pedigree or in the presence of other anomalies, particularly mental retardation.

Lack of support at the lateral canthus may also give rise to a senile or spastic blepharophimosis. Cicatrical blepharophimosis may follow destructive lesions, such as trachoma, or may occur after trauma.

THERAPY

Surgical. The goal of therapy is to create a more normal appearing eye with functional eyelids. It is usually preferable to reconstruct the medial canthal deformities 6 to 12 months before repair of the ptosis.

The upper canthal fold can be eliminated by Mustarde's double Z plasties, in which flaps are formed as rectangles and closed as triangles. This method provides needed tissue in the vertical direction. An alternative method for correction is the Y to V operation of Verwey, in which an incision in the medial canthus is created in the form of a horizontal Y and closed in the shape of a horizontal V.

If telecanthus is present, the medial canthus can be shortened before closure of the flaps in either of these procedures. To advance the angle medially, a section of the canthal tendon can be excised and the remaining edges reapproximated with a permanent suture. For larger amounts of telecanthus, transnasal wiring can be performed by creating osteotomies in the area of both anterior lacrimal crests. The medial canthal tendons are attached to each other, using wires that pass through the osteotomies and the nasal septum. The wires are tightened until the desired amount of telecanthus repair is accomplished.

Since the levator muscle is usually weak, ptosis repair is best accomplished by a tarsofrontalis suspension. Autogenous fascia lata, removed from the patient's leg and placed as a double rhomboid or double triangle, gives the best chance for permanent repair. Good alternative materials are preserved fascia lata or silicone rods.

Some types of blepharophimosis have a skin shortage instead of epicanthal folds. In these cases, full-thickness skin grafts from the retroauricular area should be placed in all four lids 6 to 12 months before the other abnormalities are corrected. Some degrees of lower lid ectropion can be repaired with rotation flaps or free skin grafts in association with the medial canthal repair.

If the lateral canthus is medially placed, a lateral canthoplasty may be required to move the lateral canthus outward. A lateral canthotomy with advancement of the conjunctiva to the new skin edges is often sufficient to increase the horizontal direction of the palpebral fissure.

Surgical repair of acquired blepharophimosis is directed at the underlying disease. Medial and lateral canthoplasties or ectropion repair may be required.

Ocular or Periocular Manifestations

Conjunctiva: Scarred or contracted in secondary blepharophimosis because of ocular pemphigus or trachoma.
Eyelids: Ectropion; epicanthus inversus; lacrimal puncta displacement; ptosis; telecanthus.

PRECAUTIONS

Some families may desire only the ptosis repair, since reconstruction of the medial canthus would cause the child to look different from other family members. Careful evaluation of eyelid excursion is important because levator function is usually so minimal that a levator resection would be insufficient to elevate the eyelids. The possibility of severe congenital deformities should be investigated in the absence of a clear dominant pedigree or if there are associated malformations or mental retardation.

COMMENTS

Congenital blepharophimosis comprises 3 to 6 per cent of congenital ptosis. The eyelid and canthal deformities can be improved by the treatment described. Repair should be done at age of 5 years or any time thereafter.

References

Beard C: Ptosis, 3rd ed. St. Louis, CV Mosby, 1981, pp 41–46, 211–225.
Callahan MA, Callahan A: Ophthalmic Plastic and Orbital Surgery. Birmingham, Aesculapius, 1979, pp 36–40.
Duke-Elder S (ed): System of Ophthalmology. St. Louis, CV Mosby, 1974, Vol XIII, pp 589–590.
Grizard WS, O'Donnell JJ, Carey JC: The cerebro-oculo-facio-skeletal syndrome. Am J Ophthalmol 89:293–298, 1980.
Kohn R, Romano PE: Blepharoptosis, blepharophimosis, epicanthus inversus, and telecanthus—a syndrome with no name. Am J Ophthalmol 72:625–632, 1971.
Mustardé JC: Repair and Reconstruction in the Orbital Region. Edinburgh, E & S Livingstone Limited, 1966, pp 338–352.
Owens N, Hadley RC, Kloepfer HW: Hereditary blepharophimosis, ptosis, and epicanthus inversus. J Int Coll Surg 33:558–574, 1960.
Sacrez R, et al: Le blépharophimosis compliqué familial. Etude des membres de la famille Ble Ann Pediatr 10:493–501, 1963.
Smith DW: Recognizable Patterns of Human Malformation: Genetic, Embryologic, and Clinical Aspects. Philadelphia, WB Saunders, 1970, pp 10–11, 54–55, 62–63, 122–125, 144–145, 240–241, 336–337, 447.

CHALAZION
HERBERT J. GERSHEN, M.D.
San Francisco, California

A chalazion is a chronic granuloma of a meibomian gland and may result from an inflammation of this gland. There is characteristic swelling caused by the retention of secretions and the formation of granulation tissue. As the gland fills with secretions and granulation tissue, it forms a tumor that can grow as large as 7 or 8 mm in diameter. It may remain contained in the tarsus or break through anteriorly beneath the skin or on the conjunctival side, possibly resulting in a fistula through which the granulation tissue protrudes. A marginal chalazion is a smaller granuloma involving the area of a meibomian gland near its marginal termination. Chalazions are more common on the upper lid, occur most often in adults, and are associated with seborrhea, chronic blepharitis, and acne rosacea.

THERAPY

Supportive. In general, most chalazions disappear in a few months without therapy. If the chalazion is small and causing no symptoms, treatment may not be required. A few seem to resolve with the use of hot packs and topical antibiotics. Systemic antibiotics are seldom indicated in the management of chalazion.
Ocular. Local injection of corticosteroids has been shown to be an effective, rapid form of treatment for chalazia. A volume of 0.5 to 2.0 ml of 5 mg/ml triamcinolone acetonide may be directly injected in the center of the chalazion. A second injection may be considered 2 to 7 days later if necessary. Topical antibiotic coverage may be given for several days after the intralesional injection.
Surgical. Surgical removal from the palpebral conjunctival side is preferred, unless a granuloma extends through skin or previous drainage has occurred externally and removal of the lesion is obviously easier by the external route. If secondarily infected, the chalazion should first be managed by heat, antibiotics, and, in selected cases, incision and drainage. A small chalazion may be treated by curettage and cauterization of the lining of the gland with phenol or trichloroacetic acid. A larger chalazion is more likely to be cured by surgical excision. Infiltration anesthesia and tarsal block are administered, and a chalazion clamp is applied. A vertical tarsal incision 2 to 3 mm from the lid margin is made. Identification and removal of the sac within its capsule are performed. Curettage and excision of the remaining tissue and sac are done carefully, being cautious not to remove normal tissue. However, in some cases, total removal of the tarsal plate within the area of the chalazion clamp without the need of curettage is the method of choice. Electrocautery may be used to prevent bleeding, although this is seldom necessary if pressure is applied for 4 to 5 minutes. A mild

pressure bandage with antibiotic ointment is applied for 4 to 6 hours. An antibiotic ointment, applied three to four times daily, may be continued for 4 to 5 days.

If the external approach is used, a horizontal incision at least 3 mm from lid margin is made in an existing crease, and the chalazion is removed. Normal lid tissue should not be sacrificed. Hemostasis is achieved with electrocautery. The wound is closed with 6-0 silk suture after the clamp is removed.

Occasionally, a chalazion involves both skin and conjunctiva; in such case, removal may be through both surfaces. A thorough-and-through hole should be avoided by offsetting the skin and conjunctival incisions.

Marginal chalazions that are improperly removed lead to notching, trichiasis, and loss of lashes. Most marginal chalazions are connected to another chalazion located farther from the lid margin. The contents may be expressed by rolling two cotton-tipped applicators toward the lid margin from both sides of the lid. If this is painful, a local anesthetic may be used. If the contents cannot be expressed, incision is made over the distal chalazion, and removal of the contents is by curettage. The marginal area of the eyelid is curetted, leaving a 3-mm bridge of normal tarsus nearest the lid margin to prevent notching. Postoperative antibiotics and a pressure patch are then applied.

Ocular or Periocular Manifestations

Eyelids: Edema; granulation tissue; mass.
Other: Astigmatism.

PRECAUTIONS

Intralesional injection of corticosteroids is particularly suitable for chalazion located near the lacrimal drainage apparatus because surgery in this area may lead to serious complications. Insoluble aqueous preparations are preferable to crystalline suspensions of corticosteroids to minimize complications of hypopigmentation and atrophy of the treated skin. A transconjunctival injection may also provide a further safeguard against these complications.

Lid incision should be made 2 to 3 mm from the lid margin to prevent notching. In general, normal lid tissue should not be sacrificed in attempting to completely remove a chalazion. A biopsy should be done on recurrent chalazions or those that appear unusual to rule out malignancy. If secondary infection exists, the pus should be evacuated, but no curettage should be performed.

COMMENTS

Conservative treatment is indicated and, in most cases, surgery should be performed only after a few weeks of hot packs. If multiple chalazions are present, they may be removed by careful dissection without fear of lid deformity, since this fibrous tissue heals without leaving gaps in the tarsal plate. Complete removal of the chalazion with the tarsal plate has not been reported to cause a lid deformity.

References

Dua HS, Nilawar DV: Nonsurgical therapy of chalazion. Am J Ophthalmol 94:424–425, 1982.
Duke-Elder S (ed): System of Ophthalmology. St. Louis, CV Mosby, 1965, Vol VIII, pp 242–247.
Epstein GA, Allen MP: Combined excision and drainage with intralesional corticosteroid injection in the treatment of chronic chalazia. Arch Ophthalmol 106:514–516, 1988.
Gershen HJ: Chalazion excision. Ophthalmic Surg 5:75–76, 1974.
King RA, Ellis PP: Treatment of chalazia with corticosteroid injections. Ophthal Surg 17:351–353, 1986.
Perry HD, Serniuk RA: Conservative treatment of chalazia. Ophthalmology 87:218–221, 1980.
Pizzarello LD, et al: Intralesional corticosteroid therapy of chalazia. Am J Ophthalmol 85:818–821, 1978.
Sloas HA Jr, et al: Treatment of chalazia with injectable triamcinolone. Ann Ophthalmol 15:78–80, 1983.
Soll DB, Winslow R: Surgery of the eyelids. In Duane TD (ed): Clinical Ophthalmology. Hagerstown, MD, Harper & Row, 1982, Vol V, pp 5:6–9.
Vidaurri LJ, Jacob P: Intralesional corticosteroid treatment of chalazia. Ann Ophthalmol 18:339–340, 1986.

DISTICHIASIS
(Districhiasis)
RICHARD L. ANDERSON, M.D., F.A.C.S.,
and JOHN B. HOLDS, M.D.
Salt Lake City, Utah

Congenital distichiasis—sometimes erroneously called "districhiasis"—is a rare condition in which an accessory row of eyelashes is present in or near the orifices of the meibomian glands. Cases have been reported with three (tristichiasis) and four (tetrastichiasis) rows of lashes. The accessory row (or rows) of lashes may consist of only a few cilia, or there may be a well-formed row. The extra cilia are generally smaller and less pigmented, although they may be as fully developed as the normal row in some cases. Abnormalities of the tarsal plate may result in slight eversion or marked ectropion of the eyelids.

Congenital distichiasis is frequently inherited as an autosomal dominant trait with high penetrance and variable expressivity. Distichiasis has also been reported in some forms of familial lymphedema (Meige disease) in association with entropion, ptosis, vertebral anomalies, extradural cysts, webbed neck, yellow nails, and other systemic anomalies. It is also associated with trisomy 18, congenital heart defects, peripheral vascular anomalies, and congenital corneal hypesthesia. The significance of distichiasis lies in the chronic irritation of the cornea and conjunctiva caused by the aberrant cilia.

Acquired distichiasis is a term that has not been widely accepted, but describes a situation in which abnormal acquired lashes appear in the same location as those aberrant lashes in congenital distichiasis. The acquired distichiatic lashes tend to be short and wiry and cause more corneal irritation than in congenital distichiasis. Acquired distichiasis occurs in cases of Stevens-Johnson syndrome, toxic epidermal necrolysis, ocular pemphigoid, and chemical and physical injuries of the eyelids. Acquired distichiasis should be distinguished from trichiasis, which implies inturned or misdirected lashes that have a normal location in the anterior lamellae of the lid, because the anatomic location and treatment of the acquired distichiatic aberrant lashes differ.

In congenital distichiasis, a developmental anomaly occurs in which a complete pilosebaceous unit (with hair and glandular structures) is present in the posterior lamella. This probably represents a failure of the primary epithelial anlage to differentiate selectively into only a sebaceous gland. If this is the case, it would not represent a true metaplasia as some have suggested. An in utero injury leading to a metaplasia inducing congenital distichiasis seems unlikely.

In acquired distichiasis, certain stimuli (immunologic, chemical, or physical) provoke metaplastic change that results in the formation of a hair follicle within or adjacent to the sebaceous meibomian gland. The clinical evidence in many cases of Stevens-Johnson syndrome, pemphigoid, and chemical or physical injuries, as well as histologic studies, provide support for this hypothesis.

THERAPY

Ocular. No treatment is required in asymptomatic individuals. Lubricating agents should be used to protect the eye from irritation until definitive treatment is performed. Therapeutic soft contact lenses may also be employed as a temporary measure.

Surgical. Although many procedures have been described for the correction of distichiasis, none has gained general acceptance. These treatment modalities can be divided into the categories of epilation, electrolysis, surgical extirpation, and cryosurgery. Epilation is only a temporizing measure and results in the recurrence of cilia that are even more irritating. Electrolysis is complicated with many recurrences, scarring, and entropion. It is virtually impossible to isolate all the distichiatic cilia, and electrolysis is only applicable in cases with very limited involvement. Procedures of microscopic identification of the follicles through a trap-door-type of posterior tarsal incision or other tarsal dissection followed by their obliteration are time consuming and tedious and fraught with recurrence because of incomplete excision. Splitting of the eyelid at the gray line with excision of the marginal portion of the tarsus can lead to entropion and trichiasis. The use of nasal mucosal, tarsoconjunctival, or buccal grafts in an attempt to reconstruct the posterior lamella is time consuming and unpredictable and results in eyelid margin disfigurement.

Cryosurgery is the most effective method available for obliterating aberrant lashes of the eyelid. Temperatures of -15 to $-20°$ C result in permanent destruction of the lash follicle; temperatures of $-30°$ C and lower cause increased necrosis and scarring. With standard forms of cryosurgical treatment, not only the abnormal posterior lashes but also the normal anterior cilia are lost. Despite efforts to limit this loss with the use of thermocouple monitoring, optimal treatment criteria have not been established. Additionally, depigmentation of the skin occurs, which is especially disfiguring in pigmented individuals. Lid splitting and posterior lamellar cryotherapy are recommended; these procedures preserve the normal anterior lashes and avoid depigmentation while obliterating the aberrant cilia in the posterior lamella.

Lidocaine with epinephrine (1 : 100,000) is injected under the skin and conjunctiva of the eyelid. Topical 2.5 per cent phenylephrine is placed in the conjunctival cul-de-sac to provide added vasoconstriction. The eyelid is split at the gray line with a No. 11 scalpel blade. Magnification, by either operating microscope or loupes, is used to verify the gray line and to ensure that all aberrant lashes are included in the posterior lamella. The incision must be made perpendicular to the lid margin. The lid splitting is continued by blunt and sharp dissection with scissors, maintaining a plane on the anterior surface of the tarsal plate. Care is taken to avoid the normal anterior lash follicles, as trauma may result in loss of normal lashes or trichiasis. The lid splitting is continued for a sufficient distance up the tarsus to ensure that the cryoprobe, when applied, will not inadvertently freeze the normal anterior cilia. Hemostasis is obtained by compression and bipolar cautery. Using the large beveled tip of the nitrous oxide eyelid cryoprobe (Cryomedics), the posterior lamella is frozen to -20 to $-25°$ C. Temperature is monitored by a thermocouple. Once experience has been gained with the technique, it may be possible to omit the thermocouple. The surgeon attempts to obtain a rapid freeze and slow thaw to room temperature, followed by a second freeze and slow thaw. Care is taken not to freeze the anterior lamella of the eyelid during this procedure.

After all areas of the posterior lamella have been treated, the anterior lamella is recessed 2 mm from the lid margin by placing 6-0 chromic horizontal mattress sutures to position the recessed anterior lamella on the tarsus. Care is taken to direct the lashes in a slightly everted position for any misdirected lashes may become trichiatic. The 2-mm anterior lamellar recession helps prevent the normal anterior lashes from misdirecting posteriorly and becoming trichiatic. Without this recession, the anterior lamella may override the posterior lamella. Within a month, the anterior lamella will have migrated toward the margin so that the anterior recession is unnoticed. Topical steroid-antibiotic ointment is an anterior and posterior lamella. The posterior lamella consists of conjunctiva and tarsus, and the anterior lamella is made up of skin, orbicularis muscle, lashes, and tarsus. Hemostasis can be obtained with a hand-held thermal cautery unit or electrocautery. If there is any significant distichiasis or trichiasis at this time, these areas can be treated with freeze-thaw-freeze-thaw cryoepilation. Monitoring tissue temperature with a thermocouple to $-20°$ C is advised by some surgeons. Following this, the lid edges are reapproximated; however, the anterior lamella is recessed superiorly relative to the posterior lamella and sutured in place with several interrupted 5-0 or 6-0 Vicryl rotational sutures. In moderate to severe cases, severing the attachments of Müller's muscle and conjunctiva from the superior border of the tarsus, has been suggested, in addition to the lid splitting and anterior lamella recession. This posterior defect is left open to re-epithelialize without contraction. One to two mm of blepharoptosis may be present postoperatively.

A buccal mucosa graft can be laid between the edge of the posterior lamella and the anterior lamella and held in place with 6-0 Vicryl sutures. The buccal mucosa graft is easily obtained from the buccal surface of the lower lip. After local infiltration, it is harvested freehand and then thinned as much as possible of its underlying subcutaneous tissue. The harvest graft bed is allowed to heal without any specific dressing or treatment. If the harvest is from the cheek area, one must be careful to avoid the opening of Stensen's duct from the parotid gland. It is usually opposite the second upper molar on either side.

In severe cases of upper lid entropion, it is often advisable to use a so-called spacer. This can be done using a composite graft of nasal septal cartilage with its overlying mucosa. It can be harvested either by an eye surgeon familiar with nasal anatomy or by an otorhinolaryngologist. For cicatricial entropion, it is suggested that the cartilage not be thinned as it sometimes is for upper eyelid reconstruction. Thinning is thought to make the cartilage graft more vulnerable to warping during the healing process, thereby increasing the chances of postoperative entropion. Once the anterior and posterior lamellae have been adequately separated, any markedly diseased, warped tarsus is resected, and the nasal composite graft is contoured to fit in the remaining space between the patient's tarsus and the margin. It is held in place with either 6-0 Vicryl sutures or a running 6-0 Prolene. The Prolene is removed about 10 days later. The mucosal surface is approximated to the lid margin on the conjunctival surfaces so that there is a moist surface in contact with the cornea. The posterior lamella spacer forces the eyelashes forward, away from the eye. For patients with Stevens-Johnson syndrome and ocular pemphigoid who have chronic epidermalization of the conjunctiva, a technique has been described that combines tarsal polishing to remove epidermalized conjunctiva with a smooth 3-mm dermabrading tip and subsequent full-thickness buccal mucous membrane graft into the prepared host bed. This procedure can be combined with the lid-splitting and spacer procedures.

Lower lid entropion can be repaired using basically the same procedures as described for the upper lid entropion; in addition to using a nasal composite graft, earlobe cartilage can be used in the lower lid to act as a spacer. Eye bank sclera has been used, but, unfortunately, it is relatively unsatisfactory as it is not stiff enough to resist the postoperative healing forces that cause the entropion to recur. In cases of mild to moderate lower lid entropion, the Wies procedure has been used. This involves a two-step transverse blepharotomy incision made through the skin, muscle (first step), and tarsus and conjunctiva (second step), 3 mm below the lid margin. Three or four double-armed mattress sutures of 5-0 silk are passed from the conjunctival fornix side of the incision into the wound, exiting the anterior surface of the proximal tarsus, and then into the superior portion of the wound and brought out through the skin near the eyelashes and tied to obtain the desired amount of overcorrection. This forces the eyelashes to rotate outward. This overcorrection will usually resolve within 1 or 2 weeks. If the overcorrection is persistent and exposure keratitis is a problem, the sutures can be removed; doing so typically reduces some of the overcorrection. This procedure can be performed for upper lid entropion, but the double-armed sutures must enter the cut edge of the tarsus, not the conjunctiva, to avoid abrading the cornea.

Ocular or Periocular Manifestations

Conjunctiva: Chemosis; chronic conjunctivitis.
Cornea: Corneal ulcer; mechanical keratitis.
Eyelids: Erythema; swelling; triachiasis.
Lacrimal System: Epiphora.

PRECAUTIONS

The keys to treatment of this disorder are accurate diagnosis and the subsequent choice of an appropriate surgical technique. The surgeon must also have a thorough knowledge of the upper and lower eyelid anatomy and try to make the surgical technique conform to that anatomy. A small amount of overcorrection postoperatively is usually desired to ensure that the entropion does not recur. If the overcorrection persists, it may require release of sutures or possibly a second procedure. It is important to operate on patients who are not on any platelet inhibitors, e.g., aspirin or nonsteroidal antiinflammatory agents or anticoagulants, such as warfarin or heparin. There is a small risk to the patient's vision with these procedures, especially in the lower lid, should they have a significant retrobulbar hemorrhage postoperatively. They should be cautioned about this complication and instructed to call the surgeon immediately if they develop significant periorbital swelling associated with pain. If this condition does develop, the incision should be opened immediately, the hematoma evacuated, and the bleeding site identified and cauterized. The wound can then be reapproximated. One should be careful not to remove too much fat because enophthalmos is often one of the contributing factors in many cases of this disease, particularly involutional entropion.

COMMENTS

The conservative treatment of taping the lower lid into position typically does not work, as the skin gets moist from epiphora and the tape slips. However, it can be used as a prognostic indicator in patients who are skeptical about having surgery. The surgical procedures are typically performed in the operating room using local infiltrative anesthesia and topical proparacaine; however, some procedures, such as the Quickert-Rathbun sutures, can still be done easily in the office or at the bedside. Secondary ocular problems typically resolve quickly with the anatomic correction of the eyelid abnormalities; however, careful monitoring of the cornea throughout the postoperative period is a priority.

References

Anderson RL: The tarsal strip. *In* Transaction of the New Orleans Academy of Ophthalmology. St. Louis, CV Mosby, 1982, pp 352–363.

Bayliss HI, Silkiss RZ: A structurally oriented approach to the repair of cicatricial entropion. Ophthalmic Plast Reconstr Surg 3:17–20, 1987.

Callahan A: Correction of entropion from Stevens-Johnson syndrome. Use of nasal septum and mucosa for severely cicatrized eyelid entropion. Arch Ophthalmol 94:1154–1155, 1976.

Jones LT, Reeh MJ, Wobig JL: Senile entropion. A new concept for correction. Am J Ophthalmol 74:327–329, 1972.

Jones LT, Wobig JL: Surgery of the Eyelids and Lacrimal System. Birmingham, Aesculapius, 1976, pp 123–131.

McCord CD, Chen WP: Tarsal polishing and mucous membrane grafting for cicatricial entropion, trichiasis, and epidermalization. Ophthalmic Surg 14:1021–1025, 1983.

Quickert MH, Wilkes DI, Dryden RM: Non-incisional correction of epiblepharon and congenital entropion. Arch Ophthalmol 101:778–781, 1981.

Tse DT, Anderson RL, Fratkin JD: Aponeurosis disinsertion in congenital entropion. Arch Ophthalmol 101:436–440, 1983.

Wies FA: Surgical treatment of entropion. J Int Coll Surg 21:758–760, 1954.

EPICANTHUS
ROGER A. DAILEY, M.D.
Seattle, Washington

The term "epicanthus" refers to a relatively vertical fold of skin that is located between the medial canthus and the nose and may cover part or all of the inner canthus of the eye. Four separate types have been described. *Epicanthus supraciliaris* is a vertical fold of skin that extends from just below the brow to an area just over the infraorbital rim, usually obscuring the caruncle. In *epicanthus palpebralis*, the skin fold extends from the medial aspect of the upper lid to the medial aspect of the lower lid in a rather symmetric fashion; the skin fold often obscures the caruncle. This is the most common configuration. *Epicanthus tarsalis* refers to a fold that begins laterally and extends over the entire lid, ending in the medial canthus. This is the typical Oriental upper lid configuration. Epiblepharon of the upper lids is distinguished from epicanthus tarsalis by its lack of a true superior palpebral fold and the presence of a fold of skin that overlaps the eyelid margin and presses the lashes against the cornea. Finally, *epicanthus inversus* is similar to epicanthus tarsalis, but involves the lower lid. It usually occurs as a part of Komoto's tetrad of blepharoptosis, blepharophimosis, telecanthus, and epicanthus inversus. Blepharophimosis is a narrowing of the palpebral aperture in its horizontal dimension. Rarely, the tetrad can occur as a developmental anomaly, but more commonly it is transmitted as an autosomal dominant trait with 100 per cent penetrance. The blepharoptosis is usually associated with poor function of the levator palpebrae superioris.

THERAPY

Surgical. In patients with these disorders, it is important to avoid early operation if possible. Many forms of epicanthus that are present when the child is young will become less apparent as the child matures and growth of the dorsum of the nose occurs. The exception is epicanthus inversus, which typically shows little improvement with age. In these children, the skin tends to be very stiff early on and difficult to work with surgically and becomes more amenable to intervention at a later age. There have never been any spinal abnormalities reported from patients going for years with blepharoptosis, and amblyopia is rare in these patients and is usually associated with other problems, such as anisometropia and astigmatism. Consideration should be given to doing surgery before the child enters school because of potential associated psychologic problems with this perceived facial anomaly.

Numerous surgical methods to correct epicanthus have been described. Most surgeons would agree that it is best to correct the epicanthus first, along with any associated telecanthus or blepharophimosis, and then at a later time correct the blepharoptosis either with a sling if the levator function is 4 mm or less or with a levator resection if the function is greater. Supramid suture slings can be performed on patients as a temporary measure if the surgery is done before 3 years of age, or banked fascia lata can be used as well. After the age of 3 years, the patient's own fascia lata can be harvested from the leg.

Several different techniques have been described to correct epicanthus: Spaeth's epicanthus operation, Verwey Y-to-V operation, double Z plasty, Mustarde's technique, the Y-to-W procedure, Roveda's technique, and, more recently, the five-flap procedure. Spaeth's technique, which involves excision of a portion of the fold of skin, is generally reserved for only mild cases of epicanthus inversus. The Verwey Y-to-V operation is more commonly used for epicanthus repair, especially epicanthus palpebralis.

Double opposing Z plasty works well for epicanthus supraciliaris or epicanthus tarsalis. It is very similar to the Mustarde procedure. It is much easier to transpose the skin flaps of this double Z if all of the incisions are made medial to the epicanthal fold and the incisions are not extended onto the lids themselves. The Mustarde technique combines a Y-to-V with double opposing Z plasty. Some surgeons feel that the measurements to set this procedure up are unduly complex, and the flaps tend to be irregular and can be difficult to transpose. The basic Y-to-W and Roveda's technique are essentially the same procedure. Roveda's technique, again, involves larger irregularly shaped flaps that can be difficult to transpose.

The five-flap technique, which is a modified Y-to-V procedure combined with a double Z plasty has been recently described. It has the advantage of being simple to mark out on the lid, and the flaps are small and relatively easy to transpose.

No matter which of the above procedures is chosen for a patient with epicanthus, some aspects of care remain generally consistent throughout. Typically, the patients who are operated on are from 3 to 5 years of age. Since epicanthus invariably occurs bilaterally, both sides can be done at the same time. A general anesthetic is used, mainly because of the child's age. Local anesthetic with epinephrine helps control hemostasis. Once the flaps are raised, any excess orbicularis muscle can be resected, and the medial canthal tendon is easily visualized. Since there is usually associated telecanthus, it can be repaired with a medial canthal tendon resection or, in severe cases, transnasal wiring. It is important to avoid injuring the canaliculus or lacrimal sac. Closure is performed with a suture of the surgeon's choice. Blepharophimosis can also be repaired at this time via a lateral canthoplasty.

Ocular or Periocular Manifestations

Conjunctiva: Hypoplasia of the caruncle; semilunar folds.
Eyelids: Blepharophimosis; blepharoptosis; telecanthus.
Lacrimal System: Lateral displacement of puncta; punctal stenosis.
Other: Amblyopia; "lop" ears; strabismus and double elevator palsy.

PRECAUTIONS

As always, accurate diagnosis is the key to a satisfactory result. Epiblepharon is essentially an exaggeration of epicanthus tarsalis. Although epicanthus is typically bilateral, epiblepharon can be unilateral. It can occur in either the upper or lower lid and usually regresses spontaneously without any surgery. Epicanthus is a cause of pseudostrabismus; therefore, it is important in these patients to check not only visual acuity but also a prism alternating cover test to rule out true strabismus.

Scarring in these patients can be quite exuberant in the initial postoperative weeks. It is important to reassure the parent that this will diminish with time. Topical steroid ointments can be massaged into the area and are felt to be of some benefit. There is no evidence that vitamin E ointment is helpful beyond the benefit gained from massaging alone. Radiation to the scarred area should not be used.

COMMENTS

Epicanthus supraciliaris, palpebralis, and tarsalis tend to regress spontaneously with age and only occasionally require surgical correction. In some patients where the epicanthus is minimal and a ptosis repair is performed, the epicanthus is exaggerated. In this instance, a Y-to-V or simple single Z plasty will often take care of the epicanthus. Amblyopia is occasionally found in these patients with epicanthus and blepharoptosis. It is important to check the visual acuity and also to rule out significant refraction errors.

References

Anderson RL, Nowinski TS: The five-flap technique for blepharophimosis. Arch Ophthalmol 107:448–452, 1989.

Beard C: Ptosis. St. Louis, CV Mosby, 1976, pp 218–235.

Callahan A: Surgical correction of the blepharophimosis syndromes. *Trans Am Acad Ophthalmol Otolaryngol* 77:687–695, 1973.

Callahan MA, Callahan A: Ophthalmic Plastic and Orbital Surgery. Birmingham, Aesculapius, 1979, pp 36–41.

Crawford JS, Apt RK: Congenital anomalies. *In* Silver B: Ophthalmic Plastic Surgery. Rochester, American Academy of Ophthalmology and Otolaryngology, 1977, pp 74–79.

Hughes WL: Surgical treatment of congenital palpebral phimosis. The Y-V operation. Arch Ophthalmol 54:586–590, 1955.

Johnson CC: Epicanthus. Am J Ophthalmol 66:939–946, 1968.

Johnson CC: Epicanthus and Epiblepharon. Arch Ophthalmol 96:1030–1033, 1978.

Kohn R, Romano PE: Blepharoptosis, blepharophimosis, epicanthus inversus and telecanthus—A syndrome with no name. Am J Ophthalmol 72:625–632, 1971.

EYELID COLOBOMA

JOHN D. BULLOCK, M.D., M.S., F.A.C.S.,
Dayton, Ohio

and STUART H. GOLDBERG, M.D.
Hershey, Pennsylvania

A coloboma is a full-thickness defect of the eyelid. Colobomas may occur congenitally or as a result of accidental or surgical trauma (secondary to excision of eyelid tumors). Congenital colobomas are most commonly unilateral, lid margin-based, triangular defects, involving the medial third of the upper lid. However, a congenital eyelid coloboma may be bilateral, rectangular, or triangular; may be found on any aspect of the lid margin; and may occur on the lower or upper lid. Lower lid lesions usually are seen laterally. A benign dermoid tumor at the limbus or apex of the coloboma is frequently encountered. A congenital eyelid coloboma may be accompanied by a variety of other facial anomalies.

THERAPY

Ocular. Corneal protection is the primary therapeutic goal. Patients with small lid defects may be adequately treated with artificial tears and ophthalmic ointments. Commercially available optical bandages that provide an airtight moist chamber have been advocated. Patching at bedtime may be required in cases where significant corneal exposure occurs during sleep.

Surgical. Corneal protection and cosmesis are indications for surgical correction. Large congenital colobomas may necessitate immediate surgical intervention to prevent corneal compromise. Small defects that are well managed with topical lubricants may have surgical correction delayed until later in childhood.

Small colobomas can be corrected by direct closure. The margins are freshened with clean incisions, and careful anastomosis of the lid margin is performed. A meticulous two-layer approximation of the incised tarsal and skin margins achieves wound closure. Lateral cantholysis and placement of a near-far, far-near suture may be necessary to minimize horizontal tension along the wound margins.

A two-stage reconstruction may be required for lid defects exceeding 40 to 50 per cent. For large lower lid colobomas, an upper lid tarsoconjunctival advancement flap with split-thickness retroauricular skin graft to the tarsal portion of the reconstructed lower lid (modified Hughes' procedure) has been recommended. Large upper lid colobomata can be reconstructed by advancement of full-thickness lower lid beneath a bridge of lower eyelid margin, with subsequent release of the flap in 8 to 12 weeks (Cutler-Beard procedure).

Alternative techniques of repairing large colobomas include use of a semicircular flap from the lateral canthal area and a full-thickness lid rotational flap from upper to lower lid for large lateral lower lid defects.

Ocular or Periocular Manifestations

Conjunctiva: Symblepharon.
Cornea: Cicatrization; exposure keratopathy.
Eyelids: Trichiasis.
Lacrimal System: Obstruction.
Sclera: Benign dermoid tumor.

PRECAUTIONS

Excision of associated limbal dermoid tumors must be undertaken with particular care. Pseudopterygium or symblepharon formation can result from attempts at simple excision. The use of lamellar grafts has been advocated.

COMMENTS

Lacrimal system obstruction is common in the setting of both upper and lower eyelid coloboma.

A complete ophthalmologic examination to rule out possible co-existing ocular anomalies should be performed at the time of surgery. Lower eyelid colobomas are characteristic of mandibulofacial dysostosis (Treacher-Collins or Franceschetti syndrome); upper eyelid colobomas are commonly seen in oculoauricular dysplasia (Goldenhar's syndrome).

References

Casey TA: Congenital colobomata of the eyelids. Trans Ophthalmol Soc UK 96:65–68, 1976.
Crawford JS: Congenital eyelid anomalies in children. J Pediatr Ophthalmol Strabismus 21:140–149, 1984.
Guibor P: Surgical repair of congenital colobomas. Trans Am Acad Ophthalmol Otolaryngol 76:671–678, 1975.
Harley RD: Disorders of the lids. Pediatr Clin North Am 30:1145–1158, 1983.
Kidwell EDR, Tenzel RR: Repair of congenital colobomas of the lids. Arch Ophthalmol 97:1931–1932, 1979.
Patipa M, Wilkins RB, Guelzow KW: Surgical management of congenital eyelid coloboma. Ophthalmic Surg 13:212–216, 1982.
Poswillo D: Pathogenesis of craniofacial syndromes exhibiting colobomata. Trans Ophthalmol Soc UK 96:69–72, 1976.

FLOPPY EYELID SYNDROME

LEE K. SCHWARTZ, M.D.
San Francisco, California

The floppy eyelid syndrome is an uncommon and frequently unrecognized cause of chronic unilateral or bilateral papillary conjunctivitis. It is frequently associated with a punctate epithelial keratitis. The syndrome is characterized by a triad of 1) diffuse papillary conjunctivitis, 2) a loose upper lid that readily everts by pulling it upward (positive lid eversion sign), and 3) a soft rubbery tarsus that can be folded on itself. The lower lids may also be involved. Both sexes are affected, but males predominate. A frequent association with obesity has been observed. Reported cases range in age between 36 and 65 years. The cause of tarsal laxity is unknown.

There is no definite association with systemic diseases of collagen or elastic tissue. Variable associations have been reported with hyperglycinemia, keratoconus, psoriasis, blepharitis, and tear dysfunction. Some authors feel that the floppy eyelid syndrome and blepharochalasis may represent a spectrum of one underlying disease.

The mechanism of the chronic conjunctivitis is thought to be eyelid eversion during sleep with corneal-conjunctival-pillow contact. An alternative explanation is that there is a poor interface between the loose upper eyelid and the underlying bulbar conjunctiva. Both, however, may be present to produce the symptoms.

Histopathologic investigations, including light and electron microscopy, have revealed chronic conjunctival inflammation with fibrosis and scarring. The appearance of tarsal collagen has been normal, with no abnormality of ultrastructure or distribution of the collagen and elastic fibers of the tarsus. Conjunctival scrapings reveal keratinized epithelial cells.

The patient's symptoms include chronic ocular irritation or foreign body sensation, red eye, and mucous discharge. They are usually worse upon awakening in the morning.

THERAPY

Supportive. Since the cause of the floppy eyelid and rubbery tarsus is unknown, therapy is aimed at preventing the probable nocturnal eyelid eversion. One method is to have the patient wear an eye shield while asleep. Not all symptoms are relieved by this treatment.

Surgical. The patients may be treated surgically by a full-thickness eyelid shortening procedure. In many cases, this produces immediate relief of symptoms. A procedure has been described utilizing a 10- to 15-mm excision of the lateral upper eyelid, followed by primary layered closure.

Another technique is to perform a full-thickness excision at the junction of the lateral middle third of the lid, beginning at the lid margin and extending vertically past the proximal margin of the tarsal plate, at which point the incision is angled medially at a 45° angle. The two cut edges of lid are overlapped with forceps. A mirror image incision is made to remove a pentagonal wedge of lid. This is large enough to allow the lid to attain a tension somewhat tighter than a normal lid after completion of the repair. After complete hemostasis is achieved, the resulting wedge defect is closed. Some authors describe the use of a 4-0 nonabsorbable nylon horizontal mattress suture placed across the wound to relieve traction on the wound. The silk and nylon sutures are removed in 7 to 10 days.

Ocular or Periocular Manifestations

Conjunctiva: Papillary conjunctivitis with mucous discharge.
Cornea: Diffuse papillary epithelial keratitis.
Eyelids: Always involves upper lids. May also involve lower lids; soft rubbery tarsus; upper lid easily everts upon itself by pulling upward.

PRECAUTIONS

In most cases, the accurate diagnosis is initially overlooked. Many patients are being inappropriately treated with various topical or systemic medications. Some patients may exhibit toxic reactions to these chronically administered but ineffective antibiotics, artificial tears, or steroids.

COMMENTS

Early recognition of this clinical entity may spare a patient many unnecessary diagnostic procedures and treatment trials. By the time some patients are appropriately diagnosed, they may have a concurrent medicamentosa conjunctivitis. The duration of symptoms before diagnosis has ranged from 8 months to 14 years.

References

Culbertson WW, Ostler HB: The floppy eyelid syndrome. Am J Ophthalmol 92:568–575, 1981.
Dutton JJ: Surgical management of floppy eyelid syndrome. Am J Ophthalmol 99:557–560, 1985.
Easterbrook M: Floppy eyelid syndrome. Can J Ophthalmol 20:264–265, 1985.
Gerner EW, Hughes SM: Floppy eyelid with hyperglycinemia. Am J Ophthalmol 98:614–616, 1984.
Goldberg R, et al: Floppy eyelid syndrome and blepharochalasis. Am J Ophthalmol 102:376–381, 1986.
Moore MB, et al: Floppy eyelid syndrome management including surgery. Ophthalmology 93:184–188, 1986.
Parunovic A: Floppy eyelid syndrome. Br J Ophthalmol 67:264–266, 1983.
Schwartz LK, Gelender H, Forster RK: Chronic conjunctivitis associated with "floppy eyelids." Arch Ophthalmol 101:1884–1888, 1983.

HEMIFACIAL SPASM
JOHN R. SAMPLES, M.D.
Portland, Oregon

Hemifacial spasm is a facial movement disorder in which there is a sporadic synchronized contraction of many muscles on one side of the face. Unlike benign essential blepharospasm, which is a bilateral disease, hemifacial spasm is confined to one side of the face. Often, it begins with twitches in a single orbicularis muscle. The twitches last from seconds to minutes and are typically irregular and clonic. The spasm may start around the eye and spread to other muscles innervated by the seventh cranial nerve. Hemifacial spasm never spreads to muscles beyond those innervated by the facial nerve. Spasms are often precipitated or made worse by fatigue and stress.

Synkinesis is observed in hemifacial spasm but not facial myokymia, from which hemifacial spasm must be differentiated. Facial myokymia is almost always a benign condition when it involves only a single muscle, such as the orbicularis oculi. However, in certain patients with multiple slcerosis or brainstem tumors, facial myokymia may be a presenting feature and may persist indefinitely. Symptomatic hemifacial spasm is caused by lesions compressing the facial nerve extra-axially, usually by aneurysm, arteriovenous malformation, or rarely a neoplasm involving the cerebellopontine angle. The majority of cases have been attributed to an aberrant blood vessel compressing the facial nerve.

THERAPY

Systemic. Hemifacial spasm is usually refractory to medical therapy, although carbamazepine[‡] has been estimated to be of benefit in up to 30 per cent of patients with this disorder. Serum levels of this drug may be obtained and followed to achieve therapeutic levels.

Botulinum A toxin[†] may be injected locally to produce a reversible neuromuscular blockade that may be useful in relieving the spasms. Many patients feel that the toxin produces significant improvement. Complications of botulinum A toxin injection into the orbicularis and adjacent muscles include ptosis, ectropion, corneal exposure, and tearing. Tolerance to the toxin does not develop. Antibodies to botulinum A toxin do not develop with the dosage commonly used in facial spasm.

Surgical. Decompression of the facial nerve in symptomatic cases has been described as being effective. Operating on cryptogenic cases and decompressing the facial nerve from aberrant blood vessels have been recommended. However, this surgical approach requires a retromastoid craniectomy and microneurosurgical techniques.

Ocular or Periocular Manifestations

Eyelids: Intermittant clonic and tonic jerks confined to the muscles about the eyelid, coupled with an ipsilateral contracture of the facial musculature.

PRECAUTIONS

Carbamazepine produces potentially alarming side effects, including hematopoietic, cardiovascular, hepatic, and renal disturbances. Careful examination and close medical supervision are required with the use of this drug. Fatal aplastic anemia, agranulocytosis, thrombocytopenia, and purpura are among the hematologic complications associated with this drug. A complete blood count, including platelet, thrombin, and reticulocyte count with serum iron determination, should be performed before initiating carbamazepine therapy and frequently throughout.

Significant risks, including ipsilateral deafness and brainstem stroke, are involved in the operative management of this condition. These major complications must be weighed against the impairment of the patient and the expected benefit of surgery; the importance of selecting a qualified neurosurgeon to perform this procedure should be emphasized.

COMMENTS

Botulinum A toxin is a new and effective treatment for this disorder. A trial with botulinum A toxin injections is indicated before undertaking surgical therapy.

References

Elston JS: Botulinum toxin therapy for involuntary facial movement. Eye 2:12–15, 1988.
Gardner WJ: Concerning the mechanism of trigeminal neuralgia and hemifacial spasm. J Neurosurg 19:947–958, 1962.
Janetta PJ: Observations on the etiology of trigeminal neuralgia, hemifacial spasm, acoustic nerve dysfunction and glossopharyngeal neuralgia. Definitive microsurgical treatment and results in 117 patients. Neurochirugia 20:145–154, 1977.
Nielsen VK: Pathophysiology of hemifacial spasm. 1. Ephaptic transmission and ectopic excitation. Neurology 34:418–426, 1984.
Savino PJ, et al: Hemifacial spasm treated with botulinum A toxin injection. Arch Ophthalmol 103:1305–1306, 1985.
Soso MJ, Nielsen VK: The lesion of hemifacial spasm is peripheral to the facial nucleus. Muscle Nerve 7:578, 1984.

HORDEOLUM
(Stye)

F.T. FRAUNFELDER, M.D.
Portland, Oregon

Hordeolum is a staphylococcal infection of the sebaceous glands of the eyelids. External hordeolum (stye) is caused by stasis with subsequent bacterial infection of the glands of Zeis or Moll. Internal hordeolum results from a secondary staphylococcal infection of a meibomian gland in the tarsal plate. Both internal and external hordeola are common sequelae of infectious blepharitis, and the most common infectious agent is *Staphylococcus aureus*. Hordeola usually begin with painful swelling and edema of the eyelid, which become localized. The purulent exudate of external hordeola often breaks through the skin near the eyelash line; however, the suppuration of the internal hordeolum occurs on the conjunctival side of the eyelid.

THERAPY

Ocular. Hordeola are usually self-limited and respond well to hot moist compresses. If applied early in the course of the infection, the hot compresses may prevent suppuration and abort the attack. To localize the infection, warm soaks administered four times daily for 15 minutes will increase the blood flow and tissue temperature so hydrolytic enzymes can break down tissue and form an abscess. Removal of the eyelashes in the affected area sometimes promotes better drainage of an external hordeolum.

After the hordeolum has started to drain or if there is a tendency to recur, topical ophthalmic antibiotics may be indicated. Tobramycin or gentamicin solution or ointment may be applied four times a day during the acute phase and continued twice daily for 1 week thereafter.

Topical ophthalmic corticosteroid therapy is rarely indicated and then only if inflammation is severe and threatening structural changes of the eyelid.

Systemic. If there are staphylococcal infections elsewhere or preauricular lymphadenopathy is present, systemic antibiotics may be necessary. Oral administration of 250 mg of erythromycin or 125 to 250 mg of dicloxacillin or cloxacillin may be given four times daily for up to 2 weeks. In chronic long-term prophylactic therapy, 250 mg of tetracycline, given orally twice daily 1 hour before meals, may be necessary for several months. Not infrequently, even antibiotic-sensitive staphylococcal organisms cannot be eradicated from the lids or nares. In these cases, lid hygiene, toxoids, a different course of systemic antibiotics, or such antiseptics as silver nitrate or gentian violet may be tried.

Surgical. After localization, these infections usually spontaneously drain, and the condition will subside. However, a stab incision in the area of the pointing abscess may occasionally be necessary. One must remember that there are frequently many pockets in large abscesses so multiple stab incisions may be necessary. If a local anesthetic is used, the injection is not given directly in the area of inflammation but either above the upper border of the upper tarsus or below the lower border of the lower tarsus. A chalazion clamp is applied, and a horizontal incision is made over the pointing area if on the skin, or a vertical incision is made if conjunctival. The lash margins should be avoided so as not to injure lash roots. The wound edges are not resutured, but postoperative warm compresses and antibiotic ointment are used until closure occurs spontaneously.

Ocular or Periocular Manifestations

Conjunctiva: Cicatrization; exudates; hyperemia.
Eyelids: Cicatrization; destruction of follicles; distortion of lid margins; edema; erythema; madarosis.

PRECAUTIONS

Attempting to excise or curette all material in the presence of an acute inflammation can result in excision of an unnecessarily large amount of tarsal tissue. Systemic antibiotics are to be avoided, unless absolutely necessary. Tetracycline may act more in changing the lipoid content of the lid secretions than as an antibiotic in chronic long-term blepharitis.

As with all penicillins, one needs to consider the adverse effects. Immediate reactions that may occur within a matter of minutes or hours include urticaria, angioneurotic edema, and anaphylaxis, with a 10 per cent mortality rate. The accelerated reactions that may occur within the first 48 hours include urticaria, laryngeal edema, fever, rash, and erythema. The delayed reactions, which usually occur 2 to 10 years later, include a delayed urticaria, drug fever, rash, serum sickness, and diarrhea. Rarely does blood dyscrasia occur with this agent.

COMMENTS

The discharge from these infections is literally loaded with pathogenic staphylococci. Treatment following subsidence of the abscess should consist of measures to keep the staphylococci count on the eyelids at a minimum. Topical ophthalmic antibiotics may be effective and may aid in preventing recurrences. Hordeola are most frequent in debilitated patients, diabetics, and patients with chronic blepharitis.

References

Briner AM: Surgical treatment of a chalazion or hordeolum internum. Aust Fam Phys 16:834–835, 1987.
Briner AM: Treatment of common eyelid cyst. Aust Fam Phys 16:828–830, 1987.
Diegel JT: Eyelid problems. Blepharitis, hordeola, and chalazia. Postgrad Med 80:271–272, 1986.

Wilson LA: Bacterial conjunctivitis. *In* Duane TD (ed): Clinical Ophthalmology. Philadelphia, Harper & Row, 1979, Vol IV, pp 4:12–16.

LAGOPHTHALMOS
RICHARD P. JOBE, M.D.
Mountain View, California

Lagophthalmos, the inability to close the eyelids fully, can result from excessive projection of the eye in the orbit, inadequate vertical dimensions of either lid, or malfunction of the orbicularis oculi. Appropriate therapy is dependent upon accurate diagnosis. Proptosis caused by congenital deformity, as in Crouzon's syndrome, requires craniofacial surgery for definitive cure. If proptosis is caused by tumor, orbital wall displacement secondary to trauma, or exophthalmos of hyperthyroidism, definitive treatment requires correction of the cause. In hyperthyroidism, surgical decompression of the orbit may perhaps be necessary if medical and radiologic treatment fail. Lid retraction caused by burns or traumatic loss of eyelid tissue requires plastic surgical reconstruction of the lids to restore the capacity to cover the eye. Paralytic lagophthalmos secondary to decreased orbicularis oculi muscle tone is commonly seen in Bell's palsy.

The presence of lagophthalmos of any origin requires prompt efforts to protect the eye because of the loss of the natural hygienic properties of lid cover. Neglect of lagophthalmos results in painful dryness and, ultimately, keratitis or corneal ulceration. Conservative measures should begin as soon as it is evident that the lids will not close, before symptoms occur, and while the cause is being determined.

THERAPY

Ocular. Maintenance of a moist surface on the eye is critical to the management of lagophthalmos. This is the purpose of the lid suture or adhesion. Petrolatum ointment for longer action or artificial tears is a critical part of the armamentarium. The addition of occlusal techniques is also helpful. A moisture chamber made of a cone of x-ray film taped over the eye is often used. Prefabricated moisture chambers of clear plastics are also available. Thin polyethylene film can be taped over the eye, or a moisture chamber or wind screen can be attached to the frame of the spectacles. One should be particularly cautious in patching the eye in lagophthalmos, because the lids can open under the patch, causing corneal abrasion. Soft contact lenses occasionally can be useful in chronic irritative conditions caused by mild or partially corrected lagophthalmos.

When the condition is severe, lid suture or lid adhesion should be promptly considered. Lid suture is usually done in the central lids, using 5-0 monofilament plastic suture material. A stitch is placed beginning about 5 mm above the upper lid margin, passed out of the lid margin at the gray line, then into the lower lid at the gray line, and out through the skin about 5 mm below the margin. It is then passed in and out of the small piece of rubber or plastic that will serve as a bolster and returns about 6 mm away from the first pass by the opposite identical route through both lids. It is then tied snugly over another bolster. This can be done quickly under local anesthesia. The lid suture can be expected to be effective for several weeks if it is not tied too tightly to avoid cutting through the tissues. If an adhesion is needed for longer or permanent use, one merely removes the epithelium from the lid margins before placing the sutures, and the sutures may be left for 12 to 14 days.

Concurrent trigeminal defects with the loss of corneal reflex or sensation add greatly to the difficulty of management of lagophthalmos. This is particularly true in the paralytic lagophthalmos of facial paralysis if one attempts to balance protection and appearance. Cooperative patients with intact corneal sensation can often be managed by techniques that allow the ocular aperture to be preserved. Where a trigeminal defect coexists, permanent tarsorrhaphy is often necessary to protect the eye, to the detriment of the patient's appearance. The temporalis muscle and fascia dynamic sling into both lids can often achieve the necessary compromise between protection and appearance in this situation.

The management of paralytic lagophthalmos involves both lids. The lower lid must be gently held against the globe. This can be accomplished temporarily by placing tapes across the lower lid just below the cilia, drawing the lid laterally and superiorly along an upper lateral crow's foot line. Similarly, the upper lid can be stiffened and held down by the application of a crescent of stiff tape between the cilia and brow.

Surgical. In studying the laxity of the lower lid, its source must be identified. In long-standing paralytic lagophthalmos, often the tendinous structure between the medial lower tarsus (punctum) and the medial canthus is stretched, allowing the punctum and tarsus to fall out and laterally. When this condition is present, a medial canthoplasty is indicated as a part of the support system for the lower lid. The usual procedures for elevation of the lower lid are less effective if this medial laxity is present. The most common useful procedure for correction of mild paralytic lagophthalmos, particularly in younger individuals where orbicularis function is in part replaced by the elasticity of the eyelid skin, is the McLaughlin lateral canthoplasty. This procedure can be done in a few minutes under local anesthesia. It consists of closure of the lateral 4 to 5 mm of the lid aperture, overlapping the upper lid with the lower lid, and attaching the two tarsal plates together, supporting the lower lid and providing a touch of animation into the lower lid as the lower tarsus rises with the upper on levator contraction. In normal lids, the tarsal plates do not contact each other. The procedure is done by incising at the gray line from a point 5 mm medial to the lateral canthus of either lid around the conjunctivo-cutaneous junction of the canthus to the same point on the opposite lid. A triangle of conjunctiva is removed along the lid margin of the upper lid, and a triangle of skin with cilia is removed from the lid margin of the lower lid. A 5-0 monofilament suture is passed from a point 5 mm above the upper cilia through the upper tarsus and both triangular wounds and then through the lower tarsus and conjunctiva. It is passed back through both lids, wounds, and skin, and it is tied over a bolster for 10 days. This procedure is useful in permanent lagophthalmos, but should be avoided in patients whose condition may be temporary, as it is difficult to restore normal canthal anatomy on release of this tarsorrhaphy. A Kuhnt-Szymanowski procedure is occasionally useful if the dimensional anatomy permits it without adding deformity.

The best durable support for the lower lid that sacrifices nothing aesthetically is a fascia lata or palmaris longus tendon sling passed through the lower lid below the margin from the medial canthal tendon to a hole drilled above the lateral canthus in the orbital rim. It should be just tight enough to hold the lid on the globe against a gentle downward pull. Such a sling will hold up well with time and will relieve many symptoms. The sling is about 3 mm wide and is sutured to the medial canthal tendon and the orbital periosteum or itself laterally after passing in and out through a small hole drilled in the bone. A third incision below the cilia in the central lower lid is helpful in passing the sling. Unless the lower lid is against the globe, measures to assist the upper lid in lagophthalmos will fail.

The upper lid in most cases of lagophthalmos has a functioning levator muscle that keeps the lids open and is the cause of most of the problems resulting from lagophthalmos. Sometimes, iatrogenic lagophthalmos, intentional or unintentional, results from overaggressive correction of ptosis. If the overcorrected ptosis causes persistent problems, a release of the correction may be warranted.

The temporalis muscle and fascia transfer of Gillies is particularly useful in lagophthalmos of Hansen's disease and where the cornea is insensitive. In this situation, the closure is active and muscular. It is a complex operation and often causes paradoxical eye closure with chewing and, uniformly, a bulge over the lateral orbit where the muscle belly is transferred toward the eye. This procedure actively replaces the orbicularis in both lids.

Foreign material placed within the lids may counteract the levator action. The use of a stainless-steel spring between the brow and upper tarsus has a few advocates who, however, seem to employ it less frequently as they accumulate experience. A silicone rubber loop around both lids has also been used to hold the lids together. In addition, magnets made of an alloy of cobalt and platinum have been placed in both lids such that the force will close the lids. The least complicated procedure and therefore the most applicable one is lid loading. It is done by addition of a gold weight to the upper lid. (Gold lid loads are available in the United States only at Meddev Corporation (415) 948-1742.) Such weights are usually about 4.5 mm high, 1 mm thick, and as long as is necessary to achieve the desired weight. As a preliminary test, weights are glued to the lid with benzoin to determine the necessary force. If the facial palsy is long standing, the weight should be about 0.2 gm greater than the ideal on testing as the levator will strengthen with the weight in place.

At surgery, the upper tarsus is exposed, and the weight is sutured in place to the orbital septum or levator aponeurosis sufficiently high in the lid that it is above the thin supraciliary lid. The orbicularis and skin are closed over the lid load, and the operation is completed in a few minutes. In the event of recovery of orbicularis function, the load can be easily removed without adverse effect.

Ocular or Periocular Manifestations

Cornea: Epithelial defects; keratitis; opacity; perforation; ulcer; xerosis.
Eyelids: Blepharochalasis (upper lid); ectropion (lower lid).
Other: Epiphora; visual loss.

Precautions

Although successful attempts at improving lid closure by weighting the upper lid or attaching springs have been reported, problems with these devices exist. Difficulties in the adjustment and tension maintenance of the stainless-steel spring may develop, and the likelihood that the spring will wear through the lid at some time necessitates the patient's continuous proximity to a surgeon familiar with the technique. Likewise, the elastic force of the silicone rubber loop may ultimately stretch the tissue through which it passes and will lose some tension. To have enough force to close the lids, the elasticity must also pull back against the eye, precluding the use of contact lenses. Although the use of magnet is a popular procedure in Germany where the magnets are made, problems have included extrusion, incorrect selection of magnets, and the weight of the lower magnet when the eye is open. The technique has been quite successful in the hands of those with experience, particularly if the magnets are placed in position before the levator muscle shortens due to myotonic contracture as a result of loss of opposing force.

Comments

Although nerve anastomosis, muscle transfers, and other more exotic and definitive measures for correction of facial paralysis are often quite successful, they do not always achieve enough ocular protection to preclude the measures outlined here. Often, surgical ocular protection is wise in contemplation of either spontaneous or postoperative nerve regeneration.

The procedures that preserve appearance may provide somewhat less protection for the eye than tarsorrhaphy and should be used only in patients who can be reliably expected to use adequate protection to achieve comfort and safety. The constant exposure of the cornea results in excessive evaporation of the tear film, dryness of the cornea, and an exposure keratitis. These conditions may progress to infection, corneal ulceration, perforation of the globe, and blindness.

References

Barclay TL, Roberts AC: Restoration of movement to the upper eyelid in facial palsy. Br J Plast Surg 22:257–261, 1969.
Beard C: Diseases of the lids. In Dunlap EA (ed): Gordon's Medical Management of Ocular Disease, 2nd ed. Hagerstown, MD, Harper & Row, 1976, p 131.
Fox SA: Ophthalmic Plastic Surgery, 5th ed. New York, Grune & Stratton, 1976, pp 279–281.
Guy CL, Ransohoff J: The palpebral spring for paralysis of the upper eyelid in facial nerve paralysis: Technical note. J Neurosurg 29:431–433, 1968.
Jobe RP: A technique for lid loading in the management of the lagophthalmos of facial palsy. Plast Reconstr Surg 53:29–32, 1974.
May M: Eyelid reanimation surgery. In The Facial Nerve, New York, Thieme-Stratton, 1986, pp 681–694.
May M: Gold weight and wire spring implants as alternatives to tarsorrhaphy. Arch Otolaryngol Head Neck Surg 113:656–660, 1987.
Mühlbauer WD: 5 Jahre Erfahrung mit der Lidmagnetimplantation beim paretischen lagophthalmus. Klin Monatsbl Augenheilkd 171:938–945, 1977.
Wood-Smith D: Experience with the Arion prosthesis. In Tessier P, et al: Plastic Surgery of the Orbit and Eyelids. New York, Masson, 1981.

LID MYOKYMIA

NORMAN S. JAFFE, M.D.,
Miami, Florida

and WILLIAM T. SHULTS, M.D.
Portland, Oregon

Myokymia is a spontaneous fascicular tremor of muscle without muscular atrophy or weakness. These irregular contractions are generally not associated with any organic disease, although precipitating factors may include fatigue, lack of sleep, bright light dazzle, irritative corneal or conjunctival lesions, debility or anemia, and occasionally excesses of alcohol, smoking, or overwork. The probable focus of irritation is in the nerve fibers within the muscle. The ocular manifestations may include contractions of the eyelids and generally are more apparent to the patient than to an observer.

THERAPY

Supportive. Inasmuch as lid myokymia is usually a self-limited condition, reassurance is the appropriate treatment for most patients.

Systemic. Lid myokymia usually resolves spontaneously, particularly when a precipitating factor is present that can be removed. However, 12.5 to 25 mg of promethazine[‡] given one to three times daily or 75 mg of tripelennamine[‡] given four times daily may be used in severe cases. Small doses of 0.2 to 0.3 gm of oral quinine[‡] may be used 1 to 3 times daily for 3 days either alone or in combination with antihistamines. Quinine should be discontinued if tinnitus or visual disturbances occur.

Ocular or Periocular Manifestations

Eyelids: Fine rippling contraction.

PRECAUTIONS

Myokymia may be caused by the topical ocular use of indirect parasympathomimetics, such as physostigmine. Myokymia followed by spastic paretic facial contracture is an important, although uncommon sign of disease in the dorsal pons in children or adults. It may also be seen in multiple sclerosis, trigeminal neuralgia, and myasthenia gravis. Myokymia must be differentiated from true fasciculation occurring with degenerative lesions in motor nerves.

COMMENTS

When involuntary twitching of the eyelids occurs over long periods of time, it produces a psychologic response that has a tendency to make the affected individual feel tense. Medical treatment may be used to alleviate this apprehension.

References

Andermann F, et al: Facial myokymia in multiple sclerosis. Brain 84:31–44, 1961.
Givner I, Jaffe NS: Myokymia of the eyelids. A suggestion as to therapy: Preliminary report. Am J Ophthalmol 32:51–55, 1949.
Lowe R: Facial twitching. Trans Ophthalmol Soc Aust 11:129–133, 1951.
Sogg RL, Hoyt WF, Boldrey E: Spastic paretic facial contracture: A rare sign of brain stem tumor. Neurology 13:607–612, 1963.

LID RETRACTION

J. TIMOTHY HEFFERNAN, M.D.,
Seattle, Washington

and RICHARD R. TENZEL, M.D.
North Miami Beach, Florida

Lid retraction is a disorder of eyelid position that can affect the upper lid, the lower lid, or both. The condition is characterized by the appearance of a band of white sclera between the limbus and the eyelid margin or margins when the eyes are in primary position.

The most common etiology of eyelid retraction is thyroid ophthalmopathy that may be present with or without exophthalmos. Other causes of upper eyelid retraction include overcorrection of ptosis repair, Marcus Gunn jaw-winking syndrome, and some lesions of the rostral midbrain. The latter condition produces a symmetric, bilateral retraction of the upper eyelids.

Lower eyelid retraction can result from thyroid eye disease or large recessions of the inferior rectus and be a complication of other surgeries in the lower lid, such as blepharoplasty and blow-out fracture repair. In this latter group of conditions, one typically finds significant scarring involving the central lamella. The anatomic basis of lower lid retraction in inferior rectus recession involves anterior extensions of tenon's capsule that surround the inferior rectus and the inferior oblique, thus forming Lockwood's ligament. Lockwood's ligament is the origin of the capsulopalpebral fascia that inserts on the lower tarsal border.

THERAPY

Surgical. Upper eyelid retraction can be corrected by recession of Müller's muscle and levator aponeurosis. This procedure is best done with local anesthesia on an awake and alert patient. Doing so allows the surgeon to lower the lid progressively while evaluating the response of the lid after each step. An incision is made through the skin at the lid crease. The orbital septum is identified and opened entirely across the lid. Protruding orbital fat can be removed as indicated. At this point, the patient is instructed to open the eyes, and the position of the lid is noted. This level is compared to the preoperative height. Any change in level is noted and if an elevation (common) or lowering (uncommon) has occurred, this amount of change is used to determine whether the lid position at the end of the procedure should be at, above, or below the desired final lid height. The levator is cut and disinserted from the tarsus. When Müller's muscle is reached, a Desmarres retractor is placed beneath the lid and the lid put on a stretch. A plane of dissection is created between the conjunctiva and Müller's muscle, which allows Müller's muscle and the levator aponeurosis to be recessed en bloc. The recession is initially confined to the temporal two thirds of the lid to prevent nasal overcorrection. During the dissection, the patient is repeatedly asked to open the eyes so the level of the lids can be evaluated. If more nasal correction is required, it is done in small segments. When the desired end point is reached, a 6-0 mersilene suture is placed partial thickness in the superior edge of the tarsus and brought through the lid retractors. This suture suspends the lid at the desired height and prevents further recession of the retractors. The lid crease is then formed at the desired height by attaching the orbicularis muscle to the tarsus with three nonabsorbable horizontal mattress sutures.

Lower eyelid retraction is approached through a conjunctival incision at the lower edge of the tarsus. The conjunctiva is dissected from the posterior surface of the lower eyelid retractors beyond the reflection of the inferior conjunctival cul-de-sac, thus cutting the connections of the capsulopalpebral fascia to the fornix. Dissection then goes through the lid retractors at the lower edge of the tarsus and continues down the anterior face of the orbital septum. This allows the lower lid retractors to recess en bloc. The orbital septum can then be opened and fat removed. If scarring from previous surgery is present, it can be excised at this point. A strip of donor sclera 2.5 times the amount of desired recession is then placed between the retractors and the tarsus and sutured into position with a running absorbable or nonabsorbable suture. Traction sutures are taped over the brow for 24 hours. An initial postoperative overcorrection is desirable.

When performing a large recession of the inferior rectus, one may avoid lid retraction by careful and complete dissection of Lockwood's ligament. If lid retraction occurs despite this procedure, a recession of the lid retractors as described earlier can be done. However, a scleral graft should not be necessary.

Ocular or Periocular Manifestations

Cornea: Exposure keratitis.
Eyelids: Lagophthalmos, ptosis.
Orbit: Exophthalmos.
Other: Chemosis, diplopia, incomitant strabismus.

PRECAUTIONS

In thyroid patients, all eyelid surgery should be postponed until the metabolic status and lid levels are stable for at least 6 months. Furthermore, if orbital decompression and strabismus repair are contemplated, these procedures should precede eyelid surgery.

Ideally, lid retraction caused by overcorrection of ptosis should be recognized and corrected in the first 10 to 14 days after the initial surgery. Doing so greatly facilitates the repair because healing has not yet occurred and one may simply reopen the wound and resuture the levator aponeurosis at the desired height.

Lids receiving scleral implants become thickened and edematous postoperatively, and the sclera resorbs in an unpredictable manner in many cases. Therefore, scleral grafts may end up less than cosmetically acceptable and require further surgery.

COMMENTS

Classically, upper eyelid retraction in thyroid eye disease was considered to be caused by increased innervation to Müller's muscle. It is now recognized, however, that many other forces are also at work, including inflammatory adhesions between the levator aponeurosis and adjacent tissues, thickening and loss of elasticity of the levator, and increased innervation of the superior rectus and levator muscle to compensate for a contracted inferior rectus. Retraction of the lids secondary to the conditions described here are amenable to correction, but each case must be individually evaluated. The patient must be warned that additional procedures may be necessary.

Lid retraction operations may be used not only to protect the cornea but to make a cosmetically deforming exophthalmos less apparent or to avoid an orbital decompression procedure with its attendant complications.

References

Dryden RM, Soll DB: The use of scleral transplantation in cicatricial entropion and eyelid retraction. Trans Am Acad Ophthalmol Otolaryngol 83:669, 1971.

Tenzel RR: Levator aponeurosis—Müller's muscle recession. In press.

MADAROSIS
(Loss of Eyelashes)
ALLEN M. PUTTERMAN, M.D.
Chicago, Illinois

Madarosis, the loss of eyelashes, can be an undesirable cosmetic deformity. It can occur from systemic or topical infections and inflammations, hysteric plucking of hairs, surgery, and trauma. The hair loss may involve the entire lid, but frequently involves only a segment.

Systemic causes of madarosis include generalized disorders, such as alopecia areata (characterized by an area or areas of sharply defined baldness) and alopecia artefacta (baldness due to neurotic plucking of hairs or cilia). Other systemic causes of madarosis are lupus erythematosus, psoriasis, and seborrhea in which loss of eyelashes follows inflammation of the lids, as well as leprosy, syphilis, tuberculosis, sickle cell anemia, and endocrine disorders. Topical infections and inflammations, such as ulcerative and allergic blepharitis, frequently lead to loss of cilia that is usually segmental.

Madarosis is also a complication of eyelid surgery. Absent lashes frequently occur when full-thickness segments of the lids are excised in the treatment of eyelid carcinoma. In other eyelid surgery, especially that related to treatment of ptosis and benign tumors, lashes can be lost because of the undermining of skin from orbicularis within 2 mm of the lid margin. Traumatic lid lacerations and avulsions are still other causes of madarosis.

THERAPY

Supportive. The treatment of absent cilia after surgery or trauma and the control of systemic and topical infections and inflammation are difficult. Certainly, the need for treatment varies, since many patients have a cosmetically acceptable appearance without lashes, especially if madarosis involves a small segment of the lid or even the entire lower lid. The easiest treatment is achieved with makeup. Eyelid liner, mascara, and false eyelashes can camouflage the defect and frequently have a better cosmetic appearance than that achieved surgically. False eyelashes can be applied to a segment of the lid. In addition, makeup experts can attach false lashes to surrounding normal cilia by a weaving process.

Systemic. Therapy for madarosis is aimed at treating the specific illnesses that are causing it. Medical management of these systemic problems, including the emotional problems of alopecia artefacta, frequently leads to regrowth of the cilia. The treatment of topical causes of madarosis, such as ulcerative and allergic blepharitis, are discussed in other areas of this book. In general, lid hygiene, lid scrubs with baby shampoo, and application of topical antibiotics (such as erythromycin) to the lid margins will control seborrheic blepharitis and prevent further loss of lashes. Allergic blepharitis is treated by eliminating the offending antigens and the application of topical steroids.

Surgical. The most pleasing surgical results are achieved in patients who have had a segmental loss of lashes. The treatment consists of an eyelid excision of a full-thickness pentagon segment in the area without lashes. The surrounding normal lid segments are then connected together. Three 6-0 black silk double-armed sutures are placed through the lid margins. One suture is placed through the squared corners where conjunctiva meets tarsus entering through the posterior aspect of the tarsus. The second suture is placed through the gray line. The third suture is placed through the most posterior row of cilia. The suture enters and exits from similar areas on each edge of the wound to avoid lid notching postoperatively. Sutures are triple-tied, and the ends of the posterior two sutures are tied over the cilia suture, so that when all six ends are cut they point away from the cornea to avoid suture keratopathy. Two to three Vicryl double-armed sutures are then passed through the pretarsal fascia and the anterior aspect of the tarsus on each side of the wound below the lid margin. The skin is closed with a continuous 6-0 black silk suture.

If the normal lid segments connect together with too much tension, a lateral canthotomy and cantholysis with or without a semicircular temporal flap may be needed. This is especially important in the upper eyelid where a tight eyelid can cause ptosis. Also, it is possible to attach a segment of the lid with normal cilia to the lid segment that has a few absent cilia. Doing so decreases the area of madarosis, and a smaller area of absent lashes is usually acceptable. The lateral canthotomy and cantholysis and semicircular flap will leave the temporal lid segment without lashes. This too is more cosmetically acceptable than absent central lashes.

Transplantation of hairs from the eyebrow to the eyelid is another alternative treatment of madarosis. An incision is made at the junction of the skin-lid margin over the absent lash area. The direction of the brow hairs is studied, and the hairs pointing in the desired direction are chosen. A portion of the eyebrow that is equivalent in length and width to the lid with absent cilia and consisting of four rows of hairs is excised from the eyebrow. The correct depth of the graft is critical; it must include the hair follicles while avoiding too much subcutaneous tissue. The graft is sutured to surrounding skin and lid margin so that the hairs are pointing away from the cornea and correspond to the direction of the adjacent normal cilia. Usually, the outer two rows of hairs eventually slough off. This procedure commonly leads to loss of hairs over parts of the graft and usually unsatisfactory cosmetic results.

Still another alternative to lash transplantation is to remove a segment of the normal temporal lashes and place them, as described above, into the area of madarosis. Naugle has advocated this approach and claims good results. Again, the cost of losing temporal lashes to create central lashes is a cosmetically desirable trade. Good results have also been achieved with the placement of individual lash grafts into areas of madarosis.

Blepharopigmentation. Blepharopigmentation is a technique in which pigment is tattooed into the eyelids. It is chiefly advocated to simulate eyeliner or to enhance the eyelashes. However, it can also be used to simulate eyelashes, and this is especially effective if the eyelashes are sparse, rather than totally absent. Equipment and pigment are available through Dioptics and Cooper-Vision. Pigment is applied beneath the skin in the desired density with a rapidly pulsating needle that is covered with pigment.

Precautions

The transplantation of eyebrow hairs into the eyelid must not be considered a cure for madarosis. The relatively high incidence of postoperative loss of transplanted brow hairs and the frequently conspicuous appearance of the brow hairs that remain should alert the surgeon to surgical failure. Blepharopigmentation was initially a popular technique, but now is used only occasionally. One of the main problems has been the difficulty of removing pigment in patients who do not like the density or areas to which it was applied.

Comments

Madarosis (loss of eyelashes) has systemic, topical, hysteric, traumatic, and surgical causes. The first three categories can be treated medically. Makeup, horizontal lid shortening, and brow and lid grafts can be used to treat traumatic and surgical causes.

References

Naugle T: Cited by Caldwell D: Eyelash loss corrected by ciliary transplantation. Ophthalmol Times 7:52–53, 1982.

Putterman AM, Migliori ME: Elective excision of permanent eyeliner. Arch Ophthalmol 106:1034, 1988.

Putterman AM: Basic oculoplastic surgery. In Peyman GA, Sanders DR, Goldberg MF (eds): Principles and Practice of Ophthalmology. Philadelphia, WB Saunders, 1980, pp 2292–2295.

MARCUS GUNN SYNDROME
(Jaw-Winking Syndrome)

JOHN S. CRAWFORD, M.D., F.R.C.S.(C)
Toronto, Ontario

and T.W. DOUCET, M.D.
Conroe, Texas

Marcus Gunn syndrome consists of blepharoptosis of the upper eyelid associated with retraction of the eyelid during stimulation of the ipsilateral pterygoid muscle. The stimulation is usually the result of chewing, opening the mouth, sucking, or contralateral jaw thrusts, but other movements have also been implicated. The natural course of the disease is not well documented, but jaw winking does not appear to lessen spontaneously with age. Although familial cases have been reported infrequently, this congenital syndrome does not appear to be hereditary. Ptosis is usually unilateral and more severe on downgaze. Amblyopia has been associated with this syndrome in 20 per cent of the patients; similarly, strabismus has occurred in 32 per cent of patients.

THERAPY

Surgical. It is important to evaluate the amount of jaw winking and the amount of blepharoptosis before deciding on the best procedure. The objective findings and subjective perceptions must be discussed with the patient preoperatively. Only then can the best surgical treatment be chosen and the best results obtained.

For patients with significant blepharoptosis (greater than 3 mm), a bilateral fascia lata sling with disinsertion of the levator muscle is the best procedure. The normal upper eyelid is everted on Desmarres retractor. The conjunctiva is incised along the upper border of the tarsus. The palpebral conjunctiva is then elevated from the under surface of Müller's muscle. The levator aponeurosis and Müller's muscle are undermined and are fixed with a ptosis clamp. They are severed from their terminal attachments and rotated downward. The orbital septum is elevated from the levator aponeurosis and is allowed to retract. The lateral and medial horns of the levator aponeurosis are cut, with care being taken not to damage the reflected tendon of the superior oblique muscle. The levator muscle is crushed with the hemostat and is severed along the crush marks. It is allowed to retract into the orbit. The conjunctiva is resutured to the upper tarsal border with a running suture of plain catgut. Immediately following a similar operation on the previously normal eyelid, a bilateral brow suspension is performed. Strips of fascia lata are used to suspend both upper eyelids by the Crawford procedure. The procedure results in two symmetrical eyelids with equal lagophthalmos on downgaze.

If patients do not want the normal lid operated on, the levator and Müller's muscle are resected as described earlier. The fascia lata should be used 1 month later to sling the lid to the frontalis muscle. During this interval, the swelling in the lid subsides and the lid can be raised to match the normal lid.

Occasionally, patient's will allow surgery to the affected lid only, but want all the surgery done at one time. In this case, the levator and Müller's muscle are resected. The fascia is placed in the lid as before, but the lid is raised 2 mm higher than normal. When the lid swelling from the levator excision has subsided, the two lids are in symmetric positions.

For patients with moderate blepharoptosis (2 to 3 mm), levator resection is used only when the patient complains that the blepharoptosis is more disturbing than the jaw winking. A minimal amount of blepharoptosis (less than 2 mm) that is more disturbing than the jaw winking is treated with a Fasanella-Servat surgical procedure (described under Ptosis) or managed without surgery.

Ocular or Periocular Manifestations

Extraocular Muscles: Superior rectus palsy.
Eyelids: Ptosis.
Other: Amblyopia; strabismus.

PRECAUTIONS

Surgical management of the Marcus Gunn phenomenon is usually less than satisfactory. Surgeons attempt to treat two separate problems (blepharoptosis and jaw winking) with an operation designed for only one problem (blepharoptosis). If levator muscle resection is done in the presence of a large ptosis, the jaw winking does not improve and frequently appears more marked. In addition, lid lag occurs in a higher percentage of patients with Marcus Gunn syndrome after levator resection than in patients with congenital ptosis only.

COMMENTS

Fascial sling with disinsertion of the levator muscle is the best procedure for individuals with significant blepharoptosis for three reasons. The blepharoptosis associated with jaw winking is difficult to cure with levator muscle resection. The postoperative appearance is unsatisfactory because the jaw winking remains or becomes cosmetically unacceptable. Also, a maximal levator muscle resection (needed in most cases) creates a moderate to severe lid lag that the patient also perceives as unsatisfactory.

References

Beard C: A new treatment for severe unilateral congenital ptosis and for ptosis with jaw-winking. Am J Ophthalmol 59:252–258, 1965.
Bradley WG, Toone BK: Synkinetic movements of the eyelid: A case with some unusual mechanisms of paradoxical lid retraction. J Neurol Neurosurg Psychiat 30:578–579, 1967.
Callahan A: Correction of unilateral blepharoptosis with bilateral eyelid suspension. Am J Ophthalmol 74:321–326, 1972.
Doucet TW, Crawford JS: The quantification, natural course, and surgical results in 57 eyes with Marcus Gunn (jaw-winking) syndrome. Am J Ophthalmol 92:702–707, 1981.
Gunn RM: Congenital ptosis with peculiar associated movements of the affected lid. Trans Ophthalmol Soc UK 3:283–287, 1883.
Kirkham TH: Paradoxical elevation of eyelid on smiling. Am J Ophthalmol 72:207–208, 1971.

MELANOCYTIC LESIONS OF THE EYELIDS
(Melanoma, Nevi, Oculodermal Melanocytosis)

VITALIANO B. BERNARDINO, JR., M.D.,
WILLIAM C. LLOYD III, M.D., F.A.C.S.
and MICHAEL A. NAIDOFF, M.D.
Philadelphia, Pennsylvania

Pigmented cutaneous eyelid lesions often arouse concern in both the patient and the ophthalmologist. The chief worry is the diagnosis of a potentially lethal cutaneous malignant melanoma. This uncommon neoplasm accounts for only 1 per cent of all primary eyelid malignancies, but nevertheless, melanoma is responsible for two thirds of all cutaneous cancer mortality. Other lesions can arise from eyelid skin with secondary pigmentation and may clinically masquerade as a more serious entity. The challenge therefore is to identify accurately the malignant and premalignant conditions.

Proper management relies on diagnostic accuracy. A complete family history is essential. Patients should be examined under ideal lighting conditions. The slitlamp is particularly useful. The ophthalmologist should palpate, measure, and record all pertinent findings. Photographic documentation should be done. When the history is unclear, the patient or guardian should be instructed to bring past photographs, if available. Full body examination is indicated in the presence of any suspicious pigmented eyelid lesion.

Eyelid skin pigmentation can only be produced by epidermal melanocytes, dermal melanocytes, and nevus cells found in both layers. This fact provides one with a useful schematic for understanding all primary pigmented lesions that affect the eyelids. Secondary pigmentation can be observed with many eyelid growths, such as seborrheic keratosis, basal cell epithelioma, inverted follicular keratosis, and others described elsewhere in this text. This secondary pigmentation has no influence on the biologic behavior of these conditions; the clinical course parallels its nonpigmented counterpart.

Epidermal melanocytes produce three common benign lesions, all of which are nonpalpable. Freckles (ephelides) are small sharply demarcated macules that appear in childhood and darken with sun exposure. Lentigo simplex is somewhat larger than the freckle, and its color is unresponsive to sunlight. Multiple facial lentigines may suggest Peutz-Jeghers syndrome, and the patient should be evaluated for the possibility of intestinal polyps and occult visceral tumors. Lentigo senilis is observed in 90 per cent of elderly Caucasians and appears as a dark brown expansile macule with an irregular border.

Dermal melanocytes are associated with lesions that have a characteristic bluish color, owing to light scattering by dermal melanin particles (Tyndall phenomenon). A blue nevus is a circumscribed papule 3 to 8 mm in diameter. Nevus of Ota represents a more diffuse dermal melanocytosis observed in conjunction with ipsilateral ocular melanocytosis (melanosis oculi), leading to the characteristic slate-gray appearance of the globe. Patients with this condition are reported to have an increased risk of developing *uveal* melanoma, and routine ophthalmoscopic examinations are warranted.

Eyelid skin nevi can be congenital or acquired. Although they share a common cytologic derivation, congenital nevi are more frequently implicated in the development of malignant melanoma, whereas acquired nevi are not more likely to undergo malignant transformation than any other melanocyte in the body. Congenital nevi are visible from birth and carry an increased risk of becoming a melanoma in the first decade of life.

Nevi are histopathologically classified based upon their location within the layers of excised tissue. Junctional nevi are purely intraepithelial and reside immediately above the epidermal-dermal junction within the epidermal basal cell layer. Junctional nevi are most often darkly pigmented, remain flat, and tend to enlarge over time. Intradermal nevi are situated exclusively within the dermis, forming an elevated mass with little, if any, pigmentation. Compound nevi are usually darkly pigmented skin lesions demonstrating minimal elevation with a velvety feel. In compound nevi, nests of nevus cells are situated among both the epithelium, as well as the dermis: in other words, a junctional and intradermal lesion. Most congenital nevi are compound nevi. A striking example of a congenital compound nevus is the split or kissing nevus wherein the areas of abnormal hyperpigmentation involve apposed eyelid skin from the upper and lower eyelids and occasionally nearby conjunctiva. It is believed that the epithelium of the fused embryonic eyelids was populated by melanocyte precursors. Intradermal nevus is the most frequently diagnosed nevus in periorbital skin, and it is commonly situated near the eyelid margins. The intradermal nevus carries the most benign prognosis. Intradermal nevi are usually pale and raised and are clinically confused with papillomata or verruca. Cilia frequently emerge from within this tumor. Because the nests of nevus cells can extend quite deep into the dermis and even into tarsus, the histopathologic appearance of this condition can masquerade as an invasive cancer.

Several unusual variant conditions deserve mention. Balloon cell nevi appear during youth and are clinically indistinguishable from a common acquired nevus; they rarely exceed 5 mm in diameter, and diagnosis is based on histologic features. The Spitz tumor (spindle-epithelioid nevus) is a weakly pigmented, benign, yet rapidly growing compound nevus seen in children and young adults. This pinkish tan mass enlarges up to 10 mm in diameter over a period of months and then ceases further growth. Dysplastic nevi are present in 8 per cent of the normal population and behave differently from most nevi. They tend to be larger, with a diameter exceeding 4 mm, and identify themselves with haphazard patches of tan, brown, and pink color. The borders of dysplastic nevi are nondistinct. Although it is reported that the risk of developing melanoma is somewhat higher in dysplastic nevi, the vast majority of these lesions will never develop into cancer; therefore, close observation, not prophylactic excision, is indicated. Dysplastic nevi can occur sporadically or follow a hereditary pattern (B-K mole syndrome). The latter group is at risk of developing multicentric cutaneous melanomas elsewhere on the body.

Nevi, as a group, pose several clinical problems. The larger and darker pigmented spots may be cosmetically unattractive. Some congenital eyelid nevi may enlarge so as to result in a mechanical ptosis and amblyopia. The hormonal influence of puberty can stimulate quiescent lesions and perturb the patient. Finally, patients may harbor fears of a malignant melanoma arising from a pre-existing eyelid nevus, despite reassurances that within the general population only a small percentage of eyelid melanomas arise from acquired nevi. The chance of any individual nevus producing a melanoma is extremely remote, and it is felt to be inappropriate to excise nevi in hopes of eliminating melanoma precursor lesions. Much of the improved survivorship for cutaneous melanoma over the past decades can be attributed directly to early detection and diagnosis. The importance of a positive family history for the disease cannot be overemphasized, since it is these patients whose nevi warrant scrupulous observation.

From the onset it should be recognized that primary eyelid melanomas are indeed rare. Lentigo maligna (Hutchinson's melanotic freckle) is a flat dark macule seen on the sun-exposed skin of elderly individuals, such as the lower eyelid and canthal angles. It is a remarkably slow-growing lesion with a prolonged horizontal (centrifugal) growth phase. In approximately 30 per cent of affected individuals, dermal invasion occurs, and the condition is transformed into lentigo maligna melanoma. Clinical signs of transformation may be absent. Five-year survival exceeds 90 per cent following treatment.

The most frequently diagnosed eyelid melanoma is the superficial spreading melanoma. This lesion is encountered even among younger individuals, affects all sun-exposed and unexposed skin surfaces, and can be palpated early in its clinical course. Its color can vary from brown, gray, or rose, and the oval configuration of superficial spreading melanoma is disrupted by protrusions and indentations. Nodules within this lesion signal vertical invasion. The characteristic histopathology of this disorder demonstrates pagetoid spread of uniformly atypical melanocytes in the epidermis combined with basal nests of atypical cells. The prognosis is worse than lentigo maligna melanoma. Nodular cutaneous melanoma is a very rare eyelid lesion. Affected individuals present with a rapidly growing palpable mass with nonuniform pigmentation. It has a short horizontal growth phase, quickly becomes invasive and, as expected, carries the poorest prognosis.

THERAPY

Supportive. Not all pigmented eyelid lesions require excision. For many patients, a clear explanation is all that is necessary. Today, those patients seeking cosmetic improvement can select from a wide variety of occlusive makeup products that are nonirritating. Photodocumentation is vital in order for the surgeon to assess the clinical course objectively. All patients need to be thoroughly advised of the warning signs that may herald the onset of a premalignant or malignant condition: changes in size, coloration, or topography and the presence of satellite lesions, ulceration, or bleeding.

Surgical. Surgical excision remains the principal treatment of pigmented eyelid lesions. Indications include clinical suspicion of melanoma, documented change or atypical behavior in an existing lesion, and a patient's preference for removal of an unsightly mass. Certainly, when the nature of a lesion is in doubt, a simple biopsy should be performed. Eyelid lesions should not receive pretreatment with cryo, dermabrasion, cauterization, laser, or radiation before biopsy, as doing so only serves to confuse the pathologist. Frozen section techniques should not be relied on for management of an initial biopsy; excisional biopsies are preferable. When an excision will result in profound lid disfigurement, shave biopsies are acceptable to establish an initial diagnosis; however, they may lead to recurrences, and specimens from second biopsies can mimic more worrisome diagnosis. All excised tissue should be forwarded for pathologic analysis, and patients should be counseled beforehand regarding the possible necessity for repeat excision. Specimen reports should include pertinent history and tissue orientation to facilitate interpretation. Tissue margins must be carefully examined for atypia. In the current management of cutaneous melanoma, the definition of "wide excision" continues to evolve. The surgeon must weigh the remote likelihood of recurrence in a biopsy with clean margins versus the morbidity associated with radical eyelid excision. Specific recommendations for every situation are beyond the scope of this article.

COMMENTS

The overall prognosis for excised primary eyelid melanoma is extremely favorable. Most melanomas are discovered before local disease can spread. Tumors excised with clean margins that are less than 2 mm deep most likely have not released micrometastasis. On the other hand, late cases of melanoma with frank preauricular and cervical adenopathy are candidates for palliative therapy.

Regardless of the specific diagnosis and whether or not surgery was performed, all patients presenting with pigmented eyelid lesions require routine follow-up examinations with photodocumentation as appropriate.

References

Elder DE, et al: Acquired melanocytic nevi and melanoma. *In* Ackerman AB (ed): Pathology of Malignant Melanomas. New York, Masson, 1981, pp 185–215.

Elder DE: Malignant melanoma. *In* Provost TT, Farmer ER (eds): Current Therapy in Dermatology-2. Toronto, BC Decker, 1988, pp 86–90.

Folberg R, Bernardino VB Jr, Bernardino EA: Pigmented eyelid lesions. *In* Hornblass A (ed): Oculoplastic, Orbital and Reconstructive Surgery. Baltimore, Williams & Wilkins, 1988, pp 259–270.

Font RL: Eyelids and lacrimal drainage system. *In* Spencer WH (ed): Ophthalmic Pathology—An Atlas and Textbook. Philadelphia, WB Saunders, 1985, pp 2183–2196.

Keeling JH III: Pigmentary problems. *In* Griffith DG, Salasche SJ, Clemons DE (eds): Cutaneous Abnormalities of the Eyelid and Face. New York McGraw-Hill, 1987, pp 169–191.

Naidoff MA, Bernardino VB Jr, Clark WH Jr: Melanocytic lesions of the eyelid skin. Am J Ophthalmol 82:371–382, 1976.

ORBITAL FAT HERNIATION
(Adipose Palpebral Bags, Baggy Eyelids)
ALLEN M. PUTTERMAN, M.D.
Chicago, Illinois

In addition to cardiorenal disease, apparent prolapses of skin around the eyes primarily represent a true herniation of encapsulated orbital fat through an opening between the rims of the orbital septum and levator aponeurosis in the upper lid or between the junction of the rim of the septum and the capculopalpebral fascia in the lower lid. These areas are anatomically weak so that orbital fat can protrude through the junctions, producing a hernia of fat. Orbital fat herniation must be distinguished from but also may be associated with dermatochalasis, which is excessive skin. These conditions pose cosmetic problems, especially in females, and may require surgical correction.

THERAPY

Surgical. At present, the only satisfactory method of treatment is surgical excision of the protruding fat. At incision is made through the upper eyelid crease or about 2 mm below the lower eyelid margin, and a skin-orbicularis flap is dissected either superiorly or inferiorly. The orbital septum is then located and tagged with 4-0 black silk sutures. The hernial sac is incised, and the fat is excised and cauterized until gentle pressure applied to the globe fails to prolapse the fat. The detached septum is not reattached to the levator or capsulopalpebral fascia, but is left to reattach spontaneously. Excessive skin and orbicularis muscle are excised as necessary, and the skin-orbicularis flaps are resutured at the original site of incision.

PRECAUTIONS

Although most cases of baggy eyelids represent true herniation, treatment, as for hernias elsewhere in the body, does not at present provide good results. If the protruding sac of fat is pushed back into place and the detached septum reattached, the problem usually recurs. Recurrence may result from the use of absorbable rather than permanent sutures. It is also possible that the exposed herniated orbital fat becomes abnormal and therefore cannot be replaced.

Lid retraction and lagophthalmos are complications of baggy eyelid surgery. Since the septum is a strong inelastic tissue, the position of its reattachment to the levator and capsulopalpebral fascia may explain these complications. Therefore, it is important that the septum is in a satisfactory position in relation to the levator and capsulopalpebral fascia before closing the wound. On the upper lid, the septum should be about 10 mm above the superior tarsal border; in the lower lid, it should be about 5 mm below the inferior tarsal border.

To avoid loss of cilia, the uppermost incision on the lower lid must not be made too close to the lid margin. Normally, the optimal position for the lower lid incision is 2 mm below the lashes. It is also important to differentiate baggy eyelids caused by herniation of orbital fat from eyelid edema secondary to metabolic problems. Pressing on the eye through the closed eyelids will lead to increased orbital fat herniation, whereas lid edema will remain unchanged.

COMMENTS

Surgical procedures for correcting baggy eyelids have been based on three different concepts regarding the pathogenesis of this condition: there is too much orbital fat, the orbital septum is absent, and the septum is thinned and degenerated with a direct herniation of the fat through it. Careful inspection shows that the condition does indeed represent a true herniation, but a thinned septum is not usually responsible for it. In most patients, the septum itself, though not its attachments, is found to be normal.

References

Putterman AM: Upper eyelid blepharoplasty. In Hornblass A (ed): Ophthalmic and Orbital Plastic and Reconstructive Surgery. Baltimore, Williams & Wilkins, 1988, pp 474–484.
Putterman AM (ed): Cosmetic Oculoplastic Surgery. New York, Grune & Stratton, 1982.
Putterman AM, Urist MJ: Baggy eyelids—A true hernia. Ann Ophthalmol 5:1029–1032, 1973.
Putterman AM, Urist MJ: Surgical anatomy of the orbital septum. Ann Ophthalmol 6:290–294, 1974.
Safian J: A late report on an early operation for "baggy eyelids." Plast Reconstr Surg 48:347–348, 1971.
Sayoc BT: Pathogenesis and management of adipose palpebral bags. Philippine J Ophthalmol 5:128–135, 1973.

PTOSIS
(Blepharoptosis)
JOHN H. SULLIVAN, M.D.
San Francisco, California

Ptosis of the upper eyelid is an uncommon disorder that is usually unilateral and may be congenital or acquired. Congenital ptosis may occasionally be associated with amblyopia secondary to ipsilateral astigmatism or myopia, but deprivation amblyopia is rare unless the lid is completely closed. Acquired ptosis is usually the result of aging or trauma.

The normal position of the upper lid is midway between the superior pupillary border and upper limbus. Elevation is accomplished by simultaneous contraction of the levator and Müller's muscle. Maximum contraction elevates the lid 8 to 15 mm, 2 to 3 mm of which are the effect of Müller's muscle. Although the diagnosis of ptosis is usually obvious, bilateral involvement may escape notice until after the more ptotic lid has been corrected. Another source of confusion can be pseudoptosis in which the lid only appears ptotic. This can occur with hypotropia, microphthalmia, dermatochalasis, and other ocular disorders.

Beard's classification of ptosis into congenital and acquired subtypes is generally accepted. The distinction between congenital and acquired is critical because much less surgery is needed for correction of acquired ptosis. The most frequent surgical errors are undercorrection of congenital and overcorrection of acquired ptosis. True "congenital ptosis" is a specific developmental anomaly of the levator muscle. Fibrous and fatty tissues replace the normal striated muscle in proportion to the severity of ptosis. Müller's muscle is usually unaffected. The result of these changes is the inability of the levator to elevate fully the lid on contraction (decreased levator function) and failure of full closure of the lid on relaxation (lid lag). Since these dystrophic changes are not found in other types of ptosis, the presence of lid lag is an important means of identifying congenital ptosis. The finding of lid lag on downgaze is always reassuring and sometimes critical in planning surgery, since it is not always possible to diagnose congenital ptosis by the date of onset. The history may be unknown, or the infant may be born with an acquired traumatic or neurogenic ptosis.

Acquired ptosis may be myogenic, neurogenic, or mechanical. It is frequently caused by disinsertion or dehiscence of the levator aponeurosis. This is believed to be the mechanism of senile (involutional) ptosis, postcataract ptosis and many instances of traumatic ptosis. Neurologic causes of acquired ptosis include Horner's syndrome, oculomotor nerve palsy, myasthenia gravis, and chronic progressive external ophthalmoplegia. Horner's syndrome causes ptosis by paresis of Müller's sympathetic muscle. The other features of the syndrome—miosis, elevation of the lower lid and anhidrosis—may be absent or so subtle that the diagnosis can be established only by testing pupillary response to topical cocaine (inhibits dilation). Ptosis from Horner's syndrome is usually mild and associated with good levator function.

THERAPY

Surgical. Proper management requires familiarity with several surgical techniques. Mild ptosis (1 to 2 mm) with good levator function (more than 8 mm) may only require shortening of Müller's muscle. Moderate ptosis (2 to 3 mm) with fair function (5 to 7 mm) is most often treated by resection of the levator. Severe ptosis (4 mm or more) with poor levator function (4 mm or less) requires a separate elevating force. The most useful alternative is suspension of the lid to the frontalis muscle; elevation of the lid is then accomplished by raising the eyebrow. Autogenous fascia lata has been found to be superior to synthetic or other biologic materials for this purpose. Another muscle that has been used is the superior rectus. However, complications of diplopia and exposure keratitis have caused virtual abandonment of this source.

Congenital ptosis may be associated with other ocular abnormalities. The most frequent, each of which occurs in approximately 5 per cent of cases, include ipsilateral superior rectus weakness, blepharophimosis syndrome, and Marcus Gunn jaw winking. Superior rectus weakness requires resection of more levator muscle. Blepharophimosis (ptosis, telecanthus, epicanthus inversus, and cicatricial ectropion) almost always requires brow suspension because of poor levator function. Ptosis with synkinetic jaw movements (Marcus Gunn syndrome) is rarely bilateral. If the normal action of the mandible in eating and speaking does not produce noticeable lid movement, surgery is limited to correction of the ptosis. To eliminate the aberrant lid movement, it is necessary to excise the levator muscle then correct the resultant complete ptosis by brow suspension. Unilateral brow suspension, however, is rarely satisfactory because there is insufficient stimulus to raise the affected brow. Bilateral suspension with excision of both levators produces the most symmetric result.

Unilateral ptosis may be the only manifestation of myasthenia gravis. Fatigue of the lid is often a clue, but intravenous edrophonium may be necessary to make the diagnosis. Surgical correction of ptosis caused by myasthenia and chronic progressive external ophthalmoplegia may be complicated by progressive deterioration and extraocular muscle involvement. A functional undercorrection is preferable to a full correction that results in exposure keratitis.

Minimal ptosis with good levator function is most easily repaired by Müllerectomy or tarsoMüllerectomy. The Fasanella-Servat procedure remains the most popular of this type because of its simplicity and predictability. In this operation, the upper lid is everted, a clamp is placed over the upper tarsus, conjunctiva, and Müller's muscle, and these tissues are resected.

Moderate or severe ptosis with good function and a high lid fold may be signs of aponeurosis disinsertion. Exploration and repair of the aponeurosis through a lid fold incision is believed to be the procedure of choice when disinsertion is suspected. Under local anesthesia, it is usually not difficult to identify the free edge of the aponeurosis and attach it to the tarsus. The lid is usually set slightly higher than the final desired result to compensate for mechanical stimulation of Müller's muscle. Because it is difficult to predict the postoperative lid position at the time of surgery, over- and undercorrections are not uncommon.

Levator resection is the mainstay of congenital ptosis surgery. An internal (conjunctival) or external (cutaneous) approach can be used. The conjunctival approach has the important advantage of adjustability in the event of overcorrection. The resected levator is secured to the tarsus by mattress sutures tied on the skin surface. Their early removal combined with manipulation allows the lid to be lowered in the immediate postoperative period. The external approach provides additional exposure, which is necessary for a maximum resection (greater than 23 mm).

The amount of levator to be resected may be determined by two methods. Predetermination can be made by Beard's guidelines of levator function and severity of ptosis. However, additional factors must also be considered, such as a 3 or 4 mm larger resection in the presence of superior rectus weakness or jaw winking. Variations in technique, such as the magnitude of tarsal resection, placement of sutures, and effect of cutting the levator horns, can also influence the final lid position. Berke's method of determining the amount of levator to be resected is based on the position of the lid during surgery. It is predicated on the knowledge that the lid will elevate or drop postoperatively in proportion to the levator function. The surgeon should be aware of both methods to predict the size of resection, confirm the choice during surgery, and anticipate postoperative changes.

Ocular or Periocular Manifestations

Eyelids: Unilateral or bilateral ptosis.
Extraocular Muscles: Superior rectus weakness.
Other: Amblyopia; astigmatism; myopia.

PRECAUTIONS

Undercorrection is the most frequent complication of surgery for congenital ptosis. Repair of undercorrection necessitates reoperation, whereas management of overcorrection is usually much easier. Early removal of sutures, massage, and stretching are sufficient for most cases of overcorrection. Levator tenotomy is used when conservative treatment fails. Lid lengthening by scleral graft is useful in the late repair of severe lagophthalmos. Eye bank sclera preserved in alcohol is used in the same manner as in correction of lid retraction from Grave's disease.

Entropion and lid contour abnormalities can be prevented by resection of no more than half the tarsal plate. Failure to remove skin from the upper lid after a large levator resection will produce a low lid fold and spoil the appearance of an otherwise excellent job. Unilateral blepharoplasty can be done later to correct this defect. Damage to the superior rectus or superior oblique can occur during ptosis surgery and may result in vertical diplopia. Caution should always be used in cutting the horns of the aponeurosis. Identification of the superior rectus can be facilitated by a bridal suture.

COMMENTS

The outcome of ptosis surgery in patients with less than good levator function is never perfect. Lid asymmetry will always be present in some position of gaze. The limitations of surgery are generally better accepted by patients with congenital defects than those whose problem has been recently acquired. In either setting, a discussion of realistic goals before surgery can prevent the problem of an unhappy patient despite the best possible result. The surgeon should be familiar with the intricate anatomy of the lid and be capable of utilizing different procedures to manage various types of ptosis.

References

Anderson RL: Age of aponeurotic awareness. Ophthalmol Plastic Reconstr Surg 1:69, 1985.
Beard C: Ptosis surgery past, present, future. Ophthalmol Plastic Reconstr Surg 1:69, 1985.
Beard C: Ptosis, 3rd ed. St. Louis, CV Mosby, 1981.
Beard C, Sullivan JH: Ptosis—Current concepts. Int Ophthalmol Clin 18:53–73, 1978.
Buckman G, Jakobiec FA, Hyde K, Lisman RD, Hornblass A, Harrison W: Success of the Fasanella-Servat operation independent of Müller's smooth muscle excision. Ophthalmology 96:413–418, 1989.
Jones LT, Quickert MH, Wobig JL: The cure of ptosis by aponeurotic repair. Arch Ophthalmol 93:629–634, 1975.
Linberg JV, Vasquez RJ, Chao GM: Aponeurotic ptosis repair under local anesthesia. Prediction of results from operative lid height. Ophthalmology 95:1046, 1988.
Merriam WW, Ellis FD, Helveston EM: Congenital blepharoptosis, anisometropia, and amblyopia. Am J Ophthalmol 89:401–407, 1980.
Putterman AM, Urist MJ: Müller muscle-conjunctiva resection. Technique for treatment of blepharoptosis. Arch Ophthalmol 93:619–623, 1975.

SEBORRHEIC BLEPHARITIS
MICHAEL HALSTED, M.D.,
and JAMES P. McCULLEY, M.D.
Dallas, Texas

Chronic blepharitis is a disease that is commonly encountered by the practicing ophthalmologist. Recently, an updated classification of chronic blepharitis based on clinical signs and symptoms has been presented. This current classification subdivides chronic blepharitis into six categories as follows: 1) staphylococcal blepharitis, 2) pure seborrheic blepharitis, 3) mixed staphylococcal/seborrheic blepharitis, 4) seborrheic blepharitis with meibomian seborrhea, 5) seborrheic blepharitis with secondary meibomianitis, and 6) meibomian keratoconjunctivitis or primary meibomianitis.

Seborrheic blepharitis commonly presents in an older age group (mean age, 50 years) and has a longer duration of symptoms than staphylococcal blepharitis. Symptoms of mattering, burning, and foreign body sensation, once present, are not associated with as frequent exacerbations as in patients with staphylococcal lid disease, but are chronic with minimal waxing and waning. The eyelids are frequently less inflamed, and the debris deposited on the eyelid margin has an oily and greasy consistency that is often called scurf. Mixed staphylococcal/seborrheic blepharitis is marked by more frequent exacerbations of symptoms and is discussed in detail in the next section.

Seborrheic blepharitis with associated meibomian seborrhea frequently presents with pronounced complaints of severe burning in the morning. Although patient symptoms are marked, the clinical signs are frequently less prominent. The foremost finding is engorged meibomian glands filled with retained secretions (meibum) that can be easily expressed on eyelid massage. The tear film has a foamy appearance that is most noticeable in the lateral canthal region.

Seborrheic blepharitis with a secondary meibomianitis presents with symptoms similar to those of seborrheic blepharitis alone, but with more significant periods of exacerbation of symptoms. The anterior/ciliary lid changes are also similar to those found in patients with seborrheic blepharitis, but examination of the posterior lid reveals patchy, scattered inflammation surrounding the meibomian glands. The affected glands are inflamed and dilated with retained solidified meibum. The involved gland orifices are blocked with inspissated secretions that are not easily expressible on massage.

Meibomian keratoconjunctivitis is distinguished from other seborrheic blepharitis by a shorter duration of symptoms at the time of presentation and a more pronounced inflammation of the eyelids. The anterior/ciliary aspect of the lids are frequently only minimally involved with deposition of an oily scurf. The prominent feature is diffuse inflammation around the meibomian glands, which are dilated with retained meibum that is not easily expressed. The orifices of the glands are obstructed and pout with inspissated secretions. There is a marked inflammation around the meibomian glands and the orifices. This constellation of findings give an overall picture of thickened and inflamed eyelids.

In addition to the lid findings, an important associated condition found in these patients is keratoconjunctivitis sicca (KCS). The symptoms of KCS are similar to and may be masked in the complaints of patients whose predominant problem is related to blepharitis. However, patients with chronic blepharitis have been shown to have changes in the composition of meibum, which may lead to alterations in the tear film, thereby predisposing these patients to associated ocular surface problems related to an unstable tear film. Nonetheless, recent studies have documented the occurrence of concurrent KCS in patients with chronic blepharitis in 25 to 60 per cent of the patients. It is imperative to look for an accompanying dry eye state in these patients and to treat it when present.

Extensive culturing, both aerobic and anaerobic of normals and patients with each form of chronic blepharitis, has revealed a significantly greater incidence of colonization by *Staphylococcus aureus* species only in the staphylococcal and mixed staphylococcal/seborrheic subgroups. There was no significant difference in the incidence of coagulase negative staphylococcus (C-NS), *Propionibacterium acnes*, or any other bacteria isolated in any of the various patient subgroups compared to normal controls. Cultures of meibum revealed no evidence to support its role as a reservoir for bacterial colonization in any form of chronic blepharitis.

The possible role of bacterial lipases in modifying the composition of meibum and differences in the biochemical composition of meibum in the various subgroups of chronic blepharitis have also been examined. Careful studies have shown that there is a higher percentage of C-NS species capable of de-esterifying fatty waxes and cholesteryl-esters in the types of chronic blepharitis with meibomian gland involvement. In addition, it has been demonstrated that the free fatty acid component of meibum in patients with meibomian gland involvement varies from that of normals. The exact role of bacterial lipases and variation in the biochemical components of meibum as factors in the pathophysiology of chronic blepharitis, as possible markers for diagnosis, or as new avenues for therapeutic intervention requires further elucidation.

THERAPY

Supportive. First and foremost in the treatment of chronic seborrheic blepharitis is the understanding by both patient and physician that the disease is chronic, occasionally marked by bothersome exacerbations of symptoms and signs, and one for which there is presently no definitive cure. The goals of therapy are to control the disease, maintain vision, and avoid secondary complications. There are characteristically two phases of therapy. The first is to bring the disease under control and then subsequently to taper the therapy to a minimum that will provide long-term control of the chronic disease process and prevent exacerbations.

Ocular. The mainstay of treatment for chronic blepharitis is lid hygiene. This must be carefully explained and demonstrated so that it will be performed properly by the patient. The aim is to remove eyelid debris adequately and restore normal meibum secretory flow.

A warm and moist compress, usually a facecloth run under a flow of water as warm as can be tolerated, should be applied to the closed eyelids for 5 to 10 minutes. As the compress cools, it should be rewarmed in a similar fashion. After the use of compresses, the tarsus containing the meibomian glands should be massaged against the globe in patients with meibomian gland involvement. This is best accomplished by rotating the tip of a finger placed just outside the lashes and applying enough pressure to the tarsus against the globe to express the contents of the glands onto the lid margin. In patients with meibomianitis, it is hoped that the warm compresses will raise the temperature of the lid sufficiently to surpass the melting point of the abnormal retained meibum. Debris is then scrubbed from the lid margin with a clean facecloth and a nonirritating baby shampoo or a commercially available eyelid scrub. The lids are then rinsed until free of shampoo. Initially, lid hygiene is required two to four times a day, but may then be tapered to once or twice a day, usually upon waking and at bedtime. The most important time to perform lid hygiene is in the morning, as the debris collects and builds up on the lids when closed during sleep.

The use of topical antibiotic is recommended in all patients except those with seborrheic blepharitis alone. The recommended topical antibiotic treatment is detailed in the next article on staphylococcal blepharitis.

Systemic. The use of systemic antibiotics in addition to local treatment is indicated in all patients with primary meibomianitis or patients with secondary meibomianitis unresponsive to local therapy. Initially, patients with meibomianitis require 250 mg of oral tetracycline four times a day to bring the inflammation under control. The mechanism of action is felt to be related to tetracycline-induced bacterial lipase inhibition and decreased free fatty acid production. In patients with secondary meibomianitis or meibomian keratoconjunctivitis without associated rosacea, the dose of tetracycline may frequently be tapered and discontinued over the course of 3 to 4 months. However, patients with meibomian keratoconjunctivitis in conjunction with rosacea frequently require a chronic low daily dose of 250 mg to control their symptoms.

In patients with seborrheic blepharitis, it is important also to look carefully for concurrent seborrheic dermatitis. The degree and distribution of involvement vary greatly from patient to patient. Involvement of the scalp, retroauricular, nasolabial, brow, and sternal regions has all been reported in patients presenting with seborrheic blepharitis. In patients who have an associated significant dermatitis, consultation with a dermatologist is prudent.

Ocular or Periocular Manifestations

Conjunctiva: Concretions; cystic changes; hyperemia; papillary hypertrophy.

Cornea: Marginal cicatrization; pannus formation; punctate epithelial erosions; punctate epithelial keratitis.

Eyelids: Chalazion; collarettes; debris; edema; erythema; hordeolum; madarosis; meibomian gland changes; poliosis; scaling.

PRECAUTIONS

In patients who require systemic tetracycline, appropriate precautions need to be taken. Tetracycline should be taken on an empty stomach, i.e., 1 hour before or 2 hours after meals. If associated gastrointestinal irritation presents as a side effect, 100 mg of doxycycline twice a day, which may be taken with food, can be substituted. Tetracycline or doxycycline should not be administered to children because of the effect on dental enamel. In addition, it is contraindicated in pregnant women and lactating mothers. When tetracycline is contraindicated, erythromycin is a suitable alternate.

COMMENTS

Although a chronic and bothersome disease, seborrheic blepharitis when correctly diagnosed and treated can usually be brought under control and the patient's symptoms reduced greatly. It is imperative that the chronic nature of the disease be explained to the patient so that false expectations may be put to rest at the onset. The close interrelationship between eyelid, tear film, and an intact and healthy ocular surface demands that careful attention to the tear film and ocular surface be paid when examining patients with blepharitis so that associated or underlying abnormalities do not go undiagnosed and untreated.

References

Bowman RW, Dougherty JM, McCulley JP: Chronic blepharitis and dry eyes. Int Ophthalmol Clin 27:27–35, 1987.

Dougherty JM, McCulley JP: Analysis of free fatty acid component of meibomian secretions in chronic blepharitis. Invest Ophthalmol Vis Sci 27:52–56, 1986.

Dougherty JM, McCulley JP: Bacterial lipases and chronic blepharitis. Invest Ophthalmol Vis Sci 27:486–491, 1986.

Leibowitz HM, Capino D: Correspondence to the editor. Arch Ophthalmol 106:720, 1988.

McCulley JP: Blepharoconjunctivitis. Int Ophthalmol Clin 24:65–77, 1984.

McCulley JP: Blepharitis associated with acne rosacea and seborrheic dermatitis. Ann Ophthalmol 17:53–57, 1985.

McCulley JP, Dougherty JM: Bacterial aspects of chronic blepharitis. Trans Ophthalmol Soc UK 105:314–318, 1986.

McCulley JP, Sciallis GF: Meibomian keratoconjunctivitis. Am J Ophthalmol 84:778–793, 1977.

McCulley JP, Dougherty JM, Deneau DG: Classification of chronic blepharitis. Ophthalmology 189:1173–1180, 1983.

Pollack FM, Goodman DF: Correspondence to the editor. Arch Ophthalmol 106:719–720, 1988.

STAPHYLOCOCCAL AND MIXED STAPHYLOCOCCAL/ SEBORRHEIC BLEPHARO- CONJUNCTIVITIS

DONNA DODSON BROWN, M.D.,
and JAMES P. McCULLEY, M.D.
Dallas, Texas

Blepharoconjunctivitis is one of the most commonly encountered diseases in ophthalmology. In 1982, a classification of chronic blepharitis was introduced that has served as a good framework on which to build our thinking about this disease. This classification scheme was based on careful ophthalmologic and dermatologic examinations, cultures of the lids and conjunctiva, and lipid studies. The categories described were 1) staphylococcal; 2) seborrheic—alone, mixed seborrheic/staphylococcal, seborrheic with meibomian seborrhea, and seborrheic with secondary meibomianitis; 3) primary meibomianitis; and 4) other, including atopic, psoriatic, fungal, etc.

Chronic staphylococcal blepharoconjunctivitis characteristically has a history of waxing and waning signs and symptoms that are usually of shorter duration than those of other types of blepharoconjunctivitis. These patients are usually younger, with a mean age of 42 compared with 51 years for other types of blepharitis. It is more common in females, with 80 per cent of cases occurring in females. Staphylococcal blepharitis is characterized by collarettes and less greasy debris than seborrheic blepharitis. The eyelids of patients with staphylococcal blepharitis alone or in association with seborrheic blepharitis are more inflamed than other subgroups. There is a lack of associated dermatologic abnormalities in the staphylococcal group. Results of aerobic and anaerobic cultures from lids and conjunctiva showed that the only blepharitis groups with a significant percentage of positive cultures for *Staphylococcus aureus* were the clinically defined groups of staphylococcal and mixed staphylococcal/seborrheic groups.

In the pure staphylococcal group, blepharitis is treatable and possibly curable, in contrast to other forms of the disease, which usually can only be controlled. Clinical features of staphylococcal blepharoconjunctivitis include inflamed eyelids with erythema and sometimes edema along the anterior ciliary portion of the lid and not uncommonly madarosis. The eyelid margin is frequently involved as well. There may be telangiectatic changes along the lid margin.

Crusting of the lashes occurs with collarettes surrounding individual cilia. Anterior or posterior hordeola intermittently occur. Fifteen per cent of patients develop bulbar and tarsal conjunctival changes, including injection, and, when chronic, papillary hypertrophy of the tarsal conjunctiva. With acute exacerbation, a follicular response may develop over the inferior tarsal plate. A keratitis characterized by punctate epithelial erosions involving the inferior one third of the cornea, which may be secondary to staphylococcal exotoxin, may occur. Other possible causes of this keratitis include an abnormal blink mechanism or destabilization of the tear film. A more severe keratitis leading to phlyctenular changes and corneal ulcers can occur. Infiltrates with a marginal keratitis may also occur. Fifty per cent of patients with staphylococcal blepharoconjunctivitis also have associated keratoconjunctivitis sicca that may have an associated corneal punctate epitheliopathy.

Forty-six per cent of eyelid cultures from patients with clinical staphylococcal blepharoconjunctivitis have been found to be positive for *Staphylococcus aureus* and 92 per cent positive for *S. epidermidis*. Conjunctival cultures were 23 per cent positive for *S. aureus* and 85 per cent positive for *S. epidermidis*. Other organisms that may be cultured are *Corynebacterium* species, *Propionibacterium acnes*, and other *Propionibacterium* species.

Mixed seborrheic/staphylococcal blepharoconjunctivitis exhibits signs of both types of blepharitis and an equal male/female distribution. The debris is characteristically an oily, greasy crusting on the anterior lid and collarettes on the lashes. Characteristically, these patients have a chronic history with periods of significant exacerbation of the inflammatory process representing the chronic seborrheic component and exacerbation occurring when the bacterial component becomes active. They typically have more inflammation than in seborrheic blepharoconjunctivitis alone.

Approximately 35 per cent of patients with mixed seborrheic/staphylococcal blepharoconjunctivitis have associated keratoconjunctivitis sicca. Most of the patients in the seborrheic/staphylococcal group also have seborrheic dermatitis. Keratoconjunctivitis is common in mixed seborrheic/staphylococcal blepharoconjunctivitis with mild inferior tarsal conjunctival papillary hypertrophy, bulbar conjunctival injection, punctate epithelial erosions over the inferior third of the cornea, and rarely follicular hypertrophy over the inferior tarsal conjunctiva.

More than 80 per cent of patients in the mixed group have positive eyelid cultures for *S. aureus*, and 50 per cent have positive conjunctival cultures. Almost all patients have positive lid cultures for *S. epidermidis*, and more than 80 per cent have positive conjunctival cultures.

THERAPY

Ocular. Although treatment for most types of chronic blepharitis is aimed at control rather than cure, treatment for staphylococcal blepharitis may be curative. There may, however, be intermittent recurrences or exacerbation of the inflammatory process after the initial treatment has led to resolution. In such patients, a less intense maintenance regimen of treatment will be required. Treatment usually requires 2 to 8 weeks of intense therapy, with lessening of treatment after the initial, more severe signs have resolved.

The most important component of the initial therapy includes the use of warm compresses aimed at loosening debris and liquefying meibomian secretions, which are followed by eyelid scrubs. It is important to instruct patients carefully in the technique of applying hot compresses and performing eyelid scrubs. The first step is to soak a clean facecloth in water as warm as the eyelids can tolerate and to apply it to the eyelid. This should be done for 5 to 10 minutes, rewarming the wash cloth as often as is necessary to maintain the warm temperature. Applying the compress loosens the debris and liquefies sebaceous secretions, which may then be removed with the lid scrubs with an innocuous soap, such as one of the baby shampoos or commercial lid scrubs. Some advise using diluted baby shampoo, but full-strength shampoo is recommended. Again, a wet facecloth is used to which shampoo has been applied, with the patient scrubbing in a left-to-right motion. Both the upper and lower lids are scrubbed, as well as the eyebrows. Excess soap is rinsed away. A facecloth is preferred over a cotton-tipped applicator because frequently either the globe is traumatized with the cotton-tipped applicator or the patient does not adequately perform scrubs because of the fear of traumatizing the globe. The patient should realize that the purpose of the compresses and scrubs is to remove the debris from the lids and lashes. The soap scrubs also help lyse bacterial membranes and thus decrease the bacterial count.

With clinical evidence of infection, cultures of the eyelids and conjunctiva may be done but are not required. Most staphylococcal species are sensitive to bacitracin, erythromycin, chloramphenicol, gentamicin, and tobramycin. In patients with clinical evidence of staphylococcal or mixed seborrheic/staphylococcal blepharoconjunctivitis, an antibiotic ointment may be used empirically after the lid scrubs. Bacitracin, which is highly effective against all staphylococci, is the first drug of choice. It is bactericidal and has a low incidence of associated allergic reactions. Erythromycin is the second drug of choice. The aminoglycosides are usually reserved for sight-threatening conditions and in treating resistant organisms.

The antibiotic ointment is rubbed into the eyelid along the lash margin after the warm compresses and scrubs have been done. One-fourth inch of ointment is also instilled into the inferior cul-de-sac at bedtime. With this approach, no ointment is instilled into the tear film during the day. If the infectious process is severe enough to cause concern about the potential for developing a corneal infection, an aminoglycoside is recommended because it is available in both ointment and drop form. This allows the use of only one antibiotic with the ointment being rubbed into the lids and lashes, as well as being instilled into the cul-de-sac at bedtime; the drops are applied to the ocular surface during the day. Tobramycin is recommended because of its broad spectrum and relative lesser toxicity.

After the initial inflammatory signs have resolved, the above regimen may be tapered to a frequency that keeps the condition stable. The compresses and lid scrubs are frequently required on a long-term basis and are most beneficial in the morning because during the night organisms and debris have accumulated on the lids. Occasionally, long-term antibiotic ointment is required, in which case the weekly alteration of antibiotic may decrease the risk of selection of resistant organisms.

Rarely, topical steroids are used when hypersensitivity infiltrates persist, but they are not recommended for routine use in acute or chronic blepharitis. Most often, eyelid hygiene and antibiotic therapy will lead to clearing of hypersensitivity keratitis. Use of steroids is risky and especially so in dry eyed patients as further suppression of the immune system may create an increased potential for infection. In any patient, severe bacterial or fungal infections may occur with long-term steroid use.

Occasionally, especially in children, systemic antibiotic therapy is necessary. Erythromycin, cephalosporin, or a penicillinase-resistant penicillin may be used in these patients.

Sensitivity testing for *Staphylococcus* species has shown some strains to be resistant to sulfonamides. Therefore, based on current knowledge of mechanisms that lead to the development of staphylococcal blepharoconjunctivitis, sulfonamides are not recommended as an antimicrobial agent.

Not uncommonly, keratoconjunctivitis sicca (KCS) coexists with staphylococcal blepharitis. It is sometimes difficult to diagnose during an acute episode of staphylococcal blepharitis, but is later discovered after the blepharitis is under control. Topical artificial tear therapy should be initiated when KCS coexists. Occasionally, other measures, such as punctal occlusion, may be required. Patients appropriately treated for KCS may be less likely to develop recurrent bacterial blepharoconjunctivitis.

Treatment of mixed seborrheic/staphylococcal blepharoconjunctivitis is aimed at control and not cure. Warm compresses followed by application of either bacitracin or erythromycin ointment two to four times daily as described for treatment of staphylococcal blepharoconjunctivitis should be done. It usually takes 2 to 8 weeks of intense therapy initially to control inflammation. After this time, tapering treatment to a frequency necessary to control inflammation is the goal. This regime, typically consists of warm compresses and lid scrubs once or twice daily. Thirty to thirty-five per cent of patients also have KCS that requires therapy.

Ocular or Periocular Manifestations

Conjunctiva: Conjunctivitis; injection; mucous or mucopurulent discharge; phlyctenules.

Cornea: Epithelial erosions; marginal infiltrates; phlyctenules; ulceration; vascularization.
Eyelids: Chalazion; collarettes; debris; edema; erythema; hordeolum; madarosis; meibomian gland changes; poliosis; scaling.
Other: Seborrheic skin changes in mixed seborrheic/staphylococcal blepharoconjunctivitis.

PRECAUTIONS

Medicamentosa conjunctivitis secondary to the topical treatment may occur, especially in patients with associated keratoconjunctivitis sicca. The patient may be reacting to the antibiotic or possibly to a preservative in a tear preparation. Discontinuation of all potentially toxic medication should result in significant improvement. Allergies to bacitracin and erythromycin are unusual but may occur, necessitating alternate therapy. Of course, patients may be allergic to a systemic antibiotic being used, especially penicillin, and a careful history to elicit this information is necessary. Chemicals present in the soaps may cause hypersensitivity and allergic reactions.

Occasionally, more severe keratitis, phlyctenular changes, and even corneal ulceration may occur that require more intensive therapy.

COMMENTS

Blepharoconjunctivitis is a condition that is commonly encountered by the ophthalmologist. Close observation of the specific eyelid, conjunctival, and corneal changes will help determine the type of blepharoconjunctivitis present, thus determining the type of treatment regimen best suited for the individual patient. With staphylococcal blepharoconjunctivitis or mixed seborrheic/staphylococcal blepharoconjunctivitis, eyelid hygiene and topical antibiotics as described earlier will cure or control the condition. When these therapies fail, attention should be given to other possible diagnoses or additional underlying problems. Occasional discontinuation of all therapy and culturing or reculturing of the eyelids and conjunctiva will aid in the diagnosis and treatment.

References

Bowman RW, Dougherty JM, McCulley JP: Chronic blepharitis and dry eyes. Int Ophthalmol Clin 27:27–35, 1987.
Bowman RW, Miller K, McCulley JP: Diagnosis and treatment of chronic blepharitis. *In* Focal Points: Clinical Modules for Ophthalmologists. in press.
Dougherty JM, McCulley JP: Comparative bacteriology of chronic blepharitis. Br J Ophthalmol 68:524–528, 1984.
McCulley JP: Blepharoconjunctivitis. Int Ophthalmol Clin 24:65–77, 1984.
McCulley JP, Sciallis GF: Meibomian keratoconjunctivitis. Am J Ophthalmol 84:788–793, 1977.
McCulley JP, Dougherty J, Deneau DG: Classification of chronic blepharitis. Ophthalmology 89:1173–1180, 1982.

Smolin G, Okumoto MA: Staphylococcal blepharitis. Arch Ophthalmol 95:812–816, 1977.
Thygeson P: Complications of staphylococcal blepharitis. Am J Ophthalmol 68:446–449, 1969.

SYMBLEPHARON
ROBERT L. STAMPER, M.D.,
and DAVID W. VASTINE, M.D.
San Francisco, California

Symblepharon is an adhesion between the palpebral conjunctiva and the bulbar conjunctiva or cornea. It may be localized and of little clinical consequence or large enough to interfere with normal eyelid function or ocular motility. Symblepharon is usually formed as a result of trauma, radiation, burns, severe inflammation, or infection. Congenital symblepharon does occur, but rarely. Chemical burns, Stevens-Johnson syndrome, ocular cicatricial pemphigoid, and recurrent pterygium are some of the more frequent conditions that cause the more severe adhesions. If the cornea is directly involved or the symblepharon leads to corneal exposure and ulceration, vision may be impaired. The pathogenesis seems to require the direct apposition of two surfaces, conjunctival or corneal, both of which have been denuded of epithelium. Disruption of a single epithelial surface rarely leads to the formation of symblepharon.

THERAPY

Ocular. Symblepharon is easier to prevent than to treat. The denuded surfaces must be separated until re-epithelialization has occurred. The classical prophylaxis and early treatment regimen is based on breaking early symblepharon with a glass rod or, if none is available, with an ordinary, rugged sterile glass rectal thermometer. Symblepharon lysis must be done at least twice daily to be effective. This regimen is difficult, if not impossible, to accomplish in children. In severe cases, despite daily lysis of adhesions, the formation of symblepharon with progressive shrinkage of the inferior or superior conjunctival cul-de-sac can occur. During the acute stages, the use of topical and systemic anti-inflammatory agents is helpful in reducing inflammation, subepithelial fibrosis, and shrinkage.

A variety of conformers and stents have been advocated to keep the raw surfaces separated. None of these devices is entirely satisfactory because none prevents subepithelial fibrosis, which may lead to shrinkage of the submucosal connective tissue and extrusion of the device. A methylmethacrylate conformer with a large central opening or vault to allow clearance of the cornea during normal ocular movement is recommended. The denuded conjunctival or corneal surfaces are separated by the plastic, and thus, healing may occur without adhesions between them. In children or uncooperative patients, a thin, flexible nonreactive material, such as a sterilized silicon sheet, plastic surgical drape, or a piece of surgical glove, can be used to separate the denuded surfaces. The material must be sutured in place so that it covers the entire involved conjunctival surface.

Surgical. Once the disease process is stabilized and quiescent, conjunctival Z plasty and other simple reconstructive procedures may be helpful in the less severely affected cases. In the more severe cases, some form of mucous membrane grafting must be utilized. The mucous membrane graft replaces the denuded epithelium of at least one of the two surfaces. Although the mucous membrane of the mouth has been the most commonly used source in the past, excellent results have been reported with autologous conjunctiva taken from the ipsilateral side when the conjunctival defect is small or from the contralateral side when the defect is large. Autologous conjunctival grafting is now the preferred technique. The donor conjunctival tissue provides more normal surface characteristics and tear function than buccal or labial mucosa. In those cases where foreshortening of the conjunctival fornices causes extrusion of a conformer, either conjunctival or mucous membrane grafting may be the only way to prevent serious lid deformity or extraocular muscle restriction. As demonstrated by long-term follow-up, eyes reconstructed with free conjunctival grafts seems to show less residual deformity and shrinkage than, the other techniques. Although heterologous donor conjunctiva has been successfully used experimentally and in rare cases of closely related patients, it is not widely used or accepted.

Ocular or Periocular Manifestations

Cornea: Exposure keratitis; keratoconjunctivitis sicca; opacity.
Eyelids: Adhesions; deformity; districhiasis; entropion; lagophthalmos; trichiasis.
Lacrimal System: Epiphora; punctal occlusion.
Other: Blindness; diplopia; restriction of extraocular motility.

PRECAUTIONS

All attempts at therapy assume that the basic disease process has become nonprogressive or is medically controlled. Control of the disease may require the use of systemic antimetabolites, such as cyclophosphamide,[‡] in ocular cicatricial pemphigoid and intense topical anti-inflammatory drugs, including steroids and nonsteroidal anti-inflammatory agents. If the process is actively progressive, almost all attempts at therapy are doomed to failure. The glass rod lysis technique should be used in the first 7 to 10 days. In mild to moderate cases, the lysis should be continued until the opposing conjunctival surfaces have re-epithelialized, as demonstrated by lack of fluorescein or rose bengal staining. If symblepharon continues to form despite repeated lysis of adhesions, a rigid donut-shaped conformer can be placed into the conjunctival fornices. If the rigid conformer is not tolerated, a soft bandage contact lens placed on the cornea before fitting may make the scleral shell more comfortable, allowing more effective long-term treatment. If the eye cannot tolerate the conformer or the newly forming symblepharon pushes the conformer out, a conjunctival or buccal mucous membrane should be considered once the active cicatricial or inflammatory reaction has subsided.

Nonsurgical therapeutic measures will not work if there is extensive subconjunctival fibrosis or the fornices have been significantly shortened. Subconjunctival fibrosis should be carefully and completely resected or lysed at the time of surgical reconstruction. If conjunctival grafts are used, only the mucosa should be transplanted, and care should be taken to leave at least 2 mm of normal conjunctiva at the limbus on the donor eye. Partial-thickness mucous membrane grafts from the mouth can be used, although this material is more likely to shrink and may produce less satisfactory cosmetic and function results than autologous conjunctiva.

COMMENTS

Symblepharon is one of the most frustrating of the eyelid problems. Progressive disease essentially prevents satisfactory therapy. Extensive scarring will hinder therapy, unless it is totally removed. However, with diligence, attention to detail, and cooperation on the part of the patient, many cases previously consigned to blindness can be helped.

References

Belin MW, Hannush SB: Mucous membrane abnormalities. *In* Abbott RL (ed): Surgical Intervention in Corneal and External Diseases. Orlando, Grune & Stratton, 1987, pp 159–176.

Demartini DR, Vastine DW: Pterygium. *In* Abbott RL (ed): Surgical Intervention in Corneal and External Diseases. Orlando, Grune & Stratton, 1987, pp 141–153.

Duke-Elder S (ed): System of Ophthalmology. St. Louis, CV Mosby, 1965, Vol VIII, pp 6–8.

Foster CS: Immunosuppressive therapy for external ocular inflammatory disease. Ophthalmology 87:140, 1980.

Kaufman HE, Thomas EL: Prevention and treatment of symblepharon. Am J Ophthalmol 88:419–423, 1979.

Schwab IR, Stamper RL: Symblepharon lysis with a thermometer. Am J Ophthalmol 90:270–271, 1980.

Vastine DW, Stewart WB, Schwab IR: Reconstruction of the periocular mucous membrane by autologous conjunctival transplantation. Ophthalmology 89:1072–1081, 1982.

TRICHIASIS
F.T. FRAUNFELDER, M.D.
Portland, Oregon

Trichiasis is a condition in which the eyelashes are directed toward the globe and irritate the cornea and the conjunctiva. The primary problem caused by trichiasis is secondary corneal ulceration with or without infection, and it may well be one of the leading causes of corneal ulcers in the older age group. The condition most often occurs secondary to chronic blepharitis, but may also be associated with trachoma, cicatricial pemphigoid, alkaline burns, and eyelid injuries. One needs to differentiate trichiasis from entropion, since the latter condition is treated with a totally different surgical procedure.

THERAPY

Surgical. Epilation provides temporary relief for trichiasis. Since the normal growth cycle of an eyelash is 6 to 8 weeks, the abnormal eyelashes usually recur within a few weeks. In general, epilation is only a temporizing measure, and a more definitive procedure usually needs to be done.

Electrolysis can be effective; however, few ophthalmologists use electrolysis for more than a few lashes. This is primarily because it takes a great deal of time to put an electrode down each individual hair follicle. In addition, scarring and secondary entropion may occur with this type of treatment. Various electrolysis instrumentations are available; some are satisfactory, whereas others, especially the battery-operated instruments, can be erratic in their function.

Cryotherapy is rapidly gaining in popularity. If at least half or the whole lid needs to be treated, cryospray is preferred. The cryoprobe is satisfactory if less than half of the lid needs to be treated.

If over half of the lid margin is to be treated, equal parts of bupivacaine and lidocaine with epinephrine are injected along the base of the hair follicles, and a topical local anesthetic is applied to the eye. A thermocouple is placed at the base of a few hair follicles, usually temporally if all the hair follicles in the lid are to be destroyed. The lid is partially everted so that the spray can be directed perpendicular to the lid margin. A Berke-Jaeger shield should be placed in the cul-de-sac to protect the eye. The area over the thermocouple is frozen to $-15°C$, and the size of the iceball to achieve this temperature is then used as a guide or template to freeze the areas away from the thermocouple. The iceball is extended along the lid margin by slowly advancing the nasal edge of the ice using an intermittent or "pulse" spray technique. The ice front (iceball on the skin) is advanced by moving the tip a little more nasally. After a complete thaw, this is repeated. Cryosurgery in this manner is used only to treat extensive trichiasis.

When treating lesions that involve less than half of the lid margin, anesthesia is rarely necessary. Under the slitlamp, a felt-tipped pen is used to mark the skin in the areas corresponding to the lashes to be destroyed. The lid is pulled away from the eye by grasping the skin with thumb and forefinger. The probe is placed on the lash line adjacent to the skin mark. The liquid nitrogen is started a second before touching the skin so the probe immediately "sticks" to the area to be frozen. Freezing is continued until a 3-mm diameter iceball (from the edge of the probe tip to the end of the ice front) forms. The area is allowed to thaw until the probe can be removed, or the ice front continues from the cryogen still in the probe, and the probe is "cracked" off the skin. The lid should be kept away from the eye to allow for a "slow" thaw. The tip of the probe is washed with sterile solution to warm the probe tip so that the tip will easily adhere or freeze to the lid on the second application. The procedure is repeated, and the involved lashes are removed manually. This procedure is repeated in multiple areas as needed.

Laser thermoablation of ciliary follicles and excision of individual follicles may be alternatives in the treatment of localized trichiasis. Argon laser treatment is performed with a spot size beam of 50 to 200 μm, of 0.1 to 0.2 second duration, and 1,000 to 1,200 mW power under local anesthesia. Approximately 12 to 15 applications are necessary to destroy the follicles. This technique is suitable when a few fine cilia are involved. Excision of individual follicles is ideal for resecting the occasional aberrant eyelash that may appear at the edge of a wound after horizontal shortening of an eyelid or eyelid laceration; however, this technique is tedious and time consuming.

Ocular or Periocular Manifestations

Conjunctiva: Chemosis; hyperemia.
Cornea: Erosion; punctate keratopathy; ulcer.
Other: Foreign body sensation; lacrimation; photophobia.

PRECAUTIONS

When using any cryogen, measures must be taken to prevent damage to the cornea and adjacent skin from either runoff or direct contact with the probe. A nonmetallic lid plate and insulating tape may be helpful. Edema of the lid and cheek may persist for as long as 1 week after treatment. Occasionally, patients may experience moderately severe pain beginning 5 to 6 hours after using the combination of a long- and short-acting local anesthetic. In general, aspirin alone is all that is necessary to control this pain. There is a loss of sensory nerves in this area within 18 to 24 hours, which may last for 6 to 12 weeks. Cutaneous depigmentation is an invariable sequela to cryotherapy, and repigmentation may take as long as 2 years to occur. Cryotherapy has not been used extensively in black patients because of the marked susceptibility of pigment cells to freezing and the subsequent problem of depigmentation. By applying the cryoprobe to the lid margin and conjunctival surface instead of to the skin, it is possible to limit the degree of depigmentation in highly pigmented lids. Thus, the complication of cosmetic blemish and the risk of actinic damage and its sequelae are decreased. However, because of the possible complication of chronic or permanent vitiligo, seldom should a darkly pigmented eyelid be treated with cryotherapy.

Lids that have been badly scarred from previous disease, prior surgery, or radiation should be treated with caution, as segmental necrosis or an aggravation of an entropion may occur. In patients with sensory or motor deprivation of the lid, care should be taken when treating with cryosurgery, since there have been reported cases of lid necrosis.

If ocular pemphigoid is in an acute phase, it should not be treated because doing so may precipitate symblepharon. However, ocular pemphigoid may be treated if the disease is in a quiescent phase.

Caution should be used when treating young patients with cryotherapy because atrophic skin in the area treated is a potential complication. In some patients, thinning of the eyelid may occur. In addition, this thinning may, in rare instances, cause problems with the tear film, since the meibomian glands are destroyed. Yet, this complication is rarely found. The main problem with freezing large areas with cryosurgery is that at each end of the areas that are not treated, there appears to be some constricture of the lid, and an entropion-type process occurs, causing trichiasis to each side of the frozen area.

Overly nervous and younger patients may not cooperate well enough for precise application of the laser, and bedridden patients are also not good candidates for this procedure.

COMMENTS

If large segments of the lashes are to be treated, cryosurgery should be done with epinephrine in the local anesthetic, since it enhances the loss of lashes. The larger lashes appear to be more cryosensitive than the fine lanugo hairs. Individual lashes can be treated by isolated refreezing with a small probe.

Cryotherapy with the retina cryoprobe instrumentation using double-freeze thaws has not been very successful. Although nitrous oxide units are satisfactory, liquid nitrogen is preferred because only one cryo unit is needed and a much smaller area of the lid is frozen, although much more intensely.

References

Awan KJ: Argon laser treatment of trichiasis. Ophthalmic Surg 17:658–660, 1986.
Delaney MR, Rogers PA: A simplified cryotherapy technique for trichiasis and distichiasis. Aust J Ophthalmol 12:163–166, 1984.
Johnson RLC, Collin JRO: Treatment of trichiasis with a lid cryoprobe. Br J Ophthalmol 69:267–270, 1985.
Majekodunmi S: Cryosurgery in treatment of trichiasis. Br J Ophthalmol 66:337–339, 1982.
Peart DA, Hill JC: Cryosurgery for trichiasis in black patients. Br J Ophthalmol 70:712–714, 1986.
Wolfley D: Excision of individual follicles for the management of congenital distichiasis and localized trichiasis. J Pediatr Ophthalmol Strabismus 24:22–26, 1987.

XANTHELASMA
(Xanthelasma Palpebrarum, Xanthoma Palpebrarum)
F.T. FRAUNFELDER, M.D.
Portland, Oregon

Xanthelasma is a form of cutaneous xanthomatosis that is characterized by the presence of rounded or oval, dull yellow, slightly elevated plaques in the skin of the eyelids. The lesions are usually located near the inner canthi and generally commence on the upper eyelid. Xanthelasma may first appear in early middle age, often in females. A minority of patients with xanthelasma have frank hyperlipidemia, although a tendency toward enhanced atherogenicity may be seen. However, these lesions commonly occur in patients with essential hyperlipidemia and in patients, such as diabetics, with secondary hyperlipidemia. Histologically, these lesions are composed of foamy histiocytes. Histochemical analysis of the lipid vacuoles in early lesions may closely resemble that of serum lipids, but the contents of older lesions differ from the composition of the serum lipids. In chronic lesions, there is an increase in the number of fibroblasts and long-spaced collagen.

THERAPY

Supportive. A serum lipid profile should be investigated to rule out hyperlipidemic syndromes and other associated diseases, such as cirrhosis, diabetes mellitus, and arteriosclerosis. Dietary treatment of hyperlipidemia may induce a regression in xanthelasma, although this response may be quite delayed.

Surgical. Cosmetic surgery on eyelids with xanthelasma can be performed. After removal of the xanthelasma from the eyelid, the defect is usually closed in a horizontal direction without causing a lid deformity. When the xanthelasma is large, a musculocutaneous flap may be used to close the defect.

An alternative method of treatment of xanthelasma is application of 75 per cent trichloroacetic acid or dichloroacetic acid. A local anesthetic is first applied beneath the lesion. Each end of a double-tipped cotton applicator is dipped into either the acidic or saturated sodium bicarbonate solution. Using the tip dipped in the acidic solution, this solution is applied in an ever-increasing circular pattern, starting from the center until the edges of the lesion are reached. After 5 to 10 seconds, the treated area turns white and bubbles. Using the tip dipped in the neutralizing solution, the treated area is sponged off with sodium bicarbonate. For 4 to 6 weeks, the treated area will form scabs, which often peel off; however, excellent cosmetic results will be attained with this method. Small areas can be retreated again, if necessary.

Precautions

If a patient with hyperlipidemia has xanthelasma, treatment of hyperlipidemia may improve the systemic disease, but will not necessarily cause the xanthelasma to regress. However, it has been noted that patients treated with the cholesterol-lowering drug, lovastatin, have experienced a decrease in intensity and possible resolution of the xanthelasma.

Cosmetic revision of the lid lesions may need to be performed, especially with recurrences of xanthelasma. It is this type of problem that may result in a lid deformity, such as ectropion.

Comments

Xanthelasma should be a signal to the physician that carbohydrate and lipid metabolism states require further investigation. Although 60 per cent of patients with xanthelasma have normal serum lipid profiles, more subtle changes in lipid composition might be found. In fact, several other abnormalities of plasma lipoproteins have been reported, which may indicate a tendency toward enhanced atherogenicity. Therefore, normolipidemic patients with xanthelasma may indeed possess a less obvious, yet potentially clinically significant disturbance of lipid metabolism.

References

Crawford JB: Neoplastic and inflammatory tumors of the eyelids. *In* Duane TD (ed): Clinical Ophthalmology. Philadelphia, Harper & Row, 1987, Vol IV, pp 3:10–12.

Depot MJ, et al: Bilateral and extensive xanthelasma palpebrarum in a young man. Ophthalmology 91:522–527, 1984.

Hosokawa K, et al: Treatment of large xanthomas by the use of blepharoplasty island musculocutaneous flaps. Ann Plast Surg 18:238–240, 1987.

Rouffy J, et al: Xanthelasma palpebrarum and dyslipoproteinaemia: Two retrospective studies. Ann Dermatol Venereol 109:231–235, 1982.

Smith RE, Lee JS: The cornea in systemic disease. *In* Duane TD (ed): Clinical Ophthalmology. Philadelphia, Harper & Row, 1980, Vol IV, pp 15:15–17.

SECTION 24

GLOBE

ANOPHTHALMOS
DANIEL MARCHAC, M.D.
Paris, France

Anophthalmos with complete absence of ectodermal and mesodermal tissues of the eye is extremely rare. In fact, microphthalmos resulting from arrest of development of the eyeball at various stages of growth of the optic vesicle is usually observed; such malformation is sometimes sporadic or congenital (autosomal dominant or recessive). External influences during pregnancy, such as rubeola or toxoplasmosis, may also play a role in some cases.

The development of the orbital region is correlated with the outgrowth of the eyeball, as demonstrated by a reduction in the volume of the orbit up to 60 per cent of the normal size after removal of eyeballs in embryos.

In microphthalmos, the orbit does not usually develop properly, with resultant loss of projection of the adjunct frontal and malar areas, particularly a small bony cavity. This small bony cavity does not allow proper fitting of a prosthesis.

THERAPY

Ocular. Anophthalmos or microphthalmos is a pediatric ocular emergency. If started in the first months of life, the use of conformers can enlarge a small cavity and allows the orbit to attain almost normal proportions. A very careful follow-up with rapidly increasing sizes of conformers will generally produce a cavity adaptable to fitting a prosthesis and a good-sized orbit.

Surgical. If the microphthalmic cavity is too small to allow for enlargement with conformers or if this treatment was not undertaken, the orbit is normally too small for a prosthesis. The lateral orbital wall needs to be displaced medially, as it is located just where the lateral part of the cavity should be created. To create a cavity in front of the bone is a poor solution, which will not give enough depth for a suitable prosthesis to project the eyelids properly. The bony orbit generally has to be enlarged in three directions: laterally, superiorly, and inferiorly. This surgical orbital expansion can be obtained by an osteotomy, dividing the existing orbital rim in three parts in a step-like fashion that allows bony contact where expanded.

A limited intracranial approach is necessary when the orbital roof has to be elevated, which is not always the case. This operation is performed through a scalp bicoronal approach. The creation of a good-sized socket is done in a second stage. Final touch-up with skin and cartilage grafts are often necessary to lengthen the eyelids.

An inflatable expander can be tried if the use of conformers was not successful. Placement of the expander to expand both the orbit and the eyelid is difficult, and trials are currently made with prostheses of various shapes—some round, some with an anterior protuberance—to expand the eyelids.

Ocular or Periocular Manifestations

Conjunctiva: Shallow lower fornix; small socket.
Extraocular Muscles: Absent.
Eyelids: Absent levator function; absent lid fold; orbicularis contraction; shortening in all directions.
Globe: Decreased or absent amount of tissue.
Lacrimal System: Absent ducts and glands.
Orbit: Medial deviation; reduced orbital rim; small optic foramen.

PRECAUTIONS

Results are often disappointing because of an immobile prosthesis, as well as such eyelid malformations as short and immobile eyelids. An early treatment is advocated for enlargement of eyelid structures.

COMMENTS

The surgical creation of a good-sized cavity and subsequent enlargement of eyelids is long and complicated. If the patient is more than a few years old, however, this is the only choice. The psychologic benefit makes this surgical reconstruction worthwhile; it should deal first with the bony problems. Early treatment with conformers should certainly be applied whenever possible to try to avoid this surgical procedure.

References

Kennedy RE: The effect of early enucleation on the orbit in animals and humans. Am J Ophthalmol 60:277–306, 1965.
Marchac D, et al: Orbital expansion for anophthalmia and micro-orbitism. Plast Reconstr Surg 59:486–491, 1977.
Mustardé JC: The orbital rim. *In* Mustardé JC, Jancsous IT (eds): Plastic Surgery in Infancy and Child-

hood. Edinburgh, Churchill Livingston, 1988, pp 150–155.

Mustardé JC: The orbital region. In Mustardé JC (ed): Plastic Surgery in Infancy and Childhood. Edinburgh, Livingstone, 1971, pp 232–237.

BACTERIAL ENDOPHTHALMITIS

SID MANDELBAUM, M.D.,
and RICHARD K. FORSTER, M.D.
Miami, Florida

Bacterial endophthalmitis is inflammation of intraocular tissues resulting from bacterial infection. The most frequent cause of bacterial endophthalmitis is recent intraocular surgery during which the organisms apparently gain access to the interior of the eye. Bacterial endophthalmitis may also occur after penetrating ocular trauma; endogenously via blood-borne spread from a site of infection elsewhere in the body; or in eyes with filtering blebs, even years after surgery, presumably by penetration of the organisms through the bleb. Infectious endophthalmitis may result from any ocular penetration, no matter how innocuous it might seem; self-sealing traumatic or surgical corneal perforations, surgical posterior capsulotomies, and even cutting of deeply placed sutures after ocular surgery have all resulted in endophthalmitis. The vitreous is the intraocular site most involved by the well-developed infectious process; this is the case even if the injury or surgery is confined to the anterior segment or the patient is phakic. Therefore, the cornerstone of laboratory evaluation is to sample and culture the vitreous if infectious endophthalmitis is considered.

Infectious endophthalmitis should be suspected whenever inflammatory signs and symptoms after intraocular surgery or penetrating trauma are out of proportion to those anticipated in the particular clinical setting. Bacterial endophthalmitis usually presents between 1 and 4 days after surgery or trauma. Pain is a prominent symptom, although it is not invariably present. Signs include lid and conjunctival edema, hyperemia, exudate, corneal edema, and especially anterior chamber reaction (often with hypopyon) and vitreitis. Less virulent bacteria, such as *Staphylococcus epidermidis* or *Propionibacterium acnes*, may incite a lower-grade reaction, often lasting weeks. Endophthalmitis caused by fungi is also indolent, often with an apparent latent period of days to weeks after surgery or trauma before the inflammation becomes evident.

Patients with blebs either as a result of glaucoma filtration surgery or that are inadvertently created during cataract extraction are susceptible to bacterial endophthalmitis months or years after their surgical procedure. Potential sources of infection include normal conjunctival flora, episodes of bacterial conjunctivitis, use of contact lenses, and contaminated medicine dropper bottle tips. Many ophthalmologists are not sensitive to the possibility of bacterial endophthalmitis in these eyes; therefore, they are often treated with steroids for presumed idiopathic uveitis until an infectious etiology is considered.

The most common organisms isolated from eyes with endophthalmitis in the postoperative period include *Staphylococcus epidermidis*, *S. aureus*, *Proteus*, and *Pseudomonas*. Organisms previously felt to be nonpathogens are increasingly being isolated, which suggests that under appropriate circumstances almost any organism is capable of causing endophthalmitis. *Bacillus cereus* has recently been associated with fulminant endophthalmitis after ocular trauma. In the group of patients with filtering blebs, streptococci appear to be responsible for the majority of cases; the most common gram-negative organism isolated has been *Hemophilus influenzae*, a very unusual cause of endophthalmitis in other circumstances.

The differential diagnosis of bacterial endophthalmitis includes the many entities causing intraocular inflammation. Postoperatively, retained lens material, incarceration of iris or vitreous in the wound, intraocular lens or other foreign body induced inflammation, and exaggerated postoperative iridocyclitis are all causes of sterile inflammation. Blood in the vitreous may simulate inflammation. An unrecognized retained foreign body is a potential cause of posttraumatic inflammation. If there is suspicion that the eye is infected, however, it is safest to culture aqueous and vitreous and begin therapy as outlined later.

THERAPY

Ocular. Patients with suspected infectious endophthalmitis require sampling and culture of at least vitreous (preferably also aqueous) and institution of broad-spectrum antibiotic therapy. There is some disagreement over the optimum route of antibiotic delivery; however, since antibiotics appropriately administered directly into the vitreous cavity appear safe both experimentally and clinically and achieve the highest intravitreal antibiotic levels, this is the preferred route. Systemic, periocular, and topical antibiotics are begun at the same time.

Patients with presumed infectious endophthalmitis should be sedated and given retrobulbar anesthesia; a beveled incision partially through peripheral clear cornea may then be made with a razor-blade knife under microscopic control. A 25-gauge needle attached to a tuberculin syringe is then utilized to enter the anterior chamber carefully through this incision, and 0.1 to 0.2 ml of aqueous is aspirated. The aqueous is immediately inoculated on fresh culture media. If the patient is aphakic, a 22-gauge needle attached to another tuberculin syringe is passed through the same keratotomy site, through the pupil, and into the midvitreous, observing the needle tip under the microscope. About 0.3 ml of vitreous is then aspirated; careful manipulation of the needle may be necessary to locate liquid vitreous. The previously prepared antibiotics, each in a separate tuberculin syringe with a 25-gauge needle, are then slowly injected into the midvitreous, inserting each needle through the keratotomy site. For initial therapy, 100 μg of gentamicin* in 0.1 ml and 1.0 mg of vancomycin* in 0.1 ml are injected. The keratotomy site is closed with one suture. The vitreous sample should immediately be inoculated on culture media.

If the patient is phakic, vitreous is aspirated through the pars plana, a sclerotomy site is prepared 4 mm posterior to the limbus, and the vitreous cavity is entered with a 22-gauge needle as above. In cases where an adequate vitreous sample cannot be obtained by simple aspiration, the entrance site should be appropriately enlarged, a vitreous cutting instrument inserted, and a localized vitrectomy performed. Intravitreal antibiotics* are injected as above. The vitrectomy sample, which must be collected in a sterile fashion, is passed through a filter system to concentrate it, and the disposable filter paper is inoculated directly onto culture media.

Broad-spectrum antibiotic therapy should begin as soon as cultures are obtained. In addition to intravitreal antibiotics, systemic, periocular, and topical antibiotics should be given. Subconjunctival injections of 40 mg of gentamicin*, 125 mg of cefazolin*, or 25 mg of vancomycin* may be repeated daily. In addition to periocular injection of antibiotics, high doses of systemic antibiotics are utilized. A combination of 1 mg/kg of gentamicin intravenously or intramuscularly every 8 hours and 1 gm of cefazolin intravenously every 6 hours should be continued for 10 to 14 days. Fortified eyedrops of gentamicin§ (9.1 mg/ml), cefazolin§ (50 mg/ml), or vancomycin§ (50 mg/ml) may be administered every hour. Topical cycloplegic agents should also be given. Adjustments in antibiotic therapy are made based on antibiotic sensitivities of the isolated organism and clinical response. If the isolated organism is virulent, an intravitreal injection may be repeated 48 hours after the initial administration. Once a susceptible organism has been exposed to appropriate antibiotics for about 24 hours, corticosteroids should be administered topically, subconjunctivally, and systemically. Oral prednisone‡ may be given in a daily dose of 40 to 80 mg, with rapid tapering after 7 to 14 days. Alternatively, steroids may be begun at the time of the diagnostic tap, if delayed infection due to fungus is not a consideration.

Surgical. The role of vitrectomy in the management of bacterial endophthalmitis remains controversial. Vitrectomy is a technically difficult procedure in infected eyes because of limited visualization of intraocular structures, uveal engorgement, and retinal edema. Nonetheless, vitrectomy may offer advantages in terms of removal of infectious organisms and inflammatory debris and elimination of loculated pockets, thus improving fluid and antibiotic circulation in the vitreous cavity. It has been shown in an experimental model of endophthalmitis that the vitreous was sterilized more frequently in eyes with combined vitrectomy and antibiotic administration than in those given antibiotics alone. The risks of vitrectomy under these circumstances must be balanced against the potential benefits for each individual case. Initial vitrectomy is recommended in advanced infections at presentation. For less advanced inflammation, initial treatment with intravitreal, systemic, periocular, and topical antibiotics is preferred. If improvement is not apparent within 36 to 48 hours or if a virulent organism, such as *Pseudomonas*, is isolated, vitrectomy is then performed, taking care to avoid the friable retinal surface. Antibiotics may be carefully injected at the completion of the vitrectomy or, alternatively, may be added to the infusion fluid as recommended by Peyman.

Precautions

Endophthalmitis is certainly a condition better prevented than treated. Careful preoperative attention to blepharitis, the lacrimal system, and infections elsewhere in the body is mandatory. Preoperative conjunctival cultures are not routinely performed, except in patients with blepharitis, extended-wear contact lenses, or wearing an ocular prosthesis on the other side; in these latter two groups, there appears to be a higher incidence of asymptomatic colonization with gram-negative bacteria than in the general population. The use of preoperative topical antibiotics seems to decrease the incidence of endophthalmitis, probably by suppressing the conjunctival flora. Periocular antibiotics may also be useful. However, antibiotics must be considered only as an adjunct to meticulous attention to sterility within the operating suite. In patients with filtering blebs, the use of contact lenses presents an additional hazard to be avoided, if at all possible. In cases of intraocular trauma, systemic and periocular antibiotics are recommended, although no firm data are available indicating their effectiveness in preventing endophthalmitis.

Clinically, the two major determinants of visual prognosis in bacterial endophthalmitis are the virulence of the infecting organism and the rapidity of institution of appropriate therapy. Most ophthalmologists are reluctant to make this diagnosis in their postoperative patients; precious time is often lost when a "wait-and-see" attitude is adopted. A hypopyon is not an invariable finding early in the course of endophthalmitis; too frequently, patients are followed with unexplained intraocular inflammation until they develop a hypopyon, at which time the diagnosis of endophthalmitis is first entertained. If infection is a possibility, the vitreous must be cultured. Aqueous cultures alone have repeatedly been shown to be inadequate; on the other hand, there are only very rare cases of positive aqueous cultures when the vitreous culture is negative. Empiric antibiotic therapy without vitreous cultures or in less than full doses is inappropriate. The response is likely to be incomplete, and further diagnostic studies and therapy are compromised. If the local environment does not provide sufficient experience or facilities to manage a case of endophthalmitis, it is in the best interest of both the patient and physician to make a prompt referral to a center where such facilities are available.

Care needs to be taken in administration of intravitreal antibiotics; dilutions must be carefully done so that the final concentration is correct. Intravitreal antibiotics must be injected slowly to avoid retinal damage from the impact of the antibiotic solution. Doses of systemic cephalosporins and aminoglycosides must be reduced if renal function is compromised. Even if renal function is normal, the serum creatinine should be checked every 2 days when systemic aminoglycosides are administered.

Comments

Although advances in the treatment of endophthalmitis in the form of more effective antibiotics, anti-inflammatory agents, and drug delivery systems may be anticipated, the greatest positive effect on the outcome of any individual case will almost certainly be that of earlier diagnosis and institution of therapy. In some respects, infectious endophthalmitis is similar to infectious meningitis; serious consideration of either diagnosis obligates the initiation of diagnostic and therapeutic measures. Although these measures are invasive, the risk/benefit ratio is such that their early application in cases of suspected endophthalmitis is a more prudent approach than observation until the diagnosis is certain.

References

Cottingham AJ Jr, Forster RK: Vitrectomy in endophthalmitis. Results of study using vitrectomy, intraocular antibiotics, or a combination of both. Arch Ophthalmol 94:2078–2081, 1976.

Diamond JG: Intraocular management of endophthalmitis. A systematic approach. Arch Ophthalmol 99:96–99, 1981.

Forster RK: Endophthalmitis. *In* Duane TD (ed) Clinical Ophthalmology. Philadelphia, Harper & Row, 1987, Vol IV, pp 24:1–21.

Forster RK, Abbott RL, Gelender H: Management of infectious endophthalmitis. Ophthalmology 87:313–319, 1980.

Jeglum EL, Rosenberg SB, Benson WE: Preparation of intravitreal drug doses. Ophthalmic Surg 12:355–359, 1981.

O'Day DM, et al: *Staphylococcus epidermidis* endophthalmitis. Visual outcome following noninvasive therapy. Ophthalmology 89:354–360, 1982.

Peyman GA, Vastine DW, Raichand M: Symposium: Postoperative endophthalmitis. Experimental aspects and their clinical application. Ophthalmology 85:374–385, 1978.

FUNGAL ENDOPHTHALMITIS
WALTER H. STERN, M.D.
San Francisco, California

Exogenous fungal endophthalmitis most often develops in healthy individuals undergoing intraocular surgery or who suffer penetrating trauma. It may also develop by spread from an infected cornea or sclera. The risk factors in *endogenous* fungal endophthalmitis include intravenous drug abuse, a compromised immune system because of disease or immunosuppressive therapy, or an infected indwelling catheter or shunt that allows hematologic seeding of the eye with fungus. Therapy should be tailored to accommodate these different infectious etiologies.

In contrast to bacterial endophthalmitis, fungal endophthalmitis is usually slowly progressive, rather than fulminant. Early symptoms may include redness of the eye with variable amounts of pain and visual loss. Physical findings may include cell and flare, hypopyon, a fibrin membrane in the anterior chamber, vitreous snowballs, and vitreous cells. If the infection is endogenous, a white fluffy retinal infiltrate may often be observed, with or without retinal hemorrhage, with variable extension into the vitreous depending on the stage of the infection.

Drug therapy of endophthalmitis depends on accurate identification of the organism. A vitreous tap or preferably a vitreous biopsy that may be positive when a vitreous tap is negative is required for identification of the organism. Filtration of the vitreous aspirate through a millipore filter accompanied by staining, or centrifugation of the aspirate followed by plating on a slide treated with gram, Giemsa, and methenamine silver stains may provide the earliest guide to treatment.

If no organism is identified on the filter or slide, it may be necessary to treat the eye empirically with antibiotics until a bacterial endophthalmitis is ruled out by culture results. If clinical suspicion of fungal endophthalmitis is high, it may be prudent to treat empirically with an intravitreal injection of 5 μg of amphotericin B* and withhold further antifungal therapy until culture results or clinical symptoms provide further guidance.

Vitreous specimens should be inoculated onto blood agar, chocolate agar, liquid brain-heart infusion, and thioglycollate broth maintained at 37°C and onto Sabouraud agar, blood agar, and brain-heart infusion with gentamicin maintained at 25°C to isolate fungi.

Anterior chamber aspirates yield a reduced incidence of positive cultures when compared to vitreous aspirates. A vitreous sample is therefore essential, whereas an anterior chamber aspirate is optional.

THERAPY

Systemic. Medical therapy should include removal of infected indwelling catheters, if present, and treatment of any predisposing systemic conditions. Drugs that have proved useful for treatment of fungal endophthalmitis include amphotericin B, flucytosine, miconazole, and ketoconazole.

Amphotericin B is effective against a wide variety of fungi and acts by binding to cell membrane sterols, thus increasing cell membrane permeability with leakage of cell contents and cell death. Although measured intraocular drug levels following intravenous administration are not very high, this fact must be interpreted cautiously because the antibiotic binds to cell membranes, in effect lowering the measured intraocular concentration.

When amphotericin B is administered intravenously, a test dose of 1 mg is first given, followed by a gradual increase in the dose up to 0.5 mg/kg per day. Complete blood counts, electrolytes, and renal function are monitored three times weekly and the dose of amphotericin B adjusted accordingly. If the decision is made to treat with intravenous amphotericin B, an attempt is made to administer a total intravenous dose in the range of 1 gm of amphotericin. This dosage, of course, may be altered by clinical events.

Flucytosine is administered orally and is converted within the fungus to fluorouracil, which inhibits DNA and RNA synthesis. Drug resistance has been noted in up to half the fungal isolates tested against this drug. Flucytosine is synergistic with amphotericin B, and a therapeutic dose can be achieved in both the aqueous and vitreous after oral administration. The daily dosage of oral flucytosine is 100 mg/kg given in four divided doses. Blood flucytosine levels should be measured and the dose of flucytosine adjusted if toxic levels (greater than 100 μg/ml) are obtained.

Ketoconazole is another drug that may be administered orally. It binds to the sterols in fungal cell membranes and is effective against a wide spectrum of fungi. Oral administration results in therapeutic drug levels in both the aqueous and vitreous. The dosage of ketoconazole is 400 to 800 mg in a single oral dose daily.

Ocular. Intraocular injection with antifungal drugs may be performed using amphotericin B and miconazole. Amphotericin B* may be safely administered intravitreally using a dose of 5 μg. This dose does not cause intraocular inflammation, which has been noted in patients receiving 10 μg of amphotericin B.

A repeat injection of amphotericin B may be administered as early as 24 hours in an eye that is aphakic and has undergone vitrectomy. If the eye is phakic or aphakic but has not undergone vitrectomy, the half-life of intraocular amphotericin B is between 5 and 9 days, and caution should be taken in administering a repeat injection until well after the half-life period has ended.

Intravitreal miconazole* (40 μg), an imidazole, has been recommended for endophthalmitis caused by *Paecilomyces lilacinous* or for amphotericin B treatment failure. Because oral ketoconazole has good ocular penetration as well as few side effects, miconazole is not frequently used.

Corticosteroids may be used to reduce intraocular inflammation after the eye has received a short period of antifungal therapy. The length of pretreatment with antifungal drugs is variable and depends on the extent of inflammation and the clinical response to treatment.

Topical and periocular antifungal therapy is indicated where the endophthalmitis is associated with a fungal keratitis. Topical ophthalmic 0.15 per cent amphotericin B*, 1 per cent miconazole,* or 5 per cent natamycin should be administered every hour, as well as subconjunctival amphotericin B* (0.5 to 1.0 mg) or miconazole* (5 to 10 mg). For the treatment of corneal, scleral, or anterior chamber involvement, oral ketoconazole (400 to 800 mg) should be administered daily, as well as intraocular amphotericin B* (5 μg), which may be repeated as described earlier.

Surgical. Vitrectomy alone in certain cases may be capable of sterilizing the vitreous cavity, removing the bulk of the infecting organisms, allowing circulation of large drug molecules, and enhancing aqueous wash-out of the vitreous cavity. Removal of the vitreous scaffold may reduce the incidence of traction retinal detachment that may be a sequela to fungal endophthalmitis. Since fungi may infiltrate intraocular tissues, vitreous surgery offers the opportunity to excise tissues, such as the iris and posterior lens capsule, in which fungus may be embedded and result in recurrent infection.

The decision to perform a vitrectomy is usually not a difficult one in eyes with fungal endophthalmitis because this procedure has many apparent advantages. The decision to remove the intraocular lens may be more difficult. In many cases, it has not been necessary to remove the intraocular lens to sterilize the eye. However, if recurrent infection or inflammation is noted, it may be prudent to remove the lens implant and the entire remaining capsular bag.

PRECAUTIONS

Systemic amphotericin B is a toxic drug, and almost all patients experience anemia and azotemia, with variable amounts of nausea, fever, chills, and diarrhea.

A small percentage of patients (1 in 10,000) may develop a transient rise in liver enzymes after treatment with ketoconazole. Nonetheless, there have been no reports of this complication in cases of fungal endophthalmitis treated with ketoconazole.

COMMENTS

There is increasing evidence that fungal endophthalmitis can be adequately treated with a combination of sequential intraocular injections of amphotericin B or miconazole (depending on the sensitivity of the organism), oral ketoconazole rather than intravenous amphotericin B, and vitrectomy surgery. This treatment course may reduce the morbidity arising from the use of intravenous amphotericin B. The timing of sequential intraocular injections of amphotericin B must take into account the presence or absence of the crystalline lens or intact lens capsule, as well as the presence or absence of an intact vitreous body.

References

Doft BH, et al: Amphotericin clearance in vitrectomized versus nonvitrectomized eyes. Ophthalmology 92:1601, 1985.
Goodman DF, Stern WH: Oral ketoconazole and intraocular amphotericin B for treatment of postoperative *Candida parapsilosis* endophthalmitis. Arch Ophthalmol 105:172, 1987.
Jones DB: Therapy of postsurgical fungal endophthalmitis. Ophthalmology 85:357, 1978.
Pflugfelder SC, et al: Exogenous fungal endophthalmitis. Ophthalmology 95:19, 1988.
Stern WH, et al: Epidemic postsurgical *Candida parapsilosis* endophthalmitis. Clinical findings and management of 15 consecutive cases. Ophthalmology 92:1701, 1985.

NANOPHTHALMOS

ROBERT J. BROCKHURST, M.D.
Boston, Massachusetts

Nanophthalmos is a rare bilateral type of microphthalmos that usually shows an autosomal recessive hereditary pattern. In contrast to the more common form of microphthalmos, which is usually unilateral and associated with poor vision and other ocular defects, the nanophthalmic eye is essentially a small eye with microcornea and a crystalline lens of normal (or slightly larger) size. Vision in younger patients who have not yet developed complications is usually normal with a strong (+10 to +20 diopters) hyperopic correction. Patients can easily be recognized by the fact that they wear "cataract glasses," but are phakic.

Since these eyes have a short axial length and diameter (14 to 20 mm), they appear deeply set in the orbits, the palpebral fissures are narrow, and it is difficult to examine and operate on the nanophthalmic eye. Because the eyeball has an overall small volume and yet the lens is of normal size, there is a lens/eye volume ratio (LEV ratio) of 10 to 30 per cent, whereas in the normal eye, LEV ratios are generally about 4 per cent. As a consequence of the large LEV ratio, the anterior chamber is compromised, and peripheral anterior synechiae gradually develop, leading to the development of "creeping" angle-closure glaucoma.

In all nanophthalmic eyes, the sclera is abnormally thick, shows larger collagen bundles, and contains an abnormally high quantity of proteoglycans. With age, the thickened sclera becomes more sclerotic and apparently offers increased resistance to venous outflow via the vortex veins as well as the transcleral passage of intraocular fluids. These changes result in congestion of the choroidal vasculature with thickening of the choroid. Clinically, this can be recognized by absence of the choroidal pattern of vessels. Gradually, the congestion becomes so severe that choroidal effusion develops—often anteriorly in a circumferential form. This phenomenon causes further embarrassment of anterior chamber angle by rotating the iris root forward. Measurement of episcleral venous pressure shows normal values.

Thus, it appears that the glaucoma that complicates nanophthalmos may be the result of a basic abnormality of the LEV ratio plus an unsuspected peripheral choroidal detachment secondary to resistance to vortex venous drainage. Ultrasound studies have confirmed the presence of a peripheral annular choroidal detachment before the development of increased intraocular pressure.

Uveal effusion with choroidal and nonrhegmatogenous retinal detachment can occur spontaneously in advanced cases because of the increasing resistance of venous drainage via the vortex veins. Moreover, in patients with glaucoma who have only limited anterior choroidal detachments, surgical procedures that result in a sudden lowering of the intraocular pressure to zero, at the time of surgery, may produce a rapid severe effusion with total retinal detachment 1 to 4 days after the operation.

THERAPY

Systemic. Medical treatment should be employed in early cases of chronic angle-closure glaucoma. Timolol in 0.25 or 0.5 per cent concentrations may be used twice a day. Carbonic anhydrase inhibitors, such as acetazolamide, may be used in doses of 250 mg four times a day.

Medical treatment of uveal effusion with nonrhegmatogenous retinal detachment has been disappointing, but occasional patients appear to respond to systemic steroid treatment. A daily dosage of 100 mg of prednisone for 1 week, followed by 100 mg every other day for 4 to 8 weeks, rarely results in improvement of the detachment.

Surgical. Argon laser is of value in chronic angle-closure glaucoma that cannot be controlled medically. Iridotomy can be performed to relieve the pupillary block. Moreover, surface treatment of the iris results in flattening of the convex iris (gonioplasty), thereby opening the angle so that medical therapy is once again effective.

Customary retinal detachment procedures for nonrhegmatogenous retinal detachment occurring in nanophthalmic eyes are ineffective. Retinal detachment repair by scleral resection and decompression of the vortex veins, combined with subretinal fluid drainage and intravitreal air injection, appears to be effective in 80 per cent of patients. However, subretinal fluid drainage with or without scleral buckling is not effective in patients with nonrhegmatogenous retinal detachment.

Ocular or Periocular Manifestations

Anterior Chamber: Narrow angle; peripheral anterior synechiae; shallow.
Choroid: Choroidal pattern not visible; peripheral detachment; thickening.
Cornea: Decreased diameter.
Eyelids: Narrowed palpebral fissures.
Iris: Forward displacement; poor pupillary dilation.
Lens: Normal or slightly larger size.
Optic Nerve: Pallor and cupping.
Orbit: Deep-set eyes.
Retina: Nonrhegmatogenous detachment.
Sclera: High concentration of proteoglycans; larger, more interwoven collagen bundles; thickening (2 to 3 mm).
Other: High hyperopia; small eye.

PRECAUTIONS

Miotics may aggravate chronic angle-closure glaucoma by increasing the degree of pupillary block. In addition, conventional glaucoma surgery should be avoided because of the danger of postoperative malignant glaucoma and total retinal detachment. The sudden decompression of the globe aggravates the uveal effusion and may lead to severe retinal detachment. Lens extraction may also result in retinal detachment; however, there is evidence that this may be prevented by prophylactic vortex vein decompression and sclerotomies. Unfortunately, choroidal detachment may be mistaken for malignant melanoma, and unnecessary enucleation may be performed. Moreover, peripheral iridectomy and filtering procedures may be followed by malignant glaucoma.

COMMENTS

A genetic predisposition causes a failure of the eye to grow to proper dimensions, resulting in narrowing of the anterior chamber angle. With age, choroidal elevation in the periphery results in forward displacement of the iris, relaxation of the zonular membrane, and further embarrassment of the angle. It is possible that vortex vein decompression would decrease the peripheral choroidal elevation and prove helpful in the control of the chronic angle-closure glaucoma.

References

Brockhurst RJ: Nanophthalmos with uveal effusion: A new clinical entity. Trans Am Ophthalmol Soc 72:371–403, 1974.
Brockhurst RJ: Vortex vein decompression for nanophthalmic uveal effusion. Arch Ophthalmol 98:1987–1990, 1980.
Calhoun FP Jr: The management of glaucoma in nanophthalmos. Trans Am Ophthalmol Soc 73:97–122, 1975.
Gass JDM: Uveal effusion syndrome: A new hypothesis concerning pathogenesis and technique of surgical treatment. Retina 3:159–163, 1983.
Kimbrough RL, et al: Angle-closure glaucoma in nanophthalmos. Am J Ophthalmol 88:572–579, 1979.
Trelstad RL, Silbermann NN, Brockhurst RJ: Nanophthalmic sclera: Ultrastructural, histo-chemical and biochemical observations. Arch Ophthalmol 100:1935–1938, 1982.

SECTION 25

INTRAOCULAR PRESSURE

APHAKIC AND PSEUDOPHAKIC PUPILLARY BLOCK

CLAUDIA U. RICHTER, M.D.,
and B. THOMAS HUTCHINSON, M.D.
Boston, Massachusetts

Pupillary block is the obstruction to aqueous humor outflow from the posterior chamber to the anterior chamber of the eye. It causes shallowing of the anterior chamber and, if untreated, the development of peripheral anterior synechiae and chronic angle-closure glaucoma. Treatment must be prompt and vigorous to prevent chronic angle-closure glaucoma. Although pupillary block may develop in the phakic and unoperated eye with iritis and posterior synechiae, it occurs more often after cataract surgery, with or without intraocular lens implantation.

Aphakic and pseudophakic pupillary block develop when the pupillary aperture and iridectomies are occluded by vitreous, inflammatory membranes, capsular or cortical remnants, or an intraocular lens. Inflammation causing iridovitreal, iridocapsular, or iridopseudophakic adhesions is the primary cause of aphakic and pseudophakic pupillary block. After intracapsular cataract extraction, vitreous alone may obstruct patent peripheral iridectomies and cause pupillary block if there is also obstruction to aqueous flow through the pupil, i.e., by vitreous or an intraocular lens.

Aphakic pupillary block classically presents with a shallow or flat anterior chamber, elevated intraocular pressure, and vitreous occluding the pupillary aperture and iridectomies in the first few days to weeks after surgery. Pseudophakic pupillary block with an anterior chamber intraocular lens has a deep central anterior chamber with the pupillary iris held posterior to the lens, but a shallow peripheral anterior chamber with an iris bombé configuration. Pseudophakic pupillary block with a posterior chamber intraocular lens may have a deep central anterior chamber and peripheral iris bombé or a more uniform shallowing of the anterior chamber with anterior displacement of the intraocular lens. The gonioscopic picture may be quite variable; the filtration angle is usually completely closed, but incomplete or early pupillary block may only cause a narrowing or partial closure of the angle. The intraocular pressure may be low or normal in early pupillary block with a wound leak or that caused by decreased aqueous production inflammation or a choroidal detachment.

Aphakic pupillary block may complicate both intracapsular and extracapsular extractions. Anterior chamber, iris plane, and posterior chamber intraocular lenses have been complicated by pupillary block. The pupil may be occluded, whether it is widely dilated or miotic. Pupillary block may occur with both peripheral and sector iridectomies.

The differential diagnosis of aphakic pupillary block includes wound leak, choroidal detachment (serous or hemorrhagic), and posterior aqueous entrapment (aphakic malignant glaucoma). A wound leak typically presents with a low intraocular pressure and a positive 2 per cent fluorescein test. A choroidal detachment may mimic pupillary block with shallowing or flattening of the anterior chamber, with or without angle closure, and with a low to normal pressure caused by decreased aqueous production. Ultrasonography may help detect peripheral choroidal effusions.

Posterior aqueous entrapment (malignant glaucoma) is similar to pupillary block in its development of a shallow or flat anterior chamber. Posterior aqueous entrapment develops when aqueous humor flow is directed into or behind the vitreous because of increased resistance through the anterior vitreous. The resistance may occur at the level of the ciliary body and has been called "ciliovitreal block." The misdirection of aqueous humor pushes the iris forward, flattens the anterior chamber, and occludes the angle. Thus, both pupillary block and posterior aqueous entrapment have shallow or flat anterior chambers and variable intraocular pressures early in their course, but both ultimately have elevated pressures. The final distinction between these two disorders can only be made by the eye's response to medical and laser treatment or surgery.

The incidence of aphakic and pseudophakic pupillary block may be minimized by careful suture placement to prevent wound leak and topical steroids to decrease inflammation and minimize synechiae. Basal peripheral iridectomies in all cataract extractions are important in preventing pupillary block. Even extracapsular cataract extraction with an intact posterior capsule and posterior chamber intraocular lens may be complicated by pupillary block, and a peripheral iridectomy in extracapsular cataract surgery is recommended. A patent peripheral iridectomy should be present or created when a posterior capsulotomy is performed, as opening the posterior capsule may allow vitreous to move anteriorly and create pupillary block.

THERAPY

Ocular. The goals of medical therapy are to break the pupillary block, deepen the anterior chamber, and prevent chronic angle-closure glaucoma. The first step has traditionally been to move the iris pharmacologically in order to break any adhesions. Cycloplegics (atropine, scopolamine, or cyclopentolate) with the addition of 2.5 per cent phenylephrine as an active mydriatic are often successful. Alternating miotics and mydriatics may be helpful: 4 per cent pilocarpine every 10 minutes for six doses followed by 2.5 per cent phenylephrine and 1 per cent cyclopentolate every half-hour for three doses.

If the intraocular pressure is elevated, topical beta-adrenergic antagonists (timolol, betaxolol, or levobunolol) and systemic carbonic anhydrase inhibitors (250 mg acetazolamide every 6 hours or 50 mg methazolamide every 8 hours) should be used. Osmotic agents are helpful if the intraocular pressure is quite high. A dosage of 120 ml of 45 per cent isosorbide may be given if the patient can tolerate oral therapy, or 1.5 gm/kg of 20 per cent mannitol may be given intravenously. Lowering the intraocular pressure makes the iris more responsive to topical medications, decreases iris congestion, and reduces the "forcefulness" of closure between the iris and the trabeculum. Corneal edema will begin to resolve as the intraocular pressure is reduced. In addition, the antiglaucomatous medications serve to protect both the recently operated wound and the optic nerve from significant compromise. Topical steroids should be used liberally to decrease the inflammatory response and inhibit synechiae formation.

Surgical. A laser iridectomy is usually successful in relieving pupillary block if medial therapy fails. Even if medical therapy relieves the pupillary block, a laser iridectomy can be performed to decrease the possibility of recurrence. Either the argon or the Neodymium YAG laser may be used. However, since the cornea may be edematous and the iris congested, the Neodymium YAG laser frequently allows more rapid iris penetration and, if available, is the laser of choice. If the cornea is edematous, topical glycerin frequently provides adequate clearing to allow a Neodymium YAG iridectomy. Two or three laser iridectomies are recommended, because even Neodymium YAG iridectomies may be occluded by iris folds as a billowing iris returns to its normal position.

If several iridectomies fail to relieve the apparent pupillary block and a wound leak and choroidal detachment have been eliminated as possible causes of the shallow anterior chamber, the diagnosis is posterior aqueous entrapment. The Neodymium YAG laser can be used to disrupt the anterior hyaloid face and relieve the posterior aqueous entrapment. It can be focused through a large peripheral iridectomy at the presumed peripheral hyaloid using low-energy (1 to 2 millijoules). If the peripheral iridectomy is too small to allow this photodisruption or the peripheral photodisruption is unsuccessful, a similar procedure to disrupt the hyaloid more centrally can be attempted.

If ocular and laser therapy fail to relieve the pupillary block or posterior aqueous diversion, surgery is necessary. If the laser is unable to establish a patent peripheral iridectomy because of total flattening of the anterior chamber or severe corneal clouding that is unresponsive to medically lowered intraocular pressure and topical glycerin, a surgical peripheral iridectomy with chamber deepening is indicated. However, if one or more patent laser iridectomies in addition to photodisruption of the hyaloid face fail to relieve the block and deepen the anterior chamber, a surgical vitrectomy or vitreous tap is necessary to relieve the posterior aqueous entrapment.

Retrobulbar anesthesia* should be used cautiously, as these eyes frequently have a recent surgical wound and a congested orbit. The orbital congestion both decreases the effectiveness of retrobulbar anesthesia and increases the risk of retrobulbar hemorrhage, a potentially devastating complication in an eye with a weak corneoscleral wound. General anesthesia is preferred if a vitrectomy is necessary.

If the patent Neodymium YAG and argon lasers have failed to establish a patent peripheral iridectomy, the surgical iridectomy is preceded by deepening the anterior chamber. A paracentesis is always performed first, employing a Wheeler knife or similar knife needle to produce a shelving tract through the peripheral cornea into the anterior chamber. The anterior chamber is reformed by injecting balanced salt solution. Posterior sclerotomies, in one or two lower quadrants, are placed to drain any suprachoroidal fluid. The anterior chamber is again reformed if significant suprachoroidal fluid is found, and removal of fluid from the sclerotomies and injection into the anterior chamber are repeated as necessary to evacuate the suprachoroidal space. If no suprachoroidal fluid is present and the intraocular pressure is elevated, vitreous aspiration may be necessary before the anterior chamber can be deepened.

If the anterior chamber remains deep after its reformation as above and communication exists between the anterior and posterior chambers with the iris in the normal aphakic position, one need not proceed further.

If pupillary block is present, the iris will not be maintained in the normal aphakic contour when the chamber is deepened with balanced salt solution, but will funnel toward the optic nerve. The pupillary block that prevents aqueous from entering the anterior chamber prevents balanced salt solution from entering the posterior chamber as well. If pupillary block persists, indicated by the funneling of the iris, a surgical peripheral iridectomy is performed at the surgical limbus away from the previous cataract wound.

If the anterior chamber is not maintained and there is no flow of aqueous from the posterior chamber after a peripheral iridectomy or if patent laser iridectomies fail to deepen the anterior chamber, posterior aqueous entrapment may be present. A pars plana vitrectomy is performed to excise the central anterior vitreous gel and any vitreous behind the iridectomies to create a pathway for normal anterior flow of aqueous. Residual cortical lens material after extracapsular cataract surgery may cause an inflammatory reaction in the lens equatorial region and contribute to the obstruction to aqueous flow. In these eyes, a small area of zonules and capsule should be removed to ensure an anterior pathway for aqueous humor. In eyes with posterior chamber intraocular lenses, one should remove as few zonules as possible to prevent lens dislocation. If a vitrectomy instrument is not available and the eye is aphakic, discission of the anterior hyaloid through an air bubble into the vitreous gel may re-establish aqueous flow. If a vitrectomy instrument is not available and the eye is pseudophakic, vitreous may be aspirated with a 19-gauge needle.

After the relief of choroidal detachment, pupillary block, or posterior aqueous entrapment, one should check the original cataract incision for wound leak that might have developed with the operative manipulation of the eye. Sterile 2 per cent fluorescein and slight pressure on the globe are recommended.

Postoperatively, cycloplegics, topical steroids, and topical broad-spectrum antibiotics are used.

Ocular or Periocular Manifestations

Conjunctiva: Variable inflammation.
Cornea: Epithelial and stromal edema; striae (if extensive iridocorneal, vitreocorneal, or pseudophakic-corneal contact or elevated intraocular pressure).
Anterior Chamber: Shallow or flat.
Iris: Bombé configuration; occluded iridectomies; peripheral anterior synechiae; posterior synechiae.
Vitreous: Anterior hyaloid or capsular-cortical remnants adherent to the borders of the pupil and all iridectomies.
Other: Choroidal detachment; elevated intraocular pressure; posterior aqueous pockets.

Precautions

It is imperative that the surgeon not become overly aggressive in the use of medical therapy, which may have significant and even catastrophic side effects. Only cautious use of 2.5 per cent phenylephrine is appropriate as this medication may cause a systemic hypertensive crisis. In addition, contraindications to topical ophthalmic beta-adrenergic antagonists, systemic osmotics, or carbonic anhydrase inhibitors must be observed carefully.

Delay in the therapy of pupillary block should be avoided, as spontaneous resolution and reformation of the anterior chamber with an open angle are rare. Furthermore, it is important to remember that a serous choroidal detachment and pupillary block may exist concurrently; the surgeon should not be lulled into complacency by a low or normal intraocular pressure that remains low only as long as the choroidal detachment persists. Although the chamber may deepen slightly after the relief of choroidal detachment, an elevated pressure will invariably result when aqueous secretion returns to normal if the pupillary block has not been treated.

The relief of pupillary block by ocular therapy or laser or surgical iridectomy does not guarantee that the angle will reopen, but only that the chamber will deepen. Gonioscopy should be repeated after resolution of pupillary block or posterior aqueous entrapment. Significant residual peripheral anterior synechiae may cause chronic angle-closure glaucoma. If more than 60 to 90 degrees of the angle remains closed by synechiae, laser gonioplasty may open the angle by causing contraction of the iris stroma. If significant angle closure is unresponsive to laser gonioplasty, especially if the intraocular pressure is elevated, then operative goniosynechialysis may open the angle adequately to minimize or prevent angle-closure glaucoma.

Comments

Visual loss from chronic angle-closure glaucoma following pupillary block can be minimized by efforts to decrease the incidence of pupillary block, prompt and vigorous treatment to ensure that the obstruction to aqueous flow is removed, gonioscopy to detect residual peripheral anterior synechiae, and laser or surgical therapy to break any synechiae. These careful and vigorous efforts will ensure that most patients who do develop aphakic or pseudophakic pupillary block will be left with a functioning trabecular meshwork.

References

Bellows AR, Chylack LT Jr, Hutchinson BT: Choroidal detachment. Clinical manifestation, therapy, and mechanism of formation. Ophthalmology 88:1107–1115, 1981.

Chandler PA: Glaucoma from pupillary block in aphakia. Trans Am Ophthalmol Soc 59:96–102, 1961.

Epstein DL, Steinert RF, Puliafito CA: Neodymium-YAG laser therapy to the anterior hyaloid in aphakic malignant (ciliovitreal block) glaucoma. Am J Ophthalmol 98:137–143, 1984.

Lynch MG, et al: Surgical vitrectomy for pseudophakic malignant glaucoma. Am J Ophthalmol 102:149–153, 1986.

Mandelcorn MS, Maatanen H: Laser iridotomy in post-traumatic and post-surgical pupillary block: A report of five cases. Can J Ophthalmol 13:163–165, 1978.

Samples JR, et al: Pupillary block with posterior chamber intraocular lenses. Arch Ophthalmol 105:335–337, 1987.

Shrader EC, et al: Pupillary block and iridovitreal block in pseudophakic eyes. Ophthalmology 91:831–837, 1984.

Simmons RJ, et al: Laser gonioplasty for special problems in angle closure glaucoma. In Symposium on Glaucoma. Transactions of the New Orleans Academy of Ophthalmology. St. Louis, CV Mosby, 1981, pp 220–235.

Van Buskirk EM: Pupillary block after intraocular lens implantation. Am J Ophthalmol 95:55–59, 1983.

Werner D, Kaback M: Pseudophakic pupillary-block glaucoma. Br J Ophthalmol 61:329–333, 1977.

CORTICOSTEROID-INDUCED GLAUCOMA

MICHAEL A. KASS, M.D.
St. Louis, Missouri

An increase in intraocular pressure may occur during topical, systemic, or periocular administration of corticosteroids. Topical glucocorticoid administration includes not only solutions and ointments applied to the eye but also creams, lotions, and ointments applied to the eyelids and face for various dermatologic disorders. These preparations may reach the eye in sufficient quantity to produce increased intraocular pressure.

The magnitude of the intraocular pressure response to corticosteroids depends on the drug administered, the route of administration, the dose, the frequency of administration, the duration of treatment, the presence of ocular disease such as uveitis, and the responsiveness of the individual to glucocorticoids. Marked elevations of intraocular pressure occur in normal individuals, but occur more frequently in patients with primary open-angle glaucoma, first-degree relatives of these patients, high myopes, diabetics, and patients with Krukenberg's spindles.

Patients receiving corticosteroid therapy may have elevated intraocular pressure without sustaining glaucomatous damage. However, if the pressure elevation has been sufficient in magnitude and duration, the clinical picture resembles primary open-angle glaucoma—elevated intraocular pressure, decreased outflow facility, open angles, optic disc cupping, and visual field loss. Patients who have been treated in the past with corticosteroids may present as if they had normal-tension glaucoma—normal intraocular pressure, normal outflow facility, optic disc cupping, and visual field loss. Only by a careful history can the physician relate the past corticosteroid treatment to the present ocular condition. Glaucoma patients started on corticosteroid therapy may become refractory to medical treatment. Infants who develop corticosteroid-induced glaucoma resemble patients with primary infantile glaucoma. The family may note tearing, photophobia, blepharospasm, and large eyes. Physical findings include increased corneal diameter, cloudy and edematous cornea, breaks in Descemet's membrane, elevated intraocular pressure, and optic disc cupping.

THERAPY

Ocular. Discontinuing glucocorticoid therapy is the most important step in managing corticosteroid-induced glaucoma. In almost all cases, the intraocular pressure elevation resolves promptly. However, there have been reports of persistent elevation of intraocular pressure after cessation of glucocorticoid therapy. It is postulated that prolonged elevation of intraocular pressure may produce permanent alterations in the outflow channels. The possibility that underlying glaucoma was unmasked or aggravated by corticosteroid administration must also be kept in mind. While awaiting resolution, treatment with standard antiglaucoma medications, such as miotics, epinephrine, dipivefrin, beta-adrenergic antagonists, or carbonic anhydrase inhibitors, may be required to control intraocular pressure. If corticosteroid therapy must continue despite elevated intraocular pressure, a weaker glucocorticoid, a lower concentration of the drug, or a steroid compound with less tendency to raise intraocular pressure may be helpful. Both medrysone and fluorometholone are thought to cause less intraocular pressure elevation for a given anti-inflammatory effect than some steroid compounds. However, both medrysone and fluorometholone can still produce elevated intraocular pressure.

Surgical. Corticosteroid-induced glaucoma resistant to medical therapy may require filtering surgery. It is reasonable to temporize in cases in which optic nerve damage is absent or minimal and in cases in which corticosteroid therapy can be discontinued even if the intraocular pressure cannot be controlled. However, such patients must be followed carefully to establish that the intraocular pressure is declining and the ocular damage is stable. If progressive optic nerve damage or visual field loss occurs or seems very likely to occur, surgical intervention is indicated.

Persistently elevated intraocular pressure related to periocular corticosteroid injections (most commonly after repository or "depo" injections) is treated by standard medical means. However, if intraocular pressure cannot be controlled and the injected drug is present beneath the conjunctiva, residual glucocorticoid material may have to be excised.

Ocular or Periocular Manifestations

Eyelids: Skin atrophy; slight ptosis.
Lens: Posterior subcapsular cataracts.
Optic Nerve: Glaucomatous cupping.
Other: Increased intraocular pressure; infection with herpes simplex or various fungi; mydriasis; visual field loss.

PRECAUTIONS

When employing corticosteroid therapy, a baseline ocular examination and close observation are mandatory. Intraocular pressure should be rechecked in 2 or 3 weeks. If the intraocular pressure has not risen and further corticosteroid therapy is needed, the ophthalmologist should re-examine the patient every 2 to 3 weeks for the first few months and every 2 to 3 months thereafter. At no point does a patient become immune from developing corticosteroid-induced glaucoma.

Not all topical corticosteroids have the same potential for elevating intraocular pressure. Dexamethasone, betamethasone, and prednisolone are among the most potent agents in this regard.

Comments

The overwhelming criterion for identification of corticosteroid-induced glaucoma is suspicion. Any patient presenting with elevated intraocular pressure or open-angle glaucoma should be questioned carefully regarding use of corticosteroid eyedrops, ointments, skin preparations, and oral medications. Physicians and other health professionals must be questioned with particular care. Unfortunately, many cases of corticosteroid-induced glaucoma result from the use of glucocorticoids for relatively minor conditions, such as eye irritation, blepharitis, or contact lens discomfort. Patients with glaucoma should be warned about the potentially dangerous effect of corticosteroids.

Once identified, most cases of corticosteroid-induced glaucoma respond promptly to cessation of the drug. The failure of physicians to recognize corticosteroid-induced glaucoma may lead to needless visual loss and difficult medicolegal problems.

References

Armaly MF: Effect of corticosteroids on intraocular pressure and fluid dynamics. I. The effect of dexamethasone in the normal eye. Arch Ophthalmol 70:482–491, 1963.
Armaly MF: Effect of corticosteroids on intraocular pressure and fluid dynamics. II. The effect of dexamethasone in the glaucomatous eye. Arch Ophthalmol 70:492–499, 1963.
Becker B, Mills DW: Corticosteroids and intraocular pressure. Arch Ophthalmol 70:500–507, 1963.
Cantrill HL, et al: Comparison of in vitro potency of corticosteroids with ability to raise intraocular pressure. Am J Ophthalmol 79:1012–1017, 1975.
Francois J, Benozzi G, Victoria-Troncoso V, Bohan W: Ultrastructural and morphometric study of corticosteroid glaucoma in rabbits. Ophthalmic Res 16:168, 1984.
Herschler J: Intractable intraocular hypertension induced by repository triamcinolone acetonide. Am J Ophthalmol 74:501–504, 1972.
Kass MA, Kolker AE, Becker B: Chronic topical corticosteroid use simulating congenital glaucoma. J Pediatr 81:1175–1177, 1972.
Weinrab RN, et al: Detection of glucocorticoid receptors in cultured human trabecular cells. Invest Ophthalmol Vis Sci 21:403, 1981.
Weinstein BI, Munnanzi P, Gordon GG, Southren AL: Defects in cortisol-metabolizing enzymes in primary open-angle glaucoma. Invest Ophthalmol Vis Sci 26:890, 1985.

EXFOLIATION SYNDROME
(Capsular Glaucoma, Pseudoexfoliation of the Lens Capsule)

AHTI TARKKANEN, M.D.
Helsinki, Finland

Exfoliation syndrome (ES) is characterized by grayish flecks that coat the surfaces of the anterior segment of the eye. The deposits can be found on the lens capsule, the ciliary processes, the zonules, and the pupillary margin. The pathologic deposits produce three different zones on the anterior lens capsule: a translucent central disc; a granular girdle around the periphery, called the peripheral band; and a clear zone separating these two areas. The central disc in the pupillary area may be quite faint and is easily missed without dilation of the pupil. Its border, however, is then seen and is more clearly outlined by a few dandruff-like deposits and a white-grayish ring at the edge. The central disc is not a constant feature of exfoliation. The peripheral band, however, is always present and shows the characteristic granular appearance. The clear intermediate zone contains no deposits. Occasionally, however, one may see some loose flakes and a bridge extending from the peripheral band to the central disc. In addition, the flakes have been observed as precipitates on the posterior surface of the cornea, floating freely in the anterior chamber, on the anterior surface of the iris, in the pupillary border, and in aphakic eyes on the hyaloid. The pupillary border may appear atrophic with a characteristic moth-eaten appearance. Transillumination of the iris in the midperiphery is often seen. On gonioscopy, the pigmentation of the trabecular meshwork may extend anterior to the Schwalbe's line (Sampaolesi's line).

Glaucoma associated with ES is called capsular glaucoma. About 20 per cent of patients with ES show abnormalities of intraocular pressure. Capsular glaucoma is often far advanced, and the progression of visual field loss is more severe than in chronic simple glaucoma. However, no difference in the degree of damage is found when intraocular pressures have been equally controlled. Intraocular pressure in capsular glaucoma is more resistant to medical therapy.

In large clinical series, ES has been found to be unilateral in approximately half of the patients, but it may progress to bilateral involvement with time. In Caucasians, it occurs more in females in a ratio about 2.3 : 1 in corrected populations. ES is known to be age dependent, and there is a clear increase with advancing age. The prevalence is low in individuals aged less than 60 years, whereas there is an increase from 1 per cent in the age group 60 to 69 years to 4.8 per cent in the group 70 to 79 years. In individuals aged 80 years or more, the prevalence has been found to be over 8 per cent. There are exceptional populations though, in which ES seems to appear about 10 years earlier. Familiar occurrence of exfoliation syndrome have been described by several authors. ES has now been described in practically all parts of the world, but recent data support the opinion that ES is not uniformly distributed in different countries.

THERAPY

Supportive. Regular follow-up examinations only are recommended for patients with ES with normal intraocular pressures and normal optic discs.

Ocular. Beta-blocking agents, such as timolol, levobunolol, or betaxolol, are used to lower intraocular pressure. These agents may be used topically every 12 to 24 hours. They lower intraocular pressure by reducing the aqueous production. Epinephrine or dipivefrin may be instilled once or twice daily to decrease the production of aqueous humour and to increase the facility of outflow. Dipivefrin is a prodrug that is converted into epinephrine within the eye. One to 4 per cent pilocarpine solution can be applied two to four times daily to decrease intraocular pressure by increasing the facility of outflow. Alternatively, 0.75 to 3.0 per cent carbachol can be instilled two to three times daily.

Systemic. Carbonic anhydrase inhibitors may be added to the treatment with topical agents. Acetazolamide may be prescribed orally from 65 to 250 mg three to four times a day. A sustained-release preparation of acetazolamide may also be tried. As alternatives to acetazolamide, methazolamide or dichlorphenamide may be used. The common dosage of methazolamide varies from 50 to 100 mg orally three times a day; the dose of dichlorphenamide ranges from 25 to 50 mg three to four times a day.

Surgical. Laser trabeculoplasty can be performed for treatment of capsular glaucoma before a filtering operation is considered. Fifty to 60 applications of 50-μm spots of the argon laser with 0.1-second duration are evenly spaced over 180° of the trabecular meshwork. Eyes with capsular glaucoma show a pigmented trabecular meshwork, which is a prerequisite for a successful operation. The reduction of intraocular pressure is caused by increase of the outflow facility. Primary success rates of 80 per cent have been reported. The greater therapeutic reduction of intraocular pressure in capsular glaucoma as compared to chronic simple glaucoma may be due to a higher pretreatment intraocular pressure level. The secondary effects of laser trabeculoplasty in capsular glaucoma include an acute undesired intraocular pressure elevation immediately posttreatment. One has to remember, that the primary success rate of 80 per cent may drop to 30 to 40 per cent in 4 years after treatment. Careful follow-up of patients with capsular glaucoma is mandatory, especially after a successful argon laser trabeculoplasty. With developing failure, another 180° of the chamber angle can be treated.

Filtering surgery is more effective in lowering intraocular pressure. The decision to operate should not be postponed until the late stage of the disease. Use of viscoelastic materials during surgery will prevent loss of anterior chamber and intraocular bleeding during operation and may prevent or lessen postoperative hypotony and cataract formation. The difficulties in the management of capsular glaucoma are illustrated by the fact that, among consecutive patients with chronic open-angle glaucoma who required filtering surgery, capsular glaucoma accounted for 62 per cent in one medical center.

Cataract surgery in ES may be linked to several problems. Eyes with ES may show spontaneous subluxation of the lens in 2 per cent of cases, which may go unnoticed because of the absence of iridodonesis. This may be explained by increased iris rigidity caused by infiltration of the iris stroma by exfoliation material. There may be a strong bonding of the posterior surface of the iris to the pre-equatorial lens capsule, preventing good pupillary dilation. The zonular fibers are known to be weak in ES and the central posterior lens capsule very thin. These features make ES a major risk factor in extracapsular cataract surgery. In a series of unselected cataract operations, the incidence of vitreous loss was 1.8 per cent in cataracts without ES and 9 per cent in those with ES. When these complications are feared, sector iridotomy is preferred, and the haptics of the intraocular lens should be placed into the ciliary sulcus. Anterior chamber intraocular lenses are not recommended in ES because the haptics in the chamber angle may further decompensate aqueous outflow.

Cataract surgery in capsular glaucoma may present further problems. If the intraocular pressure has been controlled by medication, laser therapy, or previous filtering surgery, extracapsular cataract extraction and sulcus-fixed intraocular lens implantation are recommended. If, however, the intraocular pressure cannot be brought under control, cataract surgery may be followed by very high intraocular pressures, which usually do not respond to any measures. Filtering surgery alone will not improve vision, and the patient has to face cataract surgery later. Therefore, in these cases, a glaucoma triple procedure should be considered: trabeculectomy, extracapsular cataract surgery, and posterior chamber intraocular lens implantation. The visual results are satisfactory, and immediate elevated postoperative intraocular pressures can be avoided. The long-term effects of this operation to the intraocular pressure will be known later, but the patient will have undergone only one operation. This procedure, however, is recommended only to experienced surgeons.

Ocular or Periocular Manifestations

Anterior Chamber: Exfoliation material on trabecular meshwork; pigment cells on trabecular meshwork.

Cornea: Exfoliation material or pigment granules on the endothelium.

Iris or Ciliary Body: Exfoliation material on the pupillary margin and ciliary processes; depigmentation of the pigment layer of the iris; exfoliation material or pigment granules on the iris in the pupillary border.

Lens: Exfoliation material on the anterior lens capsule; peripheral band-central disc.

Optic Nerve: Glaucomatous cupping in capsular glaucoma.

Other: Elevated intraocular pressure.

Precautions

The drugs used in the treatment of capsular glaucoma can cause undesirable side effects. Their toxic effect can be additive to systemic drugs prescribed to the patient by the family physician or internist. Timolol should be avoided in patients with a history of asthma or other lung or heart problems. Epinephrine may be associated with conjunctival irritation, allergic conjunctivitis, and even adrenochrome deposition in the conjunctiva, as well as heart arrhythmia and blood pressure elevation. Pilocarpine and carbachol may cause headache, accommodative spasm, and decreased visual acuity. Carbonic anhydrase inhibitors may be associated with malaise, fatigue, unexplained weight loss, nausea, diarrhea, depression, and paresthesias. They may further exacerbate nephrolithiasis. To avoid systemic side effects of the topical drugs, the patient can be advised to occlude the tear duct after instilling the eyedrop or to keep the eyes closed without blinking for about 2 minutes after instillation of the drops.

Comments

Exfoliation material has a fibrillar structure. The fibrils are 20 to 30 nm thick with 10-nm subunits and may be 800 to 900 nm long. Sometimes, they may show a banding periodicity of 50 nm. The material arises probably from the epithelium of the lens and the ciliary body, perhaps as the result of an unknown metabolic disorder. From these areas, the material enters the aqueous humour and is deposited on the anterior lens capsule, zonules, vitreous face, the iris, the trabecular meshwork, and the corneal endothelium. Histochemical studies have demonstrated the presence of glycosaminoglycans. Recent studies of lectin binding to the exofoliative material show that glycoconjugates present in the superficial zonular lamella, zonular fibers, and the nonpigmented epithelium of the ciliary body have a rather similar lectin-binding profile to that of exfoliative material. Of interest is that the lens capsule was essentially unreactive with all lectins used.

About 20 per cent of patients with ES show abnormalities of intraocular pressure. This data can lead to the conclusion that capsular glaucoma results from an overload of an already impaired drainage system by exfoliation material and by pigment granules. This combination is often followed by high intraocular pressures and rapid loss of visual field. Corticosteroid testing has indicated that primary open-angle glaucoma and capsular glaucoma are separate disease processes.

Exfoliation material has been shown to infiltrate even the juxtacanalicular connective tissue and to enter within the giant vacuoles of the endothelium of the Schlemm's canal. This infiltration may explain the poor response of capsular glaucoma to miotic therapy. Furthermore, the ciliary processes in eyes with ES show marked degenerative changes in addition to the exfoliative material. These changes may lead to hyposecretion of aqueous humor. Again, this phenomenon would explain why eyes with capsular glaucoma may be unresponsive to drugs that lower intraocular pressure by decreasing aqueous production.

References

Naumann GOH: Exfoliation syndrome as a risk factor for vitreous loss in extracapsular cataract surgery. Acta Ophthalmol 66(suppl 184):129–131, 1988.
Ruotsalainen J, Tarkkanen A: Capsule thickness of cataractous lenses with and without exfoliation syndrome. Acta Ophthalmol 65:444–449, 1987.
Tarkkanen A, Forsius H (eds): Exfoliation syndrome. Acta Ophthalmol 66(suppl 184):1–7, 1988.

GHOST CELL GLAUCOMA
DAVID G. CAMPBELL, M.D.
Hanover, New Hampshire

Ghost cell glaucoma is a rare form of secondary glaucoma in which elevation of intraocular pressure may occur following vitreous hemorrhage and the development of a disruption in the anterior hyaloid face that allows the contents of the vitreous cavity to pass forward into the anterior chamber. Characteristically, the main component of the vitreous hemorrhage that passes forward into the anterior chamber is degenerated red blood cells, ghost cells. Extracellular hemoglobin debris tends to remain behind in the vitreous cavity, trapped within vitreous and/or fibrin strands. The cause of the glaucoma is obstruction of the intertrabecular spaces of the trabecular meshwork by the ghost cells, which are less pliable than fresh red blood cells. Macrophages and 1 u hemoglobin particles, Heinz bodies, are found occasionally in the anterior chamber as well, although ghost cells predominate overwhelmingly.

Ghost cell glaucoma characteristically occurs in association with vitreous hemorrhage following cataract extraction, following trauma with vitreous hemorrhage and disruption of the anterior hyaloid face, and following vitrectomy for vitreous hemorrhage.

THERAPY

Supportive. If the intraocular pressure is very high and there is pain secondary to this elevation, analgesics may be valuable in controlling discomfort. Oral doses of acetaminophen, 300 to 500 mg every 4 to 6 hours, may be given. Occasionally, narcotics are necessary.

Ocular. Topical timolol, dipivefrin, and miotics should be used initially to attempt to lower intraocular pressure. Solutions of 0.1 per cent dipivefrin or 0.25 to 0.50 per cent timolol may be used every 12 hours to complement miotics, such as 1 to 4 per cent pilocarpine instilled every 6 hours.

Systemic. If topical ocular medications do not sufficiently lower the intraocular pressure, systemic therapy is indicated. Carbonic anhydrase inhibitors are used in full adult dosage; either 250 mg of acetazolamide every 6 hours or 50 mg of methazolamide every 8 hours may be administered orally. If the intraocular pressure still remains high and there is severe pain or fear of damage to the optic nerve, osmotic agents are indicated to lower the intraocular pressure. One to 1.5 gm/kg of a 50 per cent solution of glycerin mixed with fruit juice on ice can effectively lower the intraocular pressure for a few hours. If necessary, intravenous infusion of 2 gm/kg of a 20 per cent solution of mannitol may be given over a 20-minute period. If osmotic agents are contraindicated for any reason, a paracentesis procedure should be substituted at this stage.

In many cases, medical therapy may suffice to control this transient elevation of intraocular pressure. Therapy may be required for a period of weeks to months, until the point is reached at which the supply of ghost cells from the vitreous cavity is exhausted and they no longer continue to pass into the anterior chamber.

Surgical. If medical therapy fails, the intraocular pressure remains elevated, and a painful eye results, surgical therapy then becomes necessary. The first treatment advised is a paracentesis, combined with a washout or irrigation of the contents of the anterior chamber. This is accomplished through a beveled paracentesis incision that begins in the clear cornea near the limbus laterally and extends toward the inferior angle. The incision is made wide enough so that easy escape of fluid out around a cannula can occur. Then, 15 ml of balanced salt solution are passed through a small cannula without a sharp point into the anterior chamber directed toward the inferior angle. The direction of the flow is regulated around the angle so that the accumulation of ghost cells on the trabecular meshwork and within the anterior chamber is dislodged. One washout should be performed and repeated, if necessary. At the time of irrigation, the contents of the anterior chamber should be aspirated and examined histologically under phase contrast microscopy. This will allow proper histologic diagnosis of ghost cell glaucoma.

If two anterior chamber washouts are unsuccessful, a vitrectomy is indicated to irrigate and remove most, if not all, of the ghost cells and hemorrhagic debris within the vitreous cavity. If the greater portion of the ghost cells is removed, further entry into the anterior chamber will be prevented and the glaucoma will resolve. If this fails, cyclocryotherapy can be effective in lowering the intraocular pressure.

Ocular or Periocular Manifestations

Anterior Chamber: Flare; multitude of tiny, khaki-colored cells; occasional pseudohypopyon (khaki-colored, indicating ghost cell layer); open angle.

Cornea: Edema (when pressure is high).
Iris or Ciliary Body: Open trabecular meshwork (may be covered by pathognomonically khaki-colored layer of cells); signs of injury (if caused by trauma).
Optic Nerve: Atrophy without cupping (if pressure has been high for short periods of time); glaucomatous cupping (if pressure elevation is prolonged).
Vitreous: Hemorrhage (fresh or often characteristic khaki color).
Other: Elevation of intraocular pressure (moderate to marked); ocular pain (moderate to marked).

Precautions

This glaucoma must not be misdiagnosed as glaucoma secondary to uveitis or glaucoma secondary to endophthalmitis. In uveitis, keratic precipitates can be pathognomonic. In addition, there is an absence of the characteristic khaki-colored cells in the anterior chamber and vitreous and there is absence of a history of hemorrhage within the vitreous. The pseudohypopyon that occurs with ghost cell glaucoma is pathognomonically khaki-colored. A white hypopyon suggests either uveitis or endophthalmitis.

Comments

Occasionally, ghost cell glaucoma must be differentiated from neovascular glaucoma. In the latter, neovascularization at the pupillary margin and in the angle accompanied with secondary synechial closure is pathognomonic of this condition, which is often associated with vitreous hemorrhage. In ghost cell glaucoma, the angle is open, and the anterior chamber is filled with tiny, khaki-colored cells. Clearing of an edematous cornea with topical glycerin may allow new vessels to be appreciated.

Ghost cell glaucoma is a temporary glaucoma; generally, the intraocular pressure will return to normal once the supply of ghost cells from the vitreous cavity is exhausted. Permanent open-angle glaucoma secondary to the effect of ghost cells within the trabecular meshwork has not been reported.

References

Campbell DG: Ghost cell glaucoma. *In* Ritch R, Shields MB (eds): The Secondary Glaucomas. St. Louis, CV Mosby, 1982, pp 320–327.
Campbell DG, Simmons RJ, Grant WM: Ghost cells as a cause of glaucoma. Am J Ophthalmol 81:441–450, 1976.
Fenton RH, Zimmerman LE: Hemolytic glaucoma. An unusual cause of acute open-angle secondary glaucoma. Arch. Ophthalmol 70:236–239, 1963.
Phelps CD: Hemolytic glaucoma. *In* Fraunfelder FT, Roy FH: Current Ocular Therapy 2. Philadelphia, WB Saunders, 1980, pp 447–448.
Phelps CD, Watzke RC: Hemolytic glaucoma. Am J Ophthalmol 80:690–695, 1975.

GLAUCOMA AFTER OCULAR CONTUSION
(Angle Recession)

JOHN C. MORRISON, M.D.
Portland, Oregon

Blunt ocular trauma (ocular contusion) compresses the eye from front to back, forcing intraocular fluids laterally and causing lateral shearing forces between the uvea and its attachments to the corneoscleral wall. These forces cause variable damage to the angle structures, including the ciliary muscle, trabecular meshwork, and iris. Ciliary muscle tears often rupture arterioles of the ciliary vasculature, producing a hyphema, which is the most common presentation for ocular contusion.

After the hyphema resolves, several characteristic abnormalities may be found, the most common of which is angle recession. Although angle recession may present with a deepened anterior chamber, the diagnosis usually requires detailed gonioscopy of the injured eye and careful comparison with the uninjured fellow eye. Because the contusive force can tear the face of the ciliary muscle between its longitudinal and circular muscle fibers, a cleft may appear in the ciliary body band, making it appear several times wider than the trabecular meshwork and producing apparent recession of the iris root (angle recession). While sclera may occasionally appear in the depths of this cleft with an extensive tear of the ciliary muscle. Damage to the uveal meshwork may range from focal iris process tears to complete stripping away from the scleral spur, rendering it unusually white and prominent. Actual tears in the corneoscleral meshwork may also be seen, but are much more subtle. Other signs of contusion include peripheral anterior synechiae, tearing of the iris root (iridodialysis), and separation of the ciliary body from the scleral spur (cyclodialysis). A single eye can present with one or more of these signs, involving variable amounts of the angle from a single clock hour to its entire circumference.

Glaucoma following ocular contusion is also highly variable; although most eyes demonstrate elevated intraocular pressure within the first several weeks after the injury, some do not develop glaucoma until years later. Early elevations of intraocular pressure, which are often transient, may be caused by hyphema, traumatic iritis with inflammation of the trabecular meshwork, or lens dislocation with pupillary block. Alternatively, no obvious cause may be apparent. Other eyes have an initially normal or slightly low intraocular pressure, usually secondary to depressed aqueous humor formation from iridocyclitis, but occasionally from increased outflow via trabecular meshwork tears or a cyclodialysis cleft. With time, approximately 4 to 9 per cent of patients with angle recession involving more than 180° of the angle circumference will develop glaucoma. Most cases of late glaucoma arise from gradual scarring of the trabecular meshwork. Other causes include gradual closure of a cyclodialysis cleft and extension of endothelium over the chamber angle with deposition of a Descemet's-like membrane.

THERAPY

Ocular. If an early rise in intraocular pressure is felt to be caused by traumatic iritis, a trial of topical 1 per cent prednisolone four times daily with a cycloplegic, such as scopolamine, may be beneficial. Otherwise, initial treatment of elevated intraocular pressure, either of early or late onset, should begin with a beta-blocking agent, 0.25 to 0.5 per cent timolol, 0.5 per cent levobunolol, or 0.5 per cent betaxolol, used once or twice daily. Twice daily 1 per cent epinephrine and 0.1 per cent dipivefrin, 2 to 4 per cent pilocarpine four times daily, or acetylcholinesterase inhibitors (0.06 to 0.25 per cent echothiophate) twice daily may provide additional reduction of intraocular pressure. However, the effectiveness of these agents may be limited by extensive trabecular meshwork damage and disinsertion of the ciliary muscle.

Systemic. If topical medications fail to lower intraocular pressure satisfactorily, systemic carbonic anhydrase inhibitors may be necessary. These include 125 to 250 mg of oral acetazolamide four times daily or 50 to 100 mg of oral methazolamide twice daily.

Surgical. Surgery is necessary if maximally tolerated medical therapy does not lower pressure into a satisfactory range or if progressive visual field loss or disc atrophy is observed. Although generally not successful in angle-recession glaucoma, standard argon laser trabeculoplasty should precede filtering surgery if there is not extensive damage and peripheral anterior synechiae. If the optic nerve is already severely damaged, premedication with a single drop of 1 per cent apraclonidine[†] may be used to reduce the likelihood of an abrupt rise in intraocular pressure following the laser treatment. If all of the above measures are unsuccessful, a filtering procedure (trabeculectomy) is indicated to control pressure and preserve vision. Full-thickness operations, including trephination, sclerectomy, or thermal sclerostomy, are similarly effective, but have a higher complication rate, such as flat chamber and choroidal effusion.

Ocular or Periocular Manifestations

Anterior Chamber: Bare, white scleral spur; deep anterior chamber; peripheral anterior synechiae; trabecular meshwork tears.

Cornea: Blood staining.

Iris and Ciliary Body: Cyclodialysis; iridodialysis; irregular pigmentation of ciliary body band and trabecular meshwork; wide ciliary body band.

Lens: Cataract; ruptured zonules with vitreous herniation.

Retina: Commotio retinae (early); detached vitreous base; retinal holes.

Optic Nerve: Glaucomatous cupping; pallor.

Other: Elevated intraocular pressure hypotony; vitreous hemorrhages.

Precautions

The efficacy of topical and systemic agents should always be balanced against their safety and the patient's tolerance of their side effects. In patients with reactive respiratory disease, beta-blockers should be limited to betaxolol, a relatively selective $beta_1$ antagonist, with the consent of the patient's internist and careful monitoring of pulmonary functions. Echothiophate should not be used in phakic patients as they have a cataractogenic potential. Systemic carbonic anhydrase inhibitors possess many, usually self-limited side effects, including acidosis, paresthesia, and fatigue. Renal stones may accompany the acidosis, and potassium depletion may result if carbonic anhydrase inhibitors are used with diuretics. Rare, life-threatening blood dyscrasias have also been reported with carbonic anhydrase inhibitors.

Comments

Over 90 per cent of ocular contusions severe enough to cause a traumatic hyphema have gonioscopically visible angle recession or other damage to the anterior chamber angle. Since nearly 10 per cent of eyes with more than 180° of angle recession may ultimately develop glaucoma, these abnormalities should be considered evidence of concomitant injury to the trabecular meshwork. All eyes with traumatic hyphema should therefore be examined by careful gonioscopy for angle recession, iridodialysis, or cyclodialysis after the blood has completely cleared and a good view re-established. Although glaucoma is most likely to present during the first year after injury, patients with greater than 180° of angle recession should have yearly tonometry and optic nerve evaluations for the remainder of their lives.

References

Epstein DL: Chandler and Grant's Glaucoma, 3rd ed. Philadelphia, Lea and Febiger, 1986, pp 296–310.

Howard GM, Hutchinson BT, Frederick AR: Hyphema resulting from blunt trauma. Gonioscopic, tonographic, and ophthalmoscopic observations following resolution of the hemorrhage. Trans Am Acad Ophthalmol Otolaryngol 69:294–306, 1965.

Kaufman JH, Tolpin DW: Glaucoma after traumatic angle recession. A ten-year prospective study. Am J Ophthalmol 78:648–654, 1974.

Shields MB: Textbook of Glaucoma, 2nd ed. Baltimore, Williams & Wilkins, 1987, pp 328–333.

Tonjum A: Gonioscopy in traumatic hyphema. Acta Ophthalmol 44:650–664, 1966.

Wolff SM, Zimmerman LE: Chronic secondary glaucoma. Associated with retrodisplacement of iris root and deepening of the anterior chamber angle secondary to contusion. Am J Ophthalmol 54:547–562, 1962.

GLAUCOMA ASSOCIATED WITH ANTERIOR UVEITIS

M. BRUCE SHIELDS, M.D.
Durham, North Carolina

Anterior uveitis influences the intraocular pressure through effects on both aqueous humor production and resistance to aqueous outflow. Inflammation of the ciliary body usually leads to reduced aqueous production. If this reduction outweighs a concomitant increase in resistance to outflow, the intraocular pressure will be reduced, which is typically the case in acute anterior uveitis. In other cases, inflammation-induced alterations in the aqueous outflow system may be sufficient to cause pressure elevation and secondary glaucoma.

The mechanisms by which anterior uveitis increases resistance to aqueous outflow are numerous and only partially understood. They may be associated with acute, subacute, or chronic iridocyclitis. The former is characterized by ciliary flush, slight miosis, variable degrees of aqueous flare and cell, and frequent keratic precipitates. Symptoms usually include mild to moderate ocular pain, photophobia, and blurred vision, unless marked secondary intraocular pressure elevation has developed with severe pain and corneal edema. Subacute iridocyclitis produces few or no symptoms, but can have serious consequences, since complications (including secondary glaucoma) may go undetected until advanced damage has occurred. Mechanisms of increased resistance to aqueous outflow with both acute and subacute forms of anterior uveitis are usually of the open-angle type and include obstruction of the trabecular meshwork by inflammatory cells or fibrin, swelling or dysfunction of the trabecular lamellae or endothelium, and inflammatory precipitates on the meshwork. Much less commonly, these forms of uveitis may be associated with secondary angle-closure glaucoma by forward rotation of the ciliary body or by lens-iris diaphragm displacement from an associated posterior uveitis.

Chronic anterior uveitis is characterized by a protracted course of months to years, often with remissions and exacerbations, and is particularly prone to cause secondary glaucoma. The mechanisms of obstruction to aqueous outflow may be open angle, in which the meshwork is scarred or covered by a membrane, or closed angle, due to contracture of the membrane or inflammatory precipitates or following posterior synechiae formation with subsequent iris bombé. Another mechanism of secondary glaucoma to be considered during the treatment of any form of anterior uveitis is steroid-induced glaucoma.

THERAPY

Ocular. Corticosteroids constitute the first line of defense in most cases of anterior uveitis. Topical administration is usually preferred, and commonly used corticosteroids include 1 per cent prednisolone or 0.1 per cent dexamethasone. A typical maintenance dose is one drop four times daily, although more frequent instillation, such as every hour, may be required initially or in severe cases. In a rabbit model with keratitis, frequent instillation of corticosteroids every 15 minutes or five doses at 1-minute intervals each hour were more effective than an hourly regimen. If topical administration is inadequate, periocular injections of dexamethasone,* prednisolone,* or methylprednisolone* or systemic administration of prednisone may be required.

Nonsteroidal anti-inflammatory agents may be needed when corticosteroids are inadequate or contraindicated. These include prostaglandin synthetase inhibitors, such as aspirin,‡ indomethacin,‡ indoxole,† or dipyridamole,‡ and immunosuppressive agents, such as methotrexate,‡ azathioprince,‡ or chlorambucil.‡ One regimen that is reported to be effective in cases of severe chronic uveitis that have been poorly responsive or unresponsive to corticosteroid therapy is long-term daily administration of 10 to 15 mg of prednisone combined with 2.0 to 2.5 mg of azathioprine or 6 to 8 mg of chlorambucil.

In conjunction with anti-inflammatory agents, a mydriatic-cycloplegic is usually indicated to avoid the formation of posterior synechiae and to relieve the discomfort of ciliary muscle spasm. One per cent atropine, 2 to 5 per cent homatropine, or 0.5 to 1.0 per cent cyclopentolate may be used.

Antiglaucoma medication should be added to the treatment plan if the magnitude of the intraocular pressure elevation poses an immediate threat to vision or if the pressure does not respond adequately to anti-inflammatory therapy alone. Miotics are generally contraindicated in the inflamed eye because they may aggravate the inflammation, increase the chances of posterior synechiae formation, and worsen the discomfort from ciliary muscle spasm. Therefore, topical beta-blockers (0.25 or 0.5 per cent timolol or 0.5 per cent betaxolol or levobunolol), 0.5 to 2.0 per cent epinephrine, or 0.1 per cent dipivefrin twice daily are usually the initial drugs of choice. When further pressure reduction is needed, a carbonic anhydrase inhibitor, such as 25 to 50 mg of methazolamide or 500 mg of acetazolamide twice daily, may be added. Hyperosmotic agents, including oral glycerin or isosorbide and intravenous mannitol, may also be used for short-term emergency control of secondary glaucoma.

Surgical. It is a general rule that surgery should be avoided when possible in the inflamed eye. However, when surgical intervention is needed to control intraocular pressure, it is best to select the procedure with the least amount of intraocular involvement. For example, a laser iridectomy is preferable to a surgical iridectomy when a pupillary block mechanism is believed to be present. For open-angle glaucoma uncontrolled on maximum medical therapy, a filtering procedure is usually indicated. Trabeculodialysis is an alternative approach in which a goniotomy knife is used to incise above the trabecular meshwork and then to peel the meshwork downward. Laser trabeculoplasty in the management of glaucoma associated with anterior uveitis is usually ineffective and may be complicated by additional postoperative intraocular pressure increase.

Ocular or Periocular Manifestations

Anterior Chamber: Aqueous cell and flare.
Conjunctiva: Ciliary flush.
Cornea: Edema; keratic precipitates.
Iris: Inflammatory precipitates; peripheral anterior synechiae.
Other: Glaucoma.

PRECAUTIONS

Prompt, aggressive treatment of anterior uveitis is necessary to avoid serious sequelae, including complicated cataracts and chronic secondary glaucoma. However, the medications required in the treatment plan have a significant potential for adverse reactions and must be used with extreme caution. The risk of steroid-induced glaucoma exists with the use of either topical or periocular corticosteroids and, to a lesser extent, with systemic steroids. The newer progesterone-like steroids (medrysone and fluorometholone) have a lower potential for inducing pressure elevation, but are not completely devoid of this property. Care must also be taken to rule out viral or fungal infections if steroids are to be prescribed. When using nonsteroidal anti-inflammatory agents, the risk of gastrointestinal irritation must be considered with most prostaglandin synthetase inhibitors, whereas the possibility of hematologic disorders requires constant monitoring while immunosuppressive agents are being used.

The potential for angle-closure glaucoma must be assessed before prescribing a mydriatic-cycloplegic or epinephrine. With beta-blockers, the most serious potential consequences are related to systemic side effects and include bradycardia, weakened myocardial contractility, bronchospasm, and central nervous system disorders. The risk of pulmonary complications is reduced but not eliminated, with the selective beta$_1$-antagonist, betaxolol. The most significant risks of treatment with carbonic anhydrase inhibitors are electrolyte imbalance, systemic acidosis, gastrointestinal distress, genitourinary disorders, including renal calculi, and blood dyscrasias. With hyperosmotic therapy, the oral preparations may cause nausea and vomiting, which may lead to loss of any therapeutic effect; cardiovascular overload may be a problem with intravenous mannitol, particularly if there is a history of congestive heart failure.

When surgical intervention is required in the inflamed eye, a major cause of failure is excessive postoperative iridocyclitis, necessitating the use of aggressive steroid therapy during this period.

Comments

Treatment should first be directed at the underlying etiology of the ocular inflammation, such as an infectious process, if it is apparent. In the vast majority of cases, however, a definite cause for the anterior uveitis is never clearly established, and most are presumed to represent an autoimmune mechanism. The treatment in these situations is nonspecific, with anti-inflammatory agents usually constituting the first approach in the treatment plan. In many cases, resolution of the inflammatory process is sufficient to control the intraocular pressure, although other cases require medical and even surgical management of the secondary glaucoma.

References

Andrasch RH, Pirofsky B, Burns RP: Immunosuppressive therapy for severe chronic uveitis. Arch Ophthalmol 96:247–251, 1978.
Hoskins HD Jr, Hetherington J Jr, Shaffer RN: Surgical management of the inflammatory glaucomas. Perspect Ophthalmol 1:173–181, 1977.
Kanski JJ, McAllister JA: Trabeculodialysis for inflammatory glaucoma in children and young adults. Ophthalmoloy 92:927–930, 1985.
Leibowitz HM, Kupferman A: Optimal frequency of topical prednisolone administration. Arch Ophthalmol 97:2154–2156, 1979.
Luntz MH: A clinical approach to the medical treatment of uveitis. Adv Ophthalmol 36:187–196, 1978.
Roth M, Simmons RJ: Glaucoma associated with precipitates on the trabecular meshwork. Ophthalmology 86:1613–1618, 1979.
Spinelli HM, Krohn DL: Inhibition of prostaglandin-induced iritis. Topical indoxole versus indomethacin therapy. Arch Ophthalmol 98:1106–1109, 1980.
Wong VG, Hersh EM: Methotrexate in the therapy of cyclitis. Trans Am Acad Ophthalmol Otolaryngol 69:279–293, 1965.

GLAUCOMA ASSOCIATED WITH ELEVATED VENOUS PRESSURE

JOHN R. SAMPLES, M.D.
Portland, Oregon

Systemic disorders that raise the episcleral venous pressure can cause glaucoma as the increased pressure creates resistance to outflow in Schlemm's canal. Schlemm's canal is connected to the episcleral and conjunctival veins by a complicated system of vessels. Most vessels carrying aqueous humor from Schlemm's canal are directed posteriorly, with the vast majority draining into episcleral veins. A few cross the subconjunctival tissue and drain into conjunctival veins. Episcleral veins drain into the cavernous sinus via the anterior ciliary and superior ophthalmic veins, whereas the conjunctival veins drain into the superior ophthalmic or facial veins via the palpebral and angular veins. The normal episcleral venous pressure ranges between 8 and 10 mm Hg. Patients with primary open-angle glaucoma do not appear to have episcleral venous pressure elevations. In fact, there appears to be a negative correlation, with ocular hypertensive patients having significantly lower episcleral venous pressure.

Elevated venous pressure is one means by which patients with thyroid eye disease may have elevated intraocular pressure. Elevated venous pressure may occur in association with a carotid cavernous fistula. The most consistent finding in patients with an elevated episcleral venous pressure is tortuous and dilated episcleral and bulbar conjunctival vessels. When the meshwork is open, one may observe blood reflux into Schlemm's canal. Noteworthy, however, is at least one study's suggestion that elevated venous pressure may be associated with increased outflow caused by widening of Schlemm's canal. Prolonged elevation of episcleral venous pressure seems likely to lead to a reduction in outflow.

There are four categories of patients with elevated episcleral venous pressure. The first have venous obstruction. In patients with thyroid eye disease, contracture of extraocular muscles and the infiltration of plasma cells and lymphocytes into the orbit may lead to an elevated venous pressure. It must be kept in mind that thyroid dysfunction may be associated with abnormal scleral rigidity. Retro-orbital tumors, cavernous sinus thrombosis, and lesions that obstruct venous return from the head may also cause venous obstruction and elevated venous pressure.

Persons with carotid cavernous fistulas comprise the second category of patients with elevated venous pressure. The typical carotid cavernous fistula occurs as a result of severe head injury; a large fistula is created between the internal carotid artery and the surrounding cavernous sinus venous plexus. The condition is characterized by pulsating exophthalmos, a bruit over the globe, conjunctival chemosis, engorgement of episcleral venous veins, and restriction of motility with evidence of ocular ischemia. The shunting of the internal carotid cavernous fistula causes high flow and high pressure. A more recently appreciated form of carotid cavernous fistula is the "low-flow" shunt. These small fistulas may occur without a history of trauma. In these cases, the shunt is fed by a meningeal branch of the intracavernous internal carotid artery or external carotid artery that empties directly into the cavernous sinus or adjacent dural vein that connects with the cavernous sinus. Whether the patient has a high-flow or low-flow shunt, elevated pressure occurs. Venous back pressure may increase the episcleral venous pressure, which is the most common cause of intraocular pressure rise with the fistula. Angle-closure glaucoma has also been reported in association with carotid cavernous fistula.

A third condition that can lead to elevation of

episcleral venous pressure is Sturge-Weber syndrome where a hamartoma arises from the vascular tissue and produces a characteristic port-wine stain hemiangioma of the skin in a trigeminal distribution. Several mechanisms of glaucoma are possible in these patients, but at least some patients appear to have an open anterior chamber angle with small arteriovenous fistulas in the episcleral venous pressure. Orbital varices have not been associated with glaucoma, perhaps because intraocular pressure is likely to be normal between episodes. When orbital varices are present, elevated episcleral venous pressure is usually associated with stooping over or the Valsalva maneuver.

Finally, idiopathic cases of elevated episcleral venous pressure have been reported. These patients are elderly with no family history of the condition. The cause of the elevated venous pressure is unknown, and the associated glaucoma may be severe.

THERAPY

Ocular. The treatment for glaucoma associated with elevated venous pressure is no different than for other forms of glaucoma, so long as the angle is open. In cases where carotid cavernous fistula or low-flow shunt is present, pharmacologic glaucoma control should be considered before surgical intervention is contemplated when the glaucoma is the only condition prompting consideration of surgery. In some instances, angiography alone is sufficient to prompt low-flow fistulas to close spontaneously.

Surgical. If surgical intervention is necessary, a filtering procedure should be employed. There is no doubt that these patients are at substantially increased risk for uveal effusion and expulsive hemorrhage. It has been recommended that drainage of the suprachoroid be routinely performed at the time of surgery. Prophylactic sclerotomies should routinely be performed when the filtering procedure is performed.

Ocular or Periocular Manifestations

Ciliary Body: Ciliary congestion; detachment.
Conjunctiva: Dilated, tortuous bulbar conjunctival vessels.
Optic Nerve: Glaucomatous cupping.
Sclera: Dilated, tortuous episcleral veins.
Other: Increased intraocular pressure.

PRECAUTIONS

Repair of carotid cavernous fistulas may be hazardous and is at present a controversial area in neurosurgery. If glaucoma is the sole cause for intervention, one should be certain that it is significant, difficult to treat and that visual field progression is present.

COMMENTS

Elevated episcleral venous pressure as a cause of glaucoma is often overlooked. Because these patients do have increased complications at the time of filtering surgery, careful consideration of episcleral and conjunctival vessels before filtration is always indicated.

References

Barany EH: The influence of extraocular venous pressure on outflow facility in Cercopithecus ethiops Macacafascicularis. Invest Ophthalmol Vis Sci 17:711–717, 1978.
Bellows AR, et al: Choroidal effusion during glaucoma surgery in patients with prominent episcleral vessels. Arch Ophthalmol 97:493–497, 1979.
Harris GJ, Rice PR: Angle closure and carotid cavernous fistula. Ophthalmology 86:1521–1529, 1979.
Henderson JW, Schneider C: The ocular findings in carotid cavernous fistula in a series of 17 cases. Am J Ophthalmol 48:585–597, 1959.
McLenachan J, Davies DM: Glaucoma and the thyroid. Br J Ophthalmol 49:441–444, 1965.
Palestine AG, Young BR, Pipegras DG: Visual prognosis and carotid cavernous fistula. Arch Ophthalmol 99:1600–1603, 1981.
Phelps CD: The pathogenesis of glaucoma in Sturge-Weber syndrome. Ophthalmology 85:276–286, 1978.
Phelps CD, Thompson HS, Ossoinig KC: The diagnosis and prognosis of atypical carotid cavernous fistulas (Red-eyed shunt syndrome). Am J Ophthalmol 93:423–436, 1982.
Podos SM, Minas TF, MacRif J: A new instrument to measure episcleral venous pressure. Comparison of normal eyes and eyes with primary open angle glaucoma. Arch Ophthalmol 80:209–213, 1968.
Radius RL, Maumenee AE: Dilated episcleral venous vessels and open-angle glaucoma. Am J Ophthalmol 86:31–35, 1978.
Sanders MD, Hoyt WF: Hypoxic ocular sequelae of carotid cavernous fistula. The study of causes of visual failure before and after neurosurgical treatment in a series of 25 cases. Br J Ophthalmol 53:82–97, 1969.
Talusan ED, Schwartz B: Episcleral venous pressure—Differences between normal ocular hypertensive and primary open-angle glaucoma. Arch Ophthalmol 99:824–828, 1981.

GLAUCOMA ASSOCIATED WITH INTRAOCULAR LENSES

E. MICHAEL VAN BUSKIRK, M.D.
Portland, Oregon

Intraocular lenses have been welcomed by cataract patients and surgeons alike because they seem to permit better simulation of phakic vision. Despite the visual advantages offered by intraocular lenses and the technical improvements in implant design of recent years, all varieties of intraocular lenses have occasionally been associated with various forms of glaucoma.

However, complications associated with inflammation, glaucoma, and uveal decompensation are several times more common in eyes implanted with anterior chamber than with posterior chamber lenses. Despite the preponderance of posterior chamber lens implantations among cataract patients, the majority of intraocular lens-induced glaucomas in the author's experience are related to anterior chamber lenses. This higher frequency of anterior chamber lens-induced glaucoma likely relates in part to the less physiologic location of the anterior chamber lens in front of the pupil where it rests on the less hospitable structures of the anterior chamber angle. Moreover, anterior chamber lenses are often placed in eyes that have developed complications during cataract surgery, such as a ruptured capsule or vitreous loss. Such eyes are more prone to chronic inflammation and peripheral anterior synechiae and sometimes exhibit evidence of inadequate wound closure.

Glaucoma in the aphakic eye may occur both in the open- or closed-angle forms and may be related to pre-existing open-angle glaucoma, the filling of the anterior chamber with vitreous, blocking of the pupil and iridectomies by vitreous or diversion posteriorly of aqueous humor, or, most commonly, chronic peripheral anterior synechiae. All of these mechanisms can also occur in the pseudophakic eye, but additional varieties of glaucoma may be specifically attributed to the presence of the intraocular lens itself. These include chronic inflammation, mechanical distortion of the anterior chamber angle, iridociliary compression by posterior chamber lens haptics, and pseudophakic pupillary block.

Uveitis secondary to an intraocular lens is often a presumptive diagnosis because many postoperative eyes, at least acutely, have some intracameral cellular reaction as well as a partial breakdown of the blood aqueous barrier in response to the surgery itself. Moreover, the exact contribution of the intraocular lens to chronic postoperative uveitis often must be suspect, since the same condition can occur without an intraocular lens. However, in cases in which the inflammation persists beyond the usual postoperative period and no other identifiable causes for it exist, the contribution of the lens itself to the uveitis must be considered. Characteristically, these patients have a mild cellular reaction in the anterior chamber and a muddy "spattered" appearance to the trabecular meshwork; often, they do not have extensive peripheral anterior synechiae. It would appear that this form of glaucoma is more common with iris fixation or anterior chamber intraocular lenses, but can also occur with lenses placed in the posterior chamber. Chafing or even compression of the ciliary body by the lens haptics (sulcus fixation) may be a contributing factor, either from mechanical compression or disturbance of the ciliary vasculature.

Glaucoma from mechanical distortion of the anterior chamber angle can result from improper sizing or placement of rigid anterior chamber lenses that erode into the peripheral iris, trabecular meshwork, or peripheral cornea. Such improper placement may lead to bleeding, uveitis, and glaucoma—the so-called UGH syndrome. It may also lead to progressive peripheral anterior synechiae and chronic angle-closure glaucoma.

By the same token, chafing of the lens haptics against the posterior iris or ciliary body that is associated with iridociliary fixation can lead to a variety of glaucomas associated with posterior chamber intraocular lenses. Posterior chamber sulcus fixation can compress the microvasculature of the iris and ciliary body, possibly leading to ischemia and associated inflammation. Even bleeding can occur that sometimes pools in the posterior chamber or leads to chronic hyphema.

Campbell and associates have presented convincing evidence for the hypothesis that rubbing of the peripheral iris on the lens zonules may lead to the pigment dispersion syndrome in anatomically prone phakic eyes. It also appears that certain pseudophakic eyes with lenses implanted so that iris epithelium rubs on supporting structures may manifest a pigment dispersion syndrome. These patients have transillumination defects in the iris associated with supporting lens haptics, pigment granules visibly circulating in the aqueous humor, pigment dusting of the anterior iris surface, and a dense band of pigment in the filtration portion of the trabecular meshwork. As expected, this pseudophakic pigment dispersion syndrome is confined to eyes with iris plane and posterior chamber lenses.

Late-onset progressive peripheral anterior synechiae have also occasionally followed otherwise uneventful implantation of posterior chamber lenses. These patients at first exhibit peripheral anterior synechiae localized over the lens haptics, apparently from compression of the peripheral iris. Over time, these synechiae progress to include larger segments of the chamber angle.

One of the most disturbing forms of glaucoma from intraocular lenses results from pupillary block. Pupillary block has been reported in patients with all types of intraocular lenses, but seems to be most common with anterior chamber lenses where the lens haptic acts as a flap valve that occludes the pupil when the iris drifts forward. If no iridectomy is patent, pupillary block will occur, with bulging of the iris around the edges of the lens and closure of the anterior chamber angle. In some cases, the initiating factor appears to be a wound leak with forward drift of the iris diaphragm. More often, the intraocular lens has rotated to occlude the surgical peripheral iridectomy; in other cases, vitreous has come forward to block it.

Pupillary block occurs much less frequently after posterior chamber than anterior chamber lens implantation. Moreover, many of these eyes show some technical wrinkle heralding likely postoperative pupillary block, including small capsular tears during surgery. Patients with diabetes mellitus and small hyperopic eyes are already prone to angle-closure glaucoma before cataract extraction. Although the advisability of peripheral iridectomy has been debated in cataract surgery with posterior chamber lens implantation, there is little doubt that iridectomy is needed for such predisposed eyes.

Posterior diversion of aqueous humor, or malignant glaucoma, may also occur in the pseudophakic eye and may mimic simple pupillary block, especially in eyes with posterior chamber lenses. These eyes often exhibit a shallow anterior chamber, poorly controlled angle-closure glaucoma, peripheral anterior synechiae, or even a history of phakic malignant glaucoma before cataract surgery. After surgery, a shallow anterior chamber with the iris, implant, and posterior capsule appearing to bulge toward the anterior chamber may be found even in the presence of an open iridectomy. Vitreous appears to be compacted against the posterior capsule with a relatively clear aqueous-containing space deep within the posterior segment.

THERAPY

Ocular. Increased intraocular pressure should be treated as appropriate for the specific pathogenesis. Glaucomas resulting from inflammation usually respond well to topical corticosteroids, such as 1 per cent prednisolone or 0.1 per cent dexamethasone administered every 1 to 4 hours until anterior chamber inflammation has resolved and the intraocular pressure is decreasing. Depending upon the state of the optic nerve and the height of the intraocular pressure, aqueous formation inhibitors, such as 0.25 or 0.5 per cent timolol or other beta-adrenergic antagonists, may also be used to "tide" the patient through the period of increased intraocular pressure. Topical cycloplegics, such as 1 per cent atropine, are useful to produce ciliary relaxation and prevent other complications, such as pupillary block. As a last resort, an epinephrine preparation may also be added, with the knowledge that cystoid macular edema may be induced by the epinephrine or the chronic inflammation itself. Generally, glaucomas occurring on the basis of uveitis do not respond well to miotics, which themselves may exacerbate inflammation and disrupt the blood-aqueous barrier. However, if the intraocular pressure remains elevated after other ocular hypotensive agents have been employed and inflammation has subsided, a therapeutic trial with miotics, such as 4 per cent pilocarpine four times daily or 3 per cent carbachol three times daily, may be tried so long as there is a patent peripheral iridectomy and no evidence of pupillary block.

Glaucomas resulting from mechanical distortion of the anterior chamber angle generally require surgical management, but the inflammatory component may be inhibited with topical steroids as described earlier. Topical hypotensive agents, such as described above, should be used if lens removal is judged to be impracticable or dangerous.

The pseudophakic pigment dispersion syndrome often responds to conventional ocular hypotensive agents, including miotics, beta-blockers, and epinephrine. As with phakic pigment dispersion syndrome, these eyes theoretically should do well with low-dose miotics to fix the pupil and prevent the iris from rubbing on the haptic. Conventional ocular hypotensives, such as timolol, are also effective in controlling the intraocular pressure.

Pupillary block glaucoma invariably requires placement of additional iridectomies or iridotomies and, as such, is primarily a surgical condition. However, if at all possible, pupillary block should be broken medically, using topical mydriatic-cycloplegics to dilate the pupil and displace the iris diaphragm posteriorly. Short-acting mydriatics are preferred because their action can be easily reversed if the pupil becomes so dilated that one cannot readily do a laser iridotomy.

Systemic. Systemic carbonic anhydrase inhibitors may be prescribed for any of these conditions in which the intraocular pressure is unacceptably high for the optic disc. Osmotic agents are similarly useful in breaking attacks of pupillary block and as a temporary measure, for patients awaiting surgery.

Surgical. For cases of glaucoma resulting from chronic inflammation, mechanical distortion of the anterior chamber, or pigment dispersion, the primary surgical decision is whether or not to remove the intraocular lens. In many cases, the same factors that led to insertion of the intraocular lens initially make the surgeon reluctant to remove it. It is often difficult to attribute positively chronic uveitis to the presence of the intraocular lens per se. In such cases, the lens can and should often be left in place while treating the uveitis medically. However, if progressive peripheral anterior synechiae or extensive adhesions between iris and the intraocular lens itself are developing, it is preferable to remove the lens before it becomes technically dangerous to do so. The lens can sometimes be surgically manipulated into an acceptable position with mechanical distortion of the anterior chamber angle and lens subluxation.

Laser trabeculoplasty does not appear to be as successful in the aphakic or pseudophakic eye as in eyes that have not had cataract surgery. However, in medically uncontrolled open-angle glaucoma with an intraocular lens, laser trabeculoplasty should be attempted and will successfully obviate the need for surgery in many cases. The presence of active uveitis markedly worsens the prognosis for successful laser trabeculoplasty.

Cyclodestructive procedures may also be used for glaucoma, including cyclocryotherapy or transscleral ablation of the ciliary processes with the Neodymium YAG laser. Eyes with poor visual potential are often more benignly treated with less invasive procedures than the complex surgical protocols often required for eyes with multiple complications of cataract surgery. Cyclocryotherapy or probably any cyclodestructive procedure works better if there is some open angle. Unfortunately, when the anterior chamber angle is entirely closed, it is difficult to restore intraocular pressure to a physiologic range by reducing aqueous formation. The procedure may provide palliation after multiple other procedures have failed.

In the absence of extensive inflammation and conjunctival scarring and in the presence of an intact posterior capsule, conventional trabeculectomy may be used for the pseudophakic eye. Eyes with extensive conjunctival scarring after full 180° corneoscleral wounds or that have experienced vitreous loss, chronic inflammation, wound abnormalities, or other complications usually require adjunctive antimetabolite therapy, such as fluorouracil‡ or a tube or seton implant.

Precautions

The time of onset of pupillary block has been shown to be quite unpredictable, occurring as long as 3 years after the original intraocular lens implant. Hence, all patients with anterior chamber intraocular lenses require long-term careful observation and should be warned to consult their ophthalmologist promptly if unusual symptoms occur. Many such cases will already have developed extensive permanent closure of the anterior chamber angle when the pupillary block is first observed, so that the surgeon must be prepared to perform a filtration procedure to permit normalization of the intraocular pressure if insufficient open angle exists after iridotomy. All patients with pupillary block should be examined for possible wound leak, although this has only been a factor in about 10 per cent of cases seen by the author. If present, repair of the wound and, often anterior vitrectomy will be necessary. Massive suprachoroidal hemorrhage has been reported in one third of eyes after filtration surgery in aphakic or pseudophakic eyes that have had vitrectomy. A prophylactic posterior sclerotomy, a Flieringa ring, and other efforts to prevent scleral collapse during filtration surgery on such eyes may prevent this dreaded complication.

Comments

Since implantation of intraocular lenses has become a standard accompaniment to cataract surgery only within the past two decades, new varieties of pseudophakic glaucoma continue to be described. The ophthalmologist performing cataract surgery with intraocular lens implantation or seeing patients with intraocular lenses must be prepared to deal with these sequelae as they develop. For example, flexible anterior chamber lenses have many advantages over the previously used rigid varieties. However, even the closed-loop varieties of these flexible lenses have created their own complications, including erosion into anterior segment structures, bleeding, chronic uveitis, and pseudophakic bullous keratopathy. Pupillary block with a rigid anterior chamber lens leads to increased intraocular pressure, but the lens remains fixed in place. With a flexible lens, the lens optic comes forward to injure the corneal endothelium. The majority of such cases require corneal transplantation, even after correction of the pupillary block. Increased intraocular pressure commonly follows even perfect cataract surgery in patients with pre-existing open-angle glaucoma, especially during the first few days to weeks postoperatively. These patients require maximal control of intraocular pressure preoperatively, minimal intraocular manipulation during surgery, special precautions for management of the small pupil, and intensive postoperative care to prevent further compromise of the optic disc.

An ocular hypotensive response may also occur after capsulotomy with the Neodymium YAG laser in the pseudophakic eye. The mechanism of this glaucoma is not known, but the glaucoma is usually self-limited and responds to conventional hypotensive therapy. Anti-inflammatory agents should be used to diminish any inflammatory component. Apraclonidine† may diminish this complication.

References

Apple DJ, et al: Complications of intraocular lenses. A historical and histopathological review. Surv Ophthalmol 29:1, 1984.
Campbell DG: Pigmentary dispersion and glaucoma. A new theory. Arch Ophthalmol 97:1667–1672, 1980.
De Heer LJ: Glaucoma as a problem in intraocular lens implantation. Doc Ophthalmol 49:337–346, 1980.
Ellingson FT: The uveitis-glaucoma-hyphema syndrome associated with the Mark VIII anterior chamber lens implant. J Am Intraocular Implant Soc 4:50–53, 1978.
Kielar RA, Stambaugh JL: Pupillary block glaucoma following intraocular lens implantation. Ophthalmic Surg 13:647–650, 1982.
Rowsey JJ, Gaylor JR: Intraocular lens disasters. Peripheral anterior synechia. Ophthalmology 87:646–664, 1980.
Samples JR, Van Buskirk EM: Pigmentary glaucoma associated with posterior chamber intraocular lenses. Am J Ophthalmol 100:385–388, 1985.
Samples JR, et al: Pupillary block with posterior chamber intraocular lenses. Arch Ophthalmol 105:335–337, 1987.
Van Buskirk EM: Late onset, progressive, peripheral anterior synechiae with posterior chamber intraocular lenses. Ophthalmic Surg 18:115–117, 1987.
Van Buskirk EM: Pseudophakic glaucoma. In Weinstein GW: Open Angle Glaucoma. Contemporary Issues in Ophthalmology. New York, Livingstone, Vol 3, 1986, pp 133–154.
Van Buskirk EM: Pupillary block after intraocular lens implantation. Am J Ophthalmol 95:55–59, 1983.

GLAUCOMA ASSOCIATED WITH INTRAOCULAR TUMORS

CAROL L. SHIELDS, M.D.,
and JERRY A. SHIELDS, M.D.
Philadelphia, Pennsylvania

A number of intraocular tumors can produce ipsilateral elevation of the intraocular pressure.

In such instances, there may be a delay in clinical recognition of the underlying neoplasm while the patient is treated for the secondary glaucoma. In cases of malignant tumors, this delay in diagnosis can have serious consequences.

In contrast to the primary glaucomas, which are generally bilateral, tumor-induced secondary glaucomas are almost always unilateral. The mechanism of the secondary glaucomas varies with the location, size, and type of tumor. Malignant tumors in the iris and ciliary body are more likely to obstruct aqueous outflow by directly infiltrating the trabecular meshwork. More posteriorly located intraocular neoplasms can produce anterior displacement of the lens-iris diaphragm, causing angle closure; they may induce iris and angle neovascularization, causing neovascular glaucoma; or they may liberate tumor cells in the anterior chamber angle, blocking aqueous outflow.

I. PRIMARY TUMORS OF THE UVEA

Uveal nevi are benign lesions that rarely produce secondary glaucoma. Occasionally, however, localized or diffuse uveal nevi can lead to secondary glaucoma. This most often occurs with a melanocytoma or with a diffuse nevus of the iris. Melanocytoma is a specific variant of nevus that usually occurs in the optic disc, but that can arise anywhere in the uveal tract. Those located in the optic disc or choroid rarely produce secondary glaucoma, whereas those in the ciliary body or iris are more likely to produce secondary glaucoma. This tumor has an unusual tendency to undergo necrosis and fragmentation, liberating pigment into the anterior chamber and trabecular meshwork.

With regard to iris melanoma, the most common mechanism of glaucoma is direct invasion of the trabecular meshwork by tumor tissue. Occasionally the melanoma may bleed spontaneously, leading to hyphema and increased intraocular pressure. The diffuse iris melanoma produces a classic syndrome of acquired hyperchromic heterochromia and ipsilateral glaucoma.

In contrast to iris melanomas, ciliary body melanomas tend to attain a fairly large size before they are diagnosed. Ciliary body melanomas can produce secondary glaucoma by causing anterior displacement of the iris with secondary angle closure or by growing anteriorly into the trabecular meshwork and obstructing aqueous outflow. Less commonly, they can produce a hyphema, undergo necrosis, or cause iris neovascularization, all of which can lead to secondary glaucoma.

In the authors' series of 1913 eyes with choroidal melanoma, only 32 (2 per cent) had secondary glaucoma. In most prior series, the incidence of secondary glaucoma was higher, probably reflecting the earlier clinical recognition of choroidal melanomas in recent years.

Choroidal melanomas can produce secondary glaucoma from iris and angle neovascularization (56 per cent) or by causing anterior displacement of the lens-iris diaphragm and secondary angle closure (44 per cent). Large necrotic choroidal melanomas can occasionally produce intraocular inflammation or hemorrhage, which can further contribute to secondary glaucoma.

Other rare uveal tumors, such as neurilemomas, leiomyomas, or neurofibromas, can produce secondary glaucoma by the same mechanisms.

II. METASTATIC TUMORS TO THE UVEA

Malignant tumors from distant primary sites metastasize through hematogenous routes to the uveal tract and rarely to the retina or optic nerve. Choroidal metastases only produce secondary glaucoma when they attain a large size, whereas iris and ciliary body metastases frequently produce secondary glaucoma because of their tendency to involve the angle structures. In the authors' series of patients with uveal metastases, secondary glaucoma was found in 64 per cent of iris metastasis, 67 per cent of ciliary body metastasis, and 2 per cent of choroidal metastasis. Metastatic tumors to the intraocular structures most commonly occur from primary sites in breast and lung and less often from the gastrointestinal tract and kidney.

Iris and ciliary body metastases usually produce secondary glaucoma by seeding into the anterior chamber angle and trabecular meshwork, thereby mechanically blocking aqueous outflow. In some cases, a solid growth of tumor cells can assume a ring-type infiltration of the trabecular meshwork, resulting in intractable glaucoma.

Metastatic tumors to the choroid appear as single or multiple elevated or diffuse lesions that are often associated with a secondary nonrhegmatogenous retinal detachment. The most common mechanism of glaucoma with choroidal metastases is angle closure caused by anterior displacement of the lens-iris diaphragm secondary to total retinal detachment. Neovascular glaucoma can occur in advanced cases with total retinal detachment.

In general, eyes with choroidal metastases are best managed by external beam radiotherapy to the involved eye, combined with any chemotherapy that the patient may be receiving for associated systemic metastases. Such treatment may control associated secondary glaucoma, but supplemental medical treatment of the glaucoma may still be necessary. In rare instances, the associated glaucoma can produce such severe pain that palliative enucleation is necessary.

III. PRIMARY TUMORS OF THE RETINA

The most important tumors of the sensory retina are retinoblastoma, vascular tumors, and glial tumors. Retinoblastoma, the most important retinal tumor, frequently produces secondary glaucoma. In rare instances, advanced retinal capillary hemangiomas can produce secondary glaucoma in association with a total retinal detachment.

In the authors' series of 248 patients with retinoblastoma, about 17 per cent of 303 affected eyes had secondary glaucoma. The secondary glaucoma was caused by iris neovascularization in 72 per cent, angle closure secondary to anterior displacement of the lens-iris diaphragm in 26 per cent, and tumor seeding into the anterior chamber in 2 per cent of cases. In cases with iris neovascularization, secondary hyphema sometimes contributed to the mechanism of glaucoma.

IV. TUMORS OF THE NONPIGMENTED AND PIGMENTED EPITHELIUM

Tumors of the nonpigmented epithelium of the ciliary body include medulloepithelioma, adenoma, and adenocarcinoma. The medulloepithelioma (previously called diktyoma) is an embryonic ciliary body tumor that becomes clinically apparent in the first few years of life. It can be benign or malignant, but the malignancy is low grade and the systemic prognosis is generally excellent. In the five cases of this rare tumor that the authors have managed, three patients had secondary glaucoma. In a large series from the Armed Forces Institute of Pathology, glaucoma occurred in 46 per cent of cases. In these cases, glaucoma can occur secondary to iris neovascularization or from direct invasion of the anterior chamber angle structures by the tumor. In some instances, hyphema or cysts in the anterior chamber may also contribute to obstruction of aqueous outflow.

Acquired tumors of the nonpigmented ciliary epithelium are rare, slow-growing benign or lowly malignant lesions, and they rarely produce secondary glaucoma. Primary tumors of the pigmented epithelium (adenoma and adenocarcinoma) of the iris, ciliary body, and retina are rare. The mechanisms of glaucoma are the same as those of malignant melanoma.

V. LYMPHOID TUMORS AND LEUKEMIAS

Lymphoid tumors and leukemias are grouped together here because they can produce a similar infiltration of the uveal tract and retina. The most important lymphoid tumors of the intraocular structures are benign reactive lymphoid hyperplasia (BRLH) of the uvea and malignant lymphoma, particularly large cell lymphoma (histiocytic lymphoma, reticulum cell sarcoma). Secondary glaucoma most often occurs from direct infiltration of the anterior chamber angle and thickening of the iris and ciliary body by tumor cells, which result in blockage of aqueous outflow and secondary elevation of intraocular pressure.

VI. SYSTEMIC HAMARTOMATOSES (PHAKOMATOSES)

The classic phakomatoses include encephalofacial hemangiomatosis (Sturge-Weber syndrome) neurofibromatosis, retinocerebellar capillary hemangiomatosis (von Hippel-Lindau syndrome), and tuberous sclerosis. Encephalofacial hemangiomatosis and neurofibromatosis are more likely to be associated with either infantile or juvenile glaucoma.

THERAPY

Ocular. The management of glaucoma secondary to intraocular tumors depends on the type of tumor. In cases of benign tumors, it is often appropriate first to treat the glaucoma medically. In cases of malignant tumors, it may be appropriate first to treat the tumor in hopes of relieving the glaucoma. In cases of uveal melanoma, melanocytoma, metastasis, and lymphoid infiltration, the glaucoma may resolve with the primary treatment of the tumor either by surgical resection or radiotherapy. If the glaucoma persists despite effective therapy, then medical management of the secondary glaucoma is warranted. Generally, antiglaucoma eyedrops and systemic carbonic anhydrase inhibitors are instituted as necessary.

Surgical. Most melanocytic iris tumors should be managed initially by periodic observation, and any associated glaucoma should be managed medically. If the tumor shows evidence of growth or if the secondary glaucoma cannot be controlled, surgical intervention should be considered. In cases of circumscribed tumors, excision of the tumor by a partial iridectomy, sometimes with laser or surgical trabeculectomy to control the glaucoma, can be undertaken. In the case of a diffuse iris melanoma with secondary glaucoma, enucleation is generally necessary. Biopsy of the iris tumor or surgery to control the glaucoma in cases of diffuse iris melanoma can predispose to extrascleral extension of the tumor. In the case of iris melanocytoma, the liberated pigment in the trabecular meshwork may gradually disappear after complete excision of the main tumor by iridectomy or iridocyclectomy.

Small ciliary body melanomas can be managed by simple periodic observation until growth is documented before initiating treatment. Somewhat larger tumors can be managed by local resection or episcleral plaque radiotherapy. Most tumors that are large or infiltrative enough to produce secondary glaucoma are generally best managed by enucleation of the affected eye. Careful medical evaluation and follow-up are warranted because of the relatively high risk of metastatic disease in cases of ciliary body melanomas with secondary glaucoma. In the authors' series of patients with ciliary body melanomas, 50 per cent of patients with secondary glaucoma died from metastatic melanoma within 2 years of the diagnosis.

The options in management of choroidal melanomas are well outlined in the literature and include simple observation, photocoagulation, radiotherapy, local resection, enucleation, and even orbital exenteration. Unfortunately, choroidal melanomas that have produced secondary glaucoma are generally so large that enucleation is necessary.

In some cases of uveal metastases associated with secondary glaucoma, the glaucoma may ultimately require laser or surgical trabeculectomy, cyclocryotherapy, retrobulbar alcohol injection, or even enucleation. Since most affected patients have a poor systemic prognosis, enucleation should be avoided if possible, and the goal should be to make the patient comfortable.

The management of retinoblastoma should depend on the overall clinical findings and can include enucleation, radiotherapy, cryotherapy, and photocoagulation. In cases with secondary glaucoma, the tumor is usually quite advanced, and enucleation is considered the treatment of choice. In most cases of retinoblastoma associated with secondary glaucoma, the optic disc cannot be visualized ophthalmoscopically because of the large tumor within the eye. Therefore, it is particularly important in these cases to obtain a long section of optic nerve stump along with the globe at the time of enucleation, since the most important route of extraocular extension of this tumor is through the optic nerve to the central nervous system.

Management of small intraocular medulloepitheliomas consists of an attempt at local resection by a cyclectomy because the tumor is usually benign. Unfortunately, it is extremely difficult to remove such tumors completely, and recurrence is common, eventually requiring enucleation. In cases with glaucoma, enucleation is usually necessary because of pain or because malignancy cannot be excluded clinically.

Irradiation and Chemotherapy. The management of iris and ciliary body metastases should be systemic chemotherapy or other treatment that the patient is receiving for the systemic cancer. If the ocular tumor continues to proliferate, external beam radiotherapy to the eye, giving 3500 to 4000 cGy (rads) to the affected eye in divided doses over a 4-week period should be initiated. If any associated secondary glaucoma does not resolve after chemotherapy and radiotherapy, acetazolamide, timolol, or other medications should be continued to control the intraocular pressure and to keep the patient comfortable. In many instances, the glaucoma will progress relentlessly, and laser or filtering surgery can be attempted. This decision should be made in light of the patient's prognosis, and enucleation should be avoided if the systemic prognosis is dismal.

The appropriate management of intraocular lymphoid tumors and leukemias is ocular radiotherapy combined with the chemotherapy that the patient may be receiving for the systemic disease. With BRLH, about 2000 cGy (rads) is generally sufficient, whereas with malignant lymphoma about 3000 to 4000 cGy may be necessary to bring about good resolution of the tumor. Sometimes, the glaucoma resolves with the radiotherapy or chemotherapy, but in cases with severe glaucoma, this treatment may not help, and enucleation of the eye, if it is blind and painful, may be necessary.

Ocular or Periocular Manifestations

Anterior Chamber: Hyphema, hypopyon, tumor seeds in aqueous or angle.
Choroid: Tumor.
Ciliary Body: Tumor.
Conjunctiva: Injection.
Cornea: Tumor clumps on endothelium.
Episclera: Tumor sentinel vessels over ciliary body tumor.
Eyelids: Edema.
Iris: Diffuse thickening; heterochromia; neovascularization; nodules.
Lens: Subluxed lens or cataract from ciliary body tumor compression or from chronic large bullous retinal detachment.
Optic Nerve: Engorgement; glaucomatous cupping.
Retina: Endophytic or exophytic retinoblastoma; nonrhegmatogenous retinal detachment.
Vitreous: Hemorrhage; tumor seeds from retinoblastoma, melanoma, or lymphoma.

PRECAUTIONS

A patient who presents with unexplained unilateral glaucoma could be harboring an unsuspected intraocular malignant tumor. Laser surgery or filtering procedures are contraindicated until a complete ophthalmologic examination, including careful indirect ophthalmoscopy, is performed to exclude the possibility of tumor. In cases where the posterior pole or ciliary body cannot be viewed because of opaque media, ultrasonography, transillumination, or other procedures are necessary to rule out a tumor. It is particularly important not to perform glaucoma surgery or vitrectomy on a child with vitreous cells and unilateral glaucoma until the possibility of retinoblastoma is excluded.

COMMENTS

Management of tumor-induced glaucoma usually consists of enucleation because most cases are caused by advanced uveal melanoma or retinoblastoma. In cases of benign tumors, medical therapy can be attempted first, followed by laser or surgical therapy. The management of glaucoma secondary to iris tumors is a very difficult problem, because many such tumors are relatively benign histopathologically and all efforts are made to control the glaucoma by medical or laser treatment before surgical intervention. Trabeculectomy is controversial in the management of iris melanomas because of the possibility of tumor spread into the filtering bleb and episcleral tissues.

References

Broughton WL, Zimmerman LE: A clinicopathologic study of 56 cases of intraocular medulloepitheliomas. Am J Ophthalmol 85:407–418, 1978.

Duker JS, Shields JA, Ross M: Intraocular large cell lymphoma presenting as massive thickening of the uveal tract. Retina 7:41–45, 1987.
Shields CL, et al: Prevalence and mechanisms of secondary intraocular pressure elevation in eyes with intraocular tumors. Ophthalmology 94:839–846, 1987.
Shields JA: Current approaches to the diagnosis and management of choroidal melanomas. Surv Ophthalmol 21:443–463, 1977.
Shields JA: Diagnosis and Management of Intraocular Tumors. St. Louis, CV Mosby, 1983.
Shields JA, Augsburger JJ: Current approaches to the diagnosis and management of retinoblastoma. Surv Ophthalmol 25:347–372, 1981.
Shields JA, Annesley WH, Spaeth GL: Necrotic melanocytoma of iris with secondary glaucoma. Am J Ophthalmol 84:826–829, 1977.

GLAUCOMATOCYCLITIC CRISIS
(Posner-Schlossman Syndrome)
ABRAHAM SCHLOSSMAN, M.D.
New York, New York

Glaucomatocyclitic crisis is unilateral glaucoma characterized by recurrent attacks of glaucoma that are usually associated with signs of mild cyclitis. The disease generally occurs in patients between 20 to 50 years of age, with individual attacks of ocular hypertension lasting from a few hours to 1 month, but very rarely over 2 weeks. The onset of symptoms is acute with minimal ocular discomfort, blurred vision, and colored halos around lights. The intraocular pressure fluctuates, but initially is usually between 40 and 60 mm Hg. A few keratic precipitates are present, and the pupil of the affected eye is larger than that of the other. Synechiae generally do not develop. The prognosis is excellent, with no permanent changes detectable in the visual fields after an attack.

THERAPY

Ocular. Treatment of the ocular hypertension should be limited to the attack and consist of the use of mild miotics, such as 0.5 to 2.0 per cent pilocarpine or 0.25 to 0.50 per cent timolol. Topical ocular corticosteroids are used one to four times daily to control inflammation and are especially helpful during the acute phase. Occasional pupillary dilation with 10 per cent phenylephrine usually confirms that no synechiae are forming.

Supportive. Analgesics or tranquilizers may be helpful during attacks to control pain and apprehension. Follow-up examinations are important to monitor inflammation or pressure elevation.

Ocular or Periocular Manifestations

Anterior Chamber: Cells and flare.
Cornea: Epithelial edema; keratic precipitates.
Iris: Anterior and posterior synechiae (rare); ciliary flush; hypochromic heterochromia.
Optic Nerve: Glaucomatous cupping (rare).
Other: Decreased visual acuity (temporary); increased intraocular pressure; mydriasis.

PRECAUTIONS

Strong miotics and, perhaps, strong mydriatics tend to aggravate the symptoms by producing pain, congestion, and spasm of the ciliary muscle.
In view of the ineffectiveness of surgical measures and the benign and self-limited nature of the disease, there exists no indication for any surgical intervention in this syndrome. Medical therapy between attacks is not indicated.
Topical corticosteroids give good results by allaying ciliary irritability. However, corticosteroid-induced glaucoma may occur if such treatment is prolonged.

COMMENTS

The value of recognizing this syndrome lies in the fact that surgical procedures not only are unnecessary but are definitely contraindicated in this condition. Glaucomatocyclitic crises differ from acute narrow-angle glaucoma and glaucoma secondary to uveitis in that the angle of the anterior chamber is open, even at the height of an attack, and the eye is white with minimal pain during attacks. Also, facility of outflow is normal between attacks, and provocative tests give normal responses.

References

de Roetth A Jr: Glaucomatocyclitic crisis. Am J Ophthalmol 69:370–371, 1970.
Hollwich F: Zur Klinik und Therapie des Posner-Schlossman Syndroms. Klin Monatsbl Augenheilkd 172:736–744, 1978.
Posner A, Schlossman A: Syndrome of unilateral attacks of glaucoma with cyclitic symptoms. Arch Ophthalmol 39:517–535, 1948.
Posner A, Schlossman A: Further observations on the syndrome of glaucomatocyclitic crises. Trans Am Acad Ophthalmol Otolaryngol 57:531–536, 1953.
Reibaldi A, Avitabile T: Topical indomethacin in Posner and Schlossman's syndrome. J Ocular Ther Surg 4:28–31, 1985.
Theodore FH: Observations on glaucomatocyclitic crises (Posner-Schlossman syndrome). Br J Ophthalmol 36:207–210, 1952.
Varma R, Katz LJ, Spaeth GL: Surgical treatment of acute glaucomatocyclitic crisis in a patient with primary open-angle glaucoma. Am J Ophthalmol 105:99–100, 1988.

INFANTILE GLAUCOMA
(Primary Congenital Open-Angle Glaucoma)
DAVID S. WALTON, M.D.
Boston, Massachusetts

Infantile glaucoma is a specific type of childhood glaucoma and the most common cause of glaucoma in early childhood. It is caused by polygenic inheritance and is usually bilateral. The elevation of intraocular pressure is caused by a defect of the internal surface of the filtration angle. The severity of the disease is very variable, and there is a marked difference between patients in respect to the severity of symptoms and corneal signs and, subsequently, the age of diagnosis. Most patients are symptomatic before 3 months of age and diagnosed before 9 months of age. They usually possess significant light sensitivity, corneal stigmata of increased eye pressure (including defects in Descemet's membrane), and variable amounts of optic nerve cupping.

THERAPY

Surgical. The treatment of infantile glaucoma is surgical. Internal goniotomy or trabeculotomy is indicated. Surgery should be performed by surgeons experienced with these procedures and in the care of children with glaucoma. If control is not attained after repeating these procedures, filtration surgery must be considered. Cyclocryotherapy also may be employed safely and successfully, but should be reserved for use after the above surgery has failed.

Ocular. Miotics rarely are helpful for this type of glaucoma. In young children, timolol has also not proven to be a useful agent. Carbonic anhydrase inhibitors lower the eye pressure significantly in young children, but acetazolamide infrequently normalizes the pressure in infantile glaucoma. However, these agents are useful to achieve some clearing of the corneal edema and to lower the pressure before surgery is performed.

Ocular or Periocular Manifestations

Anterior Chamber: Deep; flat iris.
Ciliary Body: Poorly defined and occasionally narrow ciliary body band; poorly defined or absent scleral spur.
Cornea: Breaks in Descemet's membrane; enlargement; epithelial edema; limbal thinning; stromal edema.
Iris: Easily visible peripheral iris blood vessels and posterior pigmented epithelium.
Optic Nerve: Atrophy; glaucomatous cupping.
Other: Amblyopia; epiphora; myopia.

PRECAUTIONS

There are many causes of glaucoma in infancy and early childhood. Both primary childhood glaucomas and secondary causes of glaucoma must be considered. Careful examination of the patient with childhood glaucoma must be performed to rule out the presence of systemic or related ocular abnormalities before the diagnosis of primary congenital open-angle glaucoma can be made with confidence.

COMMENTS

The infant's eye is quickly damaged by increased intraocular pressure. The earlier the diagnosis of glaucoma is made and the more effectively pressure is brought under control, the less likely is the occurrence of secondary glaucomatous changes, such as tears in Descemet's membrane, increase in corneal size, corneal edema, damage to the optic discs, and visual field defects.

However, one must remember that vision, not pressure control, must be the goal of the ophthalmic surgeon. All children with infantile glaucoma should be examined regularly. Refraction should be part of the routine periodic examination of these children. If a child develops a deviation or a significant degree of anisometropia, treatment to prevent amblyopia should be begun promptly. Finally, the patient must have continuing examination for life to avoid the tragic loss of vision that can accompany late undetected increases in intraocular pressure.

References

Anderson DR: The development of the trabecular meshwork and its abnormality in primary infantile glaucoma. Trans Am Ophthalmol Soc 79:458–485, 1981.
DeLuise VP, Anderson DR: Review: Primary infantile glaucoma. Surv Ophthalmol 28:1–19, 1983.
Shaffer RN, Weiss DI: Congenital and Pediatric Glaucomas. St. Louis, CV Mosby, 1970, pp 37–59.
Walton DS: Primary congenital open-angle glaucoma: A study of the anterior segment abnormalities. Trans Am Ophthalmol Soc 77:746–768, 1979.
Walton DS: Primary congenital open-angle glaucoma. *In* Chandler PA, Grant WM: Glaucoma, 2nd ed. Philadelphia, Lea & Febiger, 1979, pp. 329–343.

JUVENILE GLAUCOMA
MARIANNE E. FEITL, M.D.,
and THEODORE KRUPIN, M.D.
Philadelphia, Pennsylvania

Juvenile glaucoma is not a single disease entity; rather, it is a heterogeneous grouping of glaucomas with an onset in older children and young adults. Age limits are arbitrarily set at between 3 to 5 and 30 to 35 years of age, which is after the onset of most cases of infantile glaucoma and before the manifestation of most adult primary glaucomas. In a large series of glaucoma patients, only a small number, approximately 0.02 per cent, were diagnosed within this age interval. Unfortunately, because of a low index of suspicion on the part of the physician, the diagnosis of glaucoma within this age group is easily overlooked.

Milder cases of primary congenital glaucoma may go unrecognized until later in childhood. These children show no sign of ocular discomfort and have perfectly clear corneas with only mild corneal enlargement or breaks in Descemet's membrane (Haab's striae). Progressive myopia and corneal enlargement may rarely occur in glaucoma in children over the age of 3 years, although severe buphthalmous does not generally occur. Juvenile-onset glaucoma can occur in other conditions associated with abnormal iridocorneal angles; aniridia, iridocorneal dysgenesis (Axenfeld's or Rieger's syndrome), Sturge-Weber syndrome, neurofibromatosis, and Lowe's syndrome.

Glaucoma secondary to traumatic angle recession, hyphema, glaucomatocyclitic crisis, and rubeosis iridis may occur in this age group. Neoplasia, including the phakomatoses, retinoblastoma, acute leukemia, juvenile xanthogranuloma, and medulloepithelioma, may also cause secondary glaucoma. An important cause of secondary glaucoma is previous surgery for congenital cataract. Glaucoma may also be found in patients with congenital rubella. Glaucoma in ocular rubella may be caused by iridocyclitis, angle anomalies resembling primary congenital glaucoma or mesodermal dysgenesis, an intumescent lens, or pupillary block after cataract extraction. Although the ocular abnormalities are usually noted in the neonatal period, the glaucoma may have its onset in later childhood or young adulthood. These late-onset glaucomas are most often found in eyes with microphthalmia and cataracts.

Patients with juvenile rheumatoid arthritis (JRA) have a significant incidence (8 to 24 per cent) of uveitis that may lead to glaucoma. Female patients and patients with mono- or pauciarticular JRA have a higher incidence of iridocyclitis than those with the polyarticular form. Since patients are often asymptomatic, they must be examined frequently for ocular involvement. Of note, no parallel has been found between the activity of the iridocyclitis and the joint disease. The iritis may first develop in patients over the age of 16, although an earlier onset is more common. Appropriate treatment with cycloplegics and steroids should be instituted to prevent peripheral anterior synechiae or neovascular membranes. Antiglaucoma therapy, with the avoidance of miotics, should be instituted if necessary. Other important causes of uveitis include sarcoidosis, ankylosing spondylitis, herpes zoster, syphilis, tuberculosis, and alkaline injuries.

Some cases of juvenile-onset glaucoma resemble primary open-angle glaucoma of the adult type. The possibility of secondary open-angle glaucoma related to topically applied corticosteroids, especially in contact lens wearers, must be eliminated by a careful history. In contrast to primary open-angle glaucoma, which occurs after the age of 50 years, there is a preponderance of male patients and of myopia in this condition, and also true of pigmentary glaucoma, which may have its onset during this age interval. These patients characteristically show midperipheral iris transillumination defects and pigment deposition on the corneal endothelium (Krukenberg's spindle), trabecular meshwork, iris, and lens. The disease appears to become less severe in some patients with advancing age. This decrease in severity may be due to an increase in the axial length of the lens, which elevates the peripheral iris above the lens zonules and decreases pigment liberation. Intraocular pressure in pigmentary glaucoma is subject to large spontaneous fluctuations, which must be considered in evaluating the response to medical treatment. These patients occasionally manifest the classic symptoms of an acute intraocular pressure rise, particularly after an iris pigment "shower" from mydriasis or physical exercise.

Primary angle-closure glaucoma is extremely rare in young people. When present, it is most commonly of the plateau iris type. Angle-closure glaucoma in children as a result of pupillary block is usually secondary to other ocular disorders, including microcornea, spherophakia (Marchesani's syndrome), a dislocated lens (Marfan's syndrome or homocystinuria), retrolental fibroplasia, or intraocular surgery, particularly for congenital cataracts.

THERAPY

Ocular. Most patients with juvenile open-angle glaucoma should be given a thorough trial with medical therapy. Treatment is tempered by the same consideration as with the adult glaucomas. Children are less likely than adults to complain of drug side effects and thus must be watched and questioned more carefully. The beta-adrenergic blocking drugs are not approved for use in children. Although these agents can be effective, they should be avoided in patients with asthma because of their bronchospastic effects. They also should not be used in patients with heart problems, including congestive heart failure. Topical 1 per cent epinephrine administered twice daily is an excellent hypotensive agent in juvenile patients and may be used alone or in combination with miotics or other agents. The prodrug dipivefrin is sometimes tolerated in patients who demonstrate an intolerance to topical epinephrine. Maculopathy that is reversible on stopping the topical medication can occur in aphakic eyes with either epinephrine or dipivefrin.

Oral carbonic anhydrase inhibitors are often useful and better tolerated than miotics in young glaucoma patients. Acetazolamide in daily oral doses of 15 to 30 mg/kg is administered in divided doses. Methazolamide may cause fewer side effects than acetazolamide. The possibility of renal calculi should be borne in mind and indicated to the parents. In addition, there may be a possible association of the carbonic anhydrase inhibitors with bone marrow depression and aplastic anemia.

Topical pilocarpine is an effective ocular hypotensive agent, particularly in children with open and relatively normal-appearing angles. However, despite this drug's efficacy, the induced miosis and myopia may cause sufficiently disabling symptoms to prevent its use. Occasionally, bedtime administration of pilocarpine gel is better tolerated than pilocarpine drops. Membrane-controlled pilocarpine delivery systems (Ocuserts) offer the advantages of less miosis, less induced myopia, and theoretically better diurnal intraocular pressure control. However, some patients have difficulty retaining these membranes in the cul-de-sac. Carbachol is also an excellent replacement or alternate drug for pilocarpine when resistance has developed.

Synthetic anticholinesterase agents—echothiophate, demecarium, and isofluorophate—have a long duration of action and may be better accepted than pilocarpine by young patients. Many younger patients tolerate these strong anticholinesterase drugs used as a single dose at bedtime. They produce excellent glaucoma control and a fairly constant accommodative status that can be corrected with glasses. These agents should be started in children at the lower concentrations, increasing the dosage stepwise as needed. The stronger miotics are contraindicated in the treatment of patients with narrow iridocorneal angles.

Parents of children on cholinesterase inhibitors should be warned about complications from succinylcholine administration during general anesthesia and interaction with organophosphorus insecticides. Caution regarding the development of cataracts and iris cysts is warranted in the use of these agents. Strong miotics should be temporarily discontinued at regular intervals to prevent intractable miosis, to assess the lens for cataract, and to examine the peripheral fundus for retinal pathology. Phenylephrine 2.5 per cent may be either added to the anticholinesterase preparation or used concurrently to reduce the side effect of iris cysts. The ability of the anticholinesterase agent to lower intraocular pressure is not diminished by phenylephrine.

Young patients should be examined frequently until maintenance of a satisfactory intraocular pressure level is achieved. In the absence of reliable visual fields, one must rely more heavily on correlation of intraocular pressure level and the stability of optic disc damage.

Surgical. Medical therapy is usually less effective in juvenile than in adult-onset primary glaucoma, and surgical intervention is often necessary. Iridectomy is the procedure of choice in primary or secondary angle closure. Mechanical and technical incompatibilities of the slitlamp-based laser and the need for general anesthesia may dictate a surgical rather than a laser iridectomy.

Goniotomy or ab externo trabeculotomy is indicated as the initial surgery in eyes with congenital glaucoma. Gonioscopically, the iridocorneal angle has a thick, spongy, and ground-glass uveotrabecular meshwork with poorly defined normal landmarks. The surgeon should attempt to include as many clock hours of the circumference as possible during the goniotomy incision. The same consideration applies for trabeculotomy, which functions similarly to goniotomy. Trabeculotomy is currently the preferred procedure by most surgeons and is the procedure of choice when corneal clouding prevents visualization of angle structures. Surgical results in congenital glaucoma are similar after either procedure. In addition, excellent results are claimed for trabeculotomy in infantile and juvenile glaucoma.

Filtration surgery, full or partial thickness (trabeculectomy), is less likely to be successful in juvenile than in adult glaucoma. The lower success rate in younger patients may relate both to enhanced postoperative scarring and to the types of glaucomas that tend to occur in this age group. Trabeculectomy in eyes with previous surgery or secondary glaucoma, particularly neovascular glaucoma, has a poor prognosis. The success rate for primary glaucoma in one series of young patients approached the rates quoted earlier for older patients. Trabeculectomy for primary glaucoma was successful in 25 of 30 (83 per cent) of patients aged 30 to 49 years, but only in 4 of 9 (44 per cent) patients under 30 years of age. Age as an isolated factor may have its greatest influence on surgical outcome in patients under 30 years of age. In youth, Tenon's tissue is more extensive, postoperative hypotony may be prolonged, wound healing may be more vigorous, and postoperative examination is often less than ideal. Because limbal surgical landmarks can be obscure, transillumination at the time of surgery is recommended to avoid placing the sclerostomy incision too posterior. A lamellar scleral flap helps identify the limbal surgical anatomy, in particular the scleral spur. It aids proper surgical entry into the anterior chamber. In addition, the scleral flap lowers the incidence of a postoperative flat anterior chamber and results in a thicker, more diffuse filtration bleb. However, the surgeon should remember that the sclera may be thinner in the juvenile eye, making scleral flap dissection more difficult. Corticosteroids should be used after filtration surgery to diminish postoperative inflammation and scarring of the bleb. A sub-Tenon's injection of a short-acting corticosteroid, such as dexamethasone* or triamcinolone,* at the completion of surgery and the use of topical corticosteroid drops or ointment for a minimum of 7 to 10 days after surgery are recommended. Postoperative subconjunctival injections of 5-fluorouracil* are usually impossible in young patients.

Cyclodialysis is rarely successful in children and probably should not be attempted, particularly in phakic eyes. The frequency of postoperative cataract formation, even in successful cases, is very high.

In glaucoma associated with aniridia, stripping iris stroma from the trabecular meshwork is recommended in eyes with progressive closure of the anterior chamber angle. If this approach is chosen, it should be performed before the development of complete synechial angle closure.

Cyclocryotherapy has several useful applications in the management of juvenile glaucoma. It may be effective in aphakic patients with an open or partially open anterior chamber angle. It may also be used to provide intraocular pressure control in circumstances where filtration surgery is likely to fail. This procedure has a high complication rate (e.g., phthisis bulbi and loss of vision) when used in the therapy of neovasular glaucoma and should not be used to treat this condition in eyes with visual potential. New types of cyclodestructive procedures, such as Neodymium YAG transcleral laser and therapeutic ultrasound, have limited experience in juvenile glaucoma. Their potential complications are not fully known in the young patient.

Seton devices have been used in juvenile-onset glaucoma eyes that have failed routine filtration surgery. Encouraging results have been reported using the Molteno implant and the long glaucoma valve implant. Both of these devices place an open plastic tube into the anterior chamber that is attached to an equatorial episcleral plate (Molteno) or to an encircling episcleral explant (valve implant). The resulting bleb is posterior, over the area of the encapsulated explant.

Precautions

Perhaps the saddest error in dealing with these patients is failure of early recognition. The fellow eye of patients with apparent uniocular congenital glaucoma should be followed very carefully for possible late-onset congenital glaucoma. Young patients with advancing high myopia should be regarded as potential candidates for glaucoma. Applanation tonometry is preferable to Schiötz tonometry in these patients because of their low ocular rigidity. A positive family history of glaucoma in children should suggest examination of the patient's relatives and siblings.

Comments

With the availability of hand-held portable applanation tonometers, office measurement of intraocular pressure can usually be performed on most children. It should be considered part of the complete pediatric ophthalmologic examination whenever glaucoma is suspected and should be performed in all patients who can cooperate. Gonioscopy may be performed successfully in many children, often with surprising ease; it should be attempted when gonioscopic abnormalities are suspected. Reliable visual fields are difficult to obtain in young children, placing more responsibility on the ophthalmologist for accurate assessment and recording of optic disc appearance. Routine examination of the optic disc should be done in all patients. In children on whom tonometry cannot be performed, the optic disc examination may reveal suspected or definite damage from elevated intraocular pressure. In those patients, further examination under anesthesia is warranted. If possible, the optic disc should be photographed several times yearly in individuals with suspected or proven juvenile-onset glaucoma. Rapid increase and reversal of cupping are seen much more frequently in children with glaucoma than in adults.

References

Barsoum-Homsy M, Chevrette L: Incidence and prognosis of childhood glaucoma. Ophthalmology 93:1323–1327, 1986.
Boger WP III, Walton DS: Timolol in uncontrolled childhood glaucomas. Ophthalmology 88:253–258, 1981.
Chew E, Morin JD: Glaucoma in children. Pediatr Clin North Am 30:1043–1061, 1983.
Dicken JC, Hoskins HD Jr: Diagnosis and treatment of congenital glaucoma. In Ritch R, Shields MB, Krupin T (eds): The Glaucomas, Vol II. St. Louis, CV Mosby, 1989, pp 773–785.
Gressel MG, Meuer DK, Parrish RK II, Trabeculectomy in young patients. Ophthalmology 91:1242–1246, 1984.
Hoskins HD Jr et al: Clinical experience with timolol in childhood glaucoma. Arch Ophthalmol 103:1163–1166, 1985.
Kass MA, et al: Acetazolamide and urolithiasis. Ophthalmology 88:261–265, 1981.
Krupin T: Surgical treatment of glaucoma with the Krupin-Denver valve. In Cairns JE (ed): Glaucoma. London, Grune and Stratton, 1986, Vol I, pp 239–245.
Molteno ACB: Use of Molteno implants to treat secondary glaucoma. In Cairns JE (ed): Glaucoma. London, Grune and Stratton, 1986, Vol I, pp 211–238.
Ritch R: Pigmentary glaucoma—A self-limited entity. Ann Ophthalmol 15:115–116, 1983.
Walton DS: Juvenile open-angle glaucoma. In Chandler PA, Grant WM, Glaucoma, 3rd ed. Philadelphia, Lea & Febiger, 1986, pp 528–529.

LENS—INDUCED GLAUCOMA
(Phacolytic Glaucoma)

DAVID L. EPSTEIN, M.D.

Boston, Massachusetts

Phacolytic glaucoma classically refers to a secondary open-angle glaucoma of rapid onset associated with a leaking hypermature or mature cataract. Although obstruction of the trabecular meshwork by lens-protein engorged macrophages has been postulated to be a mechanism for such glaucoma, recent studies have indicated that direct obstruction of the outflow pathways by the leaking lens proteins themselves may be an important factor.

Patients with phacolytic glaucoma present with an acute elevation of intraocular pressure, frequently to very high levels. Corneal epithelial edema is usual. The angle is open. Slitlamp examination of the anterior chamber usually reveals heavy flare but a variable cellular content. Often, chunky white particles, larger than cells, can be seen floating in the aqueous. Cellular reaction may be minimal. Although the condition is usually associated with a mature or hypermature cataract, rare cases can occur with immature cataracts, which may leak posteriorly. Patches of white material that are probably macrophages can often be seen on the lens capsule.

THERAPY

Ocular. Most often, eyes with phacolytic glaucoma show minimal response to topical ophthalmic antiglaucoma or anti-inflammatory therapy. However, other types of glaucoma caused by retained lens cortex after extracapsular cataract surgery or lens injury may respond to medical therapy. This glaucoma is probably caused by direct obstruction of the outflow channels by the liberated particulate lens material or possibly by the inflammatory reaction to such lens material. In such cases, if not too much free lens material is present, medical therapy consisting of cycloplegics, carbonic anhydrase inhibitors, timolol, and possibly corticosteroids may control the intraocular pressure until the lens material is spontaneously absorbed. If the glaucoma is severe, the residual lens material must be removed surgically.

The eye pressure in phacolytic glaucoma (leaking hypermature cataract) will usually rise progressively and may be temporarily reduced with systemic carbonic anhydrase inhibitors and osmotic therapy. Initially, 250 mg of acetazolamide should be given intravenously. This may be repeated in 30 to 60 minutes and then every 6 hours. A 50 per cent solution of glycerin in fruit juice or cola drink may be given orally in doses of 1.5 gm/kg (0.7 ml/kg), or an intravenous solution of 1 to 2 gm/kg of mannitol may be necessary in patients who are vomiting. Topical 0.5 per cent timolol may also be used every 12 hours to lower the pressure temporarily.

Pain medication is frequently necessary, and 50 mg of intramuscular meperidine may be of value.

Surgical. The intraocular pressure should be followed closely, and emergency cataract extraction may be required. Because of the fragile nature of the leaking lens capsule, chymotrypsin should be utilized in intracapsular surgery. A sector iridectomy is recommended for ease of delivery. An unplanned extracapsular extraction, in which hypermature lens material is left in the eye, may be very deleterious postoperatively, and every precaution to prevent this procedure should be employed. An intact senile nucleus should never be allowed to remain in the eye after extracapsular surgery, since it will invariably cause a severe lens reaction. Phacoanaphylaxis may result when lens material is sequestered in the eye, especially in the vitreous. When vitreous loss occurs during an extracapsular extraction in an adult, as much lens material as possible should be removed primarily at the time of the surgery.

Following uncomplicated cataract surgery, the intraocular pressure returns to normal within a few days.

A recent report suggests that planned extracapsular cataract surgery with a posterior chamber intraocular lens following thorough removal of lens material is safe and effective in phacolytic glaucoma.

PRECAUTIONS

In the differential diagnosis of phacolytic glaucoma, one must consider that a swollen cataractous lens can induce angle-closure glaucoma.

Secondary open-angle glaucoma caused by non-lens-related primary uveitis can certainly occur in patients with cataracts. Characteristic of phacolytic glaucoma is the eventual failure of response to topical ophthalmic therapy. When in doubt as to whether glaucoma is caused by phacolysis or primary uveitis, such as in the case of an immature cataract, standard medical therapy for uveitis should be tried first. Diagnostic paracentesis can establish the correct diagnosis.

In cases of phacolytic glaucoma with lenses that are dislocated into the vitreous, the presentation may be more subacute and the ocular signs more subtle. Differential diagnosis includes traumatic angle-recession glaucoma, primary open-angle glaucoma, and an idiopathic type of chronic open-angle glaucoma that is apparently not related to obvious angle recession or lens reaction.

COMMENTS

Phacolytic glaucoma usually occurs unilaterally. The preoperative vision is not indicative of the vision to be obtained postoperatively, since the postoperative results are surprisingly good if the intraocular pressure has not been elevated for significant periods of time. This is true even in patients with questionable light perception and projection preoperatively. In one series, at least 25 per cent of the eyes with phacolytic glaucoma had angle recession. The cause for this is unknown, although this may indicate that many of these eyes had trauma that led to cataract formation.

References

Epstein DL: Lens-induced glaucoma. *In* Chandler PA, Grant WM: Glaucoma, 2nd ed. Philadelphia, Lea & Febiger, 1979, pp 216–223.

Epstein DL, Jedziniak JA, Grant WM: Identification of heavy-molecular-weight soluble protein in aqueous humor in human phacolytic glaucoma. Invest Ophthalmol Vis Sci 17:398–402, 1978.

Epstein DL, Jedziniak JA, Grant WM: Obstruction of aqueous outflow by lens particles and by heavy-molecular weight soluble lens proteins. Invest Ophthalmol Vis Sci 17:272–277, 1978.

Kolker AE, Hetherington J Jr: Becker-Shaffer's Diagnosis and Therapy of the Glaucomas, 4th ed. St. Louis, CV Mosby, 1976, pp 242–244.

should be continued for 4 to 5 days, by which time approximately half of the patients will be controlled. After this time, medical therapy can be gradually withdrawn, beginning with the hyperosmotics and carbonic anhydrase inhibitors, followed by beta-blockers and mydriatics. Cycloplegics should probably be continued indefinitely, as malignant glaucoma unresponsive to medical therapy may recur if they are stopped.

Aphakic and pseudophakic eyes should also receive a trial of the same medical regimen. However, response of these eyes to medical therapy is generally poor, probably because they lack a normal crystalline lens and cycloplegics can no longer effectively counteract the anterior force of the vitreous face. If rapid improvement does not occur, surgical treatment should be begun without delay.

Surgical. Definitive surgery for malignant glaucoma involves opening the anterior vitreous face to give diverted aqueous humor direct access to the posterior chamber. This can often be accomplished with the Neodymium YAG laser using single 2- to 5-mJ pulses in aphakic and pseudophakic eyes, either through the pupil or through the peripheral iridectomy if the vitreous face can be seen between the ciliary processes. Neodymium YAG laser treatment is less successful in phakic eyes, which generally require a mechanical anterior vitrectomy.

If Neodymium YAG laser treatment to the anterior vitreous face is unsuccessful, direct argon laser photocoagulation of visible ciliary processes through the peripheral iridectomy, combined with conventional medical therapy, may occasionally eliminate the need for more invasive surgery.

If neither medical nor laser treatments are successful in relieving malignant glaucoma, surgical incision of the anterior and if possible the posterior face of the vitreous should be attempted. An ultrasound should first be done to check for suprachoroidal hemorrhage. If it is negative and a sufficient view of the posterior pole exists, the surgeon should perform a mechanical subtotal anterior vitrectomy through the pars plana.

If the view of the posterior pole is not adequate for vitrectomy, then vitreous aspiration as described by Chandler is indicated. In phakic eyes, a sclerotomy is made 3 to 3.5 mm posterior to the limbus and treated with diathermy to prevent bleeding of the underlying pars plana. An 18- to 20-gauge sharp needle is then passed 12 mm into the globe toward the optic nerve, and fluid is allowed to escape spontaneously. An additional 1 to 1.5 ml of fluid is then aspirated and the anterior chamber partially reformed by injecting balanced salt solution through a preplaced paracentesis. Air is injected to deepen the anterior chamber to myopic depth, but still leaving the eye soft. Atropine should be used for an indefinite period after the operation. Occasionally, this procedure may have to be repeated to control the attack finally.

In aphakic eyes, Neodymium YAG disruption of the anterior vitreous face often dramatically deepens the anterior chamber with lowering of intraocular pressure. If not, mechanical vitrectomy or vitreous aspiration can be performed via the limbus and through the pupil. If a posterior chamber lens is present, a pars plana anterior vitrectomy is required, with particular attention to eliminating lens capsule and cortical remnants immediately behind an otherwise patent peripheral iridectomy.

Ocular or Periocular Manifestations

Anterior Chamber: Angle closure; shallow or flat centrally.
Ciliary Body: Ciliary process apposition or overlapping of the lens equator.
Cornea: Edema (from high intraocular pressure of lenticular touch).
Lens: Anterior shift of lens; cataract (from corneal touch).
Optic Nerve: Glaucomatous cupping; Pallor.
Other: Clear spaces in vitreous; elevated intraocular pressure; thickened, glassy appearance of anterior vitreous face.

PRECAUTIONS

Patients receiving the medical regimen outlined earlier should be carefully monitored for adverse, life-threatening side effects. Hyperosmotic agents produce an osmotic diuresis with depletion of fluids and electrolytes. However, these same drugs can precipitate pulmonary edema in patients with poor cardiac or renal function. Carbonic anhydrase inhibitors can cause hypokalemia if used with diuretics and metabolic acidosis in patients with pulmonary insufficiency. Rare, life-threatening blood dyscrasias have been reported. Blood pressure should be monitored because topical 2.5 per cent phenylephrine may exacerbate pre-existing hypertension. In patients with reactive airway disease, beta-blockers should probably be limited to betaxolol with the consent of the patient's internist and close monitoring of pulmonary function.

If vitreous aspiration is required, the needle should be clamped 12 mm from its tip with a hemostat, which will thus prevent it from being inserted too far into the eye and traumatizing the retina or optic nerve head. The insertion site of the needle should be carefully placed between 3 to 3.5 mm from the limbus, since a more posterior insertion will enter through the vitreous base and not successfully incise the anterior vitreous face. A more anterior insertion may damage the lens. The eye should be moderately hypotonic at the end of the operation, since overfilling the anterior chamber may divert more fluid or air into the vitreous and the anterior chamber will once again flatten.

COMMENTS

Malignant glaucoma occurs in only 1 to 4 per cent of patients requiring surgery for pupillary block. However, this condition may also develop in apparently normal eyes after cataract extraction and posterior chamber lens implantation and should be considered whenever a shallow anterior chamber and elevated intraocular pressure coexist.

Elevated intraocular pressure with a shallow anterior chamber may also result from pupillary block, a swollen or dislocated lens, ciliochoroidal effusion, and suprachoroidal hemorrhage. Before diagnosing malignant glaucoma, one must check for a patent iridectomy. Asymmetric or extreme shallowing of the central anterior chamber also differentiates malignant glaucoma from pupillary block, since the lens is not forced anteriorly in the latter. In pseudophakia, many cases of "pupillary block" may in fact be malignant glaucoma. The appearance of vitreous bulging around the posterior chamber lens optic or through the peripheral iridectomy can clarify the diagnosis. Furthermore, an ultrasound may demonstrate a compressed anterior vitreous face and clear spaces posteriorly that presumably are filled with aqueous humor.

Although ciliochoroidal effusions are usually associated with hypotony, ciliary detachment may occasionally mechanically obstruct the chamber angle and cause glaucoma. If the fundus is not easily seen or a red reflex is absent, ultrasound may help diagnose choroidal effusions, as well as suprachoroidal hemorrhage, which is characterized by a sudden onset of severe pain.

Patients with malignant glaucoma in one eye have a significant chance of developing the same condition in the other eye if an angle closure attack requires subsequent surgery. Prophylactic laser iridotomy should therefore be done as soon as possible in all fellow eyes, and if surgery is required, cycloplegia should probably be used afterward indefinitely.

References

Chandler PA, Simmons RJ, Grant WM: Malignant glaucoma. Medical and surgical treatment. Am J Ophthalmol 66:495–502, 1968.
Epstein DL, Steinert RF, Puliafito CA: Neodymium-YAG laser therapy to the anterior gyaloid in aphakic malignant (ciliovitreal block) glaucoma. Am J Ophthalmol 98:137–143, 1984.
Hershler J: Laser shrinkage of the ciliary processes. A treatment for malignant (ciliary block) glaucoma. Ophthalmology 87:1155–1159, 1980.
Lynch MG, et al: Surgical vitrectomy for pseudophakic malignant glaucoma. Am J Ophthalmol 102:149–153, 1986.
Rieser JC, Schwartz B: Miotic-induced malignant glaucoma. Arch Ophthalmol 87:706–712, 1986.
Shaffer RN: The role of vitreous detachment in aphakic and malignant glaucoma. Trans Am Acad Ophthalmol Otolaryngol 58:217–231, 1954.
Shields MB: Textbook of Glaucoma, 2nd ed. Baltimore, Williams & Wilkins, 1987, pp 334–339.
Shrader CE, et al: Pupillary and iridovitreal block in pseudophakic eyes. Ophthalmology 91:831–837, 1984.
Simmons RJ: Malignant glaucoma. Br J Ophthalmol 56:263–272, 1972.
Weiss DJ, Shaffer RN: Ciliary block (malignant) glaucoma. Trans Am Acad Ophthalmol Otolaryngol 76:450–460, 1972.

OCULAR HYPERTENSION
STEVEN M. PODOS, M.D.,
and ROBERT RITCH, M.D.
New York, New York

It was not recognized until the middle of the 20th century that elevation of intraocular pressure is not always associated with damage to the optic nerve head and loss of vision. Ocular hypertension is not a specific disease, but a descriptive term used operationally to define the status of an eye with an open angle that has an "abnormally high" intraocular pressure but shows no clinically detectable glaucomatous damage. The adoption of the term underscored the feeling that treatment with antiglaucoma drugs was not warranted in all patients with elevated intraocular pressure. Although the term is used to differentiate patients with elevated intraocular pressure alone from those with primary open-angle glaucoma, the concept of ocular hypertension is useful also in therapeutic decisions involving those secondary entities, such as pseudoexfoliation and pigmentary dispersion syndrome, for which treatment is essentially the same as for primary open-angle glaucoma.

For large mixed populations, mean intraocular pressure is about 15.9 ± 2.9 mm Hg. Abnormally increased intraocular pressure has been arbitrarily defined as two standard deviations above the mean, so that pressures of 21.7 mm Hg or greater have been considered abnormal. The distribution of intraocular pressure within the population approximates a Gaussian curve but, rather than being symmetric about the mean, is skewed to the right. A skewed frequency distribution indicates that 95 per cent of the area under the distribution curve does not lie within two standard deviations of the mean. Therefore, the upper limit of "normal" intraocular pressure is not necessarily 21 mm Hg, nor is an eye with a "normal" intraocular pressure immune to glaucomatous damage. Consequently, the idea of a maximum "normal" intraocular pressure must be considered as only an estimation.

An intraocular pressure of 22 mm Hg is conventionally used as the dividing line in defining ocular hypertension. Included in this category are 1) eyes with an intraocular pressure that may be abnormal with regard to the mean but that may be "normal" for those particular eyes, 2) eyes that have abnormally elevated intraocular pressures but that may never (during the patients' lifetimes) develop glaucomatous damage because of the ability of the optic nerve head to withstand that particular pressure, and 3) eyes that are destined to develop damage but that have not yet done so.

Estimates of the prevalence of definite open-angle glaucoma in a number of population studies vary between 0.25 and 0.75 per cent, whereas

---

Supported in part by the Herman and Ruth Albert Educational Fund of The Glaucoma Foundation.

the prevalence of ocular hypertension is approximately 2 per cent of the population between the ages of 40 and 50 and as high as 8 per cent between 70 and 80. The prevalence of glaucoma increases with age from about 0.2 per cent of those aged 50 to 54 years to about 2 per cent of those aged 70 to 74 years. A number of studies have demonstrated that, the higher the intraocular pressure, the greater the chance of developing glaucomatous damage over a period of time. Nevertheless, the great majority of patients with intraocular pressures greater than 21 mm Hg will not develop glaucomatous damage, and pressure alone is not necessarily a sufficient criterion upon which to base the decision to institute treatment. Most long-term studies of untreated ocular hypertensives indicate that about 1 per cent per year will develop glaucomatous damage. This incidence is actually lower than the mortality rate for these patients.

Until recently, the presence or absence of glaucomatous damage was determined on the basis of the appearance of the optic nerve head and visual field. The advent of more accurate and sensitive photographic methods and psychophysical testing has enabled the detection of earlier glaucomatous changes, and it now becomes necessary to consider both what is meant by the term "ocular hypertension" and what criteria should be used to place a patient on antiglaucoma medications. Does any damage at all fulfill the criteria of the definition of glaucoma, or should the present implied definition of potentially functional loss—optic disc cupping or early visual field loss—be maintained? How useful is the concept of ocular hypertension if its meaning changes with the increasing refinement of tests? Finally, one should realize the goal in treating the patient is to prevent functional visual loss, and not necessarily the loss of each and every neuron. At present, no repeatable, reliable prognostic test exists to determine which patients with elevated intraocular pressure will go on to develop glaucomatous damage, and decisions to treat are not based on the results of psychophysical testing in the absence of disc or visual field changes.

THERAPY

Ocular. Drug treatment is similar to that of primary open-angle glaucoma. The crucial difference lies in the decision of which patients to treat and which to observe.

Certain factors have been implicated as predisposing an "ocular hypertensive" eye to glaucomatous damage. Among these are glaucomatous damage in the contralateral eye, markedly elevated intraocular pressure, recent onset of elevated intraocular pressure, myopia, congenitally large cups, family history of glaucoma, diabetes mellitus, circulatory disorders, and anemia. Black patients appear to be more likely to develop glaucomatous damage than Caucasians. A cup/disc ratio asymmetry of 0.2 or greater between the two eyes, particularly when it is associated with an afferent pupillary defect in the eye with the larger cup, is highly suspicious. The absolute number value of the intraocular pressure that the ophthalmologist feels safe not treating is also important. In the absence of other risk factors, it is recommended to institute treatment for one or both eyes at a pressure range of about 27 to 30 mm Hg, depending on the effectiveness of medications, side effects, and the age and wishes of the patient.

Observation is the simplest form of follow-up. The frequency of observation should vary directly with the level of intraocular pressure. Parameters to follow include tonometry, visual fields, and examination of the disc. Helpful adjuncts are periodic stereophotography of the discs, red-free photographs of the nerve fiber layer, and office determination of the diurnal curve to determine the time of peak pressure. In ocular hypertensive patients, office determination of intraocular pressure between 8 A.M. and 5 P.M. is usually sufficient.

Precautions

Once the decision to treat in the absence of glaucomatous damage has been made, there are several important points to consider. The drug of choice is that which effectively lowers intraocular pressure with the least amount of discomfort to the patient. A uniocular therapeutic trial should be performed when instituting therapy to ensure that it is actually the drug that is lowering intraocular pressure, rather than fluctuation due to diurnal or other variations. If a patient with symmetric elevation of intraocular pressure achieves a significant lowering of pressure in the treated eye, one may then elect to treat both eyes or to continue to treat one eye and observe the other. One is treating a patient, not a number, and one should not become obsessed with lowering the pressure to the "normal" range. A drop from 35 to 25 mm Hg may be quite sufficient to protect the patient from the future development of glaucomatous damage. Carbonic anhydrase inhibitors have significant systemic side effects, and unless intraocular pressure is extremely high, they should not be used in patients without glaucomatous damage. Laser trabeculoplasty should rarely, if ever, be used in this situation.

Comments

Certain patients merit treatment at criteria that are more liberal than those defined earlier. Monocular patients, patients who have developed a branch or central retinal vein occlusion in either eye, and patients who have evidence of systemic arterial occlusive disease should be treated if intraocular pressure is in the mid-20s or greater.

The fact that one is dealing with a physical sign and not a rigidly definable disease entity should encourage the ophthalmologist to take into account the other contributory factors mentioned in the individualization of treatment for any particular patient.

References

Chandler PA, Grant WM: "Ocular hypertension" vs. open-angle glaucoma. Arch Ophthalmol 95:585–586, 1977.

Colton T, Ederer F: The distribution of intraocular pressures in the general population. Surv Ophthalmol 25:123–129, 1980.

Graham P: Epidemiology of chronic glaucoma. In Heilmann K, Richardson KT (eds): Glaucoma. Conceptions of a disease. Philadelphia, WB Saunders, 1978, pp 7–17.

Hoskins HD Jr: Definition, classification, and management of the glaucoma suspect. In Symposium on Glaucoma. Transactions of the New Orleans Academy of Ophthalmology. St. Louis, CV Mosby, 1981, pp 19–29.

Hovding G, Aasved H: Prognostic factors in the development of manifest open-angle glaucoma. A long-term follow-up study of hypertensive and normotensive eyes. Acta Ophthalmol 64:601–608, 1986.

Kass MA, et al: Risk factors favoring the development of glaucomatous visual field loss in ocular hypertension. Surv Ophthalmol 25:155–162, 1980.

Kolker AE, Becker B: "Ocular hypertension" vs. open-angle glaucoma: A different view. Arch. Ophthalmol 95:586–587, 1977.

Krupin T, Podos SM: The glaucomas; Classification and synthesis. In Heilmann K, Richardson KT (eds): Glaucoma. Conceptions of a Disease. Philadelphia, WB Saunders, 1978, pp 348–369.

Phelps CD: Ocular hypertension: To treat or not to treat? Arch Ophthalmol 95:588–589, 1977.

Schwartz B: Roundtable discussion. Management of ocular hypertension. Surv Ophthalmol 25:215–221, 1980.

Shaffer R: "Glaucoma suspect" or "ocular hypertension"? Arch Ophthalmol 95:588, 1977.

Spaeth GL: Ocular hypertension: Reasons for abandonment of the term. Int Ophthalmol Clin 19(1):37–49, 1979.

Wilson MR, et al: A case-control study of risk factors in open-angle glaucoma. Arch Ophthalmol 105:1066–1071, 1987.

OCULAR HYPOTONY
DAVID J. WILSON, M.D.
Portland, Oregon

Ocular hypotony lacks a specific definition, but is generally considered to be present when low intraocular pressure results in demonstrable effects on the eye. The intraocular pressure at which clinical effects become apparent is variable and depends on the speed of onset and the underlying cause for the decreased intraocular pressure. Generally, no ocular effects are noted until the intraocular pressure is below 6.5 mm Hg, and usually the intraocular pressure must fall to 0 to 4 mm Hg before deleterious effects become apparent. Hypotony of this degree is usually caused by wound leaks resulting from trauma or surgery, cyclodialysis, iridocyclitis, retinal detachment, or ciliochoroidal detachment. Other less common causes of hypotony include vascular occlusive disease (carotid artery occlusive disease, temporal arteritis, and central retinal artery or vein occlusion), osmotic hypotony (dehydration, diabetic coma, and uremia), myotonic dystrophy, and pre-phthisis bulbi.

THERAPY

Ocular. The most important factor in treating ocular hypotony is recognition of the underlying cause of the low intraocular pressure. In the setting of trauma or postoperatively, it is essential to assess for the possibility of a wound leak. Seidel's test should be performed under topical anesthesia to evaluate the presence or absence of a wound leak. In this test, the lids are held in a separated position, and a fluorescein-impregnated paper is used to apply fluorescein to the area of the suspected leak. It is important to apply the fluorescein in a highly concentrated form; otherwise, small leaks may go undetected. If a leak is not detected, gentle digital pressure should be applied to the eye to see if one becomes evident. The management of postoperative wound leaks is discussed in the article of postoperative flat anterior chamber, and the repair of penetrated globes is covered under indirect global ruptures and sharp scleral injuries.

With persistent hypotony after trauma or surgery in the absence of a wound leak, a cyclodialysis should be suspected. This diagnosis may be substantiated by gonioscopy. If a cyclodialysis is identified, surgical repair may be undertaken if the hypotony is clinically significant, i.e., if it is resulting in pain or decreased vision that warrants the risks of surgical repair. Closure of cyclodialyses has been described using diathermy, cryotherapy, suturing of the ciliary body, external plombage, and argon laser photocoagulation.

Rhegmatogenous retinal detachment is frequently associated with mild hypotony, but marked hypotony may occur. The recognition and treatment of retinal detachment are covered in a separate section.

Iridocyclitis may cause mild hypotony and may be associated with any of the above conditions. Before attributing hypotony solely to iridocyclitis, other possibilities should be excluded. Likewise, if surgical intervention for cyclodialysis is contemplated and iridocyclitis is also present, a trial of topical steroids is warranted to determine if eradicating the iridocyclitis will relieve the hypotony.

Ciliochoroidal detachment or effusion is commonly associated with hypotony, but its pathogenetic role in hypotony is unclear. Pederson has demonstrated that detachment of the ciliary body with silicone oil in the monkey does not result in hypotony. However, ciliochoroidal detachment is a common accompaniment of hypotony in humans, and drainage of suprachoroidal and supraciliary fluid in some cases resolves the ocular hypotony. The indications and procedure for drainage of ciliochoroidal detachments are discussed in a separate section.

Ocular or Periocular Manifestations

Anterior Chamber: Shallow.
Ciliary Body: Ciliary congestion; cyclodialysis; detachment.
Cornea: Folds in Bowman's and Descemet's membrane.
Iris: Anterior synechia; anterior uveitis.
Retina: Detachment; folds; macular edema.
Other: Cataract; decreased vision; ocular pain; optic nerve head edema.

PRECAUTIONS

Successful treatment of ocular hypotony requires recognition of its cause. A careful eye examination, including Seidel's test for wound leaks, gonioscopy for cyclodialysis, and fundus examination to evaluate for choroidal or retinal detachment, should be conducted.

COMMENTS

In the absence of a wound leak, treatment of asymptomatic ocular hypotony may not be necessary. Therapeutic intervention in ocular hypotony should be attempted only after the physician and patient have weighed the relative risks and benefits of the planned intervention.

References

Barasch K, Galin MA, Baras I: Postcyclodialysis hypotony. Am J Ophthalmol 68:644–645, 1969.
Brubaker RF, Pederson JE: Ciliochoroidal detachment. Surv Ophthalmol 27:281–289, 1983.
Demeler U: Refixation of the ciliary body after traumatic cyclodialysis. Dev Ophthalmol 14:199–201, 1987.
Harbin TS Jr: Treatment of cyclodialysis clefts with argon laser photocoagulation. Ophthalmology 89:1082–1083, 1982.
Joondeph HC: Management of postoperative and posttraumatic cyclodialysis clefts with argon laser photocoagulation. Ophthalmic Surg 11:186–188, 1980.
Maumenee AE, Stark WJ: Management of persistent hypotony after planned or inadvertent cyclodialysis. Am J Ophthalmol 71:320–327, 1971.
Pederson JE: Hypotony. In Duane TD (ed): Clinical Ophthalmology. Philadelphia, Harper and Row, 1984, Vol 3, pp 58:1–8.
Pederson JE: Ocular hypotony. Trans Ophthalmol Soc UK 105:220–226, 1986.
Pederson JE, Gaasterland DE, MacLellan HM: Experimental ciliochoroidal detachment: Effect on intraocular pressure and aqueous humor flow. Arch Ophthalmol 97:536–541, 1979.
Portney GL, Purcell TW: Surgical repair of cyclodialysis induced hypotony. Ophthalmic Surg 5:30–32, 1974.

OPEN-ANGLE GLAUCOMA

ROBERT N. SHAFFER, M.D., F.A.C.S.
San Francisco, California

Open-angle glaucoma is usually a chronic bilateral elevation of intraocular pressure sufficient to produce damage to the optic nerve that occurs in the absence of gonioscopic evidence of a closed angle at the time of pressure elevation. In primary open-angle glaucoma, the elevated pressure is caused by increased resistance to aqueous outflow. There is no convincing evidence that hypersecretion of aqueous humor can produce increased intraocular pressure. The definitive cause of cupping of the optic disc and field loss remains to be elucidated; however, capillary disease, microinfarcts producing ischemia of the nerve fibers, mechanical damage to the fibers by slippage of the sheets of the lamina cribrosa, and interference with axoplasmic flow may all be implicated. The genetic background and general health of the patient are contributing factors. Increased intraocular pressure remains as the one definite factor contributing to nerve damage and the one factor for which definitive therapy is available.

THERAPY

Ocular. Until about 15 years ago, a finding of an intraocular pressure of 24 mm Hg or above resulted in the institution of immediate medical therapy. However, it was found that no more than 5 per cent of patients with pressures in the 24 to 30 mm Hg range would develop field defects in 10 years. Since all the drugs used in the treatment of glaucoma have undesirable and sometimes dangerous side effects, ophthalmologists have been encouraged to defer therapy in the presence of a healthy optic nerve and a reasonably healthy patient. The result—is patients who are happier and probably safer than those who are plied with a multitude of medications without certainty of their need. Glaucoma without damage is sometimes termed "ocular hypertension." However, these untreated cases are certainly at risk and must continue to be watched carefully.

Until a reliable test is developed that will predict impending nerve damage, the indications to begin therapy must remain generalized. The decision to treat depends on the height of the intraocular pressure, the appearance of the optic disc, the genetic background and general health of the patient, and the opthalmologist's intuitive feeling that damage is imminent. When in doubt, a therapeutic trial of the safer medications, such as pilocarpine, epinephrine, and beta-blocking agents, is logical. If a good reduction of intraocular pressure results and the patient has minimal side effects, the treatment should be continued. If there is little change in pressure or unpleasant side effects occur, the patient should be followed as an ocular hypertensive patient without therapy.

Any increase in optic disc cupping or any loss of field, is a clear indication that the intraocular pressures have been higher than that particular optic nerve can stand. Therapy becomes mandatory and must be sufficient to prevent any increase in damage. If medical therapy cannot reduce the pressure adequately, surgery becomes necessary.

The parasympathomimetic drugs are miotics that improve the facility of outflow, thereby lowering intraocular pressure. The resultant small pupil interferes with night vision, and in the young patient, this may cause marked myopia. Frequently, there is some discomfort when drops are started. Allergies occasionally occur, and rarely a retinal break can be produced, which can result in a retinal detachment.

Pilocarpine has been the commonly used drug for a century. It acts directly on the musculature of the iris and ciliary body. Its effect lasts 6 to 8 hours, so it must be used three to four times a day in a 1 to 4 per cent solution. A 4 per cent pilocarpine gel is now available. When used twice a day, it provides as good control as 4 per cent pilocarpine drops used four times a day. The gel occasionally causes faint superficial corneal opacities that go away when the gel is discontinued. The myopia induced in the young can be reduced by the use of pilocarpine Ocuserts. This system delivers a fixed amount of pilocarpine per day for approximately a week. It is helpful in reducing miosis, thus improving the vision when cataracts are present in the elderly. An alternative to pilocarpine is 0.75 to 3.0 per cent carbachol, which may be slightly more effective and is also useful if an allergy to pilocarpine develops.

The anticholinesterase drugs include echothiophate and demecarium, which are used in 0.06, 0.125, and 0.25 per cent solutions once or twice daily. Especially in an older population, subcapsular cataracts are frequently produced. Consequently, these agents are seldom used in phakic eyes unless there has been a failure of filtering surgery. Unless there is an obvious reason for the failure, the therapeutic armamentarium should usually be exhausted before subjecting the eye to further surgery. In aphakic eyes, the anticholinesterase drugs are particularly useful.

Sympathomimetic drugs reduce the intraocular pressure both by increasing the outflow of aqueous humor and by decreasing its production. The exact mechanism of action of epinephrine and dipivefrin is still under investigation. Epinephrine is usually used as a supplement to miotic therapy once or twice a day in 0.5 to 2 per cent solutions. Epinephrine borate has a pH close to 7.0, making it much more comfortable than the hydrochloride or the bitartrate that have a pH close to 3.5. Epinephrine can cause side effects in cardiovascular patients, with an increase in hypertension, arrhythmias, and tachycardia. Locally reactive hyperemia is common, and allergies frequently occur. The prodrug dipivefrin causes less systemic reaction than epinephrine and often can be used when allergy to epinephrine has developed.

The beta-blocking agents reduce intraocular pressure by reducing aqueous humor production. A concentration of 0.25 or 0.5 per cent may be used once or twice a day. They are of particular value in young patients, as they have no effect on the ciliary body or the pupil. They are about as effective as pilocarpine, to which their action is additive. Side effects are rare, but some are dangerous. Of particular importance is the exacerbation of pulmonary symptoms in asthma and emphysema. Like all beta-blocking agents, they reduce the heart rate and blood pressure. Syncope and collapse can occur.

The carbonic anhydrase inhibitors—acetazolamide, methazolamide, dichlorphenamide, and ethoxzolamide—are oral medications that in full dosage two to four times a day decrease some 50 per cent of the production of aqueous humor by the ciliary body. Unfortunately, they also inhibit secretion of all the glands in the body. It is not surprising that many patients find the side effects intolerable; tingling of hands and feet, loss of appetite, weight loss, fatigue, depression, disorientation, and reduced libido are common symptoms. Kidney stone formation is enhanced, although methazolamide is somewhat less likely to cause this side effect. In normal individuals, there is an early loss of serum potassium, but the level soon returns to normal. In sensitive individuals, particularly in patients using digitalis or thiazides, serious cardiac problems can arise because of potassium depletion. The acetazolamide Sequels is probably the best tolerated of the agents; however, in many instances, surgery is preferable to their many side effects.

Hyperosmotic agents increase blood osmolality, resulting in a rapid reduction of intraocular pressure. They have been of great use in the therapy of acute glaucoma and have almost eliminated the necessity of operating on an eye with markedly elevated intraocular pressure. Orally, a 50 per cent solution of glycerin is given in a dosage of 1 to 1.5 gm/kg, or 20 per cent mannitol is used intravenously in a dosage of 1.5 to 2.0 gm/kg. Mannitol has largely replaced urea as a hyperosmotic agent.

The decision to treat a patient with chronic open-angle glaucoma is based on many factors: the appearance of the optic disc, the height of the intraocular pressure, the presence of a defect in the field of vision, and demonstrated effectiveness of medication with minimal side effects. In eyes with normal optic nerves, less than one in ten of such eyes will show any damage in 10 years, even though pressures remain above 24 mm Hg. Medical management should always be thoroughly tried before resorting to surgery.

A therapeutic regimen should include a stepwise increase in therapy at 1- to 2-week intervals until satisfactory pressure control is achieved. Pilocarpine, carbachol, and carbonic anhydrase inhibitors (with the exception of acetazolamide Sequels) have a duration of action of only 6 to 8 hours and must be prescribed three to four times a day. They should be prescribed for specific times, such as on arising, lunch time, dinner time, and bedtime. Epinephrine, or the prodrug, Dipivefrin, beta-blocking agents, or acetazolamide Sequels twice a day give uniform control over a 24-hour period. Maximal medical therapy would include 4 per cent pilocarpine every 6 hours, and 2 per cent epinephrine, 0.5 per cent timolol, and acetazolamide Sequels every 12 hours. If damage to the optic nerve is continuing or if the patient cannot tolerate such intensive therapy, surgery or laser trabeculoplasty becomes necessary.

Surgical. Of increasing importance in the surgical treatment of open-angle glaucoma is laser trabeculoplasty. Between 50 and 100 applications of laser energy are made to the trabecular meshwork just above the scleral spur. The shrinkage of tissue seems to open the mesh slightly, decreasing the resistance to outflow in 70 per cent of the cases. Topical medications must be continued as a rule. In successful cases, there is an average drop of pressure of 6 to 17 mm Hg, with a greater drop in higher pressure eyes and less in lower pressure eyes. Unfortunately, over a period of weeks, months, or years, pressure tends gradually to return to the former baseline pressure. A second laser trabeculoplasty is usually much less effective. Laser trabeculoplasty is of little value in the young and in the secondary glaucomas.

When pressures cannot be held at a level low enough to protect the optic nerve from continuing damage, a filtering procedure, such as trephination, sclerectomy, or trabeculectomy, is indicated. At present, trabeculectomy is preferred because complications are somewhat fewer. The success of any of these operations depends on the healing capacity of the patient. Less success can be expected in young healthy patients because rapid healing tends to close the newly created opening. Under the age of 30, the success rate is well below 50 per cent. Over the age of 50, the success rate tends to be 65 to 75 per cent without added medication. By resuming a medical regimen, 80 to 90 per cent of these eyes can have satisfactory pressure control without additional surgery.

Added to the risk of filtration failure and the rare possibility of infection or hemorrhage is the risk of cataract formation after filtering surgery, particularly in those over the age of 65. If cataracts already exist, they can be expected to increase.

Cyclodialysis has fallen into disuse because of its unpredictability. If no suprachoroidal cleft is formed, the pressure promptly rises. When a cleft has been created, profound hypotony can occur, with macular edema and marked reduction of visual acuity, particularly in young patients. Bleeding into the anterior chamber is much more common than with trabeculectomy.

Cyclocryotherapy is used when all else fails. There is often considerable pain after the procedure. Partial ciliary body ablation can now be accomplished by YAG laser or by ultrasound. Pain is less intense with these modalities. Pressure control usually lasts only a few months at best and then must be repeated. If the treatment is too intense, phthisis bulbi can result. Occasional long-term control can be achieved, however, with this procedure.

PRECAUTIONS

All of the drugs used in the treatment of glaucoma can have undesirable side effects that can be either local or general. Their toxic effect can be additive to some systemic drug previously given to the patient by the family physician. A patient whose hypertension is being treated with beta-blocking agents can develop serious side effects if the ophthalmologist adds timolol. Timolol should also be avoided in any patient with a history of asthma or other lung or heart problems. Levobunolol and betaxolol exert less bronchial and circulatory effects than timolol. Seldom does one think of eyedrops as a possible source of systemic symptoms, yet almost half of each drop runs down the nasolacrimal duct into the nose where it is absorbed almost as rapidly as by a subcutaneous injection. Most general side effects can be avoided by teaching the patient to occlude the tear duct after instilling the eyedrop. Both the family physician and the ophthalmologist should be aware of all the medications that the patient is taking.

The frequent inclusion of a corticosteroid component in drops and ointments prescribed for conjunctivitis poses an added risk for the patient and potential legal complications for the physician if the patient happens to be a steroid responder. Too often, such medications can be continued without realizing the dangers.

The anticholinesterase drugs cause a profound drop in blood cholinesterase and pseudocholinesterase. Their synthesis resulted from the research on nerve gases during World War II. It is not surprising that toxic systemic symptoms can result. These include nausea, vomiting, diarrhea, salivation, sweating, vivid dreams, bradycardia, lowered blood pressure, and, potentially, death. Organophosphorus insecticides are also cholinesterase inhibitors. Glaucoma patients exposed to such sprays may dangerously lower their blood cholinesterase. If such patients are given general anesthesia using succinylcholine as a muscle relaxant, prolonged apnea can result because succinylcholine is destroyed by cholinesterase. When toxicity develops, atropine is an effective antidote. Toxic ocular symptoms can result as well. In phakic eyes, it is wise to avoid the use of the anticholinesterase drugs. In addition to local discomfort, almost half of such eyes will eventually develop cataracts. Also, if surgery becomes necessary, there will be more congestion of blood vessels both inside and outside the eye, decreasing the effectiveness of the surgery. It should also be remembered that the stronger the miotic, the greater is the risk of precipitating a retinal break in predisposed eyes.

COMMENTS

When glaucoma has been diagnosed, the physician should take time to explain the problem fully to the patient whose understanding and cooperation will be vital in successful therapy. The frequency of tension, disc, and field examinations depends on the amount of damage to the optic nerve and the height of the pressure. Unfortunately, occasional optic nerves suffer typical glaucomatous damage at normal intraocular pressures. These are termed "normal-tension glaucoma."

Since there is no test to tell what pressure level will damage an individual eye, one can only determine this in retrospect after damage has occurred. One then can be sure that higher intraocular pressures will continue to be damaging. The therapeutic aim is to keep pressures as low as possible without interfering unduly with the patient's health and happiness. Tensions below 18 mm Hg are unlikely to cause continuing damage; those over 30 mm Hg are very likely to cause damage at some future time. A healthy, undamaged nerve with minimal cupping may withstand increased pressures indefinitely. The more cupping and field loss that are present, the more carefully should tension be controlled.

References

Cinotti DJ, Fiore PM, Maltzman BA, Constad WH, Cinotti AA: Control of intraocular pressure in glaucomatous eyes after extracapsular cataract extraction with intraocular lens implantation. J Cataract Refract Surg 14:650–653, 1988.

Chandler PA, Grant WM: Glaucoma, 2nd ed. Philadelphia, Lea & Febiger, 1979, pp 73–110.

Hoskins HD Jr, Kass MA: Becker-Shaffer's Diagnosis and Therapy of the Glaucomas, 6th ed. St. Louis, CV Mosby, 1989, pp 277–308.

Lichter PR, Musch DC, Medzihradsky F, Standardi CL: Intraocular pressure effects of carbonic anhydrase inhibitors in primary open-angle glaucoma. Am J Ophthalmol 107:11–17, 1989.

PHACOANAPHYLACTIC ENDOPHTHALMITIS
(Endophthalmitis, Phacoanaphylactica, Phacoanaphylactic Uveitis, Phacoantigenic Uveitis)

BARTON L. HODES, M.D.

Tucson, Arizona

Phacoanaphylactic endophthalmitis is a sterile inflammatory disease of the eye that results from immunologic sensitization of a patient to lens protein after surgical, traumatic, or spontaneous disruption of the lens capsule. The inflammatory reaction may be mild, resembling anterior uveitis, or it may be severe, mimicking infectious endophthalmitis and resulting in phthisis bulbi and enucleation. The onset of the inflammation is usually 24 hours to 2 weeks after traumatic or operative perforation of the lens. Lid edema, chemosis, mutton-fat keratic precipitates, and dense posterior synechiae complete the usual clinical picture. Secondary glaucoma and cyclitic membrane formation are common. The inflammation is a frequent occurrence and tends to be chronic with relapses.

THERAPY

Ocular. Aggressive anti-inflammatory therapy should be instituted immediately. Topical 1 per cent prednisolone eyedrops should be administered every 1 to 2 hours. These drops should be tapered off as the inflammatory process decreases. An initial periocular injection of 8 mg of methylprednisolone,* followed by additional injections, may also be indicated.

Depending on the severity, daily administration of 80 to 100 mg of oral prednisone may be necessary. This should be discontinued over several weeks as the inflammation subsides.

Surgical. The treatment of choice is surgical removal of all lens material. This procedure should be performed in an eye made as free as possible from an inflammatory response. The method of surgery to be used is dependent on the age of the patient and the preference of the surgeon. Ultrasonography should also be performed so that the resorption of the lens material and the subsequent clearing of the vitreous cavity may be followed.

Ocular or Periocular Manifestations

Anterior Chamber: Cells and flare; hypopyon; mutton-fat deposits.
Conjunctiva: Chemosis; hyperemia.
Cornea: Edema; striae in Descemet's membrane.
Globe: Atropy; phthisis bulbi.
Other: Decreased visual acuity; eyelid edema; irritation; posterior synechiae; pupillary occlusion; secondary glaucoma.

PRECAUTIONS

Phacoanaphylactic endophthalmitis is easily confused with infectious endophthalmitis. In both, early etiologic diagnosis is essential, as undue prolongation of the inflammatory process usually leads to irreversible damage to the eye. The importance of early and accurate differentiation between the two cannot be overemphasized, since the therapy for each is radically different. Infectious endophthalmitis requires intensive antibiotic therapy, whereas antibiotics have no value in the treatment of phacoanaphylactic endophthalmitis.

Phacoanaphylactic endophthalmitis may occur after the extracapsular technique of phacoemulsification. Increased attention to this entity and aspiration for histopathologic diagnosis are indicated in suspected cases.

COMMENTS

Phacoanaphylactic endophthalmitis may be an autoimmune reaction to lens protein. Antilens antibodies have been reported, although their significance remains unclear. The other varieties of lens-induced inflammation include phacolytic glaucoma and nonspecific phacotoxic uveitis. To a limited extent, phacoanaphylactic endophthalmitis occurs in all patients in whom lens matter is released into the eye. As a general rule, the ocular reaction varies directly with the amount of lens material left in the eye.

References

Hodes BL, Stern G: Phacoanaphylactic endophthalmitis: Echographic diagnosis of phacoanaphylactic endophthalmitis. Ophthalmic Surg 7:60–64, 1976.

Smith RE, Weiner P: Unusual presentation of phacoanaphylaxis following phacoemulsification. Ophthalmic Surg 7:65–68, 1976.

PIGMENTARY GLAUCOMA
(Pigment Dispersion Syndrome)

DAVID G. CAMPBELL, M.D.

Hanover, New Hampshire

Pigmentary glaucoma is a form of glaucoma in which there is usually bilateral elevation of intraocular pressure, open angles, and a heavy accumulation of pigment within the trabecular meshwork. The disease most characteristically occurs in relatively young, male myopes. Initially, symptoms are usually absent due to slow and quiet elevation of intraocular pressure. Haloes due to corneal edema resulting from rapid elevation of pressure may occasionally occur, particularly after exercise. Primary findings are characteristic radial defects in the pigment epithelium in the outer periphery of the iris, seen by iris transillumination. These defects constitute the source of pigment that is dispersed throughout the posterior and anterior segments of the eye and within the trabecular meshwork. This pigmentary dispersion is noted on the posterior surface of the cornea in the form of a Krukenberg spindle, on and within the trabecular meshwork, on the anterior surface of the iris, occasionally upon the zonular fibers, characteristically as a ring on the posterior peripheral surface of the lens, and occasionally as free pigment particles within the aqueous itself. In untreated eyes, there is a characteristic posterior bowing of the peripheral iris early in the course of the disease. The cause of the syndrome may be due to mechanical rubbing between the bowed posterior surface of the iris and packets of anterior zonules in predisposed eyes. If untreated, pigmentary glaucoma can lead to optic nerve damage, visual field loss and blindness. In some cases, however, pigmentary glaucoma can resolve spontaneously. This seems to be due to forward movement of the peripheral iris off of the zonules secondary to increasing lens size and increasing relative pupillary block due to age.

THERAPY

Ocular. In these generally young patients, either timolol or epinephrine may be used as initial therapy to lower intraocular pressure. Timolol, 0.25 or 0.50 per cent, may be administered in each eye every 12 hours. One or 2 per cent epinephrine, may also be given every 12 hours to decrease aqueous secretion and increase outflow facility. Dipivefrin, 0.1 per cent, may be substituted, if ocular allergy or toxicity develops.

One to 4 per cent pilocarpine may be applied every 6 hours to decrease the intraocular pressure by increasing aqueous outflow facility. An alternative to pilocarpine can be 0.75 to 3.0 per cent carbachol instilled in each eye every 8 hours. If pigmentary glaucoma worsens and optic nerve damage results, pilocarpine should be administered to the eye with the highest intraocular pressure, even in those patients in whom pilocarpine is not tolerated bilaterally because of accommodative blurring. An increase in the number of iris transillumination defects, the dispersion of pigment in the anterior segment or the degree of darkness of pigment in the trabecular meshwork, and a decrease in the facility of outflow with increased intraocular pressure are signs of worsening of pigmentary dispersion. Early studies indicate that the flattening of the iris associated with chronic pilocarpine usage may lift the peripheral iris off the zonules, stop the abrasion to the posterior surface of the iris, and stop the alluvial flow of pigment to the trabecular meshwork, and, in some cases, allow the trabecular meshwork to begin to recover. This recovery becomes manifest as an increase in the facility of outflow and a decrease in the untreated intraocular pressure.

Systemic. When topical therapy is unsuccessful, carbonic anhydrase inhibitors may be instituted. Oral administration of 125 to 250 mg of acetazolamide may be given 4 times daily in adults; children may be given 5 mg/kg every 6 hours. Acetazolamide Sequels, 500 mg every 12 hours, are better tolerated than the tablets. Methazolamide, 50 mg orally every 8 hours, may be used instead of acetazolamide, and even lower doses, 25 mg twice daily, should be tried initially. The incidence of unwanted kidney stones may be less with methazolamide.

Surgical. If maximum tolerated medical therapy fails and cupping of the optic disc or visual field defects progress, surgical therapy is indicated. Laser trabeculoplasty is the treatment of choice if there is progressive disc and field damage or the intraocular pressure level is considered unsafe for a particular eye.

An effective laser treatment may be 80 applications spaced evenly over the circumference of the trabecular meshwork for 360°, of 0.1-second duration, and 50-micron spot size, with just enough power to cause a white blanched spot or tiny bubble formation within the mid- to upper trabecular meshwork. The treatment applications should be placed in mid- to anterior portion of the trabecular meshwork. Because it is easy to overtreat these heavily pigmented meshworks and obtain no pressure lowering or even unwanted permanent elevation, the power setting should be reduced to approximately half of the normal setting. Temporary pressure rise following laser treatment should be watched for and treated with a topical or systemic glaucoma medication, if necessary.

If laser trabeculoplasty fails, filtering surgery is the treatment of choice for progressive disc and field damage. Either a guarded filtration procedure, such as a trabeculectomy, or a thorough filtration procedure, such as a trephine or thermal sclerotomy, can be effective. Goniotomy and cyclodialysis are of low effectiveness.

Ocular or Periocular Manifestations

Anterior Chamber: Free pigment particles in aqueous, particularly after dilatation or exercise.
Cornea: Pigmentary endothelial deposits (Krukenberg spindles).
Iris: Characteristic and pathognomonic peripheral radial slit-like transillumination defects; pigment on surface of iris.
Lens: Circular pigmentary deposit on posterior peripheral lens surface; heavy pigment deposition on zonules (occasional).
Optic Nerve: Glaucomatous cupping with characteristic glaucomatous visual field loss.
Other: Increased intraocular pressure; myopia.

PRECAUTIONS

Cycloplegic therapy can cause a pressure rise in these patients, just as in most open-angle glaucomas. This is due to decreased aqueous outflow facility secondary to the loss of the normal ciliary muscle tone exerted upon the scleral spur in these predisposed eyes. If a patient has bilateral pigmentary glaucoma that is worsening in both eyes, bilateral chronic miotic therapy is recommended for the reasons given above. If the patient is young, the accommodative blurring of vision that follows parasympathomimetic therapy is often so disabling that the patient cannot maintain a normal pattern of life. This causes decreased compliance which must be watched for. If the patient cannot use bilateral therapy, at least unilateral therapy should be encouraged for the eye with the highest pressure. Prior to the institution of miotic therapy in these myopic eyes, a peripheral retinal examination should be performed, and any areas of retinal weakness should be treated to avoid induced rhegmatogenous retinal detachment.

If it is determined that the glaucoma has stabilized or perhaps begun to improve, as can happen in some cases, an occasional discontinuation of medication is in order to be certain that the medications being used are needed.

The usual precautions in regard to glaucoma medications, as described in the section on open-angle glaucoma, should be observed.

COMMENTS

Some patients with pigmentary glaucoma can develop an acute pressure rise following vigorous exercise, an increase which is due to a transient influx of released pigment to the trabecular meshwork. This pressure rise generally does not last more than a few hours but may lead to very high pressures that can damage the optic nerve. Therefore, patients should be checked following vigorous exercise; if an acute intraocular pressure rise occurs, topical pressure-lowering medications should be used whenever possible during and after exercise to avoid this increased pressure.

The prognosis for patients with pigmentary glaucoma can vary. The disease may become rapidly worse and require maximum medical or surgical therapy, or it can reach a plateau stage in which progression stops and, in some cases, spontaneous improvement follows.

References

Campbell DG: Pigmentary dispersion and glaucoma. A new theory. Arch Ophthalmol 97:1667–1672, 1979.
Epstein DL: Pigment dispersion and pigmentary glaucoma. *In* Chandler PA, Grant WM: Glaucoma. 2nd ed. Philadelphia, Lea & Febiger, 1979, pp 122–129.
Lichter PR: Pigmentary glaucoma. *In* Fraunfelder FT, Roy FH: Current Ocular Therapy 2 Philadelphia, WB Saunders, 1980, pp 465–466.
Lichter PR: Pigmentary glaucoma—Current concepts. Trans Am Acad Ophthalmol Otolaryngol 78:309–313, 1974.
Sugar HS, Barbour FA: Pigmentary glaucoma. A rare clinical entity. Am J Ophthalmol 32:90–92, 1949.

PLATEAU IRIS
ROBERT RITCH, M.D.,
and STEVEN M. PODOS, M.D.
New York, New York

Plateau iris refers to an anatomic configuration in which the iris is inserted anteriorly on the ciliary body face and the iris root angles forward and then centrally. The result is somewhat akin to a bird's-eye view of a mesa (hence the name); the iris surface appears flat and the anterior chamber deep on slitlamp examination, but the angle is narrow on gonioscopy, with a sharp dropoff of the peripheral iris. By contrast, in primary angle-closure glaucoma, the most common form of angle closure, the anterior chamber is shallow and the iris surface rounded (iris bombé).

Some patients with plateau iris develop angle-closure glaucoma. As in primary angle closure, the inciting mechanism may be development of

---

Supported in part by the Herman and Ruth Albert Educational Fund of The Glaucoma Foundation.

relative pupillary block caused by increased iris-lens contact as the lens enlarges with age. However, because of the nature of the anatomic relationships of the iridocorneal angle structures, the degree of relative pupillary block necessary to induce angle closure is less than in primary angle-closure glaucoma; this seems to account for the deeper anterior chamber and flatter iris surface in eyes with angle-closure and plateau iris. Patients with plateau iris who develop angle-closure glaucoma are somewhat younger than those with primary angle-closure glaucoma.

Most patients with plateau iris configuration who develop angle-closure glaucoma are cured by iridectomy. A minority, however, are subject to repeated attacks of angle closure despite a patent iridectomy, usually after dilation of the pupil. The term "plateau iris syndrome" is used to describe those patients in whom the angle remains capable of closure even after pupillary block has been eliminated by iridectomy. In some cases, the angle may spontaneously remain appositionally closed after iridectomy, whereas in others, it is open but closes when the pupil is dilated.

Two subtypes of plateau iris syndrome have recently been differentiated. In the complete syndrome, which comprises the classic situation, intraocular pressure rises when the angle closes with pupillary dilation. In the incomplete syndrome, intraocular pressure does not change. The important factor differentiating the complete and incomplete syndromes is the level of the iris stroma with respect to the angle structures or the "height" to which the plateau rises. If the angle closes to the upper trabecular meshwork or Schwalbe's line, intraocular pressure rises, whereas if the angle closes only the lower portion of the angle, the pressure remains unchanged.

THERAPY

Surgical. The initial treatment of choice for an angle-closure glaucoma with plateau iris configuration is laser iridectomy. If, in the presence of a patent iridectomy, the angle remains spontaneously appositionally closed and intraocular pressure is normal, there are two choices of therapy. Low-dose pilocarpine may open the angle and, if tolerated well by the patient, may be used for maintenance. In these cases, 1 per cent pilocarpine twice daily is sufficient. The alternate choice is to perform argon laser peripheral iridoplasty. This procedure alters the configuration of the plateau iris periphery to remove the sharp angulation. Laser settings of 500-μm spot size, with an exposure time of 0.5 second, and an intensity of 150 to 200 mW achieve sustained contraction of the peripheral iris. If miotics are needed for control of intraocular pressure after iridectomy, then iridoplasty is indicated only if the angle remains spontaneously appositionally closed on miotics.

If the angle is open after iridectomy but closes appositionally with pupillary dilation, treatment is indicated if intraocular pressure rises with closure. If closure is incomplete, observation for the development of future spontaneous closure is indicated.

PRECAUTIONS

If plateau iris configuration is diagnosed incidentally in an eye with an open angle, caution should be exercised in dilation and the patient followed gonioscopically at routine intervals for signs of progressive angle closure.

If the patient presents with elevated intraocular pressure, careful gonioscopy should be performed, as in all cases of glaucoma, so that the condition is not confused with open-angle glaucoma because of the normal depth of the anterior chamber and relatively flat iris surface on direct examination.

COMMENTS

The most common cause of differential diagnostic confusion on routine examination is a prominent peripheral iris roll. With this iris picture, however, the peripheral iris does not occlude the angle on dilation, and it does not predispose to angle-closure glaucoma.

If the condition was not diagnosed before iridectomy and intraocular pressure is elevated postoperatively, careful gonioscopy should be performed. If the angle is open, such diagnoses as secondary damage to the trabecular meshwork should be considered. If the angle is closed, the differential diagnosis should include ciliary block or malignant glaucoma, in which the anterior chamber is flat or extremely shallow; peripheral anterior synechiae, which can be ruled out by indentation gonioscopy; or incomplete iridectomy.

Although plateau iris syndrome usually occurs in the postoperative period, it may occur up to years later, and patients with plateau iris configuration should not be assumed to be permanently cured if plateau iris syndrome does not develop immediately.

References

Epstein DL: Chandler and Grant's Glaucoma, 3d ed. Philadelphia, Lea & Febiger, Philadelphia, 1986.

Kolker AE, Hetherington J Jr: Becker-Shaffer's Diagnosis and Therapy of the Glaucomas, 5th ed. St. Louis, CV Mosby, 1983.

Lowe RF: Primary angle-closure glaucoma: A review of ocular biometry. Aust J Ophthalmol 5:9–17, 1977.

Ritch R, Solomon IS: Glaucoma Surgery. In L'Esperance FA Jr (ed): Ophthalmic Lasers, 3rd ed. St. Louis, CV Mosby, 1989, pp 650–748.

Törnquist R: Angle-closure glaucoma in an eye with a plateau type of iris. Acta Ophthalmol 36:419–423, 1958.

Wand M, et al: Plateau iris syndrome. Trans Am Acad Ophthalmol Otolaryngol 83:122–130, 1977.

PRIMARY ANGLE-CLOSURE GLAUCOMA
(Primary Closed-Angle Glaucoma, Primary Narrow-Angle Glaucoma)

Yoshiaki Kitazawa, M.D.
Gifu, Japan

Primary angle-closure glaucoma is caused by increased intraocular pressure and obstruction of aqueous humor outflow, resulting from the closure of the angle by the peripheral root of the iris. It is a bilateral disease that affects those who are born with a narrow angle. The outflow channels of aqueous, including the trabecular meshwork, are normal before the closure of angle takes place.

In its early stage, the closure of the angle is nothing more than the contact between the trabecular meshwork and the root of the iris and is reversible once pupillary block is eliminated. However, as time goes by, the root of the iris becomes adherent to the trabeculum, forming peripheral anterior synechiae that cannot be relieved by breaking pupillary block.

Although the mechanism of pressure rise is identical in the various types of angle-closure glaucoma, symptoms vary markedly depending on the magnitude and the speed of intraocular pressure rise. With prodromal or intermittent angle-closure glaucoma, symptoms are caused by the rapid elevations and decreases of intraocular pressure. A steaminess of the cornea is caused by the abrupt rise of pressure as a result of sudden angle occlusion. Symptoms may consist of foggy or hazy vision with rainbow-colored halos around lights. Ocular congestion or discomfort may occur. Symptoms spontaneously subside in a few hours if the pupillary block is relieved by the miosis. The miosis may occur when the patient moves to a brighter environment or goes to sleep.

In the acute attack of primary angle-closure glaucoma, the symptoms are precipitated by pupillary dilation resulting from mydriatic drops, dim light, or emotional upset. Once angle closure is established, the symptoms of the intermittent or prodromal attack become more severe and permanent. Symptoms comprise blurred, foggy vision with colored halos around lights, ocular congestion, and pain. Also, nausea and vomiting may occur and are due to autonomic stimulation.

In chronic primary angle-closure glaucoma, the pressure rises insidiously as the closed area of the angle gradually increases. Patients may be totally free from symptoms or may experience some ocular discomfort and halos. Chronic primary angle-closure glaucoma cannot be differentiated from primary open-angle glaucoma on the basis of symptoms. Visual field defects are also very similar in these two basically different glaucomas.

THERAPY

Supportive. The patient with acute primary angle-closure glaucoma should be admitted to the hospital to initiate intensive medical therapy that is usually a prelude to surgery. Analgesics may be used to control pain and apprehension. Administration of 300 to 600 mg of aspirin every 6 to 8 hours is usually adequate; if not, 50 to 100 mg of meperidine may be used.

In chronic primary angle-closure glaucoma, medical therapy can be less intensive than in an acute attack. Since there is no pain, analgesics are not necessary, and patients may be treated as outpatients.

Ocular. Cholinergic agents are used to pull the iris away from the angle. In acute primary angle-closure glaucoma, one or two drops of 1 to 3 per cent pilocarpine or 0.75 to 1.5 per cent carbachol should be instilled every 5 minutes for four times, than three or four times every half-hour, and thereafter every 1 to 2 hours. Moxisylyte,[†] an alpha-adrenergic blocking agent, may be effective in breaking attacks of acute closure. Instilled topically every 10 to 15 minutes in a 0.5 per cent solution, it inhibits contraction of the dilator muscle of the iris. As a result, pilocarpine constricts the pupil more effectively when applied with moxisylyte. Twice-daily administration of adrenergic beta-blocking agents, such as 0.25 or 0.50 per cent timolol, 0.5 per cent betaxolol, or 0.5 per cent levobunolol, may be added to miotics. Corticosteroids are useful to control inflammation. One to two drops of 0.1 per cent dexamethasone are given three to four times a day. In order to obtain prompt normalization of pressure, topical drops should be used in conjunction with systemic medications.

With chronic angle-closure glaucoma, miotics are administered as for primary open-angle glaucoma. Every 4 to 6 hours, 1 to 3 per cent pilocarpine should be instilled. Twice-daily administration of adrenergic beta-blocking agents—0.25 or 0.5 per cent timolol, 0.5 per cent betaxolol, or 0.5 per cent levobunolol—may be a supplement to pilocarpine.

Systemic. In order to break an acute attack, hyperosmotic agents are used to reduce intraocular pressure promptly. Oral glycerin may be administered in a 50 or 75 per cent solution in a dosage of 1 to 1.5 gm/kg. Oral isosorbide is an alternative to oral glycerin. It is administered in doses of 1 to 2 gm/kg and is preferred in diabetics as a metabolically inactive agent. Isosorbide is usually better tolerated than glycerin. If the patient is nauseated or oral glycerin has failed to be effective, 20 per cent mannitol may be given intravenously in a dose of 1 to 2 gm/kg, or 30 per cent urea may be given intravenously in a dose of 1.0 to 1.5 gm/kg. Carbonic anhydrase inhibitors, such as acetazolamide, are given by mouth in a dose of 250 mg four times daily. If the patient cannot take oral medication because of nausea, 500 mg of acetazolamide should be injected intravenously.

With chronic primary angle-closure glaucoma,

hyperosmotic agents are of less value and are employed as a preoperative measure. Carbonic anhydrase inhibitors are used as for primary open-angle glaucoma; 250 mg of acetazolamide four times daily or 50 mg of methazolamide three times daily may be administered.

Surgical. Treatment of primary angle-closure glaucoma consists of peripheral iridectomy or laser iridotomy after the intraocular pressure has been normalized. In acute angle-closure glaucoma, the eye should be operated on promptly unless most of the angle has been confirmed to be open after the attack has been completely broken with medical measures. Iridectomy may be done surgically, or argon or Q-switched Neodymium YAG laser may be used to create an iridotomy (laser iridotomy). If the acute attack of angle closure does not respond to intensive medical therapy, filtration surgery may be considered.

In chronic primary angle-closure glaucoma, surgical iridectomy or laser iridotomy is the operation of choice. Even if intraocular pressure is normalized with medical therapy, this procedure should be done to avoid the progress of the synechial closure of the angle. Filtration surgery should not be performed unless iridectomy has failed to normalize intraocular pressure.

Ocular or Periocular Manifestations

(A) refers to acute angle-closure glaucoma; (C) indicates chronic angle-closure glaucoma.
Anterior Chamber: Closed angle (A,C).
Conjunctiva: Chemosis (A); hyperemia (A).
Cornea: Epithelial edema (A); folds in Descemet's membrane (A); hypesthesia (A); pigment on posterior surface (A).
Iris: Convex (C); forward displacement (A); peripheral anterior synechiae (A,C); posterior synechiae (A); sector atrophy, usually in the upper half (A).
Lens: Galaukomaflecken or cataracta disseminata subcapsularis glaukomatosa (A).
Optic Nerve: Atrophy (C); edema (A); glaucomatous cupping (C); hyperemia (A).
Pupil: Dilation, vertically oval, middilated and fixed (A).
Other: Increased intraocular pressure (A,C); visual field defects (A,C).

PRECAUTIONS

Intravenous hyperosmotic agents cause headache, dizziness, nausea, and vomiting; oral glycerin particularly tends to induce nausea. Urinary retention may be brought about by intense diuresis. Pulmonary edema and congestive heart failure may be precipitated in elderly patients with borderline cardiac and renal function; this is especially true with mannitol, which greatly increases blood volume. Cellular dehydration, including cerebral dehydration, may be caused more often with mannitol and results in mental disorientation. Urea can cause skin slough and phlebitis if it extravasates. Rebound elevation of intraocular pressure is common with urea.

Systemic toxicity may occur after multiple topical applications of cholinergic drops. Potent anticholinesterase inhibitors, such as echothiophate and demecarium, should not be used because of their tendency to precipitate angle closure as a result of aggravation of pupillary block and vascular congestion.

Epinephrine is contraindicated as it induces pupillary dilation. Adrenergic beta-blocking agents are considered to be supplementary to miotics as they possess no miotic effect.

COMMENTS

Acute primary angle-closure glaucoma is an ophthalmic emergency and requires immediate medical therapy. All medical measures should be used simultaneously to normalize elevated intraocular pressure. Once the pressure is brought under control, pressure gonioscopy with a Zeiss four-mirrored lens or the one devised by Nakamura and Kitazawa for this purpose is necessary to confirm the diagnosis and to evaluate the extent of peripheral anterior synechiae. If the angle is open at least one quarter of the entire circumference, a peripheral iridotomy or laser iridotomy may be postponed until the eye becomes less irritated. If the angle is closed with peripheral anterior synechiae more than three quarters in its circumference or the intraocular pressure responds poorly to maximum medical therapy, an immediate peripheral iridotomy or laser iridotomy should be performed. If the angle is open as much as half of the entire circumference, iridectomy is likely to normalize intraocular pressure without medication postoperatively. The more extensive the peripheral anterior synechiae, the more likely that antiglaucoma medications will be needed to maintain a normal intraocular pressure after surgery. The fellow eye should also be treated with topical miotics in order to avoid an acute attack. Prophylactic laser iridotomy may be preferred to surgical iridectomy because of its safety and convenience.

Chronic primary angle-closure glaucoma should be treated surgically even when the intraocular pressure is normalized with medication. Since pupillary block cannot be eliminated by medical therapy, peripheral anterior synechiae always increase in width and height, regardless of the level of intraocular pressure.

References

Drake MV: Neodymium YAG laser iridotomy. Surv Ophthalmol 32:171–177, 1987.
Forbes M: Gonioscopy with corneal indentation. A method for distinguishing between appositional closure and synechial closure. Arch Ophthalmol 76:488–492, 1966.
Halasa AH, Rutkowski PC: Thymoxamine therapy for angle-closure glaucoma. Arch Ophthalmol 90:177–179, 1973.
Lowe RF: Primary angle-closure glaucoma: Biometry and the clinician. *In* Etienne R, Paterson GD: Inter-

national Glaucoma Symposium. (XXII International Congress of Ophthalmology, Albi, France, 1974). Marseille, Diffusion Générale de Librairie, 1975, pp 247–272.

Nakamura Y, Kitazawa Y: A new goniolens for corneal indentation gonioscopy. Acta Ophthalmol 49:964–970, 1971.

Pollack IP: Laser iridotomy: Current concepts in technique and safety. Int Ophthalmol Clin 21:137–144, 1980.

Sugar HS: Surgical decision, technique and complications of peripheral iridectomy for angle-closure glaucoma. Ann Ophthalmol 7:1237–1241, 1975.

SECTION 26

IRIS AND CILIARY BODY

ACCOMMODATIVE SPASM
WILLIAM E. SCOTT, M.D.
Iowa City, Iowa

Accommodative spasm is an overactivity of accommodation wherein the refractive power of the eye is increased and the patient has an induced myopia. The tone of the ciliary muscle is increased, and a constant accommodative effort is expended by the parasympathetic nervous system to bring both the far point and near point closer. It is an involuntary action that may be constant or intermittent. Spasm of accommodation may be associated with headache, photophobia, eyestrain, defective vision for near and distance, inability to concentrate, and intermittent homonymous diplopia. The distant vision may be blurred because of the pseudomyopia. Macropsia may also occur, as well as browache, ocular fatigue, and inability to maintain visual or mental concentration. The etiology of accommodative spasm may be functional, the spasm being essentially a response to fatigue and overstrain. Spasm of accommodation occurs in patients under 40 years of age, most likely in the nervous, tense individual.

THERAPY

Ocular. Treatment of accommodative spasm is difficult and is largely based on relief of symptoms. In patients with distant blurred vision, one should not hesitate to prescribe a minus power lens, even though it is for pseudo-and not true myopia. The use of a minus lens will not influence the basic refractive error. As the patient becomes older and accommodation lessens, the spastic state will disappear, as well as the pseudomyopia. The glasses should be worn as needed.

When the complaint is blurred near vision, one should correct for near vision and inform the patient to expect distant vision to be blurred. If close work tends to cause further relapses, stronger lenses for this work may bring relief. The recommendation should be made that the glasses be worn only for prolonged near use.

A careful explanation to the patient of the condition will avoid unnecessary patient anxiety and constant lens corrections. Occasionally, a concurrent regimen of an antispasmodic, such as belladonna, and a mild sedative may be helpful to these patients.

PRECAUTIONS

Cycloplegics, such as atropine and homatropine, have been advocated for the treatment of accommodative spasm. However, the spasm is broken only during use of cycloplegics and generally recurs when the cycloplegic is discontinued. In addition, temporary reading glasses are usually needed. Such glasses are not tolerated by most patients, and it has never been shown that the spasm is influenced by them.

Accommodative spasm may be caused by miotic drugs, such as pilocarpine, physostigmine, echothiophate, neostigmine, and isoflurophate. This condition may be quite distressing to a patient beginning miotic therapy for glaucoma. Accommodative spasm may also be associated with overdosage of such drugs as morphine, alcohol, or digitalis.

COMMENTS

A tonic accommodation is a rare phenomenon in which an accommodative posture is prolonged so that the change in focus from distant to near objects or vice versa is delayed. The patient may need bifocal lenses if the defect is great. The site of the causal lesion is unknown, but has occasionally been associated with syphilis, measles, diabetes, alcoholism, Graves' disease, and trauma.

References

Dagi LR, Chrousos GA, Cogan DC: Spasm of the near reflex associated with organic disease. Am J Ophthalmol 103:582–585, 1987.
Moore S, Stockbridge L: Another approach to the treatment of accommodative spasm. Am Orthopt J 23:71–72, 1973.
Manor RS: Use of special glasses in treatment of spasm of near reflex. Ann Ophthalmol 11:903–905, 1979.
Nirankari VS, Hameroff SB: Spasm of the near reflex. Ann Ophthalmol 12:1050–1051, 1980.
Sloane AE, Kraut JA: Spasm of accommodation. Doc Ophthalmol 34:365–369, 1973.

ANIRIDIA
DAVID S. WALTON, M.D.
Boston, Massachusetts

Aniridia is a genetically determined condition with multiple congenital ocular anomalies and in which dystrophic changes progress from early childhood. Externally, there appears to be a total absence of the iris, although gonioscopy reveals some iris in all eyes. Approximately 50 per cent of patients with aniridia develop progressive glaucoma. Nearly all have visual problems. The visual acuity is usually markedly decreased (20/100 to 20/400) because of an associated foveal hypoplasia. Exceptionally, the visual acuity can be as good as 20/50. The glaucoma in aniridia characteristically develops in late childhood and seems to depend often upon the extent of the attachment of the iris stump to the trabecular meshwork. The iris deformity is always bilateral, but can show marked asymmetry. Approximately two thirds of patients with congenital aniridia have a positive family history of the autosomal dominant inheritance, whereas the remainder of cases, are sporadic. There is a significant association with Wilms' tumor, other genitourinary defects, retardation, and aniridia in certain sporadic cases that also possess a deletion of short arm of the eleventh chromosome. In glaucoma associated with aniridia, the cornea is rarely enlarged and breaks in Descemet's membrane almost never occur, unless the glaucoma occurs in infancy, which is uncommon.

THERAPY

Ocular. Miotics are used to improve outflow facility and thus lower the intraocular pressure. Also, 1 or 2 per cent epinephrine solution may be used once or twice daily to help control the pressure, but it is not consistently effective. Beta-adrenergic blockers have also been of inconsistent value.

Systemic. Carbonic anhydrase inhibitors are used to lower intraocular pressure by suppressing secretion of aqueous humor, if topical ocular miotics prove inadequate alone. The usual oral daily adult dosage of acetazolamide is 125 to 250 mg every 6 hours or 500 mg Sequels every 12 to 24 hours. Alternatively, methazolamide in doses of 25 to 100 mg every 8 to 12 hours may be used, with apparently less risk of kidney stone formation. For children, a dose of 3 mg/kg of methazolamide or 15 mg/kg of acetazolamide is used daily.

Surgical. In the majority of patients, medical therapy is helpful, but may eventually prove inadequate, and antiglaucoma surgery becomes indicated. If the glaucoma has become poorly controlled in spite of medical treatment, goniosurgery to dissect the iris stump from the trabecular meshwork may be temporarily effective in increasing the response to medical therapy, but it rarely has a lasting beneficial effect. In contrast, early prophylactic goniotomy in aniridia cases in which the iris stump is just beginning to develop synechiae to the trabecular meshwork may prove valuable in both the prevention of glaucoma and the treatment of early glaucoma, and this procedure is currently being evaluated further. Trabeculectomy may be useful in some patients, but it has not yet been adequately assessed. Classic filtration surgery also may be successful, but the risk of postoperative flat chamber and secondary corneal injury by the lens must be actively controlled. For advanced aniridia glaucoma unresponsive to other treatment, cyclocryotherapy is of value.

Cataract surgery is often necessary in time. Aspiration cataract extraction is used in the young patient, and extracapsular cataract extraction is used in older patients for removal of the opacified lens.

A peculiar corneal epithelial dystrophy usually develops, starting at the limbus and progressing centrally, but this rarely requires treatment.

Ocular or Periocular Manifestations

Conjunctiva: Hyperemia.
Cornea: Circumferential epithelial dystrophy with pannus; degeneration and progressive opacity.
Iris: Iris blockage of the trabecular meshwork; narrow peripheral rim only.
Lens: Displacement (superior); progressive opacity.
Optic Nerve: Atrophy; cupping; disc hypoplasia.
Pupil: Enlarged.
Retina: Absence of foveal reflex; foveal hypoplasia; white dots at the ora serrata.
Other: Glaucoma; nystagmus.

PRECAUTIONS

This type of glaucoma requires close follow-up, since there may be a gradual increase in intraocular pressure over a number of years. Goniosurgery is effective in some patients and is apparently best performed earlier, but the absence of iris increases the risk to the lens during the procedure. Accordingly, goniosurgery is best done by surgeons experienced in goniotomy-type surgery and thoroughly familiar with abnormalities of the angle in aniridia glaucoma.

The risks that miotics will promote lens opacities and that epinephrine will affect the macula in aniridia are unknown. Aniridic eyes nearly always undergo breakage of some of the lens zonules below, with upward displacement of the lens. These eyes also frequently develop cataracts. In aniridic eyes, it would seem unwarranted to assume that use of miotics and epinephrine involves the same risk of promoting cataract or macula edema as has been described in other kinds of eyes. Miotics may cause shallowing of the anterior chamber and blockage of the angle secondary to anterior rotation of the iris leaf circumferentially.

COMMENTS

Recognition of aniridia in the newborn is so easy that pediatricians and parents seldom fail to note this abnormality. This is important, not only because of the high risk of glaucoma but also because of the risk of associated Wilms' tumor in certain sporadic cases of aniridia. Chromosomal examination is indicated in the evaluation of all patients with aniridia and is mandatory in sporadic cases under 10 years of age. In the presence of a deletion of the short arm of the eleventh chromosome, the risk of Wilms' tumor is increased. However, the risk factor is not yet determined for these patients with abnormal chromosomes and for sporadic cases with normal chromosomes. Familial cases appear to be at no increased risk for Wilms' tumor. The average age for development of Wilms' tumor is somewhat younger in patients with aniridia (mean average, 3.6 years). The oldest age of the recognition of the development of a Wilms' tumor in a patient with sporadic aniridia has been reported at 4 years. These tumors are grossly and microscopically identical to those that appear in otherwise normal individuals. Early diagnosis and treatment of the tumor can be life saving.

The pediatrician should be alerted to the risk that Wilms' tumor might develop. These children must have a careful physical examination, and blood pressure should be measured regularly. In addition to chromosomal studies, developmental evaluation and examination for other congenital anomalies should be a part of the care of these children. Renal ultrasonography is indicated every 3 months for patients with a chromosomal deletion and at least every 6 months for sporadic cases without a detectable chromosome defect.

At 6- to 12-month intervals, an ophthalmic examination, including tonometry and gonioscopy, should be performed. If necessary, these procedures should be done under anesthesia. In some infants, it is possible to do Perkins' applanation tonometry and gonioscopy without general anesthesia while the baby is being fed.

References

Elsas FJ, et al: Familial aniridia with preserved ocular function. Am J Ophthalmol 83:718–724, 1977.

Francois J, Coucke D, Coppieters R: Aniridia-Wilms' tumour syndrome. Ophthalmologica 174:35–39, 1977.

Friedman AL: Wilms' tumor detection in patients with sporadic aniridia: Successful use of ultrasound. Am J Dis Child 140:173–174, 1986.

Grant WM, Walton DS: Progressive changes in the angle in congenital aniridia, with development of glaucoma. Am J Ophthalmol 78:842–847, 1974.

Pilling GP IV: Wilms' tumor in seven children with congenital aniridia. J Pediatr Surg 10:87–96, 1975.

Riccardi VM, et al: Chromosomal imbalance in the aniridia-Wilms' tumor association: 11p interstitial deletion. Pediatrics 61:604–610, 1978.

Walton DS: Aniridic glaucoma: The results of gonioscopy to prevent and treat this problem. Trans Am Ophthalmol Soc 84:59–70, 1986.

FUCHS' HETEROCHROMIC IRIDOCYCLITIS

THOMAS J. LIESEGANG, M.D.
Jacksonville, Florida

Fuchs' heterochromic iridocyclitis is readily recognized when it presents with its classic clinical appearance. These findings include heterochromia of the irides (usually the lighter iris is present in the involved eye), absence of conjunctival injection, specific atrophic changes on the iris surface, minimal cell and flare, widely scattered small nonconfluent keratic precipitates, vitreous cells, absence of posterior synechiae, a complicated cataract, and occasional glaucoma. It can occur at all ages in both sexes. It may present as an asymptomatic finding early in its course with minimal ocular symptoms of floaters or in some patients only after the development of a cataract. The disease is recognized in about 5 per cent of patients presenting with uveitis. In about 10 per cent of cases the disease is bilateral, and this may require an astute clinician to make the diagnosis. If the disease is unilateral at presentation, it usually remains a unilateral disease.

Fuchs' heterochromic iridocyclitis is frequently misdiagnosed by the ophthalmologist who does not see a large number of uveitis patients because of the unrecognized variants of the syndrome. The presentation, progression, and prognosis of this disease vary widely. There is a variable degree and progression of iris atrophy involving both the anterior portion of the iris and the posterior pigmented layer. This atrophy is evident as a blunting, flattening, or blurring of the surface markings of the iris crypts or rugae, especially when compared with the other eye. The whole iris tissue demonstrates rarefaction and transparency with a moth-eaten appearance and defects in the posterior pigmented layer and anterior stromal thinning with sphincter muscle atrophy. Transillumination defects are best seen with retroillumination. In a brown-eyed individual, it may be difficult to detect the iris atrophy because both layers of the iris are of the same color and texture (no heterochromia). In some individuals there is more atrophy of the anterior layer such that the iris can appear darker in the affected eye (reversed heterochromia). Daylight examination is best for detecting subtle heterochromia. Gaps or absence of the pupillary ruff is frequently seen. Gelatinous nodules are occasionally seen at the pupillary margin or on the iris surface. The iris atrophy also tends to be more prominent around the pupillary area. The absence of posterior synechiae is a constant feature of the disease, although there may be small residual pigment deposits on the anterior lens capsule from previous Koeppe nodules.

With iris atrophy, vessels within the iris stroma become more noticeable, and as the disease progresses, they become straighter and narrower. Fluorescein angiography of the iris in patients with Fuchs' heterochromic iridocyclitis has demonstrated an ischemic vasculopathy and infarction on the iris surface and the ciliary body. Over time this ischemia evolves to a fine rubeosis involving the iris surface, angle, and possible the ciliary body. Probably, this iris ischemia is also an initiating cause of the iris atrophy. The fragile blood vessels in the angle are susceptible to bleeding either spontaneously or in association with a sudden reduction of pressure in the anterior chamber. The filiform hemorrhage seen in the chamber angle or on the peripheral iris after paracentesis, glaucoma, or cataract surgery is known as Amsler's sign and is characteristic of the disease. Small peripheral anterior synechiae are occasionally seen in areas of fine rubeosis; they may be transient. In some patients a felt-like membrane develops within the angle in areas of previous fine rubeosis either with or without glaucoma. In rare cases blood-containing cysts of the ciliary body are seen and may proceed to vitreous hemorrhages upon rupture.

The cell and flare in the anterior chamber and the anterior vitreous are usually very mild. The keratic precipitates are extremely characteristic, although they are evanescent in some patients. They are small, widely scattered, round, gray-white precipitates that have a tendency to involve the whole back surface of the cornea. This is one of the only diseases in which the keratic precipitates may involve the superior part of the cornea, occasionally selectively. Between the precipitates are fine, wispy cotton-like filaments that are even more evanescent. The keratic precipitates of this disorder are never confluent, large, or greasy. Within the vitreous there may also be heavy stringy or dust-like particles adherent to a degenerative vitreous framework. After cataract surgery or occasionally spontaneously, dense vitreous veils may form, possibly related to bleeding in the ciliary body area. These may preclude vision or lead to further intraocular inflammation. The eyes with Fuchs' heterochromic iridocyclitis are usually white and quiet externally, but can be inflamed on occasion, especially in association with vitreous hemorrhage or glaucoma.

Glaucoma is a common finding in patients with long-term or more severe progression of the disease (up to 60 per cent). It is also the primary reason for permanent loss of vision with this condition. It is felt to be caused by sclerosis of the trabecular meshwork, but the findings of peripheral anterior synechiae, felt-like membrane in the angle, and trabecular spaces filled with plasma cells are alternate mechanisms of disease. Elevated intraocular pressure may be intermittent initially and may respond to topical steroids (an inflammatory glaucoma), but in many cases, it becomes recalcitrant to steroids, as well as antiglaucoma medications. Patients with this disorder are poor candidates for successful argon laser trabeculoplasty. Filtering surgery is frequently required and has a variable success rate.

Cataract is a consistent feature of Fuchs' heterochromic iridocyclitis. It begins as a posterior subcapsular cataract and has a marked tendency to progress to hypermaturity. Occasionally, the iris heterochromia becomes more obvious when the cataract matures. Patients with milder forms of the disease do well with extracapsular surgery (with or without an intraocular lens), but patients with more severe disease very frequently have anterior chamber or vitreous hemorrhage, severe glaucoma, or corneal edema in the aftermath of intraocular surgery.

The cornea in most patients with this disorder is probably normal, although patients have been noted with guttata in only the affected eye or a reduced endothelial cell count. Areas of darkness spanning several endothelial cells have been seen on specular microscopy. Some patients have demonstrated central or peripheral corneal decompensation after intraocular surgery, again suggesting poor endothelial tolerance.

Chorioretinal lesions with the distinctive appearance of focal atrophy with a hyperpigmented border have been described in a number of patients with Fuchs' uveitis. Many but not all have serologic tests confirming toxoplasmosis. A few patients have been described with a retinal vasculitis.

The pathogenesis of the condition is unknown, although for many years it was felt to be a degenerative or trophic condition, specifically of the nervous system or perhaps a vascular insufficiency. Taking all present pathologic and clinical information into account, there is significant evidence to suggest that the disease is an occlusive vasculitis as a result of a localized immunologic reaction with depression of suppressor T-cell activity. Large numbers of plasma cells, immunoglobins, and immune complexes are found locally without evidence of systemic disease. Vascular occlusion causes the hypoxia, neovascularization, and subsequent hemorrhages. It is conceivable that certain processes—for example, toxoplasmosis—may initiate the process in some patients. Early glaucoma is probably related to the obstruction of the trabecular spaces by plasma cells, but later in the course, trabecular sclerosis or vascular ischemia and rubeosis may play a more prominent role.

THERAPY

Ocular. The majority of patients with Fuchs' heterochromic iridocyclitis have few symptoms and do not require treatment other than periodic observation. Steroid drops can reduce the anterior chamber reaction and the symptoms of floaters and can occasionally lower the intraocular pressure during intermittent attacks of glaucoma. The use of topical steroids, however, is generally not indicated. Glaucoma is the most significant therapeutic problem. It may respond initially to topical steroids, but later becomes refractory to steroids. Milder cases may respond to topical or systemic antiglaucoma medications, but more severe cases will be refractory.

Surgical. Argon laser trabeculoplasty is usually not successful and probably should be avoided if there are significant peripheral anterior synechiae, fine vessels in the angle, or a felt-like membrane. Filtration surgery is frequently indicated, but anterior chamber and vitreous hemorrhage and intraocular inflammation preclude success in many cases. Light cyclocryotherapy before filtration surgery may reduce the complications that apparently are caused by neovascularization.

With milder forms of the disease, cataract surgery (even with an intraocular lens) has a good success rate. Extracapsular cataract extraction is preferred over an intracapsular cataract operation. In more severe forms of the disease, glaucoma, intraocular bleeding, and inflammation frequently preclude successful cataract surgery. Corneal transplantation has been required in only a limited number of these patients, but has met with poor success because of peripheral anterior synechiae and glaucoma in these selected patients.

Ocular or Periocular Manifestations

Angle: Felt-like membrane; fine peripheral anterior synechiae (PAS), fine rubeosis; hyphema (occasional).
Conjunctiva: Ciliary flush (occasional); quiescent (usually).
Cornea: Central or peripheral corneal edema after intraocular surgery; dark areas on specular microscopy; guttata (occasional); lower endothelial cell count.
Fundus: Focal, atrophic chorioretinal scars with pigmented borders.
Intraocular Pressure: Increased.
Lens: Posterior subcapsular cataract with tendency to progression.
Uvea: Anterior stromal and posterior pigment iris atrophy, especially in the pupillary zone; fine filaments between keratic precipitates; gaps in the pupillary ruff around the pupil with transillumination iris defects; heterochromia frequently reversed or subtle; iris vessels straight, narrow, and more evident; lack of crisp iris details; mild cell and flare; rubeosis; small, round, nonconfluent keratic precipitates, especially on the superior cornea.
Vitreous: Cells adherent to vitreous framework, condensed vitreous veils (occasional).

PRECAUTIONS

The diagnosis is frequently missed because the wide spectrum of the disease is not appreciated. The term "heterochromia" is probably inappropriate because it is frequently absent. Once the disease is confirmed, other medical workup for uveitis is not needed. If the disease is unilateral at presentation, it usually remains unilateral. Rarely, the disease is present in other family members; some patients report heterochromia since childhood. Steroid therapy is usually not successful or indicated. These patients must be followed periodically to monitor for glaucoma, cataracts, or corneal disease.

COMMENTS

The prognosis varies with the progression and severity of the clinical findings, especially with regard to iris stromal atrophy and rubeosis. The significance of toxoplasmosis-like scars is not known. In milder cases, intraocular surgery is usually successful; in more advanced cases (for example, in patients with severe glaucoma), both cataract and glaucoma surgery have a significant incidence of complications.

References

Arffa RC, Schlaegel TFJ: Chorioretinal scars in Fuchs' heterochromic iridocyclitis. Arch Ophthalmol 102:1153–1155, 1984.
Berger BB, Tessler HH, Kottow MH: Anterior segment ischemia in Fuchs' heterochromic cyclitis. Arch Ophthalmol 98:499, 1980.
Brooks AM, et al: Progressive corneal endothelial cell changes in anterior segment disease. Aust NZ J Ophthalmol 15:71–78, 1987.
Kimura SJ: Fuchs' syndrome of heterochromic cyclitis in brown-eyed patients. Trans Am Ophthalmol Soc 76:77–86, 1978.
Liesegang TJ: Clinical features and prognosis in Fuchs' uveitis syndrome. Arch Ophthalmol 100:1622–1626, 1982.
O'Connor GR: Heterochromic iridocyclitis. Trans Ophthalmol Soc UK 104:219–231, 1985.
Saari M, Vuorre I, Nieminen H: Fuchs' heterochromic cyclitis. A simultaneous bilateral fluorescein angiographic study of the iris. Br J Ophthalmol 62:715–721, 1978.

IRIDOCORNEAL ENDOTHELIAL SYNDROME
(Chandler's Syndrome, Cogan-Reese Syndrome, Progressive "Essential" Iris Atrophy)

M. BRUCE SHIELDS, M.D.
Durham, North Carolina

The iridocorneal endothelial (ICE) syndrome encompasses a spectrum of diseases, which includes Chandler's syndrome, progressive "essential" iris atrophy, and the Cogan-Reese syndrome. Common to each condition is an alteration of the corneal endothelium, which has a fine, hammered silver appearance by slitlamp biomicroscopy and typical changes by specular microscopy. In many cases, the endothelial disorder gives rise to corneal edema of variable degree. Ultrastructural studies of advanced cases reveal a multilayered Descemet's membrane lined by scant abnormal cells.

Also common throughout this spectrum of disease are peripheral anterior synechiae, which often extend to or beyond Schwalbe's line. These typically spread circumferentially around the anterior chamber angle, eventually leading to secondary glaucoma in a high percentage of cases. A third feature, and that for which the clinical variations are most easily distinguished, is change in the iris. In Chandler's syndrome, iris changes are absent or limited to mild pupillary distortion and stromal atrophy, whereas progressive iris atrophy is characterized by marked corectopia, ectropion uvea, and atrophy with hole formation. The Cogan-Reese syndrome may have any degree of iris changes, but has the additional feature of nodules on the iris. Clinically similar cases may have diffuse nevi and have been called the iris nevus syndrome. It has yet to be established whether the iris nevus syndrome is a variation of the ICE syndrome. According to the membrane theory of Campbell, endothelium from the abnormal corneal endothelium grows across the anterior chamber angle and onto the iris and subsequently undergoes contraction, leading to the aforementioned changes of both structures.

The ICE syndrome is almost always unilateral and typically becomes apparent during young adulthood, with a predilection for females. There is usually no family history of the disease or associated systemic diseases. Typical presenting complaints include visual disturbance, ranging from a mild blur in the morning hours to marked, persistent reduction of visual acuity, and alterations in the pupil or iris.

THERAPY

Ocular. Managing patients with the iridocorneal endothelial syndrome often involves treatment of corneal edema or secondary glaucoma or both. Ocular therapy may suffice for either problem, although a high percentage of patients eventually require surgical intervention.

The corneal edema is dependent to a degree on the level of intraocular pressure, although it may occur with normal pressures. Control of both corneal edema and secondary glaucoma, therefore, may be accomplished in some cases with antiglaucoma medications. Because of the obstruction of the trabecular meshwork by the membrane or synechiae, drugs that reduce aqueous production, such as beta-blockers or carbonic anhydrase inhibitors, are usually the most efficacious. Topical ophthalmic administration of 0.25 or 0.50 per cent timolol, 0.5 per cent betaxolol, or 0.5 per cent levobunolol twice daily or oral administration of 25 to 50 mg of methazolamide or 500 mg of acetazolamide twice daily may be used. However, pilocarpine or epinephrine may also be effective, especially in the early stages of the disease. In some cases, additional measures may be required for the corneal edema, such as topical hypertonic saline solutions or a soft contact lens.

Surgical. The corneal edema in some patients eventually becomes intractable to all nonsurgical measures. Glaucoma filtering surgery has been used to control the edema by further intraocular pressure reduction. However, the edema may persist despite pressures in the subteens. Penetrating keratoplasty is the preferred surgical technique for management of the corneal edema when the intraocular pressure is controlled at a level sufficient to prevent progressive glaucomatous optic atrophy. When the secondary glaucoma is uncontrolled medically, filtering surgery is the procedure of choice. Laser trabeculoplasty has not been shown to be effective in these cases.

Ocular or Periocular Manifestations

(C) indicates Chandler's syndrome; (I) refers to Cogan-Reese syndrome; and (P) indicates progressive "essential" iris atrophy.

Cornea: Edema (C,I,P); endothelial alteration (C,I,P).
Iris: Atrophy (C,I,P); ectropion uveae (P,I); holes (P,I); nodules (I); peripheral anterior synechiae (C,I,P).
Pupil: Corectopia (C,I,P); distortion (C,I,P).
Other: Secondary glaucoma (C,I,P).

PRECAUTIONS

Potential adverse reactions with beta-blockers include bradycardia, weakened myocardial contractility, bronchospasm, and central nervous system alterations. Pulmonary complications are reduced, but not eliminated, with the cardioselective beta$_1$-blocker, betaxolol. Serious side effects of carbonic anhydrase inhibitors include serum electrolyte imbalance, systemic acidosis, gastrointestinal distress, genitourinary problems, including renal calculi, and blood dyscrasias. The ICE syndrome may be confused with other disorders, which can lead to incorrect therapy. The corneal changes must be distinguished from those of Fuchs' endothelial dystrophy and posterior polymorphous dystrophy. The iris dissolution may resemble the changes in Rieger's syndrome, whereas the iris nodules may be confused with neurofibromatosis, nodular iritis, or malignant melanoma, the latter of which may mistakenly lead to enucleation.

COMMENTS

The subtle changes of Chandler's syndrome are often missed, making this a frequently overlooked cause of unilateral glaucoma. Misdiagnosis is best avoided by careful slitlamp inspection of the posterior cornea for the typical fine, hammered silver appearance, as so clearly described by Chandler.

References

Campbell DG, Shields MB, Smith TR: The corneal endothelium and the spectrum of essential iris atrophy. Am J Ophthalmol 86:317–324, 1978.
Chandler PA: Atrophy of the stroma of the iris. Endothelial dystrophy, corneal edema, and glaucoma. Am J Ophthalmol 41:607–615, 1956.
Cogan DG, Reese AB: A syndrome of iris nodules, ectopic Descemets' membrane, and unilateral glaucoma. Doc Ophthalmol 26:424–433, 1969.
Hirst LW, et al: Specular microscopy of iridocorneal

endothelial syndrome. Am J Ophthalmol 89:11–21, 1980.
Lichter PR: The spectrum of Chandler's syndrome: An often overlooked cause of unilateral glaucoma. Ophthalmology 85:245–251, 1978.
Richardson TM: Corneal decompensation in Chandler's syndrome. A scanning and transmission electron microscopic study. Arch Ophthalmol 97:2112–2119, 1979.
Scheie HG, Yanoff M: Iris nevus (Cogan-Reese) syndrome. A cause of unilateral glaucoma. Arch Ophthalmol 93:963–970, 1975.
Shields MB, Campbell DG, Simmons RJ: The essential iris atrophies. Am J Ophthalmol 85:749–759, 1978.
Shields MB, et al: Iris nodules in essential iris atrophy. Arch Ophthalmol 94:406–410, 1976.
Shields MB, et al: Corneal edema in essential iris atrophy. Ophthalmology 86:1533–1548, 1979.

IRIS BOMBÉ

LEONARD CHRISTENSEN, M.D.
Portland, Oregon

Iris bombé is a pathologic extension of pupillary block whereby the iris is bound to the lens at the pupillary border by firm fibrotic adhesions. These adhesions form most frequently, but not invariably, from chronic iridocyclitis of diverse etiology. When the adhesion is sufficiently firm and complete (seclusio or occlusio pupillae), the flow of aqueous from the posterior chamber is impeded to the extent that the pressure required to drive aqueous into the anterior chamber exceeds the pressure required to drive it out. At that level, the peripheral leaf of the iris bows forward. If the blockage is of sufficient magnitude, the iris is displaced firmly against the trabecula. In turn, the aqueous outflow from the anterior chamber is blocked, creating an acute or subacute angle-closure glaucoma. Iridolenticular adhesions are almost always related to inflammation of the iris. Initially, there is an outpouring of fibrin from the iris, creating soft adhesions to the adjacent lens. If not interrupted, this outpouring is followed by fibrocytic proliferation from the iris stroma, with consequent formation of firm, medically irreversible adhesions.

THERAPY

Ocular. Prophylaxis is most important. Initially, the iris adhesions are uniform and susceptible to medical management by mobilization of the pupil. In active iritis, the pupil should be maximally dilated to prevent iridolenticular adhesions. By alternately employing miotics occasionally, mobilization of the iris may be retained. This will further ensure against formation of adhesions.

Once formed, the fibrocytic adhesions are almost impossible to disrupt by medical means. Dilating agents, including combinations of cycloplegics and mydriatics, such as 2.5 or 10 per cent phenylephrine with 1 per cent atropine, 1 per cent cyclopentolate, or 5 per cent homatropine, may be tried. However, if the intraocular pressure is significantly high, surgical intervention should be employed as soon as possible.

Systemic. Systemic control of glaucoma may be temporarily gained by employment of osmotic agents or carbonic anhydrase inhibitors, but invariably surgery must be performed. Of the osmotic agents, 20 per cent intravenous mannitol is most effective, although oral administration of 0.75 to 1.5 gm/kg of glycerin may be sufficient temporarily.

Surgical. The aim of treatment is to re-establish communication between the posterior and anterior chamber. This may be accomplished by surgical transfixation of the iris or surgical iridectomy. The most recent innovation is iridectomy by argon or YAG laser. If the iris is in contact with the cornea at the site of perforation, heat injury to the cornea might occur. However, this injury should be discrete and at the periphery.

Surgical management consists of establishing the free flow of aqueous from the posterior chamber to the anterior chamber, thus relieving the pressure against the iris. This permits the iris to fall back from the cornea and opens the angle and escape channels. However, sometimes the iris does not spontaneously fall back. Once the anterior chamber is entered, active displacement of the iris by instrumentation is then required.

Transfixion of the iris is mentioned in the older literature. It is achieved by inserting a Graefe (or Wheeler) knife through the cornea, the iris both peripherally and centrally, and the cornea of the opposite side. Although effective, the incisions may close off because of their small size. Damage to the lens can also occur.

A peripheral iridectomy through an ab externo incision is very effective, simple, and safe. In addition, an iris spatula can be inserted between the iris and lens at the pupillary border, thus freeing up the adhesions; however, care must be taken to avoid injury to the lens. Also, the iris spatula can be employed to displace the iris from the posterior corneal surface if necessary. If recurrence is a threat, the peripheral iridectomy can be converted to a sector iridectomy, ensuring against such an event.

Ocular or Periocular Manifestations

Anterior Chamber: Cloudy aqueous.
Cornea: Keratic precipitates; thickened.
Iris: Anterior synechiae; dilated blood vessels; iridolenticular adhesions; posterior synechiae.
Lens: Anterior subcapsular opacity.
Other: Glaucoma.

PRECAUTIONS

Repeated instillation of 10 per cent phenylephrine may produce a systemic vasopressor response, particularly in very young or debilitated patients. Intravenous injections of mannitol may produce mental confusion, particularly in aged or debilitated patients. Although quite safe, this latter agent should be used with caution.

If transfixion is to be employed, care should be taken to avoid the lens, and the surgeon must appreciate that the communication can readily be closed in the face of active inflammation. With iridectomy, suction applied at the opening of the incision delivers the iris to the external surface, and the iris can be readily grasped for an iridectomy. This avoids any chance of lens injury that might occur with insertion of forceps to grasp the iris.

COMMENTS

Iris bombé is essentially the aftermath of iridocyclitis. It may be prevented by maximal pupillary dilation and active mobilization of the pupil early in the disease. Once established, it is almost always a surgical problem best resolved by peripheral or sector iridectomy.

References

Abraham RK, Miller GL: Outpatient argon laser iridectomy for angle closure glaucoma: A two-year study. Trans Am Acad Ophthalmol Otolaryngol 79:529–538, 1975.

Duke-Elder S (ed): System of Ophthalmology, St. Louis, CV Mosby, 1966, Vol IX, p 178.

Shin DH: Argon laser iris photocoagulation to relieve acute angle-closure glaucoma. Am J Ophthalmol 93:348–350, 1982.

Tomey KF, Traverso CE, Shammas IV: Neodymium-YAG laser iridotomy in the treatment and prevention of angle closure glaucoma. A review of 373 eyes. Arch Ophthalmol 105:476–481, 1987.

IRIS CYSTS
(Epithelial Cysts, Epithelial Implantation Cysts, Spontaneous Congenital Iris Cysts)

KENNETH C. SWAN, M.D.

Portland, Oregon

Iris cysts are of two general types: cysts that originate within the intraepithelium or stroma and implantation cysts from intraocular surgery or trauma. Intraepithelial cysts represent an incomplete obliteration or re-establishment of the space between the two layers of the secondary optic vessel. The outer layer is composed of pigment epithelium and presents as a black globular mass behind the iris, which does not transilluminate. Peripherally, the cysts may present as globular protrusions as the overlying iris stroma is pushed anteriorly. They may extend through the iris into the anterior chamber. Iris cysts may be concealed, unless the pupil is dilated. More than one cyst may be noted in the same eye or in the other eye. Iris nodules and cysts also may occur as a proliferative response to miotic therapy for glaucoma or accommodative esotropia. Stromal cysts typically are nonpigmented and semitransparent because they are lined by an external type of epithelium that may have goblet cells. They may be congenital or caused by implantation of corneal or conjunctival epithelium from surgery or trauma. Clinical findings may include pupillary distortion, iridocyclitis, and glaucoma. Cysts may enlarge and eventually fill the anterior chamber, with potential loss of the eye. The rate of growth of these cysts is quite variable.

THERAPY

Ocular. Iris cysts induced by miotic therapy partially recede when miotics are discontinued. In the management of accommodative esotropia, these cysts reportedly can be minimized by the concomitant use of 2.5 per cent phenylephrine given intermittently.

Surgical. The management of implantation or embryonal epithelial cysts of the iris is in a large part dependent on their growth pattern. Some small cysts will remain stationary and asymptomatic; these should only be observed. Those with evidence of growth require therapy.

For cysts that involve the corneal or limbal stroma, chemical cauterization is indicated. Retrobulbar anesthesia* is used for adults and general anesthesia for children. High magnification with the surgical microscope is essential. A discission knife is used to make a track into the cyst. The knife is withdrawn, and a short, blunt-tipped 30-gauge needle attached to a 2-ml syringe containing 0.5 ml of 20 per cent trichloroacetic acid is introduced. The cyst is aspirated, and then, without withdrawal of the needle, the mixture of cyst fluid and trichloroacetic acid is carefully injected. The clear walls of the cyst and the protein in the cyst fluid immediately turn white. The cyst contents are aspirated to collapse the cyst completely before the needle is withdrawn. Suction is maintained as the needle is withdrawn to avoid spread of the acid into the stromal tissue. Only a minimal coagulation of the conjunctiva occurs at the puncture site. Iris cysts not in contact with the wall of the eye cannot be injected safely, but simple surgical excision, performed the same way as an iridectomy, is curative.

Epithelial cysts may also be treated with xenon arc photocoagulation. Retrobulbar anesthesia* is used for adults and general anesthesia for children. A plastic water bath chamber filled with saline solution is placed between the lids. The anterior segment focusing attachment is placed on the photocoagulator. With the Zeiss unit, settings for basic intensity are (green) 1, the iris diaphragm is open, and the field diaphragm is 4.5°. The light is focused on the anterior wall of the cysts. Sufficient applications to cover the cyst in confluent fashion (usually 6 to 10) are made. There usually is little or no visible reaction. The patient is dismissed from the hospital the following day on one drop of homatropine or cyclopentolate three times daily. In patients with evidence of iridocyclitis, corticosteroid solution is used. In one month, there is usually some shrinkage of the cyst, and a second treatment is given, using the same method. During the next several weeks, the cyst usually collapses completely, but a third treatment may be necessary.

Other methods advocated include extensive surgical procedures with iridocyclectomy and corneal or corneoscleral transplants, diathermy, electrolysis, cryotherapy, and Argon laser coagulation of corneal cysts. X-ray irradiation has largely been abandoned.

Ocular or Periocular Manifestations

Lens: Cataract; subluxation (with pressure).
Pupil: Distortion; pigmented nodules.
Other: Corneal edema; decreased visual acuity; glaucoma; uveitis.

PRECAUTIONS

Therapy is not always indicated in the management of epithelial cysts of external origin; however, if one elects to observe these lesions, they must be seen at regular 6-month intervals because they may enlarge dramatically after a dormant period. After the decision to treat is made, one must treat aggressively and effectively. Incomplete management and disruption of the cyst wall can convert a localized epithelial cyst into a diffuse epithelial growth.

When injecting sclerosing fluids, such as 20 per cent trichloracetic acid, one must take great care to inject only into the cyst and not into the cornea or conjunctiva, or an opacity and severe iritis will result. Inadvertent injection of trichloroacetic acid into the anterior chamber can cause irreversible corneal, iris, and lens damage. There are usually no adverse reactions after an initial 10-day period of mild iritis. In occasional instances, a second injection has been required 1 to 6 months later.

Photocoagulation also requires great care. Inadvertent "explosions" can rupture the cyst wall, converting the cyst into an epithelial downgrowth. Cataracts or corneal and iris changes may occur with improper use of this technique. Excessive treatment may require hospitalization because postoperatively a moderately severe plastic iritis may develop, sometimes with secondary glaucoma. Photocoagulation does cause shrinkage of the iris, resulting in a slightly updrawn pupil.

It should be explained to the patient before initiating any form of therapy that multiple treatments may be necessary. These cysts may even reappear years after surgery, chemical cautery, or photocoagulation. Therefore, long-term follow-up is necessary.

COMMENTS

With renewed interest in extracapsular cataract extraction, an increased incidence of epithelial implantation or even downgrowths can be expected to result from accidental incarceration of the lens capsule in the limbal or corneal wound.

References

Cleasby GW: Photocoagulation of iris-ciliary body epithelial cysts. Trans Am Acad Ophthalmol Otolaryngol 75:638–642, 1971.
Duke-Elder S (ed): System of Ophthalmology. St. Louis, CV Mosby, 1964, Vol III, pp 603–606; 1966, Vol IX, pp 769–775.
Rosenquist RC, Fraunfelder FT, Swan KC: Treatment of conjunctival epithelial cysts with trichloracetic acid. J Ocul Ther Surg 4:51–55, 1985.
Scholtz RT, Kelley JS: Argon laser photocoagulation treatment of iris cysts following penetrating keratoplasty. Arch Ophthalmol 100:926–927, 1982.
Swan KC: Iris pigment nodules complicating miotic therapy. Am J Ophthalmol 37:886–889, 1954.
Swan KC: Epithelial cell cysts of the anterior chamber treated by acid injections. Doc Ophthalmol 18:363–370, 1979.

IRIS MELANOMA
H. JOHN SHAMMAS, M.D.
Los Angeles, California

It is generally agreed that iris melanomas are relatively benign. However, when a pigmented iris lesion is noted on slitlamp examination, it should be documented with photographs and observed at regular intervals for evidence of growth. Signs of active growth include an increase in size, new vessel formation, implantation growths, pupil distortion, and ectropion uveae. Spontaneous hyphema and secondary glaucoma occasionally complicate the course of highly vascularized melanomas. Iris melanomas grow either into the anterior chamber or along the iris surface, ultimately invading the angle and ciliary body. The iris pigment epithelium appears to be a barrier to the invasion of the posterior chamber. Diffuse iris melanomas are the result of widely scattered areas of neoplasia.

Extension of the iris melanoma into the ciliary body carries a more severe prognosis. The extension is usually not recognized early, and as a consequence, the ciliary body tumor may become quite large before it is diagnosed. The tumor's thickness can be accurately measured by ultrasonography using standardized A-scan techniques.

THERAPY

Supportive. A conservative approach is recommended at the time of initial diagnosis until definite evidence of growth is established. Iris melanomas can be followed for long periods of time because of the benign nature of these tumors.

Surgical. The surgical therapy includes iridectomy, iridocyclectomy, and enucleation. Surgery should only be considered when active signs of growth are documented over short follow-up periods.

An excisional iridectomy is indicated for melanomas localized to the iris. The specimen should be pinned to a flat surface and the borders identified so that the limits of the lesion can be determined. Measures should be taken to prevent the tissue from curling and wrinkling, which may distort the histologic findings. If there is residual tumor, it would seem safe to leave the eye alone until regrowth is evident.

If an iris melanoma has extended into the ciliary body, an iridocyclectomy can be performed. Good results can be expected because iris and ciliary body melanomas are relatively benign. There are many ways of accomplishing an iridocyclectomy; however, an en bloc excision with preservation of the outer scleral layers appears to be the safest.

Enucleation is only recommended for diffuse iris and ciliary body melanomas that cannot be managed by local excision.

Ocular or Periocular Manifestations

Anterior Chamber: Depth variations; hyphema.
Iris: Chronic uveitis; ectropion uveae; freckles; heterochromia; pigmented mass.
Other: Decreased visual acuity, glaucoma; hypotension; prominent episcleral vessels; pupillary distortion; refractive disorders.

PRECAUTIONS

Melanomas have to be differentiated from benign iris lesions, such as nevi, freckles, or melanocytomas. When making the final diagnosis, one must remember that melanomas are rare in children and non-Caucasians. A complete physical examination and laboratory studies, such as blood counts, liver function tests, and radiologic studies, should be performed to make sure that the tumor is not a metastatic lesion to the iris.

Surgical therapy is not without its risks. Most iris melanocytic lesions do not enlarge and can be safely observed. If the lesion shows only slight growth on follow-up examinations, careful observation may be recommended, but if the lesion shows more pronounced and progressive growth, then complete excision is warranted. Complications of iridectomy include hyphema, cataract, wound dehiscence, and episcleral seeding of the tumor. Complications of iridocyclectomy include vitreous loss, cataract, high astigmatism, and incomplete excision.

Radiotherapy has no place in the treatment of iris melanomas. The cytology makes it unlikely that radiation would be effective. One case of successful laser treatment of a recurrent tapioca melanoma of the iris and ciliary body has been reported.

COMMENTS

An accurate diagnosis and evidence of active growth should be established before any therapy is considered.

References

Arentsen JJ, Green WR: Melanoma of the iris: Report of 72 cases treated surgically. Ophthalmic Surg 6:23–37, 1975.
Dart JK, Marsh RJ, Garner A, Cooling RJ: Fluorescein angiography of anterior uveal melanocytic tumors. Br J Ophthalmol 72:326–336, 1988.
Demeler U: Fluorescence angiographical studies in the diagnosis and follow-up of tumors of the iris and ciliary body. Adv Ophthalmol 42:1–17, 1981.
Kersten RC, Tse DJ, Anderson R: Iris melanoma. Nevus or malignancy? Surv Ophthalmol 29:423–433, 1985.
Makley TA Jr: Management of melanomas of the anterior segment. Surv Ophthalmol 19:135–153, 1974.
Rones B, Zimmerman LE: The prognosis of primary tumors of the iris treated by iridectomy. Arch Ophthalmol 60:193–205, 1958.
Shammas HF, Blodi FC: Prognostic factors in choroidal and ciliary body melanomas. Arch Ophthalmol 95:63–69, 1977.
Shields JA, Sanborn GE, Augsburger JJ: The differential diagnosis of malignant melanoma of the iris: A clinical study of 200 patients. Ophthalmology 90:716–720, 1983.
Sunba MSN, Rahi AHS, Morgan G: Tumors of the anterior uvea. I. Metastasizing malignant melanoma of the iris. Arch Ophthalmol 98:82–85, 1980.
Territo C, Shields CL, Shields JA, Augsburger JJ, Schroeder RP: National course of melanocytic tumor of the iris. Ophthalmology 95:1251–1255, 1988.
Wilson RS, Fraunfelder FT, Hanna C: Recurrent tapioca melanoma of the iris and ciliary body treated with the argon laser. Am J Ophthalmol 82:213–217, 1976.

IRIS PROLAPSE
HAROLD C. PATTERSON, M.D.
Danbury, Connecticut

Iris prolapse is most commonly found as a complication of cataract or glaucoma surgery. It usually occurs within 48 hours after cataract extraction, but may occur 10 to 15 days later as sutures loosen and the iris slips through and becomes incarcerated between the lips of the wound protruding beneath the conjunctival flap or even escapes from beneath it. Prolapse may also occur as a result of corneal perforation, such as in acute ulcerative or degenerative conditions and injuries. Such a prolapse will involve either a portion of the body of the iris, which protrudes as a knuckle, or the free margin of the iris, in which a tag may hang freely over the cornea. When the anterior chamber reforms after corneal perforation, the iris is put under considerable pressure, and a pear-shaped or teardrop pupil may result. Alternatively, in a large central destructive process, the entire pupillary margin may be involved. A total synechia is formed, the pupil becomes completely occluded, and the whole or greater part of the iris is incorporated in the corneal scar, with grave consequences to the future of the eye.

THERAPY

Ocular. If a teardrop pupil is seen the morning after an uncomplicated intracapsular lens extraction, 250 mg of acetazolamide is given systemically to reduce intraocular volume. A topical anesthetic and potent miotic are then applied to the eye. Thirty minutes later, the portion of the cornea over the area of adhesion should be stroked with a moistened iris repositor or a blunt muscle hook.

In cases of a frank iris prolapse beneath the conjunctiva, 0.1 per cent isoflurophate or a similar strong miotic may succeed in pulling the prolapse out of the wound if it is not too large. If this is unsuccessful, a cryoprobe of controlled temperature reduction not to exceed 0° C should be applied over the base of the prolapse for about 15 seconds. This is a simple and provocative method of stimulating a contraction of the iris, and it may be applied safely after using a topical anesthetic.

If there is a proper fixation of the globe, light coagulation of prolapses of a cystic nature may be performed under topical anesthesia. Coagulation is also indicated whenever it is inadvisable to do a surgical repair for fresh iris prolapses.

Surgical. If corneal stroking and cryo stimulation fail to correct the teardrop pupil, Atkinson's procedure should be carried out. It requires a preoperative anesthesia similar to that used in the original cataract extraction. In addition, lidocaine can be injected subconjunctivally in the area of the adhesion. The spatula should then be swept down, pressing back on the iris, as in iris replacement at the time of cataract surgery. The pupil should become round immediately. A miotic should be instilled and a mild pressure bandage applied.

A frank prolapse of 2 to 3 mm may need surgical intervention to replace the iris. If the iris is strangulated and does not slip back into place after being stroked gently, it should be excised and the wound resutured under general anesthesia. If the incarceration occurs late after the patient has left the hospital, is not very large, and is covered by conjunctiva, it may be left alone.

Ocular or Periocular Manifestations

Cornea: Perforation; pseudocornea.
Iris: Anterior synechiae; exudates; fibrous tissue; granulation.
Pupil: Distortion (pear-shaped); occlusion.
Other: Decreased visual acuity; irritation.

PRECAUTIONS

Cauterization does remove the extruded iris, but does not release the incarceration. Cauterization cannot be used in the presence of iris irritation or for large prolapses, which need to be watched constantly by slitlamp for evidence of keratic precipitates. Light coagulation is much safer than cauterization, although coagulation should be used with caution in late or old iris prolapses when the iris may strongly adhere to the conjunctiva and may be burned by the coagulation. One must also be careful not to create a fistula and flat chamber.

One of the dangers of using trichloroacetic acid is adhesion of the iris to the wound, which is always a potential source of future trouble, although it may be fairly well tolerated in a high percentage of cases. General anesthesia should be used for iris excision because it is not wise to give a retrobulbar anesthetic in an eye that has recently had intraocular surgery. Topical anesthesia is not adequate to prevent pain when manipulating the iris.

COMMENTS

After all surgery in which the iris has been manipulated, the surgeon should be sure that the edges are free from the wound and that there is adequate closure. If the iris does not prolapse, it may become incarcerated. Incarceration of the iris prevents rapid healing, facilitates entrance of infection into the eye, and leads to chronic and recurrent inflammatory episodes that may ultimately destroy the function of the eye and encourage a sympathetic reaction. Preventive measures include reducing the intraocular pressure, making a slanting incision into the anterior chamber, using miotics after round pupil cataract extractions, making adequate tight closure of corneoscleral incisions, and restricting the activity of the patient. It is usually the cyclodynamics of the aqueous gushing against the posterior iris that causes it to prolapse.

References

Duke-Elder S (ed): System of Ophthalmology. St. Louis, CV Mosby, 1965, Vol VIII, pp 635–636.
Patterson HC: Complications in iris surgery and trauma. *In* Fasanella RM (ed): Management of Complications in Eye Surgery, 2nd ed. Philadelphia, WB Saunders, 1965, pp 178–180.

PARS PLANITIS
(Angiohyalitis, Chronic Cyclitis, Cyclitis, Peripheral Uveitis, Peripheral Uveoretinitis, Vitreitis)

DANIEL H. SPITZBERG, M.D.
Indianapolis, Indiana

Pars planitis is a common inflammation seen in young adults. Most cases last for decades and are usually bilateral. The minimum criterion for diagnosis is the presence of a snowbank or at least a few snowballs in the peripheral inferior retina. The cause of pars planitis is unknown. The most important guide for therapy is the degree of cystoid macular edema, and the most important feature for diagnosis is the snowbank. Pars planitis is the most commonly overdiagnosed uveitis syndrome. Ophthalmologists often make the diagnosis apparently because of cystoid macular edema; however, such macular edema is common in many different types of uveitis and is of therapeutic but not diagnostic interest.

THERAPY

Ocular. The goal of therapy is not to eradicate all signs and symptoms but to reduce the inflammation so that hypotony, cystoid macular degeneration, vitreous traction, retinal detachment, and cyclitis membrane formation will not significantly reduce visual acuity. If the disease is unilateral or asymmetric or if the patient does not tolerate systemic corticosteroids, periocular injections of methylprednisolone* may be necessary. A topical local anesthetic should be applied at least five times over the area to be injected. Some patients benefit from an oral analgesic sedative approximately 20 minutes before the injection. The head should be tilted so that gravity will pull the anesthetic into the cul-de-sac. An injectable anesthetic is neither necessary nor advisable. A 2-ml syringe is used to inject 0.5 ml of the 80 mg/ml concentration of methylprednisolone. The easiest place to make the injection is inferotemporally. The point of the needle should be placed 3 to 4 mm in front of the cul-de-sac and between blood vessels. It should be pushed into the hilt, *following the curve* of the sclera by the use of lateral motion of the needle over an area of 5 mm. This is a most valuable maneuver, since it allows one to hug the sclera as the needle goes in. The barrel of the syringe must be moved a large distance as one goes around the eyeball in order to keep the needle point near the eye. Keeping the needle near the eye with the aperture facing the sclera reduces the patient's discomfort and increases the penetration of the steroid because it keeps the medication closer to the sclera and not out in the orbital tissues. This lateral motion also avoids impaling the eyeball, since the ophthalmologist will immediately be aware that the sclera has been engaged if such a movement is used. By putting the injection far back, the side effects of chemosis and ptosis are decreased and the white material is not visible. If repeated injections are necessary, the superotemporal quadrant is usually varied with inferotemporal. If a patient develops an allergy to methylprednisolone, the diagnosis should be confirmed by 0.01 ml injected intradermally and read at 2 days, and the patient should be switched to another agent, such as triamcinolone (40 mg/ml).

These periocular injections may be given from every 2 to 26 weeks, depending on the patient's needs. At the beginning of treatment they should be given every 2 weeks until the patient's vision reaches a maximum level, and then they should be tapered to the minimal amount necessary to maintain the vision at the desired level. Since the disease lasts for decades, one should hesitate to stop medication completely, unless one can taper down to nothing without a relapse in vision. Additional topical corticosteroids or a mydriatic may not be necessary because the anterior chamber reaction is usually mild.

Systemic. Since the disease is usually bilateral and the process is extremely chronic, the systemic use of corticosteroids on an alternate-day regimen is recommended. Fifty to 100 mg of prednisone may be given every other day after breakfast, and the dosage should be adjusted depending on the therapeutic response, as well as the ocular and systemic complications of such therapy. Steroid treatment should be continued as long as ocular and systemic complications are not serious, and alternate-day administration can be continued for decades in some patients. Stopping medication will cause the cystoid changes in the macula to return and the vision to decrease. The ophthalmologist should monitor the patient's vision and should document the degree of cystoid macular edema by fluorescein angiography.

When corticosteroids are not adequate, some authorities use immunosuppressive agents. Although immunosuppressive agents are effective, they are life threatening and should not be used for mild or unilateral cases.

Surgical. Another alternative if corticosteroids are ineffective is cryotherapy. Utilizing indirect ophthalmoscopy, cryotherapy should be administered using a nitrous oxide or carbon dioxide retinal probe over the uninvolved and surrounding areas. An iceball should cover the exudative focus and then be allowed to thaw. It is then immediately refrozen to the same extent. Uninvolved ciliary body and retina are treated one probe width beyond the recognizable inflammatory reaction. A single depot injection of corticosteroids* is given to minimize the inflammatory effects of the cryotherapy. Cryotherapy may need to be repeated in 3 to 4 months.

Precautions

Immunosuppressive agents should be supervised by an oncologist, rheumatologist, hematologist, or any other expert in their use. They have an additive effect when used with corticosteroids and have the advantage of not causing glaucoma or posterior subcapsular cataracts.

Comments

About 80 per cent of cases of pars planitis do not need treatment. The patient should be treated only for a definite decrease in vision caused by cystoid macular edema and should not be treated for floaters. The level at which therapy is begun varies from a vision of 20/25 to 20/40. Evidence of the deleterious effects of smoking and pars planitis has been shown, and it is recommended that smoking be discontinued.

References

Aaberg TM, Cesarz TJ, Flickinger RR Jr: Treatment of peripheral uveoretinitis by cryotherapy. Am J Ophthalmol 75:685–688, 1973.

Aaberg TM, Cesarz TJ, Flickinger RR Jr: Treatment of pars planitis. I. Cryotherapy. Surv Ophthalmol 22:120–125, 1977.

Buckley CE III, Gills JP Jr: Cyclophosphamide therapy of peripheral uveitis. Arch Intern Med 124:29–35, 1969.

Henderly DE, Haymond RS, Rao NA, Smith RE: The significance of the pars plana exudate in pars planitis. Am J Ophthalmol 103:669–671, 1987.

Henderly DE, Genstler AJ, Rao NA, Smith RE: Pars planitis. Trans Ophthalmol Soc UK 105:227–232, 1986.

Giles CL: The use of methotrexate in the treatment of uveitis. Univ Mich Med Cent J 35:30–31, 1969.

Lazar M, Weiner MJ, Leopold IH: Treatment of uveitis with methotrexate. Am J Ophthalmol 67:383–387, 1969.

Nussenblatt RB, Palestine AG, Chan CC: Cyclosporine therapy for uveitis: Long-term followup. J Ocul Pharmacol 1:369–382, 1985.

Schlaegel TF Jr: Recent advances in uveitis. Ann Ophthalmol 4:525–552, 1972.

Schlaegel TF Jr: Peripheral uveitis. JAMA 223:696, 1973.

Schlaegel TF Jr, Weber JC: Treatment for pars planitis. II. Corticosteroids. Surv Ophthalmol 22:120–130, 1977.

Wakefield D, Dunlop I, McCluskey PJ, Penny R: Uveitis: aetiology and disease associations in an Australian population. Aust NZ J Ophthalmol 14:181–187, 1986.

Wong VG, Hersh EM: Methotrexate in the therapy of cyclitis. Trans Am Acad Ophthalmol Otolaryngol 69:279–293, 1965.

RUBEOSIS IRIDIS
(Neovascular Glaucoma)

JOHN R. SAMPLES, M.D.

Portland, Oregon

Rubeosis iridis is a condition in which the iris develops neovascularization, often starting along the pupillary margin and progressing across the root of the iris into the trabecular meshwork. It occurs as a complication of diseases in which there is retinal ischemia and is frequently associated with a severe form of secondary glaucoma, which has been termed neovascular glaucoma or rubeotic glaucoma. The growth of new blood vessels is associated with a fibrovascular membrane growing on the anterior surface of the iris and into the anterior chamber angle. These vessels can spread rapidly to cover the iris and trabecular meshwork, ultimately leading to the development of peripheral and anterior synechiae and to closure of the anterior chamber angle. The peripheral anterior synechiae gradually coalesce to close the angle in a zipper-like fashion.

About one third of patients with rubeosis iridis have diabetic retinopathy. Central retinal vein occlusion accounts for about 28 per cent of all cases of rubeosis iridis. Other causes include retinal detachment that may be chronic and may be associated with malignant melanoma. Uveitis can also cause the development of rubeosis iridis. End-stage glaucoma may result in rubeosis iridis, probably because of persistent elevated pressures leading to a central vein occlusion and its consequences. Carotid artery obstructive disease, retrolental fibroplasia, sickle-cell anemia, intraocular tumors, and carotid cavernous fistulas may lead to the development of neovascular glaucoma.

Many of the conditions that cause rubeosis share an underlying development of retinal hypoxia. It seems likely that this hypoxia leads to a "cell signal" that stimulates the angiogenesis and proliferation of new blood vessels. Similar signals may be present in uveitis, and the generation of a neovascular stimulus through a peptide signal thus seems likely. If such a peptide signal does eminate from hypoxic retina, it would be expected that removal of either vitreous or lens would increase rubeosis iridis in eyes with diabetic retinopathy. This has proven to be the case and is evidence for a diffusable angiogenic factor.

There are several stages in the development of rubeosis. At first, the intraocular pressure is normal, unless other underlying or associated abnormalities of the trabecular meshwork are present. Slitlamp biomicroscopy using high-level magnification reveals small dilated tufts of capillaries with randomly oriented vessels on the surface of the iris near the pupillary margin. These new vessels characteristically leak fluorescein. Neovascularization progresses from the pupillary margin toward the root of the iris. Initially, gonioscopy shows a normal, open anterior chamber angle, and later single vascular trunks are seen crossing and arborizing into the trabecular meshwork. In a subsequent phase, the rubeosis becomes more florid, and a fibrovascular membrane that covers the anterior chamber angle and anterior surface of the iris is appreciated. As the membrane contracts, iris pigment epithelium is everted through the pupil onto the surface of the iris, leading to ectropion uvea. Glaucoma occurs as a result of inflammatory reactions that take place in the eye, the development of subsequent hyphema, the covering of the fibrovascular membrane over the trabecular meshwork, and the development of peripheral anterior synechiae. It is important to distinguish between an open angle and an angle that is covered with synechiae; if the angle is open, there is still hope for achieving some regression of the vessels in the angle when panretinal photocoagulation is performed. In the final phase as the angle becomes completely closed, the glaucoma is quite severe, and surgical intervention is required to alleviate the pressure.

THERAPY

Ocular. The intraocular pressure should be lowered through the use of topical and systemic medications. It may be prudent to avoid miotics in these cases, since they may produce a forward shift of the lens iris diaphragm. Initial therapy should include a topical ophthalmic beta-blocker twice daily or 1 per cent epinephrine twice daily. The use of an adjunctive oral carbonic anhydrase inhibitor, such as acetazolamide, may be useful. Long-acting cycloplegics, such as 1 per cent atropine twice daily, as well as the use of the more potent topical ophthalmic steroids, are helpful in reducing pain and controlling the inflammatory response that is evident in the eye. Neovascular eyes that have reached an end stage and that are not candidates for surgical therapy require the use of chronic cycloplegics and steroids. Glycerol and mannitol, osmotic agents, can be used temporarily before surgery. Some workers have advocated radiation management in neovascular glaucoma, both for analgesia and to treat the underlying cause. Direct radiation is used, and the mechanism of action is unclear. This treatment is controversial.

Surgical. Surgical management depends on the phase at which the rubeosis is encountered. Eyes in the early phase of development of rubeosis do best with panretinal photocoagulation and carefully timed medical treatment of the glaucoma. In many instances, regression of vessels in the angle is observed after panretinal photocoagulation, and it is possible to forestall glaucoma surgery. In other instances when the pressure is quite elevated and the acuity of the eye remains at a level sufficient to retain vision, it is best to proceed with filtering surgery soon after panretinal photocoagulation. Panretinal photocoagulation inhibits the growth of rubeosis and permits the involution of active rubeosis, with subsequent improvement in outflow facility in the anterior segment. Panretinal photocoagulation is most effective when it is used prophylactically, as, for example, in a central retinal vein occlusion in which rubeosis is significantly correlated with the extent of retinal capillary nonperfusion. Fundus fluorescein angiography should be obtained whenever possible after a vein occlusion. When extensive retinal capillary nonperfusion is documented, prophylactic treatment is indicated. Because vitrectomy and lensectomy are frequently followed by the development of rubeosis, prophylactic panretinal photocoagulation after these procedures is indicated, particularly when peripupillary fluorescein leakage has been detected. In selected cases, panretinal photocoagulation may reverse intraocular pressure elevation in the early open-angle glaucoma stage of rubeosis iridis.

Goniophotocoagulation is the application of direct photocoagulation to angle vessels. It seems to be most effective for rubeosis in its earliest stages. When used and directed at the trunk vessels crossing the angle, it can provide an effective adjunct to the eventual development of intractable neovascular glaucoma. This procedure does not have any effect upon the subsequent development of rubeosis and is best regarded only as a supplement and not a replacement for a retinal ablative procedure.

Once extensive panretinal peripheral anterior synechiae or the development of a fibrovascular membrane has occurred in the angle, it is unlikely that goniophotocoagulation will have any beneficial effect upon intraocular pressure. Traditionally, filtering surgery in eyes with neovascular glaucoma has been regarded as rarely successful both because of a high risk of intraoperative bleeding and the postoperative progression of the fibrovascular membrane. However, when panretinal photocoagulation possibly combined with goniophotocoagulation is undertaken before filtration, a much more successful result may be obtained. Panretinal photocoagulation, topical steroids, cycloplegics, and the time for these measures to have an effect are important preoperative adjuncts to filtering surgery. In one report, adequate control was obtained in 67 per cent (16 of 24 eyes) after filtration surgery. In eyes that have not previously had conjunctival surgery, a trabeculectomy works well. The excised limbal block should be so anterior that one can perform a careful dissection of corneoscleral tissue away from peripheral anterior synechiae. The iris may then be inspected and surface vessels may be coagulated with a bipolar cautery as described by Herschler. Krupin has reported good results with neovascular glaucoma patients with the implantation of setons. Preliminary results have been promising with the implantation of tubes and with the Molteno seton.

The adjunctive use of fluorouracil has substantially increased the chances of success in patients undergoing routine trabecular filtering surgery for neovascular glaucoma. A variety of treatment protocols have been proposed. Optimal parameters for the treatment with fluorouracil remain to be settled. At present 0.1 ml of a solution containing 50 mg/ml of fluorouracil* is recommended for subconjunctival injection at a variety of sites, none of which is in the immediate vicinity of the filtering bleb.

A variety of cyclodestructive procedures have been advocated for some cases of neovascular glaucoma. They are usually more palliative than vision-maintaining. In addition to cyclocryotherapy, the use of both therapeutic ultrasound and of a YAG laser cyclodestructive procedure has been advocated. Since eyes with advanced rubeosis have minimal outflow, one must obliterate nearly the entire ciliary body in order to control intraocular pressure. Often, a cycloablative procedure will enable maintenance of a useful eye, staving off the need for enucleation. At present, such eyes treated with 180° of cyclocryotherapy use a 1-minute freeze at −80° C directly over the ciliary body, with a total of six applications throughout the 180°. If these fail to lower the pressure, treatment is repeated embracing 90° of previously treated ciliary body and 90° new areas.

Ocular or Periocular Manifestations

Iris: Neovascularization.

Trabecular meshwork: Neovascularization, peripheral anterior synechiae, angle closure.

Precautions

Rubeosis iridis and neovascular glaucoma develop rapidly after central retinal vein occlusion and vitrectomy. Vigilance is needed to detect these conditions early, since treatment and outcome are far better with earlier detection. Prophylactic treatment is a consideration when nonperfused ischemic areas of retina are detected on fluorescein angiogram.

Comments

Diabetic eyes that develop neovascular glaucoma have often previously undergone vitrectomy and lensectomy, making them poor candidates for limbal filtration surgery. In some instances, a Molteno implant may be useful. Alternatively, cyclodestructive procedures should be considered. When the media are too hazy and a retinal photoablative procedure is needed, a panretinal cryoablation should be considered. Neovascular glaucoma associated with retinal detachment has been reported to be associated with the development of intravitreal neovascularization from ciliary body after cyclocryotherapy.

References

Allen RC, et al: Filtration surgery in the treatment of neovascular glaucoma. Ophthalmology 89:1181–1187, 1982.
Ancker E, Molteno ACB: Molteno drainage implant for neovascular glaucoma. Trans Ophthalmol Soc UK 102:122–124, 1982.
Ehrenberg M, et al: Rubeosis iridis: Preoperative iris fluorescein angiography and periocular steroids. Ophthalmology 91:321-325, 1984.
Goldberg MF, Erickson ES: Intravitreal ciliary body neovascularization. Ophthalmic Surg 8:62–70, 1977.
Herschler J, Agness D: A modified filtering procedure for neovascular glaucoma. Arch Ophthalmol 97:2339–2341, 1979.
Heuer DK, et al: 5-fluorouracil in glaucoma filtering surgery. Ophthalmology 91:384–393, 1984.
Krupin T, et al: Long-term results of valve implants in filtering surgery for eyes with neovascular glaucoma. Am J Ophthalmol 95:775–782, 1983.
Priluch IA, Robertson DN, Hollinhorst RW: Long-term follow-up of occlusion in central retinal vein in young adults. Am J Ophthalmol 90:190–202, 1980.
Simmons RJ, Depperman SR, Dueker DK: The role of gonio-photocoagulation neovascularization of the anterior chamber angle. Ophthalmology 87:79–82, 1980.
Zegarra H, Gutman FA, Conforto J: The natural course of central retinal vein occlusion. Ophthalmology 86:1931–1939, 1979.

UVEITIS

JAMES T. ROSENBAUM, M.D.
Portland, Oregon

Many different processes, including infection, malignancy, and immune-mediated diseases, can result in inflammation of the uveal tract. These diseases can be categorized on the basis of the portion of the uveal tract that is affected. The size and distribution of keratic precipitates, the suddenness of onset, the duration of inflammation, and the association with various complications can also be helpful in categorizing uveal inflammation. The treatment of uveitis depends upon the specific diagnosis (e.g., herpes simplex keratouveitis is obviously approached differently from phacolytic glaucoma), the duration and severity of the inflammation, the location of the inflammation, and the presence of potential complications.

In designing therapy for a patient with uveitis, one must first exclude an underlying infection or malignancy. Syphilis has protean ocular manifestations and must be excluded by an appropriate serologic study, such as a fluorescent treponemal antibody absorption test. Such diagnostic entities as toxoplasmosis, herpes zoster ophthalmicus, herpes simplex keratouveitis, toxocariasis, acute retinal necrosis (which is caused by viruses from the herpes family), and infection in the immunocompromised host must be recognized and treated with specific antimicrobial therapy. Malignancies, including melanoma, lymphoma, leukemia, and retinoblastoma, may masquerade as uveitis and fail to respond to anti-inflammatory drugs.

The systemic illnesses associated with uveitis include sarcoidosis, ankylosing spondylitis, Reiter's syndrome, juvenile-onset rheumatoid arthritis, inflammatory bowel disease, interstitial nephritis, Behçet's disease, Vogt-Koyanagi-Harada syndrome, Sjögren's syndrome, and multiple sclerosis. In most cases, a careful history should lead one to suspect a related systemic disease if it is present. Of course, some of the therapeutic options for the systemic illnesses (e.g., corticosteroids for sarcoidosis or surgery for refractory inflammatory bowel disease) influence the course of the eye disease.

THERAPY

Ocular. Therapy for an acute iritis or iridocyclitis should include both a topical corticosteroid and a mydriatic or cycloplegic. By relieving spasm of the ciliary muscles, a dilating drop reduces pain. In addition, it should prevent the complication of posterior synechiae. Choices include scopolamine (0.25 to 0.5 per cent), homatropine (2 or 5 per cent), cyclopentolate (0.5 to 2.0 per cent) and atropine (0.5 to 2 per cent). Tropicamide (1 per cent) is an alternative if the inflammation is mild. The dose of the dilating drop should be adequate to reduce pain and to produce dilation without maintaining the pupil constantly in a fully dilated position.

Topical corticosteroids include dexamethasone, hydrocortisone, prednisolone, and progesterone-like compounds, including fluorometholone and medrysone. One of these should be started as soon after the onset of inflammation as possible. Often, patients with recurrent iritis experience a prodromal illness before cell and flare are detected in the anterior chamber. The initiation of topical corticosteroids at this time is optimal. Generally, the drops are given as frequently as every hour until improvement begins. Dexamethasone ointment may be added at night. Although topical steroids do vary in their tendency to elevate intraocular pressure, the rise in pressure probably correlates with the potency of the anti-inflammatory effects. Thus, the progesterone-like compounds are both less likely to elevate pressure but are also less potent in controlling inflammation.

If topical therapy is not adequate, a periocular injection of corticosteroids is an alternative. Periocular injections are an excellent choice for therapy if the disease is unilateral or posterior to the lens or both. One study has suggested that a superior, posterior, sub-Tenon's capsule approach may be more effective than an inferior approach. Corticosteroid preparations available for periocular injection include dexamethasone,* methylprednisolone,* triamcinolone,* and betamethasone.* An injection of 1.0 ml of most commercial preparations can be repeated every 2 to 6 weeks in an effort to control inflammation. The author's practice is to repeat the injection on at least one occasion before concluding that it is not effective because therapeutic benefit may vary depending on placement of the medication.

Systemic. Oral corticosteroids are indicated for intraocular inflammation that has not responded to topical or periocular medications and that is not secondary to infection or malignancy. The goal of therapy is usually not to eliminate inflammation but to reduce it to a level acceptable to the patient while using the lowest possible dose of potentially toxic medication. An amount comparable to 60 mg of prednisone taken in the morning as a single oral dose is frequently used to initiate therapy. Alternate-day therapy with corticosteroids is both less toxic and less efficacious. Dividing the daily dose is likely to increase benefit but also to increase toxicity. The dose of corticosteroids should be adjusted based on the activity of the inflammation. The benefits of corticosteroids are balanced by their risks, which are proportionate to the dosage and duration of therapy.

Four weeks of moderately high doses of corticosteroids equivalent to 40 to 60 mg of prednisone daily are generally sufficient to determine if the medication is beneficial. Oral corticosteroids should not be discontinued abruptly. A tapering schedule should be used to discontinue corticosteroids, especially if the duration of therapy has been longer than 4 weeks. Pulse therapy with corticosteroids (1 gm of methylprednisolone daily, intravenously for 3 consecutive days) has been reported to benefit a limited number of patients who do not respond adequately to oral regimens.

Guidelines for the use of systemic immunosuppressive therapy have been suggested by the International Uveitis Study Group. These guidelines include bilateral disease, best corrected vision no better than 20/50, and failure either to respond or to tolerate oral corticosteroids. Drugs within this category include cyclosporine‡ and cytotoxic medications, such as azathioprine,‡ chlorambucil,‡ cyclophosphamide,‡ and methotrexate.‡ Cyclosporine at a daily dose up to 10 mg/kg orally has resulted in improved visual acuity in many patients who have not improved with corticosteroids. However, this dose is frequently associated with nephrotoxicity. Other problems associated with cyclosporine include hepatotoxicity, hirsutism, and lymphoid malignancy. The cytotoxic drugs are all associated with cytopenias. All of these immunosuppressive agents predispose to the development of opportunistic infections.

The benefit of either oral or topical nonsteroidal anti-inflammatory drugs, such as indomethacin‡ or flurbiprofen,‡ has not been established in uveitis. Since multiple mediators undoubtedly contribute to the process of inflammation, future pharmacologic modalities may inhibit such phlogistic substances as oxygen radicals, platelet-activating factor, interleukin-1, or neuropeptides.

PRECAUTIONS

Ocular toxicity from oral, periocular, or topical corticosteroids includes posterior subcapsular cataract, raised intraocular pressure, and reduced response to infection.

An inadvertent intraocular injection of corticosteroids will normally result in permanent visual loss. Other potential hazards of periocular injections include pain or discomfort, ptosis, hemorrhage, infection, fat atrophy, and an allergic reaction to the drug vehicle. An elevation of intraocular pressure rarely occurs from a truly posterior injection of a corticosteroid. However, depot injections of corticosteroids may occasionally need to be removed in order to control intraocular pressure.

The adverse reactions from oral corticosteroids include personality changes, such as mania, psychosis, or sleep disturbance; weight gain and fat redistribution; adrenal suppression; acne; osteoporosis; avascular necrosis; immunosuppression, including reduced fever and pain from an infection, such as appendicitis; diabetes; easy bruisability; poor healing; menstrual irregularity; peptic ulcer disease; and reactivation of latent infection.

COMMENTS

The complications from uveitis may include cystoid macular edema, synechiae, band keratopathy, cataract, glaucoma, neovascularization, and retinal detachment. If therapy for the underlying inflammation cannot control or prevent a complication, the complication must obviously be addressed separately if appropriate. Band keratopathy, for example, may require chelation therapy or even corneal transplantation. Cryotherapy has been attempted for neovascularization. Vitrectomy is an option for severe vitreous opacification that has failed antiinflammatory therapy. Vitrectomy, however, may worsen underlying cystoid macular edema if that is present.

References

Andrasch RH, Pirofsky B, Burns RP: Immunosuppressive therapy for severe chronic uveitis. Arch Ophthalmol 96:247–251, 1978.

Nussenblatt RB, Palestine AG, Chan C-C: Cyclosporin A therapy in the treatment of intraocular inflammatory disease resistant to systemic corticosteroids and cytotoxic agents. Am J Ophthalmol 96:275–282, 1983.

Rubin RM, Samples JR, Rosenbaum JT: Prostaglandin-independent inhibition of ocular vascular permeability by a platelet-activating factor antagonist. Arch Ophthalmol 106:1116–1120, 1988.

Smith RE, Nozik RA: The nonspecific treatment of uveitis. In Uveitis. A Clinical Approach to Diagnosis and Management. Baltimore, Williams & Wilkins, 1989, pp 51–76.

SECTION 27

LACRIMAL SYSTEM

Lacrimal Gland

DACRYOADENITIS

JOHN L. WOBIG, M.D.
Portland, Oregon

Dacryoadenitis is an inflammatory enlargement of the lacrimal gland caused by infection, granulomatous disease of unknown cause, or a benign lymphoepithelial lesion. Acute dacryoadenitis may affect either the palpebral or orbital lobe of the gland separately or together. Acute palpebral dacryoadenitis usually presents as orbital pain followed by edema of the upper lid, which results in an S-shaped curved lid deformity and a preauricular lymph node. Palpation of the lid shows a tender nut-shaped swelling continuous with neither the orbit nor the ciliary margin. The conjunctiva may be injected and chemotic, sometimes with mucous discharge. The disease may run a brief course and then resolve, or it may progress to suppuration. Acute orbital dacryoadenitis is rarer than the palpebral form and presents with the same, although accentuated, symptoms. In addition, there is usually some proptosis as a result of the swelling extending under the orbital rim. There may be some limitation of ocular mobility with diplopia, and sometimes there is a convergent squint. Chronic dacryoadenitis usually presents as a painless swelling in the upper and outer part of the lid, accompanied by ptosis. A hard mass is palpable under the upper and outer rim of the orbit. Displacement of the globe downward and inward occurs with diplopia on looking up and out, but proptosis is rare.

THERAPY

Supportive. The therapy of dacryoadenitis is determined by the etiology. For dacryoadenitis that is a complication of systemic disease, therapy should be directed toward the overall treatment of the generalized disorder. Dacryoadenitis that is a complication of a viral disease (most commonly mumps) should be treated symptomatically. Local application of heat or cold offers some relief. Bedrest and salicylates are suggested. Dacryoadenitis secondary to sarcoidosis should be treated by systemic corticosteroids.

If the causative organism can be identified in a bacterial infection of the lacrimal gland, appropriate antibiotic therapy should be given. Hot packs followed by symptomatic therapy may give some relief.
Ocular. If discharge is present, lavage of the conjunctival sac is indicated. If lacrimal function is not adequate, replacement therapy with tear substitutes should be instituted.
Surgical. If suppuration occurs, early incision is indicated. This should be done through the conjunctiva if the palpebral lobe is involved or through the skin if the orbital lobe is affected.

Ocular or Periocular Manifestations

Conjunctiva: Chemosis; fistula; hyperemia; mucous discharge.
Eyelids: Edema; erythema; ptosis.
Globe: Proptosis.
Lacrimal System: Edema; inflammation; suppuration.
Other: Convergent squint; diplopia; ocular pain; preauricular lymphadenopathy.

PRECAUTIONS

An acute palpebral dacryoadenitis may suggest a chalazion or hordeolum. Eversion of the lid will rule out these diagnoses. Tenderness and swelling of the gland and localized chemosis are also characteristic features. Acute orbital dacryoadenitis may present a general picture suggesting orbital cellulitis.

COMMENTS

It is generally believed that lacrimal gland enlargements are caused by tumors or inflammations, with inflammations representing the more frequent cause. Among granulomatous diseases resulting in lacrimal gland inflammation, sarcoidosis and Sjögren's syndrome are the most prominent. The lacrimal gland may also experience chronic inflammation and ultimately fibrosis as sequelae to radiation or loss of innervation. However, lacrimal gland enlargement may be due to causes other than inflammation. Nutritional deficiencies, alcoholism, diabetes, tumors, and use of certain drugs may cause enlargement of the lacrimal gland. The infrequency of reported cases of dacryoadenitis reflects the fact that the lacrimal gland is housed in a bony cavity that is not regularly palpated and can conceal moderate enlargement.

References

Duke-Elder S (ed): System of Ophthalmology. St. Louis, CV Mosby, 1974, Vol VIII, pp 601–622.
Jakobiec FA, Jones IS: Orbital inflammations. In Duane TD (ed): Clinical Ophthalmology. Hagerstown, MD, Harper & Row, 1982, Vol II 35:pp 64–69.
Jakobiec FA, Gess L, Zimmerman LE: Granulomatous dacryoadenitis caused by Schistosoma haematobium. Arch Ophthalmol 95:278–280, 1977.

LACRIMAL GLAND TUMORS
(Benign Epithelial Tumors, Inflammatory or Lymphoid Tumors, Malignant Epithelial Tumors)

RICHARD D. CUNNINGHAM, M.D., M.S., and GLEN O. BRINDLEY, M.D.

Temple, Texas

The lacrimal gland lies in the superolateral portion of the orbit just behind the orbital rim. It consists of a palpebral lobe located in the temporal portion of the upper eyelid and a larger orbital lobe that lies in the lacrimal fossa. The two lobes are separated by the lateral horn of the levator aponeurosis. Fifty per cent or more of lacrimal gland swellings are lymphocytic in nature; the remainder are epithelial tumors. Half of the lymphocytic lesions are benign (infections and inflammations), and half are malignant (lymphomas).

Approximately 50 per cent of epithelial tumors of the lacrimal gland are benign mixed tumors (pleomorphic adenomas). These slow-growing tumors originate from ductular elements of the lacrimal gland. They are surrounded by an imperfect pseudocapsule that is transversed by fingers of tumor. The term "mixed tumor" arose because of the combination of unusual mesenchymal elements (myxoid, chondroid and osteoid) and double-layered tubular epithelial units. The typical presentation of a benign mixed tumor is that of a painless, slowly enlarging mass in the temporal aspect of the upper orbit without signs of inflammation. The mass effect causes inferonasal displacement of the globe and moderate proptosis. Patients tolerate the displacement of the globe very well and rarely report diplopia. In fact, most patients tolerate the presence of these tumors for several years without severe symptoms. Conventional x-ray studies usually reveal expansion of the lacrimal fossa without bone destruction. Computed tomography demonstrates the extent of the circumscribed mass and confirms the absence of destruction.

Adenoid cystic carcinoma is the most common malignant epithelial tumor of the lacrimal gland, accounting for approximately 25 per cent of all epithelial tumors of the lacrimal gland. The tumor is made up of aggregates of benign-appearing basaloid cells that proliferate around circular acellular spaces, giving the tumor an appearance similar to Swiss cheese. Adenoid cystic carcinoma may also present as a noninflammatory superior orbital mass that causes infranasal displacement of the globe, but these patients frequently complain of pain, diplopia, and visual disturbances. In contrast to benign mixed tumors, patients with adenoid cystic carcinoma become symptomatic over a short period of time, generally less than 6 months and almost always less than 1 year. X-ray studies are sometimes normal because of the short clinical course; however, enlargement of the lacrimal fossa, irregular bone destruction, bone sclerosis, or gland calcification may be noted. Computed tomography reveals a misleadingly circumscribed tumor that frequently extends medially and far posteriorly into the orbit. Periorbital and perineural invasion underlies the common symptom of pain. Multiple recurrences and a high mortality rate, approaching 90 per cent at 15 years, are the result of bone, soft tissue, and perineural extension within the orbit and cranium. The tumor does not metastasize early, but eventually will disseminate hematogenously to the lungs and lymphogenously to regional nodes. Patients can survive up to 5 years with recurrent tumor.

A malignant mixed tumor represents a benign mixed tumor that has undergone a malignant degeneration. Fewer than 10 per cent of epithelial tumors fall into this category. Patients with malignant mixed tumors tend to be older (50 to 60 years of age) when compared with those harboring benign mixed tumors or adenoid cystic carcinoma (30 to 40 years of age). There are three types of presentation of malignant mixed tumors. The first is that of a benign mixed tumor that has been incompletely excised. After several benign recurrences, the tumor ultimately degenerates into a malignant mixed tumor. The benign recurrences tend to occur over 3- to 5-year intervals, but when a malignant degeneration occurs, the patient will become symptomatic over a shorter period of time (3 to 6 months). The longer the patient has a recurrent benign mixed tumor, the more likely is the possibility for malignant transformation. Ten per cent of recurrent benign mixed tumors will become malignant after 20 years, and 20 per cent will become malignant after 30 years. This same rule probably pertains to untreated benign mixed tumors; namely, the longer the patient has the tumor, the more likely it will undergo malignant transformation. The second mode of presentation is that of a patient who has the typical history of a benign mixed tumor (painless, slow-growing, lacrimal mass without symptoms for longer than 1 year) and then suddenly over a 3- to 6-month period notices an exacerbation with more rapid growth or symptoms. The third presentation is that of a patient who has a clinical course the same as those patients with de novo malignancies, such as adenoid cystic carcinoma. These patients become symptomatic over a short period of time without a past history of long-standing benign mixed tumor. When one removes the tumor, one discovers microscopically a nidus of a benign mixed tumor out of which a malignancy has risen. The malignancy is usually a poorly differentiated carcinoma or an adenocarcinoma, although occasionally an adenoid cystic carcinoma may also be found intermixed with the pre-existent benign mixed tumor elements.

THERAPY

Systemic. Proper treatment of patients with lacrimal gland tumors is dependent on accurate categorization as to the most likely diagnosis, which is based on the clinical course, examination, and radiographs made *before treatment.* Patients with a very short history of lacrimal gland enlargement (less than 3 months) associated with inflammatory signs and without x-ray abnormalities can be treated depending upon the clinical diagnosis. Systemic antibiotics are indicated in supprative dacryoadenitis; systemic corticosteroids are recommended in treatment of inflammatory pseudotumor. There should be a progressive decrease in mass size over the next 2 to 3 weeks with eventual complete resolution. If any mass remains, the patient should then have an incisional biopsy through an anterior transeptal approach to rule out a malignant epithelial tumor. Care should be taken during this biopsy not to violate the periorbita, as this could allow potential extraperiosteal spread of malignant cells.

Surgical. Patients thought to have a benign mixed tumor based on the clinical course and typical radiographic findings (slowly progressive, noninflammatory mass lesion present for over 1 year) should not have a biopsy. Incomplete excision of a benign mixed tumor dooms the patient to multiple recurrences and the risk of malignant degeneration. The tumor should be excised in toto by a lateral orbitotomy, without disruption of its capsule, along with all surrounding tissues (lacrimal gland, conjunctiva, levator aponeurosis, and overlying periorbita). Since it has been suggested that irradiation of benign mixed tumors increases the incidence of malignant change, no benign mixed tumor, either primary or recurrent, should be irradiated.

Patients with a noninflammatory lacrimal gland mass of less than 1 year's duration should be suspected of having a malignant epithelial tumor. These patients often have pain, diplopia, vision deficit, or characteristic x-ray findings. An incisional biopsy through an anterior transeptal incision (not violating the periorbita) should be performed in order to establish the diagnosis based on permanent histologic sections. Once the diagnosis of a malignant epithelial tumor (adenoid cystic carcinoma, malignant mixed tumor, or another epithelial malignancy) is established, the patient should be thoroughly evaluated to rule out intracranial invasion or systemic metastasis. If neither of these is present, an attempt at a "curative" radical resection is performed. This should include the en bloc resection of the periorbital skin, eyelids, orbital contents, a portion of the bony lateral wall, and the roof of the orbit up to the midline. This is a major surgical undertaking and requires a neurosurgeon in addition to an orbital surgeon. Postoperative radiotherapy of 6000 rads delivered over 6 weeks is recommended. Radiotherapy alone in inoperable cases can offer palliation but not a cure. In general, the response of malignant tumors to radiation therapy is related to the histology, the extent of initial therapy, and the dose of radiation. Radical exenteration is a cosmetically disfiguring procedure, and the patient should be advised of this matter preoperatively. To date, there are too few patients who have been treated by this procedure to know if long-term survival will in fact be enhanced. Prognosis for these patients is very poor. If incisional biopsy indicates a diagnosis other than malignant epithelial tumor (e.g., lymphoma, inflammatory cellular infiltration etc.), appropriate anti-inflammatory or radiation therapy is initiated. Radiation therapy to the orbit including the conjunctiva to a tumor dose of 3000–4000 rads offers a good chance of local tumor control.

Patients who are suspected clinically of having a malignancy in a recurrent benign mixed tumor should have an anterior transeptal biopsy done on the recurrent tissue, and once malignant tissue has been discovered, radical surgery should be performed as mentioned above. The patient, of course, should first be studied for possible regional or distant metastasis. Patients who have never been treated before but present with a 2- to 3-year history of a slow-growing mass followed by a rapid acceleration of symptoms should have a biopsy through the lid, followed by radical surgery if the diagnosis of malignancy has been confirmed.

Precautions

A working diagnosis before treatment of any mass lesion of the lacrimal gland must be formulated. Inflammatory lesions of the lacrimal gland usually present with rather rapid onset of tenderness and erythema of the overlying eyelid and a painful mass without bone destruction. A biopsy must be done on any lacrimal gland mass originally thought to be inflammatory that does not completely resolve through an anterior (eyelid) incision; however, *biopsies should not be performed on suspected benign mixed tumors.*

Comments

Approximately 10 to 15 per cent of epithelial tumors of the lacrimal gland represent types of carcinoma other than malignant mixed tumors or adenoid cystic carcinomas. These cases are either de novo adenocarcinomas, squamous cell carcinomas, undifferentiated carcinomas, or mucoepidermoid carcinomas. Except for the last type these tumors have the poorest prognosis for survival of all lacrimal malignancies. These tumors tend to occur in older patients (50 to 70 years of age). The clinical presentation is usually similar to an adenoid cystic carcinoma. These tumors should be managed surgically as previously outlined. Additionally, one could entertain the possibility of performing preauricular and cervical lymph node dissections because these lesions tend to metastasize early to regional lymph nodes. The same proposal for regional lymph node dissections can be made for adenocarcinomas arising in benign mixed tumors. There is no chemotherapeutic protocol reported to be effective for treatment of primary or metastatic lacrimal gland tumors.

References

Brada M, Henk JM: Radiotherapy for lacrimal gland tumors. Radiother Oncol 9:175–183, 1987.
Byers RM, et al: Combined therapeutic approach to malignant lacrimal gland tumors. Am J Ophthalmol 79:53–55, 1975.
Font RL, Gamel JW: Epithelial tumors of the lacrimal gland: An analysis of 265 cases. In Jakobiec FA (ed): Ocular and Adnexal Tumors. Birmingham, Aesculapius, 1978, pp 787–805.
Henderson JW: Orbital Tumors, 2nd ed, New York, Brian C Decker, 1980, pp 394–423.
Jones IS: Surgical considerations in the management of lacrimal gland tumors. Clin Plast Surg 5:561–569, 1978.
Krohel GB, Steward WB, Chavis RM: Orbital Disease. A Practical Approach. New York, Grune & Stratton, 1981, pp 129–132.
Marsh JL, et al: Lacrimal gland adenoid cystic carcinoma: Intracranial and extracranial en bloc resection. Plast Reconstr Surg 68:577–585, 1981.
Perzin KH, et al: Lacrimal gland malignant mixed tumors (carcinomas arising in benign mixed tumors): A clinico-pathologic study. Cancer 45:2593–2606, 1980.
Wright JE, Stewart WB, Krohel GB: Clinical presentation and management of lacrimal gland tumours. Br J Ophthalmol 63:600–606, 1979.

MIKULICZ'S SYNDROME
(Dacryosialoadenopathy, Mikulicz-Radecki Syndrome, Mikulicz-Sjögren Syndrome)

F. HAMPTON ROY, M.D.

Little Rock, Arkansas

Mikulicz's syndrome is a symptom complex caused by a variety of systemic diseases with secondary involvement of the salivary glands with or without lacrimal gland involvement. Marked salivary gland involvement may interfere with eating and speaking. This symmetric swelling of the lacrimal gland is slow and usually painless. The swelling causes gradual difficulty in opening the eye, slight edema of the lids, and minimal congestion of the conjunctiva. Pseudoptosis may occur from narrowing of the lid of the palpebral fissures and difficulty in raising the upper lid. The enlarged lacrimal gland may cause exophthalmos with medial displacement. The primary systemic diseases implicated in this syndrome are leukemia, lymphosarcoma, tuberculosis, syphilis, sarcoidosis, mumps, and Waldenstrom's macroglobulinemia. The course of Mikulicz's syndrome is related to the systemic disorder. It occurs most commonly during the fifth and sixth decades and affects females more often than males.

THERAPY

Systemic. Systemic corticotropin and corticosteroids may decrease the lacrimal and parotid gland enlargement in Mikulicz's syndrome. Prednisone in a daily dose of 5 to 20 mg or more should be given orally to control inflammation.

Chemotherapy may be helpful in cases of malignant lymphoma. Mechlorethamine in a dose of 0.4 mg/kg should be given intravenously as a single dose or divided over 2 separate days. The total dosage for patients who have had prior radiation or chemotherapy should be limited to 0.2 to 0.3 mg/kg.

Ocular. Topical corticosteroids and cycloplegics usually control the uveitis. When there is deficient lacrimal secretion, artificial tears should also be applied several times a day. A therapeutic contact lens may also be tried with some success.

Surgical. With a proven carcinoma or a malignant mixed tumor of the lacrimal gland, exenteration is usually the treatment of choice. The bony orbital wall of the lacrimal gland fossa surrounding the orbit should be resected, even if no gross involvement can be demonstrated by x-ray. Recurrent disease is likely beyond the region of the lacrimal gland fossa, which may require a more extensive resection. In the case of a benign mixed tumor, exposure at the time of operation should be adequate to enable inspection of the contiguous bone and resection of any of the involved areas. If a dermoid cyst or cholesteatoma is present, excision or drainage with ablation is indicated.

Ocular or Periocular Manifestations

Conjunctiva: Chemosis; follicular conjunctivitis; nodules; phlyctenules.
Cornea: Infiltration; keratoconjunctivitis sicca.
Eyelids: Edema; nodules; ptosis.
Iris: Anterior uveitis; granuloma; posterior synechiae.
Lacrimal System: Dacryoadenitis; decreased tear secretion; hypertrophy of lacrimal gland.
Optic Nerve: Atrophy; optic neuritis.
Retina: Candlewax spots; periphlebitis.

Precautions

Overgrowth of bacteria, fungi, yeast, and viruses can occur with indiscriminate use of corticosteroids. Frequent blood counts, including platelets, should be done whenever the patient is on mechlorethamine.

COMMENTS

Bilateral or unilateral enlargement of the lacrimal gland, with or without enlargement of one or more of the salivary glands, is often associated with Sjögren's syndrome, keratoconjunctivitis sicca, xerostomia, or rheumatoid arthritis. The prognosis for benign mixed tumors in Mikulicz's syndrome is good; however, the prognosis for all malignant tumors is poor.

References

Lopez-Enriquez E, et al: Malignant transformation in Mikulicz's disease. Bol Assoc Med PR 72:1–6, 1980.
Meyer D, Yanoff M, Hanno H: Differential diagnosis in Mikulicz's syndrome. Mikulicz's disease, and similar disease entities. Am J Ophthalmol 71:516–524, 1971.
Penfold DN: Mikulicz's syndrome. J Oral Maxillofac Surg 43:900–905, 1985.
Som PM, et al: Manifestations of parotid gland enlargement: Radiographic, pathologic, and clinical correlations. Part II: The disease of Mikulicz's syndrome. Radiology 141:421–426, 1981.

UVEOPAROTID FEVER
(Heerfordt's Syndrome, Uveoparotitis)
R. PITTS CRICK, F.R.C.S.,
and AIDAN MURRAY, F.R.C.S.
London, England

Uveoparotid fever is a rare form of sarcoidosis that is characterized by uveitis, enlargement of the parotid and other salivary glands, and facial nerve paresis. However, the signs of the syndrome may be incomplete, and they may be associated with many other ophthalmic and general manifestations. There is an increased liability to florid forms of sarcoidosis in the black population, and when sarcoid uveitis is severe, it is particularly likely to be associated with raised intraocular pressure during the active stage. Broad adhesions across the drainage angle resulting from the fibrosis of iris nodules may later lead to chronic closed-angle glaucoma. As in any case of uveitis, secondary cataracts may form. Posterior uveitis frequently accompanies the anterior uveitis, but may appear to be present alone with snowball vitreous opacities and haze and whitish fundus lesions. Retinal vasculitis affecting the veins may be a prominent feature in some cases, but fluorescein angiography reveals that it is much more frequent than would be suspected on routine ophthalmoscopy. Only rarely are the lacrimal glands swollen, but they are frequently affected, and 65 per cent of sarcoid patients show evidence of tear deficiency, in contrast to 6 per cent of control patients. Tear deficiency tends to be severe in uveoparotid fever and may cause hyaline degeneration of the epithelial cells of the exposed conjunctiva and cornea. Conjunctival follicles with sarcoid histology are commonly present in the lower fornix and are a valuable source of biopsy material. Both the cornea and the conjunctiva may be involved in the deposits of calcium salts in exposed areas when sarcoidosis is complicated by hypercalcemia. In the cornea, this appears as a band opacity and may be associated with redness and discomfort. Such patients may become uremic from renal calcinosis. In addition to the facial palsy, in which the nerve may be involved above or below the level at which it is joined by the chorda tympani, sarcoid deposits at the base of the brain may cause other cranial nerve palsies. The optic nerve itself may be affected, with visual loss being associated with papilledema or optic atrophy. Diabetes insipidus from hypothalamic lesions may also occur. The skin of the eyelids may be affected by disfiguring sarcoid papules.

THERAPY

Systemic. Systemic treatment with corticosteroids is essential for all patients with uveoparotid fever. It will usually control the uveitis and retinal vasculitis, lead to resolution of the swollen parotid glands, improve the keratoconjunctivitis sicca by resolving lacrimal gland lesions, and restore a normal blood calcium level by increasing urinary excretion and decreasing intestinal absorption of calcium. In general, the dosage of corticosteroids is kept as low as possible to produce the desired response. Initially, daily oral administration of 40 to 60 mg of prednisone in conjunction with topical ophthalmic prednisolone, hydrocortisone, betamethasone, or dexamethasone may be necessary to control uveitis. This dosage may be slowly reduced over a period of some months, but must never be abruptly withdrawn. Central nervous system lesions usually resist treatment and may occasionally present grave therapeutic problems, especially if a large dosage is required for a long period.

Skin lesions are usually resistant to corticosteroid treatment and may be disfiguring. To avoid higher corticosteroid dosages, 200 mg of chloroquine[‡] may be given twice daily, although the cornea and retinal function must be reviewed regularly during treatment for signs of toxicity.

Ocular. The usual topical ophthalmic treatment for uveitis is mydriatic and cycloplegic medication. One per cent atropine in solution or ointment may be instilled several times daily, or 0.25 per cent scopolamine, 1 per cent cyclopentolate, or 1 per cent tropicamide may be substituted. All these parasympatholytic drugs may be aided by 10 per cent phenylephrine, which causes contraction of the sympathetically innervated dilator pupillae. In addition, local treatment with 0.1 per cent dexamethasone suspension, 0.5 per cent prednisolone solution, or 0.5

per cent hydrocortisone suspension or ointment may be used in a frequency of up to twice hourly and reduced gradually. Subconjunctival injections* are very useful in the initial treatment of severe cases. These injections may contain a long-acting corticosteroid, such as 20 mg of methylprednisolone in 0.5 ml, combined with 0.5 ml of a mixture containing 0.12 ml of a 1:1000 epinephrine solution, 1 mg of atropine, and 6 mg of procaine.

In most patients, keratoconjunctivitis sicca is not severe and requires little more than the use of methylcellulose solution every 2 to 4 hours. Only rarely is a filamentary keratitis encountered; it may require the addition of a mucolytic agent, such as 5 or 10 per cent acetylcysteine,* at intervals.

Acute corneal band opacity usually responds to a rapid reduction of the serum calcium to normal levels by the use of corticosteroids and a low calcium diet, which will lead to early resolution. It may be necessary to remove a chronic band opacity surgically after the application of a chelating agent, such as edetate disodium,* which converts it to a mush that can be wiped away. The epithelium will then regenerate and cover the denuded area. In some cases, a corneal graft is required.

Ocular or Periocular Manifestations

Conjunctiva: Follicles, hyperemia.
Cornea: Band keratopathy; keratoconjunctivitis sicca.
Eyelids: Sarcoid nodules.
Iris, Ciliary Body, or Choroid: Sarcoid nodules; uveitis.
Lacrimal System: Decreased tear secretion; infiltration of lacrimal gland.
Optic Nerve: Atrophy; papilledema.
Retina: Vasculitis.
Sclera: Episcleral nodules; episcleritis.
Vitreous: Haze; snowball opacities.
Other: Diplopia; paralysis of seventh nerve; proptosis; secondary cataract; secondary glaucoma; visual loss.

Precautions

Topical and systemic corticosteroid therapy is usually essential, but the possibility of corticosteroid-induced cataracts or glaucoma should always be borne in mind. Care must be taken to exclude other diseases, such as diabetes, tuberculosis, or peptic ulcer, before corticosteroid therapy is instituted because the usual therapy may require modification.

Comments

Uveoparotid fever must be regarded as a potentially severe form of sarcoidosis requiring prolonged energetic systemic corticosteroid therapy and close supervision. Its duration will depend on the progress of the disease. A delicate balance has to be preserved between tissue damage by sarcoidosis and the complications of corticosteroid treatment. Local therapy with mydriatics and corticosteroids alone is unlikely to control the uveitis of uveoparotid fever. However, these medications help raise intraocular concentrations even when systemic treatment is being given and may be used for local ocular defense over a long period when it is considered safe or desirable to withdraw systemic corticosteroids for the treatment of ocular or other lesions. Such patients should always be watched for signs of corticosteroid-induced glaucoma, which is more likely to be caused by local than by systemic treatment.

It is sometimes difficult to decide whether secondary glaucoma is caused by uveitis or corticosteroids. In either case, it is usually best to continue therapy and treat the raised intraocular pressure with oral acetazolamide or topical ophthalmic timolol solution, which both reduce aqueous production. Corticosteroid-induced cataracts may have to be accepted as a therapeutic risk in severe cases and should be subsequently treated with cataract extraction, although this procedure may present a difficult problem.

References

Bruins Slot WJ: Besnier-Boeck's disease and uveoparotid fever (Heerfordt). Ned Tijdschr Geneeskd 80:2859–2863, 1936.

Crick RP, Hoyle C, Smellie H: The eyes in sarcoidosis. Br J Ophthalmol 45:461–481, 1961.

Heerfordt CF: Ueber eine Febris uveo-parotidea subchronica an der Glandula parotis und der Uvea des Auges lokalisiert und häufig mit Paresen cerebrospindler Nerven Kompliziert. Arch f Ophthalmol (Leipz) 70:254–273, 1909.

James DG, et al: Ocular sarcoidosis. Br J Ophthalmol 48:461–470, 1964.

Longscope WT, Freiman DG: A study of sarcoidosis based on a combined investigation of 160 cases including 30 autopsies from the Johns Hopkins Hospital and Massachusetts General Hospital. Medicine 31:1–132, 1952.

Scadding JG: Sarcoidosis. London, Eyre & Spottiswoode, 1967.

Smellie H, Hoyle C: The natural history of pulmonary sarcoidosis. Q J Med 29:539–558, 1960.

Outflow System

ALACRIMA
TED ROSENSTOCK, M.D.,
and J.J. HURWITZ, M.D., F.R.C.S.(C)
Toronto, Ontario

The term "alacrima" is used to describe a spectrum of congenital lacrimal secretory anomalies ranging from complete absence of tears to hyposecretion to another rare condition, in which there is a selective absence of tearing to emotional stimulation while secretion remains normal to mechanical stimulation. Causes vary from failure of central connection to nuclear aplasia to failure of peripheral connections to aplasia or hypoplasia of the lacrimal gland.

Congenital alacrima is quite rare. It usually occurs in otherwise healthy individuals. However, it is known to occur in association with other congenital abnormalities, including palsies of the fifth, sixth, seventh, eighth, or twelfth cranial nerves, and as part of the symptom complex of two inherited systemic disturbances: Riley-Day syndrome (familial dysautonomia) and anhidrotic ectodermal dysplasia. There is one report of congenital alacrima with lacrimal gland hypoplasia that appeared to be inherited in an autosomal dominant fashion in an otherwise healthy family.

Characteristically, these children have a history of no tears when crying. Otherwise, these children may be asymptomatic and comfortable, and the eyes may be moist. Conversely, irritative symptoms with photophobia and conjunctival hyperemia may be present. In the latter case, a very low to absent Schirmer's test, punctate epithelial keratitis, and a sticky mucoid discharge are common findings. The absent antibacterial action of the tears makes blepharoconjunctivitis a common occurrence. Histopathology reveals hydropic degeneration of the conjunctival epithelium similar to keratoconjunctivitis sicca. Although a unilateral case in association with facial hypoplasia has occurred, most cases are bilateral.

THERAPY

Ocular. Symptomatic cases may be managed by using artificial tears as frequently as necessary to relieve ocular irritation. Petrolatum ointment, which blurs vision, should be substituted at night. Ocular inserts for sustained release of artificial tears may provide relief in more severe cases. Antibiotic drops and ointment should be added to the regimen at times when a blepharoconjunctivitis exists.

Selected cases of keratoconjunctivitis sicca, especially with corneal ulceration, may be helped by therapeutic contact lenses (used in conjunction with lubricating drops), moisture chambers, or punctal plugs.

Surgical. In severe cases, punctal occlusion or tarsorrhaphy may provide relief.

Systemic. Cases of autonomic dysfunction have been treated with subcutaneous injections of 0.25 mg of neostigmine or 3.0 mg of methacholine.

Ocular or Periocular Manifestations

Conjunctiva: Hyperemia; thick mucoid discharge.
Cornea: Hypesthesia (associated with Riley-Day syndrome); interstitial keratitis; pannus, subepithelial opacity; superficial punctate keratoconjunctivitis; ulcer.
Extraocular Muscles: Paralysis of fifth, sixth, or seventh cranial nerves.
Eyelids: Chronic or recurrent blepharoconjunctivitis.
Other: Decreased tear secretion; decreased vision; irritation; photophobia.

PRECAUTIONS

Sensitization to any of the commercially available ocular lubricants or inserts may occur. In addition, ocular inserts may cause blurring of vision in the last few hours of effectiveness.

COMMENTS

Alacrima should be considered in the differential diagnosis of red irritable eyes in young children, even without a definite history by the parents.

Long-term follow-up is indicated, even in asymptomatic cases, in view of the possible development of keratoconjunctivitis sicca.

References

Beard C: Abnormalities of eyelids, lacrimal system, and orbit. In Congenital Anomalies of the Eye. Transactions of New Orleans Academy of Ophthalmology, St Louis, CV Mosby, 1968, p 411.
Davidoff E, Friedman AH: Congenital alacrima. Surv Ophthalmol 22:113–119, 1977.
Duke-Elder S (ed): System of Ophthalmology. St Louis, CV Mosby, 1963, Vol III, pp 913–917.
Mondino BJ, Brown SI: Hereditary congenital alacrima. Arch Ophthalmol 94:1478–1480, 1976.
Murube del Castillo J: Tear production and physiology. In Smith BC, DellaRocca RC, Nesi FA, Lisman RD (ed): Ophthalmic Plastic and Reconstructive Surgery. St Louis, CV Mosby, 1987, pp 921–941.

O'Driscoll TG: Alacrima. Trans Ophthalmol Soc UK 95:13–14, 1975.

Sjögren H, Eriksen A: Alacrima congenita. Br J Ophthalmol 34:691–694, 1950.

CONGENITAL ANOMALIES OF THE LACRIMAL SYSTEM
(Anlage Duct, Closed Nasolacrimal Duct)

JOHN L. WOBIG, M.D.
Portland, Oregon

Congenital anomalies of the lacrimal system may include an absence of one or more canaliculi, multiple puncta, or anomalies of the nasolacrimal duct. The duct that ends at or near the vault of the inferior meatus and fails to perforate the nasal mucosa is by far the most common variation; however, there are a large variety of obstructions and abnormalities of the nasolacrimal outflow system. Congenital anomalies of the motor mechanism occasionally occur even when the lacrimal passages are normal. There may be paralysis of the entire orbicularis oculi muscle or only of the medial ends of the pretarsal and preseptal muscle fibers. Congenital lacrimal amniotocele occurs when the canaliculi ends in the sinus of Maier, causing infectious material to be pumped into the lacrimal sac when the eyelids close. The lacrimal anlage duct anomaly occurs when the row of cells that extend from the posterior surface of the anlage to the deeper part of the lacrimal fossa to become the origin of the tear sac proliferates and canalizes instead of degenerating. This may occur bilaterally and be inherited as an autosomal dominant trait.

THERAPY

Ocular. If inflammation is present, systemic and topical ophthalmic antibiotics may be indicated. In addition, a decongestant medication in an aqueous vehicle should be prescribed for local conjunctival use. If the inflammation is not acute, the parents should be taught to exert pressure over the top of the tear sac four or more times a day for 1 to 2 weeks.

Surgical. Unless the epiphora has subsided completely within 2 weeks, probing under local anesthesia should be considered for children under 6 months of age. A probe that will slide through the canaliculus without resistance must be chosen. A dark line should be marked at 12 mm and another at 20 mm from the tip of the silver probe by applying tincture of iodine with a toothpick. The probe should then be passed vertically through the lower punctum and then horizontally through the canaliculus, with the convex side of the curve inferiorly. As soon as the sac is entered, the probe should again be held vertically, with the convexity turned medially. If the probe stops at the 12 mm mark and upon manipulation no passage beyond is found, probing should stop there. Probably there is no nasolacrimal canal and therefore no duct. These patients should have a dacryocystorhinostomy between 6 and 12 months of age, depending on the severity of the discharge and infection. If the probe passes down to the 20-mm mark, the probe is at the level of the inferior meatus. The probe should then be passed to the obstructed end of the duct and turned, with the convex side laterally. The probe, which should be against the mucosal side of the wall, should be given a quick, sharp push. Before withdrawing the probe, a metal instrument, such as another probe, should be passed into the inferior meatus of the nose so that a "metal-to-metal" touch will prove that the tip of the first probe is in the nasal cavity.

Inferior turbinotomy under general anesthesia should be performed on all recurrent cases. When probing fails to penetrate the nasal mucosa, the surgeon should try to impale the probe between the bone and the tip of a Freer elevator, which is passed into the inferior meatus with the curved edge toward the lateral wall about 20 mm from the entrance of the nares. The sharp edge of the elevator is then moved up and down the probe, cutting and scraping through the overlying mucosa until metallic contact is made. If it does not locate the probe laterally, the elevator should be turned over and a search made for the probe on the wall of the inferior turbinate. If the mucosa of the inferior turbinate cannot be opened over the probe, a turbinate punch should be used to remove that part of the obstructing tissue. The turbinate is then infractured.

Lacrimal amniotoceles may be treated conservatively as long as there is no sign of infection. If necessary, the nasolacrimal duct may be probed and opened.

The technique for excision of the anlage duct, performed under local anesthesia, should include an injection of two or three drops of 2 per cent methylene blue into the duct. A probe should be passed in far enough to give the direction of the duct. An incision should be made only through the skin in line with the duct. The duct is then freed by blunt dissection, keeping the probe in place. When the medial canthal tendon is reached, the duct should be ligated and excised and the skin closed with interrupted sutures.

Ocular or Periocular Manifestations

Lacrimal System: Atresia; dacryoadenitis; dacryocystitis; displacement of punctum; ectasia of lacrimal passage; ectropion of punctum; epiphora; fistula; occlusion of nasolacrimal duct or canaliculi; supernumerary puncti.

Other: Paralysis of seventh nerve.

PRECAUTIONS

With the possible exception of newborn infants, there seems to be no age limit for the treatment of these anomalies. The canalicular epithelium should always be carefully handled to produce minimal trauma during manipulations. Except at the point of obstruction in the inferior meatus of the nose, the use of force during probing is contraindicated.

The earlier the obstruction is removed, the higher is the incidence of cure. This is because the vigor and growth of the lacrimal epithelium are probably greatest at birth. The more chronic the infection and the greater the fibrotic and inflammatory changes, the more difficult it is to prevent recurrence. Dilation of the punctum should not be done with a Ziegler-type dilator, as it often causes a tear.

Comments

Anomalies involving the excretory lacrimal system are much more common congenitally than are secretory anomalies. Rarely, an anomalous lacrimal secretory duct is found opening on the cutaneous surface of the upper eyelid. A secretory duct is sometimes diverted into a bulbar conjunctival nevus or dermoid. Although fistulas of the lacrimal ducts are usually acquired, they may also develop congenitally and can be excised.

In about 30 per cent of newborn infants, the duct is still closed. Apparently, the last barrier to canalization is the fibrous layer of the nasal mucoperiosteum. This should be considered a normal event, unless it fails to open within the first 2 or 3 postpartum weeks.

References

Beard C: Congenital and hereditary abnormalities of the eyelids, lacrimal system, and orbit. *In* Beard C, et al (eds): Symposium on Surgical and Medical Management of Congenital Anomalies of the Eye. St. Louis, CV Mosby, 1968, pp 411–415.
Caputo AR, et al: Definitive treatment of congenital lacrimal sac fistula. Arch Ophthalmol 96:1443–1444, 1978.
Frankel CA: The treatment of dacryostenosis (letter) JAMA 260:2666, 1988.
Jones LT, Wobig JL: Surgery of the Eyelids and Lacrimal System. Birmingham, Aesculapius, 1976, pp 157–173.
Lipton J, Jacobs N, Rosen ES: Bilateral acute dacryocystitis in an infant. Br J Hosp Med 38:251, 1987.

DACRYOCYSTITIS
ROGER A. DAILEY, M.D.
Seattle, Washington

Dacryocystitis is an inflammation of the lacrimal sac that occurs primarily because of nasolacrimal duct obstruction that is either present at birth (congenital) or acquired. Secondary dacryocystitis can be caused by the spread of infection from the nose or paranasal sinuses or trauma or be found in association with some systemic disorder, such as tuberculosis, syphilis, or Hansen's disease (leprosy).

The incidence of congenital obstruction of the nasolacrimal duct in newborn infants is approximately 2 to 6 per cent. It occurs bilaterally in one third of these cases. The formation of the lacrimal outflow system relies on canalization of an epithelial cord formed by invagination of surface ectoderm over the naso-optic fissure. This canalization occurs in a segmented fashion, which is normally completed by the time of birth or shortly thereafter. Although this canalization may fail at any point, it usually does so at the lower end, leaving an imperforate membrane where the ostium of the duct into the inferior meatus of the nose should be. Bony obstruction of the nasolacrimal duct can also occur.

Rarely, an infant is born with an amniotocele. This markedly distended lacrimal sac appears as a bluish swelling below the medial canthal tendon and can be mistaken for a hemangioma. Amniotoceles are sterile initially, but, if unresolved, can develop a secondary dacryocystitis.

Typically, infants with obstruction of the nasolacrimal duct have a history of epiphora and chronic blepharoconjunctivitis. The sac will swell if it is unable to decompress either spontaneously or with external massage.

The majority of cases of dacryocystitis are acquired, and the infection begins in the lacrimal system. Despite a protective mucosal barrier of stratified columnar epithelium and the bacteriostatic action of tear lysozymes, any stasis with accumulation of tear sac products because of partial or complete obstruction of the nasolacrimal duct will predispose the lacrimal system to infection. Idiopathic acquired closure usually occurs in middle-aged adults with a 3 : 1 preponderance among females. It is rare among black people. A heredofamilial tendency has been noted in some cases.

There are many known causes of acquired nasolacrimal duct obstruction. Intermittent or partial obstruction can be caused by a dacryolith in 15 per cent of cases. These can have associated infections with organisms, such as *Actinomyces israelii*. Many types of tumors can occur in the nasolacrimal duct or lacrimal sac. Most of these are primary tumors of epithelial origin, such as papillomas, adenomas, and carcinomas. Secondary tumors from the sinus, nose, and orbit have been reported. Metastatic disease is very rare. Both dacryoliths and tumors can be associated with bloody tears. Patients with a tumor typically have a dacryocystitis associated with an irreducible mass. Jones testing reveals a partial obstruction with an excretory system that is patent to irrigation.

THERAPY

Ocular. During the first few weeks of life, nasolacrimal duct obstruction in the majority of infants will resolve spontaneously. In the absence of spontaneous resolution, the parents are instructed to massage over the lacrimal sac in such a way as to obstruct the canaliculi and increase the hydrostatic pressure in the lacrimal sac. Occasionally, parents report a "popping" sensation when they massage the area. This sensation is followed by resolution of the epiphora. In those patients with mucopurulent discharge, parents are instructed to use an antibiotic solution. In some series, over 90 per cent of infants have cleared by 1 year of age.

Acquired dacryocystitis is initially treated with topical antibiotic or antibiotic-steroid solutions for 2 weeks. Warm compresses over the lacrimal sac are also helpful. Probing and irrigation of the canaliculi and lacrimal excretory system in the office can help, but it is not a definitive treatment.

Acute dacryocystitis is exquisitely painful for the patient. An attempt should be made to decompress the sac when the patient is first seen to relieve the pressure. After decompression, the patient is given a topical antibiotic (with or without steroid) solution. Systemic therapy in the form of 1 gm of oral dicloxacillin administered in divided doses is instituted for 10 to 14 days. Warm compresses may resolve the cellulitis, if present, but increase the chance of formation of a dacryocutaneous fistula, if one was not iatrogenically created to drain the sac. If the sac has been decompressed, the excretory system should be irrigated with a suitable topical antibiotic (with or without steroid).

Surgical. Probing is indicated any time after the infant reaches 2 months of age, either because of parental request or the surgeon's philosophy. The technique is described in the previous article on congenital anomalies of the lacrimal system. It can be done in the office before the age of 6 months. Probing in the office or hospital in experienced hands is associated with very little morbidity. After the age of 6 months, a short general anesthetic is recommended for most cases. If the dacryocystitis is allowed to persist beyond 13 months of age, the number of patients requiring a dacryocystorhinostomy at a later date increases.

If the initial office probing fails, the child is brought to the hospital operating room and probed again. If the inferior meatus is at all tight, the inferior turbinate is fractured medially with a Freer elevator or straight hemostat. The excretory system is then intubated with silicone that has been glued on the ends of Quickert probes. A square knot is tied in the silicone, and it is allowed to retract into the inferior meatus. The puncta should be checked to be sure the silicone tension is not excessive. The tube is left in place for at least 6 weeks and then removed either through the nose or the upper canalicular system.

When a patient is seen initially for an acute dacryocystitis, an attempt should be made to decompress the swollen, tender sac. Massage of the area typically elicits significant resistance from the patient because of pain. Topical proparacaine is applied to the ocular surface and then 4 per cent cocaine solution is used topically to numb the puncta, and the canaliculi may be irrigated with the 4 per cent cocaine solution. At this time, the punctum is dilated with a 1 or 2 Jones punctal dilator. The upper or lower canaliculus is probed gently with a Bowman 1 or 2 probe. Once the tip of the probe comes into contact with the common canalicular area, the probe is gently advanced past the swollen valve of Rosenmüller into the sac. It is important at this stage not to use excessive pressure and create a false passage. Often, if the probe can be placed into the lacrimal sac, the contents will drain around the probe and through the opposite canaliculus and puncta, allowing for sac decompression. If this does not happen the probe can be removed and the sac irrigated again with the 4 per cent cocaine solution. An attempt is again made to place the probe into the sac, and at this time the probe is turned 90° cephalad with the convexity of the curve in the probe against the nose. The probe is then passed toward the nasolacrimal duct, gently advanced through the duct into the nose, and removed. With a small amount of pressure externally, the sac can be decompressed into the nose and oropharynx. If this is achieved, irrigation with an antibiotic-steroid solution is helpful in resolving the acute episode of dacryocystitis.

If decompression cannot be achieved by probing, a dacryocutaneous fistula can be created by lancing the swollen sac through the overlying skin with a No. 11 Bard-Parker blade.

Dacryocystorhinostomy is performed early on infants with aminotoceles or acute dacryocystitis. It is also performed when the more conservative measures discussed earlier fail. It is best to wait until the child is at least 1 year of age. The technique is essentially the same as that used in adults with minor variations. A general anesthetic is always used, and silicone intubation is always performed. The silicone used has an outside diameter of 0.032 mm.

Dacryocystorhinostomy in an adult can be done under general anesthesia or monitored anesthesia care (MAC) with intravenous sedation. Hemostasis is not as satisfactory with general anesthesia unless hypotensive anesthesia is used. The patient is placed in a supine position on the operating table with a slight reverse Trendelenburg orientation to the table. If the dacryocystitis involves both lacrimal sacs, the surgery can be performed bilaterally. A dacryocystorhinostomy can be performed either by external skin approach or intranasal approach.

In a standard external skin approach to dacryocystorhinostomy, a local anesthetic, consisting of 2 per cent lidocaine with epinephrine 1:100,000 with hyaluronidase, is injected into the area where the skin incision will be made and also around the upper and lower canaliculus. Regional block injections of the supratrochlear nerve and the infraorbital nerve can also be used. In children, the preferred local anesthetic is 1 per cent lidocaine with epinephrine 1:200,000 and hyaluronidase. A standard facial prep with povidone-iodine solution is performed, and the patient is draped so that the nose remains out for easy access during the case. A nasal packing consisting of one-half inch packing gauze soaked first in epinephrine 1:1000 and then in 10 per cent cocaine solution is placed in the nose in the area of the anterior tip of the middle turbinate. The skin incision is initiated 11 mm medial to the medial canthus and slightly above the insertion of the medial canthal tendon and is extended approximately 18 mm inferolaterally toward the nasolabial fold. The subcutaneous tissue is opened with sharp dissection, and the orbicularis muscle fibers are separated with blunt dissection down to the periosteum over the frontal process of the maxillary bone medial to the anterior lacrimal crest. Care is taken to avoid the angular vein. The periosteum is incised vertically and spread laterally and medially until the anterior lacrimal crest can be identified. The sac is elevated out of the lacrimal fossa somewhat so that the opening of the nasolacrimal duct can be identified. It is important, at this time, to have identified the medial canthal tendon, as this is an important landmark superiorly. In general, the medial canthal tendon should not be removed from its insertion on the nose. Local anesthetic is injected into the sac at this point, and a cotton pledget, soaked first in the epinephrine and cocaine solutions, is placed into the lacrimal fossa between the lacrimal bone and the sac to allow for increased anesthesia and hemostasis. The nasal packing is removed. The bony ostium is then created medial to the anterior lacrimal crest, using a power drill and dental burr. Care is taken to avoid the nasal mucosa. The bridge of bone between the ostium and lacrimal sac can be removed with a rongeur and Kerrison punch after the cotton pledget is removed. The self-retaining retractors are relaxed, and the upper canaliculus is probed with a Bowman 1 or 2 probe; once in the sac, it is used to tent the sac medially where it can be opened with sharp dissection, creating an anterior and posterior flap. The nasal mucosa is incised as well to create an anterior and posterior flap. These posterior flaps, both from the lacrimal sac and from the nasal mucosa, are excised and not closed surgically. Once the nasal mucosa has been violated, the patient's airway is no longer protected from hemorrhage. Suction is used to avoid airway obstruction. If there is a fair amount of bleeding, an absorbable hemostatic collagen or oxidized cellulose can be placed in the area of the posterior flaps. The appropriate-sized silicone, glued on the Quickert probes, is then passed through the upper and lower canaliculi, one at a time, into the nose, posterior to the anterior flaps. The probe can be brought through the external nares using a straight hemostat. The Quickert probes are removed. The anterior flaps are then closed with two or three interrupted 5-0 Dacron sutures. The hemostatic collagen can be left in place as it will be absorbed. After closure of the anterior flaps, the periosteum and deep muscular layers can be closed with interrupted or running 6-0 Vicryl sutures, and the skin is closed with a stitch and suture of the surgeon's choice. The silicone is tied in place with a square knot and cut, and the knot is allowed to retract into the inferior meatus. It is important to check the puncta and make sure that there is no tension on the silicone that could cause a cheese-wiring of the silicone through the canaliculi.

Ocular or Periocular Manifestations

Conjunctiva: Conjunctivitis.
Cornea: Keratitis; ulceration.
Lacrimal System: Canalicular discharge (especially with digital pressure); epiphora; pain, swelling, and tenderness over the lacrimal sac.
Orbit: Cellulitis.
Other: Meningitis; panophthalmitis; periorbital edema; periorbital hyperemia; sinusitis.

PRECAUTIONS

When probing the canalicular system in either the infant or adult, the surgeon must be careful to avoid creating a false passage. This can best be avoided by maintaining good lateral pressure on the lid to avoid an accordion effect of the canaliculus as the probe is advanced. In addition, only gentle pressure should be used with the probe; it should never be forced where it will not advance easily.

It is extremely important that the silicone in the puncta is checked to ensure that canalicular erosion does not occur because of excessive tension. When removing the silicone in adults after 6 weeks, it is best to take the silicone out through the nose with a hemostat, after cutting the loop between the two puncta. Often, because this is difficult or impossible to do in the child, the knot can be rotated and brought out through the upper canaliculus, which is preferred over the lower canaliculus because of the potential for cicatricial closure. The inferior canaliculus, which is thought to be the canaliculus that is responsible for the majority of tear removal, is thus spared any possible trauma.

Dacryocystorhinostomy is successful in 90 to 95 per cent of cases; however, failures can occur. The failures are typically a result of membrane formation over the internal ostium of the surgically created fistula into the nose. This membrane can be identified by placing a 1 or 2 Bowman probe through a canaliculus into the fistular area, tenting the newly formed cicatricial membrane into the nose, and observing it through the external nares using a nasal speculum. The probe can be advanced through the membrane and identified in the nose. The membrane around the probe can then be excised and the patient reintubated with silicone. In most cases, doing so resolves the continued epiphora. In cases where the anterior tip of the middle turbinate is obstructing the ostium, it can be removed with a universal turbinate punch.

Postoperative complications include periorbital ecchymosis and swelling. A scar will form on the face, which is usually barely visible after 4 to 6 months. Silicone erosion of the canaliculus can occur if the tension on the silicone is too great.

Pyogenic granulomas can form around the silicone at the puncta and in the nose. These are easily excised and the base cauterized. The silicone tube can occasionally be caught by the patient and retracted from the puncta, leaving an externalized loop. The patient is instructed postoperatively to tape this loop onto the nose, should it occur. When the patient is seen in the office, the tube is either repositioned or removed. Cerebrospinal fluid leaks have been reported, but with careful attention to anatomy and technique, they can be avoided. They typically result from bony fracture of the floor of the anterior cranial fossa or the cribriform plate as a result of rotational force used when removing bone with the rongeur or fracturing an ethmoid air cell. Orbital hemorrhage with proptosis has also been reported, but is a very rare complication of this surgery.

Comments

As always, the appropriate management of any disease entity relies on accurate clinical diagnosis. A history of tearing with mucopurulent regurgitation from the puncta or acute inflammation in the area of the lacrimal sac, combined with Jones tests that would suggest blockage of the nasolacrimal duct, allows the surgeon to feel comfortable proceeding with probing and silicone intubation in a child or dacryocystorhinostomy in an adult.

Many authorities in this field suggest using dacryocystography in the preoperative evaluation. It is felt that this technique better delineates certain problems, such as dacryoliths and tumors, and the exact location of obstruction in some cases. Scintiscanning has also been used in the preoperative evaluation, but it is mainly confined to experimental evaluation and is rarely of clinical necessity.

Absorbable hemostatic collagen is not only helpful intraoperatively to control hemorrhage but also makes postoperative Vaseline gauze packing unnecessary. In addition, first day postoperative hemorrhage is rare. No significant complications have been encountered with collagen use.

References

Dailey RA, Wobig JL: Use of collagen absorbable hemostat in dacryocystorhinostomy. Am J Ophthalmol 106:109–110, 1988.
Font RL: Lacrimal drainage system. *In* Spencer WH (ed): Ophthalmic Pathology, 3rd ed. Philadelphia, WB Saunders, 1986, pp 2312–2336.
Hurwitz JJ, Victor WH: The role of sophisticated radiologic testing in the assessment and management of epiphora. Ophthalmology 92:407–413, 1985.
Jones LT, Wobig JL: Surgery of the Eyelids and Lacrimal System. Birmingham, Aesculapius, 1976, pp 163–167.
Kushner BJ: Congenital nasolacrimal system obstruction. Arch Ophthalmol 100:597–600, 1982.
Milder B, Demorest BH, Wobig JL: The lacrimal system. *In* Silver B (ed): Ophthalmic Plastic Surgery. Rochester, American Academy of Ophthalmology and Otolaryngology, 1977, pp 161–189.
Neuhaus RW, Baylis HI: Cerebrospinal fluid leakage after dacryocystorhinostomy. Ophthalmology 90: 1091–1095, 1983.
Paul TO: Medical management of congenital nasolacrimal duct obstruction. J Pediatr Ophthalmol Strabismus 22:68–70, 1985.
Slonim CB, Older JJ, Jones PL: Orbital hemorrhage with proptosis following a dacryocrystorhinostomy. Ophthalmic Surg 15:774–775, 1984.
Wesley RE: Inferior turbinate fracture in the treatment of congenital nasolacrimal duct obstruction and congenital nasolacrimal duct anomaly. Ophthalmic Surg 16:368–371, 1985.

DACRYOLITH
BENJAMIN MILDER, M.D.
St. Louis, Missouri

A dacryolith is a concretion or a stone in the lacrimal canaliculus or sac. The majority of dacryoliths found in the canaliculi are caused by mycotic infections and appear as doughy or granular masses made up of degenerated cells, fungi, amorphous debris and inspissated mucus. They are noncalcific and therefore not usually identifiable by x-ray. Infrequently, a foreign body within the lacrimal canaliculus may form the nidus for a dacryolith, building up strata of fibrin, necrotic cells, inspissated mucus, and occasionally calcium salts. The dacryoliths in canaliculi are usually a part of the clinical picture of mycotic canaliculitis. Ordinarily, the disease is unilateral, and only one canaliculus is involved. The clinical picture is characterized by creamy white pus, which exudes from a patulous punctum or can be expressed on light pressure. The pus may contain "sulfur granules." Frequently, there is associated chronic conjunctivitis limited to the nasal angle.

Dacryoliths in the lacrimal sac are an indication of stasis; in most instances, the excretory system is patent but nonfunctioning (functional block). The stones are noncalcific and therefore radiolucent. Although calcium salts may be present, they are rarely sufficient to produce an identifiable radiographic shadow. No systemic calcium abnormality nor hypersecretion of calcium into the tears has been found in association with dacryoliths. Dacryocystography reveals a patent system with dilation and stasis in the sac and a characteristic radiolucent central area seen in lateral views. Sixteen per cent of all functional block dacryocystitis patients are found at surgery to harbor dacryoliths within the lacrimal sac. Clinically, these patients exhibit chronic dacryocystitis, epiphora, dilation of the lacrimal sac, and mild deep tenderness. Often, one is unable to palpate a dacryolith in the lacrimal sac because they tend to be flat and lie in the sac, cradled in the lacrimal fossa.

THERAPY

Systemic. Mycotic canaliculitis may be treated systemically with 1.2 million units of intramuscular penicillin G. This is followed by 250 to 500 mg of oral penicillin V every 6 hours. Systemic antifungal agents have not proved effective.

Ocular. Cultures should be obtained and grown in thioglycollate broth (anaerobic). Nystatin is effective against *Candida* and other yeasts. A suspension of 20,000 units/ml of nystatin* may be employed topically, one drop three times daily, and irrigated into the affected canaliculus every second day. Penicillin G,* in a concentration of 50,000 units/ml, may be employed in the same manner. A 5 per cent suspension of natamycin is the treatment of choice for septate fungi, as well as *Candida*. It is nontoxic to the cornea and conjunctiva, may be administered in the form of eyedrops every 1 to 2 hours, and may be instilled into the affected canaliculus daily.

The systemic treatment of fungus canaliculitis with dacryoliths has been disappointing, and topical antifungal agents have not proved to be uniformly effective. If response is not satisfactory after a period of 2 to 3 weeks, surgical intervention is necessary.

Surgical. Surgical intervention is necessary for removal of concretions in the canaliculus. The horizontal limb of the canaliculus should be slit open on the conjunctival aspect of the lid with a lacrimal probe in place. The concretions and infected mucosa are curetted, and the remaining mucosal lining is destroyed with tincture of iodine. Dacryoliths within the lacrimal sac are a sign of lacrimal sac disease, and the removal of the dacryolith must be combined with dacryocystorhinostomy. Simple removal of the stone is not sufficient. The loss of lacrimal excretory function is remedied by the dacryocystorhinostomy.

Ocular or Periocular Manifestations

Conjunctiva: Nasal angle conjunctivitis.
Lacrimal System: Canaliculitis, dacryocystitis; distention of the sac; epiphora; moderate deep tenderness; patulous punctum; purulent discharge; "sulfur granules."

PRECAUTIONS

Topical ocular medications, such as epinephrine preparations, may cause deposits in the canaliculi, creating a nidus for dacryolith formation.

COMMENTS

The excretory system is usually patent in the presence of a dacryolith in the lacrimal sac because the dacryolith is a result of nonfunction and resulting stasis. The diagnosis can be made preoperatively by dacryocystography and the calculus identified by the radiolucent area in the lacrimal sac shadow. Lacrimal nuclear scintillography identifies the patency and functional impairment, but does not outline the dacryolith as precisely as contrast dacryocystography.

References

Bohigian GM: Handbook of External Diseases of the Eye. Fort Worth, Alcon, 1980, p 163.
Bradbury JA, Rennie IG, Parsons MA: Adrenaline dacryolith: Detection by ultrasound examination of the nasolacrimal duct. Br J Ophthalmol 72:935–937, 1988.
Duke-Elder S (ed): System of Ophthalmology. St. Louis, CV Mosby, 1974, Vol XIII, pp 768–770; 1972, Vol XIV, pp 652–655.
Herzig S, Hurwitz JJ: Lacrimal gland calculi. Can J Ophthalmol 14:17–20, 1979.
Hurwitz JJ, Welham RAN, Maisey MN: Intubation macrodacryocystography and quantitative scintillography: The "complete" lacrimal assessment. Trans Am Acad Ophthalmol Otolaryngol 81:575–582, 1976.
Jay JL, Lee WR: Dacryolith formation around an eyelash retained in the lacrimal sac. Br J Ophthalmol 60:722–725, 1976.
McCord CD Jr: The lacrimal drainage system. *In* Duane TD (ed): Clinical Ophthalmology. Hagerstown, MD, Harper & Row, 1982, Vol IV, p 13:14.

EPIPHORA

JOHN L. WOBIG, M.D.
Portland, Oregon

Epiphora is the result of hypersecretion or failure of the lacrimal excretory system to function. Many conditions cause epiphora. Stimulation of the fifth cranial nerve due to any pathologic conditions, such as corneal foreign body, corneal ulcer, or nasal pathology, will cause a reflex hypersecretion. Abnormalities of the distributional system, such as entropion or ectropion, as well as constriction or complete closure of the puncta, canaliculi, tear sac, or tear duct, may also result in epiphora.

THERAPY

Ocular. Local disorders of the eye, such as corneal ulcers, intraocular disease, allergies, and nasal pathology, are treated conservatively. The treatment is initially directed toward the cause and, when unsuccessful, toward reducing hypersecretion.

Conservative treatment of the congenitally closed nasolacrimal duct should be attempted initially. Massage of the tear sac for several weeks and instillation of antibiotic drops for infections are recommended for as long as they are effective. Canaliculitis responds temporarily to eyedrops of 10 per cent potassium iodide,* but the disease usually follows a course of remissions and exacerbations until surgical intervention prevails. Acute and chronic forms of dacryocystitis are initially managed by topical ophthalmic and systemic antibiotics. This condition also goes through periods of remission and exacerbations until resolved by a dacryocystorhinostomy.

Surgical. Hypersecretion that cannot be diagnosed or treated conservatively may be helped by a conjunctival dacryocystorhinostomy. This procedure is preferable to removal of the accessory lacrimal lobe or cautery to the ducts of the lacrimal gland. Surgery to the distributional system is generally done to correct entropion or ectropion. In order for the lacrimal pump to work, the lids must be in proper apposition to the globe. Ectropion is usually corrected by horizontal lid-shortening procedures, and entropion is repaired by reattaching the retractors of the lower eyelid to the tarsus.

The lacrimal excretory system has a number of surgical procedures employed to correct the obstruction. The punctum can be opened with a Habb needle knife under the microscope. Spastic closure of the punctum is opened by a one-snip procedure. The posterior portion of the punctum is cut vertically for approximately 2 mm. This must be dilated several times after the one-snip procedure to correct the spastic closure. If this fails, a silicone tube can be intubated through the lacrimal system. Mild eversion of the punctum is best handled by a one-snip procedure, with removal of a diamond-shaped wedge of conjunctival tissue just inferior to the punctum.

The canaliculus occludes because of flaccidity, lacerations, and cicatrization secondary to chronic use of some eyedrops and infection. The lacerations and narrowing of the canaliculus are best treated by silicone intubation. This technique is performed as described by Quickert and Dryden and gives the best anatomic repair, as well as allows the stent to remain in the canaliculus for a longer period of time than any other previously used stents. A one-snip is done on both the upper and lower punctum. Silicone wedged on a probe, such as the Quickert probe, is placed alternately through the upper and lower canaliculus, tear sac, and nasolacrimal duct. The probe is visualized in the inferior meatus and pulled out of the nose by either a grooved director or a hemostat. The probes are removed from the silicone, and the silicone is tied in a square knot and allowed to retract into the nose. Complete absence or obliteration of the canaliculus is repaired by the Jones' method of a conjunctival dacryocystorhinostomy. Concretions of the canaliculus can be removed by a small ring ear curette. If this is unsuccessful, then the canaliculus is slit open, and the concretions are removed under direct visualization. No stent is needed after removing the concretions, since the canaliculus can be primarily closed.

The tear sac obliteration can be caused by infection, dacryoliths, and, rarely, tumors. Acute and chronic dacryocystitis are best treated by dacryocystorhinostomy. Dacryocystectomy should be reserved for malignancy of the tear sac only. Dacryoliths are removed via a dacryocystorhinostomy, since there is usually an anatomic malfunction of the sac or duct that causes the stones to develop.

The nasolacrimal duct can be occluded on a congenital basis and responds best to probing. Early probing of the nasolacrimal duct with a number 0 or 00 probe before 6 months of age has an excellent cure rate. If the infant is over 1 year of age, an infracture of the turbinates should be combined with probing. Stenosis of the nasolacrimal duct in adults is treated by a dacryocystorhinostomy.

Precautions

Probing for therapeutic purposes should be confined to infants, whereas probing in adults should be limited to diagnostic tests. Dacryocystorhinostomy is the preferred treatment for most cases of epiphora, and a dacryocystectomy should be avoided. Lacrimal surgery necessitates a thorough knowledge of the lateral wall of the nose.

Comments

A lacrimal evaluation should include inspection, palpation, and the proper diagnostic tests. The lacrimal distributional, secretory, and excretory systems should all be evaluated to diagnose properly the underlying cause of epiphora.

References

Cassady JV: Developmental anatomy of nasolacrimal duct. Arch Ophthalmol 47:141–158, 1952.
Jones LT: Epiphora: Its causes and new surgical procedures for its cure; Preliminary report. Am J Ophthalmol 38:824–831, 1954.
Jones LT, Wobig JL: Surgery of the Eyelids and Lacrimal System. Birmingham, Aesculapius, 1976.
Tenzel RR: Canaliculo-dacryocystorhinostomy. Arch Ophthalmol 84:765, 1970.
Veirs ER: Lacrimal Disorders: Diagnosis and Treatment. St. Louis, CV Mosby, 1976.
Wobig JL: The office management of the lacrimal excretory system. JCE Ophthalmol December, 1978, pp 13–24.
Wobig JL: Lacerations of the Lacrimal Excretory System. Ocular Trauma. New York, Prentice Hall, 1979.
Wobig JL: Epiphora. Causes and treatment. Perspect Ophthalmol 5:177–181, 1981.

LACRIMAL HYPERSECRETION

MICHAEL A. LEMP, M.D.,
and MUNEERA A. MAHMOOD, M.D.
Washington, District of Columbia

Lacrimal hypersecretion is excessive tearing caused by increased secretion from the lacrimal glands. It must be distinguished from epiphora, which is excessive tearing caused by a blockage of the tear drainage system. High Schirmer's test values in the presence of patent drainage system indicate lacrimal hypersecretion. Lacrimal hypersecretion is usually an intermittent paroxysm without any ill effects other than social or cosmetic embarrassment. It can be divided into primary or secondary hypersecretion.

Primary lacrimal hypersecretion is very rare and is caused by a direct disturbance of the lacrimal gland. It can be initiated by strong parasympathomimetics or seen in early cases of lacrimal gland tumors or inflammation; it may also occur with thyrotoxicosis. Cases of lacrimal gland fistulas have been reported with symptomatic lacrimal hypersecretion.

Secondary lacrimal hypersecretion is more common and is either central, psychic, or neurogenic. Central or psychic hypersecretion occurs in emotional states only after the first few months of life or in physical pain, or it can be hysterical in nature. Neurogenic lacrimal hypersecretion has many different causes; reflex trigeminal irritation is the most common cause. Reflex irritation in the area of distribution of any of the three branches can cause lacrimation. Such external irritants as smog, fog, or pollutants; local inflammation; entropion; ectropion; foreign bodies; and accommodative strain all can cause lacrimation. Reflex visual irritation by bright lights causes lacrimation as well. Facial nerve or sphenopalatine ganglion irritation can cause excessive lacrimation. Paradoxical gustatory lacrimal reflexes—that is, crocodile tears—occur after aberrant regeneration of the facial nerve. Reflex lacrimation also accompanies such physiological acts as yawning, laughing, or vomiting.

THERAPY

Supportive. The first step in the treatment is to establish the etiology of lacrimal hypersecretion. Doing so requires a complete ophthalmologic examination and probably an ear, nose, and throat evaluation. Treatment should be directed to the cause, especially in local reflex irritation. When a cause cannot be determined or eliminated, mild cases might be managed by topical astringent vasoconstrictive drops.

Surgical. Partial or total extirpation of the lacrimal glands is to be considered only in the most annoying cases as there is a real and serious possibility of developing a dry eye. Surgical approach might involve removal of the palpebral lobe, which also leads to destruction of the ductules of the orbital lobe, or only the selective excision of excretory ductules subconjunctivally. In cases of lacrimal fistula, surgical redirection is performed. The sphenopalatine ganglion may also be blocked temporarily with local anesthetic injections; if it is useful, an alcohol block may be done. This is especially helpful in cases where there is nasal pathology or paradoxical weeping.

PRECAUTIONS

Surgical removal of part or all of the main lacrimal gland carries the risk of inducing a dry eye. The total mass of the accessory lacrimal glands is variable; the amount of functional lacrimal tissue remaining after surgery probably determines the adequacy of tear production. Extreme caution should be exercised in deciding to remove the main lacrimal gland.

COMMENTS

Hypersecretion of tears, which is rare, should be distinguished from epiphora caused by obstruction of the lacrimal outflow pathway. The latter is much more common, and drainage studies should yield a positive diagnosis. Other causes, such as inflammatory disease and senile ectropion, should be suspected and treated vigorously, if present.

References

Duke-Elder S (ed): System of Ophthalmology. St. Louis, CV Mosby, 1971, Vol XII, pp 959–965; 1974, Vol XIII, pp 597–599.

Gillette TE, et al: Histologic and immunohistologic comparison of main and accessory lacrimal tissue. Am J Ophthalmol 89:724–730, 1980.

Scherz W, Dohlman CH: Is the lacrimal gland dispensable? Keratoconjunctivitis sicca after lacrimal gland removal. Arch Ophthalmol 93:281–283, 1975.

LACRIMAL HYPOSECRETION

MICHAEL A. LEMP, M.D.
Washington, District of Columbia

Recent evidence suggests that all aqueous tear production by both the main and accessory lacrimal glands occurs as a result of reflex stimulation. Stimulation may be minimal, such as normal indoor air currents, or considerable, such as a surface foreign body. The previous distinction between reflex and "basal" tearing has been largely abandoned.

The tear film is composed of three components: lipid derived from the meibomian glands, mucus derived from conjunctival goblet cells, and aqueous tears produced by the main and accessory lacrimal glands. Mucus that renders the ocular surface wettable is reduced in conditions resulting in conjunctival scarring, such as erythema multiforme (Stevens-Johnson syndrome), ocular pemphigoid, chemical burns, and trachoma. Lipid production is reduced in ectodermal dysplasia. By far, the vast majority of cases of lacrimal hyposecretion, however, involve the aqueous component of tears. Decreased aqueous tear production occurs gradually with advancing age. It occurs more frequently in females and in the menopausal and postmenopausal years.

Keratoconjunctivitis sicca, the result of decreased aqueous tear production, can be seen in association with generalized collagen vascular disorders and the triad of dry eyes, dry mouth and arthritis referred to as Sjögren's syndrome. Less frequently, keratoconjunctivitis can be seen as a result of familial dysautonomia (Riley-Day syndrome). Moreover, drugs with anticholinergic side effects can also cause a decrease in aqueous tear production.

THERAPY

Ocular. Artificial tears can be used to supplement the deficient tear production. In general, nonviscous tears containing polyvinyl alcohol or adsorptive polymers form the mainstay of treatment. Frequency of dosage depends upon the severity of the condition; relatively mild conditions respond well to the use of one drop of tears two to four times a day, whereas more severe conditions require more frequent instillation. In more advanced conditions, the use of a sustained-released polymeric rod containing hydroxypropyl cellulose inserted in the inferior cul-de-sac provides relief from 6 to 12 hours. In many patients, however, this polymeric rod must be used in conjunction with artificial tears. In addition, the use of a bland lubricating ointment on retiring can be quite helpful.

Keratoconjunctivitis sicca tends to be associated with increased tear film viscosity as mucin, deprived of its normal aqueous solvent, becomes more viscous. The use of a 10 or 20 per cent acetylcysteine* solution helps reduce this viscosity.

In severe cases of keratoconjunctivitis sicca, particularly those with filamentary keratitis, a bandage soft contact lens can be particularly useful. These lenses, however, must be used in conjunction with artificial tears, and their use carries a certain risk of infection. Many clinicians prefer to use a prophylactic antibiotic drop along with these lenses. These lenses can provide a remarkable degree of comfort and melt away filaments in a very short period of time.

Systemic. In general, corticosteroids‡ and antimetabolites‡ are not useful in the treatment of keratoconjunctivitis sicca. In certain other severe inflammatory processes associated with ocular drying, such as ocular pemphigoid and Stevens-Johnson syndrome, however, they can be effective. Their use carries significant hazards; caution and close systemic monitoring are required.

In some menopausal and postmenopausal females with marked ocular surface disease associated with keratoconjunctivitis sicca, the use of systemic estrogen‡ replacement therapy can be useful. This must be done in conjunction with gynecological monitoring.

Topical. Recently, a retinoid topical ointment† has been reported to be useful in reversing conjunctival squamous cell metaplasia seen in association with dry eye conditions. Its use, however, remains experimental.

Surgical. Punctal occlusion by cautery is useful in severe cases of keratoconjunctivitis sicca, but should be used with caution because of the fluctuating nature of the condition. In general, repeated Schirmer tests of 1 mm or less or persistent ocular surface disease or both are necessary before the decision to cauterize the puncta is necessary. Too casual use of punctal cautery can cause epiphora.

A lateral tarsorrhaphy, which decreases the exposed area of the ocular surface, brings the conjunctival capillaries in constant apposition with the ocular surface, and lessens the shearing forces of the lid on the ocular surface, can be dramatically effective in reversing the ocular surface disease associated with a number of dry eye states.

Ocular or Periocular Manifestations

Cornea: Superficial punctate erosions; persistent epithelial defects; ulcer (rare).

Lacrimal System: Atrophy of the main and accessory lacrimal glands.

PRECAUTIONS

The ocular surface defense system is compromised in cases of keratoconjunctivitis sicca. These patients are therefore more prone to infections, particularly blepharitis and conjunctivitis. Exacerbations of symptoms may not be caused by a further decrease in tear production, but rather by concomitant blepharitis. Attention should be directed to the treatment of these infections when they occur.

COMMENTS

The management of a patient with moderate to severe lacrimal hyposecretion demands interest and perseverance on the part of the physician. These patients require long-term supportive help in an attempt to find which combination of treatments will provide satisfactory comfort. They should also be reassured that in the vast majority of cases this condition does not seriously affect vision.

References

Holly FJ, Lemp MA: Tear physiology and dry eyes. Surv Ophthalmol 22:69–87, 1977.
Jordan A, Baum J: Basic tear flow. Does it exist? Ophthalmology 87:920–930, 1980.
Lemp MA: Recent developments in dry eye management. Ophthalmology 94:1299–1304, 1987.
Lemp MA, Blackman HJ: Ocular surface defense mechanisms. Ann Ophthalmol 13:61–63, 1981.

SECTION 28

LENS

ADULT CATARACTS
ROBERT C. DREWS, M.D.
Clayton, Missouri

Adult cataract is not a single entity, and its different types display a wide variety of natural histories. The cataract that occurs in some alcoholics begins posterior subcapsularly and may become mature in only 6 to 12 months. Furthermore, there may be a delay in the development of cataract between the two eyes. The specific cataract of diabetes mellitus consists of cortical flakes. These may sometimes be seen in patients who have no diabetes themselves but only a family history of the disease. Unless coupled with ordinary senile cataract, these flakes are slowly progressive and seldom coalesce sufficiently to obscure vision. Diabetes mellitus may, however, hasten the progression of diffuse senile cataract. Brunescent nuclear cataract is usually a very slowly progressive condition, and good visual acuity may persist for years after the nucleus becomes so dense that direct ophthalmoscopic examination of the retina is impossible. Since many adult cataracts are of this type, treatment can appear to provide a significant delay in the need for cataract surgery. Visual acuity in this type of patient may show long periods of stabilization, even though the brunescence is increasing. Cortical cataracts (spokes and wedges) develop more rapidly than nuclear cataracts. Their course varies enough to make prediction hazardous.

THERAPY

Surgical. At the present time, cataract remains a surgical disease. Hypermaturity of a cataract with secondary uveitis or glaucoma, or swelling of the lens that threatens or has produced an angle-closure glaucoma may serve as positive indications for cataract surgery. Otherwise, cataract surgery is almost always elective. When the patient's vision is no longer sufficient to meet his or her visual needs, that individual may decide on cataract surgery. Further decisions as to intracapsular or extracapsular surgery and postoperative optical correction with glasses, contact lenses, or an intraocular lens implant depend again upon the patient's needs and the surgeon's prejudices and skills. The majority of patients in the United States now receive extracapsular surgery and a posterior chamber lens implant.

Fortunately, cataract surgery has made stunning advances so that cataract is no longer the chief cause of blindness in the United States as it was not too many years ago. When surgery is needed, rapid, full visual rehabilitation is now available for the vast majority of patients with cataract.

Precautions

The recent publication of articles on the prevention of adult cataract by aspirin has renewed interest in this country in the medical therapy of cataract. Fifty years ago, a number of nostrums were used, and even today a variety of drops are sold in most other countries with the claim that they will slow the progress of senile cataract. The public is willing to buy hope, and clinical impression is easily misled when harmless remedies are used against diseases whose natural history is only intermittently progressive.

There is a great deal of scientific interest today in the treatment of galactose cataract, since a specific metabolic defect is known. There is little evidence, however, that this defect plays any part in adult cataract; there is only the hope that similar treatable enzyme deficiencies might be found. The medical prevention of cataract has great appeal for the raising of research funds. There is little immediate promise of any efficacious solution, however.

Chronic high-dose aspirin[‡] therapy (for arthritis) has been found to be associated with a diminished incidence of senile cataract. However, the data remain somewhat soft, the connection speculative, and the possibility of other factors as a basis has not been ruled out. The risk of progression of cataract and therefore the need for therapy continue as the patient becomes more elderly. The prospective chronic use of high-dose aspirin in a large percentage of our population raises the possibility of large numbers of patients with significant aspirin side effects. Although a number of patients may choose to place themselves on such therapy, it is doubtful that the medical community will become enthusiastic about it. However, the biochemical basis, the possible relationship to tryptophan metabolism, is of fundamental importance; it is only through an understanding of the biochemical mechanisms of cataract formation that an efficacious therapy can be found.

COMMENTS

Proving the efficacy of any therapy for adult cataract may be all but impossible. Valid proof would require thousands of patients using a treatment for a minimum of 5 to 10 years, with separate bottles of eyedrops for the right and left eye (one eye serves as a control) so that neither the patient nor the physician would know which bottle of drops contained the active ingredient. Thereafter, the code could be broken and tested to see if a difference in the progression rate of cataract could be demonstrated. However, the original population would become statistically meaningless because of its hopeless decimation by death, loss to follow-up, and noncompliance. Noncompliance alone would make the study meaningless, especially when one combines informed consent with necessity for religious usage of drops forever kept separate over a test period of several years. The alternate possibility of using drops on randomly chosen patients would not change the death or dropout rate and would insufficiently increase compliance to make up for the loss of matched controls.

References

Bettman JW: General surgical concepts: Patient selection. *In* Drews RC, Steele A: Modern Trends in Cataract Surgery. West Yarmouth, MA, Butterworth, 1984.
Cotlier E, Sharma YR: Aspirin and senile cataracts in rheumatoid arthritis. Lancet 1:338–339, 1981.
Davis AE: Cataract. Its Preventive and Medical Treatment. Philadelphia, FA Davis, 1938.
Drews RC: Ethanol cataract. Act XXI Concilium Ophthalmologicum 1:753–758, 1970.
Jaffe NS, et al: A comparison of 500 Binkhorst implants with 500 routine intracapsular cataract extractions. Am J Ophthalmol 85:24–27, 1978.
Sabiston DW: Cataracts, Dupuytren's contracture, and alcohol addiction. Am J Ophthalmol 76:1005–1007, 1973.

AFTER-CATARACTS

DAVID J. McINTYRE, M.D., F.A.C.S.
Bellevue, Washington

After-cataract is a poorly defined term referring to the residual lens remnants from trauma (or incomplete surgical extraction), as well as alterations in the tissues left behind in extracapsular cataract technique, and the results of their proliferation. In the instance of trauma or incomplete surgery, the eye may undergo a period of striking inflammation. Hemorrhagic, pigmentary, and fibrotic elements may enter the field, producing multiple synechiae, distortions of the pupil, and occasionally, glaucoma or vitreous involvement with the risk of retinal detachment. Severe inflammation from this origin may result in phthisis bulbi. In the eye that is fortunate enough to avoid the inflammatory response, residual lens material may be isolated by sealing of the anterior and posterior capsular fragments. The Soemmering's ring and all of its variations result from this process. There is likely to be continued growth of new lens cortex, resulting in a slight enlargement of the Soemmering's ring over a period of years.

Currently, the greatest concern is with the after-cataract that develops after extracapsular cataract extraction. The pseudofibrotic changes in residual lens epithelial cells and the occasional growth of fibrous tissue from adhesions with the iris may ultimately result in a very heavy leathery membrane, which is a challenge in treatment.

In addition to changes in the material present at surgery, the long-term growth of secondary cortical fibers is also a problem. These fibers tend to grow across the posterior capsule in an irregular sheet or as nodular structures, classically known as Elschnig's pearls.

Severe inflammatory responses are readily apparent during the early course after trauma or surgery. In addition, those cases producing synechiae and distortion of the pupil are clearly visible at routine slitlamp examination. After-cataract is not appropriately treated unless a visual disturbance or other complication arises. The visual effect is by far the most common indication for intervention.

Early visual disturbance may result from the presence of fibrous pseudometaplasia of cortical remnants on the central posterior capsule. It may also be greatly accelerated by a fibrinous exudation during the immediate postinjury period. Wrinkling and proliferation of an irregular layer of secondary cortex may result in late changes that occur gradually over a period of several years. The incidence of clinically significant after-cataract is often reported at 40 to 50 per cent.

A recent debate has arisen regarding the effect of the posterior chamber artificial lens implant. Numerous investigators have reported that the growth of secondary cortex and the development of Elschnig's pearls are at least retarded by the contact of an artificial lens with the posterior capsule. In this author's experience with in-the-bag placement of a posterior chamber lens with its convex surface against the posterior capsule, an 11 per cent posterior capsulotomy rate at the fourth postoperative year has been found.

THERAPY

Supportive. The great majority of fibrotic after-cataracts that result from inflammation can be prevented by currently available techniques of "clean" surgery. It is now commonly taught that trauma with lens involvement should be cleaned up thoroughly at initial repair. Modern techniques for managing both lens and vitreous have greatly enhanced the outlook after trauma. Modern techniques of extracapsular cataract extraction have also sharply reduced the occurrence of postoperative inflammation. The eye without residual cortex is generally white and quiet at the first dressing.

Metaplasia and continuing growth of the lens epithelial cells do occur, and long-term clouding of vision is a potential disadvantage to the patient with extracapsular cataract surgery. In addition to an attempt to attain "clean" cataract surgery, other approaches have been made to prevent the growth of secondary cortex. Three directions of concurrent investigation have generated enthusiasm. In early clinical trials with cryotherapy, the lens epithelial cells at the midperiphery of the anterior and posterior capsule are damaged by a series of freeze-thaw cycles. This is being evaluated with the use of a modified cryoprobe and careful technique that minimizes potential damage to adjacent tissues. In a second study, antimetabolites have been placed in the anterior chamber at the conclusion of surgery to destroy the lens epithelial cells chemically. In the human, these cells are actively dividing and therefore sensitive to damage by methotrexate* during their mitotic phase. The third investigation involves an antimetabolite bound to a monoclonal antibody[†] to the lens epithelial cells. None of these techniques is currently available for widespread use, but all suggest that a preventive approach to the growth of secondary cortex will soon be possible.

Surgical. As with any intraocular procedure, it must be recognized that there are certain risks inherent in intervention directed at after-cataract. The patient must be properly informed that endophthalmitis, retinal detachment, cystoid macular edema, and intraocular hemorrhage are among the potential risks. If a surgical procedure is performed, it must be done with appropriate aseptic preparation and with the pupil dilated as needed. At the present time, the treatment of after-cataract is divided into three categories: reaspiration, discission, and excision.

Reaspiration of secondary cortical growth or "polishing" of the posterior capsule is suggested as a conservative approach to the treatment of after-cataract. It is applicable only to those cases without significant fibrosis. Those patients considered to have an unusually high risk of retinal complication may be offered reaspiration, leaving the posterior capsule intact, on the basis of intuitive logic that suggests that the capsule may then continue to protect the posterior segment.

In many cases, reaspiration is technically very similar to the aspiration of residual cortex at the time of primary extracapsular surgery. The newly grown material may be stripped from the periphery and aspirated from the eye in the usual fashion. Maintenance of the anterior chamber volume with a viscoelastic substance is an important consideration to protect the corneal endothelium during such an anterior segment procedure. The surgeon may choose instrumentation from among the modifications of the Kratz scratcher, various curettes, the coaxial cannula, or any of a variety of other aspirating devices.

The classical *surgical discission* is done with various modifications of the Ziegler knife. Alternatively, a sharp hook on the tip of a fine disposable hypodermic needle may be used to incise or tear the thin posterior capsule. If fibrotic changes have produced an irregular tough membrane, the procedure may be significantly more difficult.

Recently, the Neodymium YAG laser has become the most common instrument for posterior capsulotomy in the United States. Its astonishingly brief infrared energy creates a minute explosion in the transparent medium, thus causing a disruption of the capsular membrane. Lacking an incision, bacterial endophthalmitis is not a possible complication. However, early posttreatment secondary glaucoma is widely reported, along with cystoid macular edema, various maculopathies, and retinal detachment.

Occasionally, the after-cataract membrane may be so heavy and tough as to require *excision* with a vitreous suction/cutter. Such heavy scarring is usually associated with severe postoperative inflammation and extensive posterior synechiae formation. The individual case will dictate whether the procedure should be carried out via limbal or pars plana route.

Precautions

As previously noted, the risks of preventive techniques in current evaluation are as yet unknown. On the other hand, the risks of active surgical therapy are quite well understood. All methods of posterior capsulotomy share the risks of cystoid macular edema, retinal detachment, and accelerated macular degeneration, etc.

Endophthalmitis is a very uncommon complication of surgical discission; proper aseptic technique and close postoperative observation must be exercised. As previously noted, endophthalmitis is not a risk with laser posterior capsulotomy. A far more frequent complication is cystoid macular edema. In the past several years, it has been demonstrated that the frequency of cystoid macular edema declines as the time increases between primary cataract surgery and the posterior capsulotomy. According to some reports, discission done at the time of surgery or up until 2 months postoperatively produces a cystoid macular edema rate approximately equal to intracapsular cataract surgery. On the other hand, discission performed 12 months after the initial procedure seems to have much less effect on the macula. Therefore, to minimize cystoid macular edema the surgeon should wait as long as possible after the initial cataract operation before doing a posterior capsulotomy by any method.

In addition to cystoid macular edema, progressive macular degeneration, retinal tears, and retinal detachment occur as complications of the posterior capsulotomy. The relationship to post-cataract timing is not as yet well documented. There is a suggestion that some of these risks may be greater with laser than surgical technique.

COMMENTS

The need for management of after-cataract will probably decrease strikingly in the next several years. Techniques are available for the management of trauma, inflammation, and residual lens material with minimum risk. Similarly, currently taught techniques of extracapsular cataract extraction include very effective removal of residual cortex and, when combined with the posterior chamber artificial lens implantation, may actually retard the growth of secondary cortex.

Either chemical or cryoepithelialysis may prove so effective that management of after-cataract will become a rare task indeed. In the meanwhile, either surgical or laser posterior capsulotomy is safe and effective for the treatment of visual impairment caused by after-cataract.

References

Aron-Rosa D: Pulse Yag Laser Surgery. Thorofare, NJ, CB Slack, 1981.
Chan R, Emery JM: Mitotic inhibitors in preventing posterior capsule opacification: 2½ year follow-up. In Caldwell D: Cryotherapy of the Posterior Capsule. Current Concepts in Cataract Surgery: Selected Proceedings of the 8th Biennial Cataract Surgical Congress, 1985.
Emery JM, McIntyre DJ: Extracapsular Cataract Surgery. St. Louis, CV Mosby, 1982.
Jaffe NS: Cataract Surgery and Its Complications, 2nd ed. St. Louis, CV Mosby, 1976, pp 380–388.

CONGENITAL AND INFANTILE CATARACTS
DAVID A. HILES, M.D.
Pittsburgh, Pennsylvania

Congenital cataracts are often noted at birth or are diagnosed within the first few months of life. Infantile or juvenile cataracts may not be discovered until late childhood when progressive visual deficits or strabismus arises. Cataracts may be unilateral or bilateral, involve any part of the lens, and be stationary or progressive. Sporadic cataracts are the most common entity and constitute one third of infantile cataracts; many of these may be new autosomal dominant mutations. An additional 8 to 25 per cent of cataracts are familial. Cataracts are often associated with other ocular, systemic, chromosomal, genetic, or syndrome-related abnormalities. Cataracts are associated with craniofacial, mandibulofacial, skeletal, apical, central nervous system, muscular, dermatologic, and renal syndromes. Downs, Turner's, Patau's and Edward's chromosomal syndromes also have associated lenticular opacities. Embryopathies or nongenetic diseases affect the fetus and produce cataracts. They include the rubella syndrome, but other less common viral, bacterial, and protozoal infections also produce cataracts in infants. Deficiencies of calcium or glucose, as well as metabolic disturbances, that produce galactosemia, diabetes mellitus, homocystinuria, mannosidosis, and Wilson's, Fabry's, and Refsum's diseases also may induce lens opacities. Other cataracts seen in infants and children may be related to such ocular diseases or anomalies as retinopathy of prematurity, infantile glaucoma, retinoblastoma, microphthalmos, anterior chamber cleavage syndromes, colobomas, aniridia, ectopia lentis, persistent hyperplastic primary vitreous, retinal dysplasia, retinitis pigmentosa, and retinal detachment. Ocular trauma, ionizing radiation, and the effects of maternal or infant drug intoxication should also be considered when investigating the etiology of infantile cataracts.

Infantile cataracts are morphologically categorized according to their position within the lens. Complete cataracts are those in which no fundus reflex is visible. Partial cataracts include capsular (anterior or posterior, including lenticonus), subcapsular, lamellar, axial, cortical, nuclear, and membranous opacities.

THERAPY

Supportive. Many infantile cataracts are compatible with good vision, but frequent reevaluation of the fixation reflexes or visual acuity is indicated for these children. Refraction with the prescription of the appropriate glasses helps prevent loss of visual acuity secondary to amblyopia of anisometropia, and occlusion of the fellow eye may be necessary to prevent this complication. Atropine pupillary dilation combined with bifocals is also useful to enhance vision in patients with axial opacities. Some lens opacities increase in density with age, and surgery is required. However, the visual prognosis for these older children is often better than for children with complete cataracts discovered in the newborn period, who frequently have developed early-onset irreversible deprivation amblyopia.

Surgical. If the axial portion of the lens is obscured by an opacity 3 mm in diameter or larger, decreased visual efficiency and amblyopia may result. Patients with dense axial or complete unilateral cataracts require immediate cataract surgery to prevent deprivation amblyopia. Patients with dense bilateral cataracts require early surgery in the more involved eye; the second eye is operated on 1 to 2 weeks later, depending upon the amount of residual inflammation existing in the first eye. Other patients with bilateral cataracts may have an asymmetric onset of their cataracts, and the more severely involved eye may develop deprivation amblyopia that is further complicated by aphakia. Early optical correction and the occlusion of the sound eye help alleviate this complication. If strabismus develops, surgery is indicated as soon as a central fixation reflex is obtained in the deviating eye and the strabismic angle remains stable.

Surgery of the infantile cataracts is commonly performed through one or two small limbal incisions, but the lens may also be removed through pars plana incisions. Appropriate microsurgical skills and techniques utilizing the operating microscope facilitate surgery. Large anterior capsulectomies are performed to reduce the occurrence of dense secondary membranes. Aspiration-irrigation techniques utilize a syringe and push-pull aspiration-irrigation or mechanical suction cutting devices that fragment and aspirate the lens capsule, cortex, and nucleus as a one-stage operation. A wide posterior capsulectomy combined with an anterior vitrectomy clears the visual axis of all lens elements. This technique reduces the need for secondary membrane surgery and lessens the further risk of amblyopia by eliminating reocclusion of the visual axis with opaque tissue. The elapsed time to optical rehabilitation is also reduced.

Aphakic rehabilitation is accomplished with a contact lens placed on the eye within the first few postoperative days after cataract extraction or as soon as the surgical inflammatory response subsides. The initial contact lens K readings and trial lens fitting are accomplished under the same general anesthesia as the cataract extraction. Lens powers are based upon a postoperative refraction plus the addition of 2 to 3 more diopters to compensate for the child's near vision needs. Postoperative amblyopia therapy with light-tight part-time occlusion of the sound eye is undertaken as soon as the contact lens is in place. Repeated refractions, with modification of the contact lens, are made over the first 2 to 3 years of life to compensate for the rapid decrease in the refractive error of the infant eye. For older patients, it is suggested that the contact lens power be based upon an accurate distance refraction. The application of an over-spectacle containing the residual cylinder and a bifocal addition is prescribed. The bifocal may be of sufficient power to function as a low-vision aid, if needed.

Aphakic spectacles with a bifocal addition may be prescribed for all patients with bilateral infantile cataracts in whom contact lens compliance is reduced, the parents are reluctant to participate in their use, or other social or economic factors are present that render contact lens wear unsuccessful. Glasses, although expensive, remain a noncontact, easily modified reliable source of aphakic rehabilitation for children. To reduce the weight of aphakic spectacles in patients with very high refractive errors, a 20-diopter Fresnel power prism may be applied to a carrier spectacle lens in which residual sphere and cylinder power plus a bifocal are incorporated.

Epikeratophakia refractive techniques consist of the application of a corneal graft of human eyebank tissue lathed to proper power that is sutured over the recipient's epithelium-denuded cornea into a peripheral corneal groove. The graft may be surgically replaced if the refractive error modifies significantly with the passage of time. Epikeratophakia is indicated for patients with unilateral and bilateral, infantile or acquired (traumatic) cataracts who are older than 1 year. A rapid myopic shift is encountered before 1 year of age. Application of the epigraft after this age reduces the power inaccuracies encountered with growth. Graft failure rates approach 10 per cent, but regrafting salvages 90 per cent of the failed grafts. Visual acuities approximate those of other aphakic rehabilitation modalities for children.

Intraocular lens implantation is useful for aphakic rehabilitation of unilateral infantile cataract patients 2 to 3 years of age and older who either fail to wear a contact lens after earlier surgery, or for those patients being considered for cataract surgery for whom the parent and the ophthalmologist conclude will not successfully wear a contact lens. The intraocular lens powers implanted are the same as for the adult eye so that the child's eye grows toward adult lens powers. During the period of the child's growth and development, spectacles combined with a bifocal addition for near are prescribed for any residual distance sphere or cylinder. The visual success of this method is equal to that achieved by contact lens patients. There is, however, a reduction in anisometropia and aniseikonia with an intraocular lens, which helps reduce deprivation amblyopia. In addition, there is a constant application of the aphakic optics, as well as an absence of stress to the patient with the insertion and removal of the contact lens.

Flexible open-looped anterior chamber lenses are recommended for children 2 to 3 years of age who have had earlier cataract surgery and fail contact lens wear, and for those undergoing cataract surgery at a later age in whom a posterior capsulectomy-anterior vitrectomy procedure has been performed. Posterior chamber lenses are indicated for children 6 years of age or older who are capable of undergoing Neodymium YAG laser posterior capsulectomies.

PRECAUTIONS

Patients with an early onset of bilateral, complete, or large axial cataracts often develop nystagmus either on a familial or visual deprivation basis. Nystagmus occurs within the first 2 to 3 months of life, and cataract surgery is indicated before this time to establish secure, equal, bilateral, central fixation reflexes. If this crucial time is lost, nystagmus will persist throughout life with a coincident reduction in visual acuity.

A wide variety of lens sizes and powers must be available to the contact lens technician at the time of the lens fitting. The smaller hard lens are often superior for infants because of their ease of insertion and removal. The larger soft lens are more comfortable to wear and have a lower loss rate, but frequently break or craze with repeated bending during insertion and removal into the infant's palpebral fissures. Extended-wear lenses are used with caution because of the complications of corneal infections.

There are certain contraindications for intraocular lens implantion. Children younger than 2 to 3 years of age are not selected because of the rapid power changes associated with growth of the eye. The Food and Drug Administration regulations prohibit patients with bilateral cataracts from receiving an implant in both eyes without prior approval. Patients with bilateral cataracts with marked density asymmetry of their lens opacities may receive an intraocular lens in the eye with the denser cataract either primarily with cataract surgery or as a secondary implant. Microphthalmic eyes with corneas less than 10 mm in diameter, eyes with infantile glaucoma, and patients with chronic intraocular inflammations following the rubella syndrome, rheumatoid arthritis, pars planitis, toxoplasmosis, or toxocariasis should not be candidates for implantation. Likewise, eyes with dislocated lens that are complicated by associated retinal detachment and secondary glaucoma should not receive intraocular lens. Eyes with posterior polar defects, including posterior hyperplastic primary vitreous, macular lesions or degeneration, and optic nerve defects or atrophy, do not benefit from intraocular lens implantation. The remainder of children with unilateral cataracts may be considered for intraocular lens implantation.

The formation of secondary membranes that surround posterior chamber lenses is the major contraindication for their use in infants and young children. Postoperatively, pupillary displacement, posterior synechiae, and occlusion of the visual axis by dense membranes complicate amblyopia therapy and require frequent, often technically difficult, secondary membrane surgical procedures.

The disadvantages of epikeratophakia are that it requires human tissue, a complicated lathing technique to produce the proper aphakic power, a surgical procedure to institute or modify the graft, and a prolonged period of graft stabilization after surgery. The long-term stability of the graft appears to be excellent. An overcorrection for residual sphere or cylinder plus bifocals and amblyopia occlusion of the sound eye is still required.

COMMENTS

Unilateral infantile cataracts are most frequently sporadic in occurrence, may be part of a familial pattern, or secondary to metabolic, infectious, genetic, chromosomal diseases, drug toxicity, or other systemic syndromes.

Early discovery of a unilateral infantile cataract is dependent upon the education of nonophthalmic medical and paramedical personnel, which include obstetricians, pediatricians, family practitioners, nurses, parents, and teachers. If the axial lens opacity is greater than 3 mm in diameter, the visual axis is occluded, or a poor fundus reflex is observed, surgery is indicated at the time of discovery of the cataract. Neurophysiologic research has indicated a sensitive period for the reversal of deprivation amblyopia in kittens and monkeys. Extrapolation of this concept to the human has been made by ophthalmic surgeons, but the exact duration of the sensitive period remains unknown.

Patients with large unilateral infantile cataracts that are discovered in the neonatal period often suffer more severe deprivation amblyopia and achieve poorer visual results than those patients with small lens opacities discovered later that permit prolonged periods of visual development. However, dense, early-onset cataracts removed from the eyes of older children rarely achieve significant visual improvement. In addition, children with an early onset of infantile cataracts frequently have associated microphthalmia or other ocular defects that affect both the anterior and posterior segment. Strabismus is a frequent complication contributing to amblyopia and visual loss and must be corrected to induce binocular awareness.

Infants and children suffering ocular trauma in the amblyopia age period (birth to 8 years) also require early surgery when the visual axis becomes occluded, strabismus ensues, or there is a decrease in the quality of the fixation reflex or measured visual acuity with optical correction. These children respond to therapy in the same manner as patients with unilateral infantile cataracts and require vigorous optical rehabilitation, amblyopia occlusion, and strabismus surgery, when indicated. The visual results depend upon the age of the patient at the time of the occlusion of the visual axis, the length of time in which the opacity occludes the visual axis, the rapidity of postoperative optical correction, and the severity of the trauma to other ocular structures.

References

Hiles DA: Visual acuities of monocular IOL and non-IOL aphakic children. Ophthalmology 87:1296–1300, 1980.

Hiles DA: Part I: Cataract surgical indications in children. Cataract 1:8–12, 1984.

Hiles DA: Part II: Infantile cataracts—cataract surgery in children. Cataract 1:6–13, 1984.

Hiles DA: Part III: Infantile cataracts—aphakic optical correction. Cataract 1:20–29, 1984.

Hiles DA: Part IV: Infantile cataracts—results following surgery. Cataract 1:20–28, 1984.

Hiles DA: Intraocular lens implantation in children with monocular cataracts 1974–1983. Ophthalmology 91:1231–1237, 1984.

Hiles DA, Hered RW: Modern intraocular lens implants in children with new age limitations. J Cataract Refract Surg 13:493–497, 1987.

Morgan KS, et al: The nationwide study of epikeratophakia for aphakia in children. Am J Ophthalmol 103:366–374, 1987.

DISLOCATION OF THE LENS
(Ectopia Lentis, Luxation of the Lens, Subluxation of the Lens)

PAUL STERNBERG, JR., M.D.
Atlanta, Georgia

The crystalline lens normally occupies the pupillary space, is centered behind the iris, and is held in position by the zonules. Dislocation of the lens, or ectopia lentis, occurs when the lens is not in its proper position. A lens is subluxated when zonular fibers are broken, causing lens displacement but such that the lens remains in the pupillary aperture. Luxation of the lens implies total rupture of the zonules; such lenses are dislocated into either the vitreous cavity or anterior chamber. Progressive dislocation of the lens may occur with a subluxated lens becoming totally luxated into the vitreous cavity.

Trauma is the leading cause of lens dislocation, accounting for over half of the cases in most series. Traumatic dislocation of the lens is often accompanied by other evidence of the contusive injury to the globe, including rupture of the globe, hyphema, anterior chamber angle recession, glaucoma, iridodialysis, cyclodialysis, vitreous hemorrhage, choroidal rupture, hemorrhagic choroidal detachment, retinal dialysis, retinal tears, retinal detachment, and optic neuropathy.

Ectopia lentis is also a feature of a variety of systemic disorders, including Marfan's syndrome, Weill-Marchesani syndrome, and homocystinuria. Since Marfan's syndrome patients may have dilation or dissection of the aorta and cardiac valvular disease, and homocystinuria patients may have cardiovascular abnormalities and a tendency to thromboembolism because of platelet deficiency, it is important that the diagnosis be established before any surgical maneuvers are made that could precipitate vascular complications.

Dislocation of the lens has also been seen in some less common systemic disorders, including sulfite oxidase deficiency, hyperlysinemia, focal dermal hypoplasia, Ehlers-Danlos syndrome, aniridia, and mandibulofacial dysostosis. Ectopia lentis has been reported as an isolated autosomal dominant entity and as an autosomal recessive condition associated with corectopia (ectopia lentis et pupillae). Since these conditions are heritable, genetic counseling should be encouraged in patients with a dislocated lens.

THERAPY

Supportive. The presence of a lens displaced from its normal position does not require surgical management. In general, dislocated lenses can be tolerated well for long periods of time. If the lens is subluxated but clear, refraction usually can be accomplished satisfactorily. In some cases, dilation of the pupil or pupilloplasty may be useful. If the lens is luxated into the vitreous cavity, an aphakic correction may be used.

In some cases, a subluxated lens may cause pupillary block glaucoma. Often, this condition responds to mydriatics. If this approach is unsuccessful, laser or surgical peripheral iridectomy should be attempted before lens removal.

On occasion, lens dislocation, particularly that caused by trauma, may be accompanied by ocular inflammation. This uveitis may be managed with topical medications, including cycloplegics (1 per cent atropine twice daily), and corticosteroids (1 per cent prednisolone four times daily).

Surgical. Surgery may become necessary if the dislocated lens becomes cataractous, either preventing adequate retinoscopy in a child or causing diminished visual function. Lens extraction may also be indicated in eyes where the edge of the clear lens is in the center of the pupil, precluding suitable phakic or aphakic refraction. In rare cases, a dislocated lens may begin to leak lens protein into the eye, causing a lens-induced uveitis and glaucoma. This condition requires lens extraction if the eye is to be salvaged.

When planning surgery for a dislocated lens, the surgeon must remember that vitreous loss is likely because of the ruptured zonules; successful surgery depends on how well the vitreous is managed. A pars plana approach using vitreoretinal instrumentation decreases the risk of pulling on the vitreous with an aspiration needle, irrigation/aspiration handpiece, or cryoprobe, thereby lessening the chance of retinal tears and detachment. There is no chance of vitreous incarceration in the limbal wound with pars plana surgery.

The lens can be removed either with a vitrectomy instrument or by phacofragmentation. To prevent traction on the peripheral retina, vitreous around the lens should be managed with the cutting mode of the vitrectomy instrument. If any lens fragment falls posteriorly, a fiberoptic probe can be inserted through a sclerotomy and the lens material removed using standard vitrectomy techniques. Residual peripheral lens material can be removed by performing gentle scleral indentation to bring the pars plicata area into view.

In older patients, the lens may prove too hard to be removed by either a vitrectomy instrument or phacofragmentation probe. In these instances the lens must be removed by cryoextraction. It is important to avoid freezing the vitreous so as to prevent traction being transmitted to the peripheral retina as the lens is extracted.

In some patients, the lens may become luxated into the anterior chamber, causing secondary glaucoma and corneal edema. In these cases, efforts may be made to displace the lens into the vitreous cavity, but, in most cases, either this is unsuccessful or, if successful, luxation recurs shortly thereafter. Although pars plana surgery may be used for these lenses, intracapsular extraction through a limbal incision may be easier, particularly in the presence of corneal edema. The surgeon must anticipate the loss of vitreous and be prepared to perform an anterior vitrectomy. Preoperative placement of a Flieringa ring may prevent collapse of the globe.

PRECAUTIONS

If retinal detachment is present in a patient with a dislocated lens, removal of the lens

---

This work was supported in part by a departmental grant from Research to Prevent Blindness Inc.

should only be attempted if it precludes the surgeon's ability to visualize the retina. If it is necessary to remove the lens, pars plana surgery is preferred because of the smaller incisions and better immediate visualization of the fundus. Removal of a dislocated lens in the presence of a detached retina is hazardous; the lens must be aspirated into the vitrectomy or phacofragmentation probe and brought into the anterior vitreous away from the detached retina before attempting digestion of the lens.

COMMENTS

Occasionally, lens material or the lens nucleus may become displaced into the vitreous as a complication of extracapsular cataract extraction. In some cases, this displacement can be well tolerated, but it often results in uveitis, secondary glaucoma, and corneal edema. This complication of extracapsular cataract surgery can be managed satisfactorily with pars plana vitrectomy.

Extracapsular cataract surgery with intraocular lens implantation may also be complicated by dislocation of the pseudophakos. Partial dislocation may not require intervention; however, dislocation into the vitreous cavity can be managed successfully by pars plana vitrectomy and repositioning of the intraocular lens. In most cases, the lens should be sutured to the iris or sclera to prevent repeat dislocation.

References

Chandler PA: Choice of treatment in dislocation of the lens. Arch Ophthalmol 71:765–786, 1964.
Jarrett WH II: Dislocation of the lens. A study of 166 hospitalized cases. Arch Ophthalmol 78:289–296, 1967.
Michels RG, Shacklett DE: Vitrectomy technique for removal of retained lens material. Arch Ophthalmol 95:1767–1773, 1977.
Nelson LB, Maumenee IH: Ectopia lentis. Surv Ophthalmol 27:143–160, 1982.
Sternberg P Jr, Michels RG: Treatment of dislocated posterior chamber intraocular lenses. Arch Ophthalmol 104:1391–1393, 1986.
Treister G, Machemer R: Pars plana surgical approach for various anterior segment problems. Arch Ophthalmol 97:909–911, 1979.

LENTICONUS AND LENTIGLOBUS

MARSHALL M. PARKS, M.D.
Washington, District of Columbia

Lenticonus and lentiglobus are deformities of the anterior or posterior lens surfaces. The lens surface bows in the axial region 2 to 3 mm either forward into the anterior chamber or posteriorly into the vitreous. Lenticonus implies that the lens surface protuberance is conical; lentiglobus signifies that the lens surface is globular. The majority of cases are posterior lentiglobus. The etiology of posterior lentiglobus is unknown, but in many cases, the remnant of the hyaloid artery lies within the lentiglobus-involved portion of the posterior lens capsule. Persistent hyperplastic primary vitreous may also be associated with posterior lentiglobus. The posterior lentiglobus is presumed to result from a lens capsule weakness in the axial region that bulges increasingly with age under the intralenticular pressure. The anterior lens surface defects occur rarely and are usually bilateral, whereas the posterior lens surface defects are more common and often unilateral. Anterior lenticonus has been associated with spina bifida and Alport's and Waardenburg's syndromes.

Before cataract formation, the lentiglobus may appear as a 2- to 4-mm axial refractive defect by skiascopy; the diagnosis is proven by slitlamp biomicroscopy. Once the diagnosis is made, the progressively deteriorating character of the defect can be documented. The disrupted lens fiber lamellae become cataractous, which at first appear as a posterior axial opacity and eventually becomes a more diffuse cataract. Examination in the later stage precludes diagnosis.

THERAPY

Surgical. If visual acuity deteriorates, phacoemulsification with aspiration of the cataract associated with lenticonus and lentiglobus may be necessary. As the cataract is aspirated at surgery, the exposed diaphanous weak posterior lens capsule in the lentiglobus portion may become evident. Infusion of the irrigating solution into the anterior chamber bows the inherently defective portion of the lens capsule back into the vitreous cavity. Lowering the infusion bottle to near the level of the anterior chamber causes the lens capsule defect to bow forward toward the corneal endothelium. The lentiglobus portion of the posterior capsule often has calcium deposits within it. Usually, the diaphanous lentiglobus capsular defect tears before the lens cortex aspiration is completed, and vitreous may enter the anterior chamber.

PRECAUTIONS

Although lentiglobus usually is not detected at birth, the defect may be far advanced with rather diffuse cataracts already present. On the other hand, some early diagnosed cases without significant cataract change and with essentially clear lenses may be followed for up to 10 years. However, the majority of the cases deteriorate and require surgery.

COMMENTS

Because cataractous changes often develop during the amblyogenic age (birth to 8 years), amblyopia is probably the most serious feature associated with this disorder. Another common problem encountered in unilateral posterior lentiglobus is the mistaken impression that the poor vision associated with the unilateral cataract is unimprovable; however, because the induced poor vision may be recent, the prognosis for attaining nearly normal visual rehabilitation is good.

A good rule to follow is that, if the axial refractive defect by skiascopy is 3 mm or larger and the infant or young child is too young to test subjectively the visual acuity, amblyopia should be considered inevitable. Visual rehabilitation with lens surgery, contact lens, and occlusion therapy (if unilateral) of the good eye should seriously be considered.

References

Arnott EJ, Crawford MD'A, Toghill PJ: Anterior lenticonus and Alport's syndrome. Br J Ophthalmol 50:390–403, 1966.
Crouch ER Jr, Parks MM: Management of posterior lenticonus complicated by unilateral cataract. Am J Ophthalmol 85:503–508, 1978.
Howitt D, Hornblass A: Posterior lenticonus. Am J Ophthalmol 66:1133–1136, 1968.
Parks MM: Visual results in aphakic children. Am J Opthalmol 94:441–449, 1982.
Stafford WR: Anterior lenticonus. Posterior lentiglobus. Report of cases and review of the literature. Am J Ophthalmol 56:654–658, 1963.
Tipshus AF: Posterior traumatic lenticonus. Arch Ophthalmol 82:548–549, 1969.

MICROSPHEROPHAKIA

HAROLD E. CROSS, M.D., Ph.D.

Tucson, Arizona

Microspherophakia is a rare condition in which the lens is small in equatorial diameter and slightly increased in anteroposterior dimensions, resulting in a small spherical lens. The entire lens equator is usually visible through a dilated pupil, and the ciliary zonules are elongated and irregular. Microspherophakia is usually bilateral, and subluxation of the lens is most frequently inferior, although it can dislocate or rotate anteriorly. Cataracts are also common. Myopia is consistently high with −5.00 to −20.00 diopters. Secondary glaucoma caused by pupillary block with progressive shallowing of the anterior chamber is the most serious complication.

Ultrastructural studies reveal abnormalities in both the lens and its suspensory zonules. Cortical lens fibers in cross-section are reduced to 20 per cent of normal. Zonules on the posterior lens surface are abnormally large with no evidence of prior attachment to ciliary processes. As yet, the causes of abnormal lens-zonule development remain obscure.

THERAPY

Ocular. Intraocular pressure control is of primary concern. Mydriatics and cycloplegics, such as cyclopentolate or tropicamide, may be of value in preventing pupillary-block glaucoma, but prolonged mydriasis may allow the lens to migrate into the anterior chamber. Contact lenses should be considered in patients with high myopia.

Surgical. If the glaucoma is detected before peripheral anterior synechiae have formed, a peripheral iridectomy may be effective. If the peripheral anterior synechiae are severe, a filtration procedure may prove necessary.

Lens extraction for cataract or severe anterior displacement with intractable increased intraocular pressure may also be necessary.

Laser iridotomy may be preferable to the usual surgical approach to minimize complications. Postoperative miosis may reduce the risk of further lens dislocation, but this effect remains to be documented.

Supportive. Many ocular conditions that cause microspherophakia are hereditary. Therefore, whenever a sibling with microspherophakia is found, all other siblings in that family need to be examined, since a high frequency of visual loss occurs before diagnosis and management of unsuspected glaucoma.

Ocular or Periocular Manifestations

Lens: Anterior displacement; cataract; ectopia; inferior displacement.
Other: Decreased visual acuity; myopia; secondary glaucoma.

PRECAUTIONS

A frequent complication of microspherophakia is an atypical variety of open-angle glaucoma that has been labeled "inverse" angle-closure glaucoma. Repeated attacks may induce peripheral anterior synechiae, which complicate an already difficult situation. Mydriatics are used to relieve this condition. Because of the small lens size and high curvature of the anterior lens surface, miotics may increase the pupillary block that results if the lens becomes anteriorly displaced.

COMMENTS

Microspherophakia has been reported as an isolated familial anomaly and as a manifestation of Marfan's syndrome, homocystinuria, and most typically Weill-Marchesani syndrome. The prognosis for patients with microspherophakia is generally poor, owing to severe glaucoma resulting from peripheral anterior synechiae formation secondary to repeated asymptomatic attacks of angle-closure glaucoma.

References

Farnsworth PA, et al: Ultrastructural abnormalities in a microspherical ectopic lens. Exp Eye Res 27:399–408, 1978.

Jensen AD, Cross HE, Paton D: Ocular complications in the Weill-Marchesani syndrome. Am J Ophthalmol 77:261–269, 1974.

Johnson VP, Grayson M, Christian JC: Dominant microspherophakia. Arch Ophthalmol 85:534–537, 1971.

Kemmetmueller H: Correction of bilateral severe myopia due to spherophakia with contact lenses. A case report. Contact Lens Med Bull 3:28–29, 1970.

Ritch R, Wand M: Treatment of the Weill-Marchesani syndrome. Ann Ophthalmol 13:665–667, 1981.

Sellyei LF Jr, Barraquer J: Surgery of the ectopic lens. Ann Ophthalmol 5:1127–1133, 1973.

SECTION 29

MACULA

AGE-RELATED MACULAR DEGENERATION

MICHAEL L. KLEIN, M.D.
Portland, Oregon

Age-related macular degeneration (AMD) is the leading cause of severe, irreversible loss of vision in older Americans. The underlying pathologic changes occur primarily at the level of the retinal pigment epithelium, Bruch's membrane, and choriocapillaris in the macular region. The earliest clinical manifestations of AMD are drusen, which appear as yellow deposits beneath the pigment epithelium; they are present throughout the fundus, but are especially prominent in the macula. Drusen occur commonly in older patients, are generally not associated with visual symptoms, and are considered by some to be precursors rather than an integral component of AMD.

Some patients with drusen do develop AMD with varying degrees of visual impairment. Most develop the dry or atrophic form, which is characterized by atrophic pigment epithelial changes and is usually associated with slowly progressive, mild visual loss. A smaller number develop the wet or exudative form that results in a more rapidly progressive and severe loss of vision. These patients comprise the vast majority of those with severe visual impairment from AMD, and the most common underlying feature of their disease is the presence of subretinal neovascularization. The resulting leakage, hemorrhage, and fibrovascular scar formation produce significant loss of central vision. In occasional cases, vitreous hemorrhage may occur and produce more profound impairment of vision. Another manifestation of exudative AMD is retinal pigment epithelial detachment, which may occur independently or in association with subretinal neovascularization.

THERAPY

Ocular. No medical treatment has been proven to be effective in preventing the development or altering the natural course of AMD. Certain nutritional supplements, including zinc,[‡] selenium,[‡] and vitamins C,[‡] E,[‡] and beta carotene,[‡] have been advocated as being of possible value. However, no conclusive evidence supports their use at this time. Although long-term exposure to sunlight has been proposed as a contributing factor in the development of AMD, there is currently no evidence to demonstrate a protective effect from the routine use of any type of sunglasses.

Surgical. Laser photocoagulation has been proven to be beneficial in reducing the incidence of severe visual loss in certain patients with subretinal neovascularization and AMD. The Macular Photocoagulation Study reported favorable results using argon laser photocoagulation for subretinal neovascular membranes that lie 200 μM or more from the center of the foveal avascular zone. Principles of treatment in that trial included the use of a recent (less than 72 hours old) fluorescein angiogram; heavy, confluent burns covering the entire neovascular membrane and extending 100 μM beyond; and retrobulbar anesthesia.* Although argon blue-green laser had been used, it is now recommended that, when using argon laser photocoagulation in close proximity to the fovea, the blue component should be avoided.

Longer wavelengths, such as those produced by krypton red laser, have been shown to cause less inner retinal damage and may possibly be of value when treating subretinal neovascular membranes covered in part by blood, and in eyes with media opacities, such as cataract. However, certain complications are more common when using these wavelengths (see Precautions). The yellow wavelength of the dye laser also provides certain theoretic advantages, including excellent absorption by subretinal blood vessels, with maximum transmission through the macular xanthophyll pigment. However, the relative value of any given wavelength over another in the treatment of subretinal neovascularization has yet to be clinically demonstrated.

For neovascular membranes less than 200 μM from the center of fovea, the value of photocoagulation remains to be conclusively proven. However, some uncontrolled studies indicate that treatment does improve the very poor natural course of these lesions.

In the case of neovascularization beneath the center of the fovea, no treatment is currently indicated. A prospective, randomized clinical trial sponsored by the National Eye Institute is currently evaluating the potential benefit of limiting scotoma size by photocoagulating these lesions.

With regard to pigment epithelial detachments, the value of photocoagulation is uncertain.

Vitreous hemorrhage usually clears spontaneously, but may persist for months or more. In rare instances, vitrectomy may be indicated.

Ocular or Periocular Manifestations

Retina: Drusen; pigment epithelial atrophy; pigment epithelial detachment; subretinal exudate; subretinal fibrovascular scar; subretinal fluids; subretinal hemorrhage; subretinal neovascular membrane.

PRECAUTIONS

Complications of photocoagulation include the following: 1) inadvertent foveal photocoagulation (the likelihood is lessened by using retrobulbar anesthesia and maintaining a constant awareness of foveal location by referring to the projected fluorescein angiogram during treatment); 2) macular pucker (especially with blue-green argon laser, but is seldom of visual significance); 3) hemorrhage from the choroid or the new blood vessel membrane (the likelihood is lessened by using longer-duration burns and avoiding the use of small spot sizes); and 4) retinal pigment epithelial tears. The latter two complications are most likely to occur when using the red wavelengths.

Recurrences of subretinal neovascularization are unfortunately very common, occurring in over 50 per cent of treated eyes. Most recurrences develop within a year of treatment. Accordingly, careful postoperative follow-up is indicated to detect recurrences early, thereby allowing an opportunity for further treatment. The patient should be informed of the importance of daily monitoring of the vision in the treated eye. The use of an Amsler grid is helpful for this purpose. Frequent postoperative examinations should be carried out, using clinical signs (history of decreased vision or Amsler grid changes or the appearance of subretinal fluid or blood on clinical examination) and fluorescein angiography to detect recurrences at the earliest possible time.

COMMENTS

Patients with macular degeneration who have lost central vision in both eyes should be informed of the visual rehabilitation resources available to them. Low-vision optical aids and other devices along with a multitude of special services are available and can improve significantly the quality of life of many of these patients.

References

Bressler NM, Bressler SB, Fine SL: Age-related macular degeneration. Surv Ophthalmol 32:375–413, 1988.

Gass JDM: Stereoscopic Atlas of Macular Diseases—Diagnosis and Treatment. St. Louis, CV Mosby, 1987, pp 60–97.

Macular Photocoagulation Study Group: Argon laser photocoagulation for senile macular degeneration. Results of a randomized clinical trial. Arch Ophthalmol 100:912–918, 1982.

CYSTOID MACULAR EDEMA
(CME, Cystoid Maculopathy, Irvine-Gass Syndrome)

WAYNE E. FUNG, M.D.
San Francisco, California

Cystoid macular edema (CME) has become a term that is used everyday by clinical ophthalmologists. Yet, the condition was not discovered until 1966, when Gass and Norton studied the so-called Irvine syndrome with intravenous fluorescein. This test clearly demonstrated that the cause of decreased central vision in these aphakic eyes was fluid accumulation in intraretinal spaces within the macular region. Since then, this same alteration of macular anatomy has been recognized in many seemingly diverse clinical situations. Cystoid macular edema is advanced as the reason for decreased central vision in all cases in which it can be proven, and yet our understanding of the pathologic process underlying its production is still very incomplete.

By far, the most common condition associated with cystoid macular edema is cataract surgery. Various investigators have determined the incidence following intracapsular cataract extractions to be between 40 and 60 per cent, whereas the incidence after planned extracapsular procedures of one type or another is around 10 per cent. The role played by the presence or absence of an intraocular lens and the style of intraocular lens, combined with an intra- or extracapsular procedure, has also been the subject of investigation. It has now been well established that lenses suspended in the pupil have the worst prognosis. The next worse are anterior chamber lenses, and the lens style with the lowest incidence of CME is the posterior chamber lens implanted "in the bag." Fortunately, in the great majority of these cases, the condition resolves spontaneously within 3 to 6 months. However, if the anterior hyaloid face is disrupted or formed vitreous is incarcerated into some portion of the corneoscleral wound, the condition may become chronic.

Diabetic retinopathy is the second most common condition associated with this change. It is largely seen in adults who became diabetics after the age of 30 years and who have had the condition for more than 10 years. Concomitant hypertension or arteriosclerosis makes the presence of this condition more likely. Other conditions known to be complicated by cystoid macular edema include exudative senile maculopathy with serous detachments of the macula, vasculopathies (tributary or central vein occlusions), postscleral buckling procedures, chronic uveitis, collagen vascular disease, aphakia with topical antiglaucoma epinephrine compounds, tumors of the choroid (melanomas and capillary hemangiomas), diabetic traction detachments, retinitis pigmentosa, nicotinic acid intoxication, and perifoveal retinal telangectasia.

Based upon information produced within the past decade, the entity of cystoid macular edema may have two possible explanations: inflammation and anoxia. The inflammatory theory, proposed by Miyake, suggests that the trauma of surgery to the anterior segment during a cataract extraction either stimulates the production of prostaglandins or creates a situation that retards their reabsorption within the eye. Whichever the case, prostaglandins presumably diffuse from the anterior segment to the posterior fundus and produce increased permeability of the perifoveal capillaries. In an independent report by Martin et al., rounds cells (lymphocytes and histiocytes) were found around the small vessels in the ciliary body and the perifoveal capillaries in eyes with chronic aphakic cystoid macular edema (Irvine-Gass syndrome). In other words, abnormal uveovitreal relationships in the anterior segment can definitely influence the integrity of the perifoveal capillaries. The inflammatory theory could account for the following situations: aphakic cystoid macular edema, early and late; chronic uveitis, including pars planitis; and postscleral buckling procedures.

The vascular occlusion theory readily explains the conditions seen with obvious retinal vascular disease and detachments of the retina when one considers that the outer third of the retina derives its nourishment from the choriocapillaris. Likewise, retinitis pigmentosa seems to be a disease of the retinal pigment epithelium and the retinal arterioles, and perifoveal telangectasia produces shunts of the retinal circulation around the macula. The exact mechanism of cystoid macular edema with choroidal tumors, however, would seem obtuse were it not for the fact that Fine and Brucker's first case was precisely of this sort. Their electron microscopic examination of the retina in a nondiabetic eye containing a choroidal melanoma in the equatorial region demonstrated capillaries in the posterior pole with lumen reduced to a fine slit, secondary to swollen endothelial cells. This work conclusively showed that the macular cells most altered in these cases were the Müller cells of the central retina and that these alterations were most likely caused by occlusion of the retinal capillaries secondary to endothelial cell hypertrophy or edema. The Müller cells in Henle's layer were initially markedly swollen and later degenerated. Early in the process, the photoreceptor cells remain normal, and cystoid spaces in the retina are absent. As the condition persists, however, disruption of the Müller cells produces cystoid spaces in Henle's layer, and alteration of the microanatomy of the photoreceptors follows thereafter.

Recently, the above-mentioned intracellular theory of the *origin of the (Müller cell) cysts* has been challenged by Gass, Anderson, and Davis. They hold that the cysts arise from expansion of the extracellular spaces of the retina by serous exudates within the inner plexiform and inner nuclear layers. This theory is based on electron microscopic examination of an eye from a 67-year-old woman; this eye contained a malignant melanoma of the choroid, just posterior to the ora along the 6:00 o'clock meridian. The tumor had been treated with a cobalt[60] episcleral plaque (10,000 rads) 3 years before enucleation. Immediately after enucleation, the eye was sectioned horizontally and immersed in cold 5 per cent gluteraldehyde, thus preserving the ultrastructure of the eye as pristine as possible. These authors advance the following facts to support their hypothesis: 1) Their electron microscopic observations; 2) the highly reversible function of an aphakic CME eye, arguing against cellular death and disruption; 3) the visible lack of occluded capillaries in the macula, arguing against the presence of anoxia; 4) the orderly arrangement of the cystic spaces, as seen on fluorescein angiography, arguing for fluid being incarcerated in extracellular spaces; and 5) the absence of visibly turbid fluid in the macula of an aphakic CME eye, arguing against an increased content of lipids and proteins in the cystic spaces. They suggest that the difference in the two observations (intracellular versus extracellular) most likely is the result of slower tissue fixation in the former eyes. Indeed, two of the eyes upon which the intracellular theory is based had been fixed in formalin before being refixed in gluteraldehyde.

THERAPY

Ocular. Since the pathophysiology of this condition is still in its formative stages, the patient must understand that only an approximate risk-benefit ratio can be estimated at this time with any of the modalities.

Prophylactic treatment of cataract patients with antiprostaglandin agents appears to reduce the high incidence of transient cystoid macular edema after an intracapsular procedure. Topical ophthalmic 1 per cent indomethacin* dissolved in sesame oil or water may be administered 1 day preoperatively and three or four times daily for 4 to 6 weeks. A clinical trial of 0.5 per cent topical ophthalmic suprofen† is also in progress.

Favorable responses may also be seen with oral antiprostaglandin agents. Fenoprofen‡ may be administered in doses of 60 mg three times daily, or 400 mg of ibuprofen‡ may be given three or four times daily. Doses may be gradually reduced after 2 weeks until an effective therapeutic level is found. More recently, an encouraging report using ketoralac trimethamine† in chronic cases (6 to 24 months of aphakic and pseudophakic cystoid macular edema) has appeared. The prospective protocol called for 30 patients to apply 0.5 per cent ketoralac or placebo drops four times daily for 60 days in a double-blind randomized study. The drug group demonstrated a significant ($P = 0.005$) improvement in vision.

Corticosteroids have been shown to decrease cystoid macular edema, but it remains unknown if this is related to an anti-inflammatory effect or a rise in intraocular pressure. Topical prednisolone acetate may be administered in a concentration of one drop of 1 per cent four times daily or five drops of 0.12 per cent every 4 hours while awake. Many patients show improvement of visual acuity within 1 to 2 weeks of the initiation of intensive corticosteroid therapy. A therapeutic dose of 20 mg of oral prednisone three or four times daily should be maintained for 1 week, with gradual tapering of 20 mg per week over the next 3 weeks. Subtenon injection of 40 mg/ml of triamcinolone* may also be delivered with a 27-gauge needle under topical anesthesia.

The persistence of the cystic spaces within the retina very likely is caused by extravasation of serous fluid through damaged junctional complexes between endothelial cells of capillaries within the macula. Certainly, one sees the fluorescein accumulating in the intraretinal spaces during angiography, and it would not be difficult to believe that some, if not all, of the fluid leaks from capillaries with damaged junctional complexes.

At least two groups of investigators have reported dramatic improvement of chronic CME after treatment with hyperbaric oxygen. Ogura and colleagues reported two cases of branch vein occlusion that failed to respond to scattered laser treatment over periods ranging from 14 to 27 months, respectively. After 1 hour, twice-daily exposures to 2 atmospheres of oxygen from 4 to 14 days, retinal edema largely subsided and acuity improved from 20/70 to 20/20 and 20/25, respectively. In a randomized controlled series of eight cases of surgically aphakic eyes, all from 7 to 11 months postoperative, Ploff and Thom reported dramatic improvement in all patients receiving 2.2 atmospheres of oxygen for 1.5 hours twice daily for 7 days and then 2 hours daily for 14 days. They theorize that the beneficial effect occurs because hyperbaric oxygen may help heal the injured junctional complexes by causing constriction of the macular capillaries, along with stimulating collagen formation, which seals these spaces.

Surgical. Anterior vitrectomy through either the limbal or pars plana approach in aphakic eyes with vitreous to the wound but *without* the presence of an intraocular lens has been found to be effective in improving the patient's condition in 75 per cent of the cases. All patients had angiographically proved cystoid macular edema for 6 months or longer. The goal of surgery was to restore microsurgically the anterior segment anatomy to normal by removing all abnormal visible vitreous connections. Because significant surgical complications can and have occurred with this procedure, it is recommended that this modality be held in reserve until medical treatment fails. In cases of an uncomplicated extracapsular procedure with an "in-the-bag" posterior chamber lens, pars plana vitrectomy has proven ineffective in a handful of chronic cases. Therefore, there is no evidence that surgery is at all indicated when there is no anterior segment distortion by vitreous or when vitreous traction on the macula is absent.

Precautions

The most common adverse reactions secondary to fenoprofen or ibuprofen that patients experience are related to the gastrointestinal tract (dyspepsia, constipation, nausea, vomiting, anorexia, and flatulence). Additional adverse reactions may include headaches, somnolence, dizziness, tremor, pruritus, tinnitus, and palpitations. To minimize side effects and facilitate absorption into the serum, these drugs should be ingested 30 minutes before each meal.

Oral corticosteroids should not be given to patients with a history of peptic ulcers or osteoporosis. Before subtenon injection of corticosteroids, the patient should first be tested for possible adverse response (elevated intraocular pressure) to steroids by topical applications because the periocular injection route most likely delivers the active ingredient to the eye for 1 month.

Comments

Cystoid macular edema should be considered a *sign* of an underlying ocular disease process and not an entity in and of itself. Current investigation is aimed at testing the various hypothesis outlined earlier. Final conclusions should be forthcoming in the near future.

The role of light toxicity in causing cystoid macular edema has been considered by many clinicians. Light delivered to the retina via intravitreal fiberoptic devices has definitely been shown to be toxic to the retina, but it is unknown what role it plays in postoperative posterior vitrectomy cases with cystoid macular edema. The coaxial light of an operating microscope delivered to the posterior segment of an aphakic eye is responsible for producing a pink scotoma during the first postoperative week. Could light from the operating microscope be a cause of aphakic CME? In a prospective study by Kraff and associates, no evidence could be found to substantiate this suspicion.

References

Bresnick GH: Diabetic macular edema: A review. Ophthalmology 93:989–997, 1986.

Fine BS, Brucker AJ: Macular edema and cystoid macular edema. Am J Ophthalmol 92:466–481, 1981.

Flach AJ, Dolan BJ, Irvine AR: Effectiveness of ketorolac tromethamine 0.5% ophthalmic solution for chronic aphakic and pseudophakic cystoid macular edema. Am J Ophthalmol 104:301–302, 1987.

Fung WE, Vitrectomy-ACME Study Group: Vitrectomy for Chronic Aphakic Cystoid Macular Edema: Results of a national, collaborative, prospective, randomized investigation. Ophthalmology 92:1102–1111, 1985.

Gass JDM, Anderson DR, Davis EB: A clinical, fluorescein angiographic, and electron microscopic correlation of cystoid macular edema. Am J Ophthalmol 100:82–86, 1985.

Kraff MC, et al: Factors affecting pseudophakic CME. Five randomized trials. Am Intraocular Implant Soc J 11:380–385, 1985.

Martin NF, Green WR, Martin LW: Retinal phlebitis in the Irvine-Gass syndrome. Am J Ophthalmol 83:377–386, 1977.

Miyake K: Prevention of cystoid macular edema after lens extraction by topical indomethacin. (I). A preliminary report. Albrecht von Graefes Arch Klin Ophthalmol 203:81–88, 1977.

Ogura Y, et al: Hyperbaric oxygen treatment for chronic cystoid macular edema after branch retinal vein occlusion. Am J Ophthalmol 104:301–302, 1987.

Ploff DS, Thom SR: Preliminary report on the effect of hyperbaric oxygen on cystoid macular edema. J Cataract Refract Surg 13:136–140, 1987.

MACULAR HOLE
MARK A. BRONSTEIN, M.D.
Newport Beach, California

A macular hole is a loss of a circular or slightly oval area of retinal tissue in the macula. Typically, there is a marginal elevation of the retina around the hole that produces a gray halo or cuff, giving it the punched-out appearance of a donut. Focal vitreous changes may be observed anterior to the hole. The hole and its halo rarely reach one disc diameter in size. Yellow clumps on the surface of the pigment epithelial may be seen in the depths of the hole. Frequently, inner and external layers of the retina are absent, resulting in a full-thickness macular hole. If the inner layer is gone but the external layer surface is still intact, a lamellar hole exists. If a fine glial inner wall is present, a macular cyst is diagnosed. Biomicroscopy with a contact lens and fluorescein angiography are helpful in making these distinctions.

The vast majority of macular holes occur spontaneously in otherwise healthy elderly patients who are usually more than 50 years old. They are more common in females. Most macular holes are unilateral, and central visual loss is variable.

Macular holes can also occur secondary to blunt trauma. These macular holes may be round or oval and may also have irregular edges; they may vary in size and occasionally may be larger than a disc diameter. These holes may be seen on early examination or later with the resolution of retinal edema.

A major complication of cystoid macular edema is a spontaneous rupture at the inner wall of the large cystoid space, which leads to the formation of a lamellar hole. A round or oval one-third disc diameter defect in the center of the macula occurs. The old deposits within the hole and the gray halo of marginal retinal elevation, which is typical of the full-thickness macular hole, are not present.

Infrequently, vitreomacular traction is a cause of macular hole formation. An operculum or tractional deformity of the adjacent retina should be present to make this diagnosis. Vitreous contraction on the retinal surface may be sufficient to cause mechanically a full-thickness macular hole. The holes are oval or irregular in shape. They may resemble pseudoholes that involve epiretinal membranes alone. Fluorescein angiography differentiates between the two conditions.

Progressive myopia may also be associated with hole formation. The hole is usually quite small and round and is located in the paramacular region.

THERAPY

Ocular. No medical or surgical treatment is indicated for a macular hole without a serous retinal detachment. However, if the patient is monocular or has decreased bilateral vision, low-vision aids, microscopes for reading vision, and telescopes for distance vision can maximize residual visual function. A comprehensive ocular examination, including central visual field testing, helps in the determination and design of the needed devices.

Surgical. Surgery is indicated for serous retinal detachment caused by a macular hole. These detachments are slowly progressive, dependent in position to the hole, and do not reach the ora serrata. If these characteristics are not met, a diagnosis of peripheral retinal break is more likely.

Internal surgical treatment is the procedure of choice. If no vitreous traction is present as with a total posterior vitreous detachment, a paracentesis of the anterior chamber can be done followed by SF6 or C3F8 injection at the pars plana 4 mm behind the limbus. An alternative method is drainage of subretinal fluid externally and injection of gas. The patient is then placed in a prone position for 5 to 24 hours. In many cases, this treatment effects a cure. If the retina redetaches, the above procedure can be repeated, followed by photocoagulation or cryopexy of the macular hole when the retina is flat.

If vitreous traction is present, as with an attached or partially attached vitreous, pars plana vitrectomy is indicated. It relieves the traction on the macular hole and provides a fluid space for use of an intraocular gas bubble. The subretinal fluid can be evacuated by internal drainage. Argon laser endophotocoagulation may be used to treat the macular hole.

In severe myopia with a marked staphyloma, the above surgical procedures may fail. A lensectomy and total liquid-silicone oil exchange may be done, followed by argon endophotocoagulation.

Precautions

Retinal detachments caused by macular holes are extremely rare. If a retinal detachment has both a macular hole and a peripheral retinal break, the macular hole need not be closed. A rare exception could be a high myopic eye with a staphyloma.

Cystoid macular edema has a great propensity for spontaneous recovery unless there is a lamellar hole. If ocular inflammatory disease is present, treatment with cycloplegics, antiprostaglandins, and corticosteroids may be indicated. However, no evidence exists that pharmacologic agents can prevent or treat macular holes.

brane, although vision rarely returns to a normal level. The incidence of recurrent epiretinal membranes after vitreous surgery is low.

References

Charles S: Vitreous Microsurgery. Baltimore, Williams & Wilkins, 1981, pp 131–133.
Foos RY: Nonvascular proliferative extraretinal retinopathies. Am J Ophthalmol 86:723–725, 1978.
Francois J, Verbraeken H: Relationship between the drainage of the subretinal fluid in retinal detachment surgery and the appearance of macular pucker. Ophthalmologica 179:111–114, 1979.
Gass JDM: Stereoscopic Atlas of Macular Diseases: Diagnosis and Treatment, 2nd ed. St. Louis, CV Mosby, 1977, pp 344–366.
Kampik A, et al: Epiretinal and vitreous membranes. Comparative study of 56 cases. Arch Ophthalmol 99:1445–1454, 1981.
Machemer R: Die chirurgische Entfernung von epiretinalen Makulamembranen (macular puckers). Klin Monatsbl Augenheilkd 173:36–42, 1978.
Margherio RR, et al: The surgical management of epiretinal membranes. Ophthalmology 88(Suppl): 82, 1981.
Messner KH: Spontaneous separation of preretinal macular fibrosis. Am J Ophthalmol 83:9–11, 1977.
Michels RG: Vitreous surgery for macular pucker. Am J Ophthalmol 92:628–639, 1981.
Michels RG, Gilbert HD: Surgical management of macular pucker after retinal reattachment surgery. Am J Ophthalmol 88:925–929, 1979.
Robertson DM, Buettner H: Pigmented preretinal membranes. Am J Ophthalmol 83:824–829, 1977.
Shea M: The surgical management of macular pucker in rhegmatogenous retinal detachment. Ophthalmology 87:70–74, 1980.
Wise GN: Clinical features of idiopathic preretinal macular fibrosis. Am J Ophthalmol 79:349–357, 1975.

SOLAR RETINOPATHY
(Eclipse Burn, Foveomacular Retinitis, Photoretinitis, Solar Burn, Solar Retinitis, Sun Blindness)

ROGER A. EWALD, M.D.
Urbana, Illinois

Solar retinopathy is a pigmentary disturbance of the macula secondary to sun gazing. It is characterized by central and parafoveal depigmentation with perifoveal hyperpigmentation. The effects vary from a prolonged persistence of the negative afterimage of the sun or the appearance of scotoma to the permanent loss of central vision with objective signs of a retinal burn. In most cases of solar retinopathy, nothing abnormal is noticed immediately, except the dazzling sensation. However, shortly thereafter, a diffuse cloud floats with irregular undulations before the eyes and is usually associated with an irritating afterimage, photophobia, and occasionally photopsia and chromatopsia. Metamorphopsia, which is initially caused by displacement of the retinal elements with edema and eventually degenerative changes, may also appear in the central field. In mild cases, the macula becomes darker than usual, probably as a result of choroidal congestion. In the most severe cases, the central area may be raised and edematous, having a gray appearance and showing a dark central spot surrounded by perifoveal edema. The most striking characteristic of this disease is the development of a yellow foveal exudate. The exudate resolves in 10 to 14 days with the appearance of a reddish, foveal, "hole-like" lesion surrounded by a pale gray cuff of fine granular pigment within a larger ring of coarse pigment aggregation. Repeated sun gazing results in a mottled honeycomb pigmentary change in the macula with a dispersed light reflection.

Many investigators now believe that solar retinopathy is caused primarily by the photochemical effects of the short wavelengths in the visible spectrum of the sun, with some thermal enhancement from the longer wavelengths in the visible and near infrared. This would help explain those cases that cannot be accounted for solely on the basis of an acute thermal burn. The susceptibility of the retina to photic injury probably varies greatly among individuals.

THERAPY

Supportive. Aggressive public education about the danger of sun gazing may decrease the incidence of solar retinopathy. Emphasis should be placed on the risk inherent in gazing at the sun or other sources of bright light, particularly at the time of an eclipse. The safest advice for the public, and especially schoolchildren, is that under no circumstances should the sun be looked at directly using any type of filter whatsoever. Observing a solar eclipse through polarizing sunglasses or with photographic or x-ray film induces a false sense of security, prolongs exposure time, and results in retinal damage. Solar phenomena may be safely examined in an *indirect* manner, using a pinhole projection method with the observer's back to the sun.

Since extraction of the lens exposes the retina to near ultraviolet and short wavelength visible radiation, ophthalmic surgeons should be aware that the aphakic and pseudophakic eye is more susceptible to retinal damage from intense light sources than the phakic eye. This potential for retinal injury is clinically manifested by the complaint of erythropsia ("red vision") among aphakic and pseudophakic patients exposed to bright sunlight reflected from freshly fallen snow. Possible retinal damage can be prevented by lenses (spectacle, contact, or intraocular) with filters that absorb wavelengths shorter than 450 to 500 nm. The sensitivity of the retina to short wavelengths of light may also have clinical significance for some retinal disorders, such as senile macular degeneration and retinitis pigmentosa.

Solar retinopathy has resulted from minimal exposure, and initially, the patient may be totally unaware of the damage. Aphakic and pseudophakic patients, as well as the general public, should be encouraged to wear photoprotective lenses when engaged in such recreational activities as boating, sunbathing on bright sandy beaches, skiing, or hiking at high altitudes.

Systemic. The most useful measure after a sun gazing episode is the administration of systemic corticosteroids within 72 hours of exposure. A daily oral dosage of 60 mg of prednisone should be given and tapered over a 5-week period. A trial of systemic corticosteroids may decrease the retinal inflammatory reaction and improve the final visual result.

Ocular. In the acute stage, 20 mg of methylprednisolone* or 3 mg betamethasone* may be given by retrobulbar injection to minimize the chorioretinal reaction.

Ocular or Periocular Manifestations

Choroid: Congestion.
Retina: Absent foveal reflex; depigmentation and hyperpigmentation; foveal exudates and cyst; hyperemia; macular edema.
Other: Central scotoma; chromatopsia; frontal and temporal headaches; metamorphopsia; ocular and orbital pain; photophobia; photopsia; visual loss.

PRECAUTIONS

Cases of solar burns have occurred as a result of misconceived therapeutic measures to strengthen the eyes, as part of religious rituals, and while under the influence of psychotropic or hallucinogenic drugs. The deliberate observation of the sun with the intention of producing blindness as a means of self-mutilation has also been noted in individuals with a background of mental illness. Numerous cases of premeditated self-inflicted solar burns for secondary gain (limited duty, noncombat status, medical discharge) have been documented in military personnel. Solar retinitis associated with drug abuse should be considered in young patients who present with blurred vision, metamorphopsia, and central scotomas.

COMMENTS

In solar retinopathy, the visual prognosis is good if the central scotoma subsides or is markedly reduced during the first 4 weeks. Patients who have a final visual recovery of 20/30 or better usually do so within 6 weeks of onset. Nevertheless, some patients show gradual visual improvement for periods of as long as 1 year. Approximately 75 per cent of patients with eclipse burns or minimal solar exposure have a final visual acuity of 20/30 or better, but many have metamorphopsia or permanent central or paracentral scotoma or both. Cases of self-inflicted solar retinopathy with a background of mental illness, drug abuse, or malingering usually have more severe retinal damage, with only 35 to 50 per cent attaining a final vision of 20/30 or better.

References

Ewald RA: Sun gazing associated with the use of LSD. Ann Ophthalmol 3:15–17, 1971.
Ewald RA, Ritchey CL: Sun gazing as the cause of foveomacular retinitis. Am J Ophthalmol 70:491–497, 1970.
Gladstone GJ, Tasman W: Solar retinitis after minimal exposure. Arch Ophthalmol 96:1368–1369, 1978.
Mainster MA: Spectral transmittance of intraocular lenses and retinal damage from intense light sources. Am J Ophthalmol 85:167–170, 1978.
Penner R, McNair JN: Eclipse blindness. Report of an epidemic in the military population of Hawaii. Am J Ophthalmol 61:1452–1457, 1966.
Sadun AC, Sadun AA, Sadun LA: Solar retinopathy. A biophysical analysis. Arch Ophthalmol 102:1510–1512, 1984.
Young RW: Solar radiation and age-related macular degeneration. Surv Ophthalmol 32:252–269, 1988.
Zigman S: Photohazards of intraocular lens implants in aphakia. Am J Ophthalmol 90:114–115, 1980.

SECTION 30

OPTIC NERVE

DRUG-INDUCED OPTIC ATROPHY

ROBERTO GUERRA, M.D.,
Modena, Italy

and LUISELLA CASU, M.D.
Sassari, Italy

An increasing number of drugs are considered potential causes of optic neuropathy. Those known agents that may cause optic atrophy include amiodarone, barbiturates, chloramphenicol, chloroquine, cisplatin, corticosteroids, digoxin, disulfiram, ergotamine, ethambutol, halogenated 8-hydroxyquinolines, hexachlorophene, hexamethonium, iodide compounds, isoniazid, lithium carbonate, monoamine oxidase inhibitors, nitrosoureas, oral contraceptives, penicillamine, perhexiline, phenothiazines, streptomycin, tryparsamide, and vincristine. Renal or hepatic failure, diabetes, arteriosclerosis, and alcoholism may enhance the neuropathic effect of these drugs. Optic atrophy is often associated with deficiencies of vitamin B_{12}, aminoacids, and zinc.

The higher incidence of optic neuropathies is caused by antitubercular agents. Ethambutol-induced optic neuropathy is rare with daily doses not exceeding 25 mg/kg. Spontaneous resolution usually occurs within 3 months of its withdrawal, though this is not always the case, and the loss of central vision may be permanent.

THERAPY

Ocular. The suspected drug should be discontinued at the first sign of optic nerve dysfunction. If a chelating zinc agent, ethambutol, isoniazid, penicillamine, or quinolines are suspected, 100 to 250 mg of oral zinc sulfate[‡] three times daily may be given. Zinc does not appear to be of value if optic atrophy is far advanced. When the vision does not improve within 10 to 15 weeks after ethambutol discontinuation, the only seemingly successful treatment reported is the parenteral administration of 40 mg of hydroxocobalamin.[§] Though this dose is eight times larger than the highest amount commercially available in single vials, it should be given for 10 to 28 weeks. Most patients treated this way usually recover full vision. Low serum levels of vitamin B_{12} and zinc have been found in patients with tobacco-alcohol amblyopia and 20 mg of daily intramuscular hydroxocobalamin[§] for 4 weeks may be more effective than the usual 1-mg dose. Optic neuropathy induced by a ketogenic diet can be reversed by oral thiamine,[‡] 50 mg daily for 6 to 12 weeks.

Ocular or Periocular Manifestations

Optic Nerve: Atrophy; pallor; papilledema.
Other: Blindness; central scotoma; constriction of visual fields; dyschromatopsia; hemianopsia.

PRECAUTIONS

The protracted administration of large doses of parenteral hydroxocobalamin did not cause adverse reactions in one series of 22 cases of ethambutol optic neuropathy. Zinc therapy appears to be theoretically sound because inherited or acquired zinc deficiency causes visual impairment and optic atrophy. Although its ability to restore some visual function has not been ascertained, oral zinc administration appears to be of value in correcting many general manifestations of zinc deficiencies. Because oral supplementary zinc sulfate may cause gastrointestinal irritation, zinc gluconate may be preferred. The amount of zinc administered depends on individual tolerance. Commercial preparations of oral zinc are not available in many countries.

COMMENTS

Zinc is required for many ocular metalloenzymes, and it is well established that zinc is essential in many components of the eye. Zinc serum levels should be checked in all optic neuropathies because a close correlation exists with the clinical course of the disease. Unfortunately, oral supplementary zinc did not prove effective in restoring vision, except in tobacco-alcohol amblyopia. More clinical work is needed to establish whether different zinc compounds, doses, and routes of administration will prove more effective. Hydroxocobalamin effectiveness is based on a still small number of observations and should be confirmed by more extensive studies. Hydroxocobalamin may act by neutralizing the chelating action of ethambutol on zinc contained within the optic nerve. A prospective approach could be offered by gangliosides and glycosphingolipids, which have been reported to play a role in activating neuronal membrane enzymes. The number of toxic optic neuropathies treated with gangliosides is too small to evaluate.

References

Bechetoille A, et al: Therapeutic effects of zinc sulfate on central scotoma due to optic neuropathy in men exhibiting excessive smoking and drinking habits. J Fr Ophthalmol 6:237–242, 1983. (Cited in Surv Ophthalmol 28:420, 1984).

Derka H: Besteht Korrelation zwischen der Höhe der Myambutoldosis und der Häufigkeit der Neuritis Nervi optici? Ophthalmologica 171:123–131, 1975.

Doherty P, et al: Ganglioside GM1 does not initiate but enhances neurite regeneration of nerve growth factor dependent sensory neurons. J Neurochem 44:1259–1265, 1985.

Guerra R, Casu L: Hydroxycobalamin for ethambutol-induced optic neuropathy. Lancet 2:1176, 1981.

Karcioglu ZA: Zinc in the eye. Surv Ophthalmol 27:114–122, 1982.

ISCHEMIC OPTIC NEUROPATHY

SOHAN SINGH HAYREH, M.D., Ph.D., D.Sc., F.R.C.S.

Iowa City, Iowa

Ischemic optic neuropathy (ION) is a severe blinding disease, with sudden onset of blindness at first in one eye and then, after a variable interval, often in the other. The erroneous impression that it is a rare disease is based on frequent misdiagnosis and lack of adequate knowledge on the subject.

The disorder comprises two distinct entities: anterior (AION) and posterior (PION) ischemic optic neuropathy. The former is an occlusive disorder of the posterior ciliary artery circulation supplying the optic nerve head and retrolaminar region of the optic nerve, whereas the latter is caused by occlusion of one of more nutrient arteries to the rest of the optic nerve. The most common causes of arterial occlusion are atherosclerosis and arteriosclerosis, which explain the frequent occurrence in elderly individuals. However, particularly for posterior ciliary artery occlusion, the most important cause is temporal (giant cell or cranial) arteritis, which usually affects individuals in their sixties or older. Diabetes mellitus is the next most common and important cause and may involve not only the elderly and middle-aged but even juvenile diabetics. Other less frequent causes are collagen vascular diseases, arterial hypertension, massive systemic hemorrhages, and other systemic or local microvascular disorders. Thus, AION can be classified into 1) arteritic (due to giant cell arteritis) and 2) nonarteritic (due to other causes) types.

Usually, the onset of ischemic optic neuropathy is characterized by a sudden, painless, unilateral visual loss, mostly sectoral, although it is frequently total in temporal arteritis. Occasionally, it may be initially progressive for a few days. Visual acuity may vary from no perception of light to perfectly normal central vision. The *most important finding is the visual field defect,* and the most common field defects in AION are inferior altitudinal, inferior nasal, and central scotoma. Other types may include segmental, superior altitudinal, nerve fiber, or vertical defects and peripheral constriction. In AION, the optic disc shows on ophthalmoscopy a pink or pale-pink edema with frequent flame-shaped hemorrhages at the disc margin or adjacent retina. In half of the eyes with arteritic AION, the disc shows chalky-white swelling with only a rare hemorrhage. In diabetics, the disc may be covered with a network of prominent fine vessels, mimicking neovascularization and thus leading to the erroneous diagnosis of proliferative diabetic retinopathy. The optic disc edema usually starts to subside in a couple of weeks, completely disappears in a couple of months, and results in permanent atrophy of the involved part of the optic disc. In PION, the optic disc and fundus are normal initially, but after a month or two, disc pallor develops.

The estimated 25th-percentile time to development of bilateral AION was much shorter in patients with arteritic AION (0.4 month) than in those with nonarteritic AION (32.4 months). In the author's series of cases of arteritic AION, unilateral as well as bilateral AION had almost invariably developed before systemic steroid therapy was started and not after, indicating that this therapy is effective in preventing the development of AION in giant cell arteritis. Young diabetic males had the highest risk of developing bilateral AION. Thus, for all practical purposes, *AION is potentially a bilateral visually crippling disease.*

THERAPY

Supportive. Since ischemic optic neuropathy is a blinding disease with poor prognosis for recovery of vision and with a high risk of the second eye being involved soon after the first, particularly in temporal arteritis, it is worthwhile to consider the possible preventive measures that could be taken to lower the incidence of blindness caused by this disorder. The most important prophylactic measure is *early and correct diagnosis* of this condition. If a patient has ischemic optic neuropathy in one eye, therapy should be started immediately even if the diagnosis of temporal arteritis is not conclusive. In nonarteritic individuals, particularly those with a past history of AION in one eye, sudden falls in systemic arterial blood pressure or an increase in intraocular pressure (after cataract extraction) should be prevented. In addition, systemic circulatory hemodynamics should be improved and any hematologic abnormality corrected if possible. All patients with unilateral ischemic optic neuropathy should be warned to contact their physician immediately if there is any visual disturbance in the fellow eye. This measure will promote early diagnosis and institution of adequate and appropriate therapy.

Systemic. Ischemic optic neuropathy caused by temporal arteritis is an ocular emergency. If in doubt, AION in persons over the age of 60 years should be regarded as caused by temporal arteritis, particularly if a patient suddenly develops attacks of transient altitudinal hemianopic amaurosis or sudden complete blindness in an eye, which sometimes may be preceded by attacks of transient amaurosis. The presence of other systemic signs and symptoms of temporal arteritis may help in diagnosis. The treatment is to institute anti-inflammatory therapy *immediately* with systemic corticosteroids in *adequately high doses*, such as 80 to 100 mg (or even more) of prednisone daily. The object of the treatment is to prevent the loss of vision in the second eye. The treatment may rarely produce some visual recovery, but this tends to be insignificant. Dosage and duration of therapy are guided by the erythrocyte sedimentation rate with the goal of titrating a maintenance dose to keep a stable sedimentation rate as low as possible. These patients require prolonged corticosteroid therapy, usually for years, and suddenly reducing or stopping the drug prematurely may produce visual symptoms in the normal eye and an increase in the sedimentation rate.

Patients presenting with AION or PION caused by collagen vascular disease should be treated with high doses of systemic corticosteroids during the initial stages of the disease, before the onset of optic atrophy. The treatment regimen is a starting dose of at least 80 mg of oral prednisone daily, continuing on this dosage for 10 to 14 days, and then slowly tapering to a maintenance dose of not less than 40 mg daily so long as the disc shows edema (which lasts for a maximum of 4 to 8 weeks from its onset). There may be a significant recovery of visual function in some of these patients after instituting very early and adequate corticosteroid therapy.

There is no well-established treatment available for nonarteritic AION with diabetes mellitus; however, in a proportion of cases, there has been an excellent response with a significant visual recovery to treatment with high doses of systemic corticosteroids during the initial stages of the disease when the disc is edematous. Because the corticosteroids aggravate the diabetes, these patients require very stringent inpatient control of their diabetes by a diabetes specialist during corticosteroid therapy. Without such strict control, it may not be safe to give corticosteroid therapy to these patients.

The management of patients with nonarteritic AION due to causes other than vasculitis is highly controversial. Apart from arteriosclerosis and atherosclerosis, there is no evident abnormality. Most physicians do not treat these patients, dismissing them with philosophic advice to accept blindness as an "act of God." However, there are some reports suggesting that systemic corticosteroids in high doses during the initial stages of the disease (with optic disc edema) have a beneficial effect in a significant number of these patients.

PRECAUTIONS

Patients with ischemic optic neuropathy caused by temporal arteritis or collagen vascular disease benefit from corticosteroid treatment because of its anti-inflammatory property. In nonarteritic AION with diabetes mellitus or due to causes other than vasculitis, the rationale of corticosteroid treatment may be questioned seriously. Corticosteroids, in addition to being anti-inflammatory, have many other properties, one of which is to reduce capillary permeability. Administration of large doses of systemic corticosteroids is a standard and well-established treatment of cerebral edema of any etiology. Anoxia in ischemic optic neuropathy most probably leads to increased vascular permeability of the optic nerve head capillaries, contributing partly at least to edema of the optic disc. The edema acts as an important factor in the production of visual loss by impeding further capillary circulation in the optic nerve head. *This finding indicates that optic disc edema precedes visual loss.* The corticosteroids in ischemic optic neuropathy probably reduce edema by lowering capillary permeability and help restore the circulation and function of the still surviving, although nonfunctioning, nerve fibers.

COMMENTS

If systemic corticosteroid therapy is to show beneficial effects in ischemic optic neuropathy caused by collagen vascular diseases, diabetes mellitus, or causes other than vasculitis, the treatment must be instituted at the earliest possible moment while the optic disc still shows a fair amount of edema and recovery is still possible. The chances of visual recovery are much greater if the treatment is started within 2 weeks after the onset of AION than if treatment is started later. Once the disc has become atrophic, no treatment is worthwhile, and it is pointless to use corticosteroids. The degree of recovery depends upon the amount of ischemic damage already inflicted, as well as upon the time lapse between onset of AION and start of treatment. By no means do all cases show improvement, even if treatment is started promptly and vigorously. Since the treatment is given for no more than 4 to 6 weeks at the maximum, none of the serious side effects associated with long-term corticosteroid therapy is seen in most cases, except those with diabetes mellitus.

In addition to corticosteroid therapy, every attempt should be made to reduce the intraocular pressure to as low a level as possible in patients with AION, with a view to improving perfusion pressure in the optic disc vessels. Perfusion pressure is the mean blood pressure minus the intraocular pressure.

References

Beck RW, Servais GE, Hayreh SS: Anterior ischemic optic neuropathy. IX. Cup-to-disc ratio and its role in pathogenesis. Ophthalmology 94:1503–1508, 1987.

Beri M, et al: Anterior ischemic optic neuropathy. VII. Incidence of bilaterality and various influencing factors. Ophthalmology 94:1020–1028, 1987.

Georgiades G, Stangos N, Iliadelis E: The anterior ischemic opticopathy or vascular pseudothilitis. Ophthalmol Chron 13:32–56, 1976.

Hayreh SS: Anterior ischaemic optic neuropathy. III. Treatment, prophylaxis, and differential diagnosis. Br J Ophthalmol 58:981–989, 1974.

Hayreh SS: Anterior Ischemic Optic Neuropathy. New York, Springer-Verlag, 1975.

Hayreh SS: Ischemic optic neuropathy. Int Ophthalmol 1:9–18, 1978.

Hayreh SS: Anterior ischemic optic neuropathy: IV. Occurrence after cataract extraction. Arch Ophthalmol 98:1410–1416, 1980.

Hayreh SS: Anterior ischemic optic neuropathy. Arch Neurol 38:675–678, 1981.

Hayreh SS: Anterior ischemic optic neuropathy: V. Optic disc edema an early sign. Arch Ophthalmol 99:1030–1040, 1981.

Hayreh SS: Posterior ischemic optic neuropathy. Ophthalmologica 182:29–41, 1981.

Hayreh SS: Anterior ischemic optic neuropathy. VII. Clinical features and pathogenesis of post-hemorrhagic amaurosis. Ophthalmology 94:1488–1502, 1987.

Hayreh SS, Podhajsky P: Visual field defects in anterior ischemic optic neuropathy. In Greve EL (ed): Third International Visual Field Symposium. The Hague, Junk, 1979, pp 347–365.

Hayreh SS, Zahoruk RM: Anterior ischemic optic neuropathy: VI. In juvenile diabetics. Ophthalmologica 182:13–28, 1981.

OPTIC NEURITIS
(Papillitis, Retrobulbar Neuritis)

THOMAS C. SPOOR, M.D., M.S., F.A.C.S.,
GEOFFREY M. KWITKO, M.D.,
and JOHN M. RAMOCKI, M.D.

Detroit, Michigan

Optic neuritis is an inflammatory process affecting the optic nerve that may be secondary to viral, demyelinating, or autoimmune disease. The typical clinical picture occurs between 15 and 45 years of age and includes acute monocular loss of vision associated with retrobulbar pain, tenderness, and pain on ocular movement. These symptoms may be less severe when seen with acute retrobulbar neuritis. Examination reveals a relative afferent pupillary defect, dyschromatopsia, and a visual field defect, usually in the form of a central or cecocentral scotoma. The optic nerve head typically is swollen with edema of the surrounding nerve fiber layer. Retrobulbar neuritis, in contrast, has a normal-appearing disc during the acute episode.

Papillitis following viral respiratory infection tends to resolve and has a benign visual and neurologic prognosis without treatment. Optic neuropathies secondary to intrinsic demyelination (multiple sclerosis) result in recovery of good vision, with 75 to 90 per cent of patients achieving a visual acuity of 20/30 after 6 months. Visual recovery usually starts after 7 days, and full recovery may take weeks to months. However, studies have shown that 50 to 80 per cent of patients experience some degree of optic atrophy, and all patients reportedly develop a detectable nerve fiber layer defect after an episode of acute optic neuritis. Those patients with optic neuritis secondary to autoimmune disease, although clinically demonstrating a similar clinical picture to those described above, tend to be more likely to suffer irreversible visual loss.

The initial diagnostic workup should include complete blood count, erythrocyte sedimentation rate, antinuclear antibody test, complement (C_3, C_4), serologic test for syphilis (FTA-ABS, VDRL), chest x-ray, and formal visual fields to detect specifically treatable entities. Patients failing to improve after 10 to 14 days should undergo high-resolution CT scan of the brain and orbits or magnetic resonance imaging, neurologic consultation with lumbar puncture, and medical consultation.

THERAPY

Systemic. The use of systemic corticosteroids in the treatment of optic neuritis remains controversial. Controlled studies have failed to demonstrate any difference in the long-term outcome of patients with optic neuritis treated with pharmacologic doses of systemic corticosteroids. However, corticosteroids have been shown to shorten the duration of the acute attack in patients, presumably by decreasing the perineural inflammation, lessening axoplasmic stagnation, and reducing neuronal death.

Recent studies have shown that the clinical response to treatment with high-dose systemic corticosteroids may differ from the untreated natural course or from the clinical course of optic neuritis altered with pharmacologic doses of steroids. Visual acuity and visual fields appear to improve more rapidly (days versus weeks) in patients treated with high-dose corticosteroids. Additionally, progressive visual deterioration has not only been shown to be arrested but even reversed in some cases. The present approach to a patient referred with recent-onset "typical" optic neuritis is to obtain the blood studies mentioned earlier and a baseline visual field and to observe the patient for 7 to 14 days. If significant improvement in visual acuity or field has occurred, further observation every 1 to 2 weeks is warranted. If vision deteriorates or fails to improve, a complete neuroradiologic/neurologic evaluation is done and a course of high-dose corticosteroids is offered.

The treatment regimen consists of 500 mg of intravenous methylprednisolone every 6 hours for 5 days. Visual acuities are followed daily and visual fields tested on admission and every other day. After 5 days, corticosteroids are either abruptly discontinued, or a rapidly tapered oral course is administered. After treatment, visual acuities and visual fields are followed weekly for 1 month, monthly for 3 months, and subsequently every 3 months. The true natural course of untreated optic neuritis, as well as the role of pharmacologic and high-dose corticosteroids in altering that course, is presently being studied in a multicentered clinical trial.

Ocular. Periocular,* transeptal,* and retrobulbar* corticosteroids may also be given. Although these modes of steroid therapy may accelerate the recovery period, they offer no significant long-term benefit over untreated controls. Additionally, the potential risks of such treatment—namely, penetration of the globe or optic nerve—make local therapy less desirable than a short course of high-dose corticosteroids.

Ocular or Periocular Manifestations

Optic Nerve: Disc edema; disc hyperemia; late disc pallor; late nerve fiber layer dropout; nerve fiber layer exudates; splinter hemorrhages.

Pupil: Diminished light response; Marcus Gunn pupil.

Retina: Circinate maculopathy; exudates; hemorrhage; nerve fiber layer edema (peripapillary).

Uvea: Inflammatory cells in posterior segment.

Visual Fields: Arcuate defects; central or cecocentral scotomas; peripheral constriction.

Other: Decreased acuity; dyschromatopsia; photophobia; retrobulbar pain that increases with eye movement.

PRECAUTIONS

Since any entity that compresses the optic nerve (i.e., aneurysms, tumors, inflammatory masses) may mimic the clinical picture seen with optic neuritis, it is of paramount importance to rule these conditions out, especially because they too may respond initially to systemic high-dose corticosteroids. Additionally, steroid therapy is not innocuous. Adverse reactions to systemic corticosteroids have been reported in 16.9 per cent of consecutively monitored hospitalized patients. Daily systemic corticosteroid treatment may be complicated by multiple, potentially serious side effects, including cataract formation, superinfection, electrolyte imbalance, leukocytosis, gastrointestinal bleeding, acute psychosis, aseptic necrosis of bone, hypertension, and hyperglycemia. These side effects may produce considerable morbidity and even mortality. To minimize treatment complications, it is suggested that a thorough examination be conducted before treatment is begun, including a CT scan to detect a subtle sinusitis or mass lesion, a cerebrospinal fluid examination to detect subclinical infection, a neurologic evaluation to document mental status and detect subtle neurologic deficits, and a general medical evaluation to detect electrolyte abnormalities, renal dysfunction, or diabetes. Additionally, visual function, mental status, and levels of serum glucose, blood urea-nitrogen, creatinine, and electrolytes are determined daily once therapy is started.

COMMENTS

Although studies suggest that patients with optic neuritis treated with high-dose systemic corticosteroids tend to improve very rapidly, a randomized treatment trial is necessary to determine whether visual outcome is better than with pharmacologic doses of oral steroids or no treatment. However, since it has been shown that 50 to 80 per cent of patients have some degree of optic atrophy after an acute attack of optic neuritis and therefore have some degree of visual deficit, it seems reasonable that reducing the amount of time that the optic nerve is exposed to compressive inflammatory forces should decrease damage to intraneuronal structures. High-dose systemic corticosteroids seem to accomplish this purpose; however, the results of the optic neuritis treatment trial are awaited before altering the present treatment regimen.

References

Barnes MP, et al: Intravenous methylprednisolone infusion in multiple sclerosis. Neurology *30*:702–708, 1980.

Beck RW: The optic neuritis treatment trial. Arch Ophthalmol *106*:1051–1053, 1988.

Bird AC: Is there a place for corticosteroids in the treatment of optic neuritis? *In* Brockhurst RJ, et al (eds): Controversy in Ophthalmology. Philadelphia, WB Saunders, 1977, pp 822–829.

The Boston Collaborative Drug Surveillance Program: Acute adverse reactions to prednisone in relation to dosage. Clin Pharmacol Ther *13*:694–698, 1972.

Bowden AN, et al: A trial of corticotropin gelatin injection in acute optic neuritis. J Neurol Neurosurg Psychiatr *37*:869–873, 1974.

Bradley WG, Whitty CWM: Acute optic neuritis: Its clinical features and their relation to prognosis for recovery of vision. J Neurol Neurosurg Psychiatr *30*:531–538, 1962.

Cohen MM, Lessell S, Wolf PA: A perspective study of the risk of developing multiple sclerosis in uncomplicated optic neuritis. Neurology *29*:208–213, 1979.

Rawson MD, Liversidge LA: Treatment of retrobulbar neuritis with corticotrophin. Lancet *2*:222, 1969.

Rizzo JF, Lesell S: Risks of developing multiple sclerosis after uncomplicated optic neuritis: A long-term prospective study. Neurology *38*:185–190, 1988.

Spoor TC: Treatment of optic neuritis with megadose corticosteroids. J Clin Neuro-Ophthalmol *6*:137–143, 1986.

Spoor TC, Rockwell DL: Treatment of optic neuritis with intravenous megadose corticosteroids. Ophthalmology *95*:131–134, 1988.

Trotter JL, Garvey WF: Prolonged effects of large-dose methylprednisolone infusion in multiple sclerosis. Neurology *30*:702–708, 1980.

Wakefield D, McCluskey P, Penny R: Intravenous pulse methylprednisolone therapy in severe inflammatory eye disease. Arch Ophthalmol *104*:847–851, 1986.

PAPILLEDEMA
(Choked Disc)

THOMAS J. WALSH, M.D.
New Haven, Connecticut

Papilledema is noninflammatory congestion of the optic discs brought about by increased intracranial pressure. The most common cause of increased intracranial pressure is a space-occupying lesion, either a primary or metastatic tumor. If no mass or obstruction of cerebrospinal fluid is identified, pseudotumor cerebri should be considered. Tumors of the spinal cord and Guillain-Barré disease discharge proteins and other substances into the cerebrospinal fluid to block the absorbing channels of the cerebrospinal fluid and cause increased intracranial pressure. In addition, these substances may also be irritative or toxic and cause an arachnoiditis, which interferes with cerebrospinal fluid absorption, as well as producing an inflammatory reaction around the optic nerves that causes a decrease in vision. Certain disease states, such as nephritis, in combination with or as steroids are discontinued may cause the pseudotumor cerebri syndrome. It is therefore important not only to make the diagnosis of pseudotumor cerebri but also to try and establish the cause of it or similar nonspatial-occupying lesions.

Whatever the cause, increased pressure on the visual systems will sooner or later cause permanent loss of vision. However, vision tends to be preserved for a long period of time in the majority of patients with pseudotumor cerebri. This is not true of all cases and cannot be accurately predicted. The physician must follow these cases very carefully, since there is a fine line between judicious observation and neglect. The reason why vision tends to do better with increased intracranial pressure caused by pseudotumor cerebri than with other forms of prolonged increased intracranial pressure is not known. One theory is that the fluctuation of increased intracranial pressure from abnormal to normal, which is common in pseudotumor cerebri, may give the visual system a rest between significant rises in intracranial pressure. The periods of decrease in pressure do not last long enough, however, to clear the disc of edema.

THERAPY

Supportive. In any disease, it is important to identify the specific cause so that more appropriate and effective therapy can be administered. In the case of a tumor, the treatment is either surgical removal of the tumor, a shunting procedure to reduce the intracranial pressure, or radiation. Pseudotumor is usually treated with well-established methods of supportive therapy, rather than the direct specific treatment. However, this may not always be the proper approach. A careful history may reveal the intake of certain substances, such as tetracycline and vitamin A, which can cause pseudotumor cerebri. Obviously, discontinuance of these substances will result in a cure.

Systemic. The treatment of increased intracranial pressure depends on the specific cause. There are several therapeutic approaches to prolonged increased intracranial pressure with severe consequences to the visual system as is seen in benign intracranial hypertension.

Many patients who have mild symptoms do not require treatment. However, they need to be followed just as closely as those who have severe complaints because of possible visual system deficits. Repeated spinal fluid taps have been advocated, but are not very pleasant for the patient. Since the spinal fluid pressure usually is restored to the previous level in about 2 hours, the rationale for the use of repeated spinal taps in a chronic disease is unclear. There is also the risk of infection with multiple taps. Repeated taps may cause tears in the dura with chronic leaking of spinal fluid and perhaps worsening of the headache.

The use of carbonic anhydrous inhibitors, such as acetazolamide, decreases the production of cerebrospinal fluid, just as it reduces aqueous production in the eye. The usual dosage of acetazolamide[§] that has been shown to be effective in reducing intracranial pressure has been projected at 4 gm daily. Side effects at this dosage level or even lower include gastrointestinal symptoms, disturbances in acid-base balance, and perioral and digital paresthesias. However, in the carbonic anhydrous inhibitor group, methazolamide theoretically may be a better choice, since it is known to cross the blood-brain barrier better than acetazolamide. No studies as yet have been performed to compare the two drugs. Diuretics in classes other than carbonic anhydrous inhibitors do not work as well.

Steroids[‡] are another therapeutic possibility. Steroids in themselves have serious side effects and have been implicated in causing benign intracranial hypertension independently or in conjunction with the nephrotic syndrome. Most physicians treating benign intracranial hypertension recommend steroid use for only a short course of treatment, such as several weeks.

Oral glycerin can also be used in doses of 75 ml two to three times a day to lower intracranial pressure. However, glycerin is not always tolerated well, particularly if there is any nausea; it should be chilled and mixed with some lime juice to make it more palatable. Although it is not the first choice of an oral medication, it is an alternate therapy before moving on to intravenous urea or mannitol.

Surgical. If the disease process does not abate and the medical treatment is not effective in stopping visual loss, then surgical intervention must be considered. There are two approaches in surgical treatment. The first is the lumboperitoneal shunt. This has the advantage of rapidly normalizing the intracranial pressure and reducing the papilledema. Although any competent neurosurgeon can do this surgery, the operation, as with all operations, is not perfect, and increased intracranial pressure may recur. At the other extreme, the shunt may filter excessively and lead to increased headache because of the shifting of intracranial contents and stretching of nerves.

The second surgical approach is an optic nerve decompression. The procedure of optic nerve decompression has been well described elsewhere. The technique has had a good response in reversing visual loss from increased intracranial pressure, although the exact mechanism by which the technique accomplishes this is not well understood. One school of thought contends that an opening up of the nerve sheath may reduce pressure in the nerve and allow for better vascular profusion of the nerve. Another hypothesis is that the dural window in the optic nerve sheath may act as a draining point for cerebrospinal fluid and may therefore help reduce the intracranial pressure. Kaye and his co-workers presented a 51-year-old female with a 14-month history of papilledema and pseudotumor cerebri to refute this latter hypothesis. Because of worsening symptoms, increasing papilledema, and increasing transient obscurations, bilateral optic nerve sheath decompression was performed. Intracranial pressure was measured continuously postoperatively, and no significant lowering of intracranial pressure was recorded. However, the papilledema and symptoms decreased, and the patient was normal 2 months postoperatively. Therefore, optic nerve sheath decompression preserves optic nerve function but apparently does not treat the underlying cause of increased intracranial pressure by draining subarachnoid fluid.

Ocular or Periocular Manifestations

Optic Nerve: Blurring of disc margins (initially nasal border); hemorrhages and exudates; obscuration and displacement of vessels; subtle vertical striae on temporal side.
Retina: Absence of spontaneous venous pulse; edema; hemorrhages and exudates.
Other: Enlarged blind spot; increased intracranial pressure; permanent visual loss; visual field loss (usually the inferior nasal quadrant initially with concentric contraction later).

PRECAUTIONS

Surgical therapy for any disease always has its hazards. However, to be timid and wait until the need for surgery is obvious may still produce a visual disaster. The optimal moment to abandon medical therapy and do a surgical procedure is impossible to outline accurately. Close and careful evaluation of vision and fields is all one can do in order to time surgical intervention properly.

The criteria for surgical intervention laid down by Dandy are still valid today. They are decreasing visual acuity, progressive concentric contraction of the field, increasing transient obscurations, and gliosis of the disc. Any or all of these are signs of a nerve that is beginning to decompensate and should be viewed as an ominous prognostication for vision. Whether one chooses optic nerve decompression or a shunting procedure depends on the surgical expertise available. It is just as important to follow the fields once therapy or some definitive surgical procedure has been performed. The size of the blind spot should be measured both vertically and horizontally. The relative scotoma around and enlarging the blind spot may improve before there is visible evidence of improvement, and this is confirmed by progressive shrinking of the measurement. It is understood that these improvements should be significant and not just 3 to 5 degrees, which could easily be a variation caused by the patient's varying level of alertness and general response with repeated testing.

COMMENTS

To suggest to the physician that the first decision in observing a disc is to decide if there is true edema may appear presumptuous. However, this decision is not always that easy. Even if there is drusen of the optic nerve head, that does not preclude the patient from also having disc edema from any cause, including increased intracranial pressure. Once one decides true disc edema is present a decision as to whether it is papilledema due to increased intracranial pressure or one of the other causes needs to be made so the proper ancillary tests and treatment can be instituted promptly. An improper workup can be worse than no diagnosis at all, with this delay adding to the patient's visual deficit. A physician should constantly hone his or her clinical acumen, so that when the diagnosis of papilledema due to increased intracranial pressure is made, a proper program for patient management can be instituted promptly. The physician must walk that narrow path between reckless aggressiveness and bridled timidity.

References

Buckell M, Walsh L: Effect of glycerol by mouth on raised intracranial pressure in man. Lancet 2:1151–1152, 1964.
Davidson ST: A surgical approach to plesocephalic disc oedema. Trans Ophthalmol Soc UK 89:669–690, 1969.
Galbraith JEK, Sullivan JH: Decompression of the perioptic meningioma for relief of papilledema. Am J Ophthalmol 76:687–692, 1973.
Kaye AH, Galbraith JEK, King J: Intracranial pressure following optic nerve decompression for benign intracranial hypertension. Case report. J Neurosurg 55:453–456, 1981.
Levin BE: The clinical significance of spontaneous pulsations of the retinal vein. Arch Neurol 35:37–40, 1978.
Maren TH: Carbonic anhydrase chemistry, physiology and inhibition. Physiol Rev 47:595–781, 1967.
Maren TH, et al: The pharmacology of methazolamide in relation to the treatment of glaucoma. Invest Ophthalmol 16:730–742, 1977.

Rabinowicz IM, Ben-Sira I, Zauberman H: Preservation of visual function in papilloedema. Observed for 3 to 6 years in cases of benign intracranial hypertension. Br J Ophthalmol 52:236–241, 1968.

Van Dyk HJL: Optic nerve sheath decompression: The ophthalmic surgeon approaches papilledema. *In* Burde RM, et al: Symposium on Neuro-Ophthalmology. St. Louis, CV Mosby, 1976, pp 74–78.

Van Uitert RL, Eisenstadt ML: Venous pulsations not always indicative of normal intracranial pressure. Arch Neurol 35:550, 1978.

Walker AE, Adamkiewicz JS: Pseudotumor cerebri associated with prolonged corticosteroid therapy. Reports of four cases. JAMA 188:779–784, 1964.

SECTION 31

ORBIT

ENOPHTHALMOS

DAVID B. SOLL, M.D.
Philadelphia, Pennsylvania

Enophthalmos is a retrodisplacement of the eyeball into the orbit. It occurs in a variety of conditions when there is a disparity between the volume of the bony orbit and its contents. The most frequent cause is surgical anophthalmos. Other causes of enophthalmos may include congenital anophthalmos or microphthalmos. There is always some type of ocular remnant present in a socket, even when it is classified as congenitally anophthalmic. Phthisis of the globe secondary to trauma or disease is also usually associated with orbital fat atrophy, and the amount of enophthalmos is thus accentuated. Orbital fractures, especially unrepaired or poorly repaired blow-out fractures, are major causes of clinical enophthalmos. Sympathetic paresis, such as occurs in Horner's syndrome, often gives the appearance of enophthalmos; however, this is a pseudoenophthalmos and is secondary to a ptosis of the upper eyelid and slight elevation of the sympathetic paralysis.

Accompanying all forms of enophthalmos are usually a deep, superior eyelid sulcus and ptosis of the upper eyelid; the latter condition is secondary to inadequate support of the globe. In many cases of orbital fracture, diplopia is also present secondary to entrapment of extraocular muscles or tissue contiguous with the extraocular muscles, especially the inferior rectus-inferior oblique complex.

Enophthalmos of a prosthetic eye may be a particular problem after enucleation of the globe and may be accompanied by downward displacement of the prosthesis caused by relaxation of the lower eyelid. Following enucleation of the globe, many physiologic and functional changes occur in the orbit. The anatomic position of the levator muscle complex is changed, and some atrophy of orbital fat occurs after all enucleation procedures.

THERAPY

Surgical. In patients with anophthalmic enophthalmos after enucleation, a modification of the prosthesis should be tried first. If this proves to be ineffective, a secondary implant may be inserted. Likewise, if an implant was not used during the initial enucleation procedure or an intraorbital implant has extruded, the secondary implant is best inserted posterior to all layers of Tenon's capsule, directly within the muscle cone. The surgical procedure consists of making a horizontal conjunctival incision in the center of the posterior wall of the socket. A central vertical incision through Tenon's capsule is then made, exposing the fat of the muscle cone. A 16-mm spherical implant that has been encased in a scleral shell is inserted directly into the fatty tissue of the muscle cone. Because of the problem of AIDS, fascia, either temporalis or fascia lata, has become a popular substitute for sclera. It is also possible to use an uncovered scleral ball implant and insert the sutures directly into the substance of the silicone ball. A 5-0 Vicryl suture is placed at the apex of the implant if it covered through either the sclera or the fascia; if it is uncovered, the sutures are placed directly into the silicone ball. Two additional double-armed Vicryl sutures are placed medially and laterally in positions where the medial and lateral rectus muscles would insert if the implant were a small globe. The preplaced medial and lateral sutures are brought through Tenon's capsule and conjunctiva and tied in the medial and lateral fornices, respectively. The apical double-armed suture is used to imbricate the central portion of Tenon's capsule. Any additional defects in Tenon's capsule are closed with interrupted 5-0 Vicryl sutures. The conjunctiva is then undermined and closed with interrupted 6-0 plain gut sutures. In order to achieve good motility of the implant, it is important to ensure that the fornices are deep. If the fornices are shallow, the conjunctiva should be undermined deeply inferiorly, medially, and laterally. Conjunctival undermining superiorly has to be performed with a great deal of care in order to avoid injury to the levator muscle complex. If the fornices are shallow, the conjunctival undermining should be performed prior to the insertion of the secondary implant.

The use of de-epithelialized dermal graft as a secondary implant also works very well. The implant is obtained from the lateral buttock area. Long-term results are not as yet available concerning the eventual amount of absorption of these implants; however, their use is very valuable, especially in small orbits and in orbits where extrusion has occurred several times. Experience so far with these de-epithelialized dermal fat grafts has been very positive.

Another technique that is very useful for correcting enophthalmos and superior eyelid sulcus defects in the anophthalmic orbit is the subperiosteal insertion of Silastic RTV 382. This material is used if an intraorbital implant is already present. It is injected subperiosteally into the orbit in a semisolid state. The rate of vulcanization depends upon the amount of catalyst mixed with the RTV silicone. Once solid, the material stays in position. The surgical approach is essentially the same of that for a blow-out orbital fracture. The orbital floor periosteum is dissected free of the underlying bone with a periosteal elevator, and a ribbon retractor is used to elevate orbital contents while the Silastic material is injected. It is important that none of this Silastic material extends anterior to the anterior orbital bony rim. The long-term results of using room temperature vulcanizing Silastic material when correcting the enophthalmos in an anophthalmic orbit is very gratifying.

Because superior eyelid sulcus defects are so common in anophthalmic enophthalmic orbits, implants of de-epithelialized dermal fat placed subconjunctivally between the conjunctiva and the levator muscle with the dermal side of the graft adjacent to the subconjunctival surface have proven to be satisfactory in minimizing this defect. After the use of a de-epithelialized dermal fat graft under the upper eyelid, a smaller prosthesis is frequently required and eyelid motion is better. When enophthalmos occurs in an orbit with a seeing eye, it is much more difficult to correct. It is much easier to elevate an eye than it is to bring it forward. If there is an obvious orbital floor fracture with displacement of fragments or herniation of orbital contents into one of the sinuses, the orbital contents can be replaced in the orbit, the defect covered, and the contents supported with Supramid, silicone, or Teflon floor implants. A 0.6-mm Supramid implant tailored to be just slightly larger than the size of the defect has been found to be ideal for supporting orbital contents.

Ocular or Periocular Manifestations

Eyelids: Dropped socket appearance; inability to close eyelids; ptosis; superior eyelid sulcus.

PRECAUTIONS

The problems of epidermal cysts and fat graft absorption have been cited as reasons for the failure of dermis-fat grafts in enophthalmos. Bothersome epidermal cysts are eliminated by removal of the epidermal elements from the dermal fat graft. Fat resorption has been reduced by the use of the composite graft.

COMMENTS

Enophthalmos often develops late after unrepaired fractures and is a frequent complication of enucleation surgery. In the presence of a seeing eye, it is almost impossible to correct fully the enophthalmos as mentioned earlier. For this reason, camouflage procedures are extremely useful. In many cases of enophthalmos, there is an obvious minimal ptosis, which may be corrected by using either levator aponeurosis advancement or a tarsal conjunctival Müller's muscle resection. In addition, it is also frequently not possible to correct fully a superior sulcus defect that is present on the enophthalmic side. For this reason, an upper eyelid blepharoplasty of the normal side with excision of pre-aponeurotic fat in many cases gives better symmetry to the middle third of the face and camouflages the appearance of the enophthalmic side.

References

Bite U, Jackson IT, et al: Orbital volume measurements in enophthalmos using three dimensional CT imaging. Plast Reconstr Surg 75:502, 1985.
Bullock JD: Autogenous dermis-fat "baseball" orbital implant. Ophthal Surg 18:30, 1987.
Iverson RE, Vistnes LM, Siegel RJ: Correction of enophthalmos in the anophthalmic orbit. Plast Reconstr Surg 51:545–554, 1973.
Nunery WR, Hetzler K: Dermal-fat graft as a primary enucleation technique. Ophthalmology 92:1256, 1985 (see also Ophthalmology 93:418, 1986).
Sergott TJ, Visnes LM: Correction of enophthalmos and superior sulcus depression in the anophthalmic orbit: a longterm follow-up. Plast Reconstr Surg 79:331, 1987.
Shore JW, et al: Management of complications following dermis-fat grafting for anophthalmic socket reconstruction. Ophthalmology 92:1342, 1985.
Smith B, Petrelli R: Dermis-fat graft as a movable implant within the muscle cone. Am J Ophthalmol 85:62–66, 1978.
Smith B, Bosniak SL, Lisman RD: An autogenous kinetic dermis-fat orbital implant: An updated technique. Ophthalmology 89:1067–1071, 1982.
Soll DB: Evolution and current concepts in the surgical treatment of the anophthalmic orbit. Ophthal Plast Reconstr Surg 2:163, 1986.
Soll DB: Insertion of secondary intraorbital implants. Arch Ophthalmol 89:214–216, 1973.
Soll DB: the anophthalmic socket. *In* Soll DB, Asbell RL (eds): Management of Complications in Ophthalmic Plastic Surgery. Birmingham, Aesculapius, 1976, pp 295–344.
Soll DB: The anophthalmic socket. Ophthalmology 89:407–423, 1982.
Whitaker LA: Aesthetic augmentation of the malar midface structures. Plast Reconstr Surg 80:337, 1987.
Wojno T, Tenzel RR: Dermis grafts in socket reconstruction. Ophthal Plast Reconstr Surg 2:7, 1986.

ORBITAL CELLULITIS AND ABSCESS

GREGORY B. KROHEL, M.D.
Albany, New York

Orbital cellulitis and abscess are potentially lethal diseases that occur most frequently in conjunction with sinusitis. They may also follow trauma, other evidence of exogenous infection, or systemic disease. The diagnosis is usually made by the findings of an acute illness, proptosis, external ophthalmoplegia, visual loss, lid swelling with erythema, and frequently fever and an elevated white blood cell count. Progression is usually rapid without proper treatment. Chronic orbital infections present with a less fulminant course and are usually caused by inadequate antimicrobial therapy or by nonpurulent bacterial, fungal, or parasitic infections.

THERAPY

Systemic. Treatment of orbital infections must be instituted rapidly. High doses of intravenous antibiotics are used after cultures are obtained and before the responsible organism has been isolated.

In children, the most common etiologic agent is *Hemophilus influenzae*. Children are generally placed on 100 mg/kg of cefuroxime daily, given in divided doses every 8 hours. The total dosage given every 8 hours should not exceed 1.5 gm. Children who are allergic to cephalosporins or have had an anaphylactic reaction to penicillin can be treated with 100 mg/kg of intravenous chloramphenicol daily which is usually administered every 6 hours. Intravenous antibiotics are continued for 1 week. Oral antibiotics consisting of a daily dose of 40 mg/kg of oral cefaclor in three equally divided doses can be continued for an additional 5 to 7 days, depending on residual signs and symptoms.

The most common organisms found in adult orbital infections are streptococcus, anaerobes, and staphylococcus. Adults can be treated with 2 gm of ceftizoxime given every 8 hours. Nasal and conjunctival cultures are often inaccurate in adult orbital infections, but the antibiotic coverage can be adjusted if a positive blood culture is obtained or if a resistant organism is cultured from an orbital abscess or an adjacent infected sinus. The incidence of serious cross-reactions between cephalosporins and penicillin is very low, so penicillin-allergic patients can generally be treated with ceftizoxime unless they have had a previous anaphylactic-type response to penicillin. Patients with an anaphylactic-type allergy to penicillin can be treated with clindamycin, chloramphenicol, or vancomycin. Treatment with oral antibiotics is usually continued for another 5 to 7 days, and adults are usually treated with cephalexin, dicloxacillin, or amoxicillin/clavulanate potassium combination.

Surgical. Prompt surgical drainage with adequate exploration of the orbit is essential. Concomitant drainage of an infected sinus is imperative. Orbital foreign bodies should be searched for meticulously. Adequate postoperative drainage is maintained for several days.

Supportive. Sedatives and analgesics may be employed as needed. Such antipyretic agents as aspirin and acetaminophen should be avoided if one wishes to follow the fever curve in these patients. Antihistamines and vasoconstrictors may be used several times daily when sinus infection is present.

Ocular or Periocular Manifestations

Conjunctiva: Chemosis; hyperemia; vascular engorgement.
Eyelids: Draining abscess; edema; erythema; fluctuant abscess.
Globe: Decreased resiliency to compression; proptosis.
Optic Nerve: Atrophy; edema; ischemia.
Orbit: Abscess; edema; increased intraorbital pressure; pain on eye movement; tenderness.
Other: Anesthesia of dermatome of the first and second division of the trigeminal nerve; choroidal folds; diplopia; exposure keratitis; external ophthalmoplegia; leukocytosis; osteomyelitis; visual loss.

PRECAUTIONS

Sinus x-rays, CT scanning, and orbital ultrasound should be obtained in all cases of suspected orbital abscess. One suspects abscess formation when a patient with apparent orbital cellulitis fails to respond to high doses of intravenous antibiotics or when a relapse occurs while on therapy.

Because chloramphenicol can produce bone marrow suppression when used for long periods of time, therapy is usually limited to 7 to 10 days. Children treated longer than this period should be checked for the onset of anemia with periodic complete blood counts. The oral use of chloramphenicol is not recommended as there is a higher incidence of idiosyncratic aplastic anemia with this mode of delivery.

COMMENTS

Most patients are treated with intravenous antibiotics for 1 week, followed by 5 to 7 days of oral antibiotics. Pediatric consultation is essential for guidance in the administration of intravenous fluids and electrolytes during the acute phase of the disease. Higher dosages of antibiotics may be necessary if signs of meningitis are present. When sinus disease is evident, otolaryngologic consultation is mandatory, and infectious disease consultation is employed when dealing with an unusual organism or a resistant infection. Improvement in orbital cellulitis is usually seen within 24 to 48 hours of the initiation of therapy. Complete resolution of proptosis and motility disturbances often takes 1 to 2 weeks.

Orbital cellulitis often occurs secondary to direct extension into the orbit from an infected paranasal sinus. The ethmoid sinus is the most commonly involved. Other areas from which direct extension of the inflammatory process into the orbit can occur include the teeth, globe, middle ear, face, lids, or intracranial cavity. Superficial periorbital trauma and intraorbital foreign bodies are other important causative agents. Systemic disease, such as subacute bacterial endocarditis, influenza, scarlet fever, vaccinia, herpes simplex, or herpes zoster, may be associated with acute orbital cellulitis. Posterior extension of an orbital cellulitis may result in cavernous sinus thrombosis, meningitis, extradural abscess, brain abscess, or osteomyelitis of the skull.

References

Eustis HS, Armstrong DC, Buncic JR, et al: Staging of orbital cellulitis in children: Computerized tomography characteristics and treatment guidelines. J Pediatr Ophthalmol Strabismus 23:246–251, 1986.

Hornblass A, Herschorn BJ, Stern K, et al: Orbital abscess. Surv Ophthalmol 29:169–178, 1984.

Krohel GB, et al: Orbital abscess. Arch Ophthalmol 98:274–276, 1980.

Krohel GB, et al: Orbital abscess—Presentation, diagnosis, therapy and sequelae. Ophthalmology 89:492–498, 1982.

Rubin SE, Rubin LG, Zito J, et al: Medical management of orbital subperiosteal abscess in children. J Pediatr Ophthalmol Strabismus 26:21–27, 1989.

Schramm VL, Myers EN, Kennerdell JS: Orbital complications of acute sinusitis: Evaluation, management, and outcome. Otolaryngology 86:221–230, 1978.

ORBITAL GRAVES' DISEASE
(Autoimmune Endocrine Exophthalmos, Dysthyroid Exophthalmos, Ophthalmopathy of Graves' Disease)

J. SCOTT KORTVELESY, M.D.,
JOHN S. KENNERDELL, M.D.,
and HENRY J. L. VAN DYK, M.D.,
(Deceased)

Pittsburgh, Pennsylvania

The severity of the chronic orbital inflammation in Graves' orbitopathy may range from mild eyelid retraction to a devastating process that involves the entire orbit and culminates in gross ocular congestion, massive proptosis, and even blindness. Whether mild or severe, the clinical signs are characteristic; they may occur at any age (ranging from childhood to past the age of 70 years), but most often appear between 30 and 50 years of age. The optic neuropathy, however, is more likely to occur in patients over the age of 50. The female/male ratio is 3:1. The onset is rarely acute; typically, it is chronic and insidious, with foreign body sensation and lid fullness evolving over weeks or even months to lid retraction, exophthalmos, and diplopia. The process invariably becomes quiescent in 6 months to 3 years; however, the changes caused by fibrosis are permanent. Only 1 to 3 per cent of patients develop severe malignant exophthalmos with loss of visual acuity—the consequence of severe corneal exposure or compression of the optic nerve at the orbital apex by the thickened extraocular muscles. Occasionally, additional tests, such as forced ductions, changes in intraocular pressure with eccentric gaze, orbital ultrasound, or orbital CT scanning, are required when the diagnosis is uncertain. In the past, this condition was believed to be a complication of thyrotoxicosis. It is now known that at least 10 per cent of these patients have no abnormality of any endocrine function—past, present, or future. Indeed, some authorities now hold that the orbital process is totally unrelated to the thyroid and is a separate, organ-specific (eye muscle membranes, orbital connective tissue, lacrimal gland) autoimmune disorder. What is important to the clinician is this fact: because orbital Graves' disease is not invariably associated with a thyroid disorder, thyroid function tests cannot always be used to prove the diagnosis, since at least 10 per cent of patients with active orbital disease will have negative results.

Patients with Graves' orbitopathy are managed on an individual basis according to the predominant clinical findings, which may include 1) congestion, 2) myopathy, 3) lid retraction, 4) proptosis, or 5) optic neuropathy. Corneal involvement is secondary to lid retraction or proptosis. Therefore, management is directed at the primary cause.

THERAPY

Systemic. All patients with a clinical diagnosis of Graves' orbitopathy undergo a complete endocrinological evaluation for thyroid disease, which may include tests for T_4, T_3 uptake, T_3, TSH, and radioactive iodine uptake. The T_3 suppression and TRH stimulation tests are helpful when other tests fail to show evidence of thyroid disease.

The systemic treatment of hyperthyroidism is best managed by an internist or endocrinologist. Propylthiouracil and methimazole inhibit the synthesis of thyroid hormones within the gland itself. Radioactive iodine (Iodine[131]) accumulates in the thyroid gland and emits ionizing beta irradiation that destroys functioning thyroid cells. Propranolol[‡] suppresses some of the symptoms of hyperthyroidism, including tachycardia, palpitations, tremors, nervousness, hyperhidrosis, and spasticity.

Treatment of the orbitopathy is the domain of the ophthalmologist. Systemic corticosteroids are the mainstay of treatment for congestive symptoms and signs. Prednisone in doses of 60 to 100 mg may be useful for patients with lid edema, conjunctival chemosis and injection, tearing, and some cases of myopathy, proptosis, or optic neuropathy associated with congestion. Concomitant use of a diuretic, such as hydrochlorothiazide 50 mg a day, may help reduce orbital edema. In general, steroids should demonstrate an effect within 2 weeks if they are going to be useful; otherwise, they should be rapidly tapered and discontinued.

Other immunosuppressive agents (cyclophosphamide,[‡] azathioprine,[‡] and cyclosporine[‡]) as well as plasmapheresis, have also been used with varying success.

Ocular. Patients with Graves' orbitopathy frequently complain of grittiness and burning. Frequent lubrication of the ocular surface with artificial tears during the day and an ointment at night helps alleviate most of these symptoms. Topical vasoconstrictors (e.g., naphazoline) are of limited benefit for conjunctival chemosis and injection. Topical corticosteroids are generally not useful because of the protracted course of the disease. Most patients with Graves' orbitopathy and elevated intraocular pressure do not develop progressive optic nerve cupping. They have a pseudoglaucoma caused by a restrictive myopathy that exerts external pressure on the globe. Therefore, antiglaucoma medications are usually unnecessary. Sympatholytics, such as guanethidine,* moxisylyte,† and bethanidine,† have been administered topically in cases of eyelid retraction. Despite their documented effectiveness, these agents suffer from significant ocular surface toxicity and limited availability in the United States.

In addition to topical therapy, a variety of other approaches can help improve patient comfort. Moisture chambers and swimmers' goggles help reduce corneal exposure but have cosmetic limitations. Sunglasses reduce photophobia and tearing. Taping or patching the eyelids at night affords excellent protection in patients with lagophthalmos.

Retrobulbar corticosteroids* have been used in patients with contraindications for systemic administration; however, their effectiveness is unproven.

Small-angle tropias caused by restrictive myopathy can sometimes be treated with prisms. These are prescribed to give fusion in the primary and reading positions. Patients with large-angle or highly incomitant deviations frequently do not tolerate prism correction.

In selected cases of strabismus, botulinum toxin injections into the extraocular muscles may be of temporary benefit (2 to 3 months) before the advanced fibrotic changes occur.

Supportive. Home humidifiers may be of benefit to patients with lagophthalmos or lid retraction with corneal exposure. Elevation of the head of the bed may help reduce periorbital edema in patients with congestion.

Surgical. About 10 per cent of patients with clinical Graves' disease will need surgery for myopathy, lid retraction, proptosis, or optic neuropathy.

Orbital decompression is most beneficial in patients with lid retraction when their proptosis measures greater than 25 mm or they have compressive optic neuropathy. Coronal CT and MRI scans identify the largest muscles and help direct the ophthalmologist in planning the surgical strategy. When a decompression is performed to reduce proptosis, typically the medial or inferior walls are removed first. This removal may be augmented, if necessary, by lateral wall decompression; in exceptional cases, even the orbital roof can be safely decompressed. One wall results in a decompression of 0 to 4 mm; two wall, decompression of 3 to 6 mm; three wall, decompression of 6 to 10 mm; and four wall, decompression of 10 to 17 mm. In patients undergoing decompression for compressive optic neuropathy with or without proptosis, the medial wall of the orbital apex is the most important area to be decompressed. Surgical approaches to decompression of the orbit include the lateral (modified Kronlein), medial (Lynch), transcranial (Naffziger), antralethmoidal (translid, fornix, or Ogura), or four-wall (Kennerdell-Maroon) procedures. A variety of combinations and modifications of these techniques have also been described.

In patients with proptosis less than 25 mm that is associated with lid retraction but without optic neuropathy, orbital decompression is rarely necessary. Instead, surgery on the eyelid is usually sufficient to alleviate the corneal exposure and to mask disfiguring proptosis. For upper eyelid retraction of up to 2 mm, excision of Müllers muscle is adequate to correct the problem. For larger amounts of upper eyelid retraction, levator surgery becomes necessary. A variety of procedures have been described, including levator stripping, levator marginal myotomy, recession of the levator aponeurosis, or placement of a spacer (e.g., sclera, dura) between the aponeurosis and the upper tarsal border. Lower eyelid retraction is approached in a similar fashion. Disinsertion or extirpation of the lower lid retractors has been used with varying success. The most popular approach, however, is placement of a spacer between the disinserted capsulopalpebral fascia and the lower border of the tarsus. Sclera, cartilage, fascia, or a tarsal transplant from the upper lid have all been used successfully as spacers.

When the restrictive myopathy of Graves' orbitopathy induces a tropia that has been stable by prism measurement for 6 months or more (off of steroids), eye muscle surgery can help restore ocular alignment. The goal is to create fusion in the primary and reading positions. Adjustable suture techniques are preferable in these patients to ensure a favorable postoperative alignment. Recessions are preferred over resections because of muscle restriction and the tendency for scar formation in the orbit of patients with Graves' disease. Overcorrection is preferred because postoperative adjustment is easier when tightening the sutures, i.e., reducing the recession.

The pathologic process of dysthyroid orbitopathy will frequently lead to presenile prolapse of orbital fat in the upper and lower eyelid. This prolapse is caused by a combination of factors, including orbital congestion and inflammation, weakening of the orbital septum, and an increase in the volume of orbital fat. Cosmetic blepharoplasty should be approached with this in mind, concentrating on a more aggressive approach to fat removal while being conservative with skin excision.

When indicated, orbital decompression should be undertaken before strabismus or eyelid surgery because the decompression may alter the ocular alignment and eyelid position. Similarly, eye muscle surgery, especially inferior rectus recession, will affect the position of the eyelids. Accordingly, when eye muscle surgery is indicated, it is usually done before any contemplated eyelid surgery. Cosmetic blepharoplasty is best reserved for last when Graves' patients require more than one ophthalmic surgical procedure.

Counseling. Patients with dysthyroid orbitopathy are often quite distraught. They are beset with symptoms that may be annoying (tearing, foreign body sensation, photophobia), embarrassing (proptosis, lid retraction), or disabling (diplopia, visual loss). Usually, a careful discussion of the disease process, including reassurance that it is self-limiting, often allays many of the patient's fears. An explanation of the various medical and surgical options usually instills hope in even the most anxious patients. Careful follow-up should be emphasized to monitor progress and reinforce counseling.

Irradiation. Radiation therapy has an important role in the management of the Graves' patient. The primary indication is in patients with disabling congestive symptoms, including conjunctival chemosis, prolapse, and injection, as well as rapidly progressive proptosis or optic neuropathy. Rare cases of diplopia caused by acute congestion may also benefit from radiation. Generally, congestive symptoms are first treated with corticosteroids. Radiation is reserved for patients with contraindications to steroid therapy or those who are dependent on them but suffer from side effects. External beam radiation in doses of 20 Gy are delivered to the orbit in ten fractions. Steroid therapy is best continued for 4 to 6 weeks after completion of the radiation, since it usually takes this long for radiotherapy to be effective. Radiation will commonly induce an exacerbation of inflammatory and congestive symptoms lasting 2 to 3 weeks. In fact, it is sometimes necessary to increase the steroid dose temporarily during the radiation treatments. As a rule, patients who do not respond to steroids or are in a fibrotic, noncongestive stage of the disease process will *not* respond to radiation.

Ocular or Periocular Manifestations

Graves' disease is an orbitopathy and, as such, can affect virtually any structure of the orbit, ocular surface, or ocular adnexa. The eyeball itself is generally spared, except as a secondary effect, e.g., corneal exposure.

Conjunctiva: Chemosis; hyperemia; prolapse.

Cornea: Abscess; exposure keratopathy; perforation.

Extraocular Muscles: Infiltration and fibrosis of some or all muscles (most often inferior rectus, medial rectus, superior rectus); mild limitation of gaze to immobility of the globe.

Eyelids: Edema; lag; retraction.

Lacrimal Gland: Enlargement; infiltration; prolapse.

Optic Nerve: Apical optic nerve compression; atrophy; disc edema; disc hemorrhage.

Orbit: Axial proptosis; resistance to retrodisplacement of globe.

Other: Chorioretinal folds; increased intraocular pressure with eccentric gaze; retinal nerve fiber layer dropout; visual field defect; visual loss.

PRECAUTIONS

The first signs of orbital Graves' disease may not develop until active hyperthyroidism has been treated and the patient rendered euthyroid or even hypothyroid. Thus, the ophthalmologist should monitor patients with orbital Graves' disease closely when they are undergoing therapy for hyperthyroidism. The response of the orbital condition to the treatment of hyperthyroidism is unpredictable; the orbital changes may improve, remain stable, or worsen.

Any patient with oribtal Graves' disease who develops ptosis or fluctuating diplopia should be suspected of having coexistent myasthenia gravis.

The side effects and complications of corticosteroid therapy are well known. Chronic steroid therapy should be managed with the assistance of an internist or endocrinologist.

Orbital radiation should be performed by a radiation specialist who is experienced with irradiation of the orbit. The retrobulbar area is treated while the globe itself is shielded. Every patient should be informed of the risk, albeit very slight, of radiation-induced cataract or retinopathy.

Complications of orbital decompression include inadequate effect, loss of vision, motility disturbance, cerebrospinal fluid leaks, lacrimal outflow obstruction, sinus mucocele, sinus hematoma, oral antral fistula, infraorbital anesthesia, and eyelid malpositions.

Complications of surgery for lid retraction include ptosis (usually more prominent nasally), persistent retraction (usually more prominent temporally), contour abnormalities, ocular irritation or lid thickening induced by spacers (e.g., sclera), and damage to the lacrimal gland and its ducts.

Eye muscle surgery for restrictive myopathy has the same risks as standard strabismus surgery. However, exposure is usually more difficult because of the tethering effect of the muscles. Adhesions and scarring are more of a problem because of the orbital inflammation, especially in reoperations.

COMMENTS

CT scanning is of great value in the diagnosis of orbital Graves' disease. It is also virtually mandatory before orbital decompression is undertaken. A CT scan should be obtained with a high-resolution scanner. Thick sections through the orbit are almost useless; slice thickness should be 5 mm or thinner and must include both axial and coronal projections to permit full display of muscle enlargement and optic nerve compression. MRI scans give superb detail of intraorbital structures, but they suffer from poor delineation of the bony orbit. Orbital ultrasonography is also of great value. The best orbital assessment comes from a combination of CT scanning and orbital ultrasound.

References

Burde RM: The orbit. *In* Lessell S, van Dalen JTW (eds): Neuro-ophthalmology, 1982. Amsterdam, Excerpta Medica, 1982, Vol 2, pp 272–279.
Kennerdell JS, Maroon JC, Buerger GF: Comprehensive surgical management of proptosis in dysthyroid orbitopathy. Orbit 6:153–179, 1987.
McCord CD Jr: Current trends in orbital decompression. Ophthalmology 92:21–33, 1985.
Putterman AM: Surgical treatment of thyroid-related upper eyelid retraction. Ophthalmology 88:507–512, 1981.
Rootman J: Graves' Orbitopathy. *In* Rootman J: Diseases of the orbit. Philadelphia, JB Lippincott, 1988, pp 241–280.
Schorr N, Seiff SR: The four stages of surgical rehabilitation of the patient with dysthyroid ophthalmopathy. Ophthalmology 93:476–483, 1986.
Sergott RC, et al: The clinical immunology of Graves' ophthalmopathy. Ophthalmology 88:484–487, 1981.
Van Dyk HJL: Orbital Graves' disease: A modification of the "No Specs" classification. Ophthalmology 88:479–483, 1981.

ORBITAL HEMORRHAGES
KLAUS D. TEICHMANN, M.D., F.R.C.S.(C), F.R.A.C.O.
Kiel, West Germany

Orbital hematoma may develop spontaneously, particularly in patients with local vascular diseases (venous anomalies, advanced atherosclerosis, carotid cavernous fistula, aneurysms of the ophthalmic artery, hemangioma, arteriovenous malformations, lymphangioma), or with associated systemic diseases (scurvy, leukemia, hemophilia and various clotting disorders, anemia, sickle-cell disease, and hypertension). Most frequently, it is caused by trauma, especially orbital fractures. Hemorrhage after retrobulbar injection is also common (estimated 0.5 per cent). Surprisingly, this hemorrhage rarely leads to permanent visual impairment, despite sometimes impressive proptosis and periorbital swelling. More dangerous is hidden bleeding after orbital or lid surgery with opening of the orbital septum, removal of fat, and tight compression bandaging. The incidence of blindness following blepharoplasty is reported to be less than 1 in 1000. Prophylaxis is very important in these cases and consists of preoperative history and physical examination and the necessary laboratory tests.

THERAPY

Systemic. Control of blood pressure is important because hypertension can lead to uncontrollable hemorrhage, and hypotension may further reduce the already compromised circulation of the retina and optic nerve. Bleeding disorders should be treated as required. Intravenous acetazolamide or hyperosmotic solutions are of little use.

Supportive. Analgesics may be used generously for ocular and orbital pain while preparing for surgery; however, aspirin should be avoided.

Surgical. When vision is seriously threatened, surgical intervention is mandatory. As the survival time of vital structures during ischemia is limited (maximum, 100 minutes in complete central retinal artery occlusion), time is precious and orbital decompression should be performed rapidly. Immediate, although often short-lived relief is obtained by canthotomy or cantholysis or both. Modern imaging techniques (ultrasound, CT scan, MRI) are useful in guiding the surgeon as the hematoma may be intraconal, extraconal, or subperiosteal, but they often require too much time. Evacuation of a pocket of blood by needle aspiration or transseptal incision may sometimes gain time for more definitive treatment. Evacuation consists of exploring the orbit through previous or new incisions with drainage of fluid and blood, removal of blood clots, and meticulous cautery of bleeding points. Where necessary, the intraconal space should be entered by insertion of a fine hemostat through the intermuscular septum. The most likely cause of acute bleeding is the ophthalmic artery and its branches, including the anterior and posterior ethmoidal arteries. These can be approached through a semicircular incision medially to the nasal canthus. Removal of ethmoidal cells, including the lamina papyracea, allows access to these arteries for clamping and cautery after wide opening of the periorbita. In diffuse oozing, local application of hemostatics (topical thrombin, absorbable gelatin sponge, microfibrillar collagen) and compression can be used to achieve hemostasis. Bonewax is useful in bone bleeders. The presence of increased orbital tissue may require removal of the orbital floor together with the medial orbital wall. Pupillary response to light, visual acuity and flash visual evoked potential can serve as guides for success.

Ocular or Periocular Manifestations

Conjunctiva: Chemosis; hyperemia; hyposphagma.
Eyelids: Ecchymosis; edema; tight narrow palpebral fissure.
Other: Choroidal folds; cherry red spot; cloudy cornea; cloudy swelling of retina; disc pallor or disc edema; elevation of intraocular pressure; immobility of the globe, motor and sensory abnormalities of the pupil; ocular and periorbital pain; proptosis; pulsating or collapsed retinal arteries; vomiting.

PRECAUTIONS

Special attention should be paid preoperatively to determine the existence of hypertension, cardiovascular disease, glaucoma, or possible drug interactions with drugs, such as heparin, dicumarol, warfarin, and salicylates. If a patient is suspected of having a bleeding disorder, prothrombin time (PT), partial thromboplastin time (PTT), platelet counts, and bleeding time should be performed before surgery. During surgery, meticulous hemostasis by cautery, ligatures, hemostats, and simple compression should be achieved. Orbital fat should never be pulled forward. Prolapsing fat should be clamped, cut, and cauterized. Excessive use of epinephrine with local anesthetics is dangerous; it may provoke a marked rise in blood pressure. It can also cause a deceptively bloodless field during surgery, with diffuse oozing setting in after vasoconstriction has subsided. A rubber drain (Penrose) or a suction drain (Hemovac) is advisable for deep orbital surgery. Tight bandages should be abandoned with ice compresses applied instead. The patient's head should be elevated 45° after lid and orbital surgery. Close postoperative observation is mandatory. The patient should be asked to report the onset of severe or sudden pain. In case of doubt, one should look for proptosis, the pupils should be checked, vision tested, and the fundus examined to rule out vascular occlusion or an otherwise compromised circulation. Intraocular pressure may be measured when possible.

Orbital decompression is not free of complications. Diplopia and enophthalmos are frequent sequelae that may require additional therapy at a later date. Blindness may follow any type of orbital surgery. A conservative approach should therefore be used whenever feasible, particularly in spontaneous orbital hemorrhage and hematomas following retrobulbar injections, both of which tend to have a good prognosis.

Comments

Visual damage is caused by central retinal artery or posterior ciliary artery occlusion or optic nerve compression with disturbance of its blood supply. Optic nerve circulation seems to be more easily compromised than retinal circulation. Therefore, because of the short-lived effect and possible complications, anterior chamber paracentesis or posterior sclerotomy is not recommended. Carotid compression may help stop the bleeding, but at the same time, it reduces the perfusion of important tissues.

Despite the fact that early orbital decompression is mandatory in severe cases, occasionally, even delayed intervention (up to several days) may be beneficial. Other complications of orbital hemorrhage include delayed wound healing, infection, abscess formation, and discoloration. Fibrosis may develop later and cause motility problems, lid retraction, and ectropion.

References

Anderson RL, Edwards JJ: Bilateral visual loss after blepharoplasty. Ann Plast Surg 5:288–292, 1980.

Anderson RK, Linberg JV: Transorbital approach to decompression in Graves' disease. Arch Ophthalmol 99:120–124, 1981.

Callahan MA: Prevention of blindness after blepharoplasty. Ophthalmology 90:1047–1051, 1983.

Hayreh SS, Weingeist TA: Experimental occlusion of the central artery of the retina. I. Ophthalmoscopic and fluorescein fundus angiographic studies. Br J Ophthalmol 64:896–912, 1980.

Kelly PW, May DR: Central retinal artery occlusion following cosmetic blepharoplasty. Br J Ophthalmol 64:918–922, 1980.

Kersten RC, Rice CD: Subperiosteal orbital haematoma visual recovery following delayed drainage. Ophthalmic Surg 18:423–427, 1987.

Kraushar MF, Seelenfreud MH, Freilich DB: Central retinal artery closure during orbital hemorrhage from retrobulbar injection. Trans Am Acad Ophthalmol Otolaryngol 78:65–69, 1974.

Krohel GB, Wright JE: Orbital hemorrhage. Am J Ophthalmol 88:254–258, 1979.

McCartney DL, Char DH: Return of vision following orbital decompression after 36 hours of post-operative blindness. Am J Ophthalmol 100:602–604, 1980.

Waller RR: Is blindness a realistic complication in blepharoplasty procedures? Ophthalmology 85:730–735, 1978.

SECTION 32

REFRACTIVE DISORDERS

ANISOMETROPIA
(Asymmetropia)

MELVIN L. RUBIN, M.D.
Gainesville, Florida

In anisometropia, the refractive errors of the two eyes are unequal. The two eyes may be myopic or hypermetropic in unequal degrees; one eye may be emmetropic and the other eye ametropic, or one eye may be hypermetropic and the other myopic, a condition termed antimetropia. Except for the uncommon instances of uniocular disease or injury, anisometropia is usually genetically determined by factors related to the axial length of the eye. Anisometropia may be of varying degrees; clinically, an anisometropia of greater than 2 diopters is considered to be of high degree. However, differences up to 3 diopters are not uncommon, and disparities up to 34 diopters have been recorded. In anisometropia of significant degree, the vision may be binocular, alternating, or uniocular. Binocular vision is the rule in the lesser degrees of defect; however, since the uncorrected image of one eye is always blurred, attempts at fusion frequently bring on symptoms of accommodative asthenopia. In greater degrees of error, fusion is usually impossible, and vision is either alternating or uniocular. Alternating vision can actually be advantageous if one eye is myopic and the patient is a presbyope. The myopic eye is used for near, the other for distance. This condition is called monovision. In a hyperopic youngster, uniocular vision may cause the more hyperopic eye to become amblyopic or to deviate. These risks must be considered when deciding on an optical correction.

THERAPY

Ocular. In dealing with small degrees of anisometropia, full optical correction of both eyes is desirable. In higher degrees, however, full correction presents problems, owing to the differences in size of the images in each corrected eye and irregularities of peripheral distortion. Whenever the eyes move from the primary position, an artificial heterophoria is created with full spectacle correction in highly anisometropic eyes. Therefore, each patient must be considered a separate case, with attention given to the amount of discomfort and disability the patient is suffering without correction and the amount likely to be experienced with correction.

Full correction is especially desirable for children under the age of 12 years. If binocular vision is weak or muscular imbalance is marked, orthoptic exercises should be undertaken, and proper treatment for a squint should be given. In some young patients, temporary occlusion of the better eye may be indicated.

In adults with small degrees of anisometropia and some degree of binocular vision, an attempt should be made to use full correction spectacles. Adults who use either eye alternately for near or far work may be best left untreated, unless symptoms of eyestrain are definitely present.

Whenever possible, contact lenses should be prescribed in preference to spectacles, since contact lenses usually minimize inequality of images by bringing the lens as close as possible to the principal planes. Thus, the artificial heterophoria caused by dissimilar spectacle lenses is largely eliminated and the aniseikonia is likely to be reduced.

Precautions

With full correction in highly anisometropic eyes, prismatic imbalances may result that interfere with single binocular vision. This is particularly true for vertical imbalances that are induced when the eyes look down to read. The lines of sight pass through points on the lens that are several millimeters below the optical center, and the vertical displacement of the reading matter is greater for one eye than the other. This creates an artificial heterophoria.

Full correction spectacles, even with small degrees of anisometropia, are uncomfortable at first. However, if the spectacles are used constantly, difficulties often disappear in a few weeks' time. Every attempt should be made to see that the spectacles are worn constantly, especially in children.

Comments

Although it is difficult to assess the degree to which ametropia may be axial or refractive, it is a good assumption to consider differences in the corneal powers of the two eyes as measured by a keratometer to be indicative of refractive ametropia. Unilateral aphakia results in refractive ametropia and the formation of unequal images. This can be corrected with either a contact lens or an intraocular implant. Axial ametropia may be measured by ultrasonography.

References

Duke-Elder S (ed): System of Ophthalmology. St. Louis, CV Mosby, 1970, Vol V, pp 505–511.

Katz M: The human eye as an optical system. *In* Duane TD (ed): Clinical Ophthalmology. Hagerstown, MD, Harper & Row, 1982, Vol I, pp 33:1–52.

Milder B, Rubin ML: The Fine Art of Prescribing Glasses without Making a Spectacle of Yourself. Gainesville, Triad Scientific, 1978, pp 179–218.

Rubin ML: Optics for Clinicians, 2nd ed. Gainesville, Triad Scientific, 1974, pp 141–188.

APHAKIA

BENJAMIN F. BOYD, M.D.
Panama, Republic of Panama

Aphakia is the absence of the lens from the eye; the term also embraces those conditions in which the lens is absent from the pupillary area. Usually, the lens has been removed by operation, although it may be lost through a perforating wound or ulcer. The lens may also be absent as a congenital defect, or it may be displaced from the pupil by dislocation. An aphakic eye is strongly hypermetropic. Other things being normal, in the absence of the lens, parallel rays of light are brought to focus about 31 mm behind the cornea, whereas the average anteroposterior diameter of the eye is only between 23 and 24 mm. Astigmatism is usually present and may be a congenital abnormality before the cataract operation is performed; when significant, it is essentially related to the cataract operation itself. Accommodation is abolished in aphakic eyes. The visual field is limited, with marked diminution of peripheral vision in all directions when corrective aphakic spectacles are worn. Peripheral vision becomes almost normal when vision is corrected with contact lenses, when an intraocular lens implant has been inserted within the eye, or when a lamellar refractive keratoplasty operation is performed (keratophakia, epikeratophakia, or hypermetropic keratomileusis).

THERAPY

Ocular. When indicated, bifocal aspheric spectacles may be prescribed for some patients. Since aphakic spectacle corrections usually range from 7 to 15 diopters, special attention must be paid to the type, style, size, fit, and adjustment of the bifocals. The lenses should be made as small as acceptable, fitted as close to the face as possible, and angled in toward the face at approximately 15°. Plastic aphakic spectacles are usually preferred by patients because they are lightweight.

Astigmatism is an always present problem in postoperative aphakia. This condition diminishes rapidly over a 6-week period and then stabilizes somewhat over several months. It is therefore necessary to wait for 6 weeks after surgery before ordering a correction for an aphakic patient.

Unfortunately, only very few opticians have the technology to provide patients with distortion-free aphakic spectacles. Many of the undesirable visual effects and distortions of images from spectacles can be eliminated by wearing contact lenses or by additional surgery (secondary intraocular lens implant to render the patient pseudophakic or one of the refractive keratoplasty procedures that are not intraocular operations).

Daily-wear *contact lenses* are not usually successful in aphakic patients, particularly in older people. They are an impractical means of correcting aphakia because patients have great difficulty seeing the lenses to clean them and insert them in the eye. Many older patients have hand tremor, which increases the difficulty of handling the lenses for daily wear. This has led to the use of extended-wear soft contact lenses by some aphakic patients.

Extended-wear lenses should be removed once a week, resterilized, and treated with enzyme and surfactant cleaner to prevent inflammation and infection. The patient should remain without the lens during a 24-hour period once a week. Also available are disposable contact lenses that the patient leaves in for a week and throws away. These lenses are replaced, rather than cleaned. No sterilization or cleaning solutions are necessary, but the cost is a factor that must be considered by each patient.

Enthusiasm for extended-wear soft contact lenses has markedly diminished because they have been associated with frequent lens loss, deposits, filming, bacterial infections, *Acanthamoeba* keratitis, and fungal infections and because surgical procedures to correct aphakia have become more accepted. Very few, if any, aphakics are now fitted as *new* patients with extended-wear lenses.

In very young aphakic patients, extended-wear contact lenses constitute the treatment of choice to correct aphakia secondary to trauma or following congenital cataract surgery. One of the most successful lenses is the silicone lens of Dow Corning, which has a high oxygen transmission and corrects a fair amount of astigmatism.

Surgical. Recent advances in microsurgical techniques, design, chemical materials, and manufacturing methods now make intraocular lenses more feasible for many aphakic patients. However, the guidelines for the use of these lenses vary considerably from surgeon to surgeon.

Secondary intraocular lens implantation is probably one of the most rewarding operations that one can do in ophthalmology because patients truly appreciate the results. They know what aphakia is, whereas patients who have a primary cataract extraction and lens implantation have not gone through the problems of aphakia and do not truly appreciate the condition of pseudophakia. Secondary lens implantation is indicated for patients over 45 years of age with monocular cataract, healthy cornea and macula, and normal intraocular pressure. Its use for bilateral cataracts is still controversial.

Secondary intraocular lens implantation is also indicated for patients who obviously cannot wear contact lenses, essentially those with severe chronic blepharitis, lid abnormalities, dry eyes, or severe arthritis in the hands, Parkinson's, or hemiplegia, which would prevent them from being able to handle contact lenses. Intraocular lenses are not generally accepted for children.

If the secondary implantation is to be done after an intracapsular extraction, the surgical risk of vitreous loss is somewhat higher than if an extracapsular extraction was previously performed and the posterior capsule is intact. In most cases, an anterior chamber lens has to be used, but recently developed techniques allow the implantation of a posterior chamber lens by suture fixation.

In the preoperative evaluation, it is important to do endothelial cell counts to determine the health of the cornea before operating on a patient who has had previous intraocular surgery. When considering implantation of an anterior chamber lens, one should determine the status of the angle structures through a careful gonioscopy that assesses the type of angle present and whether there are synechiae, blood vessels, etc. In order to plan the surgery, one must also determine if the hyaloid face is intact or not, if there is vitreous in the anterior chamber or in the posterior chamber, if there is a patent iridectomy present, and how much astigmatism is present in which axis.

Surgical correction of aphakia may also be accomplished by any one of three refractive lamellar keratoplasties: keratophakia, keratomileusis, and epikeratophakia. The main indications for these extraocular procedures are 1) intolerance to the conventional methods for the correction of aphakia (eyeglasses and contact lenses), 2) a contraindication or expected high risk of a secondary lens implantation and 3) the need for better vision without the use of glasses or contact lenses.

Keratophakia induces optical correction by altering physically the shape of the cornea without changing its diameter. The correction is accomplished by interposing a homograft lenticle interlamellarly in the cornea, which is carved to increase the corneal power by the amount calculated to be necessary to correct the aphakic hypermetropia. This procedure requires a donor cornea in order to prepare the lenticle.

Keratomileusis for the correction of aphakia utilizes the patient's own cornea, therefore requiring no donor eye. It corrects less of the hypermetropic correction of the aphakic eye than does keratophakia, thereby usually requiring corrective spectacles with moderate dioptric plus power.

Epikeratophakia, another form of refractive corneal surgery for aphakia, is the surgical procedure of choice for monocular aphakia in pediatric patients, especially in the unilateral cataract patient in whom the need is much greater because of the risk of amblyopia. Clinical results with epikeratophakia in children show better predictability and faster rehabilitation of vision than in adults. Should the initial clinical outcome be insufficient, the surgical procedure can be repeated in the pediatric patient. Epikeratophakia has the following advantages: 1) it is a safe operation because it is extraocular and for the most part extracorneal, 2) it does not involve splitting the stroma or the visual axis, 3) it is easily reversible, 4) it does not require expensive instrumentation, and 5) most ophthalmic surgeons who do cataract surgery can perform this procedure.

In epikeratophakia, the "donor lenticule" tissue is reshaped to correct the refractive error of each specific patient, based on the patient's manifest refraction and K-reading. This lenticule has no living keratocytes and no living epithelial cells; it has only Bowman's membrane and the collagen of the stroma and has been cut away from Descemet's side. The tissue is sewn onto the anterior surface of the cornea after the central epithelium has been removed and a small annular keratectomy is made. The keratocytes repopulate the collagen. Eventually, the patient has someone else's Bowman's membrane and collagen on top of his or her cornea, but his or her own epithelium and keratocytes. Visual recovery is slower than with autoplastic keratomileusis, and this procedure requires donor tissue.

Comments

The basis for success in extended wear of contact lenses includes careful patient selection, meticulous fitting, diligent follow-up, and a reliable patient or family member responsible for hygiene, weekly resterilization and enzymatic cleaning, and the use of sterile solutions. Older patients who live alone or in surroundings that are unsanitary may be high risks for infection and inflammation with contact lenses. Most adult new aphakics are being managed with secondary lens implants or a refractive lamellar keratoplasty procedure if a lens implant is contraindicated. Very few new aphakic patients are being managed with contact lenses.

In pediatric aphakic patients, epikeratophakia is the treatment of choice in monocular aphakia. Silicone extended-wear lenses (Dow Corning) are the treatment of choice for bilateral aphakic children.

References

Boyd BF: Refractive surgery with the masters. *In* Boyd BF: Highlights of Ophthalmology: Atlas & Textbook, 30th ed. Panama, Highlights of Ophthalmology, Vol II, 1977.

Boyd BF, Kraff MC: The present approach to secondary lens implantation. Highlights Ophthalmol. 14:1–4, 1986.

Boyd BF, Wilson L: Infections and complications associated with extended-wear contact lenses. Highlights Ophthalmol 15:1–10, 1987.

Boyd BF, et al: Present status of refractive surgery. Highlights Ophthalmol 15:6–11, 1987.

ASTIGMATISM
SOREN S. BARNER, M.D., M.D.O.S.
Copenhagen, Denmark

Astigmatism is an optical condition in which the refractive power of the eye varies along different meridians. The resulting blurring of the image is caused by the presence of toroidal rather than spherical curvatures of the refracting surfaces. The term "astigmatism" is derived from the Greek words meaning "without a point." In *simple* astigmatism, one principal meridian is emmetropic. Both principal meridians are either myopic or hyperopic in *compound* astigmatism. In *mixed* astigmatism, one meridian is myopic, and the other is hyperopic. If the principal meridians are at right angles to each other, the astigmatism is termed *regular* and can be corrected by cylindrical lenses. In the majority of cases, the steepest meridian is vertical or "with the rule," creating *direct* astigmatism. If the horizontal curvature is steeper, the astigmatism is termed *inverse* or "against the rule." Irregular astigmatism is caused by corneal pathology (scars, keratoconus), lenticular disease (cataract), or uneven corneal pressure caused by lid tumors (chalazion). Aspherical curvature of the anterior surface of the cornea is the most common cause of astigmatism, but also curvature variations of the surfaces of the lens, cataract formation, or an improperly implanted intraocular lens may contribute to the total astigmatism. The influence of heredity in regular astigmatism is difficult to assess. Dominant inheritance with incomplete penetrance is generally accepted to be the more important means of transmission. Usually, astigmatic errors are associated with axial refractive errors. Induced meridional changes after surgery may be pronounced, especially after penetrating keratoplasty, complicated cataract extraction, and plastic surgery of the eyelids. Small degrees of direct astigmatism (<0.5 diopters) are physiologic and rarely cause any symptoms. Larger degrees, astigmatism "against the rule," or errors with an oblique axis may account for decreased visual acuity, asthenopia, frontal headaches, and tilting of the head. Estimation of the degree and axis of the toricity is carried out by keratometry, retinoscopy, and refraction.

THERAPY

Ocular. Since the purpose of refraction is to make the patients comfortable rather than to achieve theoretic optical perfection, small astigmatic errors do not require correction if they produce no symptoms. However, insufficient visual acuity or asthenopic complaints caused by astigmatism should be corrected fully by spectacles. The optical correction of astigmatism is usually achieved by a combination of spherical and cylindrical lenses, as an axial error is often present. The corrective cylinder may either be concave or convex, but it is advisable to use minus cylinders as much as possible. An initial estimation of the degree and axis is usually carried out by keratometry. After a careful refraction, the final prescription may be found to differ significantly from the keratometric measurements because of lenticular errors. It is important to assess the binocular comfort during the refraction and to measure the cylindrical error for near before prescribing glasses.

Instead of spectacles, contact lenses may be used to correct astigmatism. Mild to moderate degrees of corneal toricity are best corrected with spherical contact lenses. An ultrathin lens can be used to correct errors of 1.0 diopter or less. A conventional spherical lens may be used to correct less than 2.0 diopters if the radius of curvature of the lens is halfway between that of the steeper and flatter corneal meridian. If the astigmatism is around 3.0 diopters, a large diameter hard spherical lens may provide stability on the toric cornea. High degrees of astigmatic errors are best corrected with toric contact lenses. In order to provide stability and avoid rotation of the cylinder axis, a prism ballast may be incorporated into the lens. Truncation is another method to keep the cylinder axis and the astigmatic axis aligned. A small segment of the circular arc of the lower portion of the lens is cut off, and rotation will be stopped by the lower eyelid. Smaller degrees of meridional errors can be corrected by soft lenses. For high degrees of astigmatism, it is advisable to use hard contact lenses.

Surgical. Surgical procedures to control or eliminate excessive degrees of corneal astigmatism have been introduced, and the term "refractive keratoplasty" is used to define controlled surgical alteration of corneal curvatures or thickness in order to induce a physiologic optical correction of the refractive status. The operations have been advocated in pronounced astigmatic anisometropia and persistent high astigmatic errors postoperatively after keratoplasty, cataract extraction, or other surgical interventions involving corneal incisions. Relaxing incisions are aimed at flattening the steeper meridian in contrast to the wedge-resection technique, which is a steepening procedure. Modified radial incisions of the anterior corneal surface—radial keratotomy—is at present the most widely used surgical method to correct corneal astigmatism. A reduction of 10 diopters of astigmatism may be obtained by these operations. Thermokeratoplasty is a different method employed to correct corneal asymmetry. The induced change in corneal curvature is caused by shrinkage of collagen fibers in contact with a hot thermoprobe. Refractive keratoplasty or keratorefraction is at present considered a rather controversial method of correcting astigmatism. Various surgical keratometers have therefore been devised to prevent postoperative astigmatism by controlled suture adjustment during the operation.

Ocular or Periocular Manifestations

Cornea: Toric or irregular curvature.
Lens: Cataract; toric or irregular curvature.

Other: Amblyopia; asthenopia; decreased visual acuity; strabismus.

PRECAUTIONS

Patients with moderate or high degrees of astigmatism usually have no other ocular symptoms than insufficient visual acuity. More often, small degrees of hypermetropic or mixed astigmatism give rise to eyestrain and headache, owing to the constant accommodative effort needed to obtain a clear retinal image. It is therefore advisable to correct fully the error in order not to induce an accommodative effort. By prescribing toric spectacles, a meridional aniseikonic error and a declination error are introduced, and the patient must be warned of initial distortion of binocular single vision as compared to the accustomed uncorrected vision. As a rule, however, children adapt quickly to the new visual situation. A change in the dioptric power of the cylinder usually produces less transient symptoms than a change in the axis. If there are no ocular or visual complaints, it is unwise to change either the power of the axis or the cylinder on a routine examination, even if an improvement in visual acuity is found with a different lens. Presbyopes who do not wear spectacles for distance usually need no cylindrical correction for near. As in anisometropia of other etiology, unilateral astigmatism may be responsible for strabismus and amblyopia in childhood. In pathologic degrees of monocular corneal toricity, refractive surgery may be considered to prevent amblyopia. A transient change in astigmatism is frequently associated with uncontrolled diabetes mellitus, and metabolic regulation is necessary before a new prescription is given.

COMMENTS

Provided that there are no ocular or visual complaints, small astigmatic errors do not require correction. Far too many spectacles incorporate an unnecessary cylindrical correction as a result of a theoretic rather than a biologic refraction. It is to be remembered that 95 per cent of individuals of any population are clinically detectable as astigmatic in some degree and that the lenticular astigmatism tends to neutralize the corneal error. A small degree of astigmatism "with the rule" is the usual condition in the first few years of life. During the school years, the astigmatism changes little. From early adult life onward, there is a tendency for the direct astigmatism to decrease or even to be converted into astigmatism "against the rule." The persistent physiologic 0.5 diopter of astigmatism "with the rule" is best ignored.

References

Barner SS: Surgical treatment of corneal astigmatism. Ophthalmic Surg 7:43–48, 1976.
Barner SS: Surgical control of excessive corneal astigmatism. Experimental and clinical results. J Br Contact Lens Assoc 8:37–38, 1979.
Duke-Elder S (ed): System of Ophthalmology. St. Louis, CV Mosby, 1970, Vol V, pp 274–295.
Ellis W: Radial Keratotomy and Astigmatism Surgery, 2nd ed. Berkeley, Kugler & Ghedini, 1986.
Sloane AE, Garcia GE: Manual of Refraction, 3rd ed. Boston, Little, Brown, and Co, 1979.
Stein HA, Slatt BJ: Fitting Guide for Hard and Soft Contact Lenses. A Practical Approach, 2nd ed. St. Louis, CV Mosby, 1983, pp 222–226.
Troutman RC: Microsurgery of the Anterior Segment of the Eye. St. Louis, CV Mosby, 1977, Vol II, pp. 263–286.

HYPEROPIA
(Far-Sightedness, Hypermetropia)
GEORGE W. WEINSTEIN, M.D.
Morgantown, West Virginia

Hyperopia is a refractive error of the eye in which parallel rays of light focus behind the photoreceptor layer of the retina when the eye is at rest, resulting in a blurred image. Various optical components of this condition include flattening of the cornea or lens, a shallow anterior chamber, a low effective refractivity of the lens, and a small axial length of the eye. Classically, the hyperopic eye is smaller than normal, not only in its anteroposterior diameter but also in all its meridians. The cornea of the classical hypermetrope is small, the lens is large, and the anterior chamber is shallow. Often, the retina has a peculiar sheen (shot-silk retina), which is often associated with accentuated reflexes on the vessels. The vessels may show congenital abnormalities, such as tortuosity and abnormal branching. Symptoms vary with the amount of optical error present, but are usually absent, especially in the young with low degrees of error. In higher degrees of hyperopia, visual blurring is marked, and the patient often holds an object at a distance in order to see it more clearly. Alternatively, the patient may hold a book very close to the eye in an attempt to employ maximum accommodation. Symptoms of eyestrain frequently occur, owing to excessive accommodation and the forced disassociation between it and convergence. Headaches may be a real problem, and the patient may show an apparent divergent squint. The degree of simple hyperopia occurring without malformations of the globe or other pathologic evidences varies considerably; in the vast majority of cases, it is under 3 diopters, although very high values over 20 diopters may occur. The various ocular components that may cause hyperopia appear to be inherited as a dominant trait.

THERAPY

Ocular. As a rule, it is best to undercorrect hyperopia as long as there is some active accommodation. This is true for most young and middle-aged individuals. Since these patients unconsciously utilize accommodation, full correction would result in overcorrection. For this reason there is little need to prescribe spectacles of 1 diopter or less for young hyperopes. The asthenopic symptoms that bring these patients to the office can usually be managed more effectively in other ways. Many of these individuals are in the midst of stressful periods, such as examination times, and tire themselves by reading for long hours into the night. This eyestrain is a manifestation of their overall fatigue, and glasses are not likely to be helpful.

For older individuals who show increasing amounts of manifest hyperopia, the spectacle correction should begin to approach the full amount obtained with refraction. Even so, one should not attempt to correct any of the hyperopia "uncovered" by cycloplegics, but should rely on the "manifest refraction" for this purpose.

In hyperopia, a corrective contact lens is closer to the far point behind the eye than is a corrective spectacle lens. Therefore, the contact lens needs a higher plus power than does the spectacle lens. As the vertex distance is shifted from the usual spectacle plane (10 to 15 mm) to zero for the contact lens, negligible or small power changes are produced for low degrees of hyperopia. For larger amounts of hyperopia in aphakia, the power change is usually quite significant, and calculations or tables based on calculations must be used to determine it.

Ocular or Periocular Manifestations

Anterior Chamber: Shallow.
Ciliary Body: Failure of ciliary muscles; spasm of ciliary muscles.
Cornea: Flat; small.
Lens: Flat; large.
Retina: Macula farther than normal from optic disc; shot-silk retina; vascular tortuosity.
Other: Accommodative asthenopia; convergent squint; divergent squint; eyestrain; overaccommodation; pseudopapillitis.

Precautions

The typical hyperopic eye, with its relatively large lens and shallow anterior chamber, is of the type that is predisposed to closed-angle glaucoma. Therefore, mydriatics must be used with care in hyperopes.

Comments

Hyperopia is the normal optical condition in infants and apparently persists throughout life in some 50 per cent of the population in most areas of the world. The 2 to 3 diopters of hyperopia present in infants usually decrease steadily in the early years of life, although they may increase in some hyperopes between the ages of 5 and 14 years. Any residual hyperopia tends to remain stationary until middle age, at which time it tends to increase owing to lenticular changes.

References

Duke-Elder S (ed): System of Ophthalmology. St. Louis, CV Mosby, 1968, Vol IV, pp 257–267.

Weinstein GW: Correction of ametropia with spectacle lenses. *In* Duane TD (ed): Clinical Ophthalmology. Hagerstown, MD, Harper & Row, 1982, Vol I, pp 36:1–6.

MYOPIA

ROBERT H. BEDROSSIAN, M.D., M.Sc.,
Vancouver, Washington

and RICHARD ELANDER, M.D.
Santa Monica, California

Myopia is the optical condition of the eye in which the posterior focal point lies anterior to the retina. It is the result of an imbalance in the relationship between the refracting components (cornea and lens) and the axial length. The term "physiologic myopia" is used when these three components lie within the normal distribution curve and no pathologic process contributes to the myopia. *Physiologic myopia* usually begins during the rapid growth phase of the body, starting as early as 5 years of age. Myopia generally increases until the normal growth of the individual is completed. In females, this occurs usually between the ages of 13 and 15, and growth ends between 15 to 17 years of age in males. However, its onset may be unrelated to physical growth and not become evident until the late teens or early twenties. In such individuals, the increase in myopia occurs more likely in those who use their eyes for extensive near work.

Pathologic myopia occurs when there is excessive stretching and expansion of the posterior segment of the eye from the ora serrata posteriorly. This is a serious condition that may lead to loss of vision because of the structural changes that occur. It is usually a congenital disease and may be associated with maternal toxemia, rubella, prematurity, and congenital glaucoma. In pathologic myopia, gradual degenerative changes in the fundus occur as the sclera, choroid, and retina become thinner. These changes may occur even with a stable refraction. The earliest fundus change is a large crescent adjacent to the disc, which is followed by localized pale and tessellated patches. With continued thinning of this area, cracks appear in the retina as the posterior staphyloma enlarges. Black spots surrounded by a pale area, known as Fuch's spots, may appear centrally. These are the result of subretinal neovascularization and leakage. Sudden and permanent loss of central vision may occur with these changes. Punched-out areas of atrophy finally appear. They may coalesce and leave areas of "bare" sclera. The peripheral retina also shows areas of "white without pressure" and increasing lattice degeneration. Paving-stone degeneration, as well as pigmentary degeneration, may also occur. These changes usually correlate with axial elongation that can be seen by A- and B-scan ultrasonography. Because retinal tears and retinal detachments occur more frequently in the myopic eye compared to the hyperopic or ametropic eye, the peripheral retina should be evaluated carefully. The anterior segment is not immune from changes. Anterior insertion of the iris and remnants of mesoderm in the angle may be seen. Also associated is an increased incidence of ocular hypertension and glaucoma. Indentation tonometry is frequently inaccurate because of low scleral rigidity. These eyes may also be damaged from pressure that would be considered normal. Nuclear cataracts are a common complication of high myopia. It may be difficult to distinguish between the increasing myopia associated with nuclear sclerosis and that with active progression of pathologic myopia. Cataract surgery in the highly myopic individual has an increased incidence of retinal detachment. Topical corticosteroids should be prescribed with caution, as many high myopes respond with increased pressure. The most common course of pathologic myopia is marked by progression and additional degenerative changes. Intraocular pressures should be kept well below normal limits, if possible, to prevent increased enlargement of the scleral shell. Visual fields are also difficult to evaluate because the field defects from myopia are similar to or overlap glaucomatous changes. Fortunately, pathologic myopia is not common, but must be treated with great care when present.

Night myopia is an entity that results in increased nearsightedness when the light level is substantially reduced. The amount is variable between individuals and has been reported to be up to 6 diopters.

THERAPY

Ocular. Spectacles and contact lenses are the standard forms of correction for the visual impairment from nearsightedness. New spectacle designs and new contact lens materials are constantly being introduced into the marketplace.

Most studies on the prevention of myopia or on the alteration of the optical properties of the eye have been directed toward environmental factors that may aggravate increasing myopia. The amount of accommodation, nutrition, and posterior segment pressure are factors that are most frequently considered. Studies of this nature are frequently questioned because of the difficulty of obtaining adequately controlled human studies. There is evidence, however, that continued accommodation and close work aggravate the progression of myopia. Most medical therapy aims at relaxing accommodation. This alleviates the long sustained accommodation, which some authorities believe increases the pressure in the posterior segment of the eye, which in turn stretches the sclera. Bifocals have been advocated, and some studies suggest that they do help. The proponents of this form of treatment say that most bifocals are not high enough for children to utilize and therefore are not successful. The bifocal height must be at least to the lower edge of the pupil, and the glasses must be fitted so that they stay in position. A more recent study reported that there was no difference in the increase of myopia in three groups of individuals, one of which had only distance correction, the second with a bifocal add of 1 diopter, and the third group with a +2 add bifocal. Prisms to neutralize convergence have also been suggested. Relaxation of accommodation by periodic gaze into the distance while doing close work is advocated by the Japanese. Biofeedback to control accommodation has also been reported in some studies to be effective.

The use of 1 per cent atropine solution in the eye at night on a daily basis is effective in retarding or stopping the increase in myopia in most individuals. If atropine is used in both eyes, bifocals are also necessary. In very low myopes, the atropine can be used in one eye for several months and then in the other eye. This regimen eliminates the need for bifocals, but does not stop the progression of myopia in the untreated eye. In some individuals who have used atropine for a long time, there may be an increase or progression of the myopia despite its continued use. In these individuals, the pupil reacts, and they have partial accommodation. Occasionally, sensitivity to atropine occurs, and the eye becomes red and irritated. If this occurs, 0.25 per cent scopolamine may be substituted. Photochromic or tinted lenses are helpful in those individuals who have light sensitivity when their pupils are dilated. On rare occasions, psychologic disturbances may occur. Peer pressure on a student whose pupils are dilated may make the patient reluctant to continue using the drops. Lowering the intraocular pressure with timolol reduces the further development of myopia in a small number of patients with pathologic myopia.

Decreased scleral rigidity and elasticity may result from poor nutrition. Therefore, proper nutrition should be encouraged. The elimination of raw sugar, soda pop, candy, jelly sandwiches, and "junk foods" from the diet and the use of vitamin supplements, particularly vitamin A and vitamin C, have been reported as stabilizing the myopia. Decreased zinc utilization has also been considered as a factor in increasing myopia. The onset of juvenile diabetes may also be associated with progressive myopia and should be ruled out.

The use of contact lenses and orthokeratology as a method of stabilizing or decreasing myopia has fewer enthusiasts. Most patients are fitted with contact lenses at about the time that their nearsightedness would normally stop progressing. In many instances, it may be more a coincidence rather than a result of contact lenses that the myopia does not progress. Although some individuals appear to have a permanent decrease in their myopia after orthokeratology, the results are very unpredictable. Retainer lenses are needed in most instances after the myopia has decreased. Corneal warpage with increased astigmatism, central corneal scarring, and keratoconus have resulted from the continued use of contact lenses. Polymegathism of the corneal endothelium may represent the first stages of permanent damage to the cornea from the long continued use of contact lenses. Although these conditions may be less of a problem with the rapidly increasing use of either soft lenses or gas-permeable semirigid lenses, they may still be of concern.

Surgical. Surgically altering the cornea is becoming a more accepted option for the correction of myopia in selected individuals. Radial keratotomy continues to be, by far, the most commonly practiced surgical procedure. Since most of the effect of radial keratotomy is obtained with the first four incisions, it is increasingly common to use this number in the initial surgery in lower degrees of myopia. Eight incisions may be reserved for higher degrees of myopia in the initial surgery. Additional incisions may be added at a future time if needed. The amount of surgical correction depends primarily on the patient's age, the size of the optical zone, and the number and depth of the incisions. A central optical zone of less than 3 mm is not advisable. Cutting from the limbus toward the optical zone seems to produce more effect than cutting the optical zone outward. Corrections up to 7 and 8 diopters may be reached in older patients (40 to 50 years of age). Various computer programs and charts may be utilized to assist in determining the effects of the surgery. Late effects (2 to 3 years after surgery) can occur, which has made most operators more conservative in their approach. Transverse incisions to correct astigmatism are now made either during the initial surgical procedure or at a later date. Although still unpredictable, they can be quite effective.

The number of keratomileusis procedures appears to have leveled off. It may well be the most effective treatment of high myopia, but because of its complexity, it remains a procedure done in only a few centers. The unpredictability and late regression of epikeratophakia have limited its use in recent times. Its usefulness is continuing to be researched. Another promising development was the use of the nonfreeze technique to obtain corneal lenticules which was developed by Krumeich and Swinger. So far, it has been somewhat disappointing when practiced by others. Which of these procedures will become the dominant one in the future is difficult to predict. Perhaps a combination will be the end result.

The excimer laser has also come into increasing use. Like so many other modalities, it looks extremely promising. It may be used not only as a way to perform radial keratotomy but also as a source of resculpturing the anterior cornea. At present, many laboratories are engaged in evaluating it.

Other avenues of approach include the intrastromal use of hydrogel lenses and materials of a higher index of refraction. These include polysulfone and polycarbonate. The routine use of these materials seems several years away. More controversial is the recent interest in anterior chamber lenses in phakic eyes and clear lens extraction with or without an intraocular lens. Although these approaches are being used increasingly in Europe, it seems that their possible side effects may be too great for their widespread introduction into the correction of myopia market. Nevertheless, much activity is taking place in this field and may show promise for the future.

Thinned areas of scleral ectasia in the posterior pole may be reinforced with scleral grafts. This procedure may help prevent further degeneration in patients with pathologic myopia and degeneration.

Precautions

Patients on long-term use of cycloplegics should be adequately followed. These patients should be seen every 4 to 6 months with periodic fundus and tension examinations. If a patient has any family history of retinal disease or cone degeneration, cycloplegics on a continued basis should be used with extreme caution. Psychologic problems may also develop with the use of cycloplegics and bifocals. Fellow students may comment about the bifocals or dilated pupils.

Patients who have corneal warpage from the long-term use of contact lenses should either stop wearing the contacts and let their eyes return to a steady state or be fitted with gas-permeable lenses followed by periodic refractions and keratometer readings to determine their stability. Soft lenses may also be used, but frequently a changing degree of astigmatism occurs that may require frequent changes of toric lenses to obtain satisfactory vision. This may become an economic liability. An ideal fit with contact lenses would eliminate or minimize spectacle blur.

Surgical therapy of myopia should be considered only after an honest and fully informed consent is obtained. Patients have to be aware of the unpredictability of the procedure, as well as the side effects, such as glare and variable vision. Infections certainly can occur, but are fortunately quite rare. Concerns over long-term corneal decompensation now seem to be less important. The main advantage of epikeratophakia is its reversibility, but keratomileusis seems to give a more stable result. Irregular astigmatism is a major potential problem with both of these procedures, as well as late epithelial healing. Obviously, clear lens extraction with or without an intraocular lens has all the potential complications of cataract extraction with the added risks of operating on a highly myopic eye. Patients who are considered for this procedure should have a careful examination of the retinal periphery before any surgery. All retinal weaknesses and defects should be considered for treatment by a retinal specialist. Frequent postoperative evaluations of the retinal periphery should also be made to determine any potential hazards. In addition, cystoid macular edema, corneal dystrophy, iritis, choroidal hemorrhage, and endophthalmitis are possible complications of lens extraction with intraocular lens insertion.

COMMENTS

Spectacle glasses to correct myopia should be fitted as close to the eye as possible so that the lens strength and thickness of the glasses may be reduced, as well as changes in image size and prismatic displacement. Newer techniques of designing spectacle lenses have decreased their weight and made them much more cosmetically acceptable. Contact lenses may be a great help in patients with anisometropia. Despite the evidence that myopia may be aggravated by close work, the prohibition of all reading and close work in children with progressive myopia is unwarranted. The encouragement of participation in normal day-to-day activities and exercise, as well as good nutrition, should be given. If there are fluctuations in vision, systemic factors should be considered. Minimal diabetes without a spillover of glucose in the urine may cause a fluctuation in the refraction or an increase in myopia. A nonfasting blood sugar should be taken in situations of this nature. Early nuclear cataracts and the use of certain antihypertensive drugs, tranquilizers, and steroids must be ruled out as possible causes. Pseudomyopia and ciliary spasm can occur in individuals who are in jobs in which they use their eyes to a great extent. The use of mild cycloplegics at night may eliminate some of the ciliary spasm and permit satisfactory distance vision without glasses. The economic impact of myopia is a serious consideration. Anything that can be done to prevent severe myopia should be considered beneficial to the patient in the long run and may decrease the cost of medical eye care. Decreased visual acuity from dependence upon glasses may prevent some individuals from obtaining certain jobs and may also be a safety factor. These individuals may be candidates for refractive surgery.

References

Barraquer JI, Viteri E: Results of myopic keratomileusis. J Refract Surg 3:98–101, 1987.

Brodstein RS, et al: The treatment of myopia with atropine and bifocals. A long-term prospective study. Ophthalmology 91:1373–1379, 1984.

Grosvenor T, et al: Houston myopia control study; a randomized clinical trial. Part II. Final report by the patient care team. Am J Optom Physiol Optics 64:482–498, 1987.

Guyton DL, et al: Special symposium on radial keratotomy. J Refract Surg 3:186–199, 1987.

Hope GM, Rubin ML: Night myopia. Surv Ophthalmol 29:129–136, 1984.

Rowsey JJ, Rubin ML: Refraction problems after refractive surgery. Surv Ophthalmol 32:414–420, 1988.

Tongue AC: Refractive errors in children. Pediatr Clin North Am 34:639–643, 1987.

Trachtman JN: Biofeedback of accommodation to reduce myopia: A review. Am J Optom Physiol Optics 64:639–643, 1987.

SECTION 33

RETINA

ABETALIPOPROTEINEMIA
(Bassen-Kornzweig Syndrome)

and HOMOZYGOUS FAMILIAL HYPOBETALIPO-PROTEINEMIA

RICHARD G. WELEBER, M.D.,
and D. ROGER ILLINGWORTH, M.D., Ph.D.

Portland, Oregon

Phenotypic abetalipoproteinemia may occur on the basis of two genotypically distinct disorders in which affected patients are homozygotes. In the classic form of abetalipoproteinemia, the disorder is transmitted as an autosomal recessive trait, and obligate heterozygote parents have normal concentrations of plasma cholesterol. In contrast, the heterozygous parents of patients with homozygous hypobetalipoproteinemia display reduced levels of plasma cholesterol (70 to 120 mg/dl), and this disorder is transmitted by an autosomal dominant mode of inheritance.

The biochemical and clinical features of abetalipoproteinemia and hypobetalipoproteinemia are similar; both disorders are characterized by hypocholesterolemia (plasma cholesterol, 25 to 30 mg/dl), the presence of abnormal spiculated red cells (acanthocytes), and fat malabsorption with steatorrhea. These features are present from birth; progressive neurologic symptoms (areflexia, proprioceptive deficits, dysmetria, and ataxia) and pigmentary retinal degeneration develop insidiously in untreated patients and first become clinically evident in childhood (4 to 10 years of age). Other clinical findings that may occur in older patients include myocardial fibrosis, kyphoscoliosis, pes cavus, ophthalmoplegia, ptosis, strabismus, cataracts, and nystagmus.

The biochemical defects present in patients with abetalipoproteinemia and homozygous hypobetalipoproteinemia appear to differ, but both result in the virtual absence of lipoproteins containing apoprotein B48 and B100 from plasma. Recent studies have demonstrated that apoprotein B100 is present in increased amounts in the liver of patients with the autosomal recessive form of abetalipoproteinemia and that messenger RNA levels are increased. These data have been interpreted to indicate that this disorder is caused by an as yet undefined abnormality in the secretion of apoprotein B containing lipoproteins from the liver and intestine. In contrast, immunologically detectable apoprotein B and messenger RNA concentrations of apoprotein B are markedly reduced in the liver of patients with homozygous hypobetalipoproteinemia, inferring that this disorder results from a translational defect in the apoprotein B gene. No gross deletions in the apoprotein B gene have been observed in any of the patients with abetalipoproteinemia or homozygous hypobetalipoproteinemia studied to date. Apoprotein B48 is necessary for the assembly and secretion of chylomicrons by the intestinal mucosa, whereas apoprotein B100 is an essential component of very low (VLDL) and low density lipoproteins (LDL) that are secreted by the liver. High-density lipoproteins do not contain apoprotein B and are the only lipoproteins present in the plasma of patients with phenotypic abetalipoproteinemia. Impaired chylomicron formation in the intestinal mucosa results in malabsorption of dietary fats and the fat-soluble vitamins (particularly A, E, and K), whereas the inability to form hepatic VLDL and LDL results in hypocholesterolemia and an impaired ability to transport triglycerides from the liver. Hepatic transport of vitamin A on retinol-binding protein is normal, but the transport of vitamin E, which is normally carried on LDL, is impaired. This dual impediment in both the absorption and transport of vitamin E results in undetectably low levels of vitamin E in the plasma of untreated patients. Recent studies have shown a striking similarity between the neurologic lesions that develop in vitamin E-deficient rhesus monkeys and those that occur in untreated patients with abetalipoproteinemia. These observations, together with the documented lack of progression in neurologic or retinal pigmentary changes observed in patients with phenotypic abetalipoproteinemia who were treated for several years with high doses of vitamins E and A, support the view that these acquired degenerative changes are attributable to vitamin E deficiency.

Abetalipoproteinemia and homozygous hypobetalipoproteinemia are both rare. At present, less than 10 cases of homozygous hypobetalipoproteinemia and 60 to 80 cases of abetalipoproteinemia have been reported in the world literature. Despite similar biochemical features, clinical findings in the reported adult patients with homozygous hypobetalipoproteinemia have suggested that this disorder may be associated with less severe neuro-ophthalmologic changes than are seen in the autosomal recessive form of abetalipoproteinemia. Although the validity of these observations in a larger number of patients remains to be established, therapeutic management of both disorders is similar. Patients with heterozygous hypobetalipoproteinemia do not appear to develop any of the neurologic or retinal abnormalities seen in the homozygous state and require no specific therapy. Indeed, because of their inherently low levels of LDL cholesterol, these patients appear to have a lower than normal incidence of coronary heart disease.

THERAPY

Systemic. Supplemental high daily doses of oral water-miscible vitamin A (10,000 to 15,000 IU) have been shown to return the serum levels for this vitamin to normal and to improve dark adaptation thresholds and the electroretinogram (ERG). Although long-term vitamin A supplementation apparently has not prevented the development of retinal pigmentary degeneration in some patients, this may have been related to lack of supplemental vitamin E. Supplemental vitamin E (200 to 300 IU/kg daily) is of great importance in the prevention of neuromuscular manifestations and retinal degeneration. Plasma concentrations of vitamin E remain low in patients on supplemental therapy, but the recommended dosages have been shown to result in normal concentrations of vitamin E in adipose tissue and liver. Dietary restriction of triglycerides containing long-chain fatty acids is important to control the steatorrhea and gastrointestinal symptoms. Restriction of dietary fat to 10 to 15 per cent of calories is recommended, but this amount may be increased in older patients. Supplemental vitamin K (5 mg weekly) should be given and will correct the prolonged prothrombin time. Serum vitamin A, serum vitamin E, prothrombin time, ERG, dark adaptometry and detailed nerve conduction studies should be performed on a yearly basis to monitor the adequacy of therapy.

Medium-chain triglycerides are contraindicated in patients with phenotypic abetalipoproteinemia and may exacerbate hepatic steatosis and the development of cirrhosis. Although the lack of LDL cholesterol results in subnormal rates of production of steroid hormones by the maximally stimulated adrenal cortex or ovary, patients with phenotypic abetalipoproteinemia do not appear to be at risk for adrenal insufficiency, and coverage with exogenous corticosteroids during periods of major stress is not necessary.

Supportive. Abetalipoproteinemia is an autosomal recessive disorder. Consanguinity has been reported in up to 50 per cent of reported cases and attests to the rarity of the gene in the normal population. Parents and obligate heterozygotes are clinically and biochemically normal. Siblings may be affected, and the risk for homozygosity for each subsequent child to parents with one affected is 25 per cent. Similarly, the risk of a homozygous child in a family where both parents have heterozygous hypobetalipoproteinemia, an autosomal dominant trait, is also 25 per cent. Methods for the prenatal diagnosis of affected siblings have not been established.

Ocular or Periocular Manifestations

Choroid: Atrophy; choroiditis.
Eyelids: Epicanthal folds; ptosis.
Lens: Cataracts.
Optic Nerve: Pallor.
Retina: Abnormal dark adaptation; abnormal electrooculogram; hypopigmentation; macular degeneration; pigmentary degeneration; subnormal or undetectable electroretinogram; vascular attenuation.
Other: Cloudy vitreous; constriction of visual fields; decreased visual acuity; dyschromatopsia; nystagmus; paralysis of extraocular muscles; strabismus.

Precautions

The serum from untreated patients with abetalipoproteinemia is low in vitamins A, E, and K. Vitamin D formation in the skin is normal, so supplementation of vitamin D is not necessary.

Comments

The prognosis for patients with abetalipoproteinemia who are untreated or in whom the diagnosis is not made in childhood is poor; progressive retinal degeneration and neurologic dysfunction result. Treatment should be started early in the disease and continued on an indefinite basis. In newly diagnosed cases, the ERG may improve or even return to normal with the rise of serum vitamin A levels, and ataxia may markedly diminish with replacement vitamin E therapy. Although some patients have continued to slowly deteriorate both neurologically and ophthalmologically even while given supplemental vitamin E and A, the doses given may have been inadequate. Since careful monitoring of diet, fat-soluble vitamin levels, and clinical status is imperative in the management of these patients, they should be referred to tertiary medical care centers for evaluation and therapy.

In many cases where the diagnosis has been established in childhood and the patients treated with vitamins E and A, progressive neuro-ophthalmologic dysfunction has been averted. The prognosis for such patients appears good. Phenotypic abetalipoproteinemia must be regarded as one of the potentially treatable hereditary disorders associated with retinitis pigmentosa and spinocerebellar degeneration.

References

Biemer JJ, McCammon RE: The genetic relationship to abetalipoproteinemia and hypobetalipoproteinemia: A report of the occurrence of both diseases within the same family. J Lab Clin Med 85:556–565, 1975.

Bieri JG, et al: Vitamin A and vitamin E replacement in abetalipoproteinemia. Ann Intern Med *100*:238–239, 1984.

Carr RE: Abetalipoproteinemia and the eye. Birth Defects *12*(3):385–399, 1976.

Hegele RA, Angel A: Arrest of neuropathy and myopathy in abetalipoproteinemia with high dose vitamin E therapy. Can Med Assoc J *132*:40–45, 1985.

Herbert PN, et al: Familial lipoprotein deficiency: Abetalipoproteinemia, hypobetalipoproteinemia and Tangier disease. *In* Stanbury JB, et al (eds): The Metabolic Basics of Inherited Disease, 5th ed. New York, McGraw-Hill, 1983, pp 589–621.

Illingworth DR, Connor WE, Miller RG: Abetalipoproteinemia: Report of two cases and review of therapy. Arch Neurol *37*:659–662, 1980.

Lowry MJ, et al: Electrophysiological studies in five cases of abetalipoproteinemia. Can J Neurol Sci *11*:60–63, 1984.

Miller RG, et al: The neuropathy of abetalipoproteinemia. Neurology *30*:1286–1291, 1980.

Nelson JS, et al: Progressive neuropathologic lesions in vitamin E–deficient rhesus monkeys. J Neuropath Exp Neurol *40*:166–186, 1981.

Robison WG Jr, Kuwabara T, Bieri JG: Vitamin E deficiency and the retina: Photoreceptor and pigment epithelial changes. Invest Ophthalmol Vis Sci *18*:683–690, 1979.

Ross RS, et al: Homozygous hypobetalipoproteinemia: A disease distinct from abetalipoproteinemia at the molecular level. J Clin Invest *81*:590–595, 1988.

Traber MG, et al: Lack of tocopherol in peripheral nerves of vitamin E deficient patients with peripheral neuropathy. N Engl J Med *317*:262–265, 1987.

Von Sallmann L, Gelderman AH, Laster L: ocular histopathologic changes in a case of a-beta-lipoproteinemia (Bassen-Kornzweig syndrome). Doc Ophthalmol *26*:451–460, 1969.

Wichman A, et al: Peripheral neuropathy in abetalipoproteinemia. Neurology *35*:1279–1289, 1985.

Wolff OH, Lloyd JK, Tonks EL: A-B-lipoproteinaemia with special reference to the visual defect. Exp Eye Res *3*:439–442, 1964.

Yee RD, et al: Atypical retinitis pigmentosa in familial hypobetalipoproteinemia. Am J Ophthalmol *82*:64–71, 1976.

Yee RD, Cogan DG, Zee DS: Ophthalmoplegia and dissociated nystagmus in abetalipoproteinemia. Arch Ophthalmol *94*:571–575, 1976.

ACUTE RETINAL NECROSIS

MARK S. BLUMENKRANZ, M.D.
Royal Oak, Michigan

The acute retinal necrosis syndrome is comprised of the triad of confluent peripheral necrotizing retinitis, arteritis, and vitreitis. The disease is most commonly seen in young and middle-aged adults in the third through fifth decades of life and generally involves one eye, although bilateral disease may occur in up to one third of patients at the time of presentation. Males are slightly more commonly affected than females, and most patients are thought to be in good health with the exception of this problem. Infrequently, a patient may give a history of preceding herpes simplex or zoster mucocutaneous infection at a remote site. In addition to the triad of retinitis, arteritis, and vitreitis, most patients first come to the attention of the ophthalmologist with complaints of a red painful eye caused by granulomatous anterior uveitis, episcleritis, and often ocular hypertension. Additionally, optic nerve dysfunction may be present to a variable degree, ranging from no observable deficit to bare or no light perception, presumably on a vasculitic basis. The most serious and visually significant late complication of the disease is complex retinal detachment, which occurs in between 75 and 85 per cent of patients with this syndrome generally 45 to 60 days after the onset of the disease.

The disease has now been definitively linked to ocular infection by members of the herpes hominis group. It is likely that most cases of "typical" acute retinal necrosis are probably caused by herpes varicella zoster virus, although it is thought that retinal infection with either herpes simplex virus I and II may also produce this clinical picture. Rarely, cytomegalovirus has been implicated in the causation of this disease, although it is generally held that it affects only immunocompromised hosts, whereas most patients with acute retinal necrosis are found to be healthy on general physical and serologic examination and have no evidence of other opportunistic infections.

THERAPY

Ocular. The anterior granulomatous uveitis is treated by a combination of cycloplegics and steroids. Generally, prednisolone is administered every 2 to 6 hours, depending on the severity of the anterior inflammation, and a long-acting cycloplegic, such as 1 per cent atropine is given two to four times daily. In those patients with associated ocular hypertension, a topical oculohypotensive agent, generally a beta-blocker, such as 0.5 per cent timolol or 0.5 per cent betaxolol, is administered. The ocular hypertension is generally not severe enough to warrant the use of an oral carbonic anhydrase inhibitor, although one may be required occasionally in rare instances. The cycloplegic-steroid combination can be tapered proportional to the improvement in the anterior uveitis.

Systemic. The opaque confluent retinal lesions, which are known to be associated with active viral infection, respond promptly to treatment with systemic acyclovir. The drug is generally administered at a dosage of 1.5 gm/square meter[§] daily in three equally divided doses, for a minimum of 7 days. Although lower dosages than this have been employed for the successful treatment of other systemic herpetic infections (generally simplex), the higher dosage is recommended because of the well-documented frequency of herpes zoster varicella virus in this condition and its relatively greater resistance to acyclovir (ED-50 3 to 4 μM) compared with herpes simplex (ED-50 0.1 to 1.6 μM). The acute retinal lesions of viral origin are first noted to regress on average 4 days after the initiation of therapy, but require approximately 1 month for complete resolution. For that reason, as well as documented cases of persistence of active virus following only 1 week of intravenous therapy, supplemental therapy with oral acyclovir at a dosage of 15 to 30 mg/kg daily (usually 200 mg five times daily) is generally recommended as well.

Because of the invariable presence of retinal arteritis, frequent optic disc swelling, and vasculitis, treatment, with aspirin‡ at a dosage of 650 mg daily is also recommended for 1 to 2 months after the initiation of the disease. There is some evidence to suggest that this regimen may favorably affect abnormal platelet function that has been reported in this syndrome.

Lastly, because of the severity of vitreitis and potential optic nerve dysfunction, oral steroid therapy is also recommended. Generally it is begun 24 to 48 hours after the initiation of acyclovir therapy because of the potential risk of enhanced viral replication with steroids. Prednisone‡ at a dosage of 40 to 80 mg daily in conjunction with an antacid should be given, depending on the severity of the vitreitis and papillitis, for at least 1 week with gradual tapering depending on the response to therapy. In general, oral steroids are required for a minimum of 3 to 4 weeks. Despite specific antiviral therapy with acyclovir, many patients actually demonstrate a worsening of the vitreitis during the early phase of the disease under treatment, which can be partially ameliorated by the oral steroids. In cases where there is profound loss of vision that is presumably related to optic nerve dysfunction and in cases of recent onset, some consideration can be given to a very high-dose intravenous therapy with methylprednisolone,‡ although the benefit of this treatment remains unproven.

Surgical. Despite successful regression of the peripheral retinal lesions of viral origin, as many as 85 per cent of patients treated with acyclovir, steroids, and aspirin may still go on to develop retinal detachment, frequently associated with proliferative vitreoretinopathy (PVR). There is some evidence to suggest that, if the peripheral retinal lesions of viral etiology are surrounded by prophylactic photocoagulation (media permitting), the frequency of the incidence of retinal detachment can be reduced by approximately 50 per cent. Often, however, there is severe enough vitreous inflammation and opacification to preclude successful photocoagulation. It is recommended that, in all patients in whom the media permit, at least a triple row of argon or krypton photocoagulation be applied to the posterior extent of existing lesions as well. Prophylactic vitrectomy with photocoagulation, with or without scleral buckling, has been recommended as one means of reducing the likelihood of subsequent retinal detachment. The benefit of this form of therapy remains unproven and controversial, although it may be employed in selected cases depending on the clinical circumstances.

When prophylactic treatment is unsuccessful or cannot be employed, complicated retinal detachment frequently occurs (in up to 85 per cent of cases). This condition appears to be caused by the combination of severe vitreoretinal traction forces resulting from the vitreitis and the development of large tractional tears in postnecrotic retina. It has been established that these detachments respond poorly to conventional scleral buckling techniques and require use of a vitrectomy and long-acting vitreous substitutes for successful long-term reattachment. There is evidence to suggest that employing the additional step of scleral buckling in conjunction with vitrectomy, endophotocoagulation, and long-acting gas tamponade may actually increase the need for reoperation and the frequency of postoperative complications (choroidal detachment, ocular hypertension, fibrin syndrome).

Ocular or Periocular Manifestations

Conjunctiva: Conjunctival hyperemia without a follicular response (acute phase of disease); mild lid swelling; orbital vascular engorgement.

Cornea: Granulomatous keratic precipitates (early phases of disease).

Iris: Vascular engorgement that may be confused with rubeosis.

Vitreous: Inflammatory cells; progressive cicatrization.

Retina: Circular or nummular opacities that appear to involve the outer retina and choroid (early phase of disease); dentate or saw-toothed yellow-gray, flat, confluent infiltrates in the far periphery with their apices directed toward the optic nerve.

Optic Nerve: Hyperemia; pale.

Sclera: Episcleritis.

Other: Moderate to severe pain.

PRECAUTIONS

The major causes of permanent visual dysfunction in this syndrome are related to the sequela of retinal detachment, which still occurs at a distressingly high rate. In addition to the prompt initiation of therapy with acyclovir, oral steroids, and aspirin, photocoagulation should be promptly administered, if the ocular media permit, to reduce the likelihood of retinal detachment. Although most patients show a relatively prompt resolution of the retinal lesions on acyclovir therapy, in some instances, the lesions may actually persist or increase despite antiviral therapy. In such instances, the dosages should be carefully checked with the pharmacy to ascertain that a full complement of 1.5 gm square meter is being administered daily. It is likely that drug resistance will occur with the increased availability and treatment with various antivirals, although this response has not been well documented in the case of acute retinal necrosis. There is no evidence to suggest that treatment with topical antiviral agents, such as trifluridine or idoxuridine, is beneficial. Although other antiviral agents have been shown to be effective systemically for other herpetic infections (vidarabine and ganciclovir[†] (DHPG)), concerns regarding potential toxicity with these agents weigh against their routine use.

Because acyclovir is only converted to its active form, acycloguanosine triphosphate, in cells infected with herpes simplex or zoster varicella virus because they contain a unique thymidine kinase, the drug is remarkably nontoxic against normal human and ocular cells. Nonetheless, toxicity may occur at the highest drug levels and is generally associated with crystallization in the urinary tract. For this reason, adequate oral fluid intake is recommended with acyclovir therapy, as well as an appropriate reduction in dosage in the presence of existing renal failure or other significant medical problems.

Comments

The emergence of increasing numbers of patients with this syndrome over the past 10 years is somewhat puzzling and suggests that either the prevalence of herpes simplex and zoster infection is increasing, with the consequent increased incidence of ocular complications, or a mutant strain (e.g., herpes viruses with a predilection for retinal involvement) has evolved. Why this should result in such a high rate of retinal detachment relative to other known ocular infections, such as cytomegalovirus, toxoplasmosis, or toxocariasis, remains unknown, but the availability of specific antiviral therapy, as well as other prophylactic measures, including photocoagulation, has improved the visual prognosis of this syndrome considerably in recent years.

References

Blumenkranz MS, et al: Treatment of the acute retinal necrosis syndrome with intravenous acyclovir. Ophthalmology 93:296–300, 1986.
Blumenkranz MS, et al: Vitrectomy for retinal detachment associated with acute retinal necrosis. Am J Ophthalmol 106:426–429, 1988.
Carney MD, et al: Acute retinal necrosis. Retina 6:85, 1986.
Culbertson WW, et al: Varicella zoster virus as a cause of the acute retinal necrosis syndrome. Ophthalmology 93:559–569, 1986.
Han DP, et al: Laser photocoagulation in the acute retinal necrosis syndrome. Arch Ophthalmol 105:1051, 1987.
Young NJA, Bird AC: Bilateral acute retinal necrosis. Br J Ophthalmol 62:581, 1978.

BRANCH RETINAL VEIN OCCLUSION
FRONCIE A. GUTMAN, M.D.
Cleveland, Ohio

Occlusion of one of the tributaries of the central retinal vein produces a classic ophthalmoscopic picture that usually is easily recognized. This site of venous obstruction is at an arteriovenous crossing, and most branch vein obstructions occur in temporal retina. Superficial hemorrhages and retinal edema are invariably present in the area of the retina drained by the obstructed vein. Hemorrhage is usually moderate or heavy with a flame-shaped appearance. Cotton-wool spots usually reflect the degree of local ischemia and are transient.

Since 85 per cent of patients suffering a branch retinal vein occlusion have systemic hypertension or other signs of systemic vascular disease, a general medical evaluation is necessary to identify coincident systemic disease.

The two complications of temporal retinal branch vein occlusion usually associated with a poor visual prognosis are macular edema and preretinal neovascularization. Untreated macular edema complicating temporal retinal branch vein occlusion has an unpredictable course and frequently has a poor visual prognosis. Photocoagulation with laser paramacular grid therapy produces an improved visual prognosis in eyes with chronic macular edema and a visual acuity of 20/40 or worse. Preretinal neovascularization develops in 19 to 41 per cent of untreated eyes with temporal retinal branch vein occlusion, and 61 per cent of these eyes will develop vitreous hemorrhages. The preretinal neovascularization develops at the disc and within areas of peripheral retina drained by the obstructed vein. Only rarely does it develop in noninvolved retina.

THERAPY

Surgical. All eyes developing any form of preretinal neovascularization and all patients with macular edema and decreased visual acuity should be considered candidates for photocoagulation. Photocoagulation can be used to reverse macular edema and to induce atrophy of preretinal neovascularization. Since macular edema and preretinal neovascularization are such disparate clinical manifestations of the same disease, the indications for and the techniques of photocoagulation in these two complications must be considered separately.

Patients with macular edema are considered candidates for photocoagulation if the macular edema has been present for a minimum of 3 months and distance visual acuity is 20/40 or worse. Evaluation of these patients should include a careful refraction to determine both the best corrected distance and near visual acuities, visual fields to evaluate the density of central or paracentral scotomas, and fluorescein angiography to identify the intraretinal microvascular abnormalities and the sites of paramacular leakage. The photocoagulation technique consists of argon laser therapy to the sites of leakage associated with the paramacular intraretinal microvascular abnormalities. Sites of leakage and areas of capillary nonperfusion are readily identified on the fluorescein angiogram. Care should be taken to avoid sites of retinal hemorrhage, the capillary-free zone, and shunt vessels crossing the midline raphe. Treatment inside of the capillary-free zone causes a direct insult to the foveal cone, and treatment to the shunt vessels crossing the horizontal midline raphe may destroy collateral vessels and increase stasis within the area of retina drained by the obstructed vein. One hundred-micron spot sizes are used to create a moderate-intensity burn at the sites of intraretinal leakage. Confluent burns should be avoided to minimize the size and density of the scotoma created by destruction of the photoreceptor cells in the paramacular area. Eyes with visual loss from intraretinal hemorrhage in the fovea or foveal capillary nonperfusion are thought to have a poor visual prognosis with or without laser therapy.

A posttreatment fluorescein angiographic study will confirm the effects of treatment. If there is persistent intraretinal leakage and the visual acuity has not significantly improved, additional treatment may be considered.

Once preretinal neovascularization has been identified, photocoagulation should be considered because of the significant risk of vitreous hemorrhage. Preretinal neovascularization may develop at the disc or may present as a focal frond within the peripheral retina drained by the obstructed vein. The recommended technique for photocoagulation is argon laser therapy, utilizing large (200 to 500 μM) photocoagulation burns. If a peripheral focal frond is present, it can be treated directly with a moderate-intensity burn. For preretinal neovascularization on the disc, a pattern of scattered treatment to the peripheral retina drained by the obstructed vein is recommended. Photocoagulation burns are spaced on burn width apart and are applied to all areas of the retina drained by the obstructed vein. Contiguous burns may be applied to areas of capillary nonperfusion. If a patient has both preretinal neovascularization of the disc and peripheral preretinal neovascularization, the two techniques are combined.

After treatment, clinical examination and fluorescein angiography will document the changes in the preretinal neovascularization. Involution or atrophy of preretinal neovascularization is clinically recognized by the loss of vascularity in the preretinal frond and is confirmed by an absence of fluorescein leakage and staining. A skeleton of preretinal fibrous tissue may remain.

If initial treatment has not totally destroyed the preretinal neovascularization, an additional fluorescein angiography should be performed to identify ischemic areas of the retina. Additional treatment should be applied to those ischemic areas and to previously untreated portions of the retina drained by the obstructed vein.

Precautions

Although a thrombus within the affected vein is a consistent histopathologic finding in branch retinal vein occlusion, there is no contemporary controlled prospective study that evaluates the benefits of anticoagulant and fibrinolytic therapy. This may be partially explained by two observations. First, patients with branch retinal vein occlusion are frequently not seen for several weeks or months after the onset of symptoms. In addition, thrombus organization in the form of recanalization and endothelial cell proliferation may occur quite early (within 10 to 14 days). If thrombus organization has already commenced at the time of initial evaluation, the potential benefits of anticoagulant or fibrinolytic therapy would seem quite limited.

The complications seen after photocoagulation for preretinal neovascularization include vitreous hemorrhage, rhegmatogenous retinal detachment, traction retinal detachment, and preretinal macular fibrosis. However, since all of these complications may develop in the natural course of branch retinal venous occlusive disease, their relationship to photocoagulation treatment remains uncertain.

Comments

Although the overall visual prognosis with macular edema is favorably influenced by laser photocoagulation, only 60 per cent of treated eyes will achieve 20/40 or better visual acuity. Remission of the macular edema and improvement in visual acuity are very gradual processes, occurring over a 6- to 12-week interval. As long as there is evidence of a decrease in the paramacular leakage and improvement in visual acuity, retreatment should be deferred. If there are no signs of a remission, at least 6 weeks of observation are recommended before considering additional laser treatment. Patients with such pretreatment findings, as a visual acuity of 20/200 or worse, a dense sector scotoma, intraretinal foveal hemorrhage, and significant foveal capillary nonperfusion may have a poor visual prognosis with or without photocoagulation.

The ultimate goal in the treatment of macular edema is to improve the functional quality of central vision. For this reason, patients being considered as candidates for photocoagulation should have their distance and near visual acuities separately and carefully assessed. If a patient has only one eye with functional vision and has some level of employable reading vision, observation may be considered with deferral of photocoagulation.

Twenty-two per cent of all branch retinal vein occlusions will develop preretinal neovascularization, but significant signs of intraretinal ischemia (i.e., 5 or more disc diameters of capillary nonperfusion) double the risk of preretinal neovascularization, i.e., 41 per cent. For this reason, eyes with extensive areas of capillary nonperfusion should be frequently and prospectively watched for early signs of preretinal neovascularization.

In eyes with preretinal neovascularization, peripheral scattered laser photocoagulation promotes destruction of the neovascular fronds and reduces the incidence of vitreous hemorrhage. Atrophy of neovascular fronds is usually evident within 2 to 8 weeks after photocoagulation therapy. If a vitreous hemorrhage occurs shortly after the initial treatment, these hemorrhages may clear without recurrence. However, if vitreous hemorrhage recurs at a later time and neovascular fronds are still present, additional peripheral laser treatment should be performed.

Inferior temporal retinal branch vein occlusions with associated vitreous hemorrhage are more difficult to treat because the vitreous hemorrhage gravitates over that portion of the retina affected by the obstruction and limits the evaluation by fluorescein angiography and visualization for photocoagulation. If vitreous hemorrhage obscures the retina, laser therapy utilizing red wavelengths may be more effective than argon in producing photocoagulation burns and also may minimize thermal effects to the vitreous. Another alternative when vitreous hemorrhage obscures the involved retina is transconjunctival cryosurgery. For cases of chronic, severe, vitreous hemorrhage, vitrectomy facilitates clearing of the vitreous media and may be combined with endophotocoagulation to the involved retina.

References

Birchall CH, et al: Visual field changes in branch retinal "vein" occlusion. Arch Ophthalmol 94:747–754, 1976.
Branch Vein Occlusion Study Group: Argon laser photocoagulation for macular edema in branch vein occlusion. Am J Ophthalmol 98:271–282, 1984.
Branch Vein Occlusion Study Group: Argon laser scatter photocoagulation for prevention of neovascularization and vitreous hemorrhage in branch vein occlusion. Arch Ophthalmol 104:34–41, 1986.
Cox MS, Whitmore PV, Gutow RF: Treatment of intravitreal and prepapillary neovascularization following branch retinal vein occlusion. Trans Am Acad Ophthalmol Otolaryngol 79:387–393, 1975.
Frangieh GT, et al: Histopathologic study of nine branch retinal vein occlusions. Arch Ophthalmol 100:1132–1140, 1982.
Gutman FA: Macular edema in branch retinal vein occlusion: Prognosis and management. Trans Am Acad Ophthalmol Otolaryngol 83:488–493, 1977.
Gutman FA, Zegarra H: The natural course of temporal retinal branch vein occlusion. Trans Am Acad Ophthalmol Otolaryngol 78:178–192, 1974.
Gutman FA, et al: Photocoagulation in retinal branch vein occlusion. Ann Ophthalmol 13:1359–1363, 1981.
Michels RG, Gass JDM: The natural course of retinal vein obstruction. Trans Am Acad Ophthalmol Otolaryngol 78:166–177, 1974.
Miller SD: Argon laser photocoagulation for macular edema in branch vein occlusion. Am J Ophthalmol 99:218–219, 1985.

CENTRAL OR BRANCH RETINAL ARTERY OCCLUSION
(BRAO, CRAO)

MICHAEL H. GOLDBAUM, M.D.
San Diego, California

The significance of managing patients with central retinal artery occlusion goes beyond attempts to restore vision. Identification and treatment of associated disease may reduce morbidity or increase longevity for the patient.

The causes of obstruction of the central artery of the retina may be classified into broad groups: emboli arising spontaneously from upstream vessels or the heart, iatrogenic emboli, focal inflammation or degeneration of the retinal artery as it enters the eye, disorders of the blood or clotting mechanism, pressure to the eye, carotid insufficiency, spasm of the central retinal or ophthalmic artery, hypovolemic shock, injury to the ophthalmic or retinal artery, and anomalies or kinks in the retinal artery. Most occlusions are caused by emboli, and the remainder are probably due to locally induced thrombosis.

Embolism is the most frequent cause of occlusion of the central or branch retinal arteries. Any embolus, if small enough to enter the ophthalmic artery and large enough to obstruct the central retinal artery, may produce occlusive infarction of the retina. Platelet-fibrin clots are barely visible plugs that may originate from an ulcerated atheroma in the carotid artery, although other sources may be a mural thrombus from a myocardial infarction or a mitral valve prolapse. Bright cholesterol crystals (Hollenhorst plaques) often arise from carotid ulcerations. Calcific emboli may develop secondary to diseased aortic valves. Multiple spontaneous emboli in retinal arteries in a young person may be clumps of myxoma cells from a benign, treatable cardiac myxoma. Facial or orbital injection may inadvertently introduce into the carotid system embolic material that reaches the central retinal artery. Carotid angiography may liberate embolic material. Awareness of such iatrogenic causes may aid in their prevention.

Thrombosis of the central retinal artery occurs in patients who have degeneration or inflammation of the walls of the local artery. Atherosclerotic changes in the central retinal artery resemble the histopathologic changes in other major arteries. Turbulence in flow from irregularities in the lumen can induce thrombus formation that completes the obstruction. Giant cell arteritis, systemic lupus erythematosis, and other connective tissue disorders are able to induce an obstructive arteritis. Thrombus formation in the central retinal artery can occur from blood dyscrasias, such as hyperviscosity of the blood, disseminated intravascular coagulation, or sickle hemoglobinopathies.

Prolonged elevation of intraocular pressure above systolic pressure can result from scleral buckles or from inadvertent pressure on the eye during general anesthesia for orthopedic or neurosurgical procedures. Occlusive pressure in the central retinal or ophthalmic artery may develop from intraorbital implants or from elevated intraorbital pressure from unrelieved orbital edema, hemorrhage, or emphysema.

Acute obstruction of the retinal artery may be brief with recovery of visual function in minutes, may be transient or partial with recovery of some or all visual function in hours, or may be complete and of long enough duration to produce permanent loss of vision. The gradient of the partial pressure of oxygen from the patent choroid circulation to the inner retina after central retinal artery occlusion is insufficient to sustain viability of the inner retina, but is adequate to prolong survival of the inner retina. Experimental occlusion of the central retinal artery in monkeys for less than 100 minutes allowed full recovery of retinal function; whereas progressively longer occlusions resulted in successively less recovery of visual function. The recovery of partial or complete visual function in patients with central retinal artery occlusion may occur after several hours or days if the occlusion is not complete.

Brief slowing of the retinal blood flow or lowering of the retinal blood pressure may cause a fleeting (generally less than 10 minutes) blindness (amaurosis fugax) in the affected eye. This symptom occurs frequently in the course of stenotic carotid arterial atherosclerosis and is observed at times in valvular heart disease and systemic arteritides. Often, amaurosis fugax is caused by emboli. Residuals of such an event may persist in the retina as cholesterol emboli and cotton-wool spots. The presence of retinal emboli is evidence that the carotid artery is not totally occluded.

The main symptom of central retinal artery occlusion is a sudden, painless loss of vision in the affected eye. Sometimes, amaurosis fugax occurs hours or days before the prolonged loss of vision. If a cilioretinal artery is present, a corresponding island of visual field will remain. Conversely, occlusion of the cilioretinal artery causes a corresponding field defect.

Retinal ischemic edema becomes visible as retinal graying within 5 to 10 minutes after onset of the occlusion. At this time, the affected arteries may be thin and empty or have segments of stationary or pulsatile "box carring." The veins are darker than normal. After 70 minutes of deprivation of blood flow through the central retinal artery, the retina reaches maximal whiteness, except for the fovea, which has a cherry red or brown color because its tissue still receives adequate nutrition from the choroidal circulation.

Around one third of patients have less than complete occlusion of the central retinal artery; the presenting visual acuity in these patients may range from hand motion to 20/30. Return of circulation may be indicated by intermittent spurts of blood or slow flow. When occlusion is not complete, the final vision correlates positively with the presenting vision and negatively with the duration of visual impairment.

The electroretinogram can determine if the retinal artery occlusion is accompanied by choroidal occlusion. In pure central retinal artery occlusion, the B-wave is lost as a result of inner retinal dysfunction, but the A-wave remains because the rods and cones still function. With ophthalmic artery occlusion or pressure occlusion of both the retinal and choroidal circulations, both the B-wave and the A-wave are lost. During the fluorescein angiography, obstructed retinal circulation is slowed or stopped, and the vessels appear attenuated. With reperfusion, the fluorescein flow may appear normal. Fluorescein angiography can reveal insufficiency of preocular circulation by delay of the arm-to-retinal circulation time.

Whatever treatment is used, prompt action improves the chance for success. Complete occlusion for more than 6 hours probably produces irreversible retinal damage.

THERAPY

Supportive. The iatrogenic causes can be anticipated, and surgical procedures should be altered to reduce the risk of occlusion. For example, after a scleral buckle is placed, the central retinal artery can be checked by indirect ophthalmoscopy for patency. Retrobulbar injections into the optic nerve or its sheath can be avoided by preventing needle access to the optic nerve by having the eye look straight ahead, instead of up and nasal.

Systemic. Underlying causes of retinal artery occlusion are treated directly. For instance, sickle hemoglobinopathies may respond to exchange transfusions. Arteritides may improve with high-dose corticosteroids. For the first few days, 100 mg of oral prednisone may be administered with gradual reduction as long as the sedimentation rate is normal or manifestations are absent.

Ocular. Attempts to treat emboli are aimed at dislodging the embolus to move it downstream and providing increased oxygenation of the retina. Methods to move the embolus include trying to dilate the obstructed artery, increasing the pressure gradient across the embolus, and jarring the embolus. Supine positioning of the patient is convenient for treating the patient and may increase pressure across the embolus. Although inhaled 5 per cent carbon dioxide gas is a potent vasodilator, it has been found not to dilate the central retinal artery in normal subjects. Choroidal delivery of oxygen may be improved with 95 per cent inhaled oxygen, even though it constricts the normal central retinal artery, or with 5 per cent carbon dioxide added to the 95 per cent oxygen, which also does not reduce the vasoconstriction. Retrobulbar injection of vasodilators or smooth muscle relaxants has not been demonstrated to dilate the retinal arteries or to improve retinal blood flow. Intravenous administration of 500 mg of acetazolamide lowers intraocular pressure, thereby increasing the pressure gradient across the embolus. Ocular massage to enhance aqueous outflow, followed by abrupt release of pressure, may be as effective as anterior chamber paracentesis in increasing the pressure gradient across the embolus; in addition, ocular massage has the potential benefit of jarring the embolus. Tapping the eye also may dislodge the embolus.

The aim of treatment of a thrombus in the central retinal artery is lysis of the clot. If occlusion is incomplete, the body's natural fibrinolysis may occur in time for preservation of retinal function. Thrombolytic agents have been demonstrated to be effective in treatment of acute coronary artery occlusion. The logical extension of this concept is the intracarotid injection of urokinase[‡] or tissue plasminogen activator.[‡] Initial reports indicate that urokinase improves the visual acuity in central retinal artery occlusion; however, a controlled trial with an adequate number of patients will be necessary to evaluate the efficacy of fibrinolytic agents.

Surgical. When intraorbital pressure exceeds systolic pressure of the ophthalmic or central retinal artery, orbital decompression can be accomplished by orbital paracentesis or sectioning of canthal tendons.

Precautions

Fibrinolytic therapy should be performed by physicians experienced in this therapy.

Comments

As important as the treatment of the occlusion itself is the evaluation for systemic disease. An erythrocyte sedimentation rate can be done immediately to test for giant cell arteritis in patients over 55 years of age. Noninvasive B-scan ultrasonography and Doppler tests of the carotid circulation may reveal ulcerative plaques or significant carotid occlusion. A physician experienced in cerebrovascular disorders may be of aid in the evaluation of the patient for carotid ulcerations, giant cell arteritis, cardiac valvular disease, mural thrombosis, connective tissue diseases, and atrial myxomas. Identification and treatment of associated disorders may decrease the risk of morbidity or reduced longevity.

References

Augsburger JJ, Margargal LE: Visual prognosis following treatment of acute central retinal artery obstruction. Br J Ophthalmol 64:913–917, 1980.
Brown GC, Shields JA: Cilioretinal arteries and retinal arterial occlusion. Arch Ophthalmol 97:84–92, 1979.
Chawluk JB, et al: Atherosclerotic carotid artery disease in patients with retinal ischemic syndromes. Neurology 38:858–863, 1988.
Deutsch TA, et al: Effects of oxygen and carbon dioxide on the retinal vasculature in humans. Arch Ophthalmol 101:1278–1280, 1983.
Ffytche TJ: A rationalization of treatment of central retinal artery occlusion. Trans Ophthalmol Soc UK 94:468–479, 1974.
Hayreh SS, Weingeist TA: Experimental occlusion of the central artery of the retina. I. Ophthalmoscopic and fluorescein angiographic studies. Br J Ophthalmol 64:896–912, 1980.
Hayreh SS, Weingeist TA: Experimental occlusion of the central artery of the retina. IV. Retinal tolerance time to acute ischaemia. Br J Ophthalmol 64:818–825, 1980.
Jampol LM, et al: Ischemia of ciliary arterial circulation from ocular compression. Arch Ophthalmol 93:1311–1317, 1975.
Perkins SA, et al: The idling retina: Reversible visual loss in central retinal artery obstruction. Ann Ophthalmol 19:3–6, 1987.
Rossman H: Treatment of retinal arterial occlusion. Ophthalmologica 180:68–74, 1980.
Wise GN, Dollery CT, Henkind P: The Retinal Circulation. New York, Harper & Row, 1971.

CENTRAL SEROUS CHORIORETINOPATHY
(Central Serous Retinopathy)
JAMES C. FOLK, M.D.
Iowa City, Iowa

Central serous chorioretinopathy (CSC) is a disease in which there is a serous detachment of the neurosensory retina caused by leakage from the retinal pigment epithelium (RPE). The disease affects patients 20 to 55 years of age, with males outnumbering females by 10 to 1. Patients notice decreased vision, metamorphopsia, micropsia, and a positive central scotoma. The cause of this disease is unknown, but it typically occurs in males who are hard driving and have "type A" personalities. Often, the patient relates the onset of the disease to a time of unusual stress or anxiety, and some researchers believe the disease may be caused by higher than normal levels of circulating serum epinephrine.

THERAPY

Supportive. There is no proven medical treatment for central serous chorioretinopathy. Patients who present with their first episode can be reassured that they have at least a 90 per cent chance of retinal reattachment with an improvement of vision to 20/30 or better without treatment. Studies have shown that laser treatment directed to the site of RPE leakage hastens the resolution of the subretinal fluid and decreases the risk of recurrence, but does not improve the ultimate visual acuity. These studies contained relatively few patients and used Snellen visual acuity as an end point, which may be a relatively insensitive test of dysfunction in these patients. Although nearly all patients with a resolved episode of central serous chorioretinopathy have 20/30 or better acuity, many are persistently bothered by blurred vision, a relative scotoma, metamorphopsia, or poor color vision in the affected eye. It remains unknown whether the risk or severity of these symptoms would be decreased by a more rapid resolution of the subretinal fluid induced by laser treatment.

Surgical. A reasonable approach to patients with a first episode of central serous chorioretinopathy is to perform an initial fluorescein angiogram to rule out other causes of subretinal fluid and then to see the patient again 2 months later. If the fluid has not resolved after 2 months, treatment should be considered, especially if the leak is 300 μM or more from the foveal center. The angiogram should be repeated to locate the area(s) of RPE leakage. An appropriate frame of the angiogram should then be magnified on a viewer and the area of RPE corresponding to the leakage found by examining the patient with a contact lens at the slitlamp. A retrobulbar anesthetic* is usually unnecessary, but the patient should fixate on some target with the opposite eye and should be told not to move suddenly. Digital pressure on the fundus contact lens or the use of the larger "Yanuzzi" contact lens also helps minimize inadvertent movement of the eye being treated. Either argon green or krypton red laser can be used at a 100- to 200-μM spot size and a 0.1 second duration. The power should be set very low and increased gradually until a gray or light white burn is achieved that is sufficient. Often, only three or four gentle burns are required to treat the area of leakage.

No patching or drops are needed after treatment. The patient should return in 4 weeks or anytime either vision or metamorphopsia worsens. The fluorescein angiogram should be repeated if there is a suspicion of choroidal neovascularization or 2 months after treatment if the subretinal fluid has not resolved.

Ocular or Periocular Manifestations

Retina: Loss of foveal reflex; multiple yellow precipitates on posterior surface of detached retina, retinal pigment epithelial detachment, atrophy, and pigmentation; serous neurosensory detachment.

Other: Central scotoma; decreased color vision; decreased vision; induced hyperopia; metamorphopsia; micropsia.

PRECAUTIONS

Before making a diagnosis of central serous chorioretinopathy, other causes of a macular neurosensory retinal detachment must be ruled out. These other causes include an optic pit, a choroidal tumor, a peripheral or posterior retinal break, and a choroidal neovascular membrane. Subtle choroidal neovascularization can be easily missed in these patients. Both the fundus and the fluorescein angiogram must be studied carefully for signs of choroidal neovascularization, such as hemorrhage, a grayish color to the retinal pigment epithelium, or a vascular-like structure that fills with fluorescein dye. The risk of choroidal neovascularization increases greatly in older patients with drusen and in patients with histoplasmosis scars, angioid streaks, or high myopia. Patients with choroidal neovascular membranes have a much poorer prognosis than those with central serous retinopathy. Usually, these membranes must be treated thoroughly and promptly to decrease the risk of visual loss.

Patients with central serous chorioretinopathy must also be warned that they may have persistent symptoms of blurred vision or a scotoma even after successful treatment, that there is a small risk of developing choroidal neovascularization, and that the subretinal fluid can recur later.

COMMENTS

Patients with an acute episode of central serous chorioretinopathy can be safely followed, but laser treatment should be considered if the fluid does not resolve in 2 months. Laser treatment should be considered sooner, perhaps within a month, in patients with recurrent episodes because their risk of visual loss is greater and treatment appears to decrease the rate of recurrence. Finally, there is a small subset of patients who appear to have chronic central serous chorioretinopathy with multiple episodes of serous fluid. These patients often have gradual but progressive visual loss with RPE atrophy and pigmentation. Their serous detachment is often very shallow and difficult to detect over the atrophic RPE. These patients should have fluorescein angiography in order to determine whether there is a RPE leak. The leak may be minimal and subtle, but usually can be differentiated from the other areas of RPE atrophy or window defects, especially late in the angiogram. The leaks in these patients with chronic disease probably should be treated promptly in order to eliminate the subretinal fluid and avoid further visual loss.

References

Dellaporta A: Central serous retinopathy. Trans Am Ophthalmol Soc 74:144–153, 1976.

Folk JC, et al: Visual function abnormalities in central serous retinopathy. Arch Ophthalmol 102:1299–1302, 1984.

Frederick AR Jr: Multifocal and recurrent (serous) choroidopathy (MARC) syndrome: A new variety of idiopathic central serous choroidopathy. Doc Ophthalmologica 56:203–235, 1984.

Jalkh AE, et al: Retinal pigment epithelium decompensation. I. Clinical features and natural course. Ophthalmology 91:1544–1548, 1984.

Jalkh AE, et al: Retinal pigment epithelium decompensation. II. Laser treatment. Ophthalmology 91:1549–1553, 1984.

Klein ML, et al: Experience with nontreatment of central serous choroidopathy. Arch Ophthalmol 91:247–250, 1974.

Novak MA, et al: Krypton and argon laser photocoagulation for central serous chorioretinopathy. Retina 7:162–169, 1987.

Robertson DM, et al: Direct, indirect, and sham laser photocoagulation in the management of central serous chorioretinopathy. Am J Ophthalmol 95:457–466, 1983.

Schatz H, et al: Subretinal neovascularization following argon laser photocoagulation treatment for central serous chorioretinopathy: Complication or misdiagnosis. Trans Am Acad Ophthalmol Otolaryngol 83:893–906, 1977.

Watzke RC, et al: Ruby laser photocoagulation therapy of central serous retinopathy. Part I: A controlled clinical study. Part II: Factors affecting prognosis. Trans Am Acad Ophthalmol Otolaryngol 78:205–211, 1974.

Watzke RC, et al: Direct and indirect laser photocoagulation of central serous choroidopathy. Am J Ophthalmol 88:914–918, 1979.

Yannuzzi LA: Type-A behavior and central serous chorioretinopathy. Retina 7:111–130, 1987.

COATS' DISEASE
(Massive Exudative Retinitis, Retinal Telangiectasia)

WILLIAM TASMAN, M.D.
Philadelphia, Pennsylvania

Coats' disease is a nonhereditary abnormality of the retinal vasculature that was first described by Coats in 1908. Associated with the abnormal retinal vasculature is subretinal exudation that may involve the macula. In advanced cases, serous detachment of the sensory retina may occur. Areas of retinal ischemia characterized by capillary dropout are seen on fluorescein angiography in places where retinal telangiectasia is present. In certain cases, microaneurysmal-type changes can occur in the posterior pole, which may be associated with exudation posterior to the equator. Histologically, cholesterol crystals are seen in the retina. Although the vitreous is usually clear when the condition is mild, vitreous hemorrhage may occur in advanced cases. Optic nerve involvement in Coats' disease is rare. In the end stages of unsuccessfully treated Coats' disease, neovascular glaucoma may develop secondary to neovascularization of the iris that extends into the angle.

Coats' disease has been reported to affect both sexes, but is much more common in males than females. True instances of Coats' disease in females are exceedingly rare. The condition is unilateral in 90 per cent of cases and is diagnosed most often between the ages of 2 and 10 years.

THERAPY

Surgical. Treatment is directed at elimination of the abnormal vessels. Because the patients are in the pediatric age range, general anesthesia is required. Fluorescein angiography in the operating room helps delineate the areas of capillary nonperfusion and retinal telangiectasia that require treatment. Cryotherapy is an effective means of eliminating the abnormal vessels and can be used from the equator to the ora serrata. In patients with vascular abnormalities posterior to the equator, photocoagulation is preferable. Usually two to three treatment sessions are necessary at 4- to 6-week intervals in order to eliminate the abnormal vasculature. Those patients with involvement of two quadrants or less have the best prognosis. The prognosis becomes more guarded when three or more quadrants are involved.

Patients with marked Coats' disease may develop serous detachment of the sensory retina. In these cases, scleral buckling with drainage of subretinal fluid followed by cryotherapy to the telangiectatic vessels can lead to reattachment of the retina.

With elimination of the abnormal vessels, subretinal exudate will begin to clear. This is a slow process, and it may take as long as 1 year until all of the exudation has been absorbed. With macular involvement, a subretinal organized button may remain permanently in the fovea.

Ocular or Periocular Manifestations

Retina: Cholesterol crystals; exudate; ischemia; microaneurysms; sensory detachment; telangiectasis.
Vitreous: Hemorrhage.
Other: Neovascular glaucoma.

PRECAUTIONS

Even in patients who have been successfully treated, recurrences have been noted as much as 5 years later. It is therefore recommended that patients be followed at 6-month intervals so that if further treatment becomes necessary it can be done before the process becomes too extensive.

COMMENTS

Cryotherapy and photocoagulation have proved effective in salvaging many eyes with Coats' disease. Sometimes, however, macular vision does not return if the exudation has been present in the foveal area. It is important to consider the following conditions in the differential diagnosis of Coats' disease: angiomatosis retinae, retinoblastoma, familial exudative vitreoretinopathy, retinopathy of prematurity nematode infestation, and astrocytoma of the retina. A Coats'-type response has also been reported in 1.2 to 3.6 per cent of patients with retinitis pigmentosa.

References

Coats G: Forms of retinal disease with massive exudation. Roy Lond Ophthal Hosp Rep 18:440–525, 1907–1908.

Egerer I, Tasman W, Tomer TL: Coats' disease. Arch Ophthalmol 92:109–112, 1974.

Fox KR: Coats' disease. Metabol Pediatr Ophthalmol 4:121–124, 1980.

Harris GS: Coats' disease, diagnosis and treatment. Can J Ophthalmol 5:311–320, 1970.

Kahn JA, et al: Coats'-type retinitis pigmentosa. Surv Ophthalmol 32:317–332, 1988.

Ridley M, et al: Coats' disease: Evaluation of management. Ophthalmology 89:1381–1387, 1982.

DIFFUSE UNILATERAL SUBACUTE NEURORETINITIS (DUSN)

JOSEPH E. ROBERTSON, JR., M.D.
Portland, Oregon

Diffuse unilateral subacute neuroretinitis is a clinical syndrome characterized by visual loss, vitreitis, papillitis, and recurrent crops of gray-white retinal lesions. Progressive visual loss, optic atrophy, retinal vessel narrowing, and diffuse pigment epithelial degeneration may also develop in time. Ocular larvae migrans of nematode origin have been associated with diffuse unilateral subacute neuroretinitis. Initially, *Toxocara canis* was speculated as the nematode causing diffuse unilateral subacute neuroretinitis, but more recently, *Baylisascaris* larvae, especially *B. procyonis* from raccoons, are suspected as the probable cause of diffuse unilateral subacute neuroretinitis. When visualized, the intraocular nematodes are usually detected initially in the macular area during biomicroscopy. They range in size from 400 to 2,000 μM long, are white, often with a glistening sheen, smooth, and gently tapered at both ends. The largest diameter of the nematode is approximately 0.05 times its length. Endemic areas of the United States for this disease appear to be the Southeast and Midwest. The nematode may persist in the fundus for up to 3 years; the various sizes of worm reported are probably due to variations in its age. The nematode is actually identified in only a minority of cases, and it is the other clinical signs that usually lead to the diagnosis. Other clinical presentations include coarse clumping of subretinal pigment that is occasionally arranged in a pattern suggesting tracks and scattered focal chorioretinal atrophic scars. Progressive changes in the structure and function of the eye continue as long as the worm remains viable. There is a reduction in amplitude of both the electroretinogram and electro-oculogram that is proportional to the degree of intraocular damage. In advanced cases, both may be severely reduced or nearly extinguished. The end stage of this process may appear ophthalmoscopically similar to advanced retinitis pigmentosa. However, it is generally quite readily differentiated from retinitis pigmentosa by its unilateral presentation.

THERAPY

Surgical. Laser photocoagulation is effective in destroying the nematode and arresting the destructive process. The toxic damage and atrophic changes that have occurred before initiation of therapy are generally irreversible, although the accompanying inflammation usually slowly subsides after laser treatment.

Ocular or Periocular Manifestations

Optic Nerve: Atrophy; edema; papillitis.
Retina and Retinal Pigment Epithelium: Diffuse or focal atrophy; multifocal gray-white lesions; nematode present; vascular narrowing.
Vitreous: Vitreitis.
Other: Visual loss.

Precautions

Antihelmintic agents, such as thiabendazole and diethylcarbamazepine, are ineffective therapeutically in treating the nematodes associated with diffuse unilateral subacute neuroretinitis. The pathogenesis of this condition seems to involve a local toxic tissue effect on the outer retina caused by the worm products left in the wake and a more diffuse toxic reaction affecting both inner and outer retinal tissues. Although the variability of the inflammatory signs suggests that both the local and diffuse tissue damage are governed by the immune response of the patient, corticosteroids do not seem to have any beneficial effect in preventing this damage.

Comments

Any patient with late or early signs of the neuroretinitis should be investigated for nematodes and questioned for exposure to raccoons or skunks. Biomicroscopy and indirect ophthalmoscopy with a +15 diopter lens or a fundus camera are required to locate the smaller worms. Although inflammatory signs, particularly vitreous cells, are usually present in the late as well as the early stages of the disease, they may be absent, even in an extensively damaged eye containing a viable nematode.

References

Gass JDM, Braunstein RA: Further observations concerning the diffuse unilateral subacute neuroretinitis syndrome. Arch Ophthalmol 101:1689 1697, 1983.
Gass JDM, Scelfo R: Diffuse unilateral subacute neuroretinitis. J Roy Soc Med 71:95–111, 1978.
Gass JDM, et al: Diffuse unilateral subacute neuroretinitis. Ophthalmology 85:521–545, 1978.
Kazacos KR, et al: Diffuse unilateral subacute neuroretinitis syndrome: Probable cause. Arch Ophthalmol 102:967–968, 1984.
Oppenheim S, Rogell G, Peyser R: Diffuse unilateral subacute neuroretinitis. Ann Ophthalmol 17:336–338, 1985.

EALES' DISEASE
(Angiopathia Retinae Juvenilis, Inflammatory Disease of the Retinal Veins, Primary Perivasculitis of the Retina, Primary Retinal Hemorrhage in Young Men, Retinal Periphlebitis, Vasculitis Retinae, Vitreous Hemorrhage of Unknown Etiology)

MICHAEL L. KLEIN, M.D.
Portland, Oregon

Eales' disease was first described in 1880 as a condition in young males that was characterized by recurrent intraocular hemorrhages associated with enlarged and tortuous retinal veins and with concurrent findings of headache, constipation, and epistaxis. Soon thereafter, inflammation of the retinal veins was implicated in this disease entity, leading to subsequent recognition of periphlebitis as its most important feature. The most commonly proposed etiology has been allergy to tuberculoprotein.

In recent years, several disease entities have been identified, each having clinical features indistinguishable from Eales' disease. Thus, the diagnosis of this disease has become less common.

Today, the term "Eales' disease" refers to those cases of periphlebitis without apparent etiology. Sheathing and obstruction of retinal veins, usually in the periphery, associated with retinal hemorrhages and capillary nonperfusion, and the development of neovascularization, with its sequelae of vitreous hemorrhage, fibrous proliferation, retinal detachment in the posterior segment, and neovascular glaucoma in the anterior segment, comprise the full spectrum of changes that may be seen in this condition.

THERAPY

Surgical. Laser photocoagulation is recommended for those cases with retinal neovascularization. Scatter treatment in the nonperfused area surrounding the new vessels and in the area peripheral to them should be applied to produce regression. This may be supplemented with local treatment to the new vessels if they are lying flat on the retina. Panretinal photocoagulation is indicated for neovascular glaucoma.

Vitrectomy should be considered for those cases in which vitreous hemorrhage has remained 6 months or longer. During this waiting period, ultrasonography should be employed to establish that an accompanying retinal detachment is not present. If such is the case, immediate surgical intervention is indicated.

Ocular. No form of medical therapy has been shown to be of any benefit. Systemic corticosteroids[‡] have been used extensively, but their value has not been established.

Ocular or Periocular Manifestations

Optic Nerve: Edema.
Retina: Capillary nonperfusion; detachment; hemorrhages; neovascular glaucoma; rubeosis; perivascular exudate; perivascular sheathing; venous dilation; venous obstruction.
Vitreous: Hemorrhage.

PRECAUTIONS

Photocoagulation can be associated with complications that include hemorrhage from treated neovascular fronds, choroidal hemorrhage, choroidal vitreal neovascularization, and macular pucker.

COMMENTS

Before a diagnosis of Eales' disease can be made, patients must receive a thorough workup to rule out several known conditions that produce this clinical picture. These include varieties of hemoglobinopathies, blood dyscrasias, connective tissue disorders, and inflammatory diseases. A chest x-ray should be included in such a workup to rule out sarcoidosis and tuberculosis.

References

Elliot AJ: Periphlebitis retinae. *In* Duane TD (ed): Clinical Ophthalmology. Hagerstown, MD, Harper & Row, 1982, Vol III, pp 16:1–6.
Renie WA, et al: The evaluation of patients with Eales' disease. Retina 3:243–248, 1983.
Spitznas M: Eales' disease: Clinical picture and treatment with photocoagulation. *In* L'Esperance FA Jr (ed): Current Diagnosis and Management of Chorioretinal Diseases. St. Louis, CV Mosby, 1977, pp 513–521.
Tasman W: Eales' disease, Coats' disease and Leber's miliary aneurisms. *In* L'Esperance FA Jr (ed): Current Diagnosis and Management of Chorioretinal Diseases. St. Louis, CV Mosby, 1977, pp 159–163.
Wise GN, Dollery CT, Henkind P: The Retinal Circulation. New York, Harper & Row, 1971, pp 377–381.

GYRATE ATROPHY OF THE CHOROID AND RETINA WITH HYPERORNITHINEMIA
(Ornithine-δ-Amino Transaminase Deficiency)

RICHARD G. WELEBER, M.D.,
and NANCY G. KENNAWAY, D.Phil.
Portland, Oregon

Gyrate atrophy of the choroid and retina is a rare, autosomal recessive, progressive dystrophy that is associated with hyperornithinemia and deficient activity of ornithine-δ-amino transaminase (OAT), which is a pyridoxal phosphate-dependent enzyme required for the synthesis of proline from ornithine. The disease is characterized by circular patches of total vascular choroidal atrophy, which begin in the periphery in early childhood, enlarge and coalesce, and eventually extend toward the posterior pole. Constriction of the visual field, night blindness, cataracts, defective color vision, retinal vascular leakage, peripapillary atrophy, and macular changes develop as the disease progresses. Rarely, macular edema results. Myopia of moderate to severe degree is frequent. Legal blindness usually occurs in the fourth to fifth decade. Electroretinogram (ERG) responses and electrooculogram (EOG) light-induced rise of the resting potential of the eye, as measured by the light to dark ratios, are consistently abnormal and eventually obliterated. Seizures or abnormal electroencephalography or both have been reported. Although the neuromuscular and electromyographic examinations are normal, eosinophilic subsarcolemmal deposits, which appear as tubular aggregates on electron microscopy, are seen on muscle biopsy. They may be secondary to inhibition of creatine synthesis by ornithine.

Parents who are carriers of this condition are normal clinically. Siblings may be affected and should be evaluated by determination of serum ornithine levels and fundus examination, as eye disease may be unrecognized.

At least two forms of gyrate atrophy with hyperornithinemia are known: a vitamin B_6 nonresponsive form, and a slightly milder vitamin B_6 responsive form. An even milder form of total vascular atrophy of the peripheral choroid and retina resembling gyrate atrophy exists; these patients have normal serum ornithine levels and normal OAT activity in cultured skin fibroblasts.

THERAPY

Systemic. Supplemental pyridoxine in daily doses of 15 to 600 mg can result in over 50 per cent reduction of the serum ornithine in vitamin B_6 responsive patients; large doses (600 to 750 mg daily) have produced mild improvement in the ERG, EOG, and dark adaptometry in certain patients. However, chorioretinal atrophy has continued to progress despite partially reduced serum ornithine levels following vitamin B_6 administration.

Severe dietary arginine restriction can reduce the elevated serum ornithine levels in patients who do not respond biochemically to oral pyridoxine. Some patients have had improvements in visual acuity, ERG, visual field, color vision, and dark adaptometry after prolonged marked reduction of serum ornithine by dietary restriction of arginine. However, more recent studies have documented continual progression of atrophy of choroid and retina despite normal or near normal plasma ornithine concentrations in children 3 to 4.5 years of age.

Oral supplementation with creatine (1.5 gm daily) has been reported to reverse the muscle abnormalities but to have no effect on the retina. Supplementary proline may possibly lessen the progression of the retinal lesions in some patients.

Ocular. No known topical therapy is effective. Optical correction of myopia is indicated. Occasionally, cataract extraction is warranted.

Ocular or Periocular Manifestations

Choroid: Atrophy.
Iris: Atrophy; loss of pigment.
Lens: Subcapsular cataracts.
Optic Nerve: Pallor; peripapillary atrophy.
Retina: Abnormal dark adaptometry; abnormal EOG; atrophy; macular edema; subnormal or nonrecordable ERG; traction schisis; vascular leakage and shunt vessels; vascular sheathing and attenuation.
Vitreous: Opacity.
Other: Constriction of visual fields; decreased visual acuity; dyschromatopsia; moderate to high myopia.

PRECAUTIONS

Since pyridoxal phosphate is the co-factor for OAT, certain patients with gyrate atrophy may respond clinically and biochemically to oral pyridoxine supplementation. Short-term mild improvements in the ERG, EOG, and localized dark adaptometry have been reported with treatment. However, not all patients respond to pyridoxine; further studies will be necessary in those who do respond to determine whether the long-term course of the disease can be slowed or halted.

Vitamin B_6 is present in varying amounts in food and multiple vitamin preparations. At least one patient has been incorrectly considered a nonresponder because of failure to respond to large doses of supplemental pyridoxine at a time when the patient was already receiving supplemental pyridoxine sufficient to lower serum ornithine. Therefore, patients should be without any supplemental pyridoxine for several weeks before judging their biochemical responsiveness to oral vitamin B_6. Since high-dose pyridoxine supplementation is relatively innocuous, even nonresponders should probably be treated. Careful periodic documentation of retinal function over many years will be needed in order to determine stability or progression of the disease.

Dietary restriction of arginine requires an extremely low-protein diet that is both unpalatable and potentially dangerous. Careful monitoring of serum ammonia and nitrogen balance is essential.

Comments

Gyrate atrophy is one of the very few hereditary dystrophies of the choroid and retina that is potentially treatable. However, since treatment requires extensive clinical and biochemical evaluation and monitoring, patients should be referred to tertiary care centers, preferably those where active research on such disorders is in progress.

References

Berson EL, Schmidt SY, Shih VE: Ocular and biochemical abnormalities in gyrate atrophy of the choroid and retina. Ophthalmology 85:1018–1027, 1978.

Hayasaka S, et al: Clinical trails of vitamin B_6 and proline supplementation for gyrate atrophy of the choroid and retina. Br J Ophthalmol 69:283–290, 1985.

Kaiser-Kupfer MI, et al: Gyrate atrophy of the choroid and retina: Improved visual function following reduction of plasma ornithine by diet. Science 210:1128–1131, 1980.

Kennaway NG, Weleber RG, Buist NRM: Gyrate atrophy of choroid and retina: Deficient activity of ornithine ketoacid aminotransferase in cultured skin fibroblasts. N Engl J Med 297:1180, 1977.

McInnes RR, et al: Hyperornithinaemia is gyrate atrophy of the retina: Improvement of vision during treatment with a low-arginine diet. Lancet 1:513–517, 1981.

Shih VE, et al: Ornithine ketoacid transaminase deficiency in gyrate atrophy of the choroid and retina. Am J Hum Genet 30:174–179, 1978.

Vannas-Sulonen K, et al: Gyrate atrophy of the choroid and retina: A five-year follow-up of creatine supplementation. Ophthalmology 92:1719–1727, 1985.

Vannas-Sulonen K, Simell O, Sipilä I: Gyrate atrophy of the choroid and retina: The ocular disease progresses despite normal or near normal plasma ornithine concentration. Ophthalmology 94:1428–1433, 1987.

Weleber RG, Kennaway NG: Clinical trial of vitamin B_6 for gyrate atrophy of the choroid and retina. Ophthalmology 88:316–324, 1981.

Weleber RG, Kennaway NG: Gyrate atrophy of the choroid and retina. In Heckenlively JR (ed): Retinitis Pigmentosa. Philadelphia, JB Lippincott, 1988, pp 198–220.

Weleber RG, Kennaway NG, Buist NRM: Gyrate atrophy of the choroid and retina: Approaches to therapy. Int Ophthalmol 4:23–32, 1981.

Weleber RG, Wirtz MK, Kennaway NG: Gyrate atrophy of the choroid and retina: Clinical and biochemical heterogeneity and response to vitamin B_6. Birth Defects 18:219–230, 1982.

PERIPHERAL RETINAL BREAKS AND DEGENERATION

JULIAN J. NUSSBAUM, M.D.,
and H. MACKENZIE FREEMAN, M.D.
Boston, Massachusetts

The most common degenerative processes affecting the peripheral retina include retinal breaks, cystoid degeneration, acquired retinoschisis, paving-stone degeneration, lattice degeneration, peripheral tapetoretinal degeneration, and snowflake degeneration.

Peripheral retinal breaks may be classified into three types. The most common retinal break to cause retinal detachment is a retinal tear, which occurs as a result of increasing vitreous traction on a vitreoretinal adhesion. Tears are usually U- or V-shaped, with the base located anteriorly and the flap pointing posteriorly. Occasionally, the flap may be completely avulsed and appears as an operculum floating in the vitreous cavity. Histologic studies reveal that a retinal tear shows smooth rounded edges and a vitreoretinal adhesion. The photoreceptor layer of the retinal flap may demonstrate various stages of degeneration, depending on the age of the tear, and subretinal fluid may be seen along its margins.

Rhegmatogenous detachments caused by dialyses usually occur more slowly than those caused by other retinal breaks. There are three types of retinal dialyses. Dialysis or disinsertion of the retina occurs in utero, leading to subsequent retinal detachment at birth or in later years. A second type of dialysis accompanies blunt ocular trauma, is the most common cause of traumatic retinal detachment, and is usually found superonasally. A third type of dialysis occurs spontaneously, most often under 20 years of age and nearly always under 40 years. It affects the lower temporal quadrants, is frequently bilateral, and is occasionally familial. On pathologic examination, the dialysis is seen as a separation of the retina from the nonpigmented ciliary epithelium at the ora serrata. With trauma, an associated avulsion of the vitreous base and detachment of the ciliary epithelium may be seen as a ribbon-like structure in the vitreous.

Retinal holes are the least common retinal breaks to cause retinal detachment. They are round or oval shaped and may be seen alone or in areas of retinal degeneration. When studied pathologically, retinal holes have smooth borders without operculum or flap and are usually found within the area of the vitreous base.

Cystoid degeneration may appear as small, closely packed, parallel reddish cysts that run in a meridional direction around the peripheral retina and sometimes involve the teeth of the ora serrata. There is a greater predilection for the temporal retina. In "typical" cystoid degeneration, microcysts are located in the outer plexiform and outer nuclear layers, whereas in "reticular" cystoid degeneration, these cysts lie primarily in the nerve fiber layer. This is a benign condition seen in most eyes of patients older than 8 years of age and requires no treatment.

Acquired retinoschisis may initially appear as an exaggeration of cystoid degeneration of the peripheral retina, most often located in the inferotemporal quadrant. This degenerative process may progress nasally and, in rare cases, posteriorly, sometimes forming a large cyst-like elevation. The thin inner layer appears transparent with the exception of the retinal vessels and small snowflake-like deposits that help identify it. The outer layer may appear as a faint gray haze over the red choroidal pattern. When retinal holes occur in acquired retinoschisis, they are usually small and numerous in the inner layer, but tend to be large in the outer layer. Histologic examination shows that the splitting occurs in the outer plexiform layer, with the schisis cavity bridged by the remnants of neural processes and Müller's cells. Retinal detachment is rare in acquired retinoschisis, but may occasionally be seen when breaks are present in both layers of the schisis cavity.

Scalloped, sharply demarcated, yellow-white areas of chorioretinal atrophy characterize the lesions seen in paving-stone degeneration. Histologically, there is loss of the pigment epithelium and underlying choriocapillaris, leaving an atrophic retina opposed to Bruch's membrane. Because of this loss, the retina may remain attached in these areas, even when the remainder of the retina is detached. Tears may sometimes occur along the margin and may show degeneration.

Lattice degeneration is a circumferentially oriented lesion of retinal thinning that is usually located at or anterior to the equator. Pigment clumping is common. Its name is derived from the interlacing branching pattern of sclerotic vessels bridging the lesion. Although less than 1 per cent of patients with lattice degeneration will subsequently develop a retinal detachment, approximately one fourth to one third of retinal detachments are attributable to retinal breaks associated with lattice degeneration. These breaks are usually atrophic round holes within lattice or retinal tears along the margins where the strong vitreoretinal adhesion exists. Studied microscopically, it is an area of inner retinal atrophy with overlying vitreous liquefaction and persistent strong vitreous adhesion to its margins.

Peripheral tapetoretinal degeneration appears clinically as diffuse chorioretinal atrophy and granular pigment clumping. Histopathologically, it consists of retinal pigment epithelial and choriocapillaris atrophy with secondary photoreceptor loss. It is essentially an exaggeration of the peripheral changes seen in the normally aging eye. It is a benign process requiring no treatment.

Snowflake degeneration is characterized clinically by a myriad of yellow-white dots resembling snowflakes that are primarily located in the peripheral retina. It is a hereditary progressive process associated with vitreous degeneration, extensive whiteness from pressure, and devascularization of the affected retinal areas. The lesions become pigmented in later stages. Patients with snowflake degeneration have a higher incidence of retinal breaks and detachment, as well as presenile cataract formation.

THERAPY

Supportive. It is important to have an understanding of which retinal breaks should be treated and which can be observed. The incidence of retinal breaks without retinal detachment is approximately 7.8 per cent or about 16 million persons in the United States. Since the annual incidence of retinal detachment is about 1:9000 persons, it is obvious that the majority of retinal breaks do not result in retinal detachment and therefore do not require treatment. Therefore, when a retinal break is found, consideration should be given not only to the characteristics of the break itself but also to other ocular findings, including conditions in the other eye, and the patient's age, occupation, activity level, and family history of retinal detachment.

The characteristics of the retinal break are important factors in deciding whether treatment is indicated. All symptomatic or asymptomatic retinal tears and retinal dialyses should be treated. The larger and the greater the number of retinal breaks, the stronger and more urgent are the indications for treatment. Retinal detachment from breaks located superiorly, temporally, and posteriorly poses a greater threat to the macula than those located nasally, anteriorly, and inferiorly. For this reason, prophylactic treatment of retinal breaks with the above-mentioned characteristics is recommended.

Retinal breaks found in eyes with high myopia, retrolental fibroplasia, vitreous hemorrhage, and chronic uveitis have a greater predisposition toward retinal detachment. Treatment is indicated when breaks occur in eyes with a developing cataract because the ability to visualize an early detachment decreases as the lens becomes more cataractous. In addition, it is important to study the fellow eye for retinal breaks, and a history of retinal detachment in the fellow eye is a strong indication for treatment.

Retinal breaks found in patients with Marfan's syndrome, Wagner-Stickler syndrome, Ehlers-Danlos syndrome, and atopic dermatitis should be treated because of the poorer prognoses associated with these connective tissue diseases.

Surgical. The treatment of retinal breaks without detachment involves one or a combination of three modalities: photocoagulation, cryopexy, or scleral buckling with encircling band. Photocoagulation is a valuable tool for the nonsurgical treatment of retinal holes located posterior to the equator. It is often the treatment of choice for round holes in areas of chorioretinal degeneration without evidence of vitreous traction or hemorrhage. Photocoagulation may also be used in retinal tears with a free operculum and in the treatment of outer layer breaks in retinoschisis. Treatment of peripheral retinal breaks is done in an outpatient setting using the argon laser and three-mirror Goldmann lens. The pupil is dilated as widely as possible; only topical anesthetics are used. The patient is comfortably seated at the slitlamp delivery system, and a triple row of laser burns is placed around the posterior, lateral, and, where applicable, anterior margins of the lesion. Extensive photocoagulation may require more than one treatment session. Lesions are of moderate intensity. Average settings may vary according to the type of laser used; the presence of corneal, lenticular, or vitreous opacities; and the degree of pigment epithelial and choroidal pigmentation.

Cryotherapy is ideally suited for anteriorly located retinal breaks. It is usually carried out in an outpatient setting with topical and subconjunctival anesthesia. Subconjunctival anesthesia is preferred over retrobulbar anesthesia when treatment will not be extensive. It is a safer procedure because the needle tip is always visualized under the conjunctiva. In highly myopic eyes, retrobulbar anesthesia may be hazardous because the needle could penetrate a large posterior staphyloma. After the globe has been anesthetized topically with tetracaine or proparacaine, the bulbar conjunctiva is gently grasped with smooth forceps over the quadrant where treatment is to be performed. Two per cent lidocaine is then injected subconjunctivally, utilizing a tuberculin syringe and a short 30-gauge needle. When extensive treatment is indicated or when the patient is very young, or very old or debilitated, the procedure may be done in the operating room with cardiac monitoring. Treatment is carried out under direct visualization, utilizing indirect ophthalmoscopy and scleral depression with the tip of the cryoprobe. Pressure should be firm, and the probe tip should not be moved once freezing has commenced. Two rows of overlapping cryo lesions are placed along the posterior, lateral and, when possible, the anterior margins of the lesion, as well as freezing the break itself.

After photocoagulation or cryotherapy is completed, topical antibiotics are administered and the eye is temporarily patched for 24 hours (if not monocular). The patient is re-examined 2 weeks later, at which time pigmentation should be seen in the treated areas. If adequate treatment is noted, the patient is re-examined at 2 months and then every 6 to 12 months, depending on the nature of the underlying pathology (high myopia with lattice degeneration, history of giant tear in the fellow eye, etc.).

Scleral buckling reduces vitreous traction and is therefore beneficial in treating patients with large horseshoe tears and multiple or recurrent retinal breaks. The use of an encircling element provides permanent indentation and reduces the incidence of implant extrusion. When treating a retinal break with scleral buckling procedures, it is important to provide adequate treatment margins with cryopexy or diathermy. Two to three rows of diathermy should be placed along the posterior and lateral margins of the retinal break and, if possible, one row along the anterior border.

Precautions

Treatment must provide an adequate margin of chorioretinal adhesion along all borders of the lesion. However, excessive photocoagulation or cryotherapy should be avoided because they may cause complications of treatment, including retinal or choroidal hemorrhage, exudative choroidal and retinal detachment, and preretinal membrane formation or contracture.

Comments

It must be remembered that the great majority of peripheral retinal degenerations and breaks do not result in retinal detachment and warrant no intervention. No form of prophylactic therapy is free from the risk of complications. Therefore, when a retinal break is found, the decision "to treat or not to treat" should be made on a patient by patient basis.

References

Benson WE, Morse PH: The prognosis of retinal detachment due to lattice degeneration. Ann Ophthalmol 10:1197–1200, 1978.

Byer NE: Lattice degeneration of the retina. Surv Ophthalmol 23:213–248, 1979.

Foos RY: Retinal holes. Am J Ophthalmol 86:354–358, 1978.

Freeman HM: Fellow eyes of giant retinal breaks. Trans Am Ophthalmol Soc 76:343–382, 1978.

Freeman HM, et al: Retinal detachment in Marfans' and Marfans'-like syndromes. In press.

Hagler WS, Jarrett WH II, Chang M: Rhegmatogenous retinal detachment following chorioretinal inflammatory disease. Am J Ophthalmol 86:373–379, 1978.

Hirose T, et al: Acquired retinoschisis: Observations and treatment. In Pruett RC, Regan CDJ (eds): Retina Congress. New York, Appleton-Century-Crofts, 1974, pp 489–504.

Hirose T, Wolf E, Schepens CL: Retinal functions in snowflake degeneration. Ann Ophthalmol 12:1135–1146, 1980.

McPherson A, O'Malley R, Beltangady SS: Management of the fellow eyes of patients with rhegmatogenous retinal detachment. Ophthalmology 88:922–934, 1981.

Pollak A, Oliver M: Argon laser photocoagulation of symptomatic flap tears and retinal breaks of fellow eyes. Br J Ophthalmol 65:469–472, 1981.

Sigelman J: Vitreous base classification of retinal tears: Clinical application. Surv Ophthalmol 25:59–74, 1980.

Takahashi M, et al: Biomicroscopic evaluation and photography of liquefied vitreous in some vitreoretinal disorders. Arch Ophthalmol 99:1555–1559, 1981.

Tolentino FI, Schepens CL, Freeman HM: Vitreoretinal Disorders: Diagnosis and Management. Philadelphia, WB Saunders, 1976.

Verdaguer J, Vaisman M: Treatment of symptomatic retinal breaks. Am J Ophthalmol 87:783–788, 1979.

REFSUM'S DISEASE
(Heredopathia Atactica Polyneuritiformis, Phytanic Acid Oxidase Deficiency)

RICHARD G. WELEBER, M.D.
Portland, Oregon

Refsum's disease is a rare autosomal recessive syndrome characterized by chronic polyneuropathy, cerebellar ataxia, atypical retinitis pigmentosa, and ichthyosiform skin lesions. Raised tissue and blood levels of phytanic acid, an abnormality related to deficient phytanic acid oxidation, are present. The age of onset varies from the first to the fifth decade of life. Although phytanic acid is stored in fatty tissues, symptoms of the disease are related to the concentration of phytanic acid in the blood, rather than total body stores. The earliest symptom is almost invariably night blindness, which usually occurs before age 20. Electroretinogram responses are profoundly abnormal or nondetectable. The disturbance in retinal pigmentation, which early in the disease is often limited to the periphery, may be granular, rather than "bone-spicule." Weakness in the extremities, unsteadiness of gait, and a history of chronic exacerbations and remission are common. Complete external ophthalmoplegia has been reported. Often, the diagnosis of Friedreich's ataxia is entertained. However, tendon reflexes that are initially undetectable may return weeks or months later. Invariably, cerebrospinal fluid shows an elevation of protein content without pleocytosis. Hearing may become defective, and cataracts may occur. Orthopedic deformities of the foot and epiphyseal dysplasia have been reported. Ichthyosiform skin lesions may wax and wane with the rising and falling of serum phytanic acid level. Impairment of renal function has also been reported. Impaired atrial-ventricular conduction, bundle-branch blocks, and cardiac arrhythmia may have contributed to the occasional occurrence of sudden death. Untreated, the life expectancy is shortened.

THERAPY

Systemic. Since phytanic acid is not metabolized in patients with Refsum's disease and the only source of phytanic acid in humans in dietary, restriction of oral intake of phytanic acid and phytol (which is readily converted into phytanic acid) has been advised and found beneficial. Specifically, dietary intake of chlorophyll, dairy products, and ruminant fats, all containing phytanic acid or phytol or both, must be markedly curtailed. Caution should be observed to avoid starvation diets, as they can cause rapid mobilization of body stores of phytanic acid with marked increase in the elevation of serum phytanic levels, acute toxicity, cardiac arrhythmias, and possible cardiac arrest. Plasma exchange appears to be a very useful treatment to lower plasma phytanic acid concentrations rapidly and has a very definite role in the treatment of acute toxic states.

Supportive. Refsum's disease is an autosomal recessive genetic trait. Carriers with dietary loading may show elevated phytanic acid levels. However, carrier detection is best determined by assay of phytanic acid alpha-oxidase activity in cultured skin fibroblasts. Since cultured amniocentesis cells show that the enzyme activity, antenatal diagnosis of the affected or carrier state is theoretically possible.

Ocular or Periocular Manifestations

Optic Nerve: Partial demyelination.
Retina: Lipid deposits in pigment epithelium with degeneration of overlying photoreceptors.
Sclera: Lipid deposits.
Other: Lipid deposits in trabecular meshwork.

PRECAUTIONS

If started early, dietary restriction may possibly prevent the development of neuromuscular and retinal changes. However, no conclusive evidence of improvement in retinal function has been reported with dietary or plasma exchange therapy. This may reflect the extent of irreversible damage to the retina. Early recognition and prompt treatment may forestall the development of these irreversible visual changes, although no improvement in the vision of patients with well-advanced disease should be expected. Since careful monitoring of diet and serum phytanic levels is required, these patients should probably be referred to tertiary medical centers for medical evaluation and therapy.

COMMENTS

Definite improvement clinically and biochemically has been reported with reduction of dietary phytanic acid and plasma exchange. Muscle strength, tendon reflexes, sensory and motor nerve conduction, and certain objective tests of coordination have improved with treatment. The ichthyosiform rash and cardiac arrhythmias also clear as the serum phytanic acid decreases. One 39-year-old patient treated with diet over the past 13 years has shown only minimal progression of the visual findings during this period of time.

References

Gibberd FB, et al: Heredopathia atactica polyneuritiformis (Refsum's disease) treated by diet and plasma-exchange. Lancet *1*:575–578, 1979.

Hansen E, Bachen NI, Flage T: Refsum's disease. Eye manifestations in a patient treated with low phytol low phytanic acid diet. Acta Ophthalmol 57:899–913, 1979.

Masters-Thomas A, et al: Heredopathia atactica polyneuritiformis (Refsum's disease): 1. Clinical features and dietary management. J Hum Nutr *34*:245–250, 1980.

Masters-Thomas A, et al: Heredopathia atactica polyneuritiformis (Refsum's disease): 2. Estimation of phytanic acid in foods. J Hum Nutr 34:251–254, 1980.

Kahlke W: Refsum-Syndrome. Lipoidchemische Untersuchungen bei 9 Fällen. Klin Wochenschr 42:1011–1016, 1964.

Penovich PE, et al: Note on plasma exchange therapy in Refsum's disease. Adv Neurol 21:151–153, 1978.

Refsum S: Heredopathia atactica polyneuritiformis; familial syndrome not hitherto described; contribution to clinical study of hereditary diseases of nervous system. Acta Psychiatr Neurol 38(Suppl):1–303, 1946.

Refsum S: Heredopathia atactica polyneuritiformis phytanic acid storage disease (Refsum's disease) with particular reference to ophthalmological disturbances. Metabol Ophthalmol 1:73–79, 1977.

Steinberg D: Phytanic acid storage disease (Refsum's disease). In Stanbury JB, et al (eds): The Metabolic Basis of Inherited Diseases, 5th ed. New York, McGraw-Hill, 1983, pp 731–747.

Steinberg D, et al: Conversion of U-C^{14}-phytol to phytanic acid and its oxidation in heredopathia atactica polyneuritiformis. Biochem Biophys Res Commun 19:783–789, 1965.

Steinberg D, et al: Refsum's disease—a recently characterized lipoidosis involving the nervous system. Ann Intern Med 66:365–395, 1967.

Steinberg D, et al: Phytanic acid in patients with Refsum's syndrome and response to dietary treatment. Arch Intern Med 125:75–87, 1970.

RETINAL DETACHMENT

HARVEY LINCOFF, M.D.,
New York, New York

and INGRID KREISSIG, M.D.
Tübingen, West Germany

Retinal detachment is a separation of the sensory retina from the pigment epithelium. There are three mechanisms of detachment: rhegmatogenous or break-induced, tractional, and exudative. It is necessary to distinguish which mechanism is operative in a patient because the treatment for each is different.

Rhegmatogenous retinal detachment occurs most frequently, although its incidence is only 1 in 20,000 individuals. The retina separates because a break (tear, hole) occurs in the sensory retina that allows fluid from the vitreous to seep between the rods and cones of the retina and the villi of the pigment epithelium. The tearing of the retina is an acute episode, with symptoms of flashes as the nerve fibers part and of spots as retinal blood vessels are ruptured and bleed.

The detachment of the retina proceeds in a predictable manner from the break that has caused it. After first separating the retina around the break, subretinal fluid dissects to the ora serrata. Once a significant bulla has formed in the periphery, the effects of gravity and motion cause a rapid progression dependently and toward the disc. The patient perceives the advance as a dense curtain with a convex edge encroaching on the visual field. Detachments that originate from a break in the inferior retina progress upward toward the disc, but more slowly.

The topography of a rhegmatogenous retinal detachment is diagnostic. The elevation has convex edges and convex surfaces. If the detachment is of any duration, it will extend from ora to disc and have alternate bullae and folds (hills and valleys), all oriented in a radial direction (from ora to disc). The retina itself is edematous; it has lost the transparency that it had when attached and the "pigment epithelial pump" was clearing it. Finding a break in the retina confirms the rhegmatogenous nature of the detachment.

Tractional retinal detachment occurs in patients with an antecedent history of diabetes or other vasculopathies, perforating injury, and as a complication of retinal detachment surgery. All of these disorders can cause an abnormal bonding of the vitreous membranes to the internal surface of the retina. In the diabetic, vascular leaking seems to be the factor that incites proliferation of glial cells and fibroblasts on the surface of the retina. Actin filaments have been demonstrated in the proliferating cells, and it is believed that it is a contraction of these filaments that creates the tractional forces that detach the retina. The retinas of patients with perforating injuries detach because vitreous membranes have prolapsed through the wound and the shortened membranes that remain within the eye shrink and pull upon the retina.

Tractional detachment is a slowly progressive disorder that occasionally arrests. Rarely, a taut vitreous membrane pulls free from the surface of the retina, and the retina reattaches. Tractional detachment in the periphery may be without symptoms, unless hemorrhage on a retinal tear intervenes. The cellular structure and physiology of retinal traction, called periretinal vitreoretinopathy, are under intense investigation. Cell growth inhibitors, such as fluorouracil, have been injected into vulnerable eyes to inhibit periretinal vitreoretinopathy.

The topography of the tractional retinal detachment is diagnostic of its nature. All of its surfaces and some of its borders are concave. It can occur centrally or peripherally, but has a limited extent. In the diabetic, it tends to begin centrally around the disc and along the major vessels. Probably because the retina is thick centrally, it tends not to tear. The detachment rarely progresses beyond the equator, and peripheral vision can be maintained for years. If a retinal break does occur, peripheral vision is wiped out within hours, and examination reveals that the detachment has extended to the ora serrata and its surfaces have become convex, confirming its rhegmatogenous conversion.

Exudative retinal detachment arises from choroidal tumors (melanoma and metastatic tumors), retinal tumors (retinoblastoma and angioma), and some poorly understood inflammatory disorders, such as Coats' and Harada's diseases. The detachments become symptomatic only after they invade the macula and interfere with central vision. Like rhegmatogenous detachments, they have convex surfaces and convex borders. If the subretinal fluid is less than maximum, exudative detachments characteristically shift to that portion of the eye that is dependent. When the patient is upright, the fluid distributes symmetrically around 6 o'clock; when the patient is on the side, it runs up the dependent side. In the supine position, the fluid collects centrally, and small amounts of fluid may be overlooked. Patients with small amounts of fluid report that they have poor vision upon awakening in the morning and that their vision improves as the day progresses. Maximum exudative detachments elevate the retina in all four quadrants and detach the ciliary epithelium as well; the retina bulges anteriorly behind the lens so much as to be perceptible with a pen light.

THERAPY

Surgical. Most operations for rhegmatogenous detachment can be completed in less than 2 hours and so can be done under retrobulbar anesthesia. A lid block is not required. An adequate scleral field is made available if the conjunctival incision extends 90° to either side of the breaks. The breaks are located by directing a scleral depressor (usually a cyroprobe) to them while the retina is being observed with the indirect ophthalmoscope. The position of the break is marked on the sclera with ink or cautery. The edges of the break are treated with transcleral cryopexy.

The break is closed by compressing an elastic silicone sponge over it with a mattress suture tied under tension. One mattress suture with long intrascleral limbs (6 mm) is preferable to multiple sutures with short intrascleral passages, as the short ones tear out. Compression of the sponge causes an abrupt rise in the intraocular pressure, and it is necessary to monitor the central retinal artery to be sure that it has not closed as a result. Momentary closure of a pulsating artery is not infrequent. The artery reopens in seconds if the patient does not have glaucoma. Reopening can be accelerated by digital massage. As the eye decompresses over the ensuing hours, the sponge expands beneath the break, creating a buckle (intrusion) high enough to close it. With the pathway between the vitreous and the subretinal space closed by the buckle, the fluid beneath the retina is absorbed by the pigment epithelium, and the retina reattaches usually within 24 hours.

Whenever possible, the scleral sponge is oriented with its long axis in a radial direction. This is because the retina, fixed at the disc and the ora serrata, tends to form radial folds when detached. Circumferentially oriented buckles augment this tendency. When a fold falls into alignment with a retinal tear that is stretched across a circumferential buckle, the tear tends to open like a fish's mouth (called "fish mouthing") and enables vitreous fluid to continue to leak into the subretinal space, sustaining the detachment. Radial buckles fill the folds and prevent this complication.

There are limits to the application of radial buckles. Most retinal breaks are smaller than 3 mm and can be closed by a 5-mm radial sponge sewn in place with an 8-mm mattress suture; 8 mm is also the half circumference of the sponge and the width of the buckle. Breaks as large as 6 mm can be closed by a 7.5-mm oval sponge held in place with a 10-mm mattress suture. Breaks as large as 8 mm can be closed with two 7.5-mm overlapping sponges tied in place with a mattress suture with intrascleral limbs that are 14 mm apart. The 8-mm break and two sponges side by side mark the limit of the radial sponge operation. Three or more sponges or a mattress suture longer than 14 mm have little compression potential and make a poor buckle.

Radial buckling without drainage of subretinal fluid can be done for breaks larger than 8 mm (40° at the equator) and up to 14 mm (70°) by resorting to a scleral pouch operation. The pouch is made from a Dacron-reinforced silicone sheet cut to a radial shape and sewn over the retinal break. The elastic buckling effect is obtained by stuffing it with silicone sponge pellets. The pouch operation is time consuming, but has a reattachment rate of 95 per cent, which is as good as that of the sponge operation.

Tears longer than 70° are fortunately infrequent. When encountered, they can only be buckled circumferentially; the posterior edge of a radial pouch larger than 70° would intrude upon the posterior pole. Because circumferential buckling of long tears is especially prone to cause "fish mouthing," these tears are treated instead with intravitreal tamponades of air, gas, or silicone oil with and without vitrectomy.

The perfluorocarbon gases, which expand the injected volume by two to five times, have simplified and diminished the morbidity of intraocular gas tamponades by eliminating the need for drainage of subretinal fluid or vitrectomy to make space for an adequate gas bubble. Because of the success of the expanding gases in treating large tears (60 to 70 per cent), the gas technique has been proposed as a primary outpatient procedure for less formidable retinal detachments. The procedure is called pneumatoretinopexy. However, intraocular gas augments and may even provoke periretinal vitreoretinopathy and are not appropriate for detachments that might be treated with an external buckle, a procedure with less morbidity and a better rate of reattachment.

Ninety per cent of retinal detachments are suitable for treatment without drainage of subretinal fluid. Four per cent of these will fail to reattach completely because of another break that was undetected. Providing that the break that was buckled was the superior one, the upper border of the detachment will fall close to the level of the additional break and help detect it. Three per cent will fail because the buckle was inadequate (either too small or poorly placed). Three per cent will fail because of periretinal vitreoretinopathy. One per cent of patients will have delayed absorption because their pigment epithelium and choriocapillaris are inadequate; these patients are usually elderly or myopic. Patients in the first two categories will respond to a second buckling procedure without drainage of subretinal fluid. Elderly or myopic patients with an atrophic pigment epithelium and choriocapillaris probably ought to be drained initially if the break is in the inferior retina. If the break is above and secure on the buckle, the patient may be left to absorb the fluid over weeks or months. The patient is cautioned to sleep with the head elevated to prevent pooling of the fluid in the macula. Patients with developing periretinal vitreoretinopathy will require drainage and an operation to counteract or remove the traction on the retina. The choices for a secondary operation include encircling procedures and vitrectomy.

Less than 10 per cent of patients are selected for drainage in the primary procedure because 1) the retinal break is on the posterior slope of a bulla, and localization may be uncertain because of parallax; 2) they have glaucoma; 3) the sclera is staphylomatous and will not tolerate an increase in intraocular pressure; or 4) there is advanced periretinal vitreoretinopathy, and the break is posterior and caught up in it.

Diabetic traction detachment was refractory to treatment until the advent of vitrectomy, an operation that strips or severs the membranes on the surface of the retina. The operation has a significant morbidity, and recurrence is frequent. Vitrectomy is usually deferred until the macula becomes detached.

Peripheral traction detachments occur in eyes with retinopathy of prematurity, peripheral choroiditis, perforating injuries, or peripheral vasculopathies, such as sickle-cell disease. The loss of vision in the periphery may not be noticed by the patient. An examination of the peripheral retina reveals a concave elevation of the retina. The elevation may extend to the ora serrata, but rarely progresses posteriorly beyond the equator. Unless the detachment becomes rhegmatogenous, treatment is best deferred. Prophylactic scleral buckling has little value because the buckle cannot be made high enough to relieve traction without causing anterior chamber ischemia. Vitrectomy seems a correct approach, but is technically difficult to perform in the periphery. On the other hand, after a perforating injury, a vitrectomy that removes the central vitreous matrix and the track of the perforation reduces the incidence of traction detachment in this group of patients. A recent randomized study indicated that cryopexy to the avascular periphery of children with retinopathy of prematurity reduces the incidence of traction detachment.

If the exudating lesion in an exudative detachment can be obliterated, the subretinal fluid will be absorbed and the retina will become reattached and function again. The detachment that might accompany a melanoma will flatten within weeks after the tumor is treated with 8000 rads from a radioactive plaque, either cobalt[60] or iodine[125]. The detachment that accompanies metastatic tumor disappears after beam radiation of about 6000 rads. The same holds true for the detachment that accompanies retinoblastoma after it is treated with 3000 rads. Reattachment of the retina in a patient with angiomatosis will occur if the lesion can be destroyed with light or cryocoagulation. These tumors are difficult to manage if they are large because they tend to exudate severely as an acute response to the treatment. Preliminary coagulation around the angioma will not prevent this response. The exudative detachment that accompanies Coats' disease will regress if the vascular lesions can be obliterated with photocoagulation. The detachment that accompanies a uveitis and Harada's disease sometimes responds to steroid treatment.

The draining of subretinal fluid in an exudative detachment is to be avoided because the drainage site must be elevated for access. This causes the subretinal fluid to shift away from the drainage site so that the perforation for drainage is likely to perforate the retina or cause it to become incarcerated in the drainage site.

Precautions

The drainage of subretinal fluid is the most traumatic part of a retinal detachment procedure and has a significant intraocular morbidity; it can cause hemorrhage, retinal incarceration, choroidal effusion, and uveitis. The occurrence of hemorrhage may be minimized by transilluminating the choroid at the drainage site before perforation so as to be able to recognize and avoid perforating a choroidal vessel. Incarceration can be avoided if the retina is kept under ophthalmoscopic observation while the subretinal fluid is draining and the drainage site is closed when the retina comes in contact with it. Choroidal effusion and uveitis are the effects of temporary hypotony after drainage. Both are usually benign and recover spontaneously or with steroid therapy.

The extraocular complications of scleral buckling are infection of the buckle and diplopia. With the new silicone sponges and prophylactic subtenon gentamicin at the conclusion of the operation, the incidence of infection is less than 0.5 per cent. The manifestations of an infected explant depend upon the infecting organism. Infections caused by *Proteus* or *Staphylococcus aureus* become evident in the first to third postoperative week by a draining fistula anterior to the explant. Antibiotics will not cure the condition. The presence of pain signals uveal irritation and the need to remove the explant without delay. Most postoperative infections are however caused by *S. epidermidis* and are more benign. They manifest as pink, sticky eyes persisting for months after the operation. An examination of the conjunctival wound anterior to the buckle reveals a flat fleshy granuloma. Excision of the granuloma and the application of antibiotics ameliorate the symptoms, but they will recur. A cure can only be effected by removing the explant. The incidence of redetachment after removing a buckle is between 5 and 10 per cent. The orbit is sterile 5 days after the explant is removed and will accept rebuckling if it is required.

Diplopia occurs when a radial sponge is fixed beneath a rectus muscle, especially when it is fixed anterior to the equator. The incidence of diplopia will be reduced if the muscle is detached and transplanted adjacent to the explant. The balloon buckle causes diplopia when it is inflated beneath a muscle, but within hours after it is deflated and removed, the muscle functions normally again.

COMMENTS

Reattachment of the retina is obtained by an operation directed solely at closing the retinal breaks. Finding the breaks is done preoperatively by examination techniques that include indirect ophthalmoscopy with scleral depression and slitlamp biomicroscopy through a three-mirror contact lens, also with scleral depression. It can be a laborious task if the breaks are small. The task can be made easier by first defining the shape of the detachment, because just as the detachment proceeds in a predictable manner from the break that caused it, so the eventual shape of the detachment indicates the location of the primary break (the superior break that alone could produce the detachment).

Retinal detachments can assume three different shapes or patterns: 1) detachments that extend into the superior temporal or nasal quadrants; 2) superior detachments that cross the 12 o'clock radian and proceed down both sides of the eye to become total, and 3) inferior detachments. The analysis of a large series of retinal detachments indicates that in superior nasal or temporal detachments the primary break lies within 1.5 clock hours of the superior border of the detachment 98 per cent of the time; in superior detachments that cross the 12 o'clock radian, the break lies within a triangle whose apex is at 12 o'clock and whose sides intersect the equator 1 hour to either side of 12 o'clock 93 percent of the time; in inferior detachments, the higher border of the detachment indicates that side of the 6 o'clock radian on which the break will be found 95 per cent of the time. More than one break is present in about 70 per cent of retinal detachments. The secondary breaks tend to be located in the following order of frequency: 1) adjacent to the primary break, 2) remote from the primary break but in the same latitude, and 3) elsewhere.

Immobilization of the eye preoperatively by binocular occlusion and bedrest are useful adjuncts to therapy. Immobilization may curtail progression of the retinal detachment, a consideration that is important when the macula is still attached but threatened. Immobilization may diminish the elevation of the retinal bullae, making localization of the break at the operation more accurate. In a few patients (less than 10 per cent), it will effect complete reattachment of the retina and enable the repair to be accomplished solely by applying laser or cryopexy to the edges of the break. The earliest sign of settling of the retina is a crinkling effect on the posterior edges of the bullae. If the crinkling sign appears within 24 hours, it is worth delaying surgery in expectation of additional flattening.

References

Algvere P; Rosengren B: Immobilization of the eye. Evaluation of a new method in retinal detachment surgery. Acta Ophthalmol 55:303–316, 1977.

Blumenkranz MS, et al: Fluorouracil for the treatment of massive periretinal proliferation. Am J Ophthalmol 94:458–467, 1982.

Coleman DJ: Early vitrectomy in the management of the severely traumatized eye. Am J Ophthalmol 93:543–551, 1982.

Cryotherapy for Retinopathy of Prematurity Cooperative Group: Multicenter trial of cryotherapy for retinopathy of prematurity: Preliminary study. Arch Ophthalmol 106:471–479, 1988.

Kreissig I, et al: The treatment of difficult retinal detachments with an expanding gas bubble without vitrectomy. Graefes Arch Clin Exp Ophthalmol 224:51–54, 1986.

Lincoff H: The rationale for radial buckling. Mod Probl Ophthalmol 12:484–491, 1974.

Lincoff H, Kreissig I: Patterns of non-rhegmatogenous elevations of the retina. Br J Ophthalmol 58:899–906, 1974.

Lincoff H, Kreissig I: Results with a temporary balloon buckle for the repair of retinal detachment. Am J Ophthalmol 92:245–251, 1981.

Lincoff H, Kreissig I, Hahn YS: An elastic pouch operation for large retinal tears. Arch Ophthalmol 97:708–710, 1979.

Machemer R: Vitrectomy in diabetic retinopathy. Removal of preretinal proliferations. Trans Am Acad Ophthalmol Otolaryngol 79:394–395, 1975.

Tasman W, et al: Cryotherapy for active retinopathy of prematurity. Ophthalmology 93:580–585, 1986.

RETINAL EMBOLI
DAVID J. WILSON, M.D.
Portland, Oregon

An embolism is the sudden partial or complete obstruction of a vessel by a clot or foreign material brought to its place of lodgement by the blood current. Retinal emboli are of particular interest because the accessibility of the retinal circulation to examination permits documentation of suspected emboli.

A great variety of materials have been reported as retinal emboli, including platelets and fibrin, cholesterol, calcific material from diseased heart valves, fat following long bone fracture, air after chest compression injuries, atrial myxoma, metastatic tumor, amniotic fluid, septic emboli in bacterial endocarditis, leukocyte aggregates, talc and corn starch in intravenous drug abusers, corticosteroids after intranasal or retrobulbar steroid injections, and cloth material from prosthetic heart valves. By far, the most common source of retinal emboli is ulcerated atheromatous plaques in the carotid artery. These emboli may occur spontaneously or after manipulation of the carotid arteries during arteriography or surgery.

From a therapeutic viewpoint, retinal emboli are important because of their ocular sequelae and because they indicate the potential for emboli to the brain. Emboli are probably the most common cause of branch retinal artery occlusion and are a major cause of central retinal artery occlusion. However, other causes for arterial occlusion that should be considered in the differential diagnosis include atheromatous disease of the central retinal artery and arteritis of the retinal vessels. For additional information, see central or branch retinal artery occlusion (pp. 663–665).

THERAPY

Ocular. The goals of treatment are improvement in vision and movement of the emboli to a more distal location in the retinal circulation. Treatment should be administered without delay. It has been demonstrated in monkeys that occlusion of the central retinal artery longer than approximately 100 minutes results in irreversible retinal damage. The patient should be placed in the supine position with the legs elevated. If this is not successful, brisk tapping and massaging of the eye are performed to try and move the emboli downstream. An anterior chamber paracentesis may be done to improve the arterial perfusion pressure, and intravenous acetazolamide (0.5 to 1.0 gm) may be given to prolong ocular hypotony. If these measures are not successful, treatment with Carbogen (95 per cent oxygen and 5 per cent carbon dioxide) by mask should be tried. This therapy should be continued for 50 minutes of every hour for 24 to 36 hours if any sign of improvement is observed.

Recently, tissue plasminogen activators have been used in the treatment of occluded coronary arteries. Animal experiments have suggested that these agents may be of benefit in platelet fibrin emboli of the retinal circulation. However, use of these agents for human retinal emboli is experimental and should only be undertaken in the proper setting.

The end point of successful treatment with all of the above measures is improvement in vision and movement of the emboli to a more distal location in the retinal circulation.

Systemic. In addition to treating the ocular consequences of retinal emboli, treatment of the source of the emboli should be attempted to prevent additional retinal emboli or emboli to the brain. Consultation with an internist, neurologist, or cardiologist may be beneficial in evaluating the carotid arteries for evidence of atherosclerosis, the heart for valvular disease (including mitral valve prolapse) and atrial myxoma, and the hematologic status for evidence of a hypercoagulable state (particularly the lupus anticoagulant). Before recommending carotid endarterectomy for carotid artery disease, it is important to weigh the risks and benefits for each particular patient.

Ocular or Periocular Manifestations

Optic Nerve: Anterior ischemic optic neuropathy.
Retina: Central or branch retinal artery occlusion; retinal emboli.
Other: Cerebrovascular accident; signs of cardiac valvular disease; transient ischemic attacks.

PRECAUTIONS

Approximately 5 per cent of cases of central retinal artery occlusion are caused by giant cell arteritis. These cases should be differentiated from cases of embolic central retinal artery occlusion by history, erythrocyte sedimentation rate, and temporal artery biopsy.

COMMENTS

The treatment of retinal artery occlusion as a result of emboli is usually unsatisfactory. Few patients regain lost vision. However, in the setting of an acute embolic occlusion, the above measures should be employed to minimize the amount of visual loss. A systemic evaluation to determine the source of the emboli is important to prevent subsequent emboli.

References

Hayreh SS, Weingeist TA: Experimental occlusion of the central retinal artery of the retina. IV: Retinal tolerance time to acute ischemia. Br J Ophthalmol 64:818–825, 1980.
Levine SR, et al: Visual symptoms associated with the presence of a lupus anticoagulant. Ophthalmology 95:686–692, 1988.
Rossmann H: Treatment of retinal arterial occlusion. Ophthalmologica 180:68–74, 1980.
Trobe JD: Carotid endarterectomy: Who needs it? Ophthalmology 94:725–730, 1987.
Vine AK, et al: Recombinant tissue plasminogen activator to lyse experimentally induced retinal arterial thrombi. Am J Ophthalmol 105:266–270, 1988.
Young BR, Rosenbaum TJ: Treatment of acute central retinal artery occlusion. Mayo Clin Proc 53:408–410, 1978.

RETINAL VEIN OBSTRUCTION
LARRY E. MAGARGAL, M.D.,
and H. LOGAN BROOKS, M.D.
Philadelphia, Pennsylvania

Patients with retinal vein obstruction typically present with painless visual loss. The fundus is characterized by venous dilation and tortuosity, retinal and nerve fiber layer infarction, and retinal edema distal to the site of obstruction. Retinal vein obstructions are divided into macular, peripheral, temporal, hemispheric, and central according to the drainage area affected, and are classified as hyperpermeable, indeterminate, or ischemic according to the angiographic pattern. Hyperpermeable venous occlusive disease is characterized by vascular leakage from an intact capillary system, whereas ischemic occlusions show widespread zones of capillary dropout on fluorescein angiography. A clinically useful fluorescein angiogram may be difficult to obtain secondary to lens changes, small pupil, or extensive retinal hemorrhages. Even with a high-quality fluorescein angiogram, there can be disagreement among experienced observers concerning the amount of capillary nonperfusion. Therefore, clinical parameters, such as visual acuity, presence of an afferent pupillary defect, number of cotton-wool spots, extent of retinal hemorrhages, and visual field defects, are very important in classifying the vein occlusion clinically. In addition, electroretinography may also prove useful for determination of significant ischemia. Clinically, acute ischemic venous obstruction exhibits nerve fiber layer infarcts and more extensive retinal hemorrhages than hyperpermeable patterns.

Venous obstruction may be the result of impaired venous outflow, impaired arterial inflow, or thrombosis caused by intravascular or platelet coagulation pathway abnormalities. Impaired venous outflow is caused most often by progression of external compression of the vein by its diseased companion retinal artery at an arteriovenous crossing. For example, since the central retinal artery and vein share a common adventitial sheath as they pass through the lamina cribosa, atherosclerosis, optic disc drusen, or disc edema, or other changes in the optic nerve head architecture, such as glaucomatous disc cupping, may lead to central retinal vein occlusion. Impaired arterial inflow is usually related to ipsilateral internal carotid artery stenosis, which produces chronic ophthalmic artery insufficiency that can manifest initially as venous stasis retinopathy or as the ocular ischemic syndrome in those cases progressing to complete carotid stenosis. Stagnation thrombosis may be caused by an increase in the cellular components of the bloodstream, as in the polycythemic or leukemic states, or by an increase in the noncellular components of the bloodstream, as in the hyperglobulinemic conditions; the thrombosis may also be related to abnormalities in the size, shape, or aggregability of red blood cells and platelets. When inflammation is associated with an acute vein obstruction usually a marked cellular reaction is present in the vitreous, definite foci of inflammation are in the retina, and there is perivascular infiltration (phlebitis). Occult inflammation, if it occurs at all, is a rare cause of venous obstructive disease. Central retinal vein occlusion is bilateral in 5 per cent of cases, and bilaterality is more common if there is an underlying hyperviscosity condition.

The risk of developing complications is directly related to the type of venous obstruction and the degree and duration of retinal ischemia. In hyperpermeable patterns, the extent and duration of macular edema are the main therapeutic concerns, whereas in ischemic patterns, neovascularization and its sequelae are prominent. The principal complications of central retinal vein obstruction are iris neovascularization and secondary neovascular glaucoma, which occur in 20 per cent of cases overall (1 per cent of hyperpermeable cases and 60 per cent of ischemic ones). Retinal neovascularization, seen in 2 to 3 per cent of cases, and optic disc neovascularization, present in 25 per cent of cases, may lead to vitreous hemorrhage and traction retinal detachment. Some degree of macular edema is universal. Ischemic central retinal vein obstructions tend to progress from early stages of iris neovascularization to complete angle closure and absolute glaucoma within weeks. Patients who develop neovascular glaucoma tend to be older and have a higher incidence of pre-existent open-angle glaucoma and atherosclerotic vascular disease.

Branch retinal vein obstruction causes visual loss by associated macular edema or vitreous hemorrhage from retinal or disc neovascularization. After proliferative diabetic retinopathy, branch vein occlusion is the second leading retinal vascular cause of spontaneous vitreous hemorrhage. Neovascular glaucoma is rare, occurring in less than 1 per cent of patients with ischemic temporal branch retinal vein obstructions. Macular vein occlusion (17 per cent of all branch vein occlusions) is universally associated with macular edema. Neovascular complications do not occur in macular vein occlusions, presumably because of the small area of retina involved. Ischemic hemispheric vein occlusions have a 20 per cent risk of developing disc or retinal neovascularization and a 15 per cent risk of neovascular glaucoma. Peripheral retinal vein occlusions occur, but are rarely recognized unless there are associated retinal neovascularization and vitreous hemorrhage. Disc neovascularization and neovascular glaucoma are exceedingly rare in patients with peripheral vein occlusions.

THERAPY

Systemic. Therapy with steroids or anticoagulants (heparin or warfarin) has been unsuccessful in achieving significant visual improvement or lessening the incidence of neovascular complications. No medical therapy has proven to be of value in improving visual function in patients with venous occlusive disease associated with impaired venous outflow. In cases where a high-grade, hemodynamically significant carotid stenosis is associated with venous stasis retinopathy, carotid surgery may be of benefit. If hematologic evaluation identifies blood component pathology, the management of the venous occlusive disease should include treatment of the underlying condition. For instance, aspirin, sulfinpyrazone, or antiplatelet agents may be useful in the management of patients with increased platelet aggregability, or plasmapheresis may be indicated in certain hyperviscosity conditions. The safety and efficacy of an intravenous fibrinolytic agent (tissue plasminogen activator) are currently being prospectively evaluated.

Surgical. Argon laser panretinal photocoagulation has been proven effective in reducing the risk of neovascular glaucoma in eyes with ischemic central retinal vein obstructions. Prophylactic panretinal photocoagulation completed in two to three sessions has been shown to virtually eliminate the risk of developing neovascular glaucoma in these otherwise high-risk ischemic eyes. Although panretinal photocoagulation can cause regression of iris and angle neovascularization, the intraocular pressure will remain elevated if the anterior chamber angle has been completely obliterated by peripheral anterior synechiae. If the vision remaining is useful to the patient, consideration may be given to glaucoma surgery. The inherent difficulties in following high-risk patients clinically and angiographically at frequent intervals over extended periods of time, the tendency for rapid progression of early iris neovascularization to neovascular glaucoma, and the relatively poor results following treatment in advanced cases make the early recognition of high-risk eyes capable of developing neovascular glaucoma essential and the initiation of prophylactic panretinal photocoagulation the treatment of choice in this disorder. Hyperpermeable cases, which have only a 1 per cent risk of developing neovascular glaucoma, can be followed and treated if they convert to an ischemic pattern. Treatment with macular grid laser photocoagulation of the persistent macular edema that is seen frequently in hyperpermeable cases is currently being studied prospectively.

The Branch Vein Occlusion Study has helped clarify the criteria for management of macular edema and neovascularization associated with branch vein occlusion. Patients at least 3 months after vein occlusion with persistent macular edema and with decreased vision to the 20/40 range or worse are eligible for a grid laser photocoagulation treatment to the edematous retina outside the foveal avascular zone. Treatment benefit was noted after 3 years of follow-up, with the average visual acuity in the treatment group of 20/40 to 20/50 versus 20/70 in the untreated eyes.

The incidence of disc and retinal neovascularization at 3 years in eyes with at least 5 disc diameters of retinal involvement was reduced from 22 to 12 per cent by sector photocoagulation to the involved extrafoveal area. Three-year follow-up in eyes with posterior segment neovascularization had vitreous hemorrhage reduced from 61 to 29 per cent in cases treated with sector laser photocoagulation. Despite evidence that prophylactic laser reduces the incidence of neovascularization, there was no conclusive evidence that long-term visual acuity was improved compared to eyes receiving laser after neovascularization develops. Controversy exists because the Branch Vein Occlusion Study was not designed to study the timing of the laser photocoagulation or vitreoretinal relationships. A recent study found that 55 per cent of eyes with at least 5 disc diameters of capillary nonperfusion and no or partial vitreous detachment developed neovascularization compared to 7 per cent of eyes with equivalent nonperfusion and complete vitreous detachment. Therefore, patients with attached or incomplete vitreous detachment and significant nonperfusion must be followed more closely.

Ocular or Periocular Manifestations

Anterior Chamber: Angle closure; cells and flare (with neovascular glaucoma).
Iris: Neovascularization; peripheral anterior synechiae.
Optic Nerve: Collateral vessels; edema; glaucomatous cupping (often best seen contralaterally); hemorrhage; neovascularization; optic atrophy.
Retina: Attenuated arteries; breaks; collateral vessels; cotton-wool spots; cystic degeneration; edema; exudate; hemorrhage; microaneurysm; neovascularization; preretinal membranes; traction retinal detachment (late); venous dilation.
Vitreous: Hemorrhage; neovascularization.
Other: Afferent pupillary defect; glaucoma.

PRECAUTIONS

Retinal vein obstruction occurs with increased frequency in patients over 50 years of age with systemic hypertension and generalized vascular disease. Diabetes mellitus is also more common in patients with vein occlusions than in the general population. Pre-existing increased intraocular pressure is a risk factor in central retinal vein occlusion, with one third of patients demonstrating contralateral pressure elevation and disc cupping, but is found much less often in branch vein, macular vein, and hemispheric vein occlusions. Other systemic conditions, such as hematologic abnormalities, coagulation disorders, collagen diseases, hyperproteinemias, and hyperlipidemias, are less commonly associated with retinal vein occlusions. In young patients with vein occlusions, abnormal platelet function is common, particularly in patients with migraine syndromes and mitral valve prolapse and those on certain hormonal therapies. Because of the diversity of associated conditions, it is recommended that the ophthalmologist obtain appropriate consultations to help detect these associated conditions.

COMMENTS

Patients with an ischemic central retinal vein occlusion and a visual acuity of 20/400 or worse should receive prompt panretinal photocoagulation treatment, thereby avoiding painful neovascular glaucoma and maintaining vision. Hyperpermeable vein occlusions with good acuity should be followed, and a prospective trial is underway for grid laser photocoagulation of persistent macular edema. There is no proof that any medication, including antiplatelet agents (such as low-dose aspirin), prevents hyperpermeable patterns from progressing to ischemic ones, but there is a theoretical rationale for its use and the authors currently recommend it.

Branch vein occlusion with persistent macular edema can be treated with laser photocoagulation to improve visual acuity. Scatter laser photocoagulation in eyes with neovascularization and branch vein occlusion reduces the risk of subsequent vitreous hemorrhage. Prophylactic laser photocoagulation is controversial in branch vein occlusion at this time. Close follow-up and possible "early" laser are needed in eyes with significant capillary nonperfusion and vitreous that is attached or incompletely detached. Complete vitreous detachment markedly decreases the incidence of neovascularization, despite significant capillary nonperfusion.

References

Branch Vein Occlusion Study Group. Argon laser photocoagulation for macular edema in branch vein occlusion. Am J Ophthalmol 98:271–282, 1984.
Branch Vein Occlusion Study Group. Argon laser scatter photocoagulation for prevention of neovascularization and vitreous hemorrhage in branch vein occlusion: A randomized clinical trial. Arch Ophthalmol 104:34–41, 1986.
Brooks HL Jr, et al: More information needed regarding neovascularization and vitreous hemorrhage in branch vein occlusion. Arch Ophthalmol 105:311, 1987.
Gonder JR, et al: Central retinal vein obstruction in the young adult. Can J Ophthalmol 18:220–222, 1983.
Joffe L, et al: Macular branch vein occlusion. Ophthalmology 87:91–98, 1980.
Johnson MA, et al: Neovascularization in central retinal vein occlusion: Electroretinographic findings. Arch Ophthalmol 106:348–352, 1988.
Kado M, Trempe C: Role of the vitreous in branch retinal vein occlusion. Am J Ophthalmol 105:20–24, 1988.
Magargal LE, et al: Neovascular glaucoma following branch retinal vein obstruction. Glaucoma 3:333–335, 1981.
Magargal LE, et al: Neovascular glaucoma following central retinal vein obstruction. Ophthalmology 88:1095–1101, 1981.
Magargal LE, et al: Efficacy of panretinal photocoagulation in preventing neovascular glaucoma following ischemic central retinal vein occlusion. Ophthalmology 89:780–784, 1982.
Magargal LE, et al: Retinal ischemia and risk of neovascularization following central retinal vein obstruction. Ophthalmology 89:1241–1245, 1982.
Magargal LE, et al: Temporal branch retinal vein obstruction: A review. Ophthalmic Surg 17:240–246, 1986.
Sanborn GE, Magargal LE: Characteristics of the hemispheric retinal vein occlusion. Ophthalmology 91:1616–1624, 1984.

RETINITIS PIGMENTOSA
SAUL MERIN, M.D.
Jerusalem, Israel

Retinitis pigmentosa is an inherited progressive disease of the retina that is characterized by early and diffuse functional retinal abnormalities, a subnormal or "extinct" (nonrecordable) electroretinogram, early involvement of the retinal pigment epithelium and visual receptors, and an outcome of severely impaired vision or blindness. The symptoms of retinitis pigmentosa usually become apparent during the second decade of life, but are sometimes present in early childhood. Night blindness is usually the earliest symptom, followed by progressive loss of peripheral visual fields. Sometimes, central vision is involved early. Before the involvement of central vision, the patient may be aware of deterioration of color vision. Progression of morphologic changes of the fundus depends upon the genetic entity and varies in different types of retinitis pigmentosa.

THERAPY

Ocular. A flush-fitting, opaque scleral contact lens to produce monocular complete light deprivation has been used to slow down the degenerative changes that may occur when the eye is exposed to light, but a follow-up of two such patients for 5 years did not reveal any significant difference in the natural course of the disease. The possibility that partial and selective light restriction may be of benefit is being investigated. Until the final results of these studies become known, recommendations based on theoretical and clinical considerations suggest that patients with retinitis pigmentosa wear dark sunglasses for outdoor use, especially in bright sunlight. Side shields added to the dark sunglasses are helpful to restrict further the amount of sunlight reaching the eye. Special sunglasses that reduce considerably (more than 75 per cent) the total transmission of light and cut out the lower wavelengths of light and the ultraviolet rays are produced by several manufacturers and are commercially available.

Correction of associated refractive errors and the use of low vision aids may help improve central vision. Optical devices may be used to widen the visual fields in patients with good central vision and narrow visual fields. An image intensifier may be used to improve vision in the darkness. Early clinical trials have been encouraging. A wide-field-high-intensity lantern has also been found useful and practical for night mobility.

Surgical. Patients with advanced retinitis pigmentosa often suffer from a posterior cortical cataract. Even when the electroretinogram is very low or extinct, such patients may benefit from cataract extraction if their macular function is still preserved. In such cases, the best preoperative test is the visual evoked potential; its presence indicates good macular function. Studies indicated increased patient's satisfaction when an intraocular lens is implanted. A ultraviolet-shielded intraocular lens is advisable.

Some patients with retinitis pigmentosa develop telangiectatic capillaries in the retina, followed by extensive intraretinal and subretinal leakage of the Coats'-like variety and neovascularization on the disc and elsewhere. Panretinal photocoagulation by laser was found to be effective in reducing the complications from this condition, especially recurrent intravitreal hemorrhage.

Grid laser therapy has been used to reduce visual loss associated with cystoid macular edema, which is frequently found in retinitis pigmentosa patients. Its beneficial effect has not yet been confirmed.

Supportive. Genetic counseling should be provided. The probability of an affected person having affected children depends on the mode of inheritance if the genetic type can be accurately diagnosed. In isolated cases, the risk of affected children depends on the severity of the disease in the affected parent, the gender and the prevalence of the various types of retinitis pigmentosa in his own family population.

Ocular or Periocular Manifestations

Choroid: Disappearance of choriocapillaries; loss of larger choroidal vessels (late).
Optic Nerve: Pallor.
Retina: Attenuated arteries; depigmentation of pigmentary epithelium; edematous (tapetal) reflex of pigmentary epithelium; fine pigmentary stippling; thinning; vascular pigmentary sheathing.
Other: Dyschromatopsia; midperipheral ring scotoma; night blindness; progressive constriction of peripheral visual fields; visual loss.

PRECAUTIONS

Many drugs, operations, and bizarre procedures for the treatment of retinitis pigmentosa have been suggested. These include anticoagulants,[‡] xanthinol niacinate[‡] and other vasodilators, RNA, retrobulbar injections[*] of hyaluronidase and acid phosphates, and even subconjunctival injection[*] of peat distillate. Transplantation of human placenta, practiced for many years, continues to be used by some. Surgical transplantation of strips of extraocular muscles has been suggested to improve choroidal blood flow. It has been reported that patients responded favorably to exposure to ultrasonics and acupuncture. However, reliable evidence of the success of any of the treatments mentioned above is not available.

Vitamin A[‡] has been used for the treatment of retinitis pigmentosa, but there is no evidence of a beneficial effect from this vitamin or its derivatives; it is possible that such treatment even has a deleterious effect. Vitamin E[‡] has also been employed in the treatment of this disease; it too probably has no demonstrable benefit in the isolated form of retinitis pigmentosa.

Intramuscular injections of a ganglioside preparation were recently attempted, but their value has not yet been confirmed.

COMMENTS

Retinitis pigmentosa is associated with a variety of disease entities including lipid disorders, mucopolysaccharidosis, spinocerebellar degenerations, and other seemingly unrelated conditions. Their association with retinitis pigmentosa is still not understood, but it is conceivable that in some of these diseases, such as Refsum's syndrome, dietary control may prove useful in avoiding or retarding some of the retinal changes observed. Combined vitamin A and E therapy seems to be efficient in arresting the visual deterioration of retinitis pigmentosa associated with abetalipoproteinemia.

References

Berson EL: Experimental and therapeutic aspects of photic damage to the retina. Invest Ophthalmol 12:35–44, 1973.
Berson EL: Light deprivation and retinitis pigmentosa. Vision Res 20:1179–1184, 1980.
Bishara S, et al: Combined vitamin A and E therapy prevents retinal electrophysiological deterioration in abetalipoproteinemia. Br J Ophthalmol 66:767–770, 1982.
Lenk W: Nutritional and metabolic aspects of heredopathia atactica polyneuritiformis (Refsum's syndrome). Nutr Metab 16:366–374, 1974.
Merin S, Auerbach E: Retinitis pigmentosa. Surv Ophthalmol 20:303–346, 1976.
Muller DPR, Lloyd JK, Bird AC: Long-term management of abetalipoproteinaemia. Possible role for vitamin E. Arch Dis Child 52:209–214, 1977.
Newsome DA, Blacharski PA: Grid photocoagulation for macular edema in patients with retinitis pigmentosa. Am J Ophthalmol 103:161–166, 1987.
Noah VB: Genetic counseling in retinitis pigmentosa. Med Coll Va Q 8:283–285, 1972.
Runge P, et al: Oral vitamin E supplements can prevent the retinopathy of abetalipoproteinemia. Br J Ophthalmol 70:166–173, 1986.
Steinberg D, et al: Phytanic acid in patients with Refsum's syndrome and response to dietary treatment. Arch Intern Med 125:75–87, 1970.
Uliss AE, Gregor ZJ, Bird AC: Retinitis pigmentosa and retinal neovascularization. Ophthalmology 93:1599–1603, 1986.

RETINOPATHY OF PREMATURITY
(Retrolental Fibroplasia, RLF, ROP)
ROBERT E. KALINA, M.D.
Seattle, Washington

Retinopathy of prematurity (ROP) is a disorder of immature retinal blood vessels occurring in premature infants. The incidence is related inversely to birth weight. Oxygen in excess of need is thought to play a role by causing vaso-obliteration in the immature peripheral retina, but other factors likely also play a causative role. Presumably in response to peripheral retinal ischemia, neovascularization later develops just posterior to the junction of vascularized and nonvascularized retina. Such neovascularization most reliably is detected 6 or more weeks after birth and usually regresses spontaneously. However, in some cases, fibrous proliferation, vitreous hemorrhage, and retinal detachment supervene, and the proliferative phase leads to irreversible cicatricial changes. Cicatricial changes may range from mild dragging of the retina compatible with good visual acuity to a complete retrolental mass and phthisis bulbi. Cicatricial changes are usually completed by 15 months of age or earlier.

THERAPY

Supportive. The best therapy for ROP is prevention. The recognition of the causal relationship of oxygen in excess of need to ROP produced a dramatic decline in its incidence, but new cases continue to occur, despite the sophisticated neonatal intensive care techniques and oxygen monitoring that are available today. In general, modern-day cases appear to be less severe than those occurring in the past. However, the most severe cases now occur in very low birth weight infants (<1000 gm), a group more likely to survive with modern neonatal techniques. Since prematurity has become the most important cause of ROP, prevention ultimately rests with public health measures designed to reduce the incidence of premature birth.

Premature infants, particularly those receiving oxygen therapy, should be examined for ROP at approximately 6 weeks of age or at the time of discharge home. Infants showing ROP or those in whom vascularization of the peripheral retina is incomplete should be examined again at intervals of 1 to 6 weeks, depending upon the severity of the disease process. The binocular indirect ophthalmoscope should be used, together with an eyelid speculum, after dilation of the pupils with 2.5 per cent phenylephrine combined with either 0.5 per cent cyclopentolate or 0.5 per cent tropicamide. Children with cicatricial changes should be followed throughout life, particularly in the childhood and adolescent years, to prevent further visual loss because of amblyopia, retinal detachment, or angle-closure glaucoma.

Ocular. No topical ophthalmic preparation is known to be effective in preventing or treating ROP. However, severe proliferative ROP is associated with marked ocular inflammation, and instillation of a small amount of 0.5 per cent atropine ointment once daily may reduce posterior synechiae formation or at least allow them to form in a dilated position to permit fundus evaluation.

Surgical. Attempted treatments have included cryotherapy, laser or xenon photocoagulation, and scleral buckling, but only cryotherapy has been proven effective in a prospective controlled clinical trial. Since the proliferative changes of ROP have a remarkable propensity for regression and because cryotherapy can be associated with severe complications, treatment should be reserved for eyes with severe ROP (Stage III "plus").

In eyes in which retinal detachment has developed, cryotherapy no longer is appropriate. Scleral buckling is reasonable for rhegmatogenous retinal detachment, but definite retinal breaks rarely are confirmed in retinal detachments caused by ROP.

In eyes with chronic tractional/exudative retinal detachment, microsurgical techniques of lensectomy and vitrectomy with or without scleral buckling, usually applied between 3 and 12 months of age, have been successful in reattaching the retina in some cases. Even among eyes with initial anatomic success, however, visual results often are disappointing. Indications, timing, and techniques of surgical management continue to evolve.

Systemic. Vitamin E,[‡] an antioxidant, has been found to modify favorably the proliferative retinal vascular changes found in the kitten after oxygen exposure. Preliminary clinical reports have suggested that vitamin E may be efficacious in humans, but a committee of the Institute of Medicine determined that present evidence did not support the use of vitamin E as prophylaxis for ROP. Most institutions are withholding vitamin E supplementation in excess of the amount that is normally part of neonatal intensive care for other indications.

Ocular or Periocular Manifestations

Iris: Anterior or posterior synechiae; neovascularization.
Optic Nerve: "Dragged disc" appearance; pallor.
Retina: Attenuated vessels; detachment; dilated vessels; folds; hemorrhage; neovascularization; pigmentary changes; retrolental mass; vascular tortuosity.
Vitreous: Haze; hemorrhage; traction.
Other: Amblyopia; anisometropia; cataract; glaucoma; leukokoria; myopia; pseudostrabismus; shallow anterior chamber.

Precautions

Because topical medications may cause adverse side effects in premature infants, 10 per cent phenylephrine and 1 per cent cyclopentolate should not be used. If atropine is to be used, the concentration of 0.5 per cent is recommended, preferably in ointment form. Since absorption and systemic toxic effects of ocular medications occur mainly through the nasal mucosa, the amount applied should be minimized (never more than one drop at a time) and excess solution should be wiped away promptly. It may also be helpful to apply pressure on the closed eyelid over the area of the lacrimal sac for a few seconds after instillation of a drop.

Ophthalmoscopic examinations may be traumatic and potentially hazardous to the critically ill infant. Since ROP does not progress to clinical significance for several weeks after birth, examination should be delayed until the infant has stabilized and the risk from topical medications and eye examination can be minimized.

Comments

In addition to recommending cryotherapy for Stage III "plus" ROP, the ophthalmologist may provide a valuable service to premature infants and their families. Families deserve to learn of ROP and its potential complications from the neonatal staff, rather than to discover their infant's visual disability at home. Identification of affected infants may lead to early diagnosis and treatment of complications that threaten further visual loss.

The continuing occurrence of ROP today, despite the sophisticated medical care available, deserves emphasis. Prematurity has superseded oxygen as the prime etiologic factor. Arterial oxygen monitoring has reached a high degree of accuracy, but is limited by intermittent sampling, particularly in infants requiring chronic oxygen therapy and thus at greatest risk for ROP. Transcutaneous oxygen monitoring is helpful in neonatal care, but has not been shown to reduce the incidence of ROP.

Not all cases of proliferative vascular retinopathy in infancy and childhood are ROP. Other etiologic factors should be sought, particularly in other than very low birth weight infants.

References

Chong LP, Machemer R, de Juan E: Vitrectomy for advanced stages of retinopathy of prematurity. Am J Ophthalmol 102:710–716, 1986.
Cryotherapy for Retinopathy of Prematurity Cooperative Group: Multicentered trial of cryotherapy for retinopathy of prematurity. Arch Ophthalmol 106:471–479, 1988.
Committee for the Classification of Retinopathy of Prematurity: An international classification of retinopathy of prematurity. Arch Ophthalmol 102:1130–1134, 1984.
Flynn JT, et al: A randomized, prospective trial of transcutaneous oxygen monitoring. Ophthalmology 94:630–638, 1987.
Institute of Medicine: Vitamin E and Retinopathy of Prematurity. Report of a Study by a Committee of the Institute of Medicine, Division of Health Sciences Policy. Washington, DC, National Academy Press, 1986, pp 1–24.

RETINOSCHISIS
LOUIS DAILY, M.D., Ph.D., (Ophth)
Houston, Texas

Retinoschisis is a condition in which the sensory retina splits at any level between the inner and outer nuclear layers. This split usually occurs bilaterally at the outer plexiform layer, with the accumulation of a mucopolysaccharide-rich viscous fluid within the intervening space. As the schisis progresses, the neural elements of the retina are first stretched and finally lysed, producing absolute visual loss in the affected areas. The bulging internal wall of the cavity is thin and immobile and often has a "beaten metal" appearance. A band of prominent cystoid degeneration separating the cavity from the ora serrata is a common feature. Pigmentary lines usually are a demarcation of a secondary retinal detachment or outer layer breaks in acquired retinoschisis.

Senile (acquired) retinoschisis, which occurs as a result of a degenerative change at the periphery of the retina, affects about 3 per cent of the population and increases in frequency from the second decade onward. Retinoschisis can be a slowly progressive, self-limited disease, or it can lead to holes in both the inner and outer walls and subsequent rhegmatogenous detachment. In the rarer idiopathic or juvenile retinoschisis, a widespread vitreoretinal degeneration occurs that is characterized by onset in the first decade, a hereditary pattern (usually sex-linked and recessive), common macular involvement, and a much poorer prognosis. Unusual and anecdotal causes of clinically observed retinoschisis have been intraretinal hemorrhage in battered babies, retinoschisis secondary to retinal telangiectasia, and tractional retinoschisis in retinopathy of prematurity; the retinal elevation that communicates with optic nerve pits may be a schisis-like separation of the internal layers of the retina.

THERAPY

Surgical. Prophylactic treatment by photocoagulation or preferably by cryotherapy for senile retinoschisis is controversial when the schisis extends to no less than 20° from the macula and does not appear to be progressive. Whether and when to treat inner layer holes, outer layer holes, or the entire area of schisis is also controversial. Cryotherapy performed in two stages—the anterior two thirds first and the remainder several weeks later—probably results in fewer complications, such as macular puckering or massive vitreous or preretinal membrane contraction. The inner layer of the schisis need not be collapsed completely to prevent progression. If the macula is threatened or retinal detachment has developed in the affected eye or is attributed to retinoschisis in the fellow eye, treatment should be given. A retinal detachment associated with retinoschisis should be treated first, and then the schisis should be treated either at the conclusion of the operation or during the postoperative period. However, once the retina is reattached, retinal cysts may resolve spontaneously. When residual schisis is great, the cyst-like fluid should be evacuated during retinal detachment surgery, but the inner layer need not be collapsed completely to prevent schisis progression. Giant outer layer breaks are managed by a variety of surgical techniques, including scleral buckling, cryotherapy, or laser, together with intraocular air and postoperative positioning.

Photocoagulation can be performed with either the xenon arc coagulator or an argon (all wave or green) laser. Photocoagulation must be heavy enough to include the external plexiform layer in the final limiting scar. Settings for either type should be determined by the visible whitening effect of coagulation on the external layer. If part of the schisis is 3 disc diameters or closer to the macula's edge, the coagulation settings of the argon laser for the schisis itself should be 500 to 1000 nm beam diameters for 0.1- to 0.2-second exposure at 500 to 1200 mW power. Cryotherapy, preferably done under direct observation with an indirect ophthalmoscope, should result in whitening of the outer retinal layers and overlapping of the frozen areas.

Because x-linked juvenile retinoschisis is slowly progressive and treatment produces a high incidence of serious complications, prophylaxis to halt its progression is not indicated. The only indication for treatment is recurrent vitreous hemorrhage, for which photocoagulation could be used. The only other indication for treatment of this form of retinoschisis is a rhegmatogenous retinal detachment, for which scleral buckling is the procedure of choice. Vitreous traction on the inner wall of a raised schisis cavity can require vitrectomy, gas fluid exchange, and endolaser.

Ocular or Periocular Manifestations

Optic Nerve: Atrophy.
Retina: Atrophy; "beaten metal" appearance; cysts; deposits; detachment; holes; macular degeneration; peripheral cystoid degeneration; subretinal fibrosis; thinning; vascular sheathing.
Vitreous: Traction.
Other: Decreased visual acuity; scotoma; visual field defects.

PRECAUTIONS

Retinoschisis can be confused with rhegmatogenous retinal detachment. Clinical differentiation can nearly always be made by slitlamp examination through the three-mirror Goldmann contact lens. Focal illumination shows the inner layer of the schisis, as identified by its blood vessels, which can be seen by retroillumination or direct, diffuse, or focal illumination in wide and narrow optical sections. The origin of the schisis can be found with the focal beam. In optical section, the inner layer is thinner and more translucent than a detached retina. It is usually nonmotile, not exhibiting the undulations seen in recent retinal detachments. With the indirect ophthalmoscope, it exhibits the "beaten metal" appearance. Using these examinations, as well as transillumination, fluorescein angiography, and ultrasonography, one should easily be able to differentiate schisis from retinal detachment.

The lesion's progress should be watched carefully. If it has extended posterior to the equator, the visual field should be charted for damage, which does not arise until the central area is threatened.

COMMENTS

The prognosis for senile (acquired) retinoschisis is generally good, for it can remain stationary indefinitely or progress very slowly, and even "schisis-detachment" can remain asymptomatic and nonprogressive. Treatment for asymptomatic retinoschisis would appear to be justified very infrequently.

References

Brockhurst RJ: Comment. Should retinoschisis be treated? *In* Brockhurst RJ, et al. (eds): Controversy in Ophthalmology. Philadelphia, WB Saunders, 1977, p 562.
Brockhurst RJ: Introduction. Should retinoschisis be treated? *In* Brockhurst RJ, et al (eds): Controversy in Ophthalmology. Philadelphia, WB Saunders, 1977, p 541.
Brockhurst RJ: Reinoschisis. Complication of peripheral uveitis. Arch Ophthalmol 99:1998–1999, 1981.
Byer NE: Long-term natural history study of senile retinoschisis with implications for management. Ophthalmology 93:1127–1137, 1986.
DiSclafani M, et al: Pigmentary changes in acquired retinoschisis. Am J Ophthalmol 105:291–293, 1988.
Dobbie JG: Should retinoschisis be treated? *In* Brockhurst RJ, et al (eds): Controversy in Ophthalmology. Philadelphia, WB Saunders, 1977, pp 542–550.
Greenwald MJ, et al: Traumatic retinoschisis in battered babies. Ophthalmology 93:618–625, 1986.
Jabbour NM, et al: Stage 5 retinopathy of prematurity: Prognostic value of morphologic findings. Ophthalmology 94:1640–1645, 1987.
Lincoff H, et al: Retinoschisis associated with optic nerve pits. Arch Ophthalmol 106:61–67, 1988.
Schulman J, et al: Indications for vitrectomy in congenital retinoschisis. Br J Ophthalmol 69:482–486, 1985.
Sulonen JM, et al: Degenerative retinoschisis with giant outer layer breaks and retinal detachment. Am J Ophthalmol 99:114–121, 1985.

SUBRETINAL NEOVASCULAR MEMBRANES

HUNTER L. LITTLE, M.D., F.A.C.S.
Menlo Park, California

Subretinal neovascular membranes are proliferative blood vessels arising from the choriocapillaris and extending through breaks in Bruch's membrane into the tissue plane between Bruch's membrane and the retinal pigment epithelium (RPE). When present in the posterior pole of the eye, subretinal neovascular membranes pose a significant threat of loss of central vision. This problem is extremely common as indicated by the findings that 1) senile macular degeneration is the leading cause of legal blindness in the United States for people over 60 years of age and 2) ocular histoplasmodic choriodopathy ranks second only to diabetes as the leading cause of legal blindness for people under 50 years who live within endemic areas of histoplasmosis in the central and eastern United States. Subretinal neovascular membranes cause serous and hemorrhagic detachments of the retinal pigment epithelium and of the sensory retina in the macula in both senile macular degeneration and the presumed ocular histoplasmosis syndrome, leading to macular destruction and loss of central vision in both diseases. Furthermore, subretinal neovascularization is a frequent sequela in the natural course of serous detachment of the retinal pigment epithelium in elderly patients.

The clinical findings of subretinal neovascular membranes include hemorrhage beneath the sensory retina or beneath the retinal pigment epithelium, subretinal exudate, turbid subretinal fluid, retinal striae, and a notched contour to an RPE detachment. Angiographic findings for subretinal neovascular membranes include reticular vascular pattern; bicycle wheel pattern; serpiginous margin; bright, irregular fluorescent spots; and adjacent blocked fluorescence from hemorrhage. In addition to clinical and angiographic findings, one frequently sees a grayish discoloration at the level of the RPE that corresponds to the subretinal neovascular membrane. If the overlying RPE is atrophic, one can even see the membrane. Subretinal neovascular membranes can be multiple in origin.

Age-related macular degeneration and the ocular histoplasmosis syndrome are the most frequent causes of subretinal neovascular membranes; however, they may also occur in the following conditions: angioid streaks, traumatic ruptures of Bruch's membrane, choroidal scars (rarely with toxoplasmosis or photocoagulation scars), myopic degeneration, overlying choroidal nevi (rarely), end-stage Best's vitelliform macular degeneration, serpiginous or geographic choroiditis, acute multifocal posterior plaquoid posterior epitheliopathy, hamartoma of the retinal pigment epithelium, and optic nerve drusen.

THERAPY

Surgical. The indications for treatment include the following: 1) presence of serous or hemorrhagic detachment of the sensory retina or the RPE or both within the macula, 2) evidence of the presence of a subretinal neovascular membrane, and 3) absence of foveal involvement by the subretinal neovascular membrane.

Laser photocoagulation of subretinal neovascular membranes requires intense confluent photocoagulation burns covering the entire subretinal neovascular membrane and extending, when possible, approximately 200 μM beyond the peripheral margin of the membrane. Typical treatment parameters include a 200-μM diameter burn, 0.2-second exposure time, and 400 to 500 mW of power. These settings are typical for the green argon laser photocoagulator. The power levels for krypton laser photocoagulation are usually lower and the exposure times longer in order to minimize the risk of choroidal hemorrhage. Typical settings for the krypton laser include a 200-μM diameter burn and 0.5- to 1.0- second exposure times with 200 to 300 mW of power. Pressure may be applied to the contact lens to immobilize the eye and to minimize hemorrhage during the course of treatment. The rhodamine dye laser, using 577 to 630 nm, is used with settings ranging from those with argon green to those with krypton red. Since argon blue is absorbed by xanthophyll pigment, green, yellow, orange, and red are preferable wavelengths. Yellow to red (577 to 647 nm) wavelengths are preferable as they are totally transmitted by xanthophyll. Repeat fluorescein angiograms are done within 2 weeks, and subsequent treatment is performed if residual leakage is detected. Inadequate treatment results in hemorrhage and recurrence of the subretinal neovascular membrane.

Precautions

Photocoagulation vasculitis must be distinguished from recurrent subretinal neovascular membrane. The retinal vessels overlying subretinal neovascular membranes are damaged by argon laser photocoagulation. These retinal vessels will show fluorescence because of increased permeability during the first 3 to 4 weeks after photocoagulation. Such fluorescence from photocoagulation vasculitis must be distinguished from recurrent subretinal neovascularization.

Special mention is made of the progressive enlargement of photocoagulation scars that is noted 1 to 4 years after photocoagulation. This enlargement is evident by comparing the width of the scar shortly after photocoagulation, when it corresponds to the zone of the fresh photocoagulation burns, with the width of the scar after several years. This phenomenon explains the progressive visual loss following successful eradication of juxtafoveal subretinal neovascular membranes. The probable cause of circumferen-

Comments

The Macular Photocoagulation Study reported in a randomized control fashion that laser photocoagulation of subretinal neovascular membranes associated with senile macular degeneration reduced the loss of vision as compared with the natural course of the untreated eyes. The incidence of severe visual loss for treated eyes was 20 versus 60 per cent for untreated eyes. Successful management of subretinal neovascular membranes requires early diagnosis; proper case selection for treatment; intense, confluent photocoagulation of the entire membrane and repeat treatment until subretinal neovascular membrane is destroyed; avoidance of the fovea and preretinal blood; early and prolonged follow-up with fluorescein angiography, repeat photocoagulation (when indicated), and daily Amsler grid checks; and discontinuation of aspirin and other medications that alter coagulation.

Recurrent subretinal neovascular membranes occur in 30 to 40 per cent of eyes; for that reason, retreatment is frequently indicated within the first 2 to 3 months of follow-up. Once the membrane has been destroyed and has not recurred after 3 months, the long-term visual prognosis is good. Recurrences are more frequent when treating lesions within 300 μM of the fovea, presumably because one is restricted in the extent that one can treat around such membranes.

References

Bird AC: Treatment of senile disciform macular degeneration. Trans Ophthalmol Soc NZ 29:21–25, 1977.

Bressler, et al: Natural course of choroidal neovascular membranes within foveal avascular zone in senile macular degeneration. Am J Ophthalmol 93:157–163, 1982.

Fine SL: Macular photocoagulation study. Arch Ophthalmol 98:832, 1980.

Gutman FA: The natural course of active choroidal lesions in the presumed ocular histoplasmosis syndrome. Trans Am Ophthalmol Soc 77:515–541, 1979.

Little HL, Jack RL, Vassiliadis A: Argon laser photocoagulation of subretinal neovascular membranes. Trans Am Ophthalmol Soc 78:167–189, 1980.

Macular Photocoagulation Study Group: Argon laser photocoagulation for senile macular degeneration. Arch Ophthalmol 100:912–918, 1982.

Ryan SJ: The development of an experimental model of subretinal neovascularization in disciform macular degeneration. Trans Am Ophthalmol Soc 77:707–745, 1979.

Sabates FN, Lee KY, Ziemianski MC: A comparative study of argon and krypton laser photocoagulation in the treatment of presumed ocular histoplasmosis syndrome. Ophthalmology 89:729–734, 1982.

Sarks SH: New vessel formation beneath the retinal pigment epithelium in senile eyes. Br J Ophthalmol 57:951–965, 1973.

Teeters VW, Bird AC: The development of neovascularization of senile disciform macular degeneration. Am J Ophthalmol 76:1–18, 1973.

Trempe CL, et al: Macular photocoagulation. Optimal wavelength selection. Ophthalmology 89:721–728, 1982.

Zweng HC, Little HL: Argon Lasser Photocoagulation. St. Louis, CV Mosby, 1977, pp 127–175, 292–307.

# SECTION 34

SCLERA

EPISCLERITIS

PETER G. WATSON, M.A., M.B., B.Chir., F.R.C.S., D.O.
Cambridge, England

Episcleritis is an inflammation of the fascial coats of the eye, which lie between the conjunctiva and the sclera. It is usually a mild, self-limiting, recurrent disease that is sometimes caused by exogenous inflammatory stimuli. Episcleritis is twice as common in females as in males and has its peak incidence in the fourth decade. There are two clinical types, simple and nodular. The most common is simple episcleritis, in which there are intermittent bouts of moderate or severe inflammation at 1- to 3-month intervals. These episodes usually last 7 to 10 days and occur more commonly in the spring or fall than in summer or winter. Only rarely can the precipitating factor be found, but attacks are often precipitated by stress. Patients with nodular episcleritis give no history of periodicity, but rather of prolonged mild attacks of inflammation. Almost all the patients with this condition have some intercurrent systemic disease.

THERAPY

Supportive. Since the disease is self-limiting with little to no permanent damage to the eye, episcleritis does not generally require any treatment. However, some patients demand treatment, and a few need help because of the severity and duration of the attack. Occasionally, a clear history of an exogenous sensitization can be obtained, and removal of this agent will prevent recurrent attacks. Desensitization is not indicated in the prevention of recurrent attacks and has even precipitated attacks.

Ocular. Although simple episcleritis requires no treatment, nodular episcleritis is more indolent and may require local corticosteroid drops or anti-inflammatory agents for its control. Topical ophthalmic application of 0.5 per cent prednisolone, 0.1 per cent dexamethasone, 0.1 per cent betamethasone,* or 5 per cent oxyphenbutazone* may be indicated four times daily.

Systemic. In rare instances when nodular episcleritis is unresponsive, systemic anti-inflammatory agents may need to be given. Flurbiprofen,[‡] 100 mg three times daily, is usually effective until inflammation is suppressed. If there is no response to flurbiprofen, indomethacin[‡] should be used. This is usually administered as 100 mg daily and decreased to 75 mg when there is a response. Many patients who will not respond to one nonsteroidal anti-inflammatory agent may well respond to another.

Ocular or Periocular Manifestations

Conjunctiva: Chemosis; hyperemia.
Cornea: Diffuse stromal haze adjacent to limbus (limited to repeated episcleritis attacks in the same position); hypesthesia; vascularization.
Other: Lacrimation; ocular pain; photophobia.

PRECAUTIONS

Up to 11 per cent of patients with episcleritis may have hyperuricemia. When clinical gout gets out of control, symptoms of episcleritis may occur in some patients.

COMMENTS

Episcleritis is fairly common and seems to occur spontaneously without any known cause. It may recur in the same spot or alternate to the fellow eye or the other side of the same eye. Although nodular episcleritis is managed in the same way as simple episcleritis, it has a more protracted course. The majority of attacks last 5 to 10 days; however, there is no definite pattern. Over half of the patients have intermittent attacks that usually last 3 to 6 years, although some have been known to last up to 30 years. Episcleritis starting before puberty usually ceases at puberty; episcleritis starting before menopause usually ceases with the menopause. A hormonal factor has, however, never been demonstrated.

References

Fraunfelder FT, Watson PG: Evaluation of eyes enucleated for scleritis. Br J Ophthalmol 60:227–230, 1976.
Watson PG, Hayreh SS: Scleritis and episcleritis. Br J Ophthalmol 60:163–191, 1976.
Watson PG, Hazleman BL: The Sclera and Systemic Disorders. Philadelphia, WB Saunders, 1976.

SCLERAL STAPHYLOMA AND DEHISCENCES

BISHARA FARIS, M.D.,
Beirut, Lebanon

and H. MACKENZIE FREEMAN, M.D.
Boston, Massachusetts

Localized weakening of the sclera may lead to an oval or elliptical thin area through which the choroid is visible. When flat and meridionally oriented, such areas are termed *scleral dehiscences*; they are referred to as *staphylomas* when bulging.

Staphylomas are classified as anterior or posterior, depending on their relationship to the equator of the eye. Posterior staphylomas are found in myopes over -8 diopters, as well as in patients with the connective tissue disorders of Ehlers-Danlos' and Marfan's syndromes.

Anterior staphylomas are frequent operative findings in the nontraumatic rhegmatogenous retinal detachment population, with a reported incidence of 14 per cent. Less commonly, they occur in eyes with increased intraocular pressure and recurrent necrotizing scleritis and after deep scleral resection for episcleral malignancies. Anterior staphylomas have also been reported after subconjunctival injections of corticosteroids.

THERAPY

Supportive. Since a sustained elevation of intraocular pressure, especially in the pediatric age group, may result in anterior scleral dehiscences and staphyloma formation, the lowering of such pressure by carbonic anhydrase inhibitors and miotics is in order. Forceful rubbing of the eyeballs produces a marked elevation in pressure and should be avoided.

Surgical. When dehiscences and staphylomas are discovered in the area to be buckled during retinal detachment surgery, certain operative precautions should be taken to prevent accidental rupture of the globe. When localizing the retinal breaks, the indentation should be produced by a cotton-tipped applicator, rather than a metal electrode. Dissection of flaps in thin sclera is hazardous; therefore, the surgeon may elect to dissect small scleral flaps anterior and posterior to the dehiscence or staphyloma in order to cover the hard silicone implant and buckle the areas of retinal breaks sufficiently. The blunt edges of the implant should extend over thin scleral zones and end of healthy sclera. In cases where the thinning is extensive, it may be safer to omit undermining scleral flaps and use an episcleral silicone sponge.

Diathermy increases scleral rigidity, thereby elevating intraocular pressure. Thus, it is mandatory that chorioretinal adhesion be produced by cryoapplications, rather than by diathermy. The cryoprobe tip should be applied gently and should not be removed until it has completely thawed. Premature probe movements may rupture the sclera.

The assistant surgeon has an important role to play during surgery. Gentle exposure of the globe prevents sudden increases in intraocular pressure and subsequent rupture of the globe. It is always safer to disinsert more recti muscles to obtain good exposure of the surgical field than to resort to forceful exposure.

The use of intravenous acetazolamide and mannitol is advised in all cases, unless there is a medical contraindication. Paracentesis, as a means to lower intraocular pressure, may be used as a last resort.

When uveal tissue does bulge through dehiscences or staphylomas despite all measures taken, such areas should be immediately covered by a silicone rubber patch that is glued with cyanoacrylate adhesive.

During surgery for episcleral malignancies, scleral resection is done whenever there is evidence of scleral involvement. Deep resections involving two thirds or more of the scleral thickness may predispose to the formation of dehiscences and staphylomas. In such cases, it is wise to cover the resected zones by a preserved scleral graft.

Ocular or Periocular Manifestations

Sclera: Blue coloration; rupture; thinning.
Other: Glaucoma; myopia; retinal detachment.

PRECAUTIONS

A history of staphylomas in one eye should alert the surgeon to the possibility of their occurrence in the fellow eye. The presence or extent of a staphyloma in the fellow eye may be determined by placing a hand-held transilluminator on the cornea and observing the light transmitted through the thinned sclera.

COMMENTS

Anterior scleral staphylomas are most often located in the superior temporal quadrants. Hence, these quadrants should be avoided when subconjunctival injections of antibiotics and corticosteroids are indicated. Staphylomas may be associated with glaucoma and nontraumatic retinal detachment. When encountered during retinal detachment surgery, they can be the site of rupture of the globe unless specific operative measures are taken.

References

Edelstein AJ, Ashrafzadeh MT, Schneider J: Patch grafts for staphylomas of the anterior segment of the eye. Ophthalmic Surg 1:38–42, 1970.

Faris B, Freeman HM, Schepens CL: Scleral dehiscences, anterior staphyloma, and retinal detachment—Part 1: Incidence and pathogenesis. Trans Am Acad Ophthalmol Otolaryngol 79:851–853, 1975.

Freeman HM, Schepens CL, Faris B: Scleral dehiscences, anterior staphyloma, and retinal detachment—Part 2: Surgical management. Trans Am Acad Ophthalmol Otolaryngol 79:854–857, 1975.

Phillips CI, Dobbie JG: Posterior staphyloma and retinal detachment. Am J Ophthalmol 55:332–335, 1963.

Stewart RH, Garcia CA: Staphyloma following cyclocryotherapy. Ophthalmic Surg 5:28–29, 1974.

Watzke RC: Scleral staphylomas and retinal detachment. Arch Ophthalmol 70:796–804, 1963.

SCLERITIS

PETER G. WATSON, M.A., M.B., B.Chir., F.R.C.S., D.O.
Cambridge, England

Scleritis is a severe inflammatory process that involves the opaque collagenous outer coat of the eye. The inflammatory stimuli are almost always of endogenous origin and result in granuloma formation and a vasculitis that involves both the superficial and deeper scleral vasculature. Scleritis is often a manifestation of a chronic systemic inflammation, such as rheumatoid arthritis or other connective tissue disease. It always has a protracted course if untreated; even when well treated, recurrence is the rule. Complications are largely preventable, but if they occur, scleritis becomes one of the gravest eye diseases. Scleral inflammation usually occurs anterior to the equator, but posterior scleritis is not uncommon and often remains undiagnosed. The anterior variety is divided into diffuse, nodular, or necrotizing types. Necrotizing scleritis is further subdivided into that with inflammation and that without (scleromalacia perforans). Necrotizing scleritis has a very poor prognosis unless vigorously treated, and it usually indicates the presence of some systemic disease.

THERAPY

Systemic. Bacterial infections and other conditions for which there is a specific therapy should be treated. If no such condition is detected or the scleritis is associated with a connective tissue disease, anti-inflammatory or immunosuppressive agents should be administered. Flurbiprofen[‡] or indomethacin[‡] control most attacks of diffuse or nodular scleritis. The usual daily dosage of flurbiprofen is 300 mg daily until inflammation is suppressed and pain subsides. It is a characteristic finding in all patients with scleritis that the pain is relieved as soon as the inflammatory reaction is suppressed, even though the external appearance of the eye remains the same. The presence or absence of pain may even be used to titrate the dosage of the drug in some patients. If there is no response to flurbiprofen, indomethacin should be used. This is usually administered as 100 mg daily and decreased to 75 mg when there is a response. Many patients respond to indomethacin when they will not respond to flurbiprofen, and vice versa. Therefore, both drugs may need to be tried. If there is no response to the above anti-inflammatory medications within 1 or 2 weeks or if any avascular areas appear in the sclera or episclera, systemic corticosteroids are indicated. Initially, 80 mg of prednisolone is given daily. The dosage is then decreased according to the clinical response as rapidly as possible to a maintenance level of 15 mg a day in divided doses. At this point, an additional anti-inflammatory agent is added, and corticosteroids are further decreased in 2.5-mg steps. If inflammation recurs, increased corticosteroid dosages are required.

Immunosuppressive therapy may need to be added in patients with severe necrotizing scleritis that is not controlled by high doses of corticosteroids or in those who are developing complications with large maintenance doses of steroids. Cyclophosphamide[‡] is the drug of choice and is started at 100 mg daily, increasing the dose to 150 to 200 mg over the next 2 weeks. Side effects are frequent and severe when this drug is used for immunosuppression in this disease, and it should therefore only be used in desperate situations.

In the occasional patient who has destructive scleral disease caused by a venulitis as diagnosed on fluorescein angiography, it may be necessary to give pulse intravenous therapy. Scleromalacia perforans (necrotizing scleritis without accompanying inflammation) is caused by arteriolar obstruction and is not treatable unless caught before sequestration of tissue occurs. The cause of the necrotizing disease should be investigated. if there is evidence of a systemic vasculitis or an immune complex disorder in the presence of severe, destructive disease, a pulse dose of 500 mg of methylprednisolone should be given intravenously over 1 to 2 hours together with 500 mg of cyclophosphamide given intravenously over a period of several hours and washed through by intravenous infusion over the next 24 hours to minimize the chances of developing a hemorrhagic cystitis. This regime may be repeated at intervals dependent on the response. Oral daily therapy of 100 mg of cyclophosphamide or less may be sufficient to control the systemic manifestations if given with low maintenance doses of 15 mg of prednisolone. Pulse intravenous therapy is potentially hazardous and should only be resorted to under desperate circumstances and under the control of an internist versed in its use. It has, however, proved to be vision saving.

Ocular. Although not usually necessary, systemic anti-inflammatory drugs may be used in conjunction with topical ophthalmic corticosteroid solution or ointment or 10 per cent oxyphenbutazone* ointment. This regimen gives subjective relief and comfort to some patients. Once the disease has been suppressed, certain patients can stop the systemic therapy and keep

SECTION 35

VITREOUS

FAMILIAL EXUDATIVE VITREORETINOPATHY
(Autosomal Dominant Exudative Vitreoretinopathy, Criswick-Schepens Syndrome, FEVR)

JOSEPH E. ROBERTSON, JR., M.D.
Portland, Oregon

Familial exudative vitreoretinopathy (FEVR) is a hereditary abnormality of the peripheral retina that simulates prematurity of retinopathy in its cicatricial stage. This disorder is inherited as an autosomal dominant trait, with a high degree of penetrance and variable expressivity. The early stages of the disease indicate that it is likely a disease of small retinal vessels, rather than a true vitreoretinopathy. The developmental disorder probably affects the peripheral retinal vessels during the last few months of intrauterine life. A wide variety of retinal vascular abnormalities have been observed in the extreme fundus periphery, particularly in the temporal retinal sector. They include the presence of an avascular zone in the extreme periphery, vasodilation and arteriovenous anastomosis in the peripheral vascular zone, a V-shaped avascular zone along the temporal meridian, and neovascularization. Vitreoretinal adhesion invariably occurs along or peripheral to the equator and is often located along the peripheral margin of the vascularized retina. Other retinal abnormalities include ectopia of the macula, cystoid degeneration, falciform retinal folds, and retinoschisis. The condition is thought to be particularly stable once the patient reaches 20 years of age.

THERAPY

Supportive. Although the expression of familial exudative vitreoretinopathy may range from the extremely mild stages of the disease to the more advanced stage with visual loss, genetic counseling is indicated for patients even with the sole clinical finding of isolated intraretinal deposits. In afflicted patients, the risk of the condition developing to some degree with each pregnancy is 50 per cent. Although most patients who become blind from this disorder do so by the end of the second decade, all individuals with this disease have an ongoing increased risk of retinal detachment and deserve ongoing follow-up.

Surgical. Scleral buckling without vitreous surgery is indicated in retinal detachment without posterior tearing of fixed retinal folds. Cryopexy or laser photocoagulation of the breaks should be initiated when symptomatic tears are experienced or when new tears with persistent vitreous traction are noted.

Vitreous surgery is used when it is anticipated that 1) scleral buckling alone cannot compensate for vitreous traction sufficiently to reattach the retina, 2) dense hemorrhage accompanies the detachment, or 3) posterior breaks are involved.

Ocular or Periocular Manifestations

Cornea: Band keratopathy.
Iris: Atrophy.
Lens: Cataracts.
Macula: Cystoid degeneration; ectopia.
Retina: Detachment; exudate; hemorrhage; holes; neovascularization.
Vitreous: Hemorrhage; organization; traction.
Other: Neovascular glaucoma; phthisis bulbi; posterior synechiae; visual loss.

PRECAUTIONS

Retinopathy of prematurity and FEVR may be inseparable entities when morphologic characteristics are considered solely. Differentiation of these two disorders is most reliably achieved by a clinical history outlining the familial tendency and absence of prematurity or supplemental oxygen administration. FEVR may rank among the major causes of retinal detachment, particularly in juvenile patients.

COMMENTS

Since the disease may be transmitted by autosomal dominant inheritance, family members of the patient should be examined ophthalmoscopically. The major threats to vision are posed by retinal hemorrhages, edema, and detachment. Progression of the disease is usually limited to the early years of life. Recent evidence suggests that pathologic progression of FEVR, regardless of disease stage, is not inevitable.

References

Bergen RL, Glassman R: Familial exudative vitreoretinopathy. Ann Ophthalmol 15:275–276, 1983.

Boldrey EE, et al: The histopathology of familial exudative vitreoretinopathy. A report of two cases. Arch Ophthalmol 103:238–241, 1985.

Feldman EL, Norris JL, Cleasby GW: Autosomal dominant exudative vitreoretinopathy. Arch Ophthalmol 101:1532–1535, 1983.

Gole GA, Goodall K, James MJ: Familial exudative vitreoretinopathy. Br J Ophthalmol 69:76, 1985.

Miyakubo H, Inohara N, Hashimoto K: Retinal involvement in familial exudative vitreoretinopathy. Ophthalmologica 185:125–135, 1982.

Nicholson DH, Galvis V: Criswick-Schepens syndrome (familial exudative vitreoretinopathy). A study of a Colombian kindred. Arch Ophthalmol 102:1519–1522, 1984.

Nishimura M, et al: Falciform retinal fold as sign of familial exudative vitreoretinopathy. Jpn J Ophthalmol 27:40–53, 1983.

Ohkubo H, Tanino T: Electrophysiological findings in familial exudative vitreoretinopathy. Doc Ophthalmol 65:461–469, 1987.

Swanson D, Rush P, Bird AC: Visual loss from retinal oedema in autosomal dominant exudative vitreoretinopathy. Br J Ophthalmol 66:627–629, 1982.

Van Nouhuys CE: Dominant exudative vitreoretinopathy and other vascular developmental disorders of the peripheral retina. Doc Ophthalmol 54:1–415, 1982.

PERSISTENT HYPERPLASTIC PRIMARY VITREOUS
(PHPV)

RONALD C. PRUETT, M.D.

Boston, Massachusetts

Persistent hyperplastic primary vitreous (PHPV) is a nonhereditary congenital syndrome caused by anomalous development of the primary vitreous-hyaloid artery complex. Two clinical forms are recognized: anterior (formerly called persistent tunica vasculosa lentis) and posterior (previously known as ablatio falciformis congenita or congenital retinal fold). Intermediate forms also occur. Most commonly, the condition is unilateral and presents in an otherwise normal child, the product of an uncomplicated full-term pregnancy with no history of perinatal oxygen administration. Leukokoria, strabismus, and poor vision are frequent initial complaints.

The most common findings in anterior PHPV are microphthalmos, a shallow anterior chamber with an embryonic filtration angle, and abnormally large iris blood vessels. The lens may be small and clear initially, but a posterior capsular defect may be seen with fibrovascular invasion, hemorrhage, and cataract formation. The cataract may absorb spontaneously or swell, causing secondary angle-closure glaucoma or rarely a phacoanaphylactoid reaction. A persistent hyaloid artery with retrolental fibrovascular membrane that contracts and draws the ciliary processes centrally may also be present. The retina may be clinically normal, but can show histologic abnormalities and detachment in some eyes.

Posterior PHPV is characterized by relative microcornea and a deep anterior chamber, although the filtration angle may appear immature. The lens is usually clear and of normal size; in rare cases, the lens may be colobomatous, cataractous, or subluxated. Peripheral equatorially oriented vitreous membranes fanning out from a radially oriented vitreous stalk that emanates from the disc and contains hyaloid vascular remnants may also be present. In addition, a radial retinal fold in any meridian associated with a vitreous stalk, hypoplastic disc, attenuated and sometimes sheathed retinal vessels, pigmentation and dragging of macula, and retinal detachment are frequent signs. Histologically, the neurosensory retina is abnormal, but the retinal pigment epithelium is uninvolved.

THERAPY

Surgical. There are three objectives in the management of PHPV: avoidance of unnecessary enucleation because of incorrect diagnosis, management of complications, and improvement of visual function and ocular cosmesis.

If one is aware of the polymorphism of the syndrome and utilizes appropriate methods available for investigation, misdiagnosis in potentially useful eyes will be infrequent. Eyes with anterior PHPV and relatively clear lenses or a cataract that is undergoing spontaneous reabsorption can be followed conservatively. Those with lens swelling and actual or threatened angle closure are best managed surgically, using a closed system for fragmentation and aspiration of the cataract and fibrovascular membrane. Similar techniques are indicated for those eyes with grossly normal macula that have lens or vitreous opacities thought sufficient to threaten amblyopia. Vitreous hemorrhage, with or without suspected retinal detachment, requires careful ultrasonic evaluation, followed by closed vitrectomy and scleral buckling in selected cases. In those with posterior PHPV, progressive retinal detachment is the principal indication for surgical intervention. It may be caused by increasing vitreoretinal traction by contracting membranes associated with the persistent hyaloid vascular complex. A localized traction detachment may respond to surgery using vitreous scissors or to closed vitrectomy in more extensively involved eyes. Scleral buckling can provide further relief of vitreoretinal traction and is definitely indicated for those with rhegmatogenous detachment.

Strabismus surgery, refraction, contact lens fitting, and selective occlusion therapy can be useful in PHPV, depending upon the individual problem encountered. Although the cosmetic appearance of an eye can often be improved, the prognosis for visual function must always be guarded. Severely malformed eyes do not achieve better than 20/200 acuity. Less involved eyes can achieve more useful vision, and those with minor anomalies may have essentially normal acuity and require only long-term follow-up examinations.

Precautions

When the manifestations of PHPV are primarily anterior, the consideration of possible monocular retinoblastoma accounts for the majority of these children's eyes that are enucleated. Findings that would tend to rule out that diagnosis include microphthalmos, absence of true neovascularization of the iris, ciliary processes drawn into the pupillary aperture, and other signs of anomalous development, such as an embryonic angle configuration. Further supportive evidence for PHPV would be no family history of retinoblastoma, failure to demonstrate intraocular tumefaction by B-scan ultrasonography, and absence of tumor calcification on ocular x-ray examination. CT scan and magnetic resonance studies and cytopathologic examination of vitreous biopsy materials also can be helpful. Electroretinography, a visually evoked response, and an electrically evoked response may provide additional clues to the correct diagnosis and give some estimate of potential function.

Posterior PHPV may be confused with other conditions that produce a radial retinal fold, such as retinopathy of prematurity, chronic posterior uveitis, nematode infestation, and occult intraocular foreign body. PHPV is usually unilateral, whereas retinopathy of prematurity is bilateral. Individuals with the latter condition most often have a history of premature birth with oxygen administration. Their eyes tend to be myopic with retinal folds that are symmetric and directed temporally. Microcornea, immature angle structure, hyaloid artery remnants, and other signs of maldevelopment are lacking. These signs are also absent in eyes with other types of acquired retinal fold. A history of chronic uveitis, which may be bilateral, recent acquisition of a dog or cat, ocular trauma, or prior good vision in the involved eye would suggest noncongenital disease. Ancillary studies that can be helpful include serum antibody titers, x-rays of the eye and skull, an eosinophil count, and examination of pet stool for parasites.

Comments

This is an unusual syndrome, and its fundamental cause is still unknown. Although the majority of causes present sporadically, rare familial cases have been seen. Careful examination of immediate family members is worthwhile to search for subclinical manifestations of maldevelopment. In the absence of evidence of a hereditary factor, there is no reason at present to advise the parents of such children not to bear additional offspring. Nor would the patients be expected to produce children similarly affected.

References

Caudill JW, Streeten BW, Tso MOM: Phacoanaphylactoid reaction in persistent hyperplastic primary vitreous. Ophthalmology 92:1153–1158, 1985.

Federman JL, et al: The surgical and nonsurgical management of persistent hyperplastic primary vitreous. Ophthalmology 89:20–24, 1982.

Goldberg MF, Peyman GA: Pars plicata surgery in the child for papillary membranes, persistent hyperplastic primary vitreous, and infantile cataract. In Transactions of the New Orleans Academy of Ophthalmology. St. Louis, CV Mosby, 1983, pp 228–262.

Green WR: Diagnostic cytopathology of ocular fluid specimens. Ophthalmology 91:726–749, 1984.

Haddad R, Font RL, Reeser F: Persistent hyperplastic primary vitreous. A clinicopathologic study of 62 cases and review of the literature. Surv Ophthalmol 23:123–134, 1978.

Karr DJ, Scott WE: Visual acuity results following treatment of persistent hyperplastic primary vitreous. Arch Ophthalmol 104:662–667, 1986.

Mafee MF, Goldberg MF: Persistent hyperplastic primary vitreous (PHPV): Role of computed tomography and magnetic resonance. Radiol Clin North Am 25:683–692, 1987.

Nankin SJ, Scott WE: Persistent hyperplastic primary vitreous: Roto-extraction and other surgical experience. Arch Ophthalmol 95:240–243, 1977.

Peyman GA, Sanders DR, Nagpal KC: Management of persistent hyperplastic primary vitreous by pars plana vitrectomy. Br J Ophthalmol 60:756–758, 1976.

Pollard ZF: Treatment of persistent hyperplastic primary vitreous. J Pediatr Ophthalmol Strabismus 22:180–183, 1985.

Stark WJ, et al: Persistent hyperplastic primary vitreous. Surgical treatment. Ophthalmology 90:452–457, 1983.

PROLIFERATIVE VITREORETINOPATHY
(Massive Periretinal Proliferation, Massive Preretinal Gliosis, Massive Preretinal Organization, Massive Vitreous Retraction, Vitreoretinal Membrane Shrinkage)

STEVE CHARLES, M.D.

Memphis, Tennessee

Proliferative vitreoretinopathy is a reparative process initiated by a full- or partial-thickness retinal break or retinopexy. Loss of contact inhibition causes the surrounding glial or retinal pigment epithelial cells to migrate to both surfaces of the retina and proliferate. These cells migrate further and cover the posterior surface of the detached posterior hyaloid face. Fibronectin-lined, coated pits serve as attachments of the retinal pigment epithelium or glial cells to collagen fiber or other components of the extracellular matrix. The migration/contraction mechanism causes tangential force on the retina and multiple starfolds. Similarly, the vitreous contracts largely because of this hypocellular gel contraction.

THERAPY

Surgical. The surgical objective is to allow retinal conformation to the retinal pigment epithelium. In cases of moderate starfolds, scleral buckling without vitreous surgery is indicated. Minimal retinopexy to the breaks should be utilized to avoid inflammation and further proliferation. Retreatment of retinal pigment epithelium with overlapping rows of retinopexy should be avoided to reduce proliferative vitreoretinopathy. Postreattachment retinopexy helps reduce retinal pigment epithelium proliferation. Laser and diathermy cause less proliferative vitreoretinopathy than cryotherapy, but are more difficult to apply.

A broad, relatively high 360° encircling buckle with a smooth contour should be utilized. This is best achieved with a silicone exoplant and two or three mattress sutures per quadrant. The posterior scleral bites should be single, long, and circumferential and as posterior as possible without damage to the vortex veins. The anterior bites should be paired, radial, and placed in the condensations at the muscle ring, representing the external landmark of the ora. Elastic 5-0 monofilament sutures are preferable, with the ends cut on the knot. The broad buckle extends back to the thicker, stronger untreated retina and to the ora to prevent anterior leakage. Extensive drainage of subretinal fluid, preferably a needle drainage method, is required to achieve instant reattachment and create space for the large buckle. Anterior vitrectomy to allow paracentesis in aphakic eyes or anterior chamber paracentesis in phakic or pseudophakic eyes may be necessary to achieve volume requirements. Air (gas) injection seals the retinal breaks via a surface tension effect and allows restoration of a pressure gradient and better drainage. Because of lateral displacement of the retina, transcleral drainage of subretinal fluid should be performed very posteriorly after air injection to avoid retinal incarceration in the drainage site.

Vitreous surgery is utilized when it is anticipated that scleral buckling alone cannot compensate for vitreous traction and periretinal membrane contraction sufficiently to reattach the retina. In most instances, the lens should be removed with trans pars plana lensectomy to permit better removal of the anterior loop traction, decompartmentation, and proliferative vitreoretinopathy reduction. Trans pars plana lensectomy with the aspirating phacofragmenter and linear suction is the method of choice. The anterior and posterior hyaloid faces are usually in contact in a frontal plane configuration. This frontal plane component should be removed first, preferably with a divided 20-gauge system vitreous cutter and linear suction control using minimal suction force. The anterior loop traction then should be resected with the suction cutter if sufficient distance exists between the anterior attachment at the pars plana and the posterior attachment of this former peripheral cortical vitreous to the retina at the equator. Right-angle 20-gauge scissors should be used in most instances to resect this anterior loop component 360°.

Epiretinal membrane can then be peeled free of the retina in instances when it is minimally adherent. End-opening forceps are used for contour peeling of pits; needles and side-opening forceps cause more trauma to the internal limiting lamina. In cases of stronger adherence, it is better to use segmentation and delamination with a 20-gauge right-angle scissor with blades parallel to the retina (Charles modification of the Sutherland scissors). Segmentation of the epiretinal membrane in the center of a starfold and between each fold releases the tangential traction. If the membrane is dense and well developed, it can be delaminated from the retinal surface using both scissor blades between the retina and membrane. The goal is to release sufficient tangential traction to allow retinal conformation to the retinal pigment epithelium without necessarily removing all membranes.

Subretinal membranes can be segmented or removed with duckbill forceps if they are creating sufficient contour change in the retina to prevent reattachment. This can be accomplished through a pre-existing retinal break, or a retinotomy can be created for this purpose, using the scissors.

Incremental retinotomy after fluid/air exchange and internal drainage of subretinal fluid can be effective tools to release tangential forces on the retina when the retina is incarcerated in a wound or previous drain site or when dense membranes are strongly adherent over broad areas of atrophic retina.

Air (gas) tamponade should be used in all cases requiring vitrectomy because the tamponade effect of the posterior hyaloid face has been removed. Internal fluid gas exchange allows creation of a total fill of the vitreous space without hypotony or multiple small bubbles. A 20 per cent gaseous mixture of sulfur hexafluoride‡ may be used to prolong the absorption of the bubble. Concentrations greater than 20 per cent are not used because the expansion characteristics would cause elevation of intraocular pressure with a total fill. The gas is injected through the infusion cannula, preferably using power gas injector. Fluid egress is accomplished through a tapered, bent 20-gauge cannula held near the optic nerve and controlled by a foot-controlled linear suction system.

Internal drainage of subretinal fluid with the same tapered bent cannula placed through a convenient retinal break and held near the retinal pigment epithelium allows hydraulic reattachment. A brief, high transretinal pressure gradient forces the still foreshortened retina against the retinal pigment epithelium. The appearance of subretinal air indicates the failure to release all tangential forces on the retina and the need for further segmentation, delamination, retinotomy, scleral buckling, resection, or inoperability. Minimal transcleral diathermy or laser endophotocoagulation are then placed around each retinal break, using the operating microscope or indirect ophthalmoscope for visualization.

Scleral buckling as described earlier, using a 9- to 10 mm wide 360° silicone exoplant imbricated flush with the surface of the globe and sewed end-to-end, is utilized. It is a mistake to think of proliferative vitreoretinopathy as a localized disease and to buckle only the abnormal-appearing areas. An encircling band is not required.

Ocular or Periocular Manifestations

Retina: Epiretinal membranes; fixed folds; starfolds; subretinal placoid or dendritic proliferation.
Vitreous: Condensation; contraction; pigmentation; posterior vitreous detachment.
Other: Visual loss.

PRECAUTIONS

Vitreous (periretinal membrane) surgery should be utilized freely when it is apparent that conventional scleral buckling alone will not be effective. Vitreous surgery is a proven modality for this problem that no longer should be considered experimental. Care should be taken to minimize trauma to the internal limiting lamina by use of scissor segmentation delamination, rather than peeling. Hydraulic reattachment is preferable to the injection of an expansile sulfur hexafluoride bubble and partial drainage of subretinal fluid because it permits intraoperative recognition of the need for further mechanical release of tangential traction.

Minimal retinopexy and the liberal use of subconjunctival corticosteroids* decrease the release of fibrin and reduce proliferation along this matrix.

COMMENTS

The above techniques have a 95 per cent intraoperative anatomic success, with 65 per cent long-term anatomic success and 50 per cent long-term visual success with acuities better than 5/200. With the possibility of bilateral visual loss, it is mandatory to consider this procedure with its greater success rate and 2 to 3 hour operating time to retain an ambulatory vision eye.

Silicone oil‡ is increasingly widespread for long-term surface tension management. A combined multicenter trial has not been completed to prove its efficacy compared to gas.

Its purpose is rhegmatogenous defined and treated. No antiproliferative drugs have yet proven to be effective.

References

Charles S: Vitrectomy for retinal detachment. Trans Ophthalmol Soc UK *100*:542–549, 1980.
Charles S: Vitreous Microsurgery. Baltimore, Williams & Wilkins, 1981.
Machemer R, van Horn D, Aaberg TM: Pigment epithelial proliferation in human retinal detachment with massive periretinal proliferation. Am J Ophthalmol 85:181–191, 1978.
van Horn DL, et al: Glial cell proliferation in human retinal detachment with massive periretinal proliferation. Am J Ophthalmol 84:383–393, 1977.

VITREOUS HEMORRHAGE
RICHARD L. WINSLOW, M.D.,
and BRUCE C. TAYLOR, M.D.
Dallas, Texas

Vitreous hemorrhage, whether associated with trauma or occurring spontaneously, is a secondary diagnosis. Successful treatment depends on identifying the specific cause of the hemorrhage. In traumatic cases, one must determine if the hemorrhage has resulted from a ruptured retinal vessel, a retinal tear, or a perforating injury. The most common causes of spontaneous hemorrhage are proliferative diabetic retinopathy, posterior vitreous detachment, retinal tear without detachment, proliferative vein occlusion, retinal detachment, intraocular lens, and proliferative sickle retinopathy. Miscellaneous causes must be considered if the more common causes are absent. Occasionally, the source of the vitreous hemorrhage can never be identified. However, every attempt must be made to identify the specific cause of the vitreous hemorrhage so that specific therapy may be instituted.

THERAPY

Supportive. The patient should avoid heavy lifting, stooping, and vigorous physical activity, all of which might produce further vitreous hemorrhage. If there is no view of the retina, diagnostic ultrasonography is required to rule out a retinal detachment. Bedrest for several days with the head elevated and both eyes patched is also helpful to allow settling of the vitreous hemorrhage inferiorly so that the superior retina may be visualized. This is often diagnostic because over 80 per cent of retinal tears associated with vitreous hemorrhage occur in the superior quadrants.

Surgical. Traumatic vitreous hemorrhage may require no therapy if there is merely a ruptured retinal vessel. If a retinal tear or dialysis is noted, cryotherapy or photocoagulation should be applied to surround the retinal break. Vitrectomy and scleral buckling procedures may be required if retinal detachment occurs.

The causes of spontaneous vitreous hemorrhage may be grouped into proliferative, rhegmatogenous, and miscellaneous. The major proliferative causes include diabetic retinopathy, vein occlusion, and sickle retinopathy, which can all be treated with photocoagulation. In proliferative diabetic retinopathy, panretinal photocoagulation is extremely helpful in preventing further vitreous hemorrhage. Either xenon or argon laser photocoagulation may be used, but argon treatment is probably preferable. Laser panretinal photocoagulation is performed using a three-mirror Goldmann lens or a Rodenstock panfunduscopic lens to visualize the retina. The laser settings include a spot size of 400 to 500 μM for 0.2 seconds and a power setting adequate to produce moderate whitening of the retina. Burns are spread from 0.5 to 1 burn width apart throughout the peripheral retina, extending posteriorly no closer than 2 disc diameters from the fovea and 1 disc diameter from the disc. The total number of burns averages between 1200 to 1600, which are usually done in three to four sessions, using only topical anesthesia. Retrobulbar anesthesia may be used, but is rarely necessary. If further vitreous hemorrhage or vascular proliferation occurs, additional photocoagulation may be applied to areas between the original burns.

Argon laser photocoagulation may be used in a similar technique to prevent further vitreous hemorrhage from a proliferative branch vein occlusion. Burns are made only in the affected sector. In central retinal vein occlusion, panretinal photocoagulation is useful in preventing both recurrent vitreous hemorrhage and rubeosis iridis.

Proliferative sickle retinopathy can be treated with a scatter technique of photocoagulation applied to the peripheral areas of capillary dropout, which are present anterior to the peripheral "sea fans." The capillary dropout may be more specifically localized with fluorescein angiography.

Scatter cryotherapy may be used for proliferative diabetic retinopathy if the vitreous hemorrhage fails to clear adequately to permit photocoagulation. If the conjunctiva is not opened, two rows of three to four cryo applications are made in each quadrant 12 to 16 mm posterior to the limbus. The freeze is monitored with indirect ophthalmoscopy to produce moderate whitening of the retina. In areas where vitreous hemorrhage obscures the view, the cryo application is timed similarly to those areas that could be visualized.

Cryotherapy may also be used to treat peripheral "sea fans" in proliferative sickle retinopathy if vitreous hemorrhage prevent photocoagulation. The best technique is to use a single freeze-thaw, allowing the ice ball to extend into the vitreous until it totally engulfs the "sea fan."

In the rhegmatogenous group, no therapy is required for a posterior vitreous detachment associated with vitreous hemorrhage. Superficial retinal hemorrhages may be seen at the disc margin or equatorial region. This is a diagnosis of exclusion and can be made only after periodic examinations, performed while the vitreous hemorrhage is clearing, demonstrate a vitreous detachment but fail to show a retinal tear.

If a retinal break is present, it should be surrounded by cryotherapy so that the freezes extend into healthy retina and are contiguous. The retina should just be made to whiten. Extensive, prolonged, or repeated cryo applications are to be avoided, since they may result in excessive retinal thinning or necrosis. Posterior retinal breaks may be surrounded by photocoagulation if they cannot be reached with the cryoprobe.

In approximately 7 per cent of retinal tears, a retinal vessel bridges the tear and is not torn completely. It may be the source of recurrent vitreous hemorrhage and can usually be managed simply with cryotherapy to surround the tear, since the recurrent hemorrhage is commonly self-limiting. Laser therapy may occasionally be used to occlude the bridging vessel by applying 0.5- to 1-second burns of 400 to 500 μM in size to the vessel in an area where the vessel is in flat retina. This technique may require repeated attempts at approximately 1-week intervals to occlude the vessel. Fluorescein angiography may be helpful in demonstrating complete interruption of blood flow in the bridging vessel. Only rarely is a localized scleral buckle required to relieve the vitreous traction on the vessel to prevent further vitreous hemorrhage.

When a retinal detachment is detected, a routine scleral buckle is performed if the retinal breaks can be adequately visualized. Customarily, an encircling solid or sponge explant is sutured over the retinal break after it has been surrounded by cryotherapy and the subretinal fluid has been drained. If the retinal breaks cannot be visualized adequately, a vitrectomy must first be performed, followed by a scleral buckling procedure.

In the modern era of ophthalmology, vitreous hemorrhage associated with the use of intraocular lenses has also been seen. The hemorrhage originates in the anterior segment, but migrates into the vitreous. The source of the hemorrhage has been the angle in angle-supported lenses, the pupillary margin in iris-supported lenses (particularly those with metal loops that can erode the pupillary margin), and the ciliary body or posterior surface of the iris in posterior chamber lenses. Usually, this is self-limited, but occasionally the lens must be removed.

Ocular or Periocular Manifestations

Iris: Rubeosis iridis (with proliferative diabetic retinopathy and central retinal vein occlusion).
Lens: Posterior subcapsular cataract.
Retina: Macular pucker; traction retinal detachment.
Other: Hemolytic glaucoma (particularly in the aphakic patient).

Precautions

Patients with proliferative diabetic retinopathy are prone to develop rubeosis iridis, particularly if the lens is removed. Patients with central retinal vein occlusion are candidates for rubeosis iridis, particularly in the first 6 months after the occlusion. In the early stages, rubeosis iridis can often be controlled with panretinal photocoagulation. Patients with sickle-cell hemoglobinopathy are prone to develop anterior segment necrosis after scleral buckling. Exchange transfusion before surgery and avoidance of muscle disinsertion may be helpful in preventing this complication.

COMMENTS

Proliferative diabetic retinopathy is by far the most common cause of spontaneous vitreous hemorrhage, accounting for 32 to 54 per cent of all cases. This diagnosis can usually be made by a history of diabetes or examination of the fellow eye. Once diabetes is excluded, the most common etiology is a retinal tear with or without retinal detachment, which accounts for 33 to 64 per cent of the spontaneous vitreous hemorrhages in nondiabetic patients. The presence of a retinal tear must be ruled out by careful, repeated funduscopic examination, using indirect ophthalmoscopy and scleral indentation.

References

Blankenship GW, Okun E: Retinal tributary vein occlusion: History and management by photocoagulation. Arch Ophthalmol 89:363–368, 1973.
Branch Vein Occlusion Study Group: Argon laser scatter photocoagulation for prevention of neovascularization and vitreous hemorrhage in branch vein occlusion. Arch Ophthalmol 104:34–41, 1986.
Cox MS, Whitmore PV, Gutow RF: Treatment of intravitreal and prepapillary neovascularization following branch retinal vein occlusion. Trans Am Acad Ophthalmol Otolaryngol 79:387–393, 1975.
Davis MD: Natural history of retinal breaks without detachment. Arch Ophthalmol 92:183–194, 1974.
Diabetic Retinopathy Study Research Group: Preliminary report on effects of photocoagulation therapy. Am J Ophthalmol 81:383–396, 1976.
Diabetic Retinopathy Vitrectomy Study Research Group: Early vitrectomy for severe proliferative diabetic retinopathy in eyes with useful vision. Ophthalmology 95:1307–1320, 1988.
Diabetic Retinopathy Vitrectomy Study Research Group: Early vitrectomy for severe vitreous hemorrhage in diabetic retinopathy. Arch Ophthalmol 103:1644–1652, 1985.
DRVS Research Group: Two-year course of visual acuity in severe proliferative diabetic retinopathy with conventional management. Ophthalmology 92:492–502, 1985.
Goldbaum MH, et al: Cryotherapy of proliferative sickle retinopathy, II: Triple freeze-thaw cycle. Br J Ophthalmol 63:97–101, 1979.
Hanscom TA: Indirect treatment of peripheral retinal neovascularization. Am J Ophthalmol 93:88–91, 1982.
Jaffe NS: Complications of acute posterior vitreous detachment. Arch Ophthalmol 79:568–571, 1968.
Ross WH, Gottner MJ: Peripheral retinal cryopexy for subtotal vitreous hemorrhage. Am J Ophthalmol 105:377–382, 1988.
Schimek RA, Spencer R: Cryopexy treatment of proliferative diabetic retinopathy. Retinal cryoablation in patients with severe vitreous hemorrhage. Arch Ophthalmol 97:1276–1280, 1979.
Winslow RL, Taylor BC: Spontaneous vitreous hemorrhage: Etiology and management. South Med J 73:1450–1452, 1980.

VITREOUS WICK SYNDROME
RICHARD S. RUIZ, M.D.
Houston, Texas

The vitreous wick syndrome consists of microscopic wound breakdown with subsequent vitreous prolapse, which creates a tiny vitreous wick from the external surface to the inner eye. Severe intraocular inflammation secondary to bacterial endophthalmitis may develop. Infection appears to gain entrance into the eye by way of the vitreous wick, and the fistula fails to heal because of the external vitreous. When inflammation is present, the patient presents with sudden pain, a peaked pupil, and a rupture of the anterior hyaloid membrane. This syndrome usually occurs 2 weeks or more after uncomplicated cataract surgery.

THERAPY

Surgical. Surgical repair should be carried out without delay. At the time of surgery, an anterior chamber tap for culture and sensitivity studies is taken through the fistulous opening. Using an operating microscope, the fistulous tract is carefully examined, and the vitreous wick is identified, stretched with forceps, and excised flush with the surface of the corneoscleral wound. The wound defect is then converted to a linear incision with the razor blade knife and closed tightly with several sutures. A large air bubble is instilled in the anterior chamber to push the vitreous away from the wound. In the case of mild inflammation or no inflammation, nothing further is done. When there is severe intraocular inflammation with heavy opacification of the vitreous and hypopyon formation, an anterior vitrectomy using a suitable vitrectomy instrument should be considered. The fistulous opening is then enlarged suitably, and the vitrectomy instrument with infusion and aspiration ports is introduced into the anterior chamber. All opacified vitreous, hypopyon exudate, and other inflammatory debris are carefully removed. The instrument is then directed into the posterior segment, where an anterior vitrectomy is carried out. All aspirated material is collected and concentrated for culture and sensitivity studies. The vitrectomy instrument is then withdrawn, and depending upon the severity of the inflammation, one may consider the introduction of intraocular antibiotics. The fistulous opening, which has been enlarged, is now tightly sutured and the tone of the globe re-established with balanced salt solution.

Ocular. When intraocular inflammation is present, large doses of topical antibiotics are indicated for several weeks until the inflammation subsides.

Systemic. Large doses of systemic antibiotics and corticosteroids are used in exactly the same manner as in bacterial endophthalmitis from other causes. As soon as sensitivity and culture reports are available, antibiotics may be suitably adjusted for specific organisms.

Ocular or Periocular Manifestations

Anterior Chamber: Cells and flare; hypopyon; leak.
Pupil: Peaked.
Vitreous: Exudates; prolapse; rupture of anterior hyaloid membrane; strands.
Other: Decreased visual acuity; inflammation; ocular pain; visual loss.

PRECAUTIONS

To prevent the vitreous wick syndrome, limbus-based conjunctival flaps should be used to cover the corneoscleral sutures. These sutures should be completely buried beneath the flap. Corneoscleral sutures should not be tied tightly as they cut through the tissue, causing a fistulous opening.

If fornix-based conjunctival flaps are used, it is important to realize that careful and repeated observations are necessary for at least 1 month after routine uncomplicated cataract extraction. If peaking of the pupil is observed in the postoperative period, careful slitlamp evaluation of the vitreous face and corneoscleral wound is indicated. If vitreous adherence without wick formation is seen, the external surface of the wound should be carefully examined at close intervals in the event that vitreous prolapse develops. If a vitreous wick should develop, surgical repair should be carried out without delay.

COMMENTS

It seems reasonable that wound leakage may be largely responsible for vitreous adherence to the posterior wound following cataract surgery, particularly where definite, taut strands are noted. It is the aqueous leak that causes the vitreous to move anteriorly and become incarcerated in the fistulous opening. Often this will stop the leak, much like an iris adhesion; however, in some cases, the process progresses to frank vitreous prolapse through the wound. It seems possible that wound leak might also be responsible for anterior hyaloid rupture with or without vitreous adherence or prolapse.

Vitreous prolapsing through the fistula has the appearance of a glob of mucus on the external surface of the globe. The clinical diagnosis can be confirmed by gently stroking the externalized vitreous, which results in movement of vitreous gel in the anterior chamber and subsequent pupillary movement. A Seidel test is usually positive when gentle pressure is applied to the globe.

References

Rice TA, Michels RG: Current surgical management of the vitreous wick syndrome. Am J Ophthalmol 85:656–661, 1978.

Ruiz RS, Teeters VW: The vitreous wick syndrome. A late complication following cataract extraction. Am J Ophthalmol 70:483–490, 1970.

DRUG ROSTER

ABBREVIATIONS USED IN THE DRUG ROSTER

Arg.—Argentina
Austral.—Australia
Aust.—Austria
Belg.—Belgium
Braz.—Brazil
Canad.—Canada
Cz.—Czechoslovakia
Denm.—Denmark
Fin.—Finland
Fr.—France
G.B.—Great Britain
Germ.—Germany
Gr.—Greece
Hung.—Hungary
Ind.—India
Ire.—Ireland
Isr.—Israel

Ital.—Italy
Jap.—Japan
Mex.—Mexico
Neth.—Netherlands
Nig.—Nigeria
Norw.—Norway
N.Z.—New Zealand
Pol.—Poland
Port.—Portugal
S. Afr.—South Africa
Scand.—Scandinavia
Span.—Spain
Swed.—Sweden
Switz.—Switzerland
U.S.S.R.—Union of Soviet
Socialist Republics

ACETAMINOPHEN

Proprietary Names: Aceta, Alba-Temp, Alvedon (Swed.), Anapap, Anelix, Anuphen, Apamide, Apap, Atasol (Canad.), Ben-u-ron (Germ.), Calpol (G.B.), Campain (Canad.), Capital, Ceetamol (Austral.), Cen-Apap, Cetamol (Ire.), Chemcetaphen (Canad.), Datril, Dapa, Dimindol, Dolamin (Austral.), Dolanex, Doliprane (Fr.), Dymadon (Austral.), Febridol, Febrigesic, Febrogesic, G-1, Janupap, Korum, Lestemp, Liquiprin, Lyteca, Med-Apap, Napamol (S. Afr.), Nebs, Neopap, Nevrol (Austral.), Nilprin, Pacemol (N.Z.), Pamol (G.B.), Panado, (S. Afr.), Panadol (G.B.), Panodil (Swed.), Paracet (Austral.), Paracetamol (G.B.), Parasin (Austral.), Parmol (Austral.), Parten, Pediaphen (Canad.), Phenaphen, Phendex, Placemol (Austral.), Pirin, Proval, Pyrapap, Restin (S. Afr.), Rounox (Canad.), Salzone (G.B.), SK-Apap, Sub-Due, Taper, Temetan, Temlo, Tempra, Tenlap, Termidor (Swed.), Ticelgesic (G.B.), Tylenol, Valadol, Valorin.

Preparations

Oral: Capsules, 300 and 500 mg; drops, 60 mg/0.6 ml; elixir or syrup, 120 and 150 mg/5 ml; tablets, 300 and 325 mg; tablets (chewable), 120 mg.
Rectal: Suppositories, 120, 300, 600, and 900 mg.

Usual Dosages

Oral, Rectal: Adults, 300 to 600 mg at 4-hour intervals if necessary; total daily dose should not exceed 2.4 gm. Children 6 to 12 years of age, 150 to 300 mg; 1 to 6 years, 60 to 120 mg; under 1 year, 60 mg. These amounts are given as single doses every 4 to 6 hours, but the total dose should not exceed 1.2 gm.

ACETAMINOPHEN/CODEINE COMBINATION

Proprietary Names: Aceta with Codeine, Apap with Codeine, Empracet with Codeine, Phenaphen 2, 3, 4, Tylenol with Codeine 1, 2, 3, 4.

Preparations

Oral: Capsules, 300 mg acetaminophen with 30 to 60 mg codeine; elixir, 120 mg acetaminophen with 12 mg codeine/5 ml; tablets, 300 or 325 mg acetaminophen with 7.5, 15, 30, or 60 mg codeine.

Usual Dosages

Oral: The usual adult dose is one or two tablets or capsules every 4 hours as required.

ACETAZOLAMIDE

Proprietary Names: Defiltran (Fr.), Diamox, Diazol (S. Afr.), Didoc (Jap.), Diuramid (Pol.), Glaucomide (Austral.), Glaupax (Swed.), Hydrazol.

Preparations

Injection: Powder, 500-mg vial.
Oral: Capsules (timed-release), 500 mg; tablets, 125 and 250 mg.

Usual Dosages

Intramuscular, Intravenous: 500 mg may be administered parenterally and may be repeated in 2 to 4 hours.

---

* Route of administration not approved by FDA.
† Drug not approved by FDA for any indication.
‡ Drug not approved by FDA for this particular indication.
§ Indicated dosage above the manufacturer's recommendation.

Oral: Adults, 250 mg every 6 hours. Children, 10 to 15 mg/kg daily in divided doses. The timed-release preparation can be given every 12 hours, but may not be as effective as regular tablets. For epilepsy, the suggested total daily dose is 8 to 30 mg/kg in divided doses.

ACETOHEXAMIDE

Proprietary Names: Dimelor (G.B.), Dymelor, Ordimel (Swed.).

Preparations

Oral: Tablets, 250 and 500 mg.

Usual Dosages

Oral: Dosage should be individualized. Usual range, 0.25 to 1.5 gm daily.

ACETYLCHOLINE

Proprietary Names: Acecoline (Canad., Fr.), Covochol (S. Afr.), Miochol.

Preparations

Injection: Two-compartment vial containing 20 mg of acetylcholine chloride and 100 mg of mannitol in the lower compartment and 2 ml of sterile water in the upper compartment.

Usual Dosages

Intracameral: 0.5 to 2 ml of a freshly prepared 1:100 solution instilled in the anterior chamber.
Retrobulbar: 25 mg in 1 ml initially, 50 to 75 mg (2 to 3 ml) per injection, depending upon the response.

ACETYLCYSTEINE

Proprietary Names: Airbron (G.B., Canad.), Fluimucil (Germ., Ital., Neth., Span., Switz.), Inspir (Swed.), Lysomucil (Belg.), Mucofilm Sol (Jap.), Mucolyticum (Germ.), Mucomist (Ital.), Mucomyst, Nac (Canad.), Parvolex (G.B.).

Preparations

Topical Ophthalmic: Eyedrops containing 2, 5, 10, or 20 per cent acetylcysteine are prepared by dilution of 20 per cent solution with hydroxypropyl methylcellulose. This preparation should be adjusted to pH 9 with 4 per cent sodium hydroxide solution and prepared aseptically.

Usual Dosages

Topical Ophthalmic: Preparation may be applied up to four times daily.

---

* Route of administration not approved by FDA.
† Drug not approved by FDA for any indication.
‡ Drug not approved by FDA for this particular indication.
§ Indicated dosage above the manufacturer's recommendation.

ACETYLSALICYCLIC ACID
See Aspirin.

ACICLOVIR
See Acyclovir.

ACTH
See Corticotropin.

ACYCLOGUANOSINE
See Acyclovir.

ACYCLOVIR (ACICLOVIR, ACYCLOGUANOSINE)

Proprietary Name: Zorivax.

Preparations

Injection: Powder.
Oral: Capsules, 200 mg.
Topical: Ointment, 5 per cent.
Topical Ophthalmic: No ophthalmic preparation is commercially available, but a 3 per cent ointment in petrolatum base may be prepared.

Usual Dosages

Intravenous (Slow): 5 mg/kg (250 mg/square meter) may be infused at a constant rate over 1 hour every 8 hours (15 mg/kg, daily dose).
Oral: Usual dosage is 200 mg two to five times daily.
Topical: A sufficient quantity of ointment may be used to adequately cover all lesions every 3 hours.
Topical Ophthalmic: Approximately one-half inch of ointment is administered into the lower conjunctival sac five times daily at 3-hour intervals.

ADRENOCORTICOTROPIC HORMONE
See Corticotropin.

ALLOPURINOL

Proprietary Names: Bloxanth (Canad.), Epidropal (Germ.), Foligan (Germ.), Lopurin, Urosin (Germ.), Zyloprim, Zyloric (G.B.).

Preparations

Oral: Tablets, 100 and 300 mg.

Usual Dosages

Oral: Dose range, 100 to 800 mg daily.

ALPHA-TOCOPHEROL
See Vitamin E.

ALTEPLASE

Proprietary Name: Activase.

Preparations

Injection: Lyophilized powder, 20 mg (11.6 million IU) and 50 mg (29 million IU).

Usual Dosages

Intravenous: The usual recommended dose for coronary artery thrombus is 100 mg given as 60 mg in the first hour (of which 6 to 10 mg is given as a bolus over the first 1 to 2 minutes), 20 mg over the second hour, and 20 mg over the third hour.

ALUMINUM ACETATE

Proprietary Names: Acid Mantle, Alsol (Germ.), Domeboro, Eddikesur (Denm.), Euceta (Neth., Switz.).

Preparations

Topical: Solution, 5 per cent.

Usual Dosages

Topical: Solution may be diluted 1:10 to 1:40 and applied three to four times daily.

ALUMINUM HYDROXIDE

Proprietary Names: Adagel (Austral.), Aldrox (Arg., Belg.), Allulose (Norw.), Alterna GEL, Alu-Cap, Alugelibys (Span.), Alumag (S. Afr.), Aluminox (Neth.), Alusorb (Austral.), Alu-Tab, Amphojel, Amphotabs (Austral.), Basaljel (Austral., Canad.), Dialume, Gamma-gel (Ital.), Gastracol (Switz.), Gelox (Austral.), Minajel (Austral.), Palliacol (Germ.), Pepsamar (Span.), Uldecan (Span.).

Preparations

Oral: Suspension (gel), 320 mg/5 ml; tablets (dried gel), 300 and 600 mg.

Usual Dosages

Oral: In conjunction with dietary phosphate restriction in the management of hyperphosphatemia, 30 to 40 ml are administered three to four times daily.

AMANTADINE

Proprietary Names: Contenton (Germ.), Mantadix (Fr.), PK-Merz (Germ.), Symmetrel, Virofral (Swed.).

Preparations

Oral: Capsules, 100 mg; syrup, 500 mg/5 ml.

Usual Dosages

Oral: Range, 100 to 500 mg daily in divided doses.

---

* Route of administration not approved by FDA.
† Drug not approved by FDA for any indication.
‡ Drug not approved by FDA for this particular indication.
§ Indicated dosage above the manufacturer's recommendation.

AMIKACIN

Proprietary Names: Amikin, Amiklin (Fr.), Amukin (Belg., Neth.), BB-K8 (Ital., Mex.), Biclin (Span.), Biklin (Arg., Denm., Germ., Jap., Swed.), Pierami (Ital.).

Preparations

Injection: Solution, 50 to 250 mg/ml.

Usual Dosages

Intramuscular, Intravenous: Adults, children and older infants, 15 mg/kg daily in two or three equally divided doses. The total dose should not exceed 1.5 gm. Neonates, a loading dose of 10 mg/kg is given, followed by 7.5 mg every 12 hours. Dosage should be reduced when given to patients with impaired renal function.

AMINOBENZOIC ACID

See Para-Aminobenzoic Acid.

AMINOCAPROIC ACID

Proprietary Names: Amicar, Capracid (Ital.), Capralense (Fr.), Caprolisin (Ital.), Capramol (Belg., Fr., Ital., Switz.), Caproamin Fides (Span.), Ekaprol (Austral.), Epsamon (Switz.), Epsikapron (G.B., S. Afr., Swed., Switz.), Hemocaprol (Fr., Span., Switz.), Ipsilon (Arg.).

Preparations

Injection: Solution, 250 mg/ml.
Oral: Syrup, 1.25 gm/5 ml; tablets, 500 mg.

Usual Dosages

Intravenous, Oral: For acute bleeding syndromes caused by elevated fibrinolytic activity, 4 to 5 gm should be administered during the first hour, followed by 1 gm/hour for 8 hours or until the hemorrhagic condition is under control. When the bleeding tendency is chronic in nature, daily dosage of 5 to 30 gm administered in divided doses at 3- to 6-hour intervals has been recommended.

AMITRIPTYLINE

Proprietary Names: Amitid, Amizol (G.B.), Annolytin (Jap.), Deprex (Canad.), Domical (G.B.), Elatrol (Canad.), Elavil, Endep, Larozyl (Swed.), Lentizol (G.B.), Levate (Canad.), Mareline (Canad.), Novotriptyn (Canad.), Saroten (G.B.), SK-Amitriptyline, Tryptanol (Austral., S. Afr.), Tryptizol (G.B.).

Preparations

Injection: Solution, 10 mg/ml.
Oral: Tablets, 10, 25, 50, 75, and 100 mg; capsules, 25 and 50 mg.

Usual Dosages

Intramuscular: Adults, initially 80 to 120 mg daily in four divided doses. The oral route should be substituted as soon as possible.
Oral: Adults, initially 75 mg daily in divided doses.

A few hospitalized patients may require as much as 300 mg daily. Elderly patients and adolescents, 10 mg three times daily and 20 mg at bedtime.

AMMONIATED MERCURY

Proprietary Name: Ammoniated Mercury.

Preparations

Topical Ophthalmic: Ointment, 3 per cent.

Usual Dosages

Topical Ophthalmic: A small amount one or two times daily.

AMOBARBITAL

Proprietary Names: Amal (Austral.), Amsal (Austral.), Amylbarb (Austral.), Amylobarbitone (G.B.), Amylobeta (Austral.), Amylosol (Austral.), Amytal, Eunoctal (Fr.), Isomyl (Swed.), Isonal (Canad.), Mylodorm (Austral.), Mylosed (Austral.), Neur-Amyl (Austral.), Novamobarb (Canad.), Restal (Austral.), Schiwanox (Germ.), Sedal (Austral.), Sednotic (Austral.), Stadadorm (Germ.).

Preparations

Injection: Powder, 125, 250, and 500 mg.
Oral: Elixir, 22 and 44 mg/5 ml; tablets, 15, 30, 50, and 100 mg.; capsules, 65 and 200 mg.

Usual Dosages

Intramuscular: Adults, 65 to 500 mg. No more than 5 ml should be injected at any one site.
Oral: As a hypnotic, 100 to 200 mg. As a sedative, up to 600 mg daily in divided doses. Children up to 1 year, 15 to 50 mg; 1 to 5 years, 50 to 60 mg; 6 to 12 years, 60 to 120 mg.

AMOXICILLIN

Proprietary Names: Amoxil, Amoxycillin (G.B.), Clamoxyl (Germ., Jap.), Imacillin (Swed.), Larotid, Polymox, Pasetocin (Jap.), Robamox, Sawacillin (Jap.), Sumox, Trimox, Ulymox, Utimox.

Preparations

Oral: Capsules, 250 and 500 mg; drops for suspension (pediatric), 50 mg/ml; powder for suspension, 125 and 250 mg/5 ml; suspension, 3 gm.

Usual Dosages

Oral: Adults and children over 20 kg, 250 to 500 mg daily. Children less than 20 mg, 20 to 40 mg/kg daily. These amounts are administered in divided doses at 8-hour intervals. Larger doses may be required for persistent or severe infections. For gonorrheal or urethral infections caused by *N. gonorrhoeae,* 3 gm as a single oral dose are recommended.

AMOXICILLIN/CLAVULANATE POTASSIUM COMBINATION

Proprietary Name: Augmentin.

Preparations

Oral: Powder for suspension, 125 or 250 mg amoxicillin and 31.25 or 62.5 mg clavulanate potassium/5 ml; tablets, 250 or 500 mg amoxicillin and 125 mg clavulanate potassium; tablets (chewable), 125 or 250 mg amoxicillin and 31.25 or 62.5 mg clavulanate potassium.

Usual Dosages

Oral: For adults and children over 40 kg, usual dose is 250 mg of amoxicillin and 125 mg of clavulanate potassium every 8 hours. For more severe infections, 500 mg of amoxicillin and 125 mg of clavulanate potassium every 8 hours. In children under 40 kg, usual dose is 20 mg/kg daily in divided doses every 8 hours. For more severe infections, 40 mg/kg daily may be given in divided doses every 8 hours.

AMPHETAMINE

Proprietary Names: Badrin (Austral.), Benzedrine.

Preparations

Oral: Tablets, 5 and 10 mg.

Usual Dosages

Oral: The usual daily dose is 5 to 60 mg in divided doses. Amphetamine should be administered at the lowest effective dosage and adjusted individually.

AMPHOTERICIN B

Proprietary Names: Ampho-Moronal (Germ.), Fungilin (G.B.), Fungizone.

Preparations

Injection: Powder, 50 mg.
Topical Ophthalmic: No ophthalmic form is available, but aqueous suspension containing 0.1 to 5 mg/ml may be prepared from powder marked for intravenous use. Saline solution should *not* be used with amphotericin B, since saline solution will precipitate amphotericin B.

Usual Dosages

Intracameral: 20 to 30 µg in 0.1 to 0.2 ml of sterile 5 per cent dextrose in water.
Intrathecal: A total of 50 mg is diluted with at least 150 ml of 5 per cent dextrose injection (for intraventricular injection) or 10 per cent dextrose without preservative (for hyperbaric translumbar injection) to a final concentration of about 0.25 mg/ml. Therapy is initiated with 0.1 ml, and the dose is gradually increased until the patient can tolerate 0.5 mg, the usual maximum dose, without excessive discomfort. The

---

* Route of administration not approved by FDA.
† Drug not approved by FDA for any indication.
‡ Drug not approved by FDA for this particular indication.
§ Indicated dosage above the manufacturer's recommendation.

minimal tolerated dose is given at 48- to 72-hour intervals.

Intravenous (Slow): Dosage must be adjusted individually according to severity of the disease and tolerance of patient. Therapy is usually instituted with a daily dose of 0.25 mg/kg and *gradually* increased as tolerance permits. The optimal dose is unknown. Total daily dosage may range up to 1.0 mg/kg or alternate-day dosages ranging up to 1.5 mg/kg. *Under no circumstances* should a total daily dosage of 1.5 mg/kg be exceeded. Several months of therapy are usually necessary.

Intravitreal: 4 to 5 μg in 0.1 to 0.2 ml of sterile 5 per cent dextrose in water.

Subconjunctival: 0.75 to 3 mg in 0.5 ml of sterile 5 per cent dextrose in water. Doses as large as 5 mg in a 0.5 ml suspension have occasionally been administered.

Topical Ophthalmic: One drop of a suspension containing 0.1 to 5.0 mg/ml in sterile 5 per cent dextrose in water every 30 minutes.

AMPICILLIN

Proprietary Names: Acillin, A-Cillin, Alpen, Amblosin (Germ.), Amcill, Amipenix (Jap.), Ampen (Canad.), Amperil, Ampexin (Canad.), Ampicin (Canad.), Ampilean (Canad.), Ampilum (Ital.), Ampilux (Ital.), Ampipenin (Swed.), Austrapen (Austral.), Binotal (Germ.), D-Amp, D-Cillin, Deripen (Germ.), Doktacillin (Swed.), Domicillin (Jap.), Omnipen, Pen A or A/N, Pen-Bristol (Germ.), Penbriten, Penbritine (Fr.), Penbrock (Germ.), Penicline (Fr.), Pensyn, Pentrex (S. Afr.), Pentrexyl (G.B.), Pfizerpen A., Polycillin, Principen, Ro-ampen, Roampicillin, SK-Ampicillin, Supen, Suractin (Germ.), Synpenin (Jap.), Totacillin, Totapen (Fr.), Vidopen (G.B.).

Preparations

Injection: Powder for solution, 250 mg/ml in 2.5-gm containers; powder, 0.125, 0.25, 0.5, 1, 2, and 4 gm.

Oral: Capsules, 250 and 500 mg; drops (pediatric), 100 mg/ml; powder for suspension (pediatric), 100 mg/ml; powder for suspension, 125, 250, and 500 mg/5 ml; tablets (chewable), 125 mg.

Usual Dosages

Intracameral, Intravitreal: 500 μg in 0.1 to 0.2 ml of isotonic sodium chloride injection.

Intramuscular: Adults and children over 20 kg, 250 to 500 mg four times daily at 6-hour intervals; less than 20 kg, 25 to 50 mg/kg daily in divided doses at 6- or 8-hour intervals.

Intravenous: Adults and children over 20 kg, 250 to 500 mg four times daily at 6-hour intervals. Children under 20 kg, 25 to 50 mg/kg daily in divided doses every 6 hours. For severe infections, doses up to 2 gm every 6 hours may be used. Patients have been successfully treated for bacterial meningitis with doses of 8 to 14 gm daily; the drug is administered every 3 to 4 hours.

Oral: Adults and children over 20 kg, 250 to 500 mg four times daily at 6-hour intervals; children less than 20 kg, 25 to 50 mg/kg daily in divided doses every 6 to 8 hours. Higher doses up to 12 gm daily should be used for stubborn or severe infections. For urethritis caused by *N. gonorrhoeae*, 3.5 gm as a single oral dose are recommended. In stubborn infections, therapy may be required for several weeks.

Subconjunctival: 50 to 250 mg in 0.5 ml of isotonic sodium chloride injection or sterile water for injection.

Topical Ophthalmic: One drop of a solution containing 40 to 100 mg/ml is given every 1 to 4 hours. Fortified ampicillin eyedrops are prepared with ampicillin trihydrate.

AMPICILLIN/PROBENECID COMBINATION

Proprietary Names: Polycillin-PRB, Principen with Probenecid, Probampacin.

Preparations

Oral: Capsules, 3.5 gm ampicillin and 1 gm probenecid; powder for suspension, 3.5 mg ampicillin and 1 gm probenecid.

Usual Dosages

Oral: Usual dosage is a single dose of 3.5 gm of ampicillin and 1 gm of probenecid.

ANTIMONY MEGLUMINE

Proprietary Names: Glucantim (Ital.), Glucantime (Fr., Span.).

Preparations

Injection: Powder.

Usual Dosages

Intramuscular, Intravenous: A dose of 100 mg/kg may be administered daily for 10 to 12 days and repeated if required after an interval of 4 to 6 weeks.

APRACLONIDINE

Proprietary Name: Iopidine.

Preparations

Topical Ophthalmic: Solution, 1 per cent.

Usual Dosages

Topical Ophthalmic: One drop may be applied to the affected eye(s) once daily.

ARGENTUM NITRATE
See Silver Nitrate.

ARTIFICIAL TEARS
See Hydroxyethyl Cellulose, Hydroxypropyl Cellulose, Hydroxypropyl Methylcellulose, Methylcellulose, Polyvinyl Alcohol.

---

* Route of administration not approved by FDA.

† Drug not approved by FDA for any indication.

‡ Drug not approved by FDA for this particular indication.

§ Indicated dosage above the manufacturer's recommendation.

ASCORBIC ACID (VITAMIN C)

Proprietary Names: Ascorbef (G.B.), Ascorbicap, Cebid, Cecon, Cetane, Cevalin, Cevi-Bid, Ce-Vi-Sol, Cevita, C-Span, Dull-C, Flavorcee, Roscorbic (G.B.), Vita-C.

Preparations

Injection: Solution, 100, 250, and 500 mg/ml.
Oral: Capsules (timed-release), 500 mg; crystals, 4 gm/5 ml; liquid, 35 mg/0.6 ml; powder, 4 gm/5 ml; solution, 100 mg/ml; syrup, 500 mg/5 ml; tablets, 50, 100, 250, 500, and 1000 mg; tablets (chewable), 100, 250, and 500 mg; tablets (timed-release), 0.5 and 1.5 gm.

Usual Dosages

Intramuscular, Intravenous, Oral: Adults, average protective dose is 70 to 150 mg daily. For scurvy, 0.3 to 1.0 gm daily is recommended. To enhance wound healing, 300 to 500 mg daily for 7 to 10 days both preoperatively and postoperatively are adequate. For severe burns, 1.0 to 2.0 gm daily are recommended until healing has occurred or grafting operations are complete.

ASPIRIN (ACETYLSALICYLIC ACID)

Proprietary Names: Acetophen (Canad.), Acetylin (Germ.), Acetyl-Sal (Canad.), Albyl-Selters (Swed.), Ancasal (Canad.), Apernyl (Swed.), Aquaprin (S. Afr.), A.S.A., Asadrine (Canad.), Asagran (G.B.), Aspasol (S. Afr.), Aspegic (Fr.), Aspergum, Aspirisucre (Fr.), Aspirjen, Aspisol (Austral.), Babiprin (Ire.), Bamyl (Swed.), Bayer Aspirin, Bi-prin (Austral.), Breoprin (G.B.), Buffinol, Caprin (G.B.), Cetasal (Canad.), Chu-Pax (G.B.), Claragine (Fr.), Clariprin (Austral.), Codral Junior (Austral.), Colfarit (Germ.), Dispril (Swed.), Ecotrin, Elsprin (Austral.) Entericin, Entrophen (Canad.), Extren, Godamed (Germ.), Infatabs A (Austral.), Instantine (Swed.), Ivepirine (Fr.), Juvepirine (Fr.), Levius (G.B.), Measurin, Monasalyl (Canad.), Neopirine-25 (Canad.), Nova-Phase (Canad.), Novasen (Canad.), Novosprin (Austral.), Nu-seals Aspirin (G.B.), Premaspin (Swed.), Prodol (Austral.), Provoprin-500 (Austral.), Rhonal (Canad., Fr.), Sal-Adult/Infant (Canad.), Seclopyrine (Fr.), Solcetas (Austral.), Solusal (Austral.), St. Joseph Aspirin, Supasa (Canad.), Tasprin-Sol (G.B.), Triaphen-10 (Canad.), Zorprin.

Preparations

Oral: Capsules, 325 mg; tablets, 65, 81, 162, 325, 500, and 650 mg; tablets (buffered), 325 mg; tablets (chewable), 81 mg; tablets (enteric-coated), 300 and 600 mg; tablets (timed-release), 650 mg.

Usual Dosages

Oral, Rectal: Range, 300 mg to 8 gm daily in divided doses; children, 11 to 130 mg/kg daily.

---

* Route of administration not approved by FDA.
† Drug not approved by FDA for any indication.
‡ Drug not approved by FDA for this particular indication.
§ Indicated dosage above the manufacturer's recommendation.

ASPIRIN/CAFFEINE/BUTALBITAL COMBINATION

Proprietary Names: B-A-C, Fiorinal, Isollyl, Lanorinal, Lorprn, Marnal.

Preparations

Oral: Capsules, 325 or 650 mg aspirin, 40 or 50 mg caffeine, and 40 or 50 mg butalbital; tablets, 325 or 650 mg aspirin, 40 or 50 mg caffeine, and 40 or 50 mg butalbital.

Usual Dosages

Oral: The usual adult dose is one or two tablets or capsules every 4 hours as needed for pain. Total daily dosage should not exceed six tablets or capsules.

ASPIRIN/CODEINE COMBINATION

Proprietary Names: Ascodeen, Ascriptin with Codeine, Codasa, Codasa Forte.

Preparations

Oral: Capsules, 300 mg aspirin with 15 mg codeine, 325 mg aspirin with 15 or 30 mg codeine, 650 mg aspirin with 30 mg codeine; tablets, 325 mg aspirin with 15 or 30 mg codeine.

Usual Dosages

Oral: Two capsules or tablets every 3 or 4 hours when necessary.

ASTEMIZOLE

Proprietary Name: Hismanal (Belg.).

Preparations

Oral: Tablets, 10 mg.

Usual Dosages

Oral: A single daily dose of 10 mg is recommended. In patients with severe symptoms, a regimen of 30 mg daily for 1 week, followed by 10 mg daily, may be employed.

ATROPINE

Proprietary Names: Atropair, Atropinol (Germ.), Atropisol, Atropt (Austral.), Atroptol (Austral.), BufOpto Atropine, Isopto Atropine, Ocu-Tropine, Spersatropine (S. Afr.).

Preparations

Topical Ophthalmic: Ointment, 0.5 and 1 per cent; solution, 1, 2, 3, and 4 per cent.

Usual Dosages

Topical Ophthalmic: One drop of 1 or 2 per cent atropine solution (or 1 per cent ointment) may be instilled one to three times daily. A stronger concentration or more frequent administration may be necessary in very severe inflammations. As the inflammation subsides, the frequency of administration may be reduced to twice weekly.

AURANOFIN

Proprietary Name: Ridaura.

Preparations

Oral: Capsules, 3 mg.

Usual Dosages

Oral: Initially, 6 mg daily administered as a single dose or in two divided doses. Dosage may be increased up to 9 mg daily.

AUROTHIOGLUCOSE

Proprietary Names: Aureotan (Germ.), Solganal.

Preparations

Injection: Suspension, 50 mg/ml.

Usual Dosages

Intramuscular: Adults, initially single weekly injections of 10 mg the first week, 25 mg the second week, 25 or 50 mg the third week, and 50 mg each week thereafter until a total dosage of 0.8 to 1 gm has been administered.

AZATADINE

Proprietary Names: Idulamine (Arg.), Indulian (Fr.), Optimine, Zadine (Austral.).

Preparations

Oral: Tablets, 1 mg.

Usual Dosages

Oral: Adults, 1 to 2 mg twice daily.

AZATHIOPRINE

Proprietary Names: Imuran, Imurek (Germ.), Imurel (Aust., Fr., Swed.).

Preparations

Injection: Powder (lyophilized) equivalent to 100 mg of azathioprine.
Oral: Tablets, 50 mg.

Usual Dosages

Intravenous, Oral: The dose must be individualized. The usual initial dosage is 3 to 5 mg/kg once daily; maintenance, 1 to 4 mg/kg once daily.

AZIDOTHYMIDINE
See Zidovudine.

---

* Route of administration not approved by FDA.
† Drug not approved by FDA for any indication.
‡ Drug not approved by FDA for this particular indication.
§ Indicated dosage above the manufacturer's recommendation.

AZT
See Zidovudine.

BACITRACIN

Proprietary Name: Baciguent.

Preparations

Injection: Powder, 10,000 and 50,000 units.
Topical: Ointment, 500 units/gm.
Topical Ophthalmic: Ointment, 500 units/gm.

Usual Dosages

Intramuscular: For infants under 2.5 kg, 900 units/kg in two to three divided doses. For infants over 2.5 kg, 1000 units/kg daily in two to three divided doses.
Topical: Ointment may be applied two to three times daily.
Topical Ophthalmic: Ointment is instilled in affected eye one to three times daily or more frequently. In severe infections, one drop of solution containing 10,000 units/ml is instilled every hour until improvement occurs; the frequency of administration is then reduced.
Subconjunctival: 10,000 units in 0.5 ml of isotonic sodium chloride injection once or twice daily.

BACITRACIN/POLYMYXIN B COMBINATION

Proprietary Names: Ak-Poly-Bac, Ocumycin.

Preparations

Topical Ophthalmic: Ointment, 500 units bacitracin and 10,000 units polymyxin B/gm.

Usual Dosages

Topical Ophthalmic: A small amount every 3 or 4 hours may be applied, depending on the severity of the infection.

BACLOFEN

Proprietary Name: Lioresal.

Preparations

Oral: Tablets, 10 mg.

Usual Dosages

Oral: Initially, 5 mg three times daily, increased by 15 mg daily every fourth day to 20 mg three times daily. The total daily dose should not exceed a maximum of 80 mg daily.

BALANCED SALT SOLUTION

Proprietary Name: BSS.

Preparations

Intraocular: Ophthalmic irrigation solution, 15, 30, 250, and 500 ml bottles.

Usual Dosages

Intraocular: An adequate amount is used to irrigate the ocular tissues.

BCG VACCINE

Proprietary Name: BCG Vaccine.

Preparations

Injection: Lyophilized vaccine reconstituted with 1 ml of sterile water for injection.

Usual Dosages

Intradermal: A dose of 0.1 ml is administered.

BCNU
See Carmustine.

BELLADONNA

Proprietary Names: Belladonna Extract, Leaf, or Tincture, Bellafolin (Germ.), Bellafoline (Fr.).

Preparations

Oral: Tablets, 15 mg.

Usual Dosages

Oral: 15 mg three times daily.

BENOXINATE

Proprietary Names: Cebesine (Fr.), Conjuncain (Germ.), Dorsacaine, Novesin (Switz.), Novesina (Ital.), Novesine (Austral., Belg., Fr., Germ., Neth.), Oftalmocaina (Arg.), Oxybuprocaine (G.B.), Poen Caina (Arg.).

Preparations

Topical Ophthalmic: Solution, 0.4 per cent.

Usual Dosages

Topical Ophthalmic: One drop of solution may be instilled and may be repeated for three doses if necessary.

BENZATHINE PENICILLIN G

Proprietary Names: Ben-P (Canad.), Bicillin, Dibencil, Duapen (Canad.), Dulpecen-G (Austral.), Extencilline (Fr.), LPG (Austral.), Neolin (G.B.), Penidural (G.B.), Penilente-LA (S. Afr.), Permapen, Tardocillin (Germ.).

---

* Route of administration not approved by FDA.
† Drug not approved by FDA for any indication.
‡ Drug not approved by FDA for this particular indication.
§ Indicated dosage above the manufacturer's recommendation.

Preparations

Injection: Powder; suspension, 300,000 and 600,000 units/ml.

Usual Dosages

Intramuscular: Adults, 1.2 million units in a single dose; older children, a single injection of 900,000 units; infants and children under 27.3 kg, a single dose of 300,000 to 600,000 units. For venereal infections in adults, 2.4 million units followed by one or two doses of 2.4 million units at 7-day intervals. For congenital syphilis in children under 2 years of age, 50,000 units/kg.

BENZYLPENICILLIN POTASSIUM
See Potassium Penicillin G.

BETA CAROTENE

Proprietary Name: Solatene.

Preparations

Oral: Capsules, 30 mg.

Usual Dosages

Oral: The usual adult dosage is 30 to 300 mg administered either as a single daily dose or in divided doses, preferably with meals.

BETAINE

Proprietary Names: Acidol-Pepsin, Somatyl (Fr., Ital.), Stea-16 (Belg.).

Preparations

Oral: Tablets, 388 mg betaine and 97 mg pepsin.

Usual Dosages

Oral: One to three tablets dissolved in a glass of water three times daily, preferably after meals.

BETAMETHASONE

Proprietary Names: Bentelan (Ital.), Betapred (Swed.), Betnelan (Austral.), Betnesol (G.B.), Celestan (Germ.), Celestene (Fr.), Celestona (Swed.), Celestone.

Preparations

Injection: Solution, 3 mg/ml.
Oral: Tablets, 0.6 mg; syrup, 0.6 mg/5 ml.
Topical: Cream, 0.01, 0.2, and 0.25 per cent.
Topical Ophthalmic: No preparation is commercially available. A 0.1 per cent solution may be prepared.

Usual Dosages

Intralesional: 1.5 to 6.0 mg, depending on the size of the affected area.
Oral: Maintenance dose, 0.5 to 1.2 mg daily; dose range, 0.6 to 8.4 mg daily.

Subconjunctival: 3 to 6 mg administered in 0.5 to 1 ml.

Topical: Formulations are applied sparingly in very thin films one to four times daily.

Topical Ophthalmic: One drop of a 0.1 per cent solution every 1 to 2 hours until a response is attained.

BETANIDINE
See Bethanidine.

BETAXOLOL

Proprietary Name: Betoptic.

Preparations

Topical Ophthalmic: Solution, 0.5 per cent.

Usual Dosages

Topical Ophthalmic: The usual dose is one drop in the affected eye(s) twice daily.

BETHANECHOL

Proprietary Names: Besacolin (Jap.), Duvoid, Iricoline (Fr.), Mechothane (G.B.), Mictrol, Myotonachol, Myotonine (G.B.), Urecholine, Uro-Carb (Austral.), Urolax, Vesicholine.

Preparations

Oral: Tablets, 5, 10, 25, and 50 mg.

Usual Dosages

Oral: Adult, 5 to 50 mg three or four times daily to maximum dosage of 120 mg.

BETHANIDINE (BETANIDINE)

Proprietary Names: Batel (Span.), Benzoxine (Jap.), Betaling (Jap.), Esbaloid (Canad.), Esbatal (Arg., Austral., Belg., G.B., Ital., Neth., S. Afr., Scand.), Eusmanid (Aust.), Hypersin (Jap.), Regulin (Scand.).

Preparations

Topical Ophthalmic: No ophthalmic preparation is commercially available in the United States.

Usual Dosages

Topical Ophthalmic: One drop of a 5 to 10 per cent solution twice daily.

BLEOMYCIN

Proprietary Name: Blenoxane.

---

* Route of administration not approved by FDA.
† Drug not approved by FDA for any indication.
‡ Drug not approved by FDA for this particular indication.
§ Indicated dosage above the manufacturer's recommendation.

Preparations

Injection: Powder, 15 units.

Usual Dosages

Intramuscular, Intravenous, Subcutaneous: Because of the possibility of an anaphylactoid reaction, lymphoma patients should be treated with 2 units or less for the first two doses. If no reaction occurs, then 0.25 to 0.50 units/kg (10 to 20 units/square meter) may be given weekly or twice weekly.

BORIC ACID

Proprietary Name: Irrigate.

Preparations

Topical Ophthalmic: Crystals; granules; ointment, 5 and 10 per cent; powder; solution, 2 and 5 per cent.

Usual Dosages

Topical Ophthalmic: Solution or ointment is applied as required.

BOTULINUM A TOXIN

Proprietary Name: Oculinum.

Preparations

Injection: Powder (lyophilized), in 50-ng vials.

Usual Dosages

Intramuscular, Subcutaneous: Botulinim A toxin is diluted in normal saline without preservatives immediately before injection. To prevent breakdown of the toxin, the vial is turned gently, but should not be shaken. The usual dosage is a volume of 0.1 ml containing 0.025 to 5 units (1 unit = 1×10^{-5} μg) injected at six to ten separate sites per eye, or for a total volume of 2 ml or 20 injections per treatment. The total dose may vary in different individuals, but is usually between 12.5 and 75 units per eye.

BOTULISM ANTITOXIN

Proprietary Names: Botulinum Antiserum, Botulinus Antitoxin, Botulism Antitoxin Bivalent Type E, Trivalent Botulinus Antitoria.

Preparations

Injection: Solution containing 10,000 units of each type container (Antitoxin Bivalent Types A and B).

Usual Dosages

Intramuscular, Intravenous: Adults, 10,000 units of type A, B, and E antitoxin every 4 hours until the toxic condition has been alleviated. The antitoxin is diluted 1:10 with 10 per cent dextrose for injection prior to use. The first 10 ml is injected slowly over a 5-minute period; the remainder can be given more rapidly after 15 minutes.

BROMHEXINE

Proprietary Names: Aletor (Span.), Bisolvon (G.B.), Bromcilate (Span.), Brocokin (Ital.), Dakroy Biciron (Germ.), Ophtosol (Germ.).

Preparations

Oral: Elixir, 4 mg/5 ml; tablets, 8 mg.

Usual Dosages

Oral: The usual adult dose is 8 to 16 mg three or four times daily.

BROMOCRIPTINE

Proprietary Names: Parlodel, Pravidel (Germ., Swed.).

Preparations

Oral: Tablets, 2.5 mg.

Usual Dosages

Oral: Initially, 2.5 mg three or four times daily. The dose is increased weekly by increments of 2.5 mg over a period of 3 to 8 weeks until beneficial effects or intolerable adverse effects are noted. A total daily dose of 30 mg is generally considered minimal with a maximum daily amount of 150 mg.

BROMPHENIRAMINE

Proprietary Names: Dimegan (Fr.), Dimetane, Dimotane (G.B.), Ebalin (Germ.), Ilvin (Germ., Swed.), Rolabromophen, Symptom 3, Veltane.

Preparations

Oral: Solution, 2 mg/5 ml; tablets, 4 mg; tablets (extended-release), 8 and 12 mg.

Usual Dosages

Oral: The usual adult dosage is 4 to 8 mg three or four times daily. Alternatively, an extended-release formulation containing 8 or 12 mg may be administered every 8 to 12 hours.

BUPIVACAINE

Proprietary Names: Carbostesin (Germ.), Marcain (G.B.), Marcaine.

Preparations

Injection: Solution, 0.25, 0.5, and 0.75 per cent.

---

* Route of administration not approved by FDA.
† Drug not approved by FDA for any indication.
‡ Drug not approved by FDA for this particular indication.
§ Indicated dosage above the manufacturer's recommendation.

Usual Dosages

Injection: For retrobulbar block, 1.5 to 2 ml of a 0.5 or 0.75 per cent solution is injected inside the muscle cone behind the globe. Light pressure may be applied intermittently for 3 to 5 minutes after the injection.

BUPRENORPHINE

Proprietary Names: Buprenex, Temgesic (G.B., Norw.).

Preparations

Injection: Solution, 0.3 mg/ml in ampules of 1 and 2 ml.
Sublingual: Tablets, 200 µg.

Usual Dosages

Intramuscular, Intravenous: Adults, usual dosage is 0.3 mg given at intervals of up to every 6 hours.
Sublingual: The usual adult dosage is 200 µg.

BUROW'S SOLUTION
See Aluminum Acetate.

CALAMINE

Proprietary Name: Calamine.

Preparations

Topical: Lotion.

Usual Dosages

Topical: A sufficient amount of lotion to cover the affected area is applied twice daily.

CALCIFEDIOL

Proprietary Names: Calderol, Dédrogyl (Fr.), Hidroferol (Span.).

Preparations

Oral: Capsules, 20 and 50 µg.

Usual Dosages

Oral: Usual doses are 50 to 125 µg daily.

CALCITONIN

Proprietary Names: Calcimar, Calcitar (Fr., Ital., Jap.), Calcitare (G.B.), Cacitonina (Ital.), Calsyn (Fr.), Calsynar (G.B.), Cibacalcin (Neth., N.Z.), Miacalcic (Austral., G.B., Norw., N.Z., Swed.), Salcatonin (G.B.), Staporox (Fr.).

Preparations

Injection: Lyophilized powder, 400 MRC units/vial with 4 ml of gelatin as diluent. The final volume should be approximately 0.5 to 1.0 ml.

Usual Dosages

Intramuscular: For hypercalcemia, 100 to 400 MRC units once or twice daily.

Intramuscular, Subcutaneous: For Paget's disease, adults, initially 50 to 100 MRC units daily or three times a week until a satisfactory clinical or biochemical response is obtained. For maintenance, 50 MRC units three times a week. In patients who relapse, larger doses should be tried, but do not consistently improve the clinical response.

CALCITRIOL (1α,25 DIHYDROXYVITAMIN D$_3$)

Proprietary Name: Rocaltrol.

Preparations

Oral: Capsules, 0.25 µg.

Usual Dosages

Oral: The recommended initial dose is 0.25 µg daily. If a satisfactory response is not observed, dosage may be increased by 0.25 µg daily at 2- to 4-week intervals.

CALCIUM CARBONATE

Proprietary Names: Alka-2, Alka-Mints, Amitone, Calcilac, Calcileve (Fr.), Calglycine, Cal-tab (Austral.), Chooz, Dicarbosil, El-Da-Mint, Equilet, Mallamint, Os-Cal 500, Spar-Cal (Austral.), Spentacid, Titracid, Titralac, Trialka, Tums.

Preparations

Oral: Powder; tablets, 0.65 and 1.25 gm; tablets (chewable), 330, 350, 420, 500, 750, and 850 mg.

Usual Dosages

Oral: Adults, 1 to 2 gm three times daily with meals. The powdered preparation is mixed with water or sprinkled on food.

CALCIUM CHLORIDE

Proprietary Name: Chloro-Calcion (Fr.).

Preparations

Injection: Solution 5 and 10 per cent.
Oral: Powder.

Usual Dosages

Intravenous (Slow): Adults, 10 to 30 ml of a 5 per cent solution.
Oral: Adults, 4 to 8 gm daily in four divided doses, given with demulcent. Children, 300 mg/kg of a 2 per cent solution given daily in four divided doses.

---

* Route of administration not approved by FDA.
† Drug not approved by FDA for any indication.
‡ Drug not approved by FDA for this particular indication.
§ Indicated dosage above the manufacturer's recommendation.

CALCIUM CITRATE

Proprietary Name: Citracal.

Preparations

Oral: Tablets, 950 mg.

Usual Dosages

Oral: The usual dosage is 0.95 to 1.9 gm three to four times daily.

CALCIUM EDETATE
See Edetate Calcium Disodium.

CALCIUM GLUBIONATE

Proprietary Name: Neo-Calglucon.

Preparations

Oral: Solution, 1.8 gm/5 ml.

Usual Dosages

Oral: Adults, 20 gm daily in divided doses.

CALCIUM GLUCONATE

Proprietary Names: Sandocal (G.B.), Vical (Ital.), Weifa-Kalk (Norw.).

Preparations

Injection: Powder; solution, 10 per cent.
Oral: Tablets, 325, 500, 650 mg, and 1 gm.

Usual Dosages

Intravenous: Adults, initially, 20 ml of a 10 per cent solution injected slowly, followed by a slow infusion of a 0.3 to 0.8 per cent solution over a period of 3 to 12 hours. Children, 500 mg/kg daily in divided doses.
Oral: Adults, 15 gm daily in divided doses. Children, 500 mg/kg daily in divided doses.

CALCIUM LACTATE

Proprietary Name: Calcium Lactate.

Preparations

Oral: Powder; tablets, 325 and 650 mg.

Usual Dosages

Oral: Adults, 1.5 to 3 gm three times daily with meals. Children, 500 mg/kg daily in divided doses.

CARBACHOL

Proprietary Names: Carbacel, Isopto Carbachol, Isopto-Karbakolin (Swed.), Miostat, Mistura, PV Carbachol (Canad.).

Preparations

Topical Ophthalmic: Solution, 0.75, 1.5, 2.25, and 3 per cent.

Usual Dosages

Topical Ophthalmic: The frequency and concentration of instillation depend upon the patient's response to therapy.

CARBAMAZEPINE

Proprietary Names: Tegretal (Germ.), Tegretol.

Preparations

Oral: Tablets, 200 mg.

Usual Dosages

Oral: Adults and adolescents; initial 400 mg in two divided doses on first day, increased by 200 mg daily with the total dose divided into three or four equal portions. Doses up to 1.6 gm daily have been used in adults in rare instances. Children under 6 years, 100 mg daily initially; 6 to 12 years, 100 mg twice daily initially.

CARBENICILLIN

Proprietary Names: Anabactyl (Germ.), Carbapen (Austral.), Fugacillin (Swed.), Geocillin, Geopen, Microcillin (Germ.), Pyopen.

Preparations

Injection: Powder, 1, 2, 5, and 10 gm.
Oral: Tablets equivalent to 382 mg.

Usual Dosages

Intramuscular: Adults, 1 to 2 gm every 6 hours. Children, 50 to 200 mg/kg daily in divided doses every 4 to 6 hours.
Intravenous: For septicemia and severe systemic, respiratory, or soft tissue infections, adults, 300 to 500 mg/kg daily; children, 400 to 500 mg/kg daily. The drug can be administered in divided doses every 4 to 6 hours or by continuous or intermittent infusion. The recommended maximum intravenous dose is 40 gm per day.
Subconjunctival: 100 to 250 mg in 0.5 ml of isotonic sodium chloride injection or sterile water for injection.

CARBIDOPA/LEVODOPA COMBINATIONS

Proprietary Name: Sinemet.

Preparations

Oral: Tablets 10 or 25 mg carbidopa and 100 or 250 mg levodopa.

---

* Route of administration not approved by FDA.
† Drug not approved by FDA for any indication.
‡ Drug not approved by FDA for this particular indication.
§ Indicated dosage above the manufacturer's recommendation.

Usual Dosages

Oral: The suggested initial dosage is one tablet of Sinemet-10/100 three times daily. The amount may be increased gradually by one tablet every day or every other day up to six tablets daily. If a larger dose is needed, one tablet of Sinemet-25/250 three times daily may be administered.

CARBONIC ANHYDRASE INHIBITORS

See Acetazolamide, Dichlorphenamide, Ethoxzolamide, Methazolamide.

CARMUSTINE (BCNU)

Proprietary Name: BiCNU.

Preparations

Injection: Powder, 100 mg and 3 ml diluent.

Usual Dosages

Intravenous: The recommended dose as a single agent in previously untreated patients is 200 mg/square meter every 6 weeks. This may be given as a single dose or divided into daily injections, such as 100 mg/square meter on 2 successive days. When used in combination with other myelosuppressive drugs, dosage should be adjusted accordingly.

CEFACLOR

Proprietary Names: Ceclor, Distaclor (G.B.), Panoral (Germ.).

Preparations

Oral: Capsules, 250 and 500 mg; powder (for suspension), 125 and 250 mg/5 ml.

Usual Dosages

Oral: Adults, 250 mg every 8 hours; for severe infections, this amount may be increased to a maximum of 4 gm daily. Children, 20 to 40 mg/kg daily in equally divided doses every 8 hours.

CEFAZOLIN

Proprietary Names: Ancef, Celmetin (Swed.), Kefzol.

Preparations

Injection: Powder, 0.25, 0.5, and 1.0 gm and bulk (5 and 10 gm).
Topical Ophthalmic: No commercial preparations are available. Fortified cefazolin eyedrops can be prepared from the powder.

Usual Dosages

Intramuscular, Intravenous: Adults, 250 and 500 mg every 8 hours; in severe infections, 0.5 to 1.5 gm may be given every 6 hours. Children and infants over 1 month of age, 25 to 100 mg/kg daily in three or four divided doses. Doses of 0.5 to 1.0 gm every 12 hours may be given for pneumococcal pneumonia or acute uncomplicated urinary tract infections in either adults or children. Patients with impaired renal function should receive reduced dosages.

Intravitreal: 1.0 to 2.25 mg in 0.1 to 0.2 ml suspension.

Retrobulbar: 0.5 to 1.0 ml of a suspension containing 100 mg/ml.

Subconjunctival: 50 to 100 mg in 0.5 ml of isotonic sodium chloride injection or sterile water for injection.

Topical Ophthalmic: One drop of a solution containing 40 to 50 mg/ml every hour until improvement occurs; then reduce frequency.

CEFOTAXIME

Proprietary Name: Claforan.

Preparations

Injection: Powder, 1, 2, and 10 gm/vial.

Usual Dosages

Intramuscular, Intravenous: Adults, 2 to 12 gm daily in equally divided doses every 4 to 6 hours. The usual dosage for moderate to severe infections is 1 to 2 gm every 8 hours. The maximum daily dosage should not exceed 12 gm.

CEFOXITIN

Proprietary Names: Mefoxin, Mefoxitin (Denm. Germ., Swed. Switz.).

Preparations

Injection: Powder (equivalent to base), 1 and 2 gm.

Usual Dosages

Intramuscular, Intravenous: The usual adult dosage range is 1 to 2 gm every 6 to 8 hours. For life-threatening infections, 2 gm every 4 hours or 3 gm every 6 hours.

CEFTAZIDIME

Proprietary Names: Fortaz, Tazicef, Tazidime.

Preparations

Injection: Powder, 0.5, 1.0, and 2.0 gm/vial.

Usual Dosages

Intramuscular, Intravenous: The usual recommended dose is 1 gm every 8 to 12 hours.

CEFTIZOXIME

Proprietary Name: Cefizox.

---

* Route of administration not approved by FDA.
† Drug not approved by FDA for any indication.
‡ Drug not approved by FDA for this particular indication.
§ Indicated dosage above the manufacturer's recommendation.

Preparations

Injection: Powder, 1 or 2 gm in 28-, 50-, and 100-ml vials.

Usual Dosages

Intramuscular, Intravenous: Adults, 2 to 12 gm daily in equally divided doses every 8 to 12 hours. Children (6 months or older), 150 to 200 mg/kg daily in equally divided doses every 6 to 8 hours.

CEFTRIAXONE

Proprietary Name: Rocephin.

Preparations

Injection: Powder, 0.25, 0.5, 1, 2, and 10 gm.

Usual Dosages

Intramuscular, Intravenous: Adults, usual dose is 1 to 2 gm once daily (or in equally divided doses every 12 hours). The total daily dose should not exceed 4 gm. For uncomplicated gonococcal infections, 250 mg intramuscularly as a single dose may be administered.

CEFUROXIME

Proprietary Names: Curoxim (Ital.), Itorex (Ital.), Kefurox, Ultroxim (Ital.), Zinacef.

Preparations

Injection: Powder, 0.75, 1.5, and 7.5 gm/vial.
Oral: Tablets, 125, 250, and 500 mg.

Usual Dosages

Intramuscular, Intravenous: Adults, 2.25 to 9.0 gm daily in equally divided doses every 8 hours. Infants and children over 3 months, 50 to 100 mg/kg daily in equally divided doses every 6 to 8 hours.

Oral: Adults and children 12 years of age and over, 250 mg every 12 hours. For severe infections or infections caused by less susceptible organisms, 500 mg every 12 hours may be used.

CELLULOSE, OXIDIZED
See Oxidized Cellulose.

CEPHALEXIN

Proprietary Names: Ceporex (G.B.), Ceporexine (Fr., Swed.), Keflex, Oracef (Germ.).

Preparations

Oral: Capsules, 250 and 500 mg; drops (pediatric), 100 mg/ml (after reconstitution); suspension, 125 and 250 mg/5 ml (after reconstitution).

Usual Dosages

Oral: The daily dose should not exceed 4 gm because of possible renal damage. In adults, 250 mg every 6 hours is recommended; children, 25 to 50 mg/kg in four divided doses. For severe infections, this doses may be doubled. If more than 4 gm are needed, a parenteral cephalosporin preparation should be substituted.

CEPHALORIDINE

Proprietary Names: Ceporan (Austral., Canad., S. Afr., Swed.), Ceporin (G.B.), Keflodin (Fr.), Kefspor (Germ., Swed.), Loridine.

Preparations

Injection: Powder, 0.5 and 1 gm.

Usual Dosages

Intracameral, Intravitreal: 250 µg in 0.1 to 0.2 ml of isotonic sodium chloride injection.
Intramuscular, Intravenous: The daily dose should not exceed 4 gm because of possible renal damage. Adults, 0.5 to 1.0 gm three or four times a day at equally spaced intervals. Children, 30 to 50 mg/kg daily, preferably intramuscular, in three divided doses at equally spaced intervals. These routes should not be used in premature or full-term infants less than 1 month old. Since large doses may produce tubular necrosis, appropriate reduction in dosage should be made in patients with impaired renal function. Mixing with solutions containing other antibiotics is not recommended.
Subconjunctival: 50 to 100 mg in 0.5 ml of isotonic sodium chloride injection or sterile water for injection.
Topical Ophthalmic: One drop of solution containing 50 to 100 mg/ml is instilled every hour until improvement occurs. The frequency of administration is then reduced.

CEPHALOTHIN

Proprietary Names: Cefalotine (Fr.), Cepovenin (Germ.), Keflin.

Preparations

Injection: Powder, 0.25, 0.5, 1, 2, and 4 gm.
Topical Ophthalmic: No ophthalmic form is available, but a solution for topical use can be made from the powder.

Usual Dosages

Intramuscular, Intravenous: Adults, 1 to 2 gm every 4 to 6 hours; children, 200 mg/kg daily in four divided doses; premature and full-term newborn infants, 100 mg/kg daily in four divided doses.
Subconjunctival: 50 to 100 mg in 0.5 ml of isotonic sodium chloride injection or sterile water for injection.
Topical Ophthalmic: One drop of solution containing 50 to 100 mg/ml every hour until improvement occurs; then frequency is reduced.

CEPHAPIRIN

Proprietary Names: Ambrocef (Ital.), Ambrotina (Ital.), Brisfirina (Span.), Brisporin (Ital.), Bristocef (Germ.), Cefadyl, Cefaloject (Fr.), Cefatrexil (Arg.), Cefatrexyl (Austral., Belg., Jap., N.Z., Switz.).

Preparations

Injection: Powder, 1, 2, 4, and 20 gm.

Usual Dosages

Intramuscular, Intravenous: Adults, 0.5 to 1.0 gm every 4 to 6 hours; in severe infections, up to 12 gm daily in divided doses. Children, 40 to 80 mg/kg in four equally divided doses.

CEPHRADINE

Proprietary Names: Anspor, Cefril (S. Afr.), Eskacef (G.B.), Sefril (Germ.), Velosef.

Preparations

Injection: Powder, 0.025, 0.250, 0.5, 1, 2 and 4 gm.
Oral: Capsules, 250 and 500 mg; suspension, 125 and 250 mg/5 ml.

Usual Dosages

Intramuscular, Intravenous: Adults, 2 to 4 gm daily in equally divided doses every 6 hours. In severe infections, the dose may be increased to a maximum of 8 gm. Infants and children, 50 to 100 mg/kg daily in equally divided doses every 6 hours.
Oral: Adults, 250 to 500 mg every 6 hours or 0.5 to 1.0 gm every 12 hours. Severe infections may require large doses. Infants over 9 months and children, 25 to 50 mg/kg daily in four divided doses. The maximum daily dose should not exceed 4 gm.

CHLORAL HYDRATE

Proprietary Names: Aquachoral, Chloradorm (Austral.), Chloralate (Austral.), Chloraldurat (Germ.), Chloralex (Canad.), Chloralix (Austral.), Chloralixir (Canad.), Chloralvan (Canad.), Chloratol (Canad.), Cohidrate, Dormel (Austral.), Eudorm (Austral.), Felsules, H.S. Need, Kessodrate, Lanchloral (Austral.), Maso-Chloral, Nigracap (Canad.), Noctec, Novochlorhydrate (Canad.), Oradrate, Rectules, SK-Chloral Hydrate.

Preparations

Oral: Capsules, 225, 250, 450, and 500 mg; elixir; syrup, 250 and 500 mg/5 ml.
Rectal: Suppositories, 60, 120, 300, 460, 500, 600, and 900 mg.

Usual Dosages

Oral, Rectal: As sedative, adults, 250 mg three times daily after meals. As hypnotic, adults, 0.5 to 1.0 gm 15 to 30 minutes before bedtime. The daily dosage for adults should not exceed 2 gm.

CHLORAMBUCIL

Proprietary Names: Chloraminophene (Fr.), Leukeran.

---

* Route of administration not approved by FDA.
† Drug not approved by FDA for any indication.
‡ Drug not approved by FDA for this particular indication.
§ Indicated dosage above the manufacturer's recommendation.

716 / DRUG ROSTER

Preparations

Oral: Tablets, 2 and 5 mg.

Usual Dosages

Oral: The usual dosage is 0.1 to 0.2 mg/kg daily for 3 to 6 weeks as required.

CHLORAMPHENICOL

Proprietary Names: Ak-Chlor, Amphicol, Antibiopto, Aquamycetin (Germ.), Bipimycetin (Ind.), Catilan (Germ.), Chlomin (Austral.), Chloramex (S. Afr.), Chloramol (Austral.), Chloramphycin (Ind.), Chloramsaar (Germ.), Chlorcetin, Chlorcol (S. Afr.), Chlornicol (S. Afr.), Chlorofair, Chloromycetin, Clorfen (S. Afr.), Cloroptic, Cylphenicol, Econochlor, Enicol (Canad.), Fenicol (Canad.), Gotimycin (Germ.), Jatcetin (S. Afr.), Kamaver (Germ.), Kemicetin (G.B.), Kemicetine, Lennacol (S. Afr.), Leukomycin (Germ.), Mychel, Mycinol (Canad.), Nevimycin (Germ.), Novochlorocap (Canad.), Ocu-Chlor, Oleomycetin (Germ.), Opclor (Austral.), Ophthochlor, Pantovernil (Germ.), Paraxin, Pentamycetin (Canad.), Sintomicetine (Fr.), Solnicol (Fr.), Tifomycine (Fr.), Troymycetin (S. Afr.).

Preparations

Oral: Capsules, 50, 100, and 250 mg.
Topical Ophthalmic: Ointment, 1 per cent; solution, 0.5 per cent.

Usual Dosages

Intracameral, Intravitreal: 1 to 2 mg in 0.2 to 0.5 ml of isotonic sodium chloride injection.
Intravenous: Adults, 50 mg/kg daily in divided doses every 6 to 8 hours. Oral therapy should replace intravenous administration as soon as possible. This drug should not be used parenterally in children except to initiate therapy for meningitis or severe sepsis, when 100 mg/kg daily can be given.
Oral: Adults, children, and infants over 2 weeks of age, 50 mg/kg daily in divided doses every 6 to 8 hours. In patients in whom the half-life of the drug may be increased (e.g., those with impaired liver function), the interval between doses may have to be increased. Premature infants, 25 mg/kg daily in divided doses every 4 to 6 hours. For all infants, it is advisable to monitor chloramphenicol blood levels frequently, and ideally, to maintain the blood level of drug between 10 and 20 μg/100 ml.
Subconjunctival: 1.25 to 2 mg in 0.5 ml of isotonic sodium chloride injection.
Topical Ophthalmic: For severe conjunctivitis or corneal ulcers, one drop of a 0.5 per cent aqueous solution every 30 minutes. For mild conjunctivitis, one drop of a 0.5 per cent aqueous solution is applied at 1- to 2- hour intervals or ointment is instilled three to four times daily.

CHLORDIAZEPOXIDE

Proprietary Names: A-Poxide, Brigen-G, Calmoden (G.B.), Chemdipoxide (Canad.), Chlordiazachel, Corax (Canad.), C-Tran (Canad.), Diapax (Canad.), Elenium (Pol.), Libritabs, Librium, Lo Tense, Medilium (Canad.), Menrium, Murcil, Nack (Canad.), Novopoxide (Canad.), Protensin (Canad.), Relaxil (Canad.), Risolid (Swed.), Screen, SK-Lygen, Solium (Canad.), Tenex, Trilium (Canad.), Tropium (G.B.), Via-Quil (Canad.), Zetran.

Preparations

Injection: Powder, 100 mg in 5 ml in dry-filled containers.
Oral: Capsules, 5, 10, and 25 mg; tablets, 5, 10, and 25 mg.

Usual Dosages

Intramuscular, Intravenous: 50 to 100 mg, repeated in 2 to 4 hours or given three to four times daily, if necessary.
Oral: 10 to 100 mg daily in three or four divided doses.

CHLOROQUINE

Proprietary Names: Aralen, Arechin (Pol.), Avoclor (G.B.), Chlorocon, Chlorquin (Austral.), Malaquin (Austral.), Malarex (Denm.), Malarivon (G.B.), Nivaquine (G.B.), Resochin (G.B.), Roquine, Siragan (Aust.), Tresochin (Swed.).

Preparations

Injection: Solution, 50 mg/ml (equivalent to 40 mg of base).
Oral: Tablets, 500 mg (equivalent to 300 mg of base).

Usual Dosages

Intramuscular, Oral: 150 to 900 mg of chloroquine base daily in divided doses.

CHLOROTHIAZIDE

Proprietary Names: Diuril, Diurilix (Fr.), Flumen (Ital.), Minzil (Ital.), Salisan (Denm.), Saluren (Ital.), Saluric (G.B.), SK-Chlorothiazide, Yadalan (Span.).

Preparations

Oral: Suspension, 250 mg/5 ml; tablets, 250 and 500 mg.

Usual Dosages

Oral: Adults, initially, 500 mg twice daily. Children, 20 mg/kg daily in two divided doses.

CHLORPHENIRAMINE

Proprietary Names: Alermine, Allerbid, Allergex (Austral., S. Afr.), Allergisan (Swed.), Allerhist (S. Afr.), Allertab, Al-R, Antagonate, Ardehist, Barachlor, Chestamine, Chlo-Amine, Chlor-4/100, Chloraman, Chloramate, Chloramin (Austral.), Chloren, Chlormene, Chlorohist, Chlorophen, Chloroton, Chlorpen, Chlor-Span, Chlortab, Chlor-Trimeton, Chlor-Tripolon (Canad.), Chlortrone (Canad.), Cosea, Drize, Haynon (G.B.), Histacon, Histadur, Histaids (Austral.), Histalon (Canad.), Histaspan, Histex, Histol, H-Stadur,

---

* Route of administration not approved by FDA.

† Drug not approved by FDA for any indication.

‡ Drug not approved by FDA for this particular indication.

§ Indicated dosage above the manufacturer's recommendation.

Lorphen, Malachlor, Nasahist, Niratron, Panahist, Phenetron, Piranex (Austral.), Piriton (G.B.), Pyranistan, Rhinihist, Teldrin, Trymegen.

Preparations

Oral: Capsules (extended-release), 6 and 12 mg; solution, 2 mg/5 ml; tablets, 4 mg; tablets (timed-release), 8 and 12 mg.

Usual Dosages

Oral: Adults, 2 to 4 mg three or four times daily (tablets, syrup) or 8 to 12 mg one to three times daily (timed-release form).

CHLORPROMAZINE

Proprietary Names: Chloractil, Chlor-Promanyl (Canad.), Chlorprom-Ez-Ets (Canad.), Chlorzine, Elmarine (Canad.), Hibernal (Swed.), Klorazin (S. Afr.), Klorazine, Klorpromex (Swed.), Komazine, Largactil, Megaphen (Germ.), Onazine (Canad.), Plegomazine (Austral.), Procalm (Austral.), Promachel, Promachlor, Promacid (Austral.), Promapar, Promaz, Promosol (Canad.), Psychozine, Serazone (Austral.), Sonazine, Terpium, Thoradex, Thorazine.

Preparations

Injection: Solution, 25 mg/ml.
Oral: Capsules (sustained-release), 30, 75, 150, 200, and 300 mg; concentrate, 30 and 100 mg/ml; syrup, 10 mg/5 ml; tablets, 10, 25, 50, 100, and 200 mg.
Rectal: Suppositories, 25 and 100 mg.

Usual Dosages

Intramuscular: For emesis in adults, 25 mg initially, which may be increased to 50 mg and repeated every 3 to 4 hours if necessary; children, 0.5 mg/kg every 4 to 6 hours. For acute psychosis in hospitalized adults, 25 to 100 mg initially, repeated in 1 to 4 hours as necessary.
Oral: For emesis in adults, 10 to 25 mg every 4 to 6 hours; children, 0.5 mg/kg every 4 to 6 hours. For severe psychosis in adults, a daily dosage of 200 to 600 mg initially in divided doses may be administered and increased if necessary (maximum, 2 gm daily); children, 0.5 mg/kg every 4 to 6 hours.
Rectal: For emesis, adults, 50 to 100 mg every 6 to 8 hours; children, 1 mg/kg every 6 to 8 hours. For psychosis in children, 1 mg/kg every 6 to 8 hours.

CHLORPROPAMIDE

Proprietary Names: Chloromide (Canad.), Chloronase (Canad., Germ.), Diabetal (Swed.), Diabetoral (Germ.), Diabett, Diabines (Swed.), Diabinese, Melitase (G.B.), Novopropamide (Canad.), Stabinol (Canad.).

---

* Route of administration not approved by FDA.
† Drug not approved by FDA for any indication.
‡ Drug not approved by FDA for this particular indication.
§ Indicated dosage above the manufacturer's recommendation.

Preparations

Oral: Tablets, 100 and 250 mg.
Rectal: Suppositories, 25 and 100 mg.

Usual Dosages

Oral: Dosage must be individualized. The usual range is 100 to 500 mg daily (maximum, 750 mg).
Rectal: Adults, 50 to 100 mg every 6 to 8 hours; children, 1 mg/kg every 6 to 8 hours.

CHLORTETRACYCLINE

Proprietary Names: Aureomycin, Aureomycine (Fr.), Chlortet (Austral.), CTC, Topmycin (S. Afr.).

Preparations

Injection: Powder, 500 mg buffered with sodium glycinate.
Oral: Capsules, 50, 100, and 250 mg.
Topical Ophthalmic: Ointment, 1 per cent.

Usual Dosages

Intravenous: Adults, 500 mg every 6 to 12 hours, restricted to total daily dose of 2 gm for initiation of treatment or for very severe infections; children 10 to 20 mg/kg daily divided into two doses.
Oral: Adults, 250 to 500 mg every 6 hours (loading dose of 1 gm may be used); children, 25 to 50 mg/kg daily in four doses.
Topical Ophthalmic: Ointment applied three or four times daily.

CHLORTHALIDONE

Proprietary Names: Hygroton, Igroton (Ital.), Uridon (Canad.).

Preparations

Oral: Tablets, 50 and 100 mg.

Usual Dosages

Oral: Adults, initially 50 to 100 mg daily or 100 mg on alternate days or three times weekly; some patients may require a dose of 200 mg.

CHOLECALCIFEROL (VITAMIN D$_3$)

Proprietary Names: D-Muslin (Germ.), Provitina D$_3$ (Germ.), Ultra "D", Vigorsan D$_3$ (Germ.).

Preparations

Oral: Capsules, 0.25 and 1 μg.

Usual Dosages

Oral: Dosage must be individualized, but the following daily intakes are recommended: infants under 1 year, 7.5 μg; children 1 to 4 years, 10 μg; in pregnancy and lactation, 10 μg.

CHOLESTYRAMINE RESIN

Proprietary Names: Cuemid (Austral., Germ., Scand.), Quantalan (Aust., Germ., Port., Switz.), Questran.

Preparations

Oral: Powder or 9-gm packets containing 4 gm of cholestyramine resin.

Usual Dosages

Oral: Adults, 10 to 16 gm of resin daily in divided doses.

CHOLINE

Proprietary Name: Neurotropan (Germ.).

Preparations

Oral: Powder; tablets, 250 mg.

Usual Dosages

Oral: Adults, initially 1 gm four times daily, with the amount gradually increased over a 3- to 8-week period to a maximum of 4 to 5 gm four times daily.

CHYMOTRYPSIN

Proprietary Names: Alpha Chymar, Alphacutanee (Fr.), Aphlozyme (Fr.), Catarase, Chymar (G.B.), Chymar-Zon (G.B.), Enzeon, Kimopsin (Austral., Jap.), Quimotrase (Canad.), Zolyse, Zonulyn (Canad.), Zonulysin (G.B.).

Preparations

Injection: Powder (lyophilized), 750 units (1 mg) with 5 ml of diluent; two-compartment vial containing lyophilized powder, 300 units in lower compartment and sodium chloride injection 2 ml in upper compartment.
Topical Ophthalmic: No preparation is commercially available. A solution of 750 units dissolved in 5 ml of solvent may be prepared.

Usual Dosages

Intracameral: For enzymatic zonulolysis in intracapsular lens extraction, 0.2 to 0.5 ml of a freshly prepared 1:5000 or 1:10,000 solution is injected slowly behind the iris into the posterior chamber. One to two minutes after injection of the enzyme, the anterior chamber should be irrigated with 2 ml of the diluent, sodium chloride injection, or a balanced salt solution.
Topical Ophthalmic: Solution may be applied three to four times daily.

CIMETIDINE

Proprietary Name: Tagamet.

---

* Route of administration not approved by FDA.
† Drug not approved by FDA for any indication.
‡ Drug not approved by FDA for this particular indication.
§ Indicated dosage above the manufacturer's recommendation.

Preparations

Oral: Tablets, 200, 300, 400, and 800 mg.

Usual Dosages

Oral: The usual dosage is 300 to 400 mg two to four times daily, usually given with or immediately after meals and at bedtime for 3 to 6 weeks.

CISPLATIN

Proprietary Names: Cisplatyl (Fr.), Neoplatin (G.B.), Platinex (Germ.), Platinol.

Preparations

Injection: Powder (lyophilized), 10 mg/vial.

Usual Dosages

Intravenous: When given as a single agent, 100 mg/square meter once every 4 weeks.

CLINDAMYCIN

Proprietary Names: Cleocin, Dalacin C (G.B.), Sobelin (Germ.).

Preparations

Injection: Solution, 150 mg/ml.
Oral: Capsules, 75 and 150 mg; granules for suspensions, 75 mg/5 ml.
Topical Ophthalmic: No ophthalmic preparation is commercially available. Fortified clindamycin eyedrops may be prepared in a concentration of 50 mg/ml.

Usual Dosages

Intramuscular: Adults, 0.6 to 2.7 gm daily in two, three, or four equally divided doses; children over 1 month of age, 15 to 40 mg/kg in three or four equally divided doses.
Intravenous: Adults, 0.6 to 2.7 gm daily in two, three, or four equally divided doses; children over 1 month of age, 15 to 25 mg/kg in three or four equally divided doses.
Intravitreal: 0.1 to 1.0 mg in 0.1 to 0.2 ml of sterile solution for injection.
Oral: Adults, 150 to 450 mg every 6 hours (capsules) or 8 to 25 mg/kg daily in three or four divided doses (granules). For children 10 kg or less, 37.5 mg three times daily is minimum dose.
Subconjunctival: 15 to 40 mg in a 0.5 ml aqueous solution.
Topical Ophthalmic: One drop of a solution containing 50 mg/ml clindamycin may be given every 1 to 4 hours.

CLOBETASOL

Proprietary Names: Butavat (Gr.), Clobesol (Ital.), Dermadex (Arg.), Dermatovate (Mex.), Dermoval (Fr.), Dermovat (Scand.), Dermovate (G.B.), Dermoxin (Germ.), Dermoxinate (Germ.), Psorex (Nig.), Temovate.

Preparations

Topical: Cream, 0.05 per cent; ointment, 0.05 per cent.

Usual Dosages

Topical: Cream or ointment is applied to affected area twice daily.

CLOBETASONE

Proprietary Names: Emovat (Denm.), Enovate (Neth.), Eumovate (G.B.).

Preparations

Topical Ophthalmic: Solution, 0.1 per cent.

Usual Dosages

Topical Ophthalmic: One to two drops are applied to affected eye(s) two or three times daily.

CLOFAZIMINE

Proprietary Name: Lamprene.

Preparations

Oral: Capsules, 100 mg.

Usual Dosages

Oral: 100 to 300 mg daily, up to 1.2 gm daily has been given when required.

CLOFIBRATE

Proprietary Names: Aterosol (Swed.), Atheromide (Jap.), Atheropront (Germ.), Atromidin (Swed.), Atromid-S, Claresan (Fr.), Lipavlon (Fr.), Liprinal (G.B.), Recolip (Swed.), Regelan (Germ.), Skleromexe (Germ.).

Preparations

Oral: Capsules, 500 mg.

Usual Dosages

Oral: Adults, 500 mg two to four times daily.

CLONAZEPAM

Proprietary Names: Clonopin, Iktorivil (Swed.), Rivotril (G.B.).

Preparations

Oral: Tablets, 0.5, 1, and 2 mg.

Usual Dosages

Oral: Adults, initially 1.5 mg daily in three divided doses. Dosage then may be increased by increments of 0.5 to 1 mg every third day until seizures are adequately controlled or adverse effects intervene (maximum, 20 mg daily).

CLOTRIMAZOLE

Proprietary Names: Canastene (Belg.), Canesten (G.B.), Empecid (Arg., Jap.), Eparol (Germ.), Lotrimin, Mycelex, Panmicol (Arg.), Trimysten (Fr.).

Preparations

Oral: Powder.
Topical: Cream, 1 per cent; solution, 1 per cent.
Topical Ophthalmic: No ophthalmic preparation is commercially available. A 1 per cent solution in arachnis oil may be prepared by dissolving in chloroform, mixing with arachnis oil, and driving off the chloroform by heat. A 1 per cent suspension may also be obtained by mixing 10 mg of powder with 1 ml of artificial tears to form a suspension that must be shaken before each instillation to resuspend the drug.

Usual Dosages

Oral: Up to 54 mg/kg daily.
Topical: Sufficient amount of cream or solution to cover infected and surrounding area is applied twice daily.
Topical Ophthalmic: Drops may be instilled every 4 hours.

CLOXACILLIN

Proprietary Names: Austrastaph (Austral.), Clocillin (Jap.), Cloxapen, Cloxypen (Fr.), Ekvacillin (Swed.), Orbenin, Orbenine (Fr.), Prostaphlin-A (S. Afr.), Staphobristol (Germ.), Staphybiotic (Fr.), Tegophen.

Preparations

Oral: Capsules, 250 and 500 mg; powder for solution, 125 mg/5 ml.

Usual Dosages

Oral: Adults and children weighing 20 kg or more, 0.25 to 1.0 gm every 4 to 6 hours.

COAL TAR

Proprietary Name: Coal Tar.

Preparations

Topical: Ointment, 1, 4, and 5 per cent.

Usual Dosages

Topical: A 1 to 5 per cent concentration of coal tar in zinc oxide paste, petrolatum, or a washable base is applied two or three times daily.

COCAINE

Proprietary Name: Cocaine.

---

* Route of administration not approved by FDA.
† Drug not approved by FDA for any indication.
‡ Drug not approved by FDA for this particular indication.
§ Indicated dosage above the manufacturer's recommendation.

Preparations

Topical: No pharmaceutical dosage form is available; compounding by pharmacist is necessary.
Topical Ophthalmic: Solution, 4 and 10 per cent.

Usual Dosages

Topical: For temporary paralysis, a 10 per cent solution is placed on small cotton pledgets and applied to the nasal or punctal mucosa. No more than 200 mg should be used in a 70-kg patient over a 30-minute period.
Topical Ophthalmic: One or two drops of solution may be instilled and repeated. Care must be taken to remove excess in the fornices to prevent nasal absorption.

CODEINE

Proprietary Names: Codicept (Germ.), Codlin (Austral.), Paveral (Canad.), Tricodein (Germ.).

Preparations

Injection: Tablets (hypodermic), 15, 30, and 60 mg.
Oral: Tablets (triturates), 15, 30, and 60 mg.

Usual Dosages

Intramuscular, Oral, Subcutaneous: Adults, 30 to 60 mg four to six times daily as necessary. Children, 0.5 mg/kg four to six times daily.

COLCHICINE

Proprietary Names: Aqua-Colchin (Austral.), Colcin (Austral.), Colchineos (Fr., S. Afr.), Colgout (Austral.), Coluric (Austral.).

Preparations

Injection: Solution, 0.5 mg/ml.
Oral: Granules, 0.5 mg; tablets, 0.5 and 0.6 mg.

Usual Dosages

Intravenous: Acute attacks, 1 or 2 mg initially, followed by 0.5 mg every 3 to 6 hours as necessary (single treatment not to exceed 4 mg).
Oral: Adults, 1 or 1.2 mg initially, followed by 0.5 or 0.6 mg every 2 hours (maximum daily dose of 7 or 8 mg).

COLESTIPOL

Proprietary Name: Colestid.

Preparations

Oral: Powder in 5-gm packets and 500-gm bottles with scoop providing 5 gm/scoop.

---

* Route of administration not approved by FDA.
† Drug not approved by FDA for any indication.
‡ Drug not approved by FDA for this particular indication.
§ Indicated dosage above the manufacturer's recommendation.

Usual Dosages

Oral: Adults, 15 to 30 gm daily given with meals in two to four divided doses.

COLISTIMETHATE

Proprietary Names: Colimycine (Fr.), Colistinat (Swed.), Colistin Sulphomethate (G.B.), Coly-Mycin (Austral.), Colomycin Injection (G.B.), Coly-Mycin M.

Preparations

Injection: Powder equivalent to 150 mg colistin base.
Topical Ophthalmic: No ophthalmic form is available, but solution for topical use (1.5 to 3 mg/ml) can be made from powder.

Usual Dosages

Intramuscular, Intravenous: Adults, 2.5 to 5 mg/kg daily in two to four divided doses. Children, 5 mg/kg daily maximum, 300 mg in four divided doses. Premature and full-term newborn infants, 2.5 mg/kg daily in four divided doses.
Subconjunctival: 15 to 20 mg in 0.5 mg of isotonic sodium chloride injection or sterile water for injection. Doses as large as 37.5 mg have been used occasionally.
Topical Ophthalmic: One drop of a solution containing 1.5 to 3 mg/ml is instilled every 10 minutes for severe infections and every 1 to 4 hours for mild infections.

COLISTIN

Proprietary Names: Colimycine (Fr.), Colomycin (G.B.), Coly-Mycin (Austral.), Coly-Mycin S.

Preparations

Oral: Powder, 300 mg providing the equivalent of 25 mg of colistin base/5 ml when suspended in 37 ml of distilled water.
Topical Ophthalmic: Lyophilized powder for solution equivalent to 5 to 10 mg colistin base dissolved in 1 ml.

Usual Dosages

Oral: Infants and children, 3 to 5 mg/kg daily in three divided doses.
Topical Ophthalmic: One to two drops every 1 to 2 hours, day and night. The frequency of administration can be reduced as the infection clears.

COLLAGEN, HEMOSTATIC
See Hemostatic Collagen.

CORTICOTROPIN (ACTH)

Proprietary Names: Acortan (Germ.), Acthar, Acthelea (Arg.), Acton (Swed.), Actonar (Arg.), Cortrophin, Depot-Acethropan (Germ.), Durackin (Canad.), Reacthin (Swed.).

Preparations

Injection: Gel (repository), 40 and 80 units/ml; powder (lyophilized), 25 and 40 units; solution, 20 units/ml.

Usual Dosages

Intramuscular, Subcutaneous: For therapeutic use, 40 units of aqueous solution daily in four divided doses (10 units every 6 hours), or 40 units of gel (repository) or aqueous suspension with zinc hydroxide (repository) every 12 to 24 hours.
Intravenous: A continuous 48-hour infusion (40 units every 12 hours) may be given.

CORTISONE

Proprietary Names: Adricort, Cortal (Swed.), Cortate (Austral.), Cortelan (G.B.), Cortemel (S. Afr.), Cortilen (Ital.), Cortistab (G.B.), Cortistan, Cortisyl (G.B.), Cortogen (S. Afr.), Cortone, Pantisone.

Preparations

Injection: Suspension, 25 and 50 mg/ml.
Oral: Tablets, 5, 10, and 25 mg.
Topical Ophthalmic: Ointment, 1.5 per cent; suspension, 2.5 and 5.0 per cent.

Usual Dosages

Intramuscular: For anti-inflammatory effects, 75 to 300 mg daily for serious disease.
Oral: For anti-inflammatory effects, 25 to 50 mg daily for mild chronic diseases. In acute, life-threatening disease, 125 to 300 mg daily in at least four divided doses.
Subconjunctival: 0.5 ml of a 2.5 per cent suspension.
Topical Ophthalmic: One drop of a 0.5 per cent suspension every 1 to 2 hours until a response is obtained; the frequency then is reduced. For severe conditions, a 1.5 or 2.5 per cent suspension may be used. The ointment preparation is applied three or four times daily or as a nighttime medication when the suspension is used during the day.

COUMARIN DERIVATIVES
See Dicumarol, Warfarin.

CREDE'S SOLUTION
See Silver Nitrate.

CROMOLYN SODIUM

Proprietary Names: Opticrom, Opticron (Fr.).

Preparations

Oral: Capsules, 100 mg.
Topical Ophthalmic: Solution, 2 and 4 per cent.

Usual Dosages

Oral: The usual dosage is 400 to 800 mg equally divided in four doses.

---

* Route of administration not approved by FDA.
† Drug not approved by FDA for any indication.
‡ Drug not approved by FDA for this particular indication.
§ Indicated dosage above the manufacturer's recommendation.

Topical Ophthalmic: One or two drops in each eye four to six times daily at regular intervals.

CRYSTALLINE PENICILLIN
See Potassium Penicillin G, Sodium Penicillin G.

CYCLIZINE

Proprietary Names: Marezine, Marzine (G.B.), Valoid (G.B.).

Preparations

Injection: Solution, 50 mg/ml.
Oral: Tablets, 50 mg.

Usual Dosages

Intramuscular: Adults, 50 mg every 4 to 6 hours.
Oral: Adults, 50 mg repeated every 4 to 6 hours up to 200 mg daily. Children 6 to 12 years of age, 25 mg up to three times daily.

CYCLOGUANIL PAMOATE

Proprietary Name: Camolar (G.B.).

Preparations

Injection: Oily injection containing equivalent of 140 mg of cycloguanil base in each ml.

Usual Dosages

Intramuscular: Adults, equivalent of 350 mg or 5 to 6 mg/kg cycloguanil base every 3 or 4 months; children up to 4 years, 140 mg; children 5 to 10 years, 280 mg.

CYCLOPENTOLATE

Proprietary Names: Ak-Pentolate, Ciclolux (Ital.), Cyclogyl, Cyclopen (Austral.), Cyplegin (Jap.), Mydplegic (Canad.), Mydrilate (G.B.), Ocu-Pentolate, Pentolair, Zyklolat (Germ.).

Preparations

Topical Ophthalmic: Solution, 0.5, 1.0, and 2.0 per cent.

Usual Dosages

Topical Ophthalmic: One drop of 0.5 or 1.0 per cent solution will sustain mydriasis/cycloplegia for approximately 24 hours. In patients with darkly pigmented irides, 2 per cent solution may be necessary.

CYCLOPHOSPHAMIDE

Proprietary Names: Cytoxan, Endoxan (Austral., Fr., Germ., S. Afr.), Endoxana (G.B.), Enduxan (Braz.), Genoxal (Span.), Procytox (Canad.), Sendoxan (Norw., Swed.).

Preparations

Injection: Powder, 100, 200, and 500 mg.
Oral: Tablets, 25 and 50 mg.

Usual Dosages

Intravenous, Oral: The initial loading dose is 40 to 50 mg/kg intravenously or 1 to 5 mg/kg orally. Maintenance dosage may be started as soon as the leukocyte count returns to 3000 to 4000 cells/cubic meter. One to 5 mg/kg orally daily, 10 to 15 mg/kg intravenously every 7 to 10 days, or 3 to 5 mg/kg intravenously twice weekly may be used.

CYCLOSPORINE (CYCLOSPORIN A)

Proprietary Name: Sandimmune.

Preparations

Injection: Solution, 50 mg/ml cyclosporine with 650 mg of polyoxyethylated castor oil and 32.9 per cent alcohol.
Oral: Solution, 100 mg/ml of cyclosporine with 12.5 per cent alcohol.

Usual Dosages

Intravenous: Initially, 5 to 6 mg/kg daily.
Oral: Initially, 15 mg/kg daily, tapered to maintenance level of 5 to 10 mg/kg daily.

CYPROHEPTADINE

Proprietary Names: Antegan (Austral.), Nuran (Germ.), Periactin, Periactinol (Germ.), Vimicon (Canad.).

Preparations

Oral: Syrup, 2 mg/5 ml; tablets, 4 mg.

Usual Dosages

Oral: Adults, 4 to 20 mg daily in divided doses. Dosage must be individualized and should not exceed 0.5 mg/kg daily.

CYPROTERONE ACETATE

Proprietary Name: Androcur (Denm., G.B., Germ., Ital., Neth., Norw., Span., Swed., Switz.).

Preparations

Oral: Tablets, 50 mg.

Usual Dosages

Oral: The usual dose is 50 mg twice daily, increased if necessary after 4 weeks to 200 or 300 mg daily in divided doses until a response is achieved.

CYSTEINE

Proprietary Name: Cysteine.

Preparations

Topical Ophthalmic: Eyedrops containing 1.5 per cent cysteine are prepared by adding 1.5 gm cysteine and 10 mg benzalkonium chloride in iso-osmotic solution to 100 ml.

Usual Dosages

Topical Ophthalmic: Preparation may be applied up to four times daily.

CYTARABINE

Proprietary Names: Alexan (Belg., Germ.), Aracytine (Fr.), Cytosar.

Preparations

Injection: Powder (lyophilized), 100 and 500 mg with diluent.

Usual Dosages

Intramuscular, Subcutaneous: For maintenance of remissions, 1 mg/kg weekly.
Intravenous Infusion: 0.5 to 1 mg/kg daily infused for any desired period (1, 4, 12, or 24 hours) for 10 days, increased to 2 mg/kg until remission or hematologic toxicity.
Intravenous Injection (Rapid): 2 mg/kg daily for 10 days, increased to 4 mg/kg daily if no hematologic depression; continue until remission or hematologic toxicity.

DACARBAZINE

Proprietary Name: DTIC-Dome.

Preparations

Injection: Powder, 100 and 200 mg.

Usual Dosages

Intravenous: 2 to 4.5 mg/kg daily for 10 days every 28 days or 250 mg/square meter daily for 5 days every 3 weeks.

DACTINOMYCIN

Proprietary Name: Cosmegen.

Preparations

Injection: Powder, 0.5 mg with 20 mg of mannitol per vial.

Usual Dosages

Intravenous: Adults, 0.5 mg daily for a maximum of 5 days; single weekly doses of 2 mg for 3 weeks have been tolerated; children, 0.015 mg/kg daily for 5 days (maximum dose, 0.5 mg). Alternatively, a total dose of 2.4 mg/square meter may be given over a 1-week period to adults or children at monthly intervals.

DANAZOL

Proprietary Names: Cylomen (Canad.), Danatrol (Belg., Fr. Switz.), Danocrine, Danokrin (Aust.), Danol (G.B.), Ladogar (S. Afr.), Winobanin (Germ.).

---

* Route of administration not approved by FDA.
† Drug not approved by FDA for any indication.
‡ Drug not approved by FDA for this particular indication.
§ Indicated dosage above the manufacturer's recommendation.

Preparations

Oral: Capsules, 200 mg.

Usual Dosages

Oral: 300 to 600 mg daily with a break of 5 to 7 days every 7 days for treatment of hereditary angioedema.

DANTROLENE

Proprietary Name: Dantrium.

Preparations

Oral: Capsules, 25, 50, 75, and 100 mg.

Usual Dosages

Oral: Initial 25 mg twice daily, increased to three to four times daily and then to 100 mg or, rarely, 200 mg four times daily. Children, similar approach with 1 mg/kg once or twice daily; maximum dose is 100 mg four times daily.

DAPSONE

Proprietary Name: Avlosulfon.

Preparations

Oral: Tablets, 25 and 100 mg.

Usual Dosages

Oral: Adults, first and second weeks, 25 mg twice weekly; third and fourth weeks, 50 mg twice weekly; thereafter, 50 mg daily. A maintenance dosage of 100 to 200 mg daily also has been used. Children, 0.35 mg/kg administered in the same schedule as adults.

DAUNORUBICIN

Proprietary Names: Cerubidin (G.B.), Cerubidine, Daunoblastin (Germ.), Daunoblastina (Ital.), Ondena (Germ.).

Preparations

Injection: Powder for solutions, in vials containing the equivalent of 20 mg of daunorubicin.

Usual Dosages

Intravenous: 1 mg/kg at intervals of 1 to 4 days or 2 mg/kg at intervals of 4 to 7 days, depending on type of neoplasm.

DEFEROXAMINE

Proprietary Names: Desferal, Desferrioxamine (G.B.).

---

* Route of administration not approved by FDA.
† Drug not approved by FDA for any indication.
‡ Drug not approved by FDA for this particular indication.
§ Indicated dosage above the manufacturer's recommendation.

Preparations

Injection: Powder (lyophilized), 500 mg.
Topical Ophthalmic: No ophthalmic preparation is commercially available. Eyedrops may be prepared by dissolving 500 mg in a sterile vehicle containing 0.5 per cent methylcellulose, 1 per cent benzyl alcohol, and water for injection to 5 ml. A 5 per cent ophthalmic ointment may be prepared in a base of cetyl alcohol, wool fat, white soft paraffin, and liquid paraffin.

Usual Dosages

Intramuscular, Intravenous: An initial dose of 1 gm should be administered at a rate not to exceed 15 mg/kg/hour. This may be followed by 0.5 gm every 4 hours for two doses; subsequent doses of 0.5 gm may be necessary every 4 to 12 hours. Total amount administered should not exceed 6 gm in a 24-hour period.
Subconjunctival: For iron deposits in the deeper layers of the cornea and in the iris and lens, 0.5 ml of a 10 per cent solution is injected twice a week for 8 to 10 weeks.
Topical Ophthalmic: For treatment of superficial iron deposits in the cornea, a 10 per cent solution of deferoxamine in 1 per cent methylcellulose is used four times daily for several weeks. Alternatively, the drug may be applied in a 5 per cent concentration in any ointment base.

DEMECARIUM

Proprietary Names: Humorsol, Tosmilen (G.B.).

Preparations

Topical Ophthalmic: Solution, 0.125 and 0.25 per cent.

Usual Dosages

Topical Ophthalmic: The frequency and concentration of instillation depend upon the patient's response to therapy.

DESMOPRESSIN

Proprietary Names: Dav Ritter (Switz.), DDAVP, Minirin (Austral., Germ., Ital., Norw., Swed.), Minurin (Denm.).

Preparations

Intranasal: Solution, 0.1 mg/ml.

Usual Dosages

Intranasal: The usual dosage range in adults is 0.1 to 0.4 ml daily, either as a single dose or divided into two or three doses.

DESONIDE

Proprietary Names: Apolar (Norw., Swed.), Locapred (Fr.), PR 100 (Ital.), Prenacid (Ital.), Reticus (Ital.), Sine-Fluor (Span.), Steroderm (Ital.), Tridesilon, Tridesonit (Fr.).

Preparations

Topical: Cream, 0.05 per cent; ointment, 0.05 per cent.

Usual Dosages

Topical: Preparation is applied two or three times daily or is used under occlusive dressings.

DEXAMETHASONE

Proprietary Names: Acidocort (Fr.), Ak-Dex, Auxiloson (Germ.), Auxison (Aust., Fr.), Carulon (Jap.), Cebedex (Fr.), Corson (Jap.), Cortisumman (Germ.), Dalaron, Decacort (Swed.), Decadron, Decaesadril (Ital.), Decaject, Decameth, Decasone (Austral.), Decasterolone (Ital.), Decofluor (Ital.), Dectan (Jap.), Dectancyl (Fr.), Deksone, Delladec, Deronil, Desacort (Ital.), Desacortone (Ital.), Desalark (Ital.), Desameton (Ital.), Deseronil (Ital.), Dethamedin (Jap.), Dexacen, Dexacortal (Swed.), DexaCortisyl (Austral., G.B.), Dexair, Dexamed (Germ.), Dexamethadrone (Canad.), Dexaport, Dexa-Scheroson (Germ.), Dexa-Sine (Germ.), Dexasone, Dexinolon (Germ.), Dexmethsone (Austral.), Dexon, Dexone, Dezone, Egocort (Austral.), Fluormone (Ital.), Fluorocort (Ital.), Fortecortin (Germ.), Hexadrol, Isopto-Maxidex (Swed.), Luxazone (Ital.), Maxidex, Metasolon (Jap.), Millicorten (Germ.), Miral, Moco (Jap.), Ocu-Dex, Oradexon (Austral, G.B.), Orgadrone (Jap.), Penthasone (Canad.), Predni-F (Germ.), Savacort-D, Sawasone (Jap.), SK-Dexamethasone, Soludecadron (Fr.), Solurex, Spersadex (Germ., S. Afr.), Tendron.

Preparations

Injection: Solution, 24 mg/ml.
Injection (Subconjunctival): Solution, 0.1 per cent.
Oral: Elixir, 0.5 mg/5 ml; tablets, 0.25, 0.5, 0.75, and 1.5 mg.
Topical Ophthalmic: Ointment, 0.05 per cent; suspension, 0.1 per cent.

Usual Dosages

Intravenous, Oral: The initial dosage varies from 0.5 to 9 mg daily. Doses higher than 9 mg may be required in severe diseases.
Retrobulbar: 0.5 to 1.0 ml of a solution containing 4 mg/ml.
Subconjunctival: 0.5 ml of a 0.1 per cent solution.
Topical Ophthalmic: One drop of a 0.1 per cent suspension every 1 or 2 hours until a response is obtained. Alternatively, the ointment may be instilled three or four times daily initially and once or twice daily for maintenance.

DEXTRAN (LOW MOLECULAR WEIGHT)

Proprietary Names: Dextraven (G.B.), Gentran, Hyskon, LMD, LMWD, Lomodex (G.B.), Macrodex, Perfadex (Swed.), Rheomacrodex, Rheotran.

Preparations

Injection: Solution, 10 per cent.

---

* Route of administration not approved by FDA.
† Drug not approved by FDA for any indication.
‡ Drug not approved by FDA for this particular indication.
§ Indicated dosage above the manufacturer's recommendation.

Usual Dosages

Intravenous: 10 to 20 ml/kg should be administered; the first 500 ml rapidly infused with remainder given more slowly. Total daily dose should not exceed 20 ml/kg. If therapy is longer than 24 hours, daily dose should not exceed 10 ml/kg.

DEXTROTHYROXINE

Proprietary Names: Biotirmone (Fr.), Choloxin, Debetrol (Fr.), Dethyron (Denm.), Dynothel (Germ.), Nadrothyron (Germ.).

Preparations

Oral: Tablets, 1, 2, 4, and 6 mg.

Usual Dosages

Oral: Adults, initial daily dose should be 1 to 2 mg, increased in 1- to 2-mg increments at intervals of not less than 1 month to a maximum level of 4 to 8 mg daily.

DFP
See Isoflurophate.

DHPG
See Ganciclovir.

DHT
See Dihydrotachysterol.

DIAZEPAM

Proprietary Names: Apozepam (Swed.), Atensine (G.B.), E-Pam (Canad.), Paxel (Canad.), Relanium (Pol.), Serenack (Canad.), Stesolid (Swed.), Tensium (G.B.), Valium, Vivol (Canad.).

Preparations

Injection: Solution, 5 mg/ml.
Oral: Tablets, 2, 5, and 10 mg.

Usual Dosages

Intramuscular, Intravenous: Adults, 5 to 10 mg initially; this dose may be repeated in 2 to 4 hours if necessary, up to a maximum of 30 mg in 8 hours. Children, 0.05 to 0.2 mg/kg initially, repeated in 3 to 4 hours if necessary. The dose should not exceed 0.5 mg/kg in an 8-hour period.
Oral: Adults, 4 to 40 mg in divided doses or single dose of 2.5 to 10 mg at bedtime. Children over 12 years of age, 0.12 to 0.8 mg/kg daily, divided into three or four doses.

DIBROMOPROPAMIDINE

Proprietary Name: Brolene (Austral., G.B., S. Afr.).

Preparations

Topical Ophthalmic: Ointment, 0.15 per cent.

Usual Dosages

Topical Ophthalmic: A small quantity is applied to the affected eye(s) one to two times daily.

DICHLORPHENAMIDE

Proprietary Names: Daranide, Oralcon (Swed.), Oratrol.

Preparations

Oral: Tablets, 50 mg.

Usual Dosages

Oral: The usual initial adult dose is 100 to 200 mg, followed by 100 mg every 12 hours until the desired response is obtained. Maintenance dosage in adults is usually 25 to 50 mg one to three times daily.

DICLOFENAC

Proprietary Names: Aflamin (Ital.), Blesin (Jap.), Dichronic (Jap.), Neriodin (Jap.), Prophenatin (Jap.), Seecoren (Jap.), Sofarin (Jap.), Tsudohmin (Jap.), Voltaren (Arg., Belg., Denm., Germ., Ital., Jap., Neth., Span., Switz.), Voltarene (Fr.), Voltarol (G.B.).

Preparations

Oral: Tablets, 25 and 50 mg.

Usual Dosages

Oral: 25 to 50 mg three times daily.

DICLOXACILLIN

Proprietary Names: Constaphyl (Germ.), Dichlor-Stapenor (Germ.), Diclocil (Fr., S. Afr.), Diclocila (Swed.), Dycill, Dynapen, Pathocil, Stafopenin (Swed.), Veracillin.

Preparations

Injection: Vials, 250 mg.
Oral: Capsules, 125, 250, and 500 mg; suspension, 62.5 mg/5 ml.

Usual Dosages

Intramuscular: Adults and children weighing 40 kg or more, 125 to 250 mg every 6 hours; less than 40 kg, 12.5 to 25 mg/kg daily in four equal doses.
Oral: Adults and children weighing 40 kg or more, 125 to 250 mg every 6 hours; less than 40 kg, 12.5 to 25 mg/kg daily in four equal doses.

DICUMAROL (DICOUMAROL)

Proprietary Names: AP (Swed.), Dufalone (Canad.).

---

* Route of administration not approved by FDA.
† Drug not approved by FDA for any indication.
‡ Drug not approved by FDA for this particular indication.
§ Indicated dosage above the manufacturer's recommendation.

Preparations

Oral: Capsules, 25, 50, and 100 mg; tablets, 25, 50, and 100 mg.

Usual Dosages

Oral: Adults, 200 to 300 mg on the first day, followed by 25 to 200 mg daily, using prothrombin time determinations as a guide.

DIETHYLCARBAMAZINE

Proprietary Names: Banocide, Carbilazine (Austral.), Ethodryl (G.B.), Franocide, Hetrazan, Notezine (Fr.).

Preparations

Oral: Tablets, 50 mg.

Usual Dosages

Oral: 2 to 4 mg/kg three times daily for 1 to 4 weeks.

DIGITALIS

Proprietary Names: Digifortis, Digiglusin, Digiplex (Fr.), Digitalysat (Germ.), Pil-Digis.

Preparations

Oral: Capsules, 100 mg; tablets, 100 mg; tincture, 100 mg/ml.

Usual Dosages

Oral: Adults, initially, 1.2 to 1.5 mg over a period of 24 to 48 hours; maintenance dose, 100 mg daily.

DIHYDROTACHYSTEROL (DHT, VITAMIN D$_1$)

Proprietary Names: AT-10 (G.B.), Atecen (Swed.), Calcamine (Fr.), Dihydral (Belg., Neth., Span.), Dygratyl (Denm., Swed.), Hytakerol.

Preparations

Oral: Capsules, 0.125 mg; solution (in oil), 0.25 mg/ml; tablets, 0.125, 0.2, and 0.4 mg.

Usual Dosages

Oral: Adults, initially 0.75 to 2.5 mg daily; specific dosage is determined by frequent estimations of serum calcium levels. For maintenance, 0.25 to 1.75 mg weekly has been given. Larger doses may be required for some patients.

DIHYDROXYACETONE

Proprietary Names: Chromelin, Dy-O-Derm, Vitadye.

Preparations

Topical: Solution, 5 per cent; suspension, 5 per cent.

Usual Dosages

Topical: Solution or suspension is applied to depigmented patches of skin. This may give rise to patchy appearance which is rectified by repeated application.

1α,25 DIHYDROXYVITAMIN D₃
See Calcitriol.

DIIODOHYDROXYQUIN (DIIODOHYDROXYQUINOLINE)

Proprietary Names: Diodoquin, Direxiode (Austral., Fr.), Embequin (G.B.), Floraquin, Florequin (Swed.), Ioquin (Fr.), Moebiquin, Panaquin, Vaam-DHQ (Austral.), Yodoxin.

Preparations

Oral: Powder; tablets, 210 and 650 mg.

Usual Dosages

Oral: The usual adult dosage is 630 to 650 mg three times daily; a daily dose of 2 gm should not be exceeded.

DIMENHYDRINATE

Proprietary Names: Amosyt (Swed.), Andrumin (Austral.), Aviomarine (Pol.), Dramamine, Dramavol (Canad.), Dymenol (Canad.), Epharetard (Germ.), Gravol (G.B.), Neo-Metic (Canad.), Novodimenate (Canad.), Novomina (Germ.), Prevenause (Canad.), Travamine (Canad.), Vomex A (Germ.), Vomital (Canad.).

Preparations

Injection: Solution, 50 mg/ml.
Oral: Liquid, 12.5 mg/4 ml; tablets, 50 mg.
Rectal: Suppositories, 100 mg.

Usual Dosages

Intramuscular: Adults, 50 mg as needed; children 5 mg/kg divided into four doses during a 24-hour period (maximum, 300 mg/day).
Intravenous: Adults, 50 mg diluted in 10 ml of sodium chloride injection and injected over a period of 2 minutes.
Oral: Adults, 50 to 100 mg every 4 hours; children, 25 to 50 mg three times daily.
Rectal: Adults, 100 mg once or twice daily.

DIMETHYL SULFOXIDE (DMSO)

Proprietary Names: Domoso, Rimso-50.

Preparations

Injection: Solution, 50 per cent.

---

* Route of administration not approved by FDA.
† Drug not approved by FDA for any indication.
‡ Drug not approved by FDA for this particular indication.
§ Indicated dosage above the manufacturer's recommendation.

Usual Dosages

Intravesical: 50 ml of a 50 per cent solution may be instilled slowly by catheter directly into the bladder.

DINITROCHLOROBENZENE

Proprietary Name: Dinitrochlorobenzene.

Preparations

Topical: No topical preparations are commercially available.

Usual Dosages

Topical: Initially, 2 mg may be applied to the skin to induce a systemic hypersensitivity reaction. Later, much smaller quantities are applied to the tumor to induce local reaction and necrosis.

DIPHENHYDRAMINE

Proprietary Names: Alergicap (Austral.), Allerdryl, Baramine, Bax, Benachior, Benadryl, Benahist, Ben-Allergin, Bendylate, Benhydramil (Canad.), Bentrac, Benylin, Bonyl, Bidramine (Austral.), Dabylen (Germ.), Desentol (Swed.), Dihydral (S. Afr.), Diphen-Ex, Dyhydramine (S. Afr.), Eldadryl, Fenylhist, Histergan (G.B.), Histine, Hyrexin, Lensen, Nordryl, Notose, Phen-Amin 50, Phenamine, Rodryl, Rohydra, SK-Diphenhydramine, Span-Lanin, Tusstat.

Preparations

Injection: Solution, 10 and 50 mg/ml.
Oral: Capsules, 25 and 50 mg; elixir, 12.5 mg/5 ml.

Usual Dosages

Intramuscular: Children, 5 mg/kg divided into four doses during a 24-hour period (maximum, 300 mg/day).
Intramuscular, Intravenous: Adults, 10 mg initially. The subsequent dose may be increased to 20 to 50 mg every 2 to 3 hours (maximum, 400 mg/day).
Oral: For motion sickness, adults, 50 mg one-half hour before departure and 50 mg before each meal. Children, 5 mg/kg divided into four doses during a 24-hour period (maximum, 300 mg/day). For sedative effect, 25 to 50 mg three or four times daily.

DIPHTHERIA AND TETANUS TOXOIDS AND PERTUSSIS (DPT) VACCINE

Proprietary Names: Di-Te-Tuss (Germ.), DT Coq Adsorbe (Fr.), DT Perthydral (Fr.), Tri-Immunol, Triogen, Triple Antigen, Tri-Solgen, Trivax (G.B.), Vaccin Ipad DTC (Fr.).

Preparations

Injection: 6.7, 7.5, or 12.5 Lf units diptheria toxoid, 5 Lf units tetanus toxoid, and 4 protective units pertussis vaccine/0.5 ml.

Usual Dosages

Intramuscular: Infants 2 months of age, initially 0.5 ml followed by two more doses at 4- to 8-week intervals. A reinforcing fourth dose is given 7 to 12 months after the third, and a booster dose is given when the child is 5 to 6 years old.

DIPHTHERIA ANTITOXIN

Proprietary Name: Diphtheria Antitoxin.

Preparations

Injection: Vials of 1000, 5000, 10,000, 20,000, and 40,000 units.

Usual Dosages

Intramuscular, Intravenous: Adults and children, for prophylaxis, 1000 to 10,000 units. Adults and children, for treatment, 20,000 to 120,000 units, depending upon duration of illness, degree of toxicity, and site of membrane. The dose may be repeated as indicated.

DIPIVEFRIN (DPE)

Proprietary Name: Propine.

Preparations

Topical Ophthalmic: Solution, 0.1 per cent.

Usual Dosages

Topical Ophthalmic: The usual dosage is one drop in the eye(s) every 12 hours.

DIPYRIDAMOLE

Proprietary Names: Anginal (Jap.), Coribon (Ital.), Coronarine (Fr.), Corosan (Ital.), Coroxin (Ital.), Dipyrida (Germ.), Functiocardon (Germ.), Natyl (Fr.), Novodil (Ital.), Peridamol (Fr.), Persantin (Arg., Austral., Denm., G.B., Germ., Ital., Neth., Norw., S. Afr., Span., Switz.), Persantine, Prandiol (Fr.), Stenocardil (Ital.), Stenocor (Ital.), Stimolcardio (Ital.), Trancocard (Ital.), Viscor (Ital.).

Preparations

Oral: Tablets, 25 and 100 mg.

Usual Dosages

Oral: The recommended dosage is 50 mg three times a day, taken at least 1 hour before meals.

DMSO
See Dimethyl Sulfoxide.

---

* Route of administration not approved by FDA.
† Drug not approved by FDA for any indication.
‡ Drug not approved by FDA for this particular indication.
§ Indicated dosage above the manufacturer's recommendation.

DOXEPIN

Proprietary Names: Adapin, Aponal (Germ.), Quitaxon (Austral., Fr., S. Afr.), Sinequan, Sinquan (Germ.).

Preparations

Oral: Capsules, 10, 25, 50, 75, 100, and 150 mg; solution, 10 mg/ml.

Usual Dosages

Oral: Adults, initially 75 to 150 mg daily in divided doses. For maintenance, 25 to 150 mg daily (maximum, 300 mg daily).

DOXORUBICIN

Proprietary Names: Adriacin (Jap.), Adriamycin.

Preparations

Injection: Powder (lyophilized), 10 and 50 mg with 50 and 250 mg of lactose, respectively.

Usual Dosages

Intravenous: Adults, 60 to 75 mg/square meter, administered as a single dose at 21-day intervals. Alternatively, 25 to 35 mg/square meter may be administered daily in single doses on 2 or 3 successive days at 3- or 4-week intervals. Total dosage with either regimen should not exceed 550 mg/square meter.

DOXYCYCLINE

Proprietary Names: Doxin (Austral.), Doxy-II, Doxychel, Idocyklin (Swed.), Vibramycin, Vibramycine (Fr.), Vibra-Tabs, Vibraveineuse (Fr.), Vibravenös (Germ.).

Preparations

Injection: Powder equivalent to 100 to 200 mg of doxycycline.
Oral: Capsules, 50 and 100 mg; powder for suspension, 25 mg/5 ml after reconstitution.

Usual Dosages

Intravenous: Adults and children weighing at least 45 kg, initially, 200 mg daily given in one or two infusions, followed by 100 to 200 mg daily (depending upon the severity of infection) given in one or two infusions; children under 45 kg, 2 mg/kg daily in one or two infusions, followed by 1 or 2 mg/kg given in one or two infusions.
Oral: The usual adult dose is 100 mg at 12-hour intervals for two doses, followed by 100 mg once a day. In the management of more severe infections, up to 300 mg daily may be administered.

DPE
See Dipivefrin.

DROPERIDOL

Proprietary Names: Dridol (Swed.), Droleptan (G.B.), Inapsin (S. Afr.), Inapsine.

Preparations

Injection: Solution, 2.5 mg/ml.

Usual Dosages

Intramuscular, Intravenous: The usual dosage is 2.5 to 10 mg.

ECHOTHIOPHATE

Proprietary Names: Echodide, Echothiopate (G.B.), Phospholine.

Preparations

Topical Ophthalmic: Lyophilized sterile powder, 1.5, 3, 6.25, and 12.5 mg to make 0.03, 0.06, 0.125, and 0.25 per cent solutions, respectively.

Usual Dosages

Topical Ophthalmic: The frequency and concentration of instillation depend upon the patient's response to therapy.

ECONAZOLE

Proprietary Names: Ecostatin (G.B.), Epi-Pevaryl (Germ.), Mycopevaryl (Swed.), Pevaryl (G.B.), Skilar (Ital.), Spectazole.

Preparations

Topical: Cream, 1 per cent; lotion, 1 per cent; pessaries, 150 mg; powder, 1 per cent.
Topical Ophthalmic: No ophthalmic preparation is commercially available.

Usual Dosages

Topical Ophthalmic: A 1 per cent solution may be applied to the affected and surrounding areas twice a day for up to 8 to 12 weeks.

EDETATE CALCIUM DISODIUM

Proprietary Names: Calcium Disodium Versenate, Disodium Calcium Edetate (G.B.), Sodium Calciumedetate (G.B.).

Preparations

Topical Ophthalmic: No ophthalmic preparation is commercially available. A 4 per cent solution may be prepared with 4.1 gm of edetate calcium disodium, 10 mg of chlorhexidine acetate, and sterile water for injection to 100 ml.

Usual Dosages

Topical Ophthalmic: For the inactivation of epithelial collagenase, the eye is irrigated with 4 per cent solution.

---

* Route of administration not approved by FDA.
† Drug not approved by FDA for any indication.
‡ Drug not approved by FDA for this particular indication.
§ Indicated dosage above the manufacturer's recommendation.

EDETATE DISODIUM (EDTA, ETHYLENEDIAMINE TETRAACETIC ACID)

Proprietary Names: Chealamide, Disotate, Endrate, Sodium Versenate.

Preparations

Injection: Solution, 150 mg/ml in 20-ml vials.
Topical Ophthalmic: No ophthalmic preparation is commercially available. The intravenous solution must be diluted to the desired concentration with isotonic sodium chloride solution used for injection.

Usual Dosages

Intravenous (Slow): 15 to 50 mg/kg.
Topical Ophthalmic: The eye is irrigated with 0.35 to 1.85 per cent solution.

EDROPHONIUM

Proprietary Name: Tensilon.

Preparations

Injection: Solution, 10 mg/ml.

Usual Dosages

Intravenous: For diagnosis, adults, 3 to 4 mg injected within 15 to 30 seconds; if no response occurs within 45 seconds, additional increments up to 10 mg; children, 0.2 mg/kg, 20 per cent of total dose given within 1 minute, remainder if tolerated.

EDTA
See Edetate Disodium.

EHDP
See Etidronate Disodium.

ELEDOISIN

Proprietary Name: Eledosin.

Preparations

Topical Ophthalmic: Solution, 400 μg/ml.

Usual Dosages

Topical Ophthalmic: One to two drops are applied to each affected eye three times daily.

EPHEDRINE

Proprietary Names: Bofedrol, Ectasule Minus, Efedrinetter (Swed.), Ephedroides (Fr.), Isofedrol, Nefrytol-Junior (S. Afr.), Slo-Fedrin, Spaneph (G.B.).

Preparations

Oral: Capsules, 25 and 50 mg; syrup, 10 and 20 mg/5 ml.

Usual Dosages

Oral: Range, 25 to 400 mg daily.

EPINEPHRINE

Proprietary Names: Adremad (Fr.), Adrenalin, Adrenaline (G.B.), Adrenatrate, Asmatane, Asmolin, Asthma Meter, Bronkaid, Dysne-Inhal (Canad.), Dyspne (Austral.), E1/2, E2, Epifrin, Epinal, Epitrate, Eppy, Glaucon, Glauconin (Swed.), Glaufrin (Swed.), Glin-Epin (Austral.), Glycirenan (Germ.), Intranefrin (Canad.), Liadren (Ital.), Lyophrin (G.B.), Medihaler-Epi, Micronefrin, Mistura E, Mytrate, Primatene, Simplene (G.B.), Suprarenin, Sus-Phrine, Vaponefrin.

Preparations

Injection: Solution, 1:1000 (1 mg/ml).
Topical Ophthalmic: Solution, 0.1, 0.25, 0.5, 1.0, and 2.0 per cent.

Usual Dosages

Intramuscular, Intravenous, Subcutaneous: Adults, initially 0.5 ml of a 1:1000 solution injected intramuscularly or subcutaneously, followed by 0.25 to 0.5 ml of a 1:10,000 solution given intravenously every 5 to 15 minutes.
Topical Ophthalmic: In primary open-angle glaucoma and other chronic glaucomas, one drop of 1 or 2 per cent solution in each eye, once or twice daily.

ERGOCALCIFEROL (VITAMIN D$_2$)

Proprietary Names: Calciferol, Deltalin, Deltavit (Ital.), Drisdol, Ostelin (Austral.), Ostoforte (Canad.), Radiostol (Canad.), Savitol (Germ.), Sterogyl (G.B.).

Preparations

Oral: Capsules, 25,000 IU (0.625 mg) and 50,000 IU (1.25 mg); tablets, 50,000 IU (1.25 mg).
Injection: Solution in oil, 500,000 IU (12.5 mg)/ml.

Usual Dosages

Intramuscular, Oral: 50,000 to 400,000 IU daily; dosage must be adjusted to the needs of the patient.

ERGOTAMINE

Proprietary Names: Ergate (S. Afr.), Ergomar, Ergostat, Ergotart (Austral.), Etin (Austral.), Exmigra (Neth.), Exmigrex (Fin.), Femergin (G.B.), Gynergen, Lingraine (G.B.), Lingran (Swed.), Lingrene (Norw.), Medihaler-Ergotamine.

Preparations

Inhalation: Solution, 9 mg/ml.
Injection: Solution, 0.5 mg/ml.

---

* Route of administration not approved by FDA.
† Drug not approved by FDA for any indication.
‡ Drug not approved by FDA for this particular indication.
§ Indicated dosage above the manufacturer's recommendation.

Oral: Tablets, 1 mg.
Sublingual: Tablets, 2 mg.

Usual Dosages

Inhalation: Adults, single inhalation (0.36 mg) at onset of attack, repeated if necessary at intervals of no less than 5 minutes to a total of six inhalations in 24 hours (maximum, 12 mg in 1 week).
Intramuscular, Subcutaneous: Adults, 0.25 to 0.5 mg at onset of attack, repeated in 40 minutes if necessary; maximum of 1 mg in 1 week.
Oral: Adults, 1 to 2 mg at onset, repeated every 30 minutes; maximum of 6 mg in 24 hours and 12 mg in 1 week.
Sublingual: Adults, 2 mg at onset, repeated every 30 minutes if necessary. Dosage must not exceed 6 mg in 24 hours or 10 mg in 1 week.

ERGOTAMINE/BELLADONNA/CAFFEINE/PENTOBARBITAL COMBINATION

Proprietary Name: Cafergot P-B.

Preparations

Oral: Tablets, 1 mg ergotamine, 0.125 mg belladonna, 100 mg caffeine, and 30 mg pentobarbital.
Rectal: Suppositories, 2 mg ergotamine, 0.25 mg belladonna, 100 mg caffeine, and 60 mg pentobarbital.

Usual Dosages

Oral: Adults, two tablets at the onset of an attack. An additional tablet may be taken every 30 minutes, if needed, but the amount generally should be limited to a total of six tablets per attack or no more than ten tablets per week.
Rectal: Adults, one-half to one suppository at the onset of an attack. Another suppository may be used in 1 hour if needed; the total amount should not exceed two suppositories per attack or no more than five suppositories per week.

ERGOTAMINE/BELLADONNA/PHENOBARBITAL COMBINATION

Proprietary Name: Bellergal.

Preparations

Oral: Tablets, 0.3 mg ergotamine, 0.1 mg belladonna, and 20 mg phenobarbital; tablets (timed-release), 0.6 mg ergotamine, 0.2 mg belladonna, and 40 mg phenobarbital.

Usual Dosages

Oral: Adults, two tablets at the onset of an attack. An additional tablet may be taken every 30 minutes, if needed, but the amount generally should be limited to a total of six tablets per attack or no more than ten tablets per week.

ERGOTAMINE/CAFFEINE COMBINATION

Proprietary Name: Cafergot.

Preparations

Oral: Tablets, 1 mg ergotamine and 100 mg caffeine.

Rectal: Suppositories, 2 mg ergotamine and 100 mg caffeine.

Usual Dosages

Oral: Adults, two tablets at the onset of an attack. An additional tablet may be taken every 30 minutes, if needed, but the amount generally should be limited to a total of six tablets per attack or no more than ten tablets per week.

Rectal: Adults, one-half to one suppository at the onset of an attack. Another suppository may be used in 1 hour if needed; the total amount should not exceed two suppositories per attack or no more than five suppositories per week.

ERYTHROMYCIN

Proprietary Names: Abboject (S. Afr.), Abboticin (Swed.), Abboticine (Fr.), Bristamycin, Chemthromycin (Canad.), E-Biotic, E.E.S., Emcinka (Canad.), EMU-V (Austral., S. Afr.), E-Mycin Eratrex (Austral.), Eromel (S. Afr.), Eromycin (Austral.), Erostin (Austral.), Erycen (G.B.), Erycinum (Germ.), Erypar, Erythrocin, Erythromid (G.B.), Erythromycetine (Canad.), Erythroped (G.B.), Erythro-ST (Jap.), Ethril, Ethryn (Austral.), Ilosone, Ilotycin, Kesso-Mycin, Neo-Erycinum (Germ.), Novorythro (Canad.), Paediathrocin (Germ.), Pediamycin, Pfizer-E, Propiocine (Fr.), Retcin (G.B.), Robimycin, RP-Mycin, Rythrocaps (S. Afr.), SK-Erythromycin, Wyamycin.

Preparations

Injection: Powder, 0.5 and 1 gm; solution, 50 mg/ml.
Oral: Tablets (enteric-coated), 250 mg.
Rectal: Suppositories, 125 mg.
Topical: Ointment, 1 per cent.
Topical Ophthalmic: Ointment, 0.5 per cent.

Usual Dosages

Intramuscular (Deep): Adults, 100 mg initially, repeated a 4- to 8-hour intervals (total daily dose, 5 to 8 mg/kg). The recommended dose for children weighing over 13.6 kg is 50 mg every 4 to 6 hours, or a total of 12 mg/kg daily.
Intravenous: Adults, 1 to 4 gm daily in divided doses. Children, 50 mg/kg daily in four divided doses. Premature and full-term newborn infants, 10 mg/kg daily in four divided doses. For severe infections, 15 to 20 mg/kg may be given.
Oral: Adults, initially 500 mg followed by 250 mg every 6 hours. For severe infections, 4 gm or more daily in divided doses. Children, 30 to 50 mg/kg daily in divided doses. For severe infections, the dose may be doubled.
Subconjunctival: Up to 100 mg in 0.5 ml of isotonic sodium chloride injection.
Topical: Preparation may be applied to the affected area three or four times daily.
Topical Ophthalmic: Ointment preparation is applied one or more times daily.

---

* Route of administration not approved by FDA.
† Drug not approved by FDA for any indication.
‡ Drug not approved by FDA for this particular indication.
§ Indicated dosage above the manufacturer's recommendation.

ETHACRYNIC ACID (ETACRYNIC ACID)

Proprietary Names: Crinuryl (Isr.), Edecril (Austral., Jap.), Edecrin, Hydromedrin (Germ.).

Preparations

Injection: Powder, 50 mg/vial.
Oral: Tablets, 25 and 50 mg.

Usual Dosages

Intravenous: For adults, the usual dose is 50 mg or 0.5 to 1.0 mg/kg. In children, initially, 1 mg/kg. These doses may be increased if necessary.
Oral: Adults, initially, 50 to 100 mg daily. If an adequate response is not obtained, the daily dosage may be increased, usually in increments of 25 or 50 mg. For maintenance, the dose and frequency of administration must be determined individually. Children, initially, 25 mg daily. Dosage may be increased gradually by increments of 25 mg.

ETHAMBUTOL

Proprietary Names: Dexambutol (Fr.), Etibi (Canad.), Miambutol (Ital.), Myambutol.

Preparations

Oral: Tablets, 100 and 400 mg.

Usual Dosages

Oral: Adults, for initial treatment, 25 mg/kg daily as a single dose for 10 to 12 days, followed by 15 mg/kg daily as a single dose. For treatment, 25 mg/kg daily as a single dose. After 60 days of treatment, the dose may be reduced to 15 mg/kg daily. Therapy should be continued until bacteriologic conversion occurs or until maximal clinical improvement is noted. Information is inadequate to establish dosage for children under 13 years of age.

ETHINYL ESTRADIOL

Proprietary Names: Duramen (Switz.), Edrol (Austral.), Estigyn (Austral.), Estinyl, Eticyclin Forte (Switz.), Etifollin (Norw.), Etivex (Swed.), Farmacyrol Forte (Germ.), Feminone, Gynolett (Germ.), Linoral (Swed.), Lynoral (Austral., Belg., G.B., Germ., Neth., Switz.), Primogyn (Austral.), Progynon C or M (Austral., Germ., Span., Switz.).

Preparations

Oral: Powder, 1 gm; tablets, 0.02, 0.05, and 0.5 mg.

Usual Dosages

Oral: For hypogonadism, 0.05 mg one to three times daily for the first 2 weeks of an arbitrary cycle, with the addition of a progestin for the last 2 weeks.

ETHOXZOLAMIDE

Proprietary Names: Cardrase, Ethamide.

Preparations

Oral: Tablets, 125 mg.

Usual Dosages

Oral: In the adjunctive treatment of glaucoma in adults, 62.5 to 250 mg may be administered two to four times daily.

ETHYLENEDIAMINE TETRAACETIC ACID
See Edetate Disodium.

ETIDRONATE DISODIUM (EHDP)

Proprietary Names: Calcimux (Arg.), Didronel, Etidron (Ital.).

Preparations

Oral: Tablets, 200 mg.

Usual Dosages

Oral: For Paget's disease, a single daily dose should be given 2 hours before a meal. Initially, 5 mg/kg are given daily for a period not to exceed 6 months. Larger doses should be reserved for use when there is a need for rapid suppression of increased bone turnover or prompt reduction of elevated cardiac output. When doses greater than 10 mg/kg daily are given, the treatment period should not exceed 3 months; the daily dosage should not exceed 20 mg/kg.

ETOPOSIDE

Proprietary Name: Vepesid.

Preparations

Injection: Solution, 100 mg/5 ml.
Oral: Capsules, 50 mg.

Usual Dosages

Intravenous: 35 to 100 mg/square meter.
Oral: 100 to 200 mg/square meter.

ETRETINATE

Proprietary Names: Tegason (G.B.), Tegison.

Preparations

Oral: Capsules, 10 and 25 mg.

Usual Dosages

Oral: Initially, 0.75 to 1.0 mg/kg daily taken in divided doses. A maximum dose of 1.5 mg/kg should not be exceeded. Maintenance doses are 0.5 to 0.75 mg/kg daily.

---

* Route of administration not approved by FDA.
† Drug not approved by FDA for any indication.
‡ Drug not approved by FDA for this particular indication.
§ Indicated dosage above the manufacturer's recommendation.

FENOPROFEN

Proprietary Names: Fenopron (G.B.), Fepron (Belg., Ital., Neth.), Feprona (Germ.), Nalfon, Nalgesic (Fr.), Progesic.

Preparations

Oral: Pulvules, 300 mg; tablets, 200, 300, and 600 mg.

Usual Dosages

Oral: For osteoarthritis, the recommended initial dose is 300 to 600 mg four times daily.

FIBRINOLYSIN

Proprietary Names: Lyovac, Thrombolysin.

Preparations

Injection: Vial, 50,000 units.

Usual Dosages

Intravenous: The dosage of 50,000 to 100,000 units per hour for 1 to 6 hours each day is recommended. Dosage may be repeated for 3 or 4 consecutive days, depending on patient response. A single dose of 100,000 units may be adequate in the treatment of uncomplicated thrombophlebitis, but extensive or organized venous thrombi may require a total of 250,000 to 400,000 units.

FLUCYTOSINE

Proprietary Names: Alcobon (G.B.), Ancobon, Ancotil (Arg., Austral., Canad., Denm., Fr., Germ., Jap., Norw., Swed., Switz.).

Preparations

Oral: Capsules, 250 and 500 mg.
Topical Ophthalmic: Solution, 1 and 1.5 per cent.

Usual Dosages

Oral: Adults and children, 50 to 150 mg/kg daily in divided doses at 6-hour intervals.
Topical Ophthalmic: One or two drops of solution may be given hourly.

FLUMETHASONE

Proprietary Name: Locorten.

Preparations

Topical: Cream, 0.03 per cent.

Usual Dosages

Topical: Preparation is applied to affected area three or four times daily or is used under occlusive dressings.

FLUOCINOLONE

Proprietary Names: Flucort (Jap.), Fluonid, Jellin (Germ.), Loaclyn (Ital.), Synalar, Synamol (Canad.), Synemol.

Preparations

Topical: Cream, 0.01, 0.025, and 0.2 per cent; ointment, 0.025 per cent; solution, 0.01 per cent.

Usual Dosages

Topical: Preparation is applied three to four times daily as needed or used under occlusive dressings.

FLUOCINONIDE

Proprietary Names: Lidex, Topsyn.

Preparations

Topical: Cream, 0.05 per cent; gel, 0.05 per cent; ointment, 0.05 per cent.

Usual Dosages

Topical: Preparation is applied three or four times daily as needed.

FLUORESCEIN

Proprietary Names: Ak-Fluor, Fluor-Amps (G.B.), Fluorescite, Fluoreseptic, Fluorets (G.B.), Fluor-I-Strip, Fluoro-I-Strip (G.B.), Ful-Glo, Funduscein.

Preparations

Injection: Solution, 5 and 10 per cent.
Topical Ophthalmic: Applicators impregnated with 0.6, 1.0, and 9.0 mg/strip; solution, 2 per cent.

Usual Dosages

Intravenous: Adults, 500 mg (10 ml of a 5 per cent solution or 5 ml of a 10 per cent solution) are injected rapidly into an arm vein. The dye should appear in the central retinal artery in 9 to 15 seconds.
Topical Ophthalmic: For detection of epithelial defects, a fluorescein strip moistened with ophthalmic irrigating solution is used to touch the conjunctiva, or one drop of solution is placed in the conjunctival sac.

FLUORINATED CORTICOSTEROIDS
See Betamethasone, Dexamethasone, Flumethasone, Fluocinolone, Fluocinonide, Flurandrenolide, Halcinonide, Triamcinolone.

FLUOROMETHOLONE

Proprietary Names: FML Liquifilm, Oxylone.

Preparations

Topical Ophthalmic: Suspension, 0.1 per cent.

Usual Dosages

Topical Ophthalmic: One drop every 1 or 2 hours until response; then frequency is reduced.

FLUOROURACIL

Proprietary Names: Adrucil, Efudex, Fluoroplex, 5 FU.

Preparations

Injection: Solution, 50 mg/ml.
Topical: Cream, 5 per cent; solution, 1, 2, and 5 per cent.

Usual Dosages

Intravenous: Daily dosage is based on 12 mg/kg, but should not exceed 800 mg regardless of the patient's weight.
Subconjunctival: 0.1 ml of a solution containing 50 mg/ml.
Topical: Preparation is applied twice daily.

FLURANDRENOLIDE

Proprietary Names: Cordran, Drenison (G.B.), Drocort (Swed.), Haelen (G.B.), Sermaba (Germ.).

Preparations

Topical: Cream and ointment, 0.025 and 0.05 per cent; lotion, 0.05 per cent; tape, 4 μg/square centimeter.

Usual Dosages

Topical: Preparation is applied two or three times daily or is used under occlusive dressings. The tape is applied once every 12 hours.

FLURBIPROFEN

Proprietary Names: Ansaid, Cebutid (Fr.), Froben (G.B., S. Afr., Switz.), Ocufen.

Preparations

Oral: Tablets, 50 and 100 mg.
Topical Ophthalmic: Solution, 0.03 per cent.

Usual Dosages

Oral: 100 to 400 mg daily.
Topical Ophthalmic: A total of four drops should be administered, with instillation of one drop approximately every 30 minutes beginning 2 hours before surgery.

---

* Route of administration not approved by FDA.
† Drug not approved by FDA for any indication.
‡ Drug not approved by FDA for this particular indication.
§ Indicated dosage above the manufacturer's recommendation.

FOLIC ACID

Proprietary Names: Acfol (Span.), Folacid (Neth.), Folacin (Norw., Swed.), Folaemin (Neth.), Folasic (Austral.), Foldine (Fr.), Folettes (Austral.), Folico (Ital.), Folina (Ital.), Folsan (Germ.), Folvite, Nifolin (Denm.), Novofolacid (Canad.).

Preparations

Injection: Solution, 5 mg/ml.
Oral: Tablets, 0.1, 0.25, 0.4, 0.8, and 1 mg.

Usual Dosages

Intramuscular, Intravenous, Oral, Subcutaneous (Deep): Up to 1 mg daily. Oral dosage of 0.1 mg daily is considered sufficient as a nutritional supplement. To prevent megaloblastic anemia of pregnancy and fetal damage, up to 1 mg daily throughout pregnancy has been suggested.

F$_3$T
See Trifluridine.

FUROSEMIDE

Proprietary Names: Arasemide (Jap.), Dryptal (G.B.), Franyl (Jap.), Frusemide (G.B.), Frusid (G.B.), Furantral (Pol.), Impugan (Swed.), Lasilix (Fr.), Lasix, Seguril (Span.).

Preparations

Injection: Solution, 10 mg/ml.
Oral: Solution, 10 mg/ml; tablets, 20, 40, and 80 mg.

Usual Dosages

Intravenous: Adults, 80 to 100 mg every 1 to 2 hours until an adequate response is obtained and other therapeutic modalities can be instituted. Children, 25 to 50 mg every 4 hours.
Oral: Adults, 20 to 80 mg as a single dose initially. Children, 1 to 2 mg/kg once or twice daily initially.

GAMMA BENZENE HEXACHLORIDE
See Lindane.

GANCICLOVIR (DHPG)

Proprietary Name: Cytovene.

Preparations

Injection: Powder.

---

* Route of administration not approved by FDA.
† Drug not approved by FDA for any indication.
‡ Drug not approved by FDA for this particular indication.
§ Indicated dosage above the manufacturer's recommendation.

Usual Dosages

Intravenous: Initially, the usual daily adult dosage is 7.5 to 10 mg/kg given in divided doses at 8- to 12-hour intervals. Maintenance therapy is 5 to 6 mg/kg daily.
Intravitreal: 200 µg in 0.1 ml of aqueous solution.

GAS-GANGRENE ANTITOXIN

Proprietary Name: Gas-Gangrene Antitoxin.

Preparations

Injection: Solution, 2500 units/ml.

Usual Dosages

Intramuscular, Intravenous: The usual prophylactic dose is 25,000 units, which may be doubled or repeated if necessary. The therapeutic dose is at least 75,000 units and may be repeated every 4 to 6 hours, according to the response of the patient.

GELATIN SPONGE (ABSORBABLE)

Proprietary Name: Gelfoam.

Preparations

Topical: Sponges, sizes 12, 50, 100, and 200.

Usual Dosages

Topical: The sponges may be applied dry or saturated with sodium chloride solution for injection to the bleeding area.

GEMFIBROZIL

Proprietary Name: Lopid.

Preparations

Oral: Capsules, 300 mg.

Usual Dosages

Oral: The usual dose is 0.9 to 1.5 gm daily in divided doses.

GENTAMICIN

Proprietary Names: Cidomycin (G.B.), Garamycin, Garamycina (Swed.), Genoptic, Gentalline (Fr.), Genticin (G.B.), Geomycine (Belg.), Refobacin (Germ.), Sulmycin (Germ.), U-Gencin.

Preparations

Injection: Solution, 10 and 40 mg/ml.
Topical Ophthalmic: Ointment, 3 mg/ml; solution, 3 mg/ml.

Usual Dosages

Intramuscular, Intravenous: Adults and children (with normal renal function), 3 mg/kg daily administered in three equally divided doses. The usual dosage is 80 mg three times daily for patients weighing more than 60 kg, and 60 mg three times daily for patients weighing 60 kg or less. In serious and life-threatening infections, up to 5 mg/kg daily administered in three or four equally divided doses may be required.

Intravitreal: 100 to 400 μg in 0.1 to 0.2 ml of isotonic sodium chloride injection.

Retrobulbar: 0.5 to 1.0 ml of a solution containing 40 mg/ml.

Subconjunctival: 1.25 to 30 mg in a 0.5 ml aqueous solution. The pediatric solution for injection without preservatives is preferred for subconjunctival injections.

Topical Ophthalmic: One drop of a solution 3 to 15 mg/ml is given every 1 to 4 hours, or the ointment preparation is applied two or three times daily. Fortified gentamicin eyedrops are prepared by adding 2 ml of the parenteral preparation containing 40 mg/ml to the 5-ml dropper bottle of the gentamicin ophthalmic solution to produce a concentration of 13.6 mg/ml.

GENTIAN VIOLET

Proprietary Names: Crystal Violet (G.B.), Genapax.

Preparations

Topical: Solution, 0.5, 1.0, and 2.0 per cent.

Usual Dosages

Topical: Solution should be applied to lesions with cotton two to three times daily.

GLYCERIN (GLYCEROL)

Proprietary Names: Glyrol, Luxoral (Ital.), Ophthalgan, Osmoglyn.

Preparations

Oral: Solution, 50 (0.6 gm/ml) and 75 (0.94 gm/ml) per cent.
Topical Ophthalmic: Solution, 0.5 per cent.

Usual Dosages

Oral: One to 1.5 gm/kg usually given as a 50 or 75 per cent solution.
Topical Ophthalmic: One drop of solution may be instilled into the eye every 3 or 4 hours for reduction of corneal edema.

GOLD SALTS
See Auranofin, Aurothioglucose, Gold Sodium Thiomalate.

GOLD SODIUM THIOMALATE (SODIUM AUROTHIOMALATE)

Proprietary Names: Myochrysine, Myocrisin (G.B.), Tauredon (Germ.).

---

* Route of administration not approved by FDA.
† Drug not approved by FDA for any indication.
‡ Drug not approved by FDA for this particular indication.
§ Indicated dosage above the manufacturer's recommendation.

Preparations

Injection: Solution, 10, 25, 50, and 100 mg/ml.

Usual Dosages

Intramuscular: Adults, initially, single weekly injections of 10 mg the first week, 25 mg the second week, 25 or 50 mg the third week, and 50 mg each week thereafter until a total dosage of 0.8 to 1 gm has been administered.

GRISEOFULVIN

Proprietary Names: Fulcin (G.B.), Fulvicin-P/G, Fulvicin-U/F, Grifulvin V, Grisactin, Grisefuline (Fr.), Grisovin (G.B.), Grisowen, Gris-PEG, Lamoryl (Swed.), Likuden M (Germ.).

Preparations

Oral: Capsules, 125 and 250 mg; suspension, 125 mg/5 ml; tablets, 125, 250, and 500 mg.

Usual Dosages

Oral: Adults, 0.5 to 1 gm daily in divided doses. Children, approximately 5 to 10 mg/kg in single or divided doses.

GUANETHIDINE

Proprietary Name: Ismelin.

Preparations

Oral: Tablets, 10 and 25 mg.
Topical Ophthalmic: Preparation is not commercially available in the United States.

Usual Dosages

Oral: Adults, for ambulatory patients, initially, 10 mg daily. The dosage may be increased by increments of 10 mg every 5 to 7 days. In hospitalized patients, initial dose is 25 to 50 mg daily, increased by 25 to 50 mg daily or every other day as indicated. Because of the drug's long half-life, the maximal effect may not be observed for 7 to 14 days and it may be necessary to reduce the dose slightly after an initial antihypertensive effect has been obtained. Children, initially, 0.2 mg/kg daily, increased by the same amount every 7 to 10 days if required.
Topical Ophthalmic: One drop of a 5 to 10 per cent solution twice daily.

GUANIDINE

Proprietary Name: Guanidine.

Preparations

Oral: Tablets, 125 mg.

Usual Dosages

Oral: An initial daily test dose of 10 mg/kg is given. The total dose is arrived at by daily increments. A dosage of 10 to 58 mg/kg daily is administered in three to four divided doses.

HALCINONIDE

Proprietary Name: Halog.

Preparations

Topical: Cream, 0.1 per cent; ointment, 0.025 and 0.1 per cent; solution, 0.1 per cent.

Usual Dosages

Topical: Preparation is applied three or four times daily as needed.

HALOPERIDOL

Proprietary Names: Haldol, Serenace (G.B.).

Preparations

Injection: Solution, 5 mg/ml.
Oral: Solution, 2 mg/ml; tablets, 0.5, 1, 2, 5, and 10 mg.

Usual Dosages

Intramuscular: 1 to 5 mg given every 12 hours as needed.
Oral: 1 to 5 mg twice daily.

HALOPROGIN

Proprietary Names: Halotex, Mycanden (Arg., Germ., S. Afr.), Mycilan (Belg., Fr.), Polik (Jap.).

Preparations

Topical: Cream, 1 per cent; solution, 1 per cent.

Usual Dosages

Topical: The preparation is applied liberally to the affected area twice daily for 2 to 3 weeks.

HEMOSTATIC COLLAGEN (ABSORBABLE)

Proprietary Names: Avitene, Instat.

Preparations

Topical: Fiber squares, 70 mm × 35 or 70 mm × 1 mm.

Usual Dosages

Topical: Small squares or fibrous form may be applied directly to the source of bleeding.

HEPARIN

Proprietary Names: Calciparin (Germ.), Calciparine (Austral., Fr.), Cutheparine (Fr.), Depo-Heparin, Disebrin (Ital.), Hamocura (Germ.), Hepacarin (Jap.), Hepalean (Canad.), Hepathrom, Hep-Lock, Heprinar, Lipo-Hepin, Liquaemin, Liquemin (Germ.), Liquemine (Fr.), Norheparin (Germ.), Panheprin, Thrombophob (Germ.), Thrombo-Vetren (Germ.), Vetren (Germ.).

Preparations

Injection: Gel (for repository injection), 20,000 units/ml; solution, 200, 1000, 5000, 7500, 10,000, 15,000, 20,000, and 40,000 units/ml.

Usual Dosages

Intravenous: 10,000 USP units initially, then 5000 to 10,000 units four to six times daily. By intravenous infusion, 20,000 to 40,000 units/L at a rate of 15 to 30 units per minute.
Subcutaneous: 10,000 to 20,000 units initially, then 8000 to 10,000 units three times daily, according to prothrombin time response.

HOMATROPINE

Proprietary Names: Homatrocel, Isopto Homatropine, SMP Homatropine (G.B.).

Preparations

Topical Ophthalmic: Solution, 2 and 5 per cent.

Usual Dosages

Topical Ophthalmic: One drop instilled two to four times daily.

HYALURONIDASE

Proprietary Names: Alidase, Hyalas (Swed.), Hyalase (G.B.), Hyason (Belg.), Jalovis (Ital.), Jaluran (Ital.), Kinetin (Germ.), Permease (Aust.), Seravase (S. Afr.), Wydase.

Preparations

Injection: Powder (lyophilized), 150 and 1500 units; solution, 150 units/ml.
Topical Ophthalmic: No preparation is commercially available. A solution of 750 units dissolved in 1 ml physiologic saline may be prepared.

Usual Dosages

Infiltration: For local anesthesia of the eye, 150 units are dissolved in 1 ml of a 2 per cent procaine and 0.4 per cent potassium sulfate solution. For nerve block, 0.4 ml of this mixture is diluted to 10 ml and two drops (0.12 ml) of epinephrine are added before injection.
Topical Ophthalmic: Solution may be applied three to four times daily.

HYDROCHLOROTHIAZIDE

Proprietary Names: Aquarius (Canad.), Chemhydrazide (Canad.), Chlorzide, Delco-Retic, Direma (G.B.), Diucen-H, Diuchlor H (Canad.), Diu-Scrip, Esidrex (G.B.), Esidrix, Hydrazide (Canad.), Hydrid (Canad.), Hydro-Aquil (Canad.), Hydrodiuretex (Canad.), Hydro-

---

* Route of administration not approved by FDA.
† Drug not approved by FDA for any indication.
‡ Drug not approved by FDA for this particular indication.
§ Indicated dosage above the manufacturer's recommendation.

Diuril, Hydromal, Hydrosaluret (Canad.), HydroSaluric (G.B.), Hydrozide, Hyeloril, Hyperetic, Kenazide, Lexxor, Loqua, Mictrin, Neo-Codema (Canad.), Neoflumen (Austral.), Novohydrazide (Canad.), Oretic, Ro-Hydrazide, SK-Hydrochlorothiazide, Thiuretic, Urozide (Canad.), Zide.

Preparations

Oral: Tablets, 25, 50, and 100 mg.

Usual Dosages

Oral: Adults, initially 25 to 50 mg twice daily. Children, 2 mg/kg daily in two divided doses.

HYDROCORTISONE

Proprietary Names: Actocortin (Germ., Swed.), A-Hydrocort, Anusol-HC, Barriere-HC (Canad.), Bio-Cort (Canad.), Bio-Cortex, Biosone, Cetacort, Corlan (G.B.), Corphos, Cortamed (Canad.), Cortef, Cortenema, Cortiment (Canad., Swed.), Cortomister (Fr.), Efcortelan (G.B.), Efcortesol (G.B.), Eldecort, Emo-Cort (Canad.), Ficortril (Germ., Swed.), Flebocortid (Austral., Ital.), Heb-Cort, Hycor (Austral.), Hycorace, Hydrocort, Hydrocortal (Swed.), Hydrocortemel (S. Afr.), Hydrocortistab (G.B.), Hydrocortisone, Hydrosone, Hynax (Austral.), Hysone-A (Austral.), Idrocortisone (Ital.), Intracort (Austral.), Komed HC, Manticor (Canad.), Microcort (Canad.), Nordicort (Austral.), Novohydrocort (Canad.), Nutracort, Pabracort (G.B.), Panhydrosone, Phiacort (Austral.), Polycort (S. Afr.), Scheroson (Austral.), Scheroson F (Germ.), Sigmacort (Austral.), Siguent Hycor (Austral.), Solu-Cortef, Solu-Glyc (Swed.), Span-Ster, Squibb-HC (Austral.), Sterocort (Canad.), Tega-cort, Unicort (Canad.), Venocort (Austral.), Venocortin (S. Afri.), Wincort (Canad.).

Preparations

Injection (Ophthalmic): Suspension, 2.5 per cent.
Topical: Cream, 0.125, 0.2, 0.25, 0.5, and 1.0 per cent; lotion, 0.125, 0.25, 0.5, and 1 per cent; ointment, 1 and 2.5 per cent.
Topical Ophthalmic: Ointment, 0.5, 1.5, and 2.5 per cent; solution, 0.2 per cent; suspension, 0.5 and 2.5 per cent.

Usual Dosages

Intramuscular: For emergency situations when the intravenous route is not feasible, 100 to 250 mg initially, repeated until an adequate response is discernible. Maximum daily dose is 1 gm.
Intravenous: For conditions other than shock, 100 to 500 mg initially, repeated if necessary. Dosage may be reduced for infants and children.
Subconjunctival: 0.5 ml of a 2.5 per cent suspension.
Topical: Preparation is applied three or four times daily as required.
Topical Ophthalmic: One or two drops of a 0.2 per cent solution or 0.5 per cent suspension every 1 or 2 hours until a response is obtained; the frequency then is reduced. For severe conditions, a 2.5 per cent suspension may be used. The ointment preparation is applied three or four times daily or as a nighttime medication when the suspension is used during the day.

HYDROGEN PEROXIDE

Proprietary Name: Hydrogen Peroxide.

Preparations

Topical: Solution, 3 per cent.

Usual Dosages

Topical: Application to wounds and mucous membranes helps in debridement by loosening masses of infected detritus in wounds.

HYDROXOCOBALAMIN

Proprietary Names: Acimexan (Switz.), Acuo-Godabion B12 (Span.), Alpha Redisol, Alpha-Ruvite, Aquo-Cytobion (Germ.), Aquodavur (Span.), Axlon (Germ.), Behepan (Swed.), Berubilong (Germ.), Biocobal VCA (Ital.), Bradirubra (Ital.), Cobalidrina (Ital.), Cobalin-H (G.B.), Cobalvit (Ital.), Depo-gamma (Germ.), Docevita (Span.), Docivit Depo (Germ.), Dodecavit (Fr.), Dosixbe (Arg.), Droxodoce (Arg.), Droxofor (Arg.), Forta-B12 (Belg.), Fravit B_{12} (Ital.), Hidroxuber (Span.), Hydrocobamine (Neth.), Hydroxo B_{12}, Idrozima (Ital.), Liodozal (Switz.), Longicobal (Ital.), Macrabin H (Ind.), Mega-B12 (Belg.), Megamilbedoce (Span.), Milbedoce Depot (Span.), Natur B_{12} (Ital.), Neo-Betalin 12, Neo-Cytamen (Arg., Austral., G.B., Ital., S. Afr.), Novidroxin (Germ.), Novobedouze (Belg., Fr., Switz.), Red 1000 (Ital.), Rossobivit (Ital.), Rubesol-LA, Rubitard B_{12} (Ital.), Sytobex-H, Vibeden (Denm.), Vitarubin Depot (Switz.).

Preparations

Injection: Solution, 100, 250, and 1000 μg/ml.

Usual Dosages

Intramuscular: For patients with demonstrable neurologic damage, 1 mg may be given once weekly for several months, then once or twice monthly for another year. Neurologic damage that cannot be reversed within 12 to 18 months must be considered irreversible.

HYDROXYCHLOROQUINE

Proprietary Names: Ercoquin (Norw., Swed.), Plaquenil, Plaquinol (Port.), Quensyl (Germ.).

Preparations

Oral: Tablets, 200 mg (equivalent to 155 mg of base).

Usual Dosages

Oral: The average adult dosage is 200 mg once or twice daily.

---

* Route of administration not approved by FDA.
† Drug not approved by FDA for any indication.
‡ Drug not approved by FDA for this particular indication.
§ Indicated dosage above the manufacturer's recommendation.

HYDROXYETHYL CELLULOSE

Proprietary Names: Adsorbotear, Ciba Vision Lens Drops, Comfort Tears, Gonioscopic Prism Solution, Lens Fresh Lubricating and Rewetting Drops, Neo-Tears, Optocrymal (Canad.), TearGard.

Preparations

Topical Ophthalmic: Solution.

Usual Dosages

Topical Ophthalmic: One or two drops in the eye(s) instilled three times daily or as needed.

HYDROXYPROPYL CELLULOSE

Proprietary Name: Lacrisert.

Preparations

Topical Ophthalmic: Ophthalmic insert, 5 mg.

Usual Dosages

Topical Ophthalmic: One ophthalmic insert may be instilled in each eye one to two times daily.

HYDROXYPROPYL METHYLCELLULOSE

Proprietary Names: Celacol HPM, Contactisol (Canad.), Goniosol, Hypromellose, Isopto Alkaline, Isopt-Fluid (Germ.), Isopto Plain, Isopto Tears, Lacril, Methocel HG, Methopt (Austral.), Tearisol.

Preparations

Topical Ophthalmic: Solution, 0.5, 0.8, 1.0, and 2.5 per cent.

Usual Dosages

Topical Ophthalmic: One drop in the eye several times a day.

HYDROXYSTILBAMIDINE

Proprietary Name: Hydroxystilbamidine.

Preparations

Injection: Powder, 225 mg.

Usual Dosages

Intravenous (Slow Infusion): The daily dose range for adults is 225 mg in 200 ml of 5 per cent dextrose injection or sodium chloride injection, up to a total of 5 to 25 gm. In most cases, a maximum of 8 gm is recommended.

---

* Route of administration not approved by FDA.
† Drug not approved by FDA for any indication.
‡ Drug not approved by FDA for this particular indication.
§ Indicated dosage above the manufacturer's recommendation.

HYDROXYUREA

Proprietary Names: Hydrea, Litalir (Germ.).

Preparations

Oral: Capsules, 500 mg.

Usual Dosages

Oral: 80 mg/kg as a single dose every 3 days or 20 to 30 mg/kg daily.

HYDROXYZINE

Proprietary Names: Atarax, Atazina (Ital.), Aterax (S. Afr.), Masmoran (Germ.), Neocalma (Ital.), Neurozina (Ital.), Paxistil (Belg.), Sedaril, Vistaril.

Preparations

Injection: Solution, 25, 50, and 100 mg/ml.
Oral: Capsules, 25, 50, and 100 mg; suspension, 25 mg/ml; syrup, 10 mg/5 ml; tablets, 10, 25, 50, and 100 mg.

Usual Dosages

Intramuscular: Adults, for serious psychiatric conditions, 50 to 100 mg initially and every 4 to 6 hours as needed.
Oral: For anxiety, adults, 225 to 400 mg daily divided in three or four doses. For pruritus in adults, 25 mg three to four times daily; children over 6 years, 50 to 100 mg daily in divided doses; children under 6 years, 50 mg daily in divided doses.

HYOSCINE
See Scopolamine.

HYPEROSMOTIC AGENTS
See Glycerin, Isosorbide, Mannitol, Urea.

IBUPROFEN

Proprietary Names: Brufen (G.B.), Motrin.

Preparations

Oral: Tablets, 300 and 400 mg.

Usual Dosages

Oral: 300 or 400 mg three or four times daily may be administered.

IDOXURIDINE (IDU)

Proprietary Names: Dendrid, Herpid (G.B.), Herpidu (S. Afr.), Herplex, Iduridine (Germ., Swed.), Iduviran (Fr.), Kerecid (G.B.), Ophthalmadine (G.B.), Stoxil, Synmiol (Germ.), Virunguent (Germ.).

Preparations

Topical Ophthalmic: Ointment, 0.5 per cent; solution, 0.1 per cent.

Usual Dosages

Topical Ophthalmic: One drop of the solution instilled every hour during the day and every 2 hours at night. The ointment is applied four or five times daily or as nighttime medication when the solution is used during the day. Treatment should be continued for at least 2 weeks.

IFOSFAMIDE

Proprietary Names: Cyfos, Holoxan (Fr., Germ., Neth.), Ifex, Mitoxana, Naxamide.

Preparations

Injection: Powder in vials of 0.5, 1.0 and 2.0 gm.

Usual Dosages

Intravenous: A total dose for each course is 8 to 10 gm/square meter administered as a single daily dose over 3 to 10 days.

IMIPENEM/CILASTATIN COMBINATION

Proprietary Name: Primaxin.

Preparations

Injection: Powder (equivalent to base), 250 mg of imipenem and 250 mg of cilastatin.

Usual Dosages

Intravenous: The daily dosage should not exceed 50 mg/kg or 4 gm, whichever is lower. The usual adult dosage is 500 mg every 6 hours.

IMIPRAMINE

Proprietary Names: Berkomine (G.B.), Censtim (Austral.), Chemipramine (Canad.), Co-Caps Imipramine (G.B.), Dimipressin (G.B.), Imavate, Imiprin (Austral.), Impranil (Canad.), Impril (Canad.), Iramil (Austral.), Janimine, Melipramine (Austral.), Norpramine (G.B.), Novopramine (Canad.), Oppanyl (G.B.), Panpramine (S. Afr.), Praminil (G.B.), Presamine, Prodepress (Austral.), SK-Pramine, Somipra (Austral.), Thymopramine (S. Afr.), Tofranil, W.D.D.

Preparations

Injection: Solution, 12.5 mg/ml.
Oral: Capsules, 75, 100, 125, and 150 mg; tablets, 10, 25, and 50 mg.

Usual Dosages

Intramuscular: Adults, initially up to 100 mg daily in divided doses. The oral route should be substituted as soon as possible.

---

* Route of administration not approved by FDA.
† Drug not approved by FDA for any indication.
‡ Drug not approved by FDA for this particular indication.
§ Indicated dosage above the manufacturer's recommendation.

Oral: Adults (hospitalized), initially, 100 mg daily in divided doses, increased gradually to 200 mg daily; 250 to 300 mg daily may be given if there is no response after 2 weeks. Adults (outpatients), initially, 75 mg increased to 150 mg daily in divided doses; for maintenance, 50 to 150 mg daily at bedtime (maximum, 300 mg daily). Adolescents and elderly patients, initially, 30 to 40 mg daily (maximum, 100 mg daily).

INDOMETHACIN (INDOMETACIN)

Proprietary Names: Amuno (Germ.), Confortid (Swed.), Imbrilon (G.B.), Inacid (Span.), Indacin (Jap.), Indocid (G.B.), Indocin, Indomee (Swed.), Infrocin (Canad.), Metindol (Pol.), Mezolin (Jap.).

Preparations

Oral: Capsules, 25 and 50 mg.
Topical Ophthalmic: No commercial preparations are available. A 1 per cent solution may be prepared by dissolving 10 mg of indomethacin in 1 ml of sesame oil or water.

Usual Dosages

Oral: 50 to 200 mg daily in divided doses.
Topical Ophthalmic: Solution may be administered three or four times daily.

INFLUENZA VIRUS VACCINE

Proprietary Names: Fluax, Fluogen, Fluvirin (G.B.), Fluzone, Influvac (G.B.), MFV-Ject (Fr., G.B.).

Preparations

Injection: Suspension, 100 μg/ml.

Usual Dosages

Intramuscular: For adults and children older than 12 years of age, the usual dosage is 0.5 ml administered as a single dose.

INSULIN

Proprietary Names: Actrapid, Deposulin (Germ.), Endopancrine (Fr.), Insulatard NPH, Lentard, Lente (Iletin or Insulin), Mixtard, Monotard, NPH Iletin, Protamine (Zinc and Iletin), Regular (Iletin or Insulin), Semilente (Iletin or Insulin), Semitard, Ultralente (Iletin or Insulin), Ultratard, Velosulin.

Preparations

Injection: Solution and suspension, 40, 80, 100, and 500 units/ml.

Usual Dosages

Intramuscular, Intravenous, Subcutaneous: The number and size of daily doses are dependent upon patient's need.

INTERFERON-ALPHA

Proprietary Names: Alferon, Intron A, Roferon-A, Wellferon.

Preparations

Injection: Powder, 18 million units/vial; solution, 3 or 6 million units/ml.
Topical Ophthalmic: No ophthalmic preparation is commercially available. A solution containing 30 million units/ml may be prepared by using parenteral preparations.

Usual Dosages

Intramuscular, Subcutaneous: Initially, the usual dose is 3 million units daily. The recommended maintenance dose is 3 million units 3 times weekly. Doses higher than 3 million units are not recommended.
Topical Ophthalmic: Two drops may be applied to the eye(s) daily.

INTERFERON GAMMA

Proprietary Name: Interferon Gamma.

Preparations

Injection: Lyophilized powder for reconstitution with sterile water. One mg is equivalent to 20 million units.

Usual Dosages

Intramuscular, Subcutaneous: The usual daily dose is 1 to 10 million units (0.125 to 0.5 mg)/square meter. Depending on the severity, the duration of administration may last several months.

INTERLEUKIN-2

Proprietary Name: Cetus.

Preparations

Injection: Solution.

Usual Dosages

Intravenous: Initially, the usual dose is 30,000 to 100,000 units/kg every 8 hours.

ISOFLUROPHATE (DFP)

Proprietary Names: Diflupyl (Fr.), Dyflos (G.B.), Floropryl.

Preparations

Topical Ophthalmic: Ointment, 0.025 per cent; solution, 0.1 per cent.

Usual Dosages

Topical Ophthalmic: One drop daily or 1/4-inch strip of ointment every 12 to 72 hours.

---

* Route of administration not approved by FDA.
† Drug not approved by FDA for any indication.
‡ Drug not approved by FDA for this particular indication.
§ Indicated dosage above the manufacturer's recommendation.

ISOMETHEPTENE/DICHLORALPHENAZONE COMBINATION

Proprietary Name: Midrin.

Preparations

Oral: Capsules, 65 mg isometheptene and 100 mg dichloralphenazone.

Usual Dosages

Oral: At first sign of a migraine attack, two capsules should be taken, followed by one capsule every hour until migraine is relieved. Maximum dose is five capsules in a 12-hour period.

ISONIAZID

Proprietary Names: Cedin (Germ.), Cotinazin, Dinacrin, Dow-Isoniazid, Hydronsan (Jap., S. Afr.), Hyzyd, INH, Isobicina (Ital.), Isotamine (Canad.), Isotinyl (Austral.), Isozid (Germ.), Laniazid, Neoteben (Germ.), Niconyl, Nidaton, Nydrazid, Panazid, Rimifon (G.B.), Rolazid, Tb-Phlogin (Germ.), Teebaconin, Tibinide (Swed.), Triniad, Uniad.

Preparations

Injection: Solution, 100 mg/ml.
Oral: Syrup, 50 mg/5 ml; tablets, 100 and 300 mg.

Usual Dosages

Intramuscular, Oral: Adults, 5 mg/kg daily in a single dose (maximum, 300 mg daily). Children inactivate this drug faster than adults and may be given 30 mg/kg daily in a single dose (maximum, 300 mg daily). The larger doses should be used for atypical infection. For prophylactic use, adults, 300 mg daily in a single dose; children, 10 mg/kg daily in a single dose (maximum, 300 mg daily).

ISOPROTERENOL

Proprietary Names: Aerolone, Isoprenaline (G.B.), Isuprel, Norisodrine, Vapo-Iso.

Preparations

Inhalation: Aerosol, 0.2 and 0.25 per cent; solution for nebulization, 0.031, 0.062, 0.25, 0.5, and 1.0 per cent.
Injection: Solution, 0.02 and 0.2 mg/ml.
Sublingual: Tablets, 10 and 15 mg.

Usual Dosages

Inhalation: For treatment of bronchospasm during mild acute asthmatic attacks, the usual dose is 120 to 262 μg (one or two inhalations of a 0.25 per cent solution) administered via a metered aerosol.
Intramuscular, Intravenous, Subcutaneous: The usual adult bolus dose is 0.02 to 0.06 mg, with subsequent doses ranging from 0.01 to 0.2 mg.
Sublingual: Adults, usual dose is 10 to 20 mg. Daily dosage should not exceed 60 mg. Children, usual dose is 5 to 10 mg. Daily dosage should not exceed 30 mg.

ISOSORBIDE

Proprietary Name: Isosorbide.

Preparations

Oral: Solution, 45 per cent.

Usual Dosages

Oral: Adults, initially, 1.5 gm/kg may be given up to four times daily. The usual dose range is 1 to 3 gm/kg two to four times a day as needed.

IVERMECTIN

Proprietary Names: Cardomec, Eqvalan, Heartgard-30, Ivomec (G.B.), Zimecterin.

Preparations

Oral: Tablets.

Usual Dosages

Oral: A single oral dose of 12 mg annually.

KANAMYCIN

Proprietary Names: Kamycine (Fr.), Kanabristol (Germ.), Kanasig (Austral.), Kanmy (S. Afr.), Kannasyn (G.B.), Kantrex, Kantrox (Swed.), Klebcil.

Preparations

Injection: Solution, 37.5, 250, and 333 mg/ml.

Usual Dosages

Intramuscular: To achieve continuously high blood levels, 15 mg/kg daily in divided doses every 6 to 8 hours. Otherwise, a dose of 7.5 mg/kg every 12 hours should not be exceeded.
Intravenous: This route is used only if intramuscular route is not possible. The dose should not exceed 15 mg/kg daily and must be administered slowly.

KETOCONAZOLE

Proprietary Name: Nizoral.

Preparations

Oral: Suspension, 100 mg/5 ml; tablets, 200 mg.
Topical: Cream, 2 per cent.
Topical Ophthalmic: No ophthalmic preparation is commercially available.

Usual Dosages

Oral: The recommended starting dose is 200 mg in a single daily dose. In very serious infections, the dose may be increased up to 1.2 gm daily.

---

* Route of administration not approved by FDA.
† Drug not approved by FDA for any indication.
‡ Drug not approved by FDA for this particular indication.
§ Indicated dosage above the manufacturer's recommendation.

Topical Ophthalmic: A 1 to 2 per cent solution may be applied to the affected and surrounding areas twice a day for up to 8 to 12 weeks.

KETOTIFEN

Proprietary Names: Zaditen (Belg., G.B., Germ., Lux., Neth., Switz.).

Preparations

Oral: Capsules, 1 mg; elixir, 1 mg/5 ml; tablets, 1 mg.

Usual Dosages

Oral: The usual daily dose is 1 mg twice daily.

LEUCOVORIN

Proprietary Names: Lederfoline (Fr.), Ledervorin (Neth.), Ledervorin Calcium (Belg.).

Preparations

Injection: Powder, 50 mg; solution, 3 mg/ml.

Usual Dosages

Intramuscular, Intravenous, Oral, Subcutaneous (Deep): Up to 1 mg daily; maintenance dose of 0.1 to 0.25 mg daily.

LEVAMISOLE

Proprietary Names: Decaris (Denm., Hung.) Ergamisol (Belg., Ital, S. Afr.), Ketrax (G.B.), Meglum (Arg.), Solaskil (Fr.), Stimamizol (Arg.).

Preparations

Oral: Syrup, 40 mg/5 ml; tablets, 40 mg.

Usual Dosages

Oral: An initial daily dose of 40 mg is recommended, increasing the amount by 40 mg every 2 weeks to a maximum of 150 mg.

LEVOBUNOLOL

Proprietary Name: Betagan.

Preparations

Topical Ophthalmic: Solution, 0.5 per cent.

Usual Dosages

Topical Ophthalmic: The usual dose is one drop in the affected eye(s) one to two times daily.

LEVODOPA

Proprietary Names: Bendopa, Berkdopa (G.B.) Bio Dopa, Brocadopa (G.B.), Dopar, Dopastral (Swed.), Emeldopa (S. Afr.), Helfo-dopa (Germ.), Larodopa, Le-dopa (Fr.), Levopa (G.B.), Parda, Parkidopa (Swed.), Rio-Dopa, Sobiodopa (Fr.), Speciadopa (Fr.), Syndopa (Austral.), Veldopa (G.B.).

Preparations

Oral: Capsules, 100, 250, and 500 mg; tablets, 100, 250, and 500 mg.

Usual Dosages

Oral: The usual initial dosage is 0.5 to 1.0 gm daily, divided into two or more doses. The usual optimal therapeutic dosage should not exceed 8 gm daily.

LEVOTHYROXINE

Proprietary Names: Cytolen, Eltroxin (G.B.), Euthyrox (Germ.), Letter, Levaxin (Swed.), Levoid, Levothroid, Noroxine, Oroxine (Austral.), Percutacrine, Thyroxinique (Fr.), Synthroid, Thyratabs (Swed.), Thyrine (Austral.), Thyroxevan (Austral.), Thyroxinal (Austral.), Thyroxine (G.B.).

Preparations

Oral: Tablets, 0.025, 0.05, 0.1, 0.15, 0.175, 0.2, and 0.3 mg.

Usual Dosages

Oral: Initially, 0.05 to 0.1 mg daily, increased by increments of 0.05 to 0.1 mg at 2- to 3-week intervals until the desired response is maintained. Most patients can be maintained in a full clinical euthyroid state with doses of 0.1 to 0.2 mg daily.

LIDOCAINE

Proprietary Names: Anaesthol (Germ.), Anestacon, Ardecaine, Canocaine, Dolicaine, Indolor (S. Afr.), L-Caine, Leostesin (S. Afr.), Lida-Mantle, Lidocaton (G.B.), Lidothesin (G.B.), Lignane (S. Afr.), Lignocaine (G.B.), Lignostab (G.B.), Nervocaine, Norocaine, Nurocain (Austral.) Rocaine, Sarnacaine (Austral.), Stanacaine, Ultracaine, Xylestesin (Germ.), Xylocaine, Xylocard (G.B.), Xylotox (G.B.).

Preparations

Injection: Solution, 0.5, 1.0, 1.5, 2.0, 4.0, and 5.0 per cent.
Topical: Jelly, 2 per cent; ointment, 2.5 and 5.0 per cent; solution, 2 and 4 per cent.

Usual Dosages

Infiltration: Without epinephrine, for extensive procedures, 25 to 60 ml of a 0.5 per cent solution or 10 to 30 ml of a 1 per cent solution; for minor surgery and relief of pain, 2 to 50 ml of a 0.5 per cent solution. With epinephrine 1:200,000, up to 50 ml of a 1 per cent solution.

---

* Route of administration not approved by FDA.
† Drug not approved by FDA for any indication.
‡ Drug not approved by FDA for this particular indication.
§ Indicated dosage above the manufacturer's recommendation.

Topical: The 2 per cent solution is generally recommended for topical anesthesia. The 4 per cent solution should be used only when the lower concentration does not provide adequate anesthesia. The maximum dose is 10 ml of the 2 per cent or 5 ml of the 4 per cent concentration.

LINCOMYCIN

Proprietary Names: Albiotic (Germ.), Cillimycin (Germ.), Lincocin, Mycivin (G.B.).

Preparations

Injection: Solution, 300 mg/ml.
Oral: Capsules, 250 and 500 mg.

Usual Dosages

Intramuscular: Adults, 0.6 to 1.2 gm daily. Children and infants over 1 month, 10 to 20 mg/kg daily.
Intravenous: Adults, 0.6 to 1.0 gm every 8 to 12 hours. Maximum daily dose should not exceed 8 gm. Children and infants over 1 month, 10 to 20 mg/kg daily in two or three divided doses.
Oral: Adults, 500 mg three or four times daily. Children and infants over 1 month, 30 to 60 mg/kg in three or four divided doses.
Subconjunctival: 150 mg in a 0.5 ml aqueous solution.

LINDANE (GAMMA BENZENE HEXACHLORIDE)

Proprietary Names: Aphtiris (Fr.), Elentol (Fr.), Gamene, Jacutin (Germ.), Lorexane (G.B.), Kevellada (Canad.), Kwell.

Preparations

Topical: Cream, lotion, and shampoo, 1 per cent.

Usual Dosages

Topical: Cream or lotion is applied with soft brush and washed off thoroughly after 24 hours using a soft brush. For head lice, shampoo is applied, lathered, and rinsed thoroughly after 5 minutes; this may be repeated in 1 week if indicated. For pubic lice, shampoo applied as above, or after a scrub bath as outlined previously, thin layer of lotion is applied to affected area and washed off 24 hours later.

LIOTHYRONINE

Proprietary Names: Cynomel (Fr.), Cytomel, Tertroxin (G.B.), Triiodothyronine (G.B.), Trithyrone (Fr.).

Preparations

Oral: Tablets, 5, 25, and 50 μg.

Usual Dosages

Oral: Initially, 25 μg daily, increased by increments of 12.5 to 25 μg at intervals of 1 to 2 weeks until the desired response is maintained. The usual maintenance dose is up to 75 to 100 μg daily.

LITHIUM

Proprietary Names: Camcolit (G.B.), Carbolith (Canad.), Eskalith, Hypnorex (Germ.), Lithane, Lithicarb (Austral.), Lithionit (Swed.), Lithium Duriles (Germ.), Lithium Oligosol (Fr.), Lithobid, Litho-Carb (Canad.), Lithonate, Lithotabs, Maniprex (Belg.), Neurolithium (Fr.), Pfi-Lith, Phasal (G.B.), Priadel (G.B.), Quilonum (Germ., S. Afr.).

Preparations

Oral: Capsules, 300 mg; syrup, 8 mEq/5 ml; tablets, 300 mg.

Usual Dosages

Oral: Dosage should be individualized on the basis of serum levels and response.

LOVASTATIN (MEVINOLIN)

Proprietary Name: Mevacor.

Preparations

Oral: Tablets, 20 mg.

Usual Dosages

Oral: The dose range is 20 to 80 mg daily in single or divided doses.

LUBRICANTS

See Petrolatum, Artificial Tears.

MALATHION

Proprietary Names: Derbac (G.B.), Noury Hoofdlotion (Neth.), Prioderm.

Preparations

Topical: Liquid, 0.05 per cent; lotion, 0.05 per cent; shampoo, 1 per cent.

Usual Dosages

Topical: The recommended treatment for head lice is two applications 1 week apart.

MANNITOL

Proprietary Names: Manicol (Fr.), Osmitrol, Osmosol (Austral.), Resectisol.

Preparations

Injection: Solution, 5, 10, 15, and 20 per cent.

Usual Dosages

Intravenous: 0.5 to 2 gm/kg given as a 20 per cent solution is infused slowly over a period of 30 to 60 minutes.

MEASLES, MUMPS, AND RUBELLA VIRUS VACCINE LIVE

Proprietary Name: M-M-R.

Preparations

Injection: 1000 $TCID_{50}$ measles virus vaccine live, 5000 $TCID_{50}$ mumps virus vaccine live, and 1000 $TCID_{50}$ rubella virus vaccine live/0.5 ml.

Usual Dosages

Subcutaneous: The usual dose is 0.5 ml administered as a single dose.

MEBENDAZOLE

Proprietary Names: Mebendacin (Span.), Mebutar (Arg.), Nemasole (Arg.), Vermox.

Preparations

Oral: Tablets (chewable), 100 mg.

Usual Dosages

Oral: Adults and children, 100 mg given morning and evening for 3 consecutive days for most infections. Enterobiasis can usually be treated with a single 100-mg dose; if a cure is not achieved with initial therapy, a second course 3 weeks later may be beneficial.

MECHLORETHAMINE

Proprietary Names: Caryolysine (Fr.), Cloramin (Ital.), Erasol (Denm.), Mustargen, Mustine (G.B.).

Preparations

Injection: Powder, 10 mg.
Topical: No topical preparations are commercially available, but a 0.02 to 0.1 per cent solution can be prepared.

Usual Dosages

Intravenous: The usual dosage is 0.4 mg/kg per course of therapy, given in a single dose or on 2 separate days. The interval between courses of therapy is usually 3 to 6 weeks.
Topical: Solution may be applied daily for 4 weeks in treatment of mycosis fungoides.

MECLIZINE (MECLOZINE)

Proprietary Names: Antivert, Antrizine, Bonamine (Canad., Germ.), Bonine, Calmonal (Germ.), Dizmiss, Eldezine, Lamine, Mecazine (Canad.), Motion Cure, Navicalm (S. Afr.), Postafen (Germ., Swed.), Roclizine, Ru-Vert-M, Veritab, Vertizine, Vertrol, Wehvert.

---

* Route of administration not approved by FDA.
† Drug not approved by FDA for any indication.
‡ Drug not approved by FDA for this particular indication.
§ Indicated dosage above the manufacturer's recommendation.

Preparations

Oral: Tablets, 12.5, 25, and 50 mg; tablets (chewable), 25 mg.

Usual Dosages

Oral: The daily dose is 25 to 50 mg in single or divided doses.

MEDRYSONE

Proprietary Name: HMS Liquifilm.

Preparations

Topical Ophthalmic: Suspension, 1 per cent.

Usual Dosages

Topical Ophthalmic: One drop of suspension every 1 or 2 hours until response is obtained; frequency then reduced.

MELPHALAN

Proprietary Name: Alkeran.

Preparations

Oral: Tablets, 2 mg.

Usual Dosages

Oral: The usual dosage is 6 mg daily.

MENADIOL

Proprietary Names: Kappadione, Synkayvite.

Preparations

Injection: Solution, 5, 10, and 37.5 mg/ml.
Oral: Tablets, 5 mg.

Usual Dosages

Intramuscular, Intravenous, Oral, Subcutaneous: The usual adult therapeutic dose is 5 to 15 mg.

MENADIONE

Proprietary Name: Menadione.

Preparations

Oral: Powder; tablets, 5 mg.

---

* Route of administration not approved by FDA.
† Drug not approved by FDA for any indication.
‡ Drug not approved by FDA for this particular indication.
§ Indicated dosage above the manufacturer's recommendation.

Usual Dosages

Oral: The usual adult therapeutic dose is 2 to 10 mg.

MEPERIDINE (PETHIDINE)

Proprietary Names: Demerol, Dolantin (Germ.), Dolosal (Fr.), Pethoid (Austral.), Phytadon (Canad.), Suppolosal (Fr.).

Preparations

Injection: Solution, 50, 75, and 100 mg/ml.
Oral: Elixir, 50 mg/5 ml; tablets, 50 and 10 mg.

Usual Dosages

Intramuscular, Intravenous (Slow), Oral, Subcutaneous: Adults, 50 to 150 mg every 3 to 4 hours as necessary. Children, 1 to 1.5 mg/kg (maximum dose, 100 mg) administered orally, subcutaneously, or intramuscularly. The dose may be repeated at intervals of 3 to 4 hours if necessary.

MERCAPTAMINE

Proprietary Names: Cysteamine (G.B.), Lambratene (Ital.).

Preparations

Injection, Oral: Powder.
Topical Ophthalmic: No ophthalmic preparation is commercially available.

Usual Dosages

Oral: A 5 per cent solution may be given in an initial daily dose of 30 mg/kg, divided into four equal parts. This may be increased to 60 mg/kg after 4 weeks, to 90 mg/kg after a further 4 weeks, and then maintained at this dose.
Topical Ophthalmic: A solution containing 0.1 per cent mercaptamine may be prepared with the powder for injection.

METHACHOLINE

Proprietary Name: Methacholine.

Preparations

Injection: Ampule, 1 and 10 gm.

Usual Dosages

Subcutaneous: 10 to 25 mg.

METHAZOLAMIDE

Proprietary Name: Neptazane.

Preparations

Oral: Tablets, 50 mg.

Usual Dosages

Oral: The usual adult dosage is 50 to 100 mg two or three times daily.

METHICILLIN

Proprietary Names: Azapen, Belfacillin (Swed.), Celbenin, Cinopenil (Germ.), Flabelline (Fr.), Lucopenin (Denm.), Metin (Austral.), Penistaph (Fr.), Staphcillin, Synticillin (Denm.).

Preparations

Injection: Powder (buffered), 1, 4, and 6 gm (900 mg methicillin base/gm).

Usual Dosages

Intracameral: 1 mg in 0.2 to 0.5 ml of isotonic sodium chloride injection.
Intramuscular: Adults, 1 gm every 6 hours. Infants and children, 25 mg/kg every 6 hours.
Intravenous: Adults, 1 gm every 6 hours. Higher doses may be required in the treatment of severe infections, and intramuscular doses of up to 8 gm a day and intravenous doses of 8 to 24 gm a day have been used.
Subconjunctival: 50 to 150 mg in 0.5 ml of isotonic sodium chloride injection or sterile water for injection.

METHIMAZOLE

Proprietary Name: Tapazole.

Preparations

Oral: Tablets, 5 and 10 mg.

Usual Dosages

Oral: Adults, 15 to 60 mg daily for initial treatment of hyperthyroidism and 5 to 15 mg daily for maintenance.

METHOCARBAMOL

Proprietary Names: Delaxin, Lumirelax (Fr.), Metho-500, Methocabal (Jap.), Parabaxin, Robaxin, Romethocarb, SK-Methocarbamal, Tresortil (Denm.).

Preparations

Injection: Solution, 100 mg/ml.
Oral: Tablets, 500 and 750 mg.

Usual Dosages

Intravenous: Adults, 1 to 3 gm daily at a rate not exceeding 3 ml/min.
Oral: Adults, initially, 1.5 to 2 gm four times daily for 48 to 72 hours; for maintenance, 1 gm four times daily.

---

* Route of administration not approved by FDA.
† Drug not approved by FDA for any indication.
‡ Drug not approved by FDA for this particular indication.
§ Indicated dosage above the manufacturer's recommendation.

METHOTREXATE

Proprietary Names: Ledertrexate (Fr.), Mexate.

Preparations

Injection: Solution, 2.5, 20, 25, 50, 100, and 250 mg/ml.
Oral: Tablets, 2.5 mg.

Usual Dosages

Intramuscular: In the management of rheumatoid arthritis, parenteral dosage regimen often consists of 7.5 to 15 mg given intramuscularly once weekly.
Oral: For psoriasis chemotherapy, divided dose schedule recommends 2.5 mg at 12-hour intervals for 3 doses or at 8-hour intervals for 4 doses each week. When remission is achieved and supportive care in antineoplastic chemotherapy has produced general clinical improvement, maintenance therapy of 30 mg/square meter is administered 2 times weekly either by mouth or intramuscularly. In the management of rheumatoid arthritis, oral dosage regimen often consists of 2.5 mg administered at 12-hour intervals for three doses each week.

METHOXSALEN

Proprietary Names: Oxsoralen, Oxsoralen Ultra, Soloxsalen (Canad.).

Preparations

Oral: Capsules, 10 mg.
Topical: Lotion, 1 per cent.

Usual Dosages

Oral: 20 to 70 mg followed by UV irradiation.
Topical: Application followed by UV irradiation.

METHYLCELLULOSE

Proprietary Names: BFL (Canad.), Cellulone (Austral.), Cologel, Hydrolose, Isopto-Plain, Lacril (Canad.), Methocel A, Methulose, Tearisol, Viscosae (Denm.), Visulose.

Preparations

Topical Ophthalmic: Solution, 0.25, 0.5, and 1 per cent.

Usual Dosages

Topical Ophthalmic: One drop as needed.

METHYLENE BLUE (METHYLTHIONINE)

Proprietary Names: Desmoidpillen (Germ.), M-B Tabs, Urolene Blue, Wright's Stain.

Preparations

Injection: Solution, 1 to 5 per cent.

Usual Dosages

Injection: In the form of a 2 per cent sterile solution, it is used to outline various body cavities.

METHYLPREDNISOLONE

Proprietary Names: A-Methapred, Depo-Medrate (Germ.), Depo-Medrol, Depo-Medrone (G.B.), Depo-Pred, Dura-Meth, Medralone, Medrate (Germ.), Medrol, Medules, Mepred, Rep-Pred, Solu-Medrol, Solu-Medrone (G.B.), Urbason (Germ., Swed.).

Preparations

Injection: Aqueous suspension, 20, 40 and 80 mg/ml; powder, 40, 125, 500 mg, and 1 gm. The aqueous suspension for injection may be used for subconjunctival injection.
Oral: Capsules, 2 and 4 mg; tablets, 2, 4, 8, 16, 24, and 32 mg.

Usual Dosages

Intravenous: Initially, 10 to 40 mg. For high dose therapy, 30 mg/kg infused over 10 to 20 minutes.
Oral: The initial dosage may vary from 4 to 48 mg daily depending on the specific disease entity being treated. It should be emphasized that dosage requirements are variable and must be individualized on the basis of the disease under treatment and the response of the patient.
Subconjunctival: 0.5 ml of a suspension containing 20, 40, or 80 mg/ml. This dose may be repeated every 3 to 5 weeks.

METHYLTESTOSTERONE

Proprietary Names: Android, Glosso-Sterandryl (Fr.), Mesteron (Pol.), Metandren, Neohombreol M, Oreton Methyl, Testin (Norw.), Testomet (Austral.), Testred, Virilon.

Preparations

Oral: Tablets, 5 and 10 mg.

Usual Dosages

Buccal: 10 mg sublingually may reduce the frequency and severity of angioedema attacks.

METHYLTHIONINE
See Methylene Blue.

METHYSERGIDE

Proprietary Names: Deseril (G.B.), Desernil (Fr.), Sansert.

Preparations

Oral: Tablets, 2 mg.

Usual Dosages

Oral: Adults, 2 to 8 mg daily in divided doses.

---

* Route of administration not approved by FDA.
† Drug not approved by FDA for any indication.
‡ Drug not approved by FDA for this particular indication.
§ Indicated dosage above the manufacturer's recommendation.

METRONIDAZOLE

Proprietary Names: Clont (Germ.), Debetrol (Arg.), Deflamon (Ital.), Elyzol (Scand.), Entizol (Pol.), Flagyl, Fossyol (Germ.), Gineflavir (Ital.), Kreucosan (Germ.), Meronidal (Jap.), Metrolag (Switz.), Nalox (Arg.), Neo-Tric (Canad.), Nida (Jap.), Novonidazol (Canad.), Rathimed N (Germ.), Salandol (Jap.), Sanatrichom (Germ.), Tranoxa (Arg.), Trichocide (Jap.), Tricho-Gynaedron (Germ.), Trichos Cordes (Germ.), Trichomal (Denm.), Trichozole (Austral.), Tricocet (Ital.), Tricofin (Arg.), Tricowas (Span.), Trikacide (Canad.), Trivazol (Ital.), Vagilen (Ital.), Vaginyl (G.B.).

Preparations

Oral: Tablets, 200 and 250 mg.

Usual Dosages

Oral: Adults, 250 mg three times daily for 7 days; course may be repeated if needed after interval of 4 to 6 weeks.

MEVINOLIN
See Lovastatin.

MICONAZOLE

Proprietary Names: Albistat (Belg., Neth.), Andergin (Ital.), Daktar (Germ., Norw., Swed.), Daktarin (G.B.), Deralbine (Arg.), Dermonistat (G.B.), Epi-Monistat (Germ.), Fungisidin (Span.), Micatin, Micotef (Ital.).

Preparations

Injection: Solution, 10 mg/ml in 20-ml ampules.
Oral: Available from Centers for Disease Control.
Topical: Cream, 2 per cent.
Topical Ophthalmic: No ophthalmic preparation is commercially available. A 1 per cent solution in arachnis oil may be prepared by dissolving in chloroform, mixing with arachnis oil, and driving off chloroform by heat. A 2 per cent ointment form may also be prepared. A 1 per cent solution may also be obtained by using the intravenous preparation containing 10 mg/ml.

Usual Dosages

Intravenous: A daily dosage of 25 to 30 mg/kg in two or three equally divided doses at 8- or 12-hour intervals.
Intravitreal: 40 μg in 0.1 to 0.2 ml of sterile aqueous solution.
Subconjunctival: 5 to 10 mg in a 0.5 ml aqueous solution.
Topical: A sufficient amount of cream to cover the affected area is applied twice daily.
Topical Ophthalmic: Preparation is applied to affected and surrounding areas twice a day. Ophthalmic form is applied up to 8 to 12 weeks.

MINOCYCLINE

Proprietary Names: Klinomycin (Germ.), Minocin, Minomycin (Austral., S. Afr.), Mynocine (Fr.), Ultramycin (Canad.), Vectrin.

Preparations

Injection: Powder, 100 mg (of base).
Oral: Capsules, 50 and 100 mg (of base); syrup, 50 mg (of base)/5 ml.

Usual Dosages

Intravenous: Adults, 200 mg followed by 100 mg every 12 hours (maximum, 400 mg daily). Children 8 to 12 years of age, 4 mg/kg initially followed by 2 mg/kg every 12 hours.
Oral: Adults and children over 12 years of age, 200 mg initially, followed by 100 mg every 12 hours. Children 8 to 12 years of age, 4 mg/kg daily in divided doses every 12 hours.

MITHRAMYCIN
See Plicamycin.

MONOBENZONE

Proprietary Names: Aloquin (Austral.), Benoquin, Depigman (Germ., Neth., Switz.), Dermochinona (Ital.), Leucodinine (Belg.).

Preparations

Topical: Cream, 20 per cent; ointment, 20 per cent.

Usual Dosages

Topical: Preparation is applied to the affected area two or three times daily.

MOXISYLYTE

Proprietary Names: THY (G.B.), Thymoxamine (G.B.).

Preparations

Topical Ophthalmic: Solution, 0.1, 0.2, and 0.5 per cent.

Usual Dosages

Topical Ophthalmic: The frequency and concentration of instillation depend upon the patient's response to therapy.

MUMPS VIRUS VACCINE LIVE

Proprietary Name: Mumpsvax.

Preparations

Injection: 5000 TCID$_{50}$/0.5 ml.

---

* Route of administration not approved by FDA.
† Drug not approved by FDA for any indication.
‡ Drug not approved by FDA for this particular indication.
§ Indicated dosage above the manufacturer's recommendation.

Usual Dosages

Subcutaneous: The usual dosage is 0.5 ml administered as a single dose.

MUPIROCIN

Proprietary Name: Bactroban.

Preparations

Topical: Ointment, 2 per cent.

Usual Dosages

Topical: A small amount of ointment is applied to the affected area three times daily.

NAFCILLIN

Proprietary Names: Nafcil, Unipen.

Preparations

Injection: Powder, 0.5, 1, and 2 gm.
Oral: Capsules, 250 mg; powder for solution, 250 mg/5 ml; tablets, 500 mg.

Usual Dosages

Intramuscular: Adults, 500 mg every 4 to 6 hours; children, 25 mg/kg twice daily; newborn infants, 10 mg/kg twice daily.
Intravenous: Adults, 0.5 to 1.0 gm in 15 to 30 ml of water for injection or sodium chloride injection infused over a 10-minute period for 4 hours or dissolved in 150 ml of sodium chloride injection and given by slow intravenous drip. Up to 8 gm daily can be given for serious infections. Older infants and children, 50 mg/kg daily in six divided doses.
Oral: Adults, 0.25 to 1.0 gm every 4 to 6 hours, preferably 2 hours before meals. Children, 25 to 50 mg/kg daily in four divided doses. Newborn infants, 10 mg/kg twice daily.

NALOXONE

Proprietary Name: Narcan.

Preparations

Injection: Solution, 0.02, 0.4, and 1.0 mg/ml.

Usual Dosages

Intramuscular, Intravenous, Subcutaneous: For narcotic overdose in adults, the initial dose is 0.4 to 2.0 mg intravenously, which may be repeated at 2- to 3-minute intervals up to 10 mg. For pruritus, and intravenous infusion of 2.0 to 6.4 mg may be administered over a 4-hour period.

NAPHAZOLINE

Proprietary Names: Ak-Con, Albalon, Allerest, Clear Eyes, Degest, Naphcon, Opticon, Vasoclear.

Preparations

Topical Ophthalmic: Solution, 0.012 and 0.1 per cent.

Usual Dosages

Topical Ophthalmic: One drop is instilled every 2 to 3 hours or as needed until symptoms subside.

NAPROXEN

Proprietary Names: Anaprox, Naprosyn, Naxen (Mex.), Proxen (Aust., Germ., Switz.).

Preparations

Oral: Tablets, 250 mg.

Usual Dosages

Oral: Adults, 500 to 750 mg daily in divided doses.

NATAMYCIN

Proprietary Names: Myprozine, Natacyn.

Preparations

Topical Ophthalmic: Suspension, 5 per cent.

Usual Dosages

Topical Ophthalmic: One drop of a 5 per cent suspension every 1 to 2 hours. The effect may be enhanced by concomitant treatment with 1 per cent potassium iodide solution, also applied topically.

NEOARSPHENAMINE

Proprietary Name: Collunovar (Fr.).

Preparations

Injection: Powder.

Usual Dosages

Intravenous: Usual dosage is 150 to 600 mg.

NEOMYCIN

Proprietary Names: Bykomycin (Germ.), Emelmycin (S. Afr.), Herisan Antibiotic (Canad.), Myacyne (Germ.), Mycifradin, Myciguent, Neobiotic, Neobram (Austral.), Neocin (Canad.), Neomate (Austral.), Neomin (G.B.), Neo Morrhuol (Austral.), Neopan (S. Afr.), Neopt (Austral.), Nivemycin (G.B.).

---

* Route of administration not approved by FDA.
† Drug not approved by FDA for any indication.
‡ Drug not approved by FDA for this particular indication.
§ Indicated dosage above the manufacturer's recommendation.

Preparations

Injection: Powder, 500 mg.
Oral: Solution, 125 mg/5 ml; tablets, 500 mg.
Topical: Cream, 5 mg/gm; ointment, 5 mg/gm.
Topical Ophthalmic: Ointment, 3.5 and 5.0 mg/ml.

Usual Dosages

Oral: For diarrhea caused by enteropathogenic *E. coli*, adults, 50 mg/kg daily in four divided doses; newborn and premature infants, 10 to 50 mg/kg daily in four divided doses; older infants and children, 50 to 100 mg/kg daily in four divided doses.
Topical: Preparation may be applied two to three times daily.
Topical Ophthalmic: Ointment is applied one to three times daily.

NEOMYCIN/HYDROCORTISONE COMBINATION

Proprietary Names: AK-Neo-Cort, Neo-Cortef.

Preparations

Topical Ophthalmic: Ointment, 0.5 per cent neomycin and 1.5 per cent hydrocortisone; solution, 0.5 per cent neomycin and 1.5 per cent hydrocortisone.

Usual Dosages

Topical Ophthalmic: Preparation is applied two to three times daily.

NEOMYCIN/POLYMYXIN B COMBINATION

Proprietary Names: Polyspectin Liquifilm, Statrol.

Preparations

Topical Ophthalmic: Ointment, 5 mg neomycin and 6000 units/gm polymyxin B; solution, 5 mg neomycin and 5000 units/ml polymyxin B.

Usual Dosages

Topical Ophthalmic: One drop of solution in lower conjunctival sac(s) several times daily as required. A 0.5-inch ribbon of ointment is instilled in conjunctival sac(s) at night when used adjunctively with the solution.

NEOMYCIN/POLYMYXIN B/BACITRACIN COMBINATION

Proprietary Names: Mycitracin, Neo-Polycin, Neosporin, Polyspectrin S.O.P., Pyocidin.

Preparations

Topical Ophthalmic: Ointment, 5000 units/gm polymyxin B, 400 units/gm bacitracin, and 5 mg/gm neomycin.

Usual Dosages

Topical Ophthalmic: A small amount of ointment may be applied to conjunctival sac several times daily or as required until favorable response is observed.

The number of daily applications may then be reduced until the disorder is under control.

NEOMYCIN/POLYMYXIN B/GRAMICIDIN COMBINATION

Proprietary Name: Neosporin.

Preparations

Topical Ophthalmic: Solution, 1.75 mg neomycin, 10,000 units polymyxin B, and 0.025 mg gramicidin/ml.

Usual Dosages

Topical Ophthalmic: One or two drops of solution in the affected eye(s) are instilled two to four times daily, or more frequently as required, for 7 to 10 days. In acute infections, drops may be applied every 15 to 30 minutes.

NEOSTIGMINE

Proprietary Name: Prostigmin.

Preparations

Injection: Solution, 0.25, 0.50, and 1 mg/ml.
Topical Ophthalmic: Solution, 5 per cent.

Usual Dosages

Intramuscular: Adults, 15 mg/kg daily in divided doses every 6 hours. The total daily dose should not exceed 1 gm.
Subcutaneous: 0.5 to 2 mg.
Topical Ophthalmic: A dosage of one to two drops may be applied two to six times daily.

NIACIN (NICOTINIC ACID)

Proprietary Names: Acidemel (S. Afr.), Diacin, Efacin, Niac, Nicangin (Swed.), Nico-400, Nicobid, Nicocap, Nicolar, Niconacid (Germ.), Ni Cord, Nico-Span, Nicotinex, Nicyl (Fr.), Ni-Span, SK-Niacin, Span Niacin, Vasotherm, Wampocap.

Preparations

Oral: Tablets, 500 mg.

Usual Dosages

Oral: Adults, initially, 100 mg three times daily, increased to 1.5 to 6 gm divided into three doses given with or after meals.

NIFEDIPINE

Proprietary Names: Adalat, Adalate (Fr.), Nifelate (Arg.), Procardia.

---

* Route of administration not approved by FDA.
† Drug not approved by FDA for any indication.
‡ Drug not approved by FDA for this particular indication.
§ Indicated dosage above the manufacturer's recommendation.

Preparations

Oral: Capsules, 10 and 20 mg.

Usual Dosages

Oral: The usual dosage range is 10 to 20 mg three times daily. The maximum daily dose is 180 mg.

NIRIDAZOLE

Proprietary Name: Ambilhar.

Preparations

Oral: Tablets, 500 mg.

Usual Dosages

Oral: Adults and children, 25 mg/kg daily in two divided doses for 5 to 7 days in schistosomiasis and 7 to 10 days in dracunculiasis.

NITROGEN MUSTARD
See Mechlorethamine.

NITROGLYCERIN

Proprietary Names: Anginine (Austral.), Angised (S. Afr.), Ang-O-Span, Cardabid, Corobid, Gilucor Nitro (Germ.), Glyceryl Trinitrate (G.B.), Glynite (Canad.), Gly-Trate, Klavi Kordal, Lenitral (Fr.), Niglycon, Niong, Nitora, Nitrangin (Germ.), Nitrine, Nitro-Bid, Nitrocap, Nitrocels, Nitrocontin (G.B.), Nitro-Dial, Nitrodyl, Nitroglyn, Nitrol, Nitrolar, Nitrolex TD, Nitrolingual (Germ.), Nitro-Lyn, Nitro Mack Retard (Germ.), Nitronet, Nitrong, Nitroprn, Nitrorectal (Germ.), Nitroretard (Swed.), Nitro-SA, Nitrospan, Nitrostabilin (Canad.), Nitrostat, Nitro-TD, Nitrotym, Nitrozell Retard (Germ.), Sustac (G.B.), Trates, Triagin (Austral.), Vasitrin (Austral.), Vasoglyn.

Preparations

Oral: Capsules (extended-release), 2.5, 6.5, and 9 mg; tablets (extended-release), 1.3, 2.6, and 6.5 mg.
Sublingual: Tablets, 0.15, 0.3, 0.4, and 0.6 mg.

Usual Dosages

Oral: 1.3 to 9 mg of extended-release formulation may be administered every 8 to 12 hours.
Sublingual: 0.15 to 0.6 mg repeated in 5 minutes if necessary, but no more than 1.8 mg should be used within a 15-minute period.

NYSTATIN

Proprietary Names: Candex, Candio-Hermal (Germ.), Canstat (S. Afr.), Diastatin (Austral.), Fungalex (S. Afr.), Fungistatin (S. Afr.), Korostatin, Moronal (Germ.), Mycostatin, Mycostatine (Fr.), Nilstat, Nystan (G.B.), Nystavescent (G.B.), O-V Statin.

Preparations

Injection: Powder, 100,000 units/gm.
Topical: Cream, 100,000 units/gm; ointment, 100,000 units/gm.

Topical Ophthalmic: No ophthalmic form is available, but preparations for parenteral administration or dermatologic use may be applied. Powder should be reconstituted with isotonic sodium chloride injection to make suspension containing 25,000 units/ml for topical ophthalmic use or 10,000 units/ml for subconjunctival injection.

Usual Dosages

Subconjunctival: 5000 units in 0.5 ml of isotonic sodium chloride injection.
Topical Ophthalmic: One drop of a suspension containing 25,000 units/ml may be applied every 15 minutes or powder may be dusted onto the lesion. Alternatively, an ointment preparation containing 100,000 units/gm may be applied four times daily.

OSMOTIC AGENTS
See Glycerin, Isosorbide, Mannitol, Urea.

OXACILLIN

Proprietary Names: Bactocill, Bristopen (G.B., Fr.), Cryptocillin (Germ.), Prostaphlin, Staphenor (Germ.).

Preparations

Injection: Powder, 0.25, 0.5, 1, 2, and 4 gm.

Usual Dosages

Intramuscular: Adults and children weighing more than 40 kg, 0.25 to 1.0 gm every 4 to 6 hours (up to 8 gm daily may be given for severe infections). Children weighing less than 40 kg, 50 to 100 mg/kg daily (or more in severe infections) in equal doses every 4 to 6 hours. Newborns and premature infants, 25 mg/kg daily.
Intravenous: When administered by direct infusion, the dose should be well diluted and given over a period of approximately 10 to 15 minutes. Doses should be comparable to those administered intramuscularly; for severe infections, 1 gm or more may be given intravenously every 3 to 4 hours.

OXAMNIQUINE

Proprietary Names: Mansil (Braz.), Vansil (S. Afr.).

Preparations

Oral: Powder.

Usual Dosages

Oral: Adults, 15 mg/kg as a single dose; children, 20 mg/kg in two equally divided doses 2 to 8 hours apart.

---

* Route of administration not approved by FDA.
† Drug not approved by FDA for any indication.
‡ Drug not approved by FDA for this particular indication.
§ Indicated dosage above the manufacturer's recommendation.

OXIDIZED CELLULOSE

Proprietary Names: Hemo-Pak, Oxycel, Surgicel.

Preparations

Topical: Pads, 3″ × 3″; pledgets, 2″ × 1″ × 1″; strips, 5″ or 36″ × 0.5″, 0.5″, 3″, 14″, or 18″ × 2″, and 4″ × 8″.

Usual Dosages

Topical: Minimal amounts of an appropriate size are laid on the bleeding site.

OXYMETHOLONE

Proprietary Names: Adroyd, Anadrol-50, Anadroyd (Belg.), Anapolon (G.B.), Anasteron (Denm., Norw., Swed.), Anasteronal (Span.), Nastenon (Fr.), Oxitosona-50 (Span.), Pardroyd (Germ.), Plenastril (Germ., Switz.), Synasteron (Belg.), Zenalosyn (Neth.).

Preparations

Oral: Tablets, 5, 10, and 50 mg.

Usual Dosages

Oral: The usual adult dose is 5 to 10 mg daily.

OXYPHENBUTAZONE

Proprietary Names: Butapirone (Ital.), Iridil (Ital.), Oxalid, Phlogase (Germ.), Rheumapax (Swed.), Tandacote (G.B.), Tandearil, Tanderil (G.B.).

Preparations

Oral: Tablets, 100 mg.
Topical Ophthalmic: No ophthalmic preparation is available commercially. A 5 per cent solution or 10 per cent ointment may be prepared by the pharmacist.

Usual Dosages

Oral: Range, 100 to 600 mg.
Topical Ophthalmic: Preparation is applied three to four times daily.

OXYTETRACYCLINE

Proprietary Names: Abbocin (G.B.), Berkmycen (G.B.), Biotet (S. Afr.), Bobbamycin (Austral.), Chemocycline (G.B.), Clinimycin (G.B.), Dalimycin, Galenomycin (G.B.), Imperacin (G.B.), Lenocycline (S. Afr.), Macocyn (Germ.), 0-4-cycline (S. Afr.), Oppamycin (G.B.), Otetryn, Oxamycen (Jap.), Oxlopar, Oxycycline (Austral.), Oxydon (G.B.), Oxy-Dumocyclin (Swed.), Oxyject, Oxy-Kesso-Tetra, Oxymycin (G.B.), Oxytetral (Swed.), Roxy (S. Afr.), Stecsolin (G.B.), Terramycin, Terravenös (Germ.), Tetlong (S. Afr.), Tetramel (S. Afr.), Tetramine, Tetra-Tablinen (Germ.), Unimycin (G.B.), Uri-Tet, Vendarcin (Austral., Germ., Neth., S. Afr.).

Preparations

Oral: Tablets, 250 mg.
Topical Ophthalmic: Ointment, 0.5 per cent.

Usual Dosages

Oral: Adults, 1 gm daily in divided doses; a total of 2 to 4 gm may be given to severely ill patients. Children, 25 to 50 mg/kg daily in four divided doses.

Topical Ophthalmic: Ointment preparation may be applied two to three times daily.

PAPAVERINE

Proprietary Names: Artegodan (Germ.), Cerebid, Cerespan, Dilaspan, Dipav, Dylate, Kavrin, Myobid, P-200, Pameion (Ital.), Panergon (Germ., Switz.), Papaverlumin Fuerte (Span.), Pavabid, Pava-2 Caps, Pavacap, Pavacen, Pavakey, Pavased, Pavatran, Pava-Wol, Paverine, Paveron (Germ.), Pavine TD, Qua-Bid, Sustaverine, Therapav, Vasal, Vasocap, Vaso-Pav, Vasospan.

Preparations

Oral: Capsules (timed-release), 150 mg; tablets, 30, 60, 100, and 200 mg.

Usual Dosages

Oral: The usual dosage range for adults is 60 to 300 mg one to five times daily. Timed-release capsules may be given every 8 to 12 hours.

PARA-AMINOBENZOIC ACID

Proprietary Names: PABA, pabaGel, Pabanol, Pre Sun, Sunbrella.

Preparations

Topical: Jelly, 5 per cent; solution, 5 per cent; suspension, 5 per cent.

Usual Dosages

Topical: Preparation should be applied uniformly and generously to all exposed skin surfaces before exposure to UVB light.

PAROMOMYCIN

Proprietary Names: Aminoxidin (Ital.), Gabbromicina (Arg.), Gabbromycin (Germ.), Gabbroral (Arg., Belg., Ital.), Gabromicina (Span.), Gaboral (Span.), Humagel (Fr.), Humatin, Paramicina (Ital.), Sinosid (Ital.).

Preparations

Oral: Capsules, 250 mg.
Topical Ophthalmic: No ophthalmic preparation is commercially available.

Usual Dosages

Oral: For intestinal amebiasis, 25 to 35 mg/kg daily in three divided doses for 5 to 10 days.

---

* Route of administration not approved by FDA.
† Drug not approved by FDA for any indication.
‡ Drug not approved by FDA for this particular indication.
§ Indicated dosage above the manufacturer's recommendation.

Topical Ophthalmic: A 0.1 per cent solution may be applied to affected eye(s) twice daily.

PENICILLAMINE

Proprietary Names: Cuprenil (Pol.), Cuprimine, Depamine (G.B.), Depen, Distamine (G.B.), D-Penamine (Austral.), Metalcaptase (Germ.), Trolovol (Germ.).

Preparations

Oral: Capsules, 250 mg.

Usual Dosages

Oral: Adults, for cystinuria, 2 gm daily, with a range of 1 to 4 gm daily in divided doses. For rheumatoid arthritis, 125 to 250 mg initially as a single daily dose; the amount may be increased by increments of 250 mg/day at 2- to 3-month intervals with the average daily maintenance dose at 500 to 750 mg. The maximum daily dosage is usually 1 gm, but up to 1.5 gm may be required in some patients.

PENICILLIN G
See Benzathine Penicillin G, Potassium Penicillin G, Procaine Penicillin G, Sodium Penicillin G.

PENICILLIN V

Proprietary Names: Acipen-V (Neth.), Biotic, Fenospen (Ital.), Oracilline (Belg., Fr.), Penbec-V (Canad.), Pengrocill (Switz.), Penoral (S. Afr.), Tripapenicillina (Ital.), V-Cillin, Veekay (S. Afr.), V-Pen, Widocillin (Switz.).

Preparations

Oral: Capsules, 250 mg; suspension, 125 to 250 mg/5 ml; tablets, 125, 250, and 500 mg.

Usual Dosages

Oral: Adults, for mild to moderate infections, 125 to 250 mg three times daily; for severe infections, 500 mg three times daily or 250 mg every 4 hours. Children, for mild to moderate infections, 125 to 250 mg three times daily; for severe infections, 250 mg four times daily. Infants, 12.5 to 50 mg/kg daily in three to six divided doses.

PENTAMIDINE

Proprietary Names: Lomidine (Fr., Germ.), Pentam.

Preparations

Injection: Powder, 200 and 300 mg/vial.
Topical Ophthalmic: No ophthalmic preparation is commercially available. A 1 per cent solution may be prepared with 10 mg pentamidine powder mixed with 1 ml artificial tears.

Usual Dosages

Intramuscular, Intravenous: The usual dosage is 300 mg daily or on alternate days until 12 to 15 doses are given; a second course can be administered 1 or 2 weeks later.

Topical Ophthalmic: One or two drops of 1 per cent solution may be instilled in the affected eye(s) one to four times daily.

PENTAZOCINE

Proprietary Names: Fortal (Belg., Fr.), Fortalgesic (Swed., Switz.), Fortral (G.B.), Fortralin (Scand.), Talwin.

Preparations

Injection: Solution, 30 mg/ml.
Oral: Tablets, 50 mg.

Usual Dosages

Intramuscular, Intravenous, Subcutaneous: Adults, 30 mg every 3 to 4 hours as necessary; single doses in excess of 30 mg intravenously or 60 mg intramuscularly or subcutaneously are not advisable. The total daily dose should not exceed 360 mg. Children under 12 years of age, dosage is not established.

Oral: Adults, 50 mg every 3 or 4 hours as necessary. This may be increased to 100 mg if necessary. The daily dose should not exceed 600 mg. Children under 12 years of age, dosage is not established.

PERMETHRIN

Proprietary Name: Nix.

Preparations

Topical: Liquid, 1 per cent.

Usual Dosages

Topical: A sufficient volume to saturate the hair and scalp should be applied and allowed to remain on the hair for 10 minutes before rinsing off with water.

PETHIDINE
See Meperidine.

PETROLATUM (WHITE PETROLATUM)

Proprietary Names: Duolube, Duratears, Lacri-Lube, Moroline, Refresh PM.

Preparations

Topical: Ointment.
Topical Ophthalmic: Ointment.

Usual Dosages

Topical: Small amount of ointment may be applied as needed.

---

* Route of administration not approved by FDA.
† Drug not approved by FDA for any indication.
‡ Drug not approved by FDA for this particular indication.
§ Indicated dosage above the manufacturer's recommendation.

Topical Ophthalmic: Small amount of ointment may be applied as needed.

PHENOXYMETHYLPENICILLIN POTASSIUM
See Potassium Penicillin V.

PHENYLBUTAZONE

Proprietary Names: Algoverine (Canad.), Artrizin (Denm.), Artropan (Ital.), Azolid, Butacal (Austral.), Butacote (G.B.), Butagesic (Canad.), Butalan (Austral.), Butalgin (Austral.), Butaphen (Austral.), Butapirazol (Pol.), Butarex (Austral.), Butazolidin, Butazone (G.B.), Butina (S. Afr.), Butoroid (Austral.), Butoz (Austral.), Butozone (S. Afr.), Butrex (S. Afr.), Buzon (Austral.), Chembutazone (Canad.), Diossidone (Ital.), Ecobutazone (Canad.), Elmedal (Germ.), Eributazone (Canad.), Ethibute (G.B.), Flexazone (G.B.), Intrabutazone (Canad.), Kadol (Ital.), Malgesic (Canad.), Merizone (Canad.), Nadozone (Canad.), Neo-Zoline (Canad.), Novophenyl (Canad.), Oppazone (G.B.), Panazone (S. Afr.), Phenbutazol (Canad.), Phenybute (Austral.), Phenylbetazone (Canad.), Praecirheumin (Germ.), Tazone (Canad.), Tetnor (G.B.), Ticinil (Ital.), Wescozone (Canad.).

Preparations

Oral: Tablets, 100 mg.

Usual Dosages

Oral: Initially, 300 to 600 mg daily in divided doses. A 1-week trial period is considered adequate to determine response. If symptoms can be controlled with a maintenance dose of 100 to 200 mg daily, the drug may be given for longer periods under careful supervision.

PHENYLEPHRINE

Proprietary Names: Ak-Dilate, Ak-Nefrin, Alcon-Efrin, Degest (Austral., Canad.), Dilatair, Efricel, I-Care (Austral.), Isopto Frin, Isopto Phenylephrine (Austral.), Mistura D, Mydfrin, Neo-Synephrine, Ocu-Phrin, Ocugestrin, Prefrin, Tear-Efrin.

Preparations

Topical Ophthalmic: Solution, 0.12, 0.125, 0.2, 2.5, and 10 per cent.

Usual Dosages

Topical Ophthalmic: Solution may be applied one to three times daily.

PHENYTOIN

Proprietary Names: Dantoin (Canad.), Difhydan (Swed.), Dihycon, Di-Hydan (Fr.), Dilabid, Dilantin, Di-Phen, Diphentyn (Canad.), Diphenyl, Diphenylan, Ditoin (Austral.), Divulsan (Canad.), Ekko, Epanutin (G.B.), Fenantoin (Swed.), Kessodanten, Novodiphenyl (Canad.), Phenhydan (Germ.), Phentoin (Austral.), Pyoredol (Fr.), Solantyl (Fr.), Toin, Zentropil (Germ.).

Preparations

Injection: Powder for solution containing approximately 50 mg/ml when diluted with special solvent provided.
Oral: Capsules, 30 to 100 mg; suspension, 30 mg/5 ml (pediatric) and 125 mg/5 ml; tablets (pediatric), 50 mg.

Usual Dosages

Intramuscular, Intravenous: Adults, 150 to 250 mg followed if necessary by 100 to 150 mg 30 minutes later. The rate of administration should not exceed 50 mg/minute. Higher doses may be required to control seizures.
Oral: Dosage must be individualized. Adults, initially, 300 mg daily. The maintenance dose is usually 100 mg three to four times daily.

PHOSPHATE SALTS

Proprietary Names: K-Phos, Neutra-Phos.

Preparations

Oral: Capsules, 250 mg phosphorus, 7.125 or 14.25 mEq potassium, and 0 or 7.125 mEq sodium; solution, 250 mg phosphorus, 7.125 or 14.25 mEq potassium, and 0 or 7.125 mEq sodium/75 ml; tablets, 114, 126, or 250 mg phosphorus, 45, 90, or 144 mg potassium, and 0, 67, 134, or 298 mg sodium.

Usual Dosages

Oral: Adults, 2 to 4 gm of phosphorus daily in divided doses.

PHYSOSTIGMINE

Proprietary Name: Isopto Eserine.

Preparations

Topical Ophthalmic: Ointment, 0.25 per cent; solution, 0.1, 0.25, and 0.5 per cent.

Usual Dosages

Topical Ophthalmic: In primary open-angle and other chronic glaucomas, one drop of 0.25 or 0.5 per cent solution in each eye every 4 to 6 hours; ointment is used at night.

PHYTONADIONE (VITAMIN K$_1$)

Proprietary Names: AquaMEPHYTON, Konakion, MEPHYTON.

Preparations

Injection: Solution, 2 and 10 mg/ml.
Oral: Tablets, 5 mg.

---

* Route of administration not approved by FDA.
† Drug not approved by FDA for any indication.
‡ Drug not approved by FDA for this particular indication.
§ Indicated dosage above the manufacturer's recommendation.

Usual Dosages

Intramuscular, Intravenous, Oral, Subcutaneous: In the treatment of hypoprothrombinemia resulting from malabsorption syndromes, 2 to 25 mg may be administered to adults initially and repeated if necessary, depending on the severity of the deficiency and the response to the drug.

PILOCARPINE

Proprietary Names: Adsorbocarpine, Akarpine, Almocarpine, Isopto Carpine, Isopto-Pilocarpine (Fr.), Licarpin (Swed.), Marticarpine (Fr.), Mio-Carpine-SMP (S. Afr.), Mistura P, Nova-Carpine (Canad.), Ocu-Carpine, Ocusert, Pilocar, Pilocarpina Lux (Ital.), Pilocel, Pilokair, Pilomiotin, Pilopine, Pilopt (Austral.), Piloptic, PV Carpine, Spersacarpine (S. Afr., Swed.).

Preparations

Topical Ophthalmic: Gel, 4 per cent; ocusert, 20 to 40 µg of pilocarpine released each hour for 1 week; solution, 0.25, 0.5, 1.0, 2.0, 3.0, 4.0, 5.0, 6.0, 8.0, and 10 per cent.

Usual Dosages

Topical Ophthalmic: The frequency and concentration of instillation depend upon the patient's response to therapy.

PIPERACILLIN

Proprietary Names: Pentcillin (Jap.), Pipracil, Pipril (G.B., Germ.).

Preparations

Injection: Powder, 2, 3, 4, and 40 gm.

Usual Dosages

Intramuscular, Intravenous: For serious infections, the usual dosage is 3 to 4 gm administered every 4 to 6 hours as a 20- to 30-minute infusion. The maximum dose is 24 gm, although higher doses have been used. Intramuscular injections should be limited to 2 gm/site.

PIPERAZINE

Proprietary Names: Adipalit (Ital.), Ancazine (Canad.), Antelmina (Fr.), Antepar, Antivermine (Pol.), Ascalix (G.B.), Bryrel, Citrazine (Austral.), Dietelmin (Fr.), Divermex (Austral.), Entacyl (G.B.), Eraverm (Germ.), Helmezine (G.B.), Lumbrioxyl (Fr.), Multifuge, Oxucide, Oxypel (Canad.), Paravermin (Germ.), Perin, Pinsirup, Pin-Tega, Pipenin (Jap.), Piperasol (Pol.), Piperol (Fr.), Piperzinal (Canad.), Pipril, Piprosan (Austral.), Razine, Stavermol (Germ.), Tasnon (Germ.), Ta-Verm, Uvilon (Germ.), Vermago, Vermicompren (Germ.), Vermolina (Austral.).

Preparations

Oral: Syrup, 500 mg/5 ml; tablets, 500 mg (in terms of hexahydrate salt).

Usual Dosages

Oral: For roundworms, adults, 3.5 gm once daily for 2 consecutive days; children, 75 mg/kg (maximum, 3.5 gm) once daily for 2 consecutive days. For pinworms, adults and children, 65 mg/kg (maximum, 2.5 gm) once daily for 7 consecutive days. In severe infections, the above doses may be repeated at a 1-week interval.

PIROXICAM

Proprietary Name: Feldene.

Preparations

Oral: Capsules, 10 and 20 mg.

Usual Dosages

Oral: The usual daily dosage is 20 mg administered as a single or divided dose.

PLICAMYCIN (MITHRAMYCIN)

Proprietary Name: Mithracin.

Preparations

Injection: Powder (for solution) in vials containing 2500 µg plicamycin, 100 mg mannitol, and sufficient disodium phosphate to adjust pH to 7.

Usual Dosages

Intravenous: 25 µg/kg as a single dose by direct injection or added to 5 per cent dextrose in water and infused gradually over a 4- to 8-hour period.

PNEUMOCOCCAL VACCINE

Proprietary Names: Pneumovax, Pnu-Imune.

Preparations

Injection: 25 µg/0.5 ml.

Usual Dosages

Intramuscular, Subcutaneous: A single dose of 0.5 ml is injected.

POLYMYXIN B

Proprietary Names: Aerosporin, Polmix (Austral.)

Preparations

Injection: Powder, 500,000 units (equivalent to polymyxin standard 50 mg).

---

* Route of administration not approved by FDA.
† Drug not approved by FDA for any indication.
‡ Drug not approved by FDA for this particular indication.
§ Indicated dosage above the manufacturer's recommendation.

Topical Ophthalmic: For ophthalmic administration, the sterile powder is reconstituted by adding 20 to 50 ml of sterile water for injection or 0.9 per cent sodium chloride injection to a vial labeled as containing 500,000 units of polymyxin B. This provides solutions containing approximately 10,000 to 25,000 units/ml (10,000 units = 1 mg).

Usual Dosages

Intravenous: 15,000 to 25,000 units/kg daily. Infants may tolerate up to 40,000 units/kg daily if needed.
Subconjunctival: Up to 10,000 units daily.
Topical Ophthalmic: One drop of solution every hour as frequently as needed. The interval between doses may be increased if a favorable therapeutic response occurs.

POLYVINYL ALCOHOL

Proprietary Names: AKWA Tears, Barnes-Hind Wetting Solution, Contique Artificial Tears, Hypotears, Liquifilm Forte, Liquifilm Tears, Pre-Sert, Total.

Preparations

Topical Ophthalmic: Solution, 1.4, 2, and 3 per cent.

Usual Dosages

Topical Ophthalmic: Solution may be used as a substitute for tears, and one or two drops may be applied to the eyes as needed.

POTASSIUM IODIDE

Proprietary Names: Jodetten (Germ.), KI-N, Pherajod (Germ.), Pima, Solvejod (Swed.), SSKI.

Preparations

Oral: Solution, 300 mg/0.3 ml and 1 gm/ml.
Topical Ophthalmic: No ophthalmic preparation is commercially available. A 10 per cent solution can be prepared by dilution.

Usual Dosages

Oral: For use as an antifungal agent, 0.6 to 1 ml of a saturated solution (100 per cent) three times daily; amount is increased by 0.06 ml at each dose until the maximum tolerated dose is reached. Maximum daily dose is 12 to 15 ml.
Topical Ophthalmic: For fungal ulcers, 1 to 10 per cent solutions may be instilled in the conjunctival sac four to six times daily.

POTASSIUM PENICILLIN G (BENZYLPENICILLIN POTASSIUM)

Proprietary Names: Abbocillin (Canad.), Abbocillin-G (Austral.), Arcocillin, Biotic-T, Burcillin-G, Cilloral, Cryspen, Crystapen (G.B.), Deltapen, Dymocillin (Canad.), Eskacillin 100 (G.B.), Falapen (G.B.), Fivepen (Canad.), Forpen (Canad.), G-Recillin-T, Hyasorb, Hylenta (Canad.), Ka-Pen (Canad.), K-Cillin, Kesso-Pen, K-Pen, Lanacillin, Lemicillin, Liquapen, Nece-Pen (Fr.), Neo-Pens (Canad.), Novopen (Canad., S. Afr.), P-50 (Canad.), Paclin G, Palocillin, Parcillin,

Penalev, Pencitabs (Canad.), Penevan (Austral.), Penioral (Canad.), Peniset (Austral.), Pensol (Austral.), Pensorb, Pentids, Pfizerpen G, Pharmacillin (Germ.), Purapen G (G.B.), SK-Penicillin G, Solupen (G.B.), Specilline G (Fr.), Sugracillin, Tabillin (G.B.), Therapen-K (Canad.), Tu Cillin, Wescopen (Canad.).

Preparations

Injection: Powder; suspension for injection.

Usual Dosages

Intramuscular, Intravenous: Adults, 300,000 to 1.2 million units daily. Doses as large as 60 million units daily have been infused for certain serious infections. Children, 300,000 to 1.2 million units daily. Doses as large as 10 million units daily may be necessary (by intravenous infusion). Premature or full-term newborn infants, 600,000 units daily in two divided doses.

Oral: Adults and children, 600,000 to 3 million units daily.

POTASSIUM PENICILLIN V
(PHENOXYMETHYLPENICILLIN POTASSIUM)

Proprietary Names: Abbocillin VK (Austral.), Acocillin (Swed.), Apopen (Swed.), Apsin VK (G.B.), Arcasin (Germ.), Beromycin (Germ.), Betapen-VK, Biotic-V, Bopen V-K, Bramcillin (Austral.), Calciopen (Swed.), Calcipen (Austral., Norw.), Caps-Pen V (Austral.), Cilicaine-V or VK (Austral.), Cillaphen (Austral.), Co-Caps Penicillin V-K (G.B.), Cocillin V-K, Compocillin-VK, Corcillin V (S. Afr.), Crystapen V (G.B.), Crystapen-VK (Austral.), CVK (G.B.), CVL (Austral.), Darocillin (S. Afr.), Deltacillin (S. Afr.), Diacipen-VK (S. Afr.), Distaquaine V or V-K (G.B.), Dowpen VK, Econocil-VK (G.B.), Econopen V (G.B.), Falcopen V or VK (Austral.), Fenoxicillin (Denm.), Fenoxypen (Germ., S. Afr., Swed.), GPV (G.B.), Hi-Pen (Canad.), Ia-pen (G.B.), Icipen (G.B.), Isocillin (Germ.), Ispenoral (Germ.), Jatcillin (S. Afr.), Kabipenin (Germ.), Kavepenin (Swed.), Kesso-Pen-VK, Lanacillin VK, Ledercillin VK, LPV (Austral.), LV, Meropenin (Swed.), Nadopen-V (Canad.), Norcillin (G.B.), Novopen-V (Canad.), Nutracillin (S. Afr.), Oracilline (Fr.), Orapen (S. Afr.), Oratren (Germ.), Orvepen (Neth.), Ospen (Fr., Germ.), Ospeneff (G.B.), Paclin VK, Pancillen (Austral.), Penaper VK, Pencompren (Germ.), Pengen-VK, Penicals (G.B.), Penicillin V-K (Austral.), Peni-Vee (K) (Austral.), Penoxyl VK (G.B.), Pen-Vee (Canad.), Pen-Vee K, Pfipen V (Austral.), Pfizerpen VK, Phenethicillin, P-Mega-Tablinen (Germ.), Propen-VK (Austral.), PVF K (Canad.), PVK (Austral.), PVO (Austral.), QIDpen VK, Repen-VK, Robicillin VK, Rocilin (Austral., Norw.), Ro-Cillin VK, Roscopenin (Swed.), Saropen-VK, SK-Penicillin VK, Stabillin V-K (G.B.), Suspen V (Austral.), Ticillin V-K (G.B.), Tikacillin (Swed.), Uticillin VK, V-Cil-K (G.B.), V-Cillin K, VC-K (Canad.), Veecillin (Austral.), Veekay (S. Afr.), Veetids, Vepen (Swed.), Viacillin (Swed.), Vicin (Austral.), Vikacillin (S. Afr.), Viraxacillin-V (Austral.), V-Pen, VPV (Austral.), Weifapenin (Scand.), Win-V-K (Canad.).

---

* Route of administration not approved by FDA.
† Drug not approved by FDA for any indication.
‡ Drug not approved by FDA for this particular indication.
§ Indicated dosage above the manufacturer's recommendation.

Preparations

Oral: Granules for solution, 125 and 250 mg/5 ml; powder for drops, 125 mg/2.5 ml; powder for solution, 125 and 250 mg/5 ml; tablets, 125, 250, and 500 mg.

Usual Dosages

Oral: Adults and children over 12 years of age, 125 to 500 mg (200,000 to 800,000 units) every 6 to 8 hours for 10 days. Infants and small children, 25,000 to 100,000 units/kg daily in three to six divided doses.

POVIDONE-IODINE

Proprietary Names: ACU-dyne, Betadine, Betaisodona (Germ.), Betiadine (Arg.), Biodine, Bridine (Canad.), Disadine (G.B.), Efodine, Final Step, Frepp, Frepp/Sepp, Iodex, Iso-Betadine (Belg.) Isobetadine (Denm.), Isodine, Jodocur (Ital.), Mallisol, Neojodin (Jap.), Nutradine (S. Afr.), Operand, Pervinox (Arg.), Pevidine (G.B.), Pharmadine Polydine, Povadyne, Proviodine (Canad.), PV-I (G.B.), Savlon Dry (Austral.), Surgi-Sep, Topionic (Span.), Videne (G.B.).

Preparations

Topical: Ointment, 1 per cent; solution, 1, 7.5, and 10 per cent.

Usual Dosages

Topical: Preparation is applied directly to the affected area(s) as needed.

PRAZIQUANTEL

Proprietary Names: Cesol (Germ.), Biltricide (Germ.).

Preparations

Oral: Powder.

Usual Dosages

Oral: 40 to 60 mg/kg administered as a single or multiple dose.

PRAZOSIN

Proprietary Names: Hypovase (G.B.), Minipres (Arg.), Minipress, Peripress (Scand.).

Preparations

Oral: Capsules, 1, 2, and 5 mg.

Usual Dosages

Oral: Initially, 1 mg two or three times daily. The usual maintenance dosage is 6 to 15 mg daily in divided doses.

PREDNISOLONE

Proprietary Names: Adnisolone (Austral.), Ak-Pred, Ak-Tate, Alto-Pred (G.B.), Bio-Pred, Codelcortone (G.B.), Codelsol (G.B.), Cordrol, Dacortin H (Span.),

Decortin-H (Germ.), Delcort-E, Delcortol (Denm.), Delta-Cortef, Deltacortenolo (Ital.), Delta-cortilen (Ital.), Deltacortril (G.B.), Deltalone (G.B.), Delta Phoricol (G.B.), Deltasolone (Austral.), Deltastab (G.B.), Deltidrosol (Ital.), Di-Adreson-F (G.B.), Di-Pred, Donisolone (Jap.), Dua-Pred, Duo-Cort, Durapred, Econopred, Encortolone (Pol.), Endoprenovis (Ital.), Erbacort (Fr.), Fernisolone-P, Hostacortin-H (Germ.), Hydeltra, Hydeltrasol, Hydrocortancyl (Fr.), Hydrosol, Inflamase, Jectasone, Keteocort H (Germ.), Key-Pred, Lenisolone (S. Afr.), Marsolone (G.B.), Mecortolon (Pol.), Meticortelone, Metreton, Nisolone, Nor-Pred, Nova-Pred (Canad.), Ocu-Pred, Ocu-Pred-A, Ocu-Pred Forte, Optocort (Austral.), Panacort, Panafcortelone (Austral.), Panisolone, Paracortol (Austral.), Phortisolone (Fr.), Poly-Pred (S. Afr.), Precortalon (Swed.), Pre-Cortisyl (G.B.), Predair, Predair-A, Predair Forte, Predalone, Pred-Clysma (Swed.), Predeltilone (S. Afr.), Predenema (G.B.), Pred Forte, Predicort, Pred Mild, Prednelan (N.Z.), Prednesol (G.B.), Predni-Coelin (Germ.), Predni-H (Germ.), Predniretard (Fr.), Prednisol (Ital.), Predonine (Jap.), Predoxine, Predsol (G.B.), Predulose, Prelone (Austral.), PSP-IV, Rolesone (Fr.), Ropredlone, Savacort-50/100, Scherisolon (Austral., Germ.), Sigpred, Sintisone (G.B.), Sodasone, Solone (Austral.), Sol-Pred, Solucort (Fr.), Solu-Dacortin (Aust., Austral., Swed.), Solu-Decortin-H (Germ.), Solu-Pred, Solu Predalone, Ster-5, Steraject-50, Sterane, Sterofrin (Austral.), Ulacort, Ultracorten-H (Germ.), Ultracortenol (Austral., Germ.).

Preparations

Injection: Powder, 66.9 mg equivalent to 50 mg prednisolone; solution equivalent to 20 mg/ml prednisolone; suspension, 20, 25, 50, and 100 mg/ml.
Oral: Tablets, 5 mg.
Topical Ophthalmic: Ointment, 0.25 per cent; solution, 0.125, 0.5, and 1.0 per cent; suspension, 0.12, 0.125, and 1.0 per cent.

Usual Dosages

Intramuscular, Intravenous: 4 to 60 mg daily.
Oral: The initial dosage may vary from 5 to 60 mg daily, depending on the specific disease entity being treated. Higher initial dosage may be required in selected patients. It should be emphasized that dosage requirements are variable and must be individualized on the basis of the disease under treatment and the response of the patient.
Retrobulbar: 0.5 to 1.0 ml of solution containing 25 mg/ml.
Topical Ophthalmic: One drop of 0.12 to 1 per cent suspension every 2 to 4 hours until a response is obtained. The frequency is then reduced. The ointment preparation is applied three to four times daily or as a nighttime medication when the solution is used during the day.

PREDNISONE

Proprietary Names: Adasone (Austral.), Ancortone (Ital.), Colisone (Canad.), Cortancyl (Fr.), Dabroson

---

* Route of administration not approved by FDA.
† Drug not approved by FDA for any indication.
‡ Drug not approved by FDA for this particular indication.
§ Indicated dosage above the manufacturer's recommendation.

(Germ.), Dacortin (Span.), Decortin (Germ.), DeCortisyl (G.B.), Delcortin (Denm.), Deltacortene (Ital.), Deltacortone (G.B.), Delta Prenovis (Ital.), Deltasone, Deltison (Swed.), Di-Adreson (G.B.), Encorton (Pol.), Erftopred (Germ.), Hostacortin (Germ.), Inocortyl (Fr.), Keteocort (Germ.), Keysone, Lisacort, Marsone (G.B.), Maso-Pred, Meticorten, Nisone (Span.), Orasone, Panafcort (Austral., S. Afr.), Pan-Sone, Paracort (Canad.), Parmenison (Aust.), Pred-5, Predeltin (S. Afr.), Prednicen-M, Prednilong (S. Afr.), Prednilonga (Germ.), Predniment (Germ.), Predni-Tablinen (Germ.), Prednital (Ital.), Presone (Austral.), Propred (Austral.), Rectodelt (Germ.), Ropred, Sarogesic, Servisone, SK-Prednisone, Sone (Austral.), Sterapred, Ultracorten (Germ.), Urtilone (Fr.), Wescopred (Canad.), Winpred (Canad.).

Preparations

Oral: Tablets, 1, 2.5, 5, 10, 20, 25, and 50 mg.

Usual Dosages

Oral: The initial dosage may vary from 5 to 60 mg daily, depending upon the specific disease entity being treated. Higher initial dosages may be required in selected patients. It should be emphasized that dosage requirements are variable and must be individualized on the basis of the disease under treatment and the response of the patient.

PRIMAQUINE

Proprietary Name: Primaquine.

Preparations

Oral: Tablets, 26.3 mg (equivalent to 15 mg of base).

Usual Dosages

Oral: (Doses expressed in terms of the base). To prevent relapses, adults, 15 mg; children, 1.75 mg/4.5 kg. The dose is given daily for 14 days, concomitantly with other antimalarial drugs given on the first 3 days of an acute attack.

PROBENECID

Proprietary Names: Benacen, Benemid, Benemide (Fr.), Benn, Benuryl (Canad.), Panuric (S. Afr.), Probalan, Probecid (Norw., Swed.), Probemid (Span.), Proben (S. Afr.), Prebenid (Belg.), Procid (Austral.), Robenecid, SK-Probenecid, Solpurin (Ital.), Uroben (Ital.), Urocid (Ital.).

Preparations

Oral: Tablets, 500 mg.

Usual Dosages

Oral: Adults, for treatment of gout, 250 mg twice daily for 1 week, followed by 500 mg twice daily thereafter. When used in combination with penicillin therapy, the recommended dosage is 2 gm daily in divided doses.

PROBUCOL

Proprietary Name: Lorelco.

Preparations

Oral: Tablets, 250 mg.

Usual Dosages

Oral: Adults, 500 mg twice daily taken with meals.

PROCAINE

Proprietary Names: Anucaine, Durathesia, Neocaine, Novocain, P45 (Austral.), Planocaine (S. Afr.), Rectocaine, Unicaine, Westocaine (Canad.).

Preparations

Injection: Solution, 1, 2, and 10 per cent.

Usual Dosages

Nerve Block: With or without epinephrine 1:200,000, up to 50 ml of the 1 per cent or 25 ml of the 2 per cent solution.

PROCAINE PENICILLIN G (AQUEOUS)

Proprietary Names: Almopen (S. Afr.), Aquacaine G (Austral.), Aquacillin (Austral.), Ayercillin (Canad.), Cilicaine (Austral.), Crysticillin AS, Depocillin, Depocillin (S. Afr.), Duracillin AS, Eskacillin (G.B.), Evacilin (Austral.), Flo-Cillin, Flocilline (Fr.), Francacilline (Canad.), Hostacillin (Austral.), Hydracillin (Swed.), Ibacillin (Canad.), Megapen (Austral.), Novocillin (S. Afr.), Parencillin, Penlator, Pentids-P, Pfizerpan-AS, Procillin (Austral., S. Afr.), Pro-Stabillin AS (G.B.), Suspenin (Swed.), Therapen (Canad.), Viraxacillin (Austral.), Wycillin.

Preparations

Injection: Powder; suspension for injection.

Usual Dosages

Intramuscular: Adults and children, 600,000 to 1 million units daily in one or two doses, depending upon the condition being treated. Doses as large as 4.8 million units divided into at least two doses have been injected at different sites at one visit for certain serious infections. Ten days to 2 weeks of therapy are usually sufficient.

PROCARBAZINE

Proprietary Names: Matulane, Natulan (G.B.), Natulanar (Swed.).

Preparations

Oral: Capsules, 50 mg.

Usual Dosages

Oral: Single or divided doses of 2 to 4 mg/kg daily are recommended for the first week. Daily doses should then be maintained at 4 to 6 mg/kg daily until the white blood count falls below 4000/cubic millimeter or the platelets fall below 100,000/cubic millimeter.

PROCHLORPERAZINE

Proprietary Names: Anit-Naus (Austral.), Compazine, Stemetil (G.B.), Tementil (Fr.), Vertigon (G.B.).

Preparations

Injection: Solution, 5 mg/ml.
Oral: Capsules (sustained-release), 10, 15, and 30 mg; syrup, 5 mg/5 ml; tablets, 5, 10, and 25 mg.
Rectal: Suppositories, 2.5, 5.0, and 25.0 mg.

Usual Dosages

Intramuscular: Adults, 5 to 10 mg every 3 to 4 hours (maximum, 40 mg daily).
Oral: Adults, 5 to 10 mg three to four times daily.
Rectal: Adults, 25 mg twice daily.

PROMETHAZINE

Proprietary Names: Atosil (Germ.), Avomine (G.B.), Fellozine, Ganphen, Histantil (Canad.), K-Phen, Lemprometh, Lenazine (S. Afr.), Lergigan (Swed.), Methazine, Meth-Zine (Austral.), Pentazine, Phenergen, Phenerhist, Phenerject, Progan (Austral.), Promethapar, Prorex, Prothazine (Austral.), Provigan, Quadnite, Remsed, Rolamethazine, Sigazine, ZiPan.

Preparations

Injection: Solution, 25 and 50 mg/ml.
Oral: Syrup, 6.25 and 25 mg/5 ml; tablets, 12.5, 25, and 50 mg.
Rectal: Suppositories, 25 and 50 mg.

Usual Dosages

Intramuscular, Intravenous, Rectal: Adults, 25 mg repeated in 2 hours if necessary.
Intramuscular, Oral: Children, 0.5 mg/kg at bedtime or 0.13 mg/kg in the morning or when necessary.
Oral: Adults, 25 mg at bedtime or 12.5 mg four times daily.

PROPAMIDINE

Proprietary Name: Brolene (Austral., G.B.).

Preparations

Topical Ophthalmic: Solution, 0.1 per cent.

Usual Dosages

Topical Ophthalmic: One or two drops of solution in the affected eye(s) are instilled two to four times daily, or more frequently as required, for 7 to 10 days.

---

* Route of administration not approved by FDA.
† Drug not approved by FDA for any indication.
‡ Drug not approved by FDA for this particular indication.
§ Indicated dosage above the manufacturer's recommendation.

In acute infections, drops may be applied every 15 to 30 minutes. Treatment should not be prolonged for longer than 1 week.

PROPARACAINE (PROXYMETACAINE)

Proprietary Names: Ak-Taine, Alcaine, Kainair, Keracaine (Fr.), Ocu-Caine, Ophthaine, Ophthetic.

Preparations

Topical Ophthalmic: Solution, 0.5 per cent.

Usual Dosages

Topical Ophthalmic: For minor procedures, one drop of solution is instilled before the procedure. For deeper anesthesia, more frequent instillation is required.

PROPOXYPHENE

Proprietary Names: Algaphan (Austral.), Antalvic (Fr.), Darvon, Depronal SA (G.B.), Develin (Germ.), Dextropropoxyphene (G.B.), Dolene, Dolocap, Dolotard (Swed.), Doloxene, Erantin (Germ.), Harmar, Mardon, Pro-65 (Canad.), Propox 65, Propoxychel, Proxagesic, Ropoxy, Scrip-Dyne, SK-65, S-Pain-65.

Preparations

Oral: Capsules, 32 and 65 mg; suspension, 50 mg/5 ml; tablets, 100 mg.

Usual Dosages

Oral: 65 (hydrochloride salt) or 100 mg (napsylate salt) three or four times daily.

PROPRANOLOL

Proprietary Names: Dociton (Germ.), Herzul (Jap.), Inderal, Kemi (Jap.).

Preparations

Injection: Solution, 1 mg/ml.
Oral: Tablets, 10, 40, 80, and 160 mg.

Usual Dosages

Intravenous (Slow): 1 to 10 mg.
Oral: 20 mg to 2 gm daily in divided doses; the initial dose should not exceed 40 mg.

PROPYLTHIOURACIL

Proprietary Names: Propacil, Propycil (Germ.), Propyl-Thyracil (Canad.), Thyreostat II (Germ.), Tiotil (Swed.).

---

* Route of administration not approved by FDA.
† Drug not approved by FDA for any indication.
‡ Drug not approved by FDA for this particular indication.
§ Indicated dosage above the manufacturer's recommendation.

Preparations

Oral: Tablets, 50 mg.

Usual Dosages

Oral: For management of hyperthyroidism, adults, initially 300 to 400 mg daily in divided doses every 8 hours. Some patients may require as much as 900 mg daily for initial control. For maintenance, 100 to 300 mg is given daily in three divided doses.

PSORALENS
See Methoxsalen, Trioxsalen.

PYRANTEL

Proprietary Names: Antiminth, Aut (Arg.), Cobantril (Switz.), Combantrin (Arg., Austral., Belg., Canad., Fr., Ital., Neth., S. Afr.), Helmex (Germ.), Lombriareu (Span.), Trilombrin (Span.).

Preparations

Oral: Suspension, 250 mg/5 ml.

Usual Dosages

Oral: Adults and children, for roundworms and pinworms, 11 mg/kg (maximum, 1 gm); for hookworms, this dose is given for 3 consecutive days. Repeated in 1 month if indicated.

PYRAZINAMIDE

Proprietary Names: Piraldina (Ital.), Pyrafat (Germ.), Pyrazide (S. Afr.), Tebrazid (Belg., Canad.), Zinamide (Austral., G.B.).

Preparations

Oral: Tablets, 500 mg.

Usual Dosages

Oral: Adults, 20 to 35 mg/kg daily in one or more doses (maximum, 3 gm daily).

PYRETHRINS

Proprietary Names: A-200 Pyrinate, Barc, Blue, Licetrol, Pyrinyl, R&C, RID, Tisit, Tisit Blue, Triple X.

Preparations

Topical: Gel, 0.18, 0.3, or 0.33 per cent pyrethrins, 2.2, 3.0, or 4.0 per cent piperonyl butoxide, and 1, 2, or 4.8 per cent petrolatum; liquid, 0.18, 0.2, or 0.3 per cent pyrethrins, 2.0, 2.2, or 3.0 per cent piperonyl butoxide, 0.8, 1.2, or 5.5 per cent petrolatum, and 2.4 per cent benzyl alcohol, 0.2 per cent pyrethrins, 20 per cent piperonyl butoxide, and 0.8 per cent kerosene, 0.3 per cent pyrethrins and 2 per cent piperonyl butoxide; shampoo, 0.17 or 0.3 per cent pyrethrins, 2 or 3 per cent piperonyl butoxide, 1.2 per cent petrolatum, and 2.4 per cent benzyl alcohol.

Usual Dosages

Topical: Preparation is applied undiluted to infected areas, allowed to remain no longer than 10 minutes, and rinsed thoroughly with warm water and soap or shampoo; no more than two consecutive applications within 24 hours.

PYRIDOSTIGMINE

Proprietary Names: Mestinon, Regonol.

Preparations

Oral: Syrup, 60 mg/5 ml; tablets, 60 mg; tablets (timed-release), 180 mg.

Usual Dosages

Oral: Range, 0.06 mg to 1.5 gm daily.

PYRIDOXINE (VITAMIN B$_6$)

Proprietary Names: B$_6$-Vicotrat (Germ.), Becilan (Fr.), Bedoxine (Belg.), Beesix, Benadon (G.B.), Bivit-6 (Ital.), Complement (G.B.), Dermo 6 (Fr.), Dextamina B6 (Span.), Farmobion B$_6$ (Ital.), Gonabion B6 (Span.), Gravidox, Hexa-Betalin, Hexapyral (Swed.), Hexavibex, Hexobion (Germ., Span.), Lactosec 200 (S. Afr.), Pan B-6, Pydox (Austral.), Pyricamphre (Fr.), Pyroxin (Austral.), Rodex, Seibion (Ital.), Sibevit B6 (Span.), Vitanoxi B6 (Span.), Xanturenasi (Ital.).

Preparations

Injection: Solution, 50 and 100 mg/ml.
Oral: Tablets, 10, 25, 50, and 100 mg.

Usual Dosages

Intramuscular, Intravenous, Oral: In cases of dietary deficiency, 10 to 20 mg daily for 3 weeks. For drug-induced deficiency, 100 mg daily for 3 weeks followed by a 30-mg maintenance dose daily. For inborn errors of metabolism, as much as 600 mg a day and a daily intake of 30 mg for life.

PYRIMETHAMINE

Proprietary Names: Daraprim, Erbaprelina (Ital.), Tindurin (Hung.).

Preparations

Oral: Tablets, 25 mg.

Usual Dosages

Oral: For treatment of chloroquine-resistant *P. falciparum* malaria, adults 25 mg twice daily for the first 3 days of treatment with quinine and sulfadiazine. For ocular toxoplasmosis, adults, initially 100 to 150 mg. Then 25 mg are administered twice daily for 8 weeks, followed by 25 mg once daily for an additional 8 weeks. Finally, 25 mg are given every other day until a total of 6 months of therapy has been completed. Sulfadiazine should be given concomitantly.

QUININE

Proprietary Names: Bi-quinate (Austral.), Coco-Quinine, Dentojel (Canad.), Quinamm, Quinate (Austral.), Quinbisan (Austral.), Quine, Quinsan (Austral.).

Preparations

Injection: Powder.
Oral: Capsules, 130, 200, and 325 mg; tablets, 325 mg.

Usual Dosages

Intravenous: Adults, 600 mg every 8 hours until a clinical response is obtained (usually at least 3 days).
Oral: For treatment of chloroquine-resistant *P. falciparum* malaria, adults, 650 mg every 8 hours for 14 days in combination with pyrimethamine and sulfadiazine.

RABIES IMMUNE GLOBULIN (RIG)

Proprietary Name: Hyperab.

Preparations

Injection: Vial, 2 ml (300 IU) and 10 ml (1500 IU).

Usual Dosages

Intramuscular: 20 IU/kg; half of materials should be infiltrated around the wound if possible. Used in conjunction with 14 or 21 doses of rabies vaccine; when this serum is used for immediate delivery of preformed antibody, a total of 21 doses of rabies vaccine is preferred, either as 21 daily doses or 14 doses in the first 7 days followed by 7 daily doses; three booster doses of vaccine follow: one 10 days after completion of the series, the second 20 days later, and the third 90 days later.

RABIES VACCINE

Proprietary Name: Rabies Vaccine.

Preparations

Injection: Powder.

Usual Dosages

Subcutaneous: Adults and child for pre-exposure immunoprophylaxis, two 1-ml doses administered in outer aspect of the upper arm at approximately 1-month intervals, followed by booster dose after 6 or 7 months; booster doses repeated until antibody response detectable; persons in high-risk occupations should be given booster dose at least every 2 years; if bitten by rabid animal, five daily doses of vaccine, followed by booster dose 20 days after last injection. For postexposure immunoprophylaxis, when given without rabies immune globulin or antiserum, 14 daily injections should be administered, using doses recommended by manufacturer; when given with rabies immune globulin or anti-

---

* Route of administration not approved by FDA.
† Drug not approved by FDA for any indication.
‡ Drug not approved by FDA for this particular indication.
§ Indicated dosage above the manufacturer's recommendation.

serum, 21 doses are administered; these may be given as 21 daily doses or 14 doses during the first 7 days and then 7 daily doses; three supplemental doses of vaccine should be given 10, 20, and 90 days after completion of 14- or 21-day course.

RETINOL
See Vitamin A.

RIFAMPIN (RIFAMPICIN)

Proprietary Names: Rifa (Germ.), Rimactane, Rifadin.

Preparations

Oral: Capsules, 300 mg.
Topical Ophthalmic: Ointment, 1 per cent.

Usual Dosages

Oral: Adults, 600 mg in a single daily administration. In serious infections, a maximum daily dose of 1.2 gm may be given. Children, 10 to 20 mg/kg (not to exceed 600 mg) daily.
Topical Ophthalmic: Ointment preparation may be applied two to three times daily.

SALICYLATES
See Aspirin, Sodium Salicylate.

SCOPOLAMINE (HYOSCINE)

Proprietary Names: Isopto Hyoscine, Scopolamina Lux (Ital.), Scopos (Fr.).

Preparations

Injection: Solution, 0.3, 0.4, 0.5, 0.6, and 1 mg/ml.
Oral: Tablets, 0.4 and 0.6 mg.
Topical Ophthalmic: Ointment, 0.2 per cent; solution, 0.2, 0.25, 0.3, 0.5, and 1.0 per cent.

Usual Dosages

Intramuscular: Adults, 0.4 mg; infants 4 to 7 months, 0.1 mg; 7 months to 3 years, 0.15 mg; 3 to 8 years, 0.2 mg; 8 to 12 years, 0.3 mg.
Oral, Subcutaneous: Adults, 0.6 to 1 mg; children, 0.006 mg/kg.
Topical Ophthalmic: One drop applied in the eyes three to four times daily or more frequently if required.

SELENIUM

Proprietary Names: Selenitrace, Selepen.

Preparations

Injection: 40 and 50 µg/ml in 10- and 30-ml vials.

---

* Route of administration not approved by FDA.
† Drug not approved by FDA for any indication.
‡ Drug not approved by FDA for this particular indication.
§ Indicated dosage above the manufacturer's recommendation.

Usual Dosages

Intravenous: Adults, recommended daily intake is 20 to 50 µg. In deficiency states, 100 µg daily for 1 month reverses the deficiency symptoms without toxicity.

SILVER NITRATE (ARGENTUM NITRATE, CREDE'S SOLUTION)

Proprietary Name: Mova Nitrat (Germ.).

Preparations

Topical Ophthalmic: Solution, 0.5, 0.67 and 1 per cent.

Usual Dosages

Topical Ophthalmic: One drop may be applied to each eye.

SITOSTEROLS

Proprietary Name: Cytellin.

Preparations

Oral: Suspension, 3 gm/15 ml.

Usual Dosages

Oral: Adults, 12 to 24 gm daily, given in divided doses immediately before meals.

SODIUM ASCORBATE

Proprietary Names: Cenolate, Cevita.

Preparations

Injection: Solution, 250 and 562.5 mg/ml.
Oral: Crystals, 1020 mg/1.25 ml; powder, 1020 mg/1.25 ml; tablets, 585 mg.

Usual Dosages

Intramuscular, Intravenous, Oral: Adults, the average protective dose is 70 to 150 mg daily. For scurvy, 0.3 to 1.0 gm daily is recommended. To enhance wound healing, 300 to 500 mg daily for 7 to 10 days both preoperatively and postoperatively are adequate. For severe burns, 1.0 to 2.0 gm daily are recommended until healing has occurred or grafting operations are complete.

SODIUM AUROTHIOMALATE
See Gold Sodium Thiomalate.

SODIUM CHLORIDE

Proprietary Names: Adsorbonac, Hyperopto, Hypersal, Muro-128, Ocean, Ocurins.

Preparations

Injection: Solution, 0.45, 0.9, 3, and 5 per cent.
Topical Ophthalmic: Ointment, 5 per cent; solution, 2 and 5 per cent.

Usual Dosages

Intravenous: Adults and children, as required to correct dehydration and increase calcium excretion.
Topical Ophthalmic: One drop in eye(s) every 3 or 4 hours. Ointment may be applied as necessary as directed by the physician.

SODIUM CITRATE/CITRIC ACID COMBINATION

Proprietary Name: Bicitra.

Preparations

Oral: Liquid, 500 mg sodium citrate and 334 mg citric acid/5 ml.

Usual Dosages

Oral: Adults, 10 to 30 ml diluted in 30 to 90 ml water after meals and at bedtime.

SODIUM HYALURONATE

Proprietary Names: Connettivina (Germ., Ital.), Healon.

Preparations

Injection: Syringes, 10 mg/ml.
Topical Ophthalmic: No ophthalmic preparation is commercially available. The preparation intended for injection may be used to obtain the desired concentration.

Usual Dosages

Intracameral: A sufficient amount is slowly and carefully introduced.
Topical Ophthalmic: For treatment of keratoconjunctivitis sicca, 0.1 to 0.2 per cent may be applied two to four times daily or more frequently if needed.

SODIUM IODIDE[131]

Proprietary Names: Iodotope I-131, Oriodide-131, Theriodide-131.

Preparations

Oral: Capsules, 1, 3, 5, 6, 7, 8, 9, and 10 millicuries; solution, 1 to 200 millicuries.

Usual Dosages

Oral: For treatment of suitable patients with Graves' disease and hyperthyroidism, the usual dose is 4 to 10 millicuries. If the first treatment is not successful, retreatment after an interval of 3 or 4 months is usually recommended. Larger doses are required for suitable patients with toxic nodular goiter.

SODIUM PENICILLIN G

Proprietary Names: Gonopen (N.Z.), Novopen (S. Afr.), Specilline (Fr.).

Preparations

Injection: Powder (for solution), 1 and 5 million units.
Topical Ophthalmic: Ointment, 1000 units/gm.

Usual Dosages

Intracameral: 1000 to 4000 units in 0.2 to 0.5 ml of isotonic sodium chloride injection.
Intravenous: Adults, 8 to 20 million units daily; children, 200,000 to 400,000 units/kg daily in four divided doses; premature and full-term newborn infants, 40,000 to 80,000 units/kg daily in four divided doses.
Subconjunctival: 500,000 to 1 million units in 0.5 ml of isotonic sodium chloride injection or sterile water for injection.
Topical Ophthalmic: Ointment may be used several times daily. Fortified sodium penicillin G eyedrops are prepared by adding 15 to 600 mg (25,000 to 1 million units) with 50 mg of sodium citrate and 0.002 per cent phenylmercuric nitrate to 10 ml sterile water for injection.

SODIUM SALICYLATE

Proprietary Names: Alysine, Ancosal (Austral.), Ensalate (Austral.), Enterosalicyl (Fr., Swed.), Enterosalyl (G.B.), Idocyl (Swed.), Klev (Canad.), Rhumax (Austral.), Uracel.

Preparations

Oral: Tablets, 300 and 600 mg.

Usual Dosages

Oral: 600 mg every 4 to 6 hours as necessary (range, 300 mg to 4 gm daily).

SODIUM STIBOGLUCONATE
See Stibogluconate Sodium.

SPECTINOMYCIN

Proprietary Names: Actinospectacin, Trobicin.

Preparations

Injection: Powder, 2 and 4 gm (supplied with 3.5 and 6.5 ml of diluent, respectively.)

Usual Dosages

Intramuscular: Adults, 2 to 4 gm. The larger doses are indicated for retreatment after other antibiotic therapy has failed or for patients living in areas where resistance to penicillin is known to be prevalent. The larger dose should be divided between two gluteal injection sites.

---

* Route of administration not approved by FDA.
† Drug not approved by FDA for any indication.
‡ Drug not approved by FDA for this particular indication.
§ Indicated dosage above the manufacturer's recommendation.

SPIRAMYCIN

Proprietary Names: Rovamycin (G.B.), Selectomycin (Germ.).

Preparations

Oral: Syrup, 125 mg/5 ml; tablets, 250 mg.

Usual Dosages

Oral: 2 to 4 gm daily in divided doses.

SPIRONOLACTONE

Proprietary Name: Aldactone.

Preparations

Oral: Tablets, 25 mg.

Usual Dosages

Oral: Adults, 50 to 100 mg daily; children, 3.3 mg/kg daily in divided doses.

STIBOCAPTATE

Proprietary Name: Astiban (G.B.).

Preparations

Injection: Powder, 0.5 and 10 gm.

Usual Dosages

Intramuscular: A 10 per cent solution is prepared in water for injection and should be used in 24 hours if unrefrigerated; refrigerated solution may be used if colorless and clear. The total dose is divided into five equal amounts and given once or twice a week or, in hospitalized patients, as often as every day, depending upon tolerance of patient. Adults, 40 mg/kg in five divided doses; children 6 years and older, 50 mg/kg in five divided doses.

STIBOGLUCONATE SODIUM

Proprietary Name: Pentostam.

Preparations

Injection: Solution, 330 mg/ml.

Usual Dosages

Intramuscular, Intravenous (Slow): A course of treatment consists of six to ten daily injections, each of 6 ml, repeated if necessary on two occasions after 10-day intervals.

---

* Route of administration not approved by FDA.
† Drug not approved by FDA for any indication.
‡ Drug not approved by FDA for this particular indication.
§ Indicated dosage above the manufacturer's recommendation.

STREPTOKINASE

Proprietary Names: Kabikinase, Streptase.

Preparations

Injection: Powder, 100,000, 250,000, 600,000 and 750,000 IU.

Usual Dosages

Intravenous: A loading dose of 250,000 IU is administered over a 30-minute period. Following the loading dose, a maintenance infusion is given for 24 to 72 hours.

STREPTOMYCIN

Proprietary Names: Darostrep (S. Afr.), Isoject-Streptomycin Injection, Novostrep (S. Afr.), Orastrep (G.B.), Strepolin (Austral., S. Afr.), Streptevan (Austral.), Strept-evanules (Austral.), Streptosol (Canad., S. Afr.), Strycin.

Preparations

Injection: Powder (for solution), 1 and 5 gm; solution, 200, 400, and 500 mg/ml.

Usual Dosages

Intramuscular: Adults, 0.5 to 2 gm daily in two divided doses for 7 to 10 days and 1 gm daily thereafter for no longer than 3 weeks. Children, 20 to 30 mg/kg daily in divided doses. In severe infections, 2 to 4 gm daily (adults) or 20 to 40 mg/kg (children) in divided doses every 6 to 12 hours.

SUCCINYLCHOLINE (SUXAMETHONIUM)

Proprietary Names: Anectine, Brevidil E/M (G.B.), Celocurin-Klorid (Swed.), Lysthenon (Germ.), Pantolax (Germ.), Quelicin, Scoline (Austral., Canad., S. Afr.), Succinyl (Germ.), Sucostrin, Sux-Cert.

Preparations

Injection: Powder, 0.5 and 1.0 gm; solution, 20 mg/ml.

Usual Dosages

Intramuscular: The usual dosage is 2.5 mg/kg, but single doses should not exceed 150 mg.
Intravenous: For short procedures, 10 to 30 mg given over 10 to 30 seconds. Up to 80 mg may be required by some patients.

SULFACETAMIDE

Proprietary Names: Acetopt (Austral.), Ak-Sulf, Albucid (G.B.), Bleph-10, Cetamide, Isopto Cetamide, Ocu-Sul-10/15/30, Op-Sulfa, Optamide (Austral.), Optiole S (Canad.), Sulamyd, Sulf-10, Sulfacel, Sulfair, Sulphacalyre (G.B.), Sulphacetamide (G.B.), Sulten-10, Vasosulf (G.B.).

Preparations

Topical Ophthalmic: Ointment, 10 and 30 per cent; solution, 10, 15, and 30 per cent.

Usual Dosages

Topical Ophthalmic: For acute cases, frequent administration of 10 or 15 per cent solution every 10 to 30 minutes. For chronic cases, 10 per cent ointment applied three or four times daily or 30 per cent solution three or four times daily in combination with 10 per cent ointment used at bedtime.

SULFADIAZINE

Proprietary Names: Adiazine (Fr.), Coco-Diazine, Diazyl (Austral.), Microsulfon, Solu-Diazine (Canad.), Sulfadets (Canad.), Sulphadiazine (G.B.).

Preparations

Oral: Suspension, 500 mg/5 ml; tablets, 500 mg; tablets (chewable), 300 mg.

Usual Dosages

Oral: The usual loading dose in adults is 2 to 4 gm, with a maintenance dose of 2 to 4 gm daily in three to six divided doses. For treatment of chloroquine-resistant *P. falciparum* malaria, adults, 2 gm daily for the first 6 days of therapy with pyrimethamine and quinine. For ocular toxoplasmosis, adults, 4 gm daily in four divided doses for 1 to 3 weeks, then 2 gm daily in four divided doses until a total of 6 weeks of therapy has been completed.

SULFAFURAZOLE
See Sulfisoxazole.

SULFALENE

Proprietary Names: Kelfizina (Arg., Belg., Ital., Neth.), Kelfizine (G.B.), Longum (Arg., Belg., Germ., Neth.), Policydal (Jap.).

Preparations

Oral: Suspension, 100 mg/ml in 10- and 20-ml bottles; tablets for suspension, 2 gm.

Usual Dosages

Oral: In adults, 2 gm once a week in a single dose. For children, the dose is 30 mg/kg once a week.

SULFAMETHOXAZOLE

Proprietary Name: Gantanol.

Preparations

Oral: Suspension, 500 mg/5 ml; tablets, 500 mg.

Usual Dosages

Oral: Adults, 2 gm initially, then 1 gm two or three times daily. Children over 2 months of age, initially 60 mg/kg (maximum, 2 gm), then half of this amount every 12 hours.

SULFAMETHOXAZOLE/TRIMETHOPRIM COMBINATION
See Trimethoprim/Sulfamethoxazole Combination.

SULFASALAZINE

Proprietary Names: Azulfidine, Salazopyrin, Salazopyrine (Fr.), Salicylazosulfapyridine, S.A.S.-500, S.A.S.P., Sulcolon, Sulphasalazine (G.B.).

Preparations

Oral: Tablets, 500 mg.

Usual Dosages

Oral: Initially, adults, 1 to 4 gm daily in four to eight divided doses; for maintenance, up to 2 gm daily in four divided doses. To prevent attacks of chronic ulcerative colitis, 3 gm may be necessary daily in divided doses.

SULFINPYRAZONE

Proprietary Names: Anturan (Agr., Austral., Belg., Canad., Denm., G.B., S. Afr., Span., Switz.), Anturane, Anturano (Germ.), Enturen (Ital., Neth.), Zynol (Canad.).

Preparations

Oral: Capsules, 200 mg; tablets, 100 mg.

Usual Dosages

Oral: Dose range, 200 to 800 mg daily.

SULFISOXAZOLE (SULFAFURAZOLE)

Proprietary Names: Gantrisin, Gantrisine (Fr.), Lipo Gantrisin, Novosoxazole (Canad.), SK-Soxazole, Sosol, Soxomide, Sulfagen (Canad.), Sulfalar, Sulfizin, Sulfizole (Canad.), Sulphafurazole (G.B.), US-67 (Canad.).

Preparations

Oral: Liquid (timed-release), 1 gm/5 ml; suspension (pediatric), 500 mg/5 ml; syrup, 500 mg/5 ml; tablets, 500 mg.
Topical Ophthalmic: Ointment, 4 per cent; solution, 4 per cent.

Usual Dosages

Oral: Adults, 2 to 4 gm initially, then 1 to 2 gm every 4 to 6 hours.
Topical Ophthalmic: Ointment is applied three or four times daily.

---

* Route of administration not approved by FDA.
† Drug not approved by FDA for any indication.
‡ Drug not approved by FDA for this particular indication.
§ Indicated dosage above the manufacturer's recommendation.

SULINDAC

Proprietary Names: Arthrocine (Fr.), Artribid (Port.), Citireuma (Ital.), Clinoril, Imbaral (Germ.).

Preparations

Oral: Tablets, 150 and 200 mg.

Usual Dosages

Oral: The usual maximum dosage is 400 mg/day.

SUPROFEN

Proprietary Name: Surfrex (Belg.).

Preparations

Topical Ophthalmic: No commercial preparation is available, but a 0.5 per cent solution may be prepared.

Usual Dosages

Topical Ophthalmic: Solution may be administered three to four times daily.

SUXAMETHONIUM
See Succinylcholine.

TERBUTALINE

Proprietary Names: Brethine, Bricanyl (G.B.), Bristurin (Jap.), Feevone (Austral.), Filair (G.B.), Terbasmin (Ital., Span.).

Preparations

Injection: Solution, 1 mg/ml.
Oral: Tablets, 2.5 and 5 mg.

Usual Dosages

Oral: Adults, initially, 2.5 mg three times daily at approximately 8-hour intervals, increased gradually over a period of 2 to 4 weeks to 5 mg three times daily. Children 12 years and under, 1.25 to 2.5 mg three times daily at approximately 6- to 8-hour intervals, increasing the dose, if needed and tolerated, to a maximum of 5 mg daily.
Subcutaneous: Adults, 0.25 mg repeated in 15 to 30 minutes if necessary; no more than 0.5 mg should be administered in any 4-hour period. Children, 0.01 mg/kg (maximum total dose, 0.25 mg). The dose may be repeated once in 30 minutes if necessary, but usually is effective for 4 hours.

TERFENADINE

Proprietary Name: Seldane.

---

* Route of administration not approved by FDA.
† Drug not approved by FDA for any indication.
‡ Drug not approved by FDA for this particular indication.
§ Indicated dosage above the manufacturer's recommendation.

Preparations

Oral: Tablets, 60 mg.

Usual Dosages

Oral: Adults, 60 mg twice daily.

TETANUS AND DIPHTHERIA TOXOIDS (TD) ADSORBED

Proprietary Name: Tetanus and Diphtheria Toxoid.

Preparations

Injection: 5 Lf units tetanus toxoid and 1.4, 1.5, or 2 Lf units diphtheria toxoid/0.5 ml or 10 Lf units tetanus toxoid and 2 Lf units diphtheria toxoid/0.5 ml.

Usual Dosages

Intramuscular: Adults and children 7 years and older, two injections of 0.5 ml with an interval of at least 4 weeks between injections. A reinforcing dose to complete basic immunization is given 6 to 12 months later and every 10 years thereafter.

TETANUS ANTITOXIN (EQUINE OR BOVINE)

Proprietary Name: Tetanus Antitoxin.

Preparations

Injection: Ampules of 1500, 10,000, 15,000, and 50,000 units.

Usual Dosages

Intramuscular: Adults and children, for prophylaxis 5000 to 10,000 units within 24 hours after injury. If 48 hours have elapsed between the time of injury and treatment, a dose of 10,000 to 20,000 units is recommended.
Intravenous: Adults and children, for treatment, 40,000 to 100,000 units or more.

TETANUS IMMUNE GLOBULIN (TIG)

Proprietary Names: Homo-Tet, Hyper-Tet, Tet-Conn-G.

Preparations

Injection: Syringe, 250 unit; vial, 250 unit.

Usual Dosages

Intramuscular: For prophylaxis, adults and children, 250 units as a single dose. For treatment, the optimal therapeutic dose has not been established; 3000 to 6000 units are usually cited, but doses as large as 10,000 units have been used.

TETANUS TOXOID

Proprietary Names: Tetanol (Germ.), Tetatoxoid (Germ.), Tetavax (Fr.), T-Immun (Germ.).

Preparations

Injection: Ampules, 0.5 ml; vials, 5 ml.

Usual Dosages

Intramuscular: Adults and children, 0.5 ml for three injections; second injection given 4 to 6 weeks after first, and third given 6 months to 1 year after second. A booster dose is given every 10 years.

TETRACYCLINE

Proprietary Names: Achromycin, Ambramycin-P (S. Afr.), Amer-Tet, Amtet, Austramycin (Austral.), Bicycline, Bristacycline, Bristrex, Capcycline (S. Afr.), Cefracycline (Canad.), Centet, Chemcycline (Canad.), Co-Caps Tetracycline (G.B.), Cycline, Cyclopar, Decabiotic (Canad.), Decycline (Canad.), Dema, Desamycin, Dumocyclin (Swed.), Economycin (G.B.), Fed-Mycin, Fermentmycin (S. Afr.), Florocycline (Fr.), Gene-Cycline (Canad.), G-Mycin, GT-250/500 (Canad.), GT-Liquid (Canad.), Hexacycline (Fr.), Hostacyclin (Germ.), Hostacycline (Austral., S. Afr.), Hydracycline (Austral.), Kesso-Tetra, Lemtrex, Lexacycline, Maso-Cycline, Maytrex, Mericycline, Miriamycine (Fr.), Muracine (Canad.), Neo-tetrine (Canad.), Nor-Tet, Novotetra (Canad.), Oppacyn (G.B.), Paltet, Panmycin, Partrex, Pexobiotic (Canad.), Phosmycine (S. Afr.), Piracaps, Polycycline, QIDtet, Quadcin (N.Z.), Quadracycline-V (Austral.), Quatrax (Austral.), Retet, Rexamycin, Robitet, Ro-Cycline, Sanclomycine (Fr.), Sarocycline, Scotrex, Sifacycline (Fr.), SK-Tetracycline, Steclin, Sumycin, Supramycin N (Germ.), Sustamycin (G.B.), Svedocyklin (Swed.), T-125/250, T-Caps, Tet-Cy, Tetrabiotic (Canad.), Tetra-C, Tetracap (Austral., Canad.), Tetrachel, Tetracitro S (Germ.), Tetraclor, Tetra-Co, Tetracrine (Canad.), Tetracyn, Tetracyne (Fr.), Tetradecin Novum (Swed.), Tetral (Canad.), Tetralan, Tetralean (Canad.), Tetralution (Germ.), Tetram, Tetramax, Tetramykoin (Austral.), Tetrex, Tetrosol (Canad.), T-Liquid (Canad.), Totomycin (G.B.), Trexin, Triacycline (Canad.), T-Tabs (Canad.), U-Tet, Wintracin (Canad.).

Preparations

Injection: Solution, 100, 250, and 500 mg.
Oral: Capsules, 100, 125, 250, and 500 mg; syrup, 125 mg/5 ml; tablets, 50, 100, 125, and 250 mg.
Topical: Powder with diluent to make solution, 2.2 mg/ml.
Topical Ophthalmic: Ointment, 1 and 3 per cent; suspension in oil, 1 per cent.

Usual Dosages

Intramuscular: Children, 25 mg/kg daily in four divided doses (intravenous route preferred). This route should not be used in newborn infants.
Intravenous: Children, 15 mg/kg daily in four divided doses. This route should not be used in newborn infants.
Oral: Adults, 1 to 4 gm daily divided into three to four doses.

---

* Route of administration not approved by FDA.
† Drug not approved by FDA for any indication.
‡ Drug not approved by FDA for this particular indication.
§ Indicated dosage above the manufacturer's recommendation.

Subconjunctival: 2.5 to 5.0 mg in 0.5 ml of isotonic sodium chloride injection.
Topical: 0.5 to 1.0 ml of the prepared solution is applied twice daily.
Topical Ophthalmic: One drop of a 0.5 per cent solution is instilled every 30 minutes to 2 hours. Solutions should be freshly prepared every 24 to 48 hours and kept refrigerated. Ointment may be applied directly to the affected area every 2 hours or more often, as the severity of the infection and the degree of response indicate. Severe or stubborn ocular infections may require treatment for many days.

TETRAHYDROZOLINE

Proprietary Names: Murine Plus, Soothe, Tetracon, Visine.

Preparations

Topical Ophthalmic: Solution, 0.05 per cent.

Usual Dosages

Topical Ophthalmic: One or two drops are instilled every 2 to 3 hours or as needed until symptoms subside.

THIABENDAZOLE

Proprietary Names: Mintezol, Minzolum (Germ.).

Preparations

Oral: Suspension, 500 mg/5 ml; tablets (chewable), 500 mg.
Topical Ophthalmic: No ophthalmic preparation is commercially available. A 1 to 4 per cent solution in a cremophore base or in arachnis oil may be prepared.

Usual Dosages

Oral: 25 to 100 mg/kg, up to a maximum of 3 gm, in two divided doses daily, for 2 to 7 days.
Topical Ophthalmic: Solution is applied to affected and surrounding areas twice a day.

THIAMINE (VITAMIN B$_1$)

Proprietary Names: B-1, Betalin S, Bewon.

Preparations

Oral: Tablets, 100, 250, and 500 mg.

Usual Dosages

Oral: For thiamine deficiency syndromes, 5 to 10 mg three times daily.

THIOTEPA

Proprietary Names: Thio-Tepa (G.B.), Tifosyl (Swed.).

Preparations

Injection: Vial, 15 mg.

Usual Dosages

Topical Ophthalmic: For the treatment of pterygium, a solution of 0.05 per cent may be administered to the eye every 3 hours during the waking period for 6 to 8 weeks.

THROMBIN

Proprietary Names: Thrombinar, Thrombostat.

Preparations

Topical: Powder, 1000, 5000, 10,000 and 20,000 units.

Usual Dosages

Topical: For general use, concentrations of 1000 units/10 ml are used on the bleeding site. When bleeding is profuse, concentrations as high as 1000 to 2000 units/ml may be required.

THYROGLOBULIN

Proprietary Names: Proloid, Thyractin.

Preparations

Oral: Tablets, 16, 32, 65, 100, 130, 200, and 325 mg (1 gr = 65 mg).

Usual Dosages

Oral: Dosage should be started in small amounts and increased gradually with increments at intervals of 1 to 2 weeks. Usual maintenance dose is 0.5 to 3.0 gr (32 to 200 mg) daily.

TICARCILLIN

Proprietary Names: Aerugipen (Germ.), Tarcil (Austral.), Ticar, Ticarpen (Neth., Switz.).

Preparations

Injection: Powder, 1, 3, and 6 gm (equivalent to base).

Usual Dosages

Intramuscular, Intravenous: The usual adult dose in the treatment of severe gram-negative infections is the equivalent of 15 to 20 gm daily in divided doses every 4 to 8 hours, although 3 gm may be given every 3 hours in very severe infection. Children may be given 200 to 300 mg/kg daily in divided doses. In the treatment of uncomplicated urinary tract infections, the usual dosage is equivalent to 3 to 4 gm in divided doses daily intramuscularly or by slow intravenous infusion.

---

* Route of administration not approved by FDA.
† Drug not approved by FDA for any indication.
‡ Drug not approved by FDA for this particular indication.
§ Indicated dosage above the manufacturer's recommendation.

TIMOLOL

Proprietary Names: Timoptic, Timoptol (Austral., Fr., G.B., Neth., N.Z., S. Afr.).

Preparations

Topical Ophthalmic: Solution, 0.25 and 0.5 per cent.

Usual Dosages

Topical Ophthalmic: One drop of solution may be applied to each eye twice daily. If systemic side effects occur, punctal occlusion should be done.

TISSUE PLASMINOGEN ACTIVATOR
See Alteplase, Streptokinase, Urokinase.

TITANIUM DIOXIDE

Proprietary Name: Titanium Dioxide.

Preparations

Topical: Ointment, 20 per cent; paste, 20 per cent.

Usual Dosages

Topical: Preparation may be applied two or three times daily as needed.

TOBRAMYCIN

Proprietary Names: Brulamycin (Hung.), Gernebcin (Germ.), Nebcina (Denm., Norw., Swed.), Nebcin, Nebcine (Fr.), Nebicina (Ital.), Obracin (Belg., Neth., Switz.), Tobra (Arg.), Tobracin (Jap.), Tobradistin (Span.), Tobrex.

Preparations

Injection: Solution, 10 to 40 mg/ml.
Topical Ophthalmic: Ointment, 0.3 per cent; solution, 0.3 per cent.

Usual Dosages

Intramuscular, Intravenous: According to the severity of infection, a total daily dose of 3 to 5 mg/kg is usually given in equally divided amounts every 8 hours. Daily dosage should not exceed 5 mg/kg unless serum levels are monitored.
Subconjunctival: 2.5 to 40 mg in 0.5 ml of isotonic sodium chloride injection or sterile water for injection.
Topical Ophthalmic: In mild to moderate disease, drug may be instilled two to three times daily. In severe infections, hourly applications may be used until improvement, after which treatment should be reduced before discontinuation. Fortified tobramycin eyedrops may be prepared to produce a concentration of 15 mg/ml.

TOLBUTAMIDE

Proprietary Names: Arcosal (Denm.), Artosin (Austral., Germ., S. Afr., Swed.), Chembutamide (Canad.), Dolipol (Fr.), Insilange-D (Jap.), Ipoglicone (Ital.), Mellitol (Canad.), Mobenol (Canad.), Neo-Dibetic

(Canad.), Nigloid (Jap.), Novobutamide (Canad.), Oramide (Canad.), Oribetic, Orinase, Pramidex (G.B.), Rastinon (G.B.), SK-Tolbutamide, Tolbutol (Canad.), Tolbutone (Canad.), Wescotol (Canad.).

Preparations

Oral: Tablets, 500 mg.

Usual Dosages

Oral: Dosages should be individualized. Usual dose is 500 mg twice daily with a range of 0.25 to 3 gm daily.

TOLMETIN

Proprietary Names: Tolectin, Tolmex (Ital.).

Preparations

Oral: Capsules, 400 mg; tablets, 200 mg.

Usual Dosages

Oral: The recommended starting dose for adults is 400 mg three times daily, preferably including a dose on arising and a dose at bedtime.

TOLNAFTATE

Proprietary Names: Aftate, Focusan (Swed.), Sporiderm (Fr.), Sporiline (Fr.), Tinacidin (Austral.), Tinactin, Tonoftal (Germ.).

Preparations

Topical: Cream, 1 per cent; gel, 1 per cent; powder, 1 per cent; solution, 1 per cent.

Usual Dosages

Topical: One to two drops of solution or a small amount of cream or powder is rubbed into lesions twice daily for 2 to 3 weeks.

TRANEXAMIC ACID

Proprietary Names: Amcacid (Ital.), Amchafibrin (Span.), Amstat (Span.), Anvitoff (Germ., Switz.), Carxamin (Jap.), Cyclokapron (Arg., Belg.), Cyklokapron (Denm., G.B., Germ., Neth., Norw., S. Afr., Swed., Switz.), Exacyl (Fr.), Frenolyse (Fr.), Hexapromin (Jap.), Hexatron (Jap.), Tranex (Ital.), Tranexan (Jap.), Transamin (Jap.), Trasmalon (Jap.), Ugurol (Ital.).

Preparations

Injection: Solution, 100 mg/ml.
Oral: Syrup, 500 mg/5 ml; tablets, 500 mg.

---

* Route of administration not approved by FDA.
† Drug not approved by FDA for any indication.
‡ Drug not approved by FDA for this particular indication.
§ Indicated dosage above the manufacturer's recommendation.

Usual Dosages

Intravenous (Slow): 0.5 to 1.0 gm given two to three times daily over a period of at least 5 minutes.
Oral: 1.0 to 1.5 gm two to three times daily.

TRETINOIN

Proprietary Names: A-Acido (Arg.), Aberel, Aberela (Norw.), Acid A Vit (Belg., Neth.), Acnavit (Denm.), Acretin (Belg.), Airol (Arg., Austral., Denm., Germ., Ital., Norw., S. Afr., Switz.), A-vitaminsyre (Denm.), Avitoin (Norw.), Cordes VAS (Germ.), Dermairol (Swed.), Dermojuventus (Span.), Effederm (Fr.), Epi-Aberel (Germ.), Eudyna (Germ.), Retin-A.

Preparations

Topical: Cream, 0.05 and 0.1 per cent; gel, 0.01 and 0.025 per cent; liquid, 0.05 per cent.
Topical Ophthalmic: No ophthalmic preparation is commercially available. A preparation of 0.1 per cent tretinoin in arachnis oil may be prepared.

Usual Dosages

Topical: One application daily to the involved areas.
Topical Ophthalmic: One application of 0.1 per cent tretinoin in arachnis oil may be applied three times daily.

TRIAMCINOLONE

Proprietary Names: Acetospan, Adcortyl (G.B.), Amcort, Aristocort, Aristo-Pak, Aristosol, Aristospan, Cenocort, Cino-40, Delphicort (Germ.), Kenacomb (Austral.), Kenacort, Kenalog, Kenalone (Austral.), Ledercort (G.B.), Lederspan (G.B.), Rocinolone, SK-Triamcinolone, Solodelf (Germ.), Solutedarol (Fr.), Spencort, Tedarol (Fr.), Tracilon, Triamalone (Canad.), Triamcin, Triamcort (Ital.), Triam Forte, Triamolone, Tri-Kort, Vertalog, Volon (Germ.), Volonimat (Germ.).

Preparations

Injection: Suspension (aqueous), 10 and 40 mg/ml.
Topical: Cream, 0.025, 0.1, and 0.5 per cent; lotion, 0.025 and 0.1 per cent; ointment, 0.025 and 0.1 per cent; suspension, 0.007 and 0.1 per cent.

Usual Dosages

Intralesional: The size of the lesion will determine the total amount of drug needed, the concentration used, and the number and pattern of injection sites utilized. (For small lesions, 5 mg/2 ml divided over several locations.)
Retrobulbar: 10 to 40 mg/ml in 0.5 to 1.0 ml.
Topical: Preparation is applied three or four times daily.

TRICHLOROACETIC ACID

Proprietary Name: Trichloroacetic Acid.

Preparations

Topical: Solution, 15 to 100 per cent.

Usual Dosages

Intralesional: After removal of the contents of an epithelial implantation cyst of the anterior chamber, the cyst may be injected with 10 to 20 per cent trichloroacetic acid. This is allowed to remain from 30 to 120 seconds before it is withdrawn.

Topical Ophthalmic: A 10 to 25 per cent aqueous solution has been used to cauterize the surface of the cornea in treatment of recurrent erosion, bullous keratopathy, and other painful corneal diseases. The corneal epithelium may first be scraped with a knife. The solution should be applied to the surface of the eye for 15 seconds and then flushed with water or saline.

TRIFLURIDINE (F_3T)

Proprietary Names: Bephen (Germ.), TFT (Neth.), Triherpine (Lux.), Viroptic.

Preparations

Topical Ophthalmic: Solution, 1 per cent.

Usual Dosages

Topical Ophthalmic: One drop in the eye(s) every 2 hours while awake until herpetic lesion is completely re-epithelized, then one drop every 4 hours for 7 days.

TRIHEXYPHENIDYL

Proprietary Names: Anti-Spas (Austral.), Antitrem, Aparkane (Canad.), Artane, Benzhexol (G.B.), Hexyphen, Novohexidyl (Canad.), Pargitan (Germ., Swed.), Peragit (Denm., Norw.), Pipanol, Tremin, Trihexy (Canad.), Trixyl (Canad.).

Preparations

Oral: Capsules (timed-release), 5 mg; elixir, 2 mg/5 ml; tablets, 2 and 5 mg.

Usual Dosages

Oral: The total daily dosage usually ranges between 5 and 15 mg and is administered in divided doses according to the patient's need.

TRIMEPRAZINE

Proprietary Names: Penectyl (Canad.), Repeltin (Germ.), Temaril, Theralen (Swed.), Theralene (Fr., Germ.), Vallergan (G.B.).

Preparations

Oral: Capsules (timed-release), 5 mg; syrup, 2.5 mg/5 ml; tablets, 2.5 mg.

Usual Dosages

Oral: Adults, 10 mg daily divided into two to four doses.

---

* Route of administration not approved by FDA.
† Drug not approved by FDA for any indication.
‡ Drug not approved by FDA for this particular indication.
§ Indicated dosage above the manufacturer's recommendation.

TRIMETHOPRIM/SULFAMETHOXAZOLE COMBINATION

Proprietary Names: Abacin (Ital.), Abactrim (Span.), Ampliespectrum (Span.), Bacterial (Ital.), Bacticel (Arg.), Bactifor (Span.), Bactramin (Jap.), Bactrim, Bactrimel (Neth.), Baktar (Jap.), Biosulten (Span.), Brogenit (Span.), Chemitrin (Ital.), Co-Trim (S. Afr.), Cotrim (Germ.), Cotrimox (G.B.), Co-Trimoxazole (G.B.), Dhas (Span.), Drylin (Germ.), Duratrimet (Germ.), Espectrin (Braz.), Eusaprim (Aust., Belg., Fin., Fr., Germ., Ital., Neth., Norw., Swed., Switz.), Fectrim (G.B.), Gantaprim (Ital.), Gantrim (Ital.), Helveprim (Switz.), Hulin (Span.), Isotrim (Ital.), Ixazolina (Span.), Kepinol (Germ.), Kitaprim (Span.), Lescot (Arg.), Magisprim (Ital.), Medixin (Ital.), Metroprin (Span.), Mezenol (S. Afr.), Microtrim (Germ.), Missile (Arg.), Nodilon (G.B.), Nopil (Switz.), Omsat (Germ.), Oxaprim (Ital.), Paitrin (Ital.), Purbac (S. Afr.), Septocid (Ital.), Septra, Septran (S. Afr.), Septrin, Sigaprim (Germ.), Sinerbactin (Span.), Soifasul (Span.), Sulfacet (Germ.), Sulfotrim (Denm., Neth., Switz.), Sulfotrimin (Germ.), Suprim (Ital.), System (Ital.), Tacumil (Span.), Teleprim (Ital.), Thoxaprim (S. Afr.), TMS (Germ.), Trib (Austral.), Trigonyl (Germ.), Trim (Ital.), Trimesulf (Ital.), Trimetoprim-Sulfa (Norw., Swed.), Trisazol (Span.), Trisural (Denm.), Ultrasept (S. Afr.), Uro-Septra (Braz.).

Preparations

Injection: Solution, 80 mg trimethoprim and 400 mg sulfamethoxazole/5 ml.

Oral: Suspension, 40 mg trimethoprim and 200 mg sulfamethoxazole/5 ml; tablets, 80 mg trimethoprim and 400 mg sulfamethoxazole or 160 mg trimethoprim and 800 mg sulfamethoxazole.

Topical Ophthalmic: No ophthalmic preparation is commercially available.

Usual Dosages

Intravenous: Total daily dose of 8 to 20 mg/kg (based on trimethoprim component) may be given in three or four equally divided doses over a period of 60 to 90 minutes.

Oral: Adults and children over 12 years of age, two tablets every 12 hours for 12 to 14 days for urinary tract infections. For severe infections, the daily amount may be increased by half and given in three divided doses. For patients with impaired renal function, the usual dose may be given initially and subsequent doses reduced by one third to one half with a 12-hour interval between doses.

Topical Ophthalmic: One drop of a solution containing 16 mg trimethoprim and 80 mg sulfamethoxazole may be administered every 1 to 4 hours.

TRIOXSALEN

Proprietary Name: Trisoralen.

Preparations

Oral: Tablets, 5 mg.

Usual Dosages

Oral: 20 to 80 mg daily followed by UV irradiation.

TRIPELENNAMINE

Proprietary Names: PBZ, Pyribenzamine, Ro-Hist.

Preparations

Oral: Tablets, 25 and 50 mg.

Usual Dosages

Oral: 25 to 600 mg daily.

TRISULFAPYRIMIDINES

Proprietary Names: Neotrizine, Quadetts, Quadramoid, Sulfonsol, Sulfose, Triple Sulfas, Terfonyl, Trisem.

Preparations

Oral: Suspension, 500 mg/5 ml; tablets, 500 mg.

Usual Dosages

Oral: Adults, 3 to 4 gm initially, then 1 gm every 6 hours. Children and infants over 2 months, 75 mg/kg initially, then 150 mg/kg daily in four to six divided doses.

TROPICAMIDE

Proprietary Names: Mydriacyl, Mydriafair, Mydriaticum (Germ.), Myriaticum (S. Afr.), Ocu-Tropic, Tropicacyl.

Preparations

Topical Ophthalmic: Solution, 0.5 and 1 per cent.

Usual Dosages

Topical Ophthalmic: For ophthalmoscopy, one drop of 0.5 or 1 per cent tropicamide may be supplemented with 10 per cent phenylephrine. For refraction, one drop of 1 per cent tropicamide repeated in 5 minutes.

TYPHOID VACCINE

Proprietary Name: Typhoid Vaccine.

Preparations

Injection: Suspension, 8 units/ml in vials of 5, 10, and 20 ml.

Usual Dosages

Subcutaneous: For primary immunization of adults and children over 10 years of age, two doses of 0.5 ml may be administered at an interval of 4 or more weeks. For children under 10 years of age, two doses of 0.25 ml may be administered at an interval of 4 or more weeks.

UREA

Proprietary Names: Aquacare, Aqua Lacten, Carmol, Nutraplus, U-Lactin, Ureaphil, Urevert (G.B.).

Preparations

Injection: Powder (lyophilized), 40 and 90 gm.
Topical: Cream, 2, 10, and 20 per cent; lotion, 2 and 10 per cent.

Usual Dosages

Intravenous: Adults, 0.5 to 2 gm/kg given as a 30 per cent solution, administered at a rate of 60 drops/minute. Children, 0.5 to 1.5 gm/kg infused over 30-minute period.
Topical: Preparation may be applied two or three times daily.

UROKINASE

Proprietary Names: Abbokinase, Breokinase, Win-Kinase.

Preparations

Injection: Powder, 250,000 IU.

Usual Dosages

Intravenous: Using a solution containing 50,000 IU/ml, the usual priming dose is 4400 IU/kg at a rate of 90 ml/hour for 10 minutes, followed by continuous infusion of 4400 IU/kg at a rate of 15 ml/hour for 12 hours.
Intravitreal: 25,000 IU in 0.3 ml of distilled water.

VACCINIA IMMUNE GLOBULIN (HUMAN)

Proprietary Name: Vacciniabulin (Germ.).

Preparations

Injection: A sterile solution of globulins derived from blood plasma of adult human donors who have been vaccinated against smallpox. Each 100 ml contains 15 to 19 gm of protein of which not less than 90 per cent is globulin.

Usual Dosages

Intramuscular: Adults, prophylactic, 0.3 ml/kg; therapeutic, 0.6 ml/kg. Children, prophylactic, 0.3 to 0.5 ml/kg; therapeutic, 0.6 to 1 ml/kg.

VANCOMYCIN

Proprietary Names: Diatracin (Span.), Vancocin.

Preparations

Injection: Powder, 500 mg.
Oral: Powder, 10 gm.
Topical Ophthalmic: No ophthalmic preparation is commercially available.

---

* Route of administration not approved by FDA.
† Drug not approved by FDA for any indication.
‡ Drug not approved by FDA for this particular indication.
§ Indicated dosage above the manufacturer's recommendation.

Usual Dosages

Intravenous: Adults, 2 gm daily in two to four divided doses. Doses of 3 to 4 gm daily are used for seriously ill patients with normal renal function. Children, 40 mg/kg daily. The dose should be diluted with 100 to 200 ml of sodium chloride injection or 5 per cent dextrose injection and given slowly to lessen the possibility of thrombophlebitis.
Intravitreal: 0.1 to 1.0 mg in 0.1 ml of isotonic sodium chloride for injection.
Oral: Adults, maximum daily dose of 4 gm in aqueous solution in doses of 0.5 to 1.0 gm every 6 hours.
Subconjunctival: 25 mg in a 0.5 ml aqueous solution.
Topical Ophthalmic: One drop of a solution containing 50 mg/ml of vancomycin may be given every 1 to 4 hours.

VASOPRESSIN

Proprietary Name: Pitressin.

Preparations

Injection: Solution, 10 pressor units/0.5 ml.

Usual Dosages

Intramuscular, Subcutaneous: For the treatment of diabetes insipidus, the dosage is 5 to 10 units repeated two or three times daily as needed.

VIDARABINE

Proprietary Name: Vira-A.

Preparations

Topical Ophthalmic: Ointment, 3 per cent.

Usual Dosages

Topical Ophthalmic: Approximately one-half inch of ointment is administered into the lower conjunctival sac five times daily at 3-hour intervals.

VINBLASTINE

Proprietary Names: Velban, Velbe (G.B.).

Preparations

Injection: Powder (lyophilized), 10 mg.

Usual Dosages

Intravenous: To initiate therapy for adults, 3.7 mg/square meter is administered. The following dosages are given at weekly intervals: 5.5, 7.4, 9.25, and 11.1 mg/square meter. The maximum adult dose should not exceed 18.5 mg/square meter. For most adult patients, the weekly dosage will prove to be 5.5 to 7.4 mg/square meter.

VINCRISTINE

Proprietary Name: Oncovin.

Preparations

Injection: Powder, 1 and 5 mg with diluent.

Usual Dosages

Intravenous: A usual dose of 1.4 mg/square meter is recommended, with a pediatric dosage of 2 mg/square meter. Vincristine is usually administered as a single dose at weekly intervals.

VITAMIN A (RETINOL)

Proprietary Names: A 313 (Fr.), Acon, Alphalin, A-Mulsin (Germ.), Anatola (Canad.), Arovit (Fr., Germ., Swed.), Aquasol A, Atamin Forte (Austral.), Avibon (Fr.), A-Vicotrat (Germ.), Avita (S. Afr.), A-Vitan, Carotin (Austral.), Dispatabs, Fab-A-Vit (S. Afr.), Halivite (Fr.), Ido-A (Swed.), Ro-A-Vit (G.B.), Solatene, Solu-A, Vi-Alpha, Vogan (Germ.).

Preparations

Injection: Solution, 50,000 and 100,000 IU/ml.
Oral: Capsules, 5000, 25,000, 50,000 and 100,000 IU; solution (in oil), 50,000 IU/ml; tablets, 50,000, 75,000, and 150,000 IU.

Usual Dosages

Intramuscular: In severe vitamin A deficiency, adults and children over 8 years of age, 50,000 to 100,000 IU daily for 3 days, followed by 50,000 IU daily for 2 weeks.
Oral: In severe vitamin A deficiency, adults and children over 8 years, 100,000 IU daily for 3 days, followed by 50,000 IU daily for 2 weeks and 10,000 to 20,000 IU daily for another 2 months.

VITAMIN B_1
See Thiamine.

VITAMIN B_6
See Pyridoxine.

VITAMIN B COMPLEX

Proprietary Names: B-50/100/125, Becotin, Bejectal, Betalin, Mega-B, Orexin, Solu-B.

Preparations

Injection: Ampules; two separate vials of sterile solution, the contents of which when mixed provide 10 ml of solution; vials.
Oral: Pulvules, 10 mg B_1, 10 mg B_2, 4.1 mg B_6, 50 mg niacinamide, 25 mg pantothenic acid, and 1 μg B_{12}; softab, 10 mg B_1, 5 mg B_6, and 25 μg B_{12}; tablets, 100 mg B_1, 100 mg B_6, 100 μg B_{12}, 100 mg niacinamide, 100 μg folic acid, and 100 mg pantothenic acid.

---

* Route of administration not approved by FDA.
† Drug not approved by FDA for any indication.
‡ Drug not approved by FDA for this particular indication.
§ Indicated dosage above the manufacturer's recommendation.

Usual Dosages

Intramuscular, Intravenous: Before administration, 4 ml of solution no. 2 should be aseptically withdrawn and added to solution no. 1 vial if using two separate vial preparations. Ordinarily 2 ml at each injection should be adequate, although 5 ml or even more may be given if indicated.

Oral: Usual dosage is one pulvule or tablet daily.

VITAMIN C
See Ascorbic Acid.

VITAMIN D$_1$
See Dihydrotachysterol.

VITAMIN D$_2$
See Ergocalciferol.

VITAMIN D$_3$
See Calcitriol or Cholecalciferol.

VITAMIN E (ALPHA-TOCOPHEROL)

Proprietary Names: Aquasol E, Dalfatol, Dextamina-E Fuerte (Span.), Dif-Vitamin E (Span.), E-Ferol, Egermol (Belg.), Eprolin, Epsilan-M, E Sir (Ital.), Esorb, Eta-Monovit (Ital.), E-Toplex, Everol (Span.), Evion (Span.), E-Vites, Fertilvit (Ital.), Godabion E (Span.), Ilitia (Ital.), Invite E (Austral.), Lan-E, Lethopherol, Na-To-Caps, Natopherol, Pertropin, Propan E (S. Afr.), Solucap E, Tocerol (Austral.), Tocopher, Tocopherex, Tocopherol, Tocovite (Austral.), Vascuals, Viteril (Ital.).

Preparations

Injection: Solution, 100, 200, 220, and 500 units/ml.
Oral: Capsules, 30, 50, 100, 200, 400, 500, 600, 800, and 1000 units; elixir, 333 units/5 ml; solution, 50 units/ml; tablets, 100, 200, 300, and 400 units.
Topical: Cream, 30, 60, and 120 gm; liquid, 10, 15, 30, and 60 ml; oil, 15, 30, and 60 ml; ointment, 45 and 60 gm.

Usual Dosages

Intramuscular, Oral: Four to five times RDA in suspected deficiency.
Topical: A thin layer is applied over the affected area(s).

VITAMIN K
See Menadiol, Menadione, Phytonadione.

---

* Route of administration not approved by FDA.
† Drug not approved by FDA for any indication.
‡ Drug not approved by FDA for this particular indication.
§ Indicated dosage above the manufacturer's recommendation.

WARFARIN

Proprietary Names: Athrombin-K, Coumadin, Coumadine (Fr.), Marevan (G.B.), Panwarfin, Waran (Swed.), Warfilone (Canad.), Warnerin (Canad.).

Preparations

Injection: Powder (lyophilized), 50 mg with 2 ml of diluent and 75 mg with 3 ml of diluent.
Oral: Tablets, 2, 2.5, 5, 7.5, 10 and 25 mg.

Usual Dosages

Intramuscular, Intravenous, Oral: 30 to 50 mg initially; subsequent doses, 3 to 10 mg daily, according to prothrombin activity of the blood.

WHITE PETROLATUM
See Petrolatum.

YELLOW MERCURIC OXIDE

Proprietary Name: Yellow Mercuric Oxide.

Preparations

Topical Ophthalmic: Ointment, 1 and 2 per cent.

Usual Dosages

Topical Ophthalmic: A small quantity is applied one to two times daily.

ZIDOVUDINE (AZIDOTHYMIDINE, AZT)

Proprietary Name: Retrovir.

Preparations

Oral: Capsules, 100 mg.

Usual Dosages

Oral: The usual dose is 200 mg administered every 4 hours around the clock.

ZINC GLUCONATE

Proprietary Name: Zinc.

Preparations

Oral: Tablets, 10, 25, 50, and 100 mg.

Usual Dosages

Oral: As a dietary adjunct, two to three tablets daily.

ZINC OXIDE

Proprietary Names: Continuous Coverage, Covermark, Dermablend.

Preparations

Topical: Ointment, 20 per cent; paste, 25 per cent.

Usual Dosages

Topical: Preparation may be applied two to three times daily as needed.

ZINC SULFATE

Proprietary Names: Bufopto Zinc Sulfate, Medizinc, Op-Thal-Zin, Orazinc, Scrip-Zinc, Solvezinc (Austral.), Solvezink (Denm., Norw., Swed.), Verazinc, Zinc-200, Zincaps (Austral.), Zinc-Glenwood, Zincomed (G.B.), Zin-Cora, Zinc Sulphate (G.B.), Zinklet (Denm.).

Preparations

Oral: Capsules, 220 mg (50 mg zinc); tablets, 66 mg (15 mg zinc).
Topical Ophthalmic: Ointment, 0.5 per cent; solution, 0.1, 0.2, and 0.25 per cent.

Usual Dosages

Oral: 66 to 220 mg daily.
Topical Ophthalmic: Application of the solution or ointment is required two to four times a day.

---

* Route of administration not approved by FDA.
† Drug not approved by FDA for any indication.
‡ Drug not approved by FDA for this particular indication.
§ Indicated dosage above the manufacturer's recommendation.

INDEX

Abducens (sixth nerve) paralysis, 460–461
Abetalipoproteinemia, 244–245, 657–659
Abiotrophic ophthalmoplegia, 243–245
Abrasion, corneal, 343–344
Abscess, orbital, 641–643
  with sporotrichosis, 66
AC/A ratio, high, esotropia with, 476–477
Acanthamoebae infection, 98–100
Accommodative effort syndrome, 464–465
Accommodative esotropia, 461–463
Accommodative insufficiency, 464–465
Accommodative spasm, 580
Acid burns, 312–313
Acinetobacter infection, 3–4
Acne rosacea
  keratitis, phlyctenulosis associated with, 455
  with chalazions, 497
Acquired epithelial inclusion cyst, 440–441
Acquired fixation nystagmus, 482–486
Acquired immunodeficiency syndrome (AIDS), 43–44, 72–76
Acquired lues, 4–6
Acquired nonaccommodative esotropia, 465–466
Acquired ptosis, 521–522
Acquired retinoschisis, 672
Acquired strabismus, 461–463
Acquired syphilis, 4–6
Acrodermatitis enteropathica, 174–175
Actinic keratosis, 267–268
  with ultraviolet radiation, 315
Actinomycosis, 53–54
Acute febrile polyneuritis, 233–234
Acute follicular conjunctivitis, 92–93
Acute hemorrhagic conjunctivitis, 76–77
Acute idiopathic polyneuritis, 233–234
Acute infectious polyneuritis, 233–234
Acute interstitial keratitis, 14
Acute retinal necrosis, 659–661
Addison's disease, with candidiasis, 57
Adenovirus conjunctivitis, 92–93
Adenovirus infection, 78–79, 92
Adult cataract, 613–614
African *Loa loa* eye-worm disease, 111–112
After-cataract, 614–616
Age-related macular degeneration, 623–627
Alacrima, 603–604
Albers-Schönberg disease, 220–222
Alkaline burns, 313–315
  trichiasis with, 529
Allergic conjunctivitis, 400–402
Allergy, contact dermatitis, 190
Alternating nystagmus, periodic, 482–486
Alternating sursumduction, 474–475
Amblyopia, 465–466
  functional, 250–251
  in acquired nonaccommodative esotropia, 465
  in capillary hemangioma, 268
  in cerebral palsy, 242

  in Duane's retraction syndrome, 475
  in Marcus Gunn syndrome, 516
American mucocutaneous leishmaniasis, 100–101
Amyloidosis, 358–359
Anderson-Fabry disease, 156–157
Anemia
  Cooley's, 171–172
  sickle cell, 167–169, 387, 515, 598
Aneurysm, 164–165
Angiitis, necrotizing, 198–200
Angioblastic hemangioma, 268–270
Angioedema, hereditary, 192–194
Angioendotheliomatosis pseudolymphoma, neoplastic, 297–299
Angiohyalitis, 590–592
Angioid streaks, 387–388
  with subretinal neovascular membrane, 687
Angiokeratoma corporis diffusum universale, 156–157
Angioma, arteriovenous, 164–165
Angiomatosis retinae, 228–229
Angioneurotic edema, 192–194
  with anxiety states, 255
Angiopathic retinae juvenilis, 669
Angle recession, 547–548
Angle-closure glaucoma, 537, 541, 577–579
Aniridia, 580–582
Anisometropia, 648–649
  with acquired nonaccommodative esotropia, 465
  with Duane's retraction syndrome, 475
  with functional amblyopia, 250
Ankyloblepharon, 313, 493
Ankylosing spondylitis, 219–220
Anophthalmos, 532–533
Anterior chamber, postoperative flat, 380–383
Anterior granulomatous uveitis, 659
Anterior ischemic optic neuropathy, 633–635
Anterior uveitis, glaucoma with, 548–550
Anxiety states, 255–256
A-pattern esotropia, 466–467
A-pattern exotropia, 467–468
Apert's syndrome, 211–212
Aphakia, 649–650
  glaucoma with, 552
Aphakic pupillary block, 539–541
Aqueous diversion, posterior, 565–567
Arteriovenous fistula, 164–165
Arteriovenous malformation, 164–166
Arteritis, temporal, 169–171, 633
Artery, retinal, occlusion of, 663–665
Arthritis, rheumatoid, 204–206. See also *Rheumatoid arthritis*
Ascariasis, 101–103
Aspergillosis, 54–55
Aspergillus infection, in cavernous sinus thrombosis, 166
Asthenopia, 464–465
  with high AC/A ratio, 476–477
Asthenovergence of Stutterheim, 472–474

Astigmatism, 651–652
  in aphakia, 649
  in congenital fibrosis of extraocular muscles, 470
  in pellucid marginal corneal degeneration, 425
  in Weill-Marchesani syndrome, 209–210
Asymmetropia, 648–649
Atopic cataract, 175–176
Atopic conjunctivitis, 400–402
Atopic dermatitis, 175–176, 183–184
Atopic ectropion, 500
Atopic eczema, 175–176
Atrophy
  of choroid, gyrate, 670–671
  of iris, progressive, essential, 584–586
  of retina, gyrate, 670–671
  optic. See *Optic atrophy.*
Attention deficit syndrome, 249
Autoimmune deficiency syndrome, 59, 295
Autoimmune endocrine exophthalmos, 643–646
Autosomal dominant exudative vitreoretinopathy, 694–695
Avulsion, of eyelid, 345–347
Azobacter infection, 6–7

Bacillus cereus infection, 7–8
Bacillus subtilis infection, 8–10
Bacterial conjunctivitis, 402–403
Bacterial corneal ulcer, 439–440
Bacterial endophthalmitis, 379, 533–535
Bacterial infection, 3–50, 312, 416–418
Bacterial keratitis, 415, 439–440
Bacteroides fragilis infection, 20
Baggy eyelid, 520
Band keratopathy, 408–409, 453
Basal cell carcinoma, 288–289
Basic exotropia, 468–469
Bassen-Kornzweig syndrome, 243, 657–659
Beal, syndrome of, 92–93
Bee sting, of cornea, 355–356
Behçet's disease, 359–360
Bell's palsy, 234–236
  chronic progressive external ophthalmoplegia with, 244
  lagophthalmos with, 511
Benign congenital melanosis, 406–408
Benign epithelial tumor, 598–600
Benign essential blepharospasm, 494–495
Benign intracranial hypertension, 236–240
  with papilledema, 637
Benign mucous membrane pemphigoid, 403–406
Benign neoplasm, 267–268
Benign reactive lymphoid hyperplasia, 556–557
Berlin's edema, with ciliary body concussions and lacerations, 339
Berry syndrome, 223–224
Besnier's prurigo, 175–176
Beta-glucuronidase deficiency, 154–155
Bilharziasis, 117–118
Bird-headed dwarfism, 216
Bite, spider, 356–357
B-K mole syndrome, 518
Blackwater fever, 114
Blastomycosis, 55–56
Bleb, filtering, 410–411
  in bacterial endophthalmitis, 533
  in Fuchs' dellen, 423
Bleeding. See also *Hemorrhage; Vitreous hemorrhage.*
  late, recurrent, from focal wound vascularization, 383–384
  traumatic, 384–386
Blepharitis
  seborrheic, 522–524
  staphylococcal, with corneal mucous plaques, 422–423
  with candidiasis, 57
  with chalazion, 497
  with demodicosis, 106
  with Down's syndrome, 217
  with hordeolum, 510
  with madarosis, 515
  with neurodermatitis, 183
  with ocular rosacea, 184
  with ocular vaccinia, 90
  with trichiasis, 529
Blepharochalasis, 495–496
Blepharoconjunctivitis, mixed staphylococcal/seborrheic, 525–527
  staphylococcal, 456, 525–527
Blepharophimosis, 496–497
  in systemic sclerosis, 210
  in Waardenburg's syndrome, 160
Blepharopigmentation, 516
Blepharoptosis, 520–522
  epicanthus inversus in, 505
  in chronic progressive external ophthalmoplegia, 244
Blepharospasm, 255
  essential, benign, 494–495
  in anxiety states, 256
  in filamentary keratitis, 444
  in poison ivy, oak, or sumac dermatitis, 187
Blindness, 240–241
  eclipse, 630–631
  in age-related macular degeneration, 623
  in angioid streaks, 387–388
  in bacterial keratitis, 439–440
  in carotid cavernous fistula, 165
  in chronic angle-closure glaucoma, 541
  in cicatricial pemphigoid, 403–404
  in craniopharyngioma, 272–273
  in Creutzfeldt-Jakob disease, 247–248
  in cysticercosis, 106
  in diabetes mellitus, 144–146
  in dry eye syndrome, 450
  in erythema multiforme, 178
  in entropion, secondary to trachoma, 563
  in expulsive hemorrhage, 394
  in glaucoma, 209–210
  in gyrate atrophy, 670
  in Hodgkin's disease, 293–294
  in hysteria, 255
  in ischemic optic neuropathy, 633–635
  in juvenile rheumatoid arthritis, 198
  in listeriosis, 29
  in measles, 95
  in migraine, 251
  in onchocerciasis, 114
  in optic glioma, 632
  in orbital Graves' disease, 643
  in osteopetrosis, 221
  in papilledema, 637–639
  in retinitis pigmentosa, 682–683
  in temporal arteritis, 170
  in toxocariasis, 120–121
  in trachoma, 52
  in tyrosinemia II, 142–143
  in Vogt-Koyanagi-Harada syndrome, 372–373

Blindness (cont'd.)
  in Weill-Marchesani syndrome, 209
  night, 132–134, 670, 674, 682
  snow, 315
  sun, 630–631
  word, 248–249
Blowout fracture, 335–337
  with enophthalmos, 641
Blurred vision, transient, 252–253
Borrelia infection, 37
Botulism, 10–11
Bowen's disease, 289–291
Brain damage syndrome, 241–243
Brain dysfunction syndrome, minimal, 249
Branch retinal artery occlusion, 663–665
Branch retinal vein occlusion, 661–663
Brazilian purpuric fever, 24
Brown's superior oblique tendon sheath syndrome, 469–470
Brown's syndrome, 204, 469–470
Brucellosis, 11–12
Bücklers' type I dystrophy, 431–432
Bullous keratopathy, 442
Burns, 312–326
  from acid, 312–313
  from alkali, 313–315
  from eclipse, 630–631
  from electricity, 320–322
  thermal, 324–326, 511, 527

Calcification
  conjunctival, 408–409
  corneal, 408–409
  metastatic, in hyperparathyroidism, 125
Calcium deposition, in familial dysautonomia, 363
Camurati-Englemann disease, 212–213
Canaliculitis, in *Fusobacterium* infection, 20
Cancer, of skin, from phototherapy, 192
Cancerous melanosis, 406–408
Candida albicans infection, 56–59
  with fungal keratitis, 446
  with phlyctenulosis, 455
  with thermal burns, 325
Capillary hemangioma, 268–270
Capsular glaucoma, 543–545
Carbohydrate metabolism disorders, 144–155
Carcinoma. See also *Neoplasm; Tumor;* specific neoplasm.
  basal cell, 288–289
  of sebaceous gland, 310–311
  squamous cell, 276, 289–291, 305–306
Cardiovascular disorders, 164–173
Carotid cavernous fistula, 165–166
Cataract
  adult, 613–614
  after-, 614–616
  atopic, 175–176, 183–184
  bleb after surgery for, 410–411
  congenital, 141, 616–618
  congenital rubella, 94
  from electrical burn, 321
  from radiotherapy, 310
  from ultraviolet radiation, 316–317
  in Cockayne's syndrome, 216
  in Down's syndrome, 217
  in Fuchs' heterochromic iridocyclitis, 583
  in gyrate atrophy, 671
  in Hallermann-Streiff-Francois syndrome, 222
  in hypocalcemia, 128–130
  in hypoparathyroidism, 129
  in juvenile rheumatoid arthritis, 197–198
  in microspherophakia, 621
  in myopia, 653
  in oculocerebrorenal syndrome, 141
  in pseudoxanthoma elasticum, 203
  in Werner's syndrome, 218–219
  infantile, 616–618
  oil drop, 146
  traumatic, 354–355
Cataract surgery
  cystoid macular edema with, 624–627
  Descemet's membrane detachment during, 353
  in capsular glaucoma, 544
Cataractogenesis, 161
Cat-scratch disease, 77–78
Cavernous carotid fistula, 165–166
Cavernous hemangioma, 270–271
Cavernous sinus thrombosis, 166–167
Cellophane maculopathy, 628–630
Cellulitis, orbital, 641–643
Central nervous system, angiomatosis of, 228–229
  disease of, pruritis in, 188
Central retinal artery occlusion, 663–665
Central retinal vein occlusion, 679–682
Central serous chorioretinopathy, 665–667
Cephalalgia, paroxysmal nocturnal, 246–247
Cerebral palsy, 241–243
Chalazion, 497–498
  with blepharitis, 497
  with ocular rosacea, 184
Chalcosis, 326–329
Chamber, anterior, 377–386
  postoperative flat, 380–383
Chandler's syndrome, 584–586
Chiasmal glioma, 285
Chickenpox, 96–97
Chlamydial infection, 50–53
Choked disc, 637–639
Chorioretinal concussions and lacerations, 338–339
Chorioretinopathy, serous, central, 665–667
Choristoma, dermoid, 273–274
Choroid, 387–399
  gyrate atrophy of, 670–671
Choroidal detachment, 381–382, 388–390
Choroidal effusion, intraoperative, 389
Choroidal melanoma, 394–398, 555
Choroidal neovascular membrane, 390–392
Choroidal rupture, 392
Chronic cyclitis, 590–592
Chronic progressive external ophthalmoplegia, 243–245
Chrono-osteodystrophy, 152–153
Cicatricial ectropion, 500
Cicatricial entropion, 563
Cicatricial pemphigoid, 403–406
Ciliary block glaucoma, 565–567
Ciliary body, 580–596
  concussions of, 339–341
  lacerations of, 339–340
  melanoma, 394–398, 555
Ciliary neuralgia, 246–247
Ciliochoroidal detachment, 388–390, 569–570
Cirsoid aneurysm, 164–165
Clostridium botulinum infection, 10
Clostridium difficile infection, 8
Clostridium perfringens infection, 12–13
Clostridium tetani infection, 42–43
Cluster headache, 246–247
Coats' disease, 667–668

Coccidioidomycosis, 59–61
Cockayne's syndrome, 215–216
Coenurosis, 103–104
Cogan-Reese syndrome, 584–586
Cogan's microcystic corneal dystrophy, 427–428
Cogan's syndrome, 360–362
Coloboma, in Goldenhar's syndrome, 224–225
   of eyelid, 507
Compression injuries, 343
Concussion, chorioretinal, 338–339
   in ciliary body, 339–341
Congenital alacrima, 603–604
Congenital anomalies, of lacrimal system, 604–605
Congenital cataract, 141, 616–618
Congenital enophthalmos, with ocular muscle fibrosis and ptosis, 470–471
Congenital esotropia, 463
Congenital fibrosis, 470–471
Congenital hereditary endothelial dystrophy, 435
Congenital iris cyst, spontaneous, 587–588
Congenital melanosis, benign, 406–408
Congenital nystagmus, 482–486
Congenital ptosis, 521–522
Congenital rubella cataract, 94
Congenital syphilis, 13–15
Conjunctiva, 400–421
   calcifications of, 408–409
   contusions of, 342–343
   cysts of, 440–441
   intraepithelial neoplasia of, 289–291
   lacerations of, 342–343
   melanotic lesions of, 406–408
Conjunctivitis. See also *Blepharoconjunctivitis*; *Keratoconjunctivitis*.
   acute follicular, 92–93
   acute hemorrhagic, 76–77
   acute solar, 184–185
   adenovirus, 92–93
   allergic, 400–402
   atopic, 400–402
   bacterial, 402–403
   chronic, 508
   giant papillary, 400–402, 411–413
   gonococcal, 21–22
   gonorrheal, 417
   hay fever, 400–402
   in *Acinetobacter* infection, 3–4
   in *Bacillus subtilis* infection, 9
   in brucellosis, 11
   in candidiasis, 57
   in cat-scratch disease, 78
   in chylamidial infections, 50–51
   in coccidiodomycosis, 59
   in contact dermatitis, 177
   in diphtheria, 15
   in Down's syndrome, 217
   in *Escherichia coli* infection, 18
   in *Fusobacterium* infections, 20
   in gonorrhea, 21
   in gout, 160
   in *Hemophilus influenzae* infection, 23
   in infectious mononucleosis, 84
   in influenza, 85
   in Koch-Weeks bacillus infection, 24
   in leishmaniasis, 100
   in lice infestation, 116
   in Lyme disease, 86
   in molluscum contagiosum, 87–88
   in *Moraxella* infection, 29
   in mumps, 88
   in newborns, 416–418
   in Newcastle disease, 89
   in ophthalmia neonatorum, 32
   in papilloma, 286
   in Reiter's disease, 367–369
   in Rocky Mountain spotted fever, 69
   in rubeola, 95
   in schistosomiasis, 117–118
   in scrub typhus, 70
   in sporotrichosis, 66
   in *Staphylococcus* infection, 38
   in *Streptococcus* infection, 41
   in sunburn, 185
   in trachoma, 51
   in tuberculosis, 44
   in tularemia, 45
   in typhoid fever, 46
   in vaccinia, 90
   in Wegener's granulomatosis, 172
   in yersinosis, 48–49
   inclusion, 416–418
   irritative, 413–414
   ligneous, 414–415
   medicamentosa, 527
   mucopurulent, 402–403
   pink eye, 24, 78
   purulent, 402–403, 416
   swimming pool, 92
   toxic, 413–414
Connective tissue disorders, 197–210
Contact dermatitis, 176–177
   ectropion with, 500
   neurodermatitis with, 183
   pruritis with, 188
Contact lenses
   Acanthamoebae contamination of, 98–99
   giant papillary conjunctivitis with, 411–413
   in aphakia, 649
   in corneal erosion, 427–428
   in erythema multiforme, 178
   in idiopathic facial paralysis, 234–236
   in myopia, 653–656
   in Sjögren's syndrome, 207
   Pseudomonas infection with, 35–37
Contact urticaria, pruritis in, 188
Contusion, 338–355
   conjunctival, 342–343
   corneal, 343–344
   ocular, glaucoma after, 547–548
   of eyelid, 345–347
   of lacrimal system, 351–352
Convergence insufficiency syndrome, 471–472
Convergence-retraction nystagmus, 484
Cooley's anemia, 171–172
Copper foreign body, intraocular, 326–329
Cornea, 422–459
   bee sting of, 355–356
   ectatic conditions of, 438–439
Corneal abrasion, 343–344
Corneal calcification, 408–409
Corneal contusion, 343–344
Corneal cyst, 440–441
Corneal degeneration, 422–426
Corneal dystrophy
   dot, 427
   endothelial, 435–437
   epithelial, 427–430
   Fehr's, 433
   fingerprint, 427
   Fuchs', 435–436
   granular, 431–432
   Groenouw's type II, 433

Corneal dystrophy (cont'd.)
  hereditary, deep, 437
  in angiokeratoma corporis diffusum universale, 156
  in Cockayne's syndrome, 215
  in xeroderma pigmentosum, 161
  juvenile, 428–429
  lattice, 432–433
  macular, 433–434
  map, 427
  polymorphous, posterior, 437
  Reis-Bücklers', superficial, 429–430
  Schnyder's crystalline, 430–431
  stromal, 430–434
Corneal ectasia, 438–439
Corneal edema, 442
  with filamentary keratitis, 444
  with bee sting, 355
  with fibrous ingrowth, 379
  with stripping or detachment of Descemet's membrane, 352
Corneal erosion
  in Bell's palsy, 234
  in ocular rosacea, 184
  recurrent, 427–428
Corneal hypesthesia, in familial dysautonomia, 363
Corneal intraepithelial neoplasia, 289–291
Corneal keloid, in oculocerebrorenal syndrome, 141
Corneal laceration, 343–344
Corneal melt, in rheumatoid arthritis, 205–206
Corneal mucous plaque, 422–423
Corneal neovascularization, 443–444
Corneal opacity
  with alkaline burns, 314
  with corneal abrasion, 343
  with corneal calcification, 408
  with Fabry's disease, 156
  with functional amblyopia, 250
  with hyperparathyroidism, 126
  with ichthyosis, 181
  with intraocular inert foreign body, 329
  with intraocular steel or iron, 331
  with ligneous conjunctivitis, 414
  with mucopolysaccharidosis I-H, 147
  with mucopolysaccharidosis I-H/S, 148
  with mucopolysaccharidosis I-S, 149
  with mucopolysaccharidosis IV, 152
  with mucopolysaccharidosis VI, 153
  with mucopolysaccharidosis VII, 154
Corneal perforation, 343–344
  in ocular rosacea, 184
Corneal piriformis, 425
Corneal transplantation
  Creutzfeldt-Jakob disease spread by, 247–248
  in xeroderma pigmentosum, 162
  rabies transmission by, 93–94
Corneal ulcer, 9
  bacterial, 439–440
  fungal, 445–448
  in acid burns, 312
  in *Acinetobacter* infection, 3
  in actinomycosis, 53
  in alkaline burns, 313
  in asperigillosis, 54
  in *Bacillus subtilis* infection, 8
  in blastomycosis, 55
  in candidiasis, 57–58
  in cicatricial pemphigoid, 404
  in dacryocystitis, 607
  in diphtheria, 15
  in erythema multiforme, 178
  in *Fusobacterium* infection, 19
  in gonorrhea, 22
  in herpes simplex, 79
  in hypovitaminosis A, 134
  in lagophthalmos, 512
  in leishmaniasis, 100
  in measles, 95
  in *Pneumococcus* infection, 32
  in *Pseudomonas* infection, 35–36
  in rheumatoid arthritis, 205
  in rubeola, 95
  in sporotrichosis, 66
  in *Streptococcus* infection, 41
  in trichiasis, 529
  in tularemia, 45
  in typhoid fever, 47
  in tyrosinemia II, 142–143
  in yersiniosis, 49
Corticosteroid-induced glaucoma, 542–543
Corynebacterium diphtheriae infection, 15
Cotton wool spots, in systemic lupus erythematosus, 209
Coxiella burnetti, 68–69
Cranial neuralgia, 253
Craniofacial dyostosis, 211–212
  with basic exotropia, 468
  with eyelid coloboma, 507
Craniopharyngioma, 271–273
Craniostenosis, 211–215
CREST syndrome, 200
Cretinism, 130–131
Creutzfeldt-Jakob disease, 247–248
Criswick-Schepens syndrome, 694–695
Crohn's disease, 132–134
Crouzon's disease, 211–212
  with lagophthalmos, 511
  with orbital hypertelorism, 214
Cryoinjury, 322–323
Crystal deposits, in cystinosis, 136
Crystalline corneal dystrophy, Schnyder's, 430–431
Crystalline keratopathy, infectious, 448–449
Cutaneous leishmaniasis, 104–105
Cutaneous T-cell lymphoma, 300–301
Cyclitis, chronic, 590–592
Cyclops infection, 110
Cyst
  acquired epithelial inclusion, 440–441
  conjunctival, 440–441
  corneal, 440–441
  dermoid, 273–274
  epithelial, 377–378, 440–441, 587–588
  hydatid, 110–111
  intraocular, 103, 377–378
  on iris, 587–588
  scleral, 440–441
Cysticercosis, 105–106
Cystinosis, 136–137
Cystoid degeneration, 671–672
Cystoid macular edema, 624–627
Cystoid maculopathy, 624–627
Cytomegalovirus retinopathy, in AIDS, 72–75

Dacryoadenitis, 597–598
  in erysipelas, 17
  in mumps, 89
Dacryocystitis, 605–608
  in actinomycosis, 54
  in candidiasis, 58
  in dacryolith, 609
  in *Fusobacterium* infection, 20

Dacryocystitis (cont'd.)
  in lacrimal system lacerations, 352
  in *Pneumococcus* infection, 33
  in rhinosporidiosis, 65–66
  in sporotrichosis, 67
  in *Streptococcus* infection, 41
  in tularemia, 45
  in Waardenburg's syndrome, 227
  in Wegener's granulomatosis, 173
Dacryolith, 608–609
Dacryosialoadenopathy, 600–601
Deerfly tularemia, 45–46
Degeneration
  corneal, 425
  cystoid, 671–672
  Koeppe's posterior polymorphous, 437
  macular, age-related, 623–627
    disciform, 390–392
  retinal. See *Retinal degeneration.*
  snowflake, 672
  Terrien's marginal, 426
Dehiscence, scleral, 690–691
Dellen, Fuchs', 423
Demodicosis, 106–108
Depigmentation, retinal, 195
Dermatitis
  atopic, 175–176, 183–184
  contact, 176–177
  poison ivy, oak, and sumac, 187–188
  Rhus, 187–188
  venenata, 176–177
Dermatologic disorders, 174–196
Dermatophytosis, 61–62
Dermoid, 273–274
Dermolipoma, 273–274
  in oculoauriculovertibral dysplasia, 224
Descemet's membrane, stripping or detachment of, 352–354
Detachment, choroidal, 381–382, 388–390
  ciliochoroidal, 388–390, 569–570
  disciform, 390–392
  of Descemet's membrane, 352–354
  retinal. See *Retinal detachment.*
  rhegmatogenous, 671
Diabetes insipidus, in histiocytosis X, 367
Diabetes mellitus, 144–146
  accommodative spasm with, 580
  Bell's palsy with, 236
  cataract with, 613, 616
  dacryoadenitis with, 597
  filamentary keratitis with, 444
  hyperlipoproteinemia with, 157
  hypotony with, 569
  ischemic optic neropathy with, 633
  low tension glaucoma with, 564
  muromycosis with, 62
  neovascular glaucoma with, 594
  retinal detachment with, 675, 677
  rubeosis iridis with, 592
  vein occlusion with, 681
  vitiligo with, 194
  Werner's syndrome with, 218
Diabetic retinopathy, 144–146, 218
  with cystoid macular edema, 624–627
Dialysis, retinal breaks from, 671
Diaphyseal dysplasia, 212–213
Diastrophic dwarfism, with Robin sequence, 225
Diffuse unilateral subacute neuroretinitis, 668–669
Diktyoma, 279–280
Dimples, Fuchs', 423

Diphtheria, 15–16
  with ankyloblepharon, 493
Diplopia, 397
  in abducens paralysis, 461
  in chronic progressive external ophthalmoplegia, 243
  in dacryoadenitis, 597
  in high AC/A ratio, 476
  in internal orbital fracture, 335
  in iridodialysis, 350
  in mucocele, 282
  in myasthenia gravis, 262
  in neurilemoma, 284
  in superior oblique palsy, 488
  in temporal arteritis, 170
Dirofilariasis, 108–109
Disc, choked, 637–639
Disc neovascularization, in diabetes mellitus, 144–146
Disciform herpetic disease, 80
Disciform macular degeneration, 390–392
Dislocation, of lens, 618–620
Dissociated nystagmus, 482–486
Dissociated vertical deviation and divergence, 472–473
Distichiasis, 498–500
  in symblepharon, 528
Dot dystrophy, 427–428
Downbeat nystagmus, 482–486
Downgrowth, epithelial, 378–379
Down's syndrome, 216–218
Dracontiasis, 109–110
Dracunculiasis, 109–110
Dracunculosis, 109–110
Drug-induced optic atrophy, 632–633
Dry eye syndrome, 449–452
  in familial dysautonomia, 363
Duane's retraction syndrome, 474–475
  with abducens paralysis, 460
  with V-pattern exotropia, 492
Dwarfism, 215–219
Dysautonomia, familial, 362–364
Dyscephaly, mandibulo-oculofacial, 222–223
Dyslexia, 248–249
Dysmorphia, mandibulo-oculofacial, 222–223
Dysostosis, craniofacial, 211–212
  mandibulofacial, 222–227
  multiplex, 147–148
Dysplasia, diaphyseal, 212–213
  intraepithelial, 289–291
  oculoauriculovertebral, 224–225
Dysthyroid exophthalmos, 643–646
Dysthyroidism, 245

Eales' disease, 669
Echinococcosis, 110–111
Eclipse burn, 630–631
Ectasia, corneal, 438–439
  marginal, 426
Ectodermal dysplasia, with filamentary keratitis, 444
Ectopia lentis, 618–620
  with congenital cataract, 616
Ectropion, 500–502
  in Bell's palsy, 234
  in epiphora, 610
  in ichthyosis, 182
  in mycosis fungoides, 300
  in thermal burns, 325
Eczema, atopic, 175–176

Edema
    angioneurotic, 192–194
    Berlin's, 339
    bilateral, in trichinosis, 123
    corneal, 442
    giant, 192–194
    macular, cystoid, 624–627
    orbital, 193–194
Electrical injury, 320–322
Embolus, retinal, 678–679
Encephalitis
    granulomatous, 98
    Guillain-Barré, 94
    with leptospirosis, 26
Encephalopathy, perinatal, 241–243
Encephalotrigeminal syndrome, 231–232
Endocrine disorders, 125–131
Endocrine exophthalmos, autoimmune, 643–646
Endophthalmitis
    bacterial, 379, 533–535
    fungal, 535–537
    nocardial, 31
    phacoanaphylactic, 573–574
    with aspergillosis, 55
    with *Bacillus subtilis* infection, 9
    with candidiasis, 58, 132
    with *Clostridium perfringens* infection, 12–13
    with coccidioidomycosis, 59–60
    with corneal abrasion, 313
    with erythema multiforme, 178
    with *Escherichia coli* infection, 18–19
    with fungal keratitis, 447
    with intraocular copper foreign body, 328
    with *Listeria monocytogenes* infection, 28
    with ophthalmic neonatorum, 416
    with *Pneumococcus* infection, 32
    with *Propionibacterium acnes* infection, 33
    with *Proteus* infection, 34
    with sporotrichosis, 67
    with *Staphylococcus* infection, 38
    with *Streptococcus* infection, 40
    with thermal burns, 326
    with tularemia, 45
    with typhoid fever, 47
    with vitreous wick syndrome, 700
    with yersinosis, 48
Englemann's disease, 212–213
Enophthalmos, 640–641
    congenital, with muscle fibrosis and ptosis, 470–471
    with internal orbital fracture, 335
    with neurofibromatosis, 230
Enteritis, regional, 132–134
Entropion, 52, 502–505, 529
    with distichiasis, 500
    with epiphora, 610
    with erythema multiforme, 178
    with thermal burns, 325
    with trachoma, 52
Eosinophilic granuloma, 364–367
Ephelides, 518
Epiblepharon, 506
Epicanthus, 505–506
Epidemic hemorrhagic keratoconjunctivitis, 76–77
Epidemic keratoconjunctivitis, 78–79
Epidermolytic hyperkeratosis, 181–182
Epidermomycosis, 61–62
Epidermophytosis, 61–62
Epikeratophakia, 650
Epiphora, 609–610

Episcleral venous pressure, elevated, with glaucoma, 550–551
Episcleritis, 689
    in coccidioidomycosis, 59
    in Crohn's disease, 132
    in gout, 160
    in relapsing polychondritis, 203
    in rheumatoid arthritis, 204
Epithelial basement membrane dystrophy, 427–428
Epithelial cyst, 377–378, 440–441, 587–588
Epithelial downgrowth, 378–379
Epithelial edema, 442
Epithelial erosion, recurrent, 427–428
Epithelial implantation cyst, 587–588
Epithelial ingrowth, 377–378
Epithelial tumor, 556, 598–600
Epithelioma, intraepithelial, 289–291
Epitheliopathy, 453
Epstein-Barr virus, 84
Erysipelas, 17–18
Erythema multiforme, 177–179
Erythema nodosum leprosum, 25–26
Escherichia coli infection, 18–19
Esotropia
    accommodative, 461–463
    A-pattern, 466–467
    congenital, 463
    essential-infantile, 471–472
    nonaccommodative, acquired, 465–466
    V-pattern, 490–491
    with abducens paralysis, 460
    with high AC/A ratio, 475–476
Essential-infantile esotropia, 476–477
Ewing's sarcoma, 291–292, 304, 310
Exfoliation syndrome, 543–545
Exophthalmos
    dysthyroid, 643–646
    endocrine, autoimmune, 643–646
    in Crouzon's disease, 211
    in Englemann's disease, 211
    in histiocytosis X, 366
    in neurofibromatosis, 230
    in orbital Graves' disease, 643
Exotropia
    A-pattern, 467–468
    basic, 468–469
    intermittent, 478–481
    V-pattern, 491–492
Expulsive hemorrhage, 392–394
Extraocular muscles, 460–492
    congenital fibrosis of, 470–471
    lacerations of, 344–345
Exudative vitreoretinopathy, familial, 694–695
Eyelashes, loss of, 515–516, 530
Eyelid, 493–531
    avulsions of, 345–347
    baggy, 520
    bilateral edema of, in trichinosis, 123
    coloboma of, 507
    contusions of, 345–347
    floppy, 507–508
    lacerations of, 345–347
    melanocytic lesions of, 517–520
    myokymia of, 513
    retraction of, 514–515
Eye-worm disease, African *Loa loa*, 111–112

Fabry's disease, 156–157, 616
Facets, 423

Facial paralysis, idiopathic, 234–236
Familial dysautonomia, 362–364
　alacrima with, 603
　neuroparalytic keratitis with, 452
Familial exudative vitreoretinopathy, 694–695
Far-sightedness, 652–653
Fat, orbital, herniation of, 520
Febrile polyneuritis, acute, 233–234
Fehr's macular dystrophy, 433–434
Fever, blackwater, 114
　Brazilian prupuric, 24
　Japanese river, 70–72
　Malta, 11–12
　Mediterranean, 11–12, 358
　pharyngoconjunctival, 92–93
　Q, 68–69
　query, 68–69
　rabbit, 45–46
　recurrent, 37–38
　relapsing, 37–38
　Rocky Mountain spotted, 69–70
　typhoid, 46–48
　typhus, 70–72
　undulent, 11–12
　uveoparotid, 601–602
Fiber, ragged red, chronic progressive external ophthalmoplegia with, 243–245
Fibroblastic ingrowth, 379–380
Fibrocytic ingrowth, 379–380
Fibroplasia, retrolental, 683–685
Fibrosarcoma, 292–293
Fibrosis, congenital, of extraocular muscles, 470–471
　of inferior rectus, with ptosis, 470–471
　macular, preretinal, 628–630
Fibrous ingrowth, 378–379
Filamentary keratitis, 444–445
Filtering blebs, 410–411
Fingerprint dystrophy, 427–428
Fisher's syndrome, 233–234
Fistula
　arteriovenous, 164–166
　carotid cavernous, 165–166
Floppy eyelid syndrome, 507–508
Foreign body, intraocular
　conjunctival lacerations from, 342
　copper, 326–329
　corneal abrasions from, 343
　inert, 329–330
　iron, 330–332
　nonmagnetic, 329–330
　orbital cellulitis with, 642
　steel, 330–332
Foveomacular retinitis, 630–631
Fractures, 333–338
　blowout, 335–337, 641
　external orbital, 333–335
　internal orbital, 335–337
　LeFort, 333
　of optic foramen, 337–338
Fragile bone disease, 219–222
Franceschetti syndrome, 223–224
Francisella tularensis infection, 45–46
Francois syndrome, 222–223
Francois-Hallermann-Streiff syndrome, 222–223
Freckles, on eyelid, 518
Frostbite injury, 322–323
Fuchs' corneal dystrophy, 435–436
Fuchs' dellen, 423
Fuchs' dimples, 423
Fuchs' heterochromic iridocyclitis, 582–584
Functional amblyopia, 250–251

Fungal endophthalmitis, 535–537
Fungal keratitis, 445–448
Furrow dystrophy, 426
Fusobacterium infection, 19–20

Galactosemias, 146–147
Gamma ray injury, 323–324
Gaze paresis, 233–234
Gaze-evoked nystagmus, 482–486
General fibrosis syndrome, 470–471
German measles, 94–95
Ghost cell glaucoma, 545–546
Giant cell arteritis, 169–171
　with ischemic optic neuropathy, 633
　with retinal artery occlusion, 663
Giant edema, 192–194
Giant papillary conjunctivitis, 400–402, 411–413
Giant urticaria, 192–194
Glaucoma. See also *Aniridia*.
　after ocular contusion, 547–548
　angle-closure, 537, 541, 577–579
　aphakic pupillary block, 539–541
　capsular, 543–545
　chronic angle-closure, 541
　ciliary block, 565–567
　closed angle, 337, 541, 577–579
　congenital, 435
　corticosteroid-induced, 542–543
　expulsive hemorrhage in, 393–394
　ghost cell, 545–546
　infantile, 559
　juvenile, 559–562
　lens-induced, 562–564
　low-tension, 564–565
　malignant, 565–567
　narrow-angle, 577–579
　neovascular, 145, 592–594
　open-angle, 559, 562–565, 570–573
　phacolytic, 562–564
　pigmentary, 574–575
　primary angle-closure, 577–579
　primary narrow-angle, 577–579
　pupillary block, 553
　with anterior uveitis, 548–550
　with aphakic eye, 552
　with blindness, 541
　with elevated episcleral venous pressure, 550–551
　with Englemann's disease, 213
　with epithelial ingrowth, 378–379
　with exfoliation syndrome, 543
　with familial dysautonomia, 363–364
　with fibrous ingrowth, 379
　with Fuchs' heterochromic iridocyclitis, 583
　with Hallermann-Streiff-Francois syndrome, 222–223
　with homocystinuria, 137–138
　with intraocular lenses, 551–554
　with intraocular tumors, 554–558
　with juvenile rheumatoid arthritis, 198
　with juvenile xanthogranuloma, 274
　with leiomyoma, 277–278
　with lens dislocation, 618
　with medulloepithelioma, 279
　with microspherophakia, 621–622
　with mucopolysaccharidosis I-S, 149–150
　with myopia, 653
　with neurofibromatosis, 230
　with oculocerebrorenal syndrome, 141
　with postoperative flat anterior chamber, 380–381
　with rheumatoid arthritis, 204–205

Glaucoma (cont'd.)
  with Robin sequence, 225–226
  with rubeosis iridis, 592
  with sarcoidosis, 369–371
  with scleral staphyloma, 690
  with sickle cell disease, 168
  with Sturge-Weber syndrome, 231–232
  with Weill-Marchesani syndrome, 209–210
Glaucomatocyclitic crisis, 558
Glioma, optic, 284–286
Gliosis, preretinal, massive, 696–698
Global rupture, indirect, 348–349
  with lens dislocation, 619
Globe, 532–538
Glycolipid lipidosis, 156–157
Goiter, hypothyroid, 130–131
Goldenhar's syndrome, 224–225
  with dermoid, 274
Gonococcal ocular disease, 20–22
Gonorrhea, 20–22
Gonorrheal ophthalmia neonatorum, 417
Gougerot-Sjögren syndrome, 206–207
Gout, 160–161
Granular corneal dystrophy, 431–432
Granuloma, eosinophilic, 365–367
Granulomatosis, Wegener's 172–173
Graves' disease, 643–646
  accommodative spasm with, 580
Greig's syndrome, 213–215
Groenouw's type I dystrophy, 431–432
Groenouw's type II dystrophy, 432–434
Grönblad-Strandberg syndrome, 202–203
Guillain-Barré encephalitis, 94
Guillain-Barré syndrome, 10, 26, 233–234
Guinea worm infection, 109–110
Gyrate atrophy, of choroid, 670–671

Hallermann-Streiff syndrome, 222–223
Hallermann-Streiff-Francois syndrome, 222–223
Hamartomatoses, systemic, 556
Hand-Schüller-Christian disease, 364–367
Hansen's disease, 24–26
  lagophthalmos in, 512
Harada's syndrome, 372–373
  with retinal detachment, 675
Hay fever conjunctivitis, 400–402
Headache, 251–255
  cluster, 246–247
  histamine, 246–247
  in intracranial hypertension, 237–238
  migraine, 252, 254
  tension, 253–254
  vascular, 251
Heerfordt's syndrome, 601–602
Hemangioblastoma, 268–270
  retinal, 228–229
Hemangio-endothelioma, benign, 268–270
Hemangioma
  angioblastic, 268–270
  capillary, 268–270
  cavernous, 270–271
  of optic disc, 228–229
  racemose, 164–165
  strawberry, 268–270
Hematologic disorders, 164–173
Hematopoietic disorder, pruritus in, 188
Hemifacial spasm, 509
Hemophilus aegyptius infection, 24
Hemophilus influenzae infection, 22–23

Hemorrhage. See also *Bleeding; Vitreous hemorrhage.*
  expulsive, 392–394
  orbital, 646–647
  retinal, primary, in young men, 669
Hemorrhagic choroidal detachment, 381–382, 389
Hemorrhagic disciform detachment, 390–392
Hereditary angioedema, 192–194
Hereditary deep dystrophy, 437
Hereditary diaphyseal dysphasia, 212–213
Hereditary endothelial dystrophy, congenital, 435
Hereditary mesodermal dystrophy, 437
Hereditary multiple diaphyseal sclerosis, 212–213
Heredopathia atactica polyneuritiformis, 674–675
Herellea vaginicola infection, 3–4
Herniation, of orbital fat, 520
Herpes keratoconjunctivitis, in newborns, 416–417
Herpes simplex, 79–82, 456
  erythema multiforme with, 177
  malaria with, 113
  ophthalmia neonatorum with, 416
Herpes zoster, 82–84
  corneal mucous plaques with, 422
  neuroparalytic keratitis with, 452
Herpetic keratitis, recurrent, 80
  with corneal edema, 442
Heterochromia iridis, with Waardenburg's syndrome, 227
Heterochromic iridocyclitis, Fuchs', 582–584
Hirschsprung's disease, 226–227
Hirsutism, 179–181
Histamine headache, 246–247
Histiocytosis X, 364–367
Histoplasmosis, ocular, 63–64
Hives, 192–194
HLA-B27, 367
HLA-BW51, 359
Hodgkin's disease, 293–294
Holes, in iris, 349–350
  macular, 627–628
  retinal, 671
Homocystinuria, 137–138
  with congenital cataracts, 616
  with lens dislocation, 619
  with microspherophakia, 621
Homozygous familial hypobetalipoproteinemia, 657–659
Hordeolum, 510–511
Horner's syndrome, 246
  with cluster headache, 246
  with Hodgkin's disease, 293
  with ptosis, 521
Human immunodeficiency virus, type 1, 72–73, 75–76
Hunter syndrome, 150–151
Hurler syndrome, 147–148
Hurler/Scheie syndrome, 148–149
Hydatid cyst hydatidosis, 110–111
Hydrophobia, 93–94
Hyperkeratosis, epidermolytic, 181–182
Hyperlipidemia, 157–159
  retinal vein obstruction with, 681
  xanthelasma with, 531
Hyperlipoproteinemia, 157–159
Hypermetropia, 652–653
  functional amblyopia with, 250
Hyperopia, 652–653
Hyperornithinemia, 670–671
Hyperostosis, progressive, 212–213
Hyperparathyroidism, 125–126
  corneal calcification with, 408

Hyperplasia, lymphoid, benign, 298, 556–557
  reactive, 297–299, 556–557
Hyperproteinemia, with retinal vein obstruction, 681
Hypersecretion, lacrimal, 610–611
Hyperstosis corticalis generalisata familiaris, 212–213
Hypertelorism, orbital, 213–215
Hypertension, benign, intracranial, 236–240
  ocular, 567–569
Hypertrichosis, 179–181
Hypertropia, 474–475
Hyperuricemia, 160–161
Hypesthesia, corneal, in familial dysautonomia, 363
Hyphema. See *Bleeding*; *Hemorrhage*; *Vitreous hemorrhage*.
Hypobetalipoproteinemia, familial, homozygous, 657–659
Hypocalcemia, 126–129
Hypoparathyroidism, 129–130
Hyposecretion, lacrimal, 611–612
Hypothermal injury, 322–323
Hypothyroid goiter, 130–131
Hypothyroidism, 130–131
Hypotony, 569–570
Hypovitaminosis A, 134–135
Hysteria, 255–256

Ichthyosis, 181–182
Idiopathic facial paralysis, 234–236
Idiopathic intracranial hypertension, 236–240
Idiopathic multiple pigmented sarcoma, 294–296
Idiopathic orbital inflammation, 298
Idiopathic polyneuritis, acute, 233–234
Ileitis, terminal, 132–134
Ileocolitis, granulomatous, 132–134
Ill-sustained accommodation, 464–465
Impetigo, 182–183
  ankyloblepharon with, 493
Implant, orbital, extrusion of, 332–333
Implantation. See also *Lens implantation*.
  cyst, epithelial, 587–588
Inclusion conjunctivitis, 50–51, 416–418
Infantile cataract, 616–618
Infantile essential esotropia, 471–472
Infantile glaucoma, 559
Infection
  bacterial, 3–97, 312, 416–418
  chlamydial, 50–53
  mycotic, 53–68
  rickettsial, 68–72
  staphylococcal, of eyelid, 510–511
  viral, 72–97
  with adenovirus, 92
  with guinea worm, 109–110
Infectious crystalline keratopathy, 448–449
Infectious mononucleosis, 84–85
Infectious polyneuritis, acute, 233–234
Inflammation, orbital, idiopathic, 298
Inflammatory disease, of retinal vein, 669
Inflammatory polyradiculoneuropathy, 233–234
Inflammatory pseudotumor, 297–299
Inflammatory tumor, 598–600
Influenza, 85–86
  orbital cellulitis and abscess with, 642
Infrared ray injury, 323–324
Ingrowth
  epithelial, 378–379
  fibrous, 379–380
  stromal, 379–380
Injuries
  from burns, 312–325
  from foreign bodies, 326–333
  from fractures, 333–338
  from lacerations, tears, and contusions, 338–355
  from venom, 355–357
  mechanical and nonmechanical, 312–357
  scleral, sharp, 348–349
Insufficiency
  accommodative, 464–465
  of convergence, 472–474
Intermittent exotropia, 478–481
Intestinal parasites, phlyctenulosis with, 456
Intracranial hypertension
  benign, 236–240
  with abducens paralysis, 460
Intraocular epithelial cyst, 379–381
Intraocular lenses
  glaucoma with, 551–554
  uveitis with, 552
  vitreous hemorrhage with, 698
Intraocular pressure, 539–579
Intravitreous cysticercosis, 105
Iridocorneal endothelial syndrome, 584–586
Iridocyclitis, 569. See also *Uveitis*.
  chronic, in Crohn's disease, 132–133
  heterochromic, Fuchs', 582–584
  toxoplasmic, 121–123
  with ankylosing spondylitis, 219–220
  with juvenile rheumatoid arthritis, 197–198
  with leptospirosis, 27
Iridodialysis, 349–350
  with lens dislocation, 619
Iridovitreal block, 565–567
Iris, 580–596
  atrophy of, essential, progressive, 584–586
  bombé, 586–587
  cysts on, 587–588
  holes in, 349–350
  lacerations of, 349–350
  melanoma of, 555, 588–589
  plateau, 575–576
  prolapse of, 589–590
Iritis
  with Behçet's disease, 359
  with Crohn's disease, 132
  with intraocular inert foreign body, 329
  with leprosy, 25
  with malaria, 113
  with Moore's ulcer, 424
  with rheumatoid arthritis, 205
Iron, intraocular, injury from, 330–332
Irritative conjunctivitis, 413–414
Irvine-Gass syndrome, 624–627
Ischemic optic neuropathy, 633–635
  in temporal arteritis, 170

Japanese river fever, 70–72
Jaw-winking syndrome, 516–517
Juvenile cerebral palsy, 242–243
Juvenile corneal epithelial dystrophy, 428–429
Juvenile glaucoma, 559–562
Juvenile hypothyroidism, 130–131
Juvenile Paget's disease, 212–213
Juvenile rheumatoid arthritis, 197–198
  juvenile glaucoma with, 560
Juvenile xanthogranuloma, 274–275, 364

Kaposi's sarcoma, 294–296
Kearns-Sayre-Daroff syndrome, 243–245
Kearns-Shy syndrome, 243–245

Keloid, corneal, 141
Keratitis
  acne rosacea, 455
  acute, interstitial, 14
  bacterial, 415, 439–440
  bullosa interna, 437
  epithelial, dendritic, 84
  filamentary, 444–445
  fungal, 445–448
  furrow, 426
  herpetic epithelial recurrent, 80
  mucosa, 422–423
  neuroparalytic, 452–454
  neurotropic, 452–454
  pseudodendritic, 142–143
  sicca, 449–452
  stromal herpetic, 80
  with *Acanthamoebae* infection, 98
  with acute idiopathic polyneuritis, 233–234
  with aspergillosis, 55
  with *Azobacter* infection, 7
  with *Candida* infection, 57
  with Cogan's syndrome, 362
  with congenital syphilis, 13–14
  with herpes simplex, 113
  with herpes zoster, 82–83
  with hypoparathyroidism, 129
  with inclusion conjunctivitis, 416
  with influenza, 85
  with lagophthalmos, 511
  with molluscum contagiosum, 68
  with mumps, 88
  with Newcastle disease, 89
  with ocular vaccinia, 90
  with papilloma, 287
  with pharyngoconjunctival fever, 92
  with sporotrichosis, 66
  with *Staphylococcus* infection, 39
  with *Streptococcus* infection, 40
  with systemic sclerosis, 201
  with tuberculosis, 43
  with tyrosinemia II, 142
  with varicella, 96
Keratoacanthoma, 275–276
Keratoconjunctivitis. See also *Conjunctivitis*.
  atopic, 175–176, 400–401
  chronic, 51–52
  epidemic, 78–79
  hemorrhagic epidemic, 76–77
  herpetic, in newborn, 416–417
  limbic, 457–458
  meibomian, 523–524
  phlyctenular, 44, 454–456
  superior limbic, 444–445, 457–458
  vernal, 400–401, 420–421
  with *Acinetobacter* infection, 4
  with atopic dermatitis, 175
  with candidiasis, 57
  with contact dermatitis, 176
  with hypoparathyroidism, 129
  with neurodermatitis, 183
  with psoriasis, 191–192
  with rheumatoid arthritis, 204, 206
  with Sjögren's syndrome, 206–207
  with systemic lupus erythematosus, 208–209
  with systemic sclerosis, 201
  with trachoma, 51–53
Keratoconjunctivitis sicca, 449–452
  with Cockayne's syndrome, 215–216
  with corneal mucous plaques, 422–423
  with erythema multiforme, 177–179
  with filamentary keratitis, 444–445
  with hypothyroidism, 130–131
  with lacrimal hyposecretion, 611–612
  with Mikulicz's syndrome, 600
  with relapsing polychondritis, 203–204
  with rheumatoid arthritis, 204–206
  with Sjögren's syndrome, 206
Keratoconus, 438–439
  with astigmatism, 651
  with Down's syndrome, 217
Keratomileusis, 650
Keratomycosis, 445–448
  with *Aspergillus* infection, 55
  with stripping or detachment of Descemet's membrane, 353
Keratopathy
  band, 125–126, 198, 408–409, 453
  bullous, 442
  exposure, in chronic progressive external ophthalmoplegia, 244
  in ankylosing spondylitis, 219–220
  infectious crystalline, 448–449
  neuropathic, trigeminal, 452–454
  Thygeson's superficial punctate, 458–459
Keratophakia, 650
Keratosis
  actinic, 267–268
  recessive, palmoplantaris, 142–143
  seborrheic, 267–268
  with ultraviolet radiation, 315
Keratosulfaturia, 152–153
Ketoaciduria, branched-chain, 138–140
Klein-Waardenburg syndrome, 226–227
Koch-Weeks bacillus, 24
Koeppe's posterior polymorphous degeneration, 437
Komoto's tetrad, 505

Lacerations, 338–355
  chorioretinal, 338–339
  of ciliary body, 339–341
  of conjunctiva, 342–343
  of cornea, 343–344
  of extraocular muscle, 344–345
  of eyelid, 345–347
  of iris, 349–350
  of lacrimal system, 351–352
Lacrimal gland, 597–602
  tumors of, 598–600
Lacrimal hypersecretion, 610–611
Lacrimal hyposecretion, 611–612
Lacrimal system, 597–612
  congenital anomalies of, 604–605
  contusions of, 351–352
  lacerations of, 351–352
Lagophthalmos, 511–512
  with Bell's palsy, 511
Lamellar ichthyosis, 181–182
Landry-Guillain-Barré-Strohl syndrome, 233–234
Landry's paralysis, 233–234
Lashes. See *Eyelashes*.
Lattice corneal dystrophy, 432–433
Leaking, 410–411
LeFort fracture, 333
Leiomyoma, 277–278
Leishmaniasis
  cutaneous, 104–105
  mucocutaneous, American, 100–101
  Old World, 104–105

Lens, 613–622
Lens capsule, pseudoexfoliation of, 543–545
Lens dislocation, 618–620
Lens implantation
 in aphakia, 649–650
 in glaucoma, 551–554
 -induced glaucoma, 562–564
 -induced uveitis, 552
 post-cataract surgery, for low vision, 257
Lens luxation, 618–620
Lenticonus, 620–621
Lentiglobus, 620–621
Lentigo senilis, on eyelid, 518
Lentigo simplex, on eyelid, 518
Leprosy, 24–26
 lagophthalmos in, 512
Leptospirosis, 26–28
Lesions
 corneal, in tyrosinemia II, 142–143
 melanocytic, of eyelid, 517–520
Letterer-Siwe disease, 364–367
Leukemia, 556
 Midulicz's syndrome in, 600
 mucormycosis in, 62
 T-cell lymphoma-, 300–301
Lice, 115–117
Lichen simplex chronicus, 183–184
Lid. See *Eyelid*.
Ligneous conjunctivitis, 414–415
 with filamentary keratitis, 444
Limbic keratoconjunctivitis, superior, 457–458
Lipid metabolism disorders, 156–159
Lipodermoid, 273–274
Liposarcoma, 296
Listeriosis, 28–29
Liver disease, pruritus in, 188
Loa loa, 111–112
Lockjaw, 42–43
Loiasis, 111–112
Low vision, 256–259
Lowe's syndrome, 141–142
Low-tension glaucoma, 564–565
Lues, 4–6
Lupus erythematosus, systemic, 207–209
Luxation, of lens, 618–620
Lyme disease, 86–87
Lymphangioma, 278–279
Lymphoid hyperplasia, benign, 298
Lymphoid tumor, 297–299, 556, 598–600
Lymphoma
 cutaneous, 300–301
 intraocular, 297–299
 malignant, 297–299
 systemic, 298
 T-cell, 300–301
Lymphomatoid papulosis, 300–301

Macula, 623–631
Macular corneal dystrophy, 433–434
Macular degeneration, age-related, 623–627
 disciform, 390–392
Macular edema
 cystoid, 624–627
 with gyrate atrophy, 670
 with retinal vein obstruction, 679–682
Macular fibrosis, preretinal, 628–630
Macular hole, 627–628
Macular pucker, 628–630

Maculopathy, cellophane, 628–630
 cystoid, 624–627
Madarosis, 515–516
 in acrodermatitis enteropathica, 174
 in dermatophytosis, 62
Malaria, 112–114
Malignancy, pruritus in, 188
Malignant epithelial tumor, 598–600
Malignant glaucoma, 565–567
 with postoperative flat anterior chamber, 380
Malignant lymphoma, 297–299
Malignant melanoma, of posterior uvea, 394–398
Malingering, 255–256
Malta fever, 11–12
Malum venereum, 4–6
Mandibulofacial dysostosis, 222–227
 with congenital cataract, 616
Mandibulo-oculofacial dyscephaly, 222–223
Mandibulo-oculofacial dysmorphia, 222–223
Map dystropy, 427–428
Maple syrup urine disease, 138–140
Marble bone disease, 220–222
Marachesani's syndrome, with juvenile glaucoma, 560
Marcus Gunn syndrome, 516–517
Marfan's syndrome
 juvenile glaucoma in, 560
 lens dislocation in, 619
 microspherophakia in, 621
 scleral staphyloma in, 690
Marginal corneal degeneration, pellucid, 425
Marginal ectasia, 426
Marie-Strumpell disease, 219–220
Maroteau-Lamy syndrome, 153–154
Massive exudative retinitis, 667–668
Massive preretinal gliosis, 696–698
Massive preretinal proliferation, 696–698
Massive vitreous retraction, 696–698
Measles, 95–95
 accommodative spasm with, 580
 German. See *Rubella*.
Medicamentosa conjunctivitis, 527
Mediterranean fever, 11–12, 358
Medulloepithelioma, 279–280
Meesmann's corneal dystrophy, 428–429
Meibomian gland granuloma, 497–498
Meibomian keratoconjunctivitis, 523–524
Melanocytic lesion of eyelid, 517–520
Melanoma
 choroidal, 394–398, 555
 malignant, of posterior uvea, 394–398
 of ciliary body, 394–398, 555
 of eyelid, 517–520
 of iris, 555, 588–589
Melanosis, 406–408
Melitococcosis, 11–12
Meningioma, 280–282
Meningismus, 26
Meningitis, bacterial, of childhood, 22–23
Meretoja's syndrome, 432–433
Metabolic disease, pruritus in, 188
Metabolic disorders, 160–163
 of carbohydrates, 144–155
 of lipid, 156–159
 of protein, 136–143
Metaplasia, fibrous, 379–380
 of lens, 615
Metastatic calcification, in hyperparathyroidism, 125
Metastatic neuroblastoma, 301–302
Metastatic ocular tuberculosis, 44

Metastatic tumor. See also *Tumor*.
  ocular, 302–303
  orbital, 304–305
  to uvea, 555
Microgliomatosis, 298
Microphthalmos, 532–533
  with congenital cataracts, 618
  with endophthalmos, 640
Microspherophakia, 621–622
  in Weill-Marchesani syndrome, 209
Microstrabismus, 481–482
Microtropia, 481–482
Microwave injury, 323–324
Migraine, 251–252
  isolated ophthalmic, 252, 254
  pediatric, 254
Migrainous neuralgia, periodic, 246–247
Mikulicz's syndrome, 600–601
Mikulicz-Radecki syndrome, 600–601
Mikulicz-Sjögren syndrome, 600–601
Mima polymorpha infection, 3–4
Minimal brain dysfunction syndrome, 249
Mite-bourne typhus, 70–72
Mixed staphylococcal/seborrheic blepharoconjunctivitis, 525–527
Molluscum contagiosum, 87–88
Mongolism, 216–218
Monofixation syndrome, 481–482
Mononucleosis, infectious, 84–85
Mooren's ulcer, 424
Moraxella infection, 7, 29–30
Morbilli, 95–96
Morquio syndrome, 152–153
Morquio-Brailsford syndrome, 152–153
Mucocele, 282–283
Mucopolysaccharidosis
  I-H, 147–148
  I-H/S, 148–149
  I-S, 149–150
  II, 150–151
  III, 151–152
  IV, 152–153
  VI, 153–154
  VII, 154–155
Mucopurulent conjunctivitis, 402–403
Mucormycosis, 62–63
  with thermal burns, 325
Mucous membrane, pemphigoid, benign, 403–406
Mucous plaque, corneal, 422–423
Multiceps infection, 103
Multiple sclerosis, 259–261
  optic neuritis in, 635
Mumps, 88–89
  Mikulicz's syndrome in, 600
Muscles, extraocular, 460–492
  congenital fibrosis of, 470–471
  lacerations of, 344–345
  progressive dystrophy of, 243–245
Muscles, ocular, fibrosis and ptosis of, 470–471
Muscular dystrophy, 243–245
Myasthenia gravis, 245, 261–262
  progressive external ophthalmoplegia in, 243
  ptosis in, 521
Mycobacterium leprae infection, 24
Mycosis fungoides, 300–301
Mycotic infection, 533–68
Myokymia
  of eyelid, 513
  superior, oblique, 488
Myopathy, ocular and oculoskeletal, 243–245

Myopia, 580, 653–656
  choroidal neovascular membranes with, 390
  gyrate atrophy with, 670
  high AC/A ratio with, 476–477
  lenticular, in Weill-Marchesani syndrome, 209–210
  macular hole with, 627–628
  microspherophakia with, 621
  pathologic, 653
  physiologic, 653
Myxedema, 130–131

Nanophthalmos, 537–538
Narrow-angle glaucoma, primary, 577–579
Necrosis, retinal, acute, 659–661
Necrotizing angiitis, 198–200
Neisseria gonococcus infection, 4
Neisseria gonorrhoeae infection, 20–22
Neonatal ophthalmia, 416–418
Neoplasm, 267–311. See also *Carcinoma; Tumor;* specific neoplasm.
  benign, 267–288
  invasive, 289–291
  malignant, 288–311
Neoplastic angioendotheliomatosis pseudolymphoma, 297–299
Neovascular glaucoma, 592–594
Neovascularization
  corneal, 443–444
  of disc, in diabetes mellitus, 144–146
  retinal. See *Retinal neovascularization*.
  subretinal, 390–392
Nerve
  third (oculomotor), paralysis of, 486–487
  sixth (abducens), paralysis of, 460–461
Nettle rash, 192–194
Neuralgia
  ciliary, 246–247
  cranial, 253
  migrainous, periodic, 246–247
  trigeminal, 265–266
Neurilemoma, 283–284
Neurinoma, 283–284
Neuritis, optic, 259–260, 635–636
  retrobulbar, 635–636
Neuroblastoma, metastatic, 301–302
Neurodermatitis, 183–184
Neurofibromatosis (NF-1), 229–231
Neurologic disorders, 233–266
Neuromuscular disease, oculocraniosomatic, 243–245
Neuroparalytic keratitis, 452–454
Neuropathic keratopathy, trigeminal, 452–454
Neuropathy, optic, in Crohn's disease, 132
  ischemic, 633–635
Neuroretinitis, diffuse unilateral subacute, 668–669
Neurosyphilis, 5
  in AIDS, 73
Neurotropic keratitis, 452–454
Nevoxanthoendothelioma, 274–275
Nevus
  benign, 406–408
  of eyelid, 517–520
  of Ota, 518
Newcastle disease, 89–90
Night blindness
  in Crohn's disease, 132–133
  in gyrate atrophy, 670
  in hypovitaminosis A, 134

Night blindness (cont'd.)
  in Refsum's disease, 674
  in retinitis pigmentosa, 682
Nocardiosis, 30–31
Nocturnal cephalalgia, proxysmal, 246–247
Nonmagnetic chemically inert foreign body, intraocular, 329–330
Nutritional disorders, 132–135
Nystagmus, 482–486
  in abetalipoproteinemia, 657
  in cerebral palsy, 242
  in Down's syndrome, 217
  in maple syrup urine disease, 139
  in rubella, 94
  in toxoplasmosis, 121–123
  rebound, 482–486
  with congenital cataracts, 617

Obstruction, of retinal vein, 679–682
Occlusion
  of branch retinal vein, 661–663
  of retinal artery, 663–665
Occlusion hypertropia, 474–475
Ocular contusion, glaucoma after, 547–548
Ocular histoplasmosis, 63–64
Ocular hypertension, 567–569
Ocular hypotony, 569–570
Ocular metastatic tumor, 302–303
Ocular muscle fibrosis and ptosis, with congenital enophthalmos, 470–471
Ocular myopathy, 243–245
Ocular rosacea, 184–185
Ocular syphilis, in AIDS, 73
Ocular toxoplasmosis, 121–123
Ocular vaccinia, 90–91
Oculoauriculovertebral dysplasia, 224–225
Oculocerebrorenal syndrome, 141–142
Oculocraniosomatic neuromuscular disease, 243–245
Oculodermal melanocytosis, 517–520
Oculomotor (third nerve) paralysis, 486–487
Oculopharyngeal muscular dystrophy syndrome, 243–245
Oculoskeletal myopathy, 243–245
Oil drop cataract, 146
Old World leishmaniasis, 104–105
Onchocerciasis, 114–115
Open-angle glaucoma, 559, 562–565, 570–573
Ophthalmia, sympathetic, 398–399
Ophthalmia neonatorum, 32, 416–418
  chlamydial, 50
  gonococcal, 21
  gonorrheal, 417
Ophthalmic migraine headache, 252, 254
Ophthalmopathy
  of Graves' disease, 643–646
  thyroid, 514
Ophthalmoplegia
  abiotrophic, 243–245
  chronic progressive external, 243–245
  in abetalipoproteinemia, 657
  in acute idiopathic polyneuritis, 233
  in amyloidosis, 358
  in maple syrup urine disease, 140
  in orbital cellulitis, 342
  in Tolosa-Hunt syndrome, 264
  in toxoplasmosis, 121–123
  painful, 264–265
  plus, 243–245
Optic atrophy
  drug-induced, 632–633
  with cerebral palsy, 242
  with congenital syphilis, 13
  with Crouzon's disease, 211
  with Englemann's disease, 211
  with hyperparathyroidism, 125
  with maple syrup urine disease, 139
  with meningioma, 281
  with mucopolysaccharidosis I-H, 147
  with mucopolysaccharidosis VI, 153
  with optic foramen fractures, 337
  with osteoporosis, 221
Optic disc, capillary hemangiomas of, 228–229
Optic foramen fracture, 337–338
Optic glioma, 284–286
Optic nerve, 632–639
Optic neuritis, 635–636
  with infectious mononucleosis, 84
  with multiple sclerosis, 259–260
  with mumps, 88
  with systemic lupus erythematosus, 207
Optic neuropathy, in Crohn's disease, 132
  ischemic, 633–635
Orbit, 640–647
Orbital abscess, 641–643
  with sporotrichosis, 66
Orbital anomalies, in Crouzon's disease, 211
Orbital cellulitis, 641–643
  with *Clostridium perfringens* infection, 12
  with dacryocystitis, 607
  with *Hemophilus influenzae* infection, 23
  with mucormycosis, 62
  with ocular vaccinia, 90
  with *Pneumococcus* infection, 32
  with *Staphylococcus* infection, 38
  with *Streptococcus* infection, 40
Orbital edema, 193–194
Orbital fat herniation, 520
Orbital fractures, 333–335
Orbital Graves' disease, 643–646
Orbital hemorrhage, 646–647
Orbital hypertelorism, 213–215
Orbital implant extrusion, 332–333
Orbital metastases, 304–305
Oriental sore, 104–105
Ornithine ketoacid transaminase deficiency, 670–671
Orthophoria, monofixational, 481–482
Oscillation, saccadic, 482–486
Osteopathia hyperostotica sclerotisans multiplex infantilis, 212–213
Osteopetrosis, 220–222
Osteosclerosis congenita diffusa, 220–222
Osteosclerosis fragilis generalista, 220–222
Otitis media, in histiocytosis X, 367
Outflow system, 603–612
Overgrowth, stromal, 379–380

Paget's disease
  angioid streaks in, 387
  juvenile, 212–213
Pahvant Valley plague, 45–46
Painful ophthalmoplegia, 264–265
Palsy
  Bell's, 234–236, 511
  cerebral, 241–243
  of sixth nerve, 460–461
  progressive supranuclear, 263–264
  superior, oblique, 488–490
Panophthalmitis, in *Proteus* infection, 34.
  See also *Endophthalmitis*.

Papilledema, 637–639
  with acute idiopathic polyneuritis, 233
  with benign intracranial hypertension, 637
  with craniopharyngioma, 272
  with Englemann's diséase, 212
  with Hodgkin's disease, 293
  with hyperparathyroidism, 125
  with hypocalcemia, 127
  with hypoparathyroidism, 129
  with meningioma, 281
  with mucopolysaccharidosis II, 150
  with mucopolysaccharidosis VI, 154
  with osteopetrosis, 221
  with pseudotumor cerebri, 237
Papillitis, 635–636
Papilloma, 286–288
Papulosis, lymphomatoid, 300–301
Paralysis, facial, idiopathic, 234–236
    Landry's, 233–234
    of sixth nerve, 460–461
    of third nerve, 486–487
Parasitic disease, 98–124
Parinaud's oculoglandular syndrome
  in cat-scratch disease, 77–78
  in yersiniosis, 48
Parkinson's disease, 263–264
Paroxysmal nocturnal cephalalgia, 246–247
Pars planitis, 590–592
Pediatric migraine headache, 252–254
Pediculosis, 115–117
Pellucid marginal corneal degeneration, 425
Pemphigoid, cicatricial, 403–406
Perforation, corneal, 343–344
Periarteritis nodosa, 198–200
Perinatal encephalopathy, 241–243
Periocular squamous cell carcinoma, 305–306
Periodic alternating nystagmus, 482–486
Peripheral retinal breaks and degeneration, 671–673
Peripheral uveitis, 590–592
Peripheral uveoretinitis, 590–592
Periphlebitis, retinal, 669
Perivasculitis, retinal, primary, 669
Persistent hyperplastic primary vitreous, 695–696
    functional amblyopia with, 250
    lenticonus with, 620
Peutz-Jeghers syndrome, 518
Pfaudnler-Herler syndrome, 147–148
Phacoanaphylactic endophthalmitis, 573–574
Phacolytic glaucoma, 562–564
Phakomatoses, 228–232, 556
Pharyngoconjunctival fever, 92–93
Phlyctenular keratoconjunctivitis, 454–456
Phlyctenulosis, 454–456
Phoria, monofixational, 481–482
Photokeratitis, 185
    ultraviolet, 315
Photokeratoconjunctivitis, 185
Photophobia, in cystinosis, 136
Photoretinitis, 630–631
Photosensitivity, 185–186
    in xeroderma pigmentosum, 161
Photosensitized ultraviolet radiation, 315–320
Phototherapy, skin cancer from, 192
Phototoxicity, chemical, 185
Phthiriasis, 115–117
Phythanic acid oxidase deficiency, 674–675
Pierre Robin syndrome, 225–226
Pigment dispersion syndrome, 574–575
Pigmentary glaucoma, 574–575
Pink eye, 24, 78
Placental shock, 14

Plaque, mucous, corneal, 422–423
Plateau iris, 575–576
Pneumococcus infection, 31–33, 40–41
  in bacterial conjunctivitis, 402
  in ophthalmia neonatorum, 416
Poison ivy dermatitis, 176–177, 187–188
Poison oak and sumac dermatitis, 187–188
Polyarteritis nodosa, 198–200
Polychondritis, relapsing, 203–204
Polyneuritis, idiopathic, acute, 233–234
Polyradiculoneuropathy, inflammatory, 233–234
Posner-Schlossman syndrome, 558
Postcataract bleb, 410–411
Postcataract extraction syndrome, 33
Posterior aqueous diversion, 565–567
Posterior ischemic optic neuropathy, 633–635
Posterior polymorphous corneal dystrophy, 437
Postinfectious polyneuritis, 233–234
Postoperative flat anterior chamber, 380–383
Precancerous melanosis, 406–408
Prematurity, retinopathy of, 683–685
Preretinal macular fibrosis, 628–630
Pressure
    intraocular, 539–579
    venous, episcleral, glaucoma with, 550–551
Presumed ocular histoplasmosis syndrome, 63–64
Primary acquired melanosis, 406–408
Primary angle-closure glaucoma, 577–579
Primary congenital open-angle glaucoma, 559
Primary perivasculitis of retina, 669
Primary retinal hemorrhage, in young men, 669
Progeria, 216
Progressive essential iris atrophy, 584–586
Progressive hyperostosis, 212–213
Progressive supranuclear palsy, 263–264
Prolapse, of iris, 589–590
Proliferative vitreoretinopathy, 696–698
Propionibacterium acnes infection, 33–34
Protein metabolism disorders, 136–143
Proteus infection, 34–35
  with bacterial endophthalmitis, 533
  with electrical injury, 321
Pruritis, 188–191
Pseudodendritic keratitis, 142–143
Pseudoexfoliation, of lens capsule, 543–545
Pseudolymphoma, neoplastic angioendotheliomatosis, 297–299
Pseudomonas aeruginosa infection, 35–37
  with bacterial corneal ulcer, 439
  with bacterial endophthalmitis, 533
  with electrical injury, 321
Pseudophakic pigment dispersion syndrome, glaucoma with, 533
Pseudophakic pupillary block, 539–541
Pseudostrabismus, from epicanthus, 506
Pseudopterygium, 418–420
Pseudotumor, inflammatory, 297–299
Pseudotumor cerebri, 236–240
Pseudoxanthoma elasticum, 200–201
Psoriasis, 191–192
Pterygtium, 418–420
Ptosis, 520–522
    in acute idiopathic polyneuritis, 234
    in botulism, 10
    in chronic progressive external ophthalmoplegia, 244
    in extraocular muscle fibrosis, 471
    in internal orbital fractures, 336
    in maple syrup urine disease, 140
    in Marcus Gunn syndrome, 516
    in mucormycosis, 62

Ptosis (cont'd.)
  in myasthenia gravis, 521
  in neuilemoma, 284
  in oculomotor paralysis, 487
  in rhabdomyosarcoma, 310
  in tetanus, 42
  of ocular muscle, 470–471
  repair of, 495
  traumatic, 344
Pucker, macular, 628–630
Pupillary block glaucoma, 552–553
  aphakic, 539–541
  pseudophakic, 539–541
  with intraocular lenses, 532
  with microspherophakia, 621
Purulent conjunctivitis, 402–403, 416
PUVA therapy
  cataract formation from, 317
  for psoriasis, 191–192
Pyocele, 282–283

Query fever (Q fever), 68–69
Quincke's disease, 192–194

Rabbit fever, 45–46
Rabies, 93–94
Racemose hemangioma, 164–165
Radiation
  injury from, 323–324
  ultraviolet, direct and photosensitized, 315–320
Radiowave injury, 323–324
Raeder's paratrigeminal syndrome, benign, 246–247
Ragged red fibers, chronic progressive external ophthalmoplegia with, 243–245
Rash, from nettle, 192–194
Reactive lymphoid hyperplasia, 297–299
Rebound nystagmus, 482–486
Recess-angle glaucoma, 547–548
Recessive keratosis palmoplantaris, 142–143
Rectus, inferior, congenital fibrosis of, with ptosis, 470–471
Recurrent epithelial erosion, 427–428
Recurrent fever, 37–38
Recurrent herpetic epithelial keratitis, 80
Recurrent late hyphema, from focal wound vascularization, 383–384
Refractive disorders, 648–656
  in cerebral palsy, 242
  in Down's syndrome, 217
  in homocystinuria, 137–138
Refsum's disease, 674–675
  chronic progressive external ophthalmoplegia with, 245
  congenital cataracts with, 616
Reis-Bücklers' superficial corneal dystrophy, 429–430
Reiter's disease, 367–369
Relapsing fever, 37–38
Relapsing polychondritis, 201–202
Renal disease, pruritis in, 188
Reticulum cell sarcoma, 298
Retina, 657–688
  gyrate atrophy of, 670–671
  primary perivasculitis of, 669
  primary tumors of, 555–556
  spectral sensitivitiy of, 317
Retinal angiomatosis, 228–229
Retinal artery occlusion, 663–665
Retinal breaks, peripheral, 671–673

Retinal degeneration
  in chronic progressive external ophthalmoplegia, 244
  in intraocular steel or iron foreign body, 350
  in mucopolysaccharidosis, 147–152
  in myopia, 653
  in osteopetrosis, 221
  peripheral, 671–673
Retinal depigmentation, 195
Retinal detachment, 569–570, 675–678
  in AIDS, 74
  in chorioretinal concussions and lacerations, 338–339
  in choroid rupture, 392
  in congenital cataracts, 616
  in Crohn's disease, 132
  in cysticercosis, 105–106
  in fibrous ingrowth, 379
  in homocystinuria, 138
  in intraocular inert foreign body, 329
  in intraocular steel or iron foreign body, 330–332
  in lens dislocation, 619
  in macular hole, 627
  in macular pucker, 629
  in myopia, 653
  in nanophthalmos, 537
  in ocular hypotony, 569
  in retinal breaks, 672
  in retinopathy of prematurity, 684
  in sickle cell disease, 168
  in toxocariasis, 120–121
  in Vogt-Koyanagi-Harada syndrome, 372–373
Retinal emboli, 678–679
Retinal hemangioblastoma, 228–229
Retinal hemorrhage, primary, in young men, 669
Retinal hole, 671
Retinal necrosis, acute, 659–661
Retinal neovascularization
  in retinal vein obstruction, 680
  in sarcoidosis, 370
  in sickle cell disease, 168
  in thalassemia, 171
Retinal periphlebitis, 669
Retinal revascularization, in angioid streaks, 387–388
Retinal telangiectasia, 667–668
Retinal vein, engorgement of, in scrub typhus, 71
  inflammation of, 669
  obstruction of, 679–682
  occlusion of, 661–663
Retinitis
  exudative, massive, 667–668
  foveomacular, 630–631
Retinitis pigmentosa, 682–683
  with abetalipoproteinemia, 658
  with chronic progressive external ophthalmoplegia, 243
  with cystoid macular edema, 624
  with Refsum's disease, 674
Retinoblastoma, 306–399, 556–557
  with congenital cataracts, 616
  with fibrosarcoma, 292
  with retinal detachment, 675
Retinochoroiditis, toxoplasmic, 121–123
Retinopathy
  cytomegalovirus, in AIDS, 72–75
  diabetic, 144–146, 624–627
  in systemic lupus erythematosus, 208
  in systemic sclerosis, 201
  in Werner's syndrome, 218
  of prematurity, 683–685
  serous, central, 665–667

Retinopathy (cont'd.)
  solar, 630–631
  surface-wrinkling, 628–630
  with vitreous hemorrhage, 684
Retinoschisis, 685–686
Retraction
  Duane's, 475–476
  of eyelid, 514–515
  vertical, 470–471
  vitreous, massive, 696–698
Retrobulbar neuritis, 635–636
Retrolental fibroplasia, 683–685
Rhabdomyosarcoma, 309–310
Rhegmatogenous detachment, 671
Rheumatoid arthritis, 203–205
  juvenile, 197–198, 560
  keratoconjunctivitis sicca in, 204–206
  Miculicz's syndrome in, 601
  Mooren's ulcer in, 424
  scleritis in, 205
  Sjögren's syndrome in, 206
Rhinosporidiosis, 65–66
Rhus dermatitis, 187–188
Richner-Hanhart syndrome, 142–143
Rickettsial infection, 68–72
Riley Day syndrome, 362–364
Robin anomalad, 225–226
Robin sequence, 225–226
Rocky Mountain spotted fever, 69–70
Rosacea
  acne, 455
  ocular, 184–185
Rubella, 94–95
  cerebral palsy with, 241
  congenital cataracts in, 616
  myopia in, 653
Rubeola, 95–96
  anophthalmos with, 378
Rubeosis iridis, 592–594
Rubrophytia, 61–62
Rupture
  choroidal, 392
  global, indirect, 348–349
Rural typhus, 70–72

Saccadic oscillations, 482–486
St. Anthony's fire, 17–18
Salmonella typhi infection, 46
Sandboxes, toxocariasis spread in, 121
Sanfilippo syndrome, 151–152
Sarcoidosis, 369–372
  filamentary keratitis in, 444
  Miculicz's syndrome with, 600
Sarcoma
  Ewing's, 291–292, 304, 310
  idiopathic multiple pigmented, 294–296
  Kaposi's, 294–296
  reticulum cell, 298
Scheie syndrome, 149–150
Schistosomiasis, 117–118
Schlichting's dystrophy, 437
Schnyder's crystalline corneal dystrophy, 430–431
Schwannoma, 283–284
Sclera, 689–693
Scleral cysts, 440–441
Scleral dehiscences, 690–691
Scleral injuries, sharp, 348–349
Scleral perforation, with conjunctival laceration, 342
Scleral staphyloma, 690–691

Scleritis, 691–692
  in ankylosing spondylitis, 219–220
  in choroidal detachment, 388
  in coccidioidomycosis, 61
  in Cogan's syndrome, 361
  in mumps, 88
  in relapsing polychondritis, 203
  in rheumatoid arthritis, 205
  in sporotrichosis, 67
  in Wegener's granulomatosis, 172
Scleroderma, 200–202
Scleromalacia perforans, 692–693
Sclerosis
  hereditary multiple diaphyseal, 212–213
  multiple, 259–261
  systemic, 200–202
Scotoma
  arcuate, 387
  with migraine, 251
Scrub typhus, 70–72
Sebaceous gland carcinoma, 310–311
Seborrhea
  chalazion with, 497
  madarosis with, 515
Seborrheic blepharitis, 522–524
Seborrheic blepharoconjunctivitis, 525–527
Seborrheic keratosis, 267–268
Seckle dwarfism, 216
Serous chorioretinopathy, central, 665–667
Sézary syndrome, 300–301
Shock, placental, 14
Sickle cell disease, 168–169
  angioid streaks in, 387
  madarosis in, 515
  vitreous hemorrhage in, 598
Siderosis, 330–332
Silk Road disease, 359–360
Sinus thrombosis, cavernous, 166–167
Sjögren's syndrome, 205–206, 449–452
  dacryoadenitis with, 597
  filamentary keratitis with, 444
  keratoconjunctivitis sicca with, 206
  lacrimal hyposecretion with, 612
  Miculicz's syndrome with, 601
  systemic lupus erythematosus with, 208
Skeletal disorders, 211–227
Skin cancer, from phototherapy, 192
Snow blindness, 315
Snowflake degeneration, 672
Solar burn, 630–631
  keratosis with, 315
  photokeratitis with, 185
  urticaria with, 193
Solar retinopathy, 630–631
Sore, 104–105
Sparganosis, 118–119
Spasms, 508–509
Spider bites, 356–357
Spontaneous congenital iris cyst, 587–588
Sporotrichosis, 66–68
Squamous cell carcinoma, 276, 289–291
  periocular, 305–306
Staphylococcal blepharoconjunctivitis, 525–527
Staphylococcus infection, 38–39
  in bacterial conjunctivitis, 402
  in bacterial corneal ulcer, 439
  in bacterial endophthalmitis, 533
  in electrical injury, 321
  in erythema multiforme, 178
  in hordeolum, 510
  in impetigo, 182–183

Staphylococcus infection (*cont'd.*)
  in ophthalmia neonatorum, 416
  in seborrheic blepharitis, 522
  -induced phylctenulosis, 455–456
  of eyelid, 510–511
Staphyloma, scleral, 690–691
Steel, intraocular, injury from, 330–332
Stevens-Johnson syndrome, 177–179
  with distichiasis, 499
  with entropion of eyelid, 563
  with lacrimal hyposecretion, 611
  with symblepharon, 527
Stickler syndrome, 225–226
Sticky eye, 416–418
Sting, of bee, 355–356
Strabismus, 465–466. See also *Exotropia*.
  acquired, 461–463
  fixus, 470–471
  in abetalipoproteinemia, 658
  in amblyopia, 250–251
  in cerebral palsy, 242
  in Crouzon's disease, 211
  in maple syrup urine disease, 140
  in Marcus Gunn syndrome, 516
  in optic glioma, 285
  in orbital hypertelorism, 214
  in persistent hyperplastic primary vitreous, 695
  in Robin sequence, 225
  in rubella, 94
Strawberry hemangioma, 268–270
Strephosymbolia, 248–249
Streptococcus infection, 31–33, 39–40
  in bacterial corneal ulcer, 439
  in bacterial endophthalmitis, 379
  in electrical injury, 321
  in impetigo, 182–183
Stripping, of Descemet's membrane, 352–354
Stromal edema, 442
Stromal herpetic keratitis, 80
Stromal ingrowth, 379–380
Stromal overgrowth, 379–380
Stromal ulceration, indolent, 80–81
Sturge-Weber syndrome, 231–232
  with arteriovenous fistula, 164
  with juvenile glaucoma, 560
Stye, 510–511
Subchoroidal expulsive hemorrhage, 392–394
Subluxation, of lens, 618–620
Subretinal cysticercosis, 106
Subretinal neovascular membranes, 687–688
Subretinal neovascularization, 390–392
Sun blindness, 630–631
Sunburn, 185–186, 191
Superficial puntate keratopathy, Thygeson's, 458–459
Superior limbic keratoconjunctivitis, 444–445, 457–458
Superior oblique myokymia, 488
Superior oblique palsy, 488–490
Surface-wrinkling retinopathy, 628–630
Sursumduction, alternating, 474–475
Swimming pool conjunctivitis, 92
Symblepharon, 527–528
  with thermal burns, 324
Sympathetic ophthalmia, 398–399
  with vitiligo, 194
Sympathetic uveitis, 398–399
Synkinesis, 509
Syphilis, accommodative spasm with, 580
  acquired, 4–6
  AIDS with, 73
  congenital, 13–15
  late (tertiary), 4
  latent, 3–4
  Mikulicz's syndrome with, 600
  ocular, 5, 73
  primary, 4–5
  secondary, 4–5
Systemic hamartomatoses, 556
Systemic lupus erythematosus, 206–208
Systemic lymphoma, 298
Systemic sclerosis, 208–209

T-cell lymphoma, 300–301
T-cell lymphoma-leukemia, 300–301
Tear secretion, abnormal, in systemic sclerosis, 201
Tears, 338–355
Telangiectasia, retinal, 667–668
Temporal arteritis, 169–171, 633
Tendon sheath, superior, oblique, 469–470
Tension, low-, glaucoma, 564–565
Tension headache, 253–254
Terrien's marginal degeneration, 426
Tetanus, 42–43
  with eyelid laceration, 346
Thalassemia, 171–172
Thelaziasis, 119
Theodore's superior limbic keratoconjunctivitis, 457–458
Thermal burns, 324–326
  ankyloblepharon in, 493
Thrombosis, cavernous sinus, 166–167
Thygeson's superficial punctate keratopathy, 458–459
Thyroid ophthalmopathy, 514
Tic doloureux, 265–266
Tinea, 61–62
Tolosa-Hunt syndrome, 264–265
Toxic conjunctivitis, 413–414
Toxocariasis, 120–121
Toxoplasmic iridocyclitis, 121–123
Toxoplasmic retinochoroiditis, 121–123
Toxoplasmosis, 121–123
  anophthalmos with, 532
Trachoma, 51–53
  with blepharophimosis, 496
  with blindness, 52
  with entropion, 52
Transplantation, corneal, Creutzfeldt-Jakob disease spread by, 247–248
  in xeorderma pigmentosum, 162
  rabies spread by, 93–94
Traumatic cataract, 354–355
Traumatic hyphema, 384–386
  recessed-angle glaucoma after, 547
Treacher Collins syndrome, 223–224
Treponema pallidum infection, 4–5, 13–15
Trichiasis, 52, 529–530
  with cicatricial pemphigoid, 289
  with symblepharon, 528
Trichinellosis, 123–124
Trichinosis, 123–124
Trichophytosis, 61–62
Trigeminal neuralgia, 265–266
Trigeminal neuropathic keratopathy, 452–454
Trisomy 21, 216–218
Tropical sore, 104–105
Tropical typhus, 70–72
Tsutsugamushi disease, 70–72
Tuberculosis, 43–44
  madarosis with, 515
  metastatic ocular, 44

Tuberculosis (cont'd.)
  Mikulicz's syndrome with, 600
  phlyctenulosis with, 454
Tularemia, 45–46
Tumor. See also *Carcinoma*; *Neoplasm*; specific neoplasm.
  inflammatory, 598–600
  intraocular, glaucoma with, 554–558
  lymphoid, 297–299, 556, 598–600
  metastatic, ocular, 302–303
  metastatic, orbital, 304–305
  metastatic, to uvea, 555
  of epithelium, 556, 598–600
  of lacrimal gland, 598–600
  of retina, 228–229, 555–556
  of uvea, 555
Typhoid fever, 46–48
Typhus, 70–72
Tyrosinosis, 142–143

Ulcer, corneal. See *Corneal ulcer.*
Ultraviolet radiation, direct and photosensitized, 315–320
Unclassified diseases, 358–373
Undulant fever, 11–12
Unilateral rotary nystagmus, 488
Upbeat nystagmus, 484
Urticaria, 192–194
  contact, pruritis in, 188–189
  giant, 192–194
Uvea
  metastatic tumors to, 555
  posterior, malignant melanoma of, 394–398
  primary tumors of, 555
  reactive lymphoid hyperplasia of, 299
Uveal tract, metastasis in, 302–303
Uveitis, 546, 594–596
  anterior, glaucoma with, 548–550
  granulomatous, anterior, 659
  in acanthamoebae, 98
  in ankylosing spondylitis, 219
  in ascariasis, 102
  in brucellosis, 11
  in candidiasis, 37
  in coenurosis, 103
  in Cogan's syndrome, 361
  in congenital syphilis, 13
  in cystoid macular edema, 624
  in dirofilariasis, 108
  in electrical injury, 321
  in eptospirosis, 27
  in fibrous ingrowth, 379
  in glaucoma, 548–550
  in gout, 160
  in juvenile glaucoma, 560
  in Hallermann-Streiff-Francois syndrome, 222
  in histiocytosis X, 364
  in inclusion conjunctivitis, 51
  in influenza, 85
  in iris cysts, 587
  in juvenile rheumatoid arthritis, 197
  in mumps, 88
  in psoriasis, 191–192
  in Reiter's disease, 367–369
  in relapsing fever, 37
  in relapsing polychondritis, 203
  in Rocky Mountain spotted fever, 69
  in sarcoidosis, 369–371
  in scrub typhus, 71
  in sporotrichosis, 67
  in sympathetic ophthalmia, 399
  in tuberculosis, 43
  in typhoid fever, 47
  in varicelola, 96
  in Vogt-Koyanagi-Harada syndrome, 372
  in Wegener's granulomatosis, 172
  peripheral, 590–592
  phacoanaphylactic, 573–574
  sympathetic, 398–399
  secondary to intraocular lens, 552
Uveitis-vitiligo-alopecia-poliosis syndrome, 372–373
Uveoparotid fever, 601–602
Uveoparotitis, 601–602
Uveoretinitis, peripheral, 590–592

Vaccinia, ocular, 90–91
Varicella, 96–97
Varicose aneurysm, 164–165
Vascular headache, 251
Vascular occlusion, with cystoid macular edema, 624–627
Vasculitis retinae, 669
Vein, retinal. See *Retinal vein.*
Venom, injuries from, 355–357
Venous pressure, episcleral, glaucoma with, 550–551
Vernal keratoconjunctivitis, 400–401, 420–421
Verruca, 286–288
Vertical deviation and divergence, dissociated, 474–475
Vertical retraction syndrome, 470–471
Vestibular nystagmus, 482–486
Viral infection, 72–97
Vision, blurred, transient, 252–253
  low, 256–259
Visual obscuration, transient, in intracranial hypertension, 237
Vitiligo, 194–196
Vitretis, 590–592
Vitreolenticular ciliary block, 565–567
Vitreoretinal membrane shrinkage, 696–698
Vitreoretinopathy
  exudative, familial, 694–695
  proliferative, 696–698
Vitreous, 694–701
  persistent hyperplastic primary, 695–696
Vitreous hemorrhage, 545, 669, 698–700. See also *Bleeding; Hemorrhage.*
  of unknown etiology, 669
  with ciliary body concussions and lacerations, 339
  with conjunctival lacerations and contusions, 342
  with corneal abrasions, 343
  with dislocation of lens, 619
  with ghost cell glaucoma, 545
  with intraocular inert foreign body, 329
  with retinal vein obstruction, 680
  with retinal vein occlusion, 661
  with retinopathy of prematurity, 684
  with sickle cell disease, 168
  with typhoid fever, 46
Vitreous retraction, massive, 696–698
Vitreous wick syndrome, 700–701
Vogt-Koyanagi-Harada syndrome, 372–373
  with vitiligo, 194
von Hippel-Lindau disease, 228–229
von Hippel's disease, 228–229
von Recklinghausen's disease, 229–231
  with neurilemoma, 284
V-pattern esotropia, 490–491
V-pattern exotropia, 491–492

Waardenburg's syndrome, 226–227
Waldenstrom's macroglobulinemia, with Mikulicz's syndrome, 600
Wart, 286–288
Wegener's granulomatosis, 172–173
Weill-Marchesani syndrome, 209–210
　lens dislocation with, 618
　microspherophakia with, 621
Weil's syndrome, 26
Werner's syndrome, 218–219
Wilm's tumor, 304
Word blindness, 248–249
Wound vascularization, focal, recurrent late hyphema from, 383–384

Xanthelasma, 530–531
　in crystalline corneal dystrophy, 430
　in hyperlipoproteinemia, 157
　palpebrarum, 530–531
Xanthogranuloma, juvenile, 274–275, 364
Xanthoma palpebrarum, 530–531
Xeroderma pigmentosum, 161–163
　with keratoacanthoma, 275
Xerophthalmia, 134–135
X-ray injury, 323–324

Yersiniosis, 48–50